Reproduction

From contraception to cloning and from pregnancy to populations, reproduction presents urgent challenges today. This field-defining history synthesizes a vast amount of scholarship to take the long view. Spanning from antiquity to the present day, the book focuses on the Mediterranean, western Europe, North America and their empires. It combines history of science, technology and medicine with social, cultural and demographic accounts. Ranging from the most intimate experiences to planetary policy, it tells new stories and revises received ideas. An international team of scholars asks how modern 'reproduction' – an abstract process of perpetuating living organisms – replaced the old 'generation' – the active making of humans and beasts, plants and even minerals. Striking illustrations invite readers to explore artefacts, from an ancient Egyptian fertility figurine to an announcement of the first test-tube baby. Authoritative and accessible, *Reproduction* offers students and non-specialists an essential starting point and sets fresh agendas for research.

Nick Hopwood is Professor of History of Science and Medicine at the University of Cambridge. He is the author of *Haeckel's Embryos: Images, Evolution, and Fraud* (2015), which won the Suzanne J. Levinson Prize of the History of Science Society.

Rebecca Flemming is Senior Lecturer in Ancient History at the University of Cambridge. She has published widely on medicine and gender in antiquity, including *Medicine and the Making of Roman Women: Gender, Nature, and Authority from Celsus to Galen* (2000).

Lauren Kassell is Professor of History of Science and Medicine at the University of Cambridge and directs the Casebooks Project. Her publications include *Medicine and Magic in Elizabethan London: Simon Forman, Astrologer, Alchemist, and Physician* (2005).

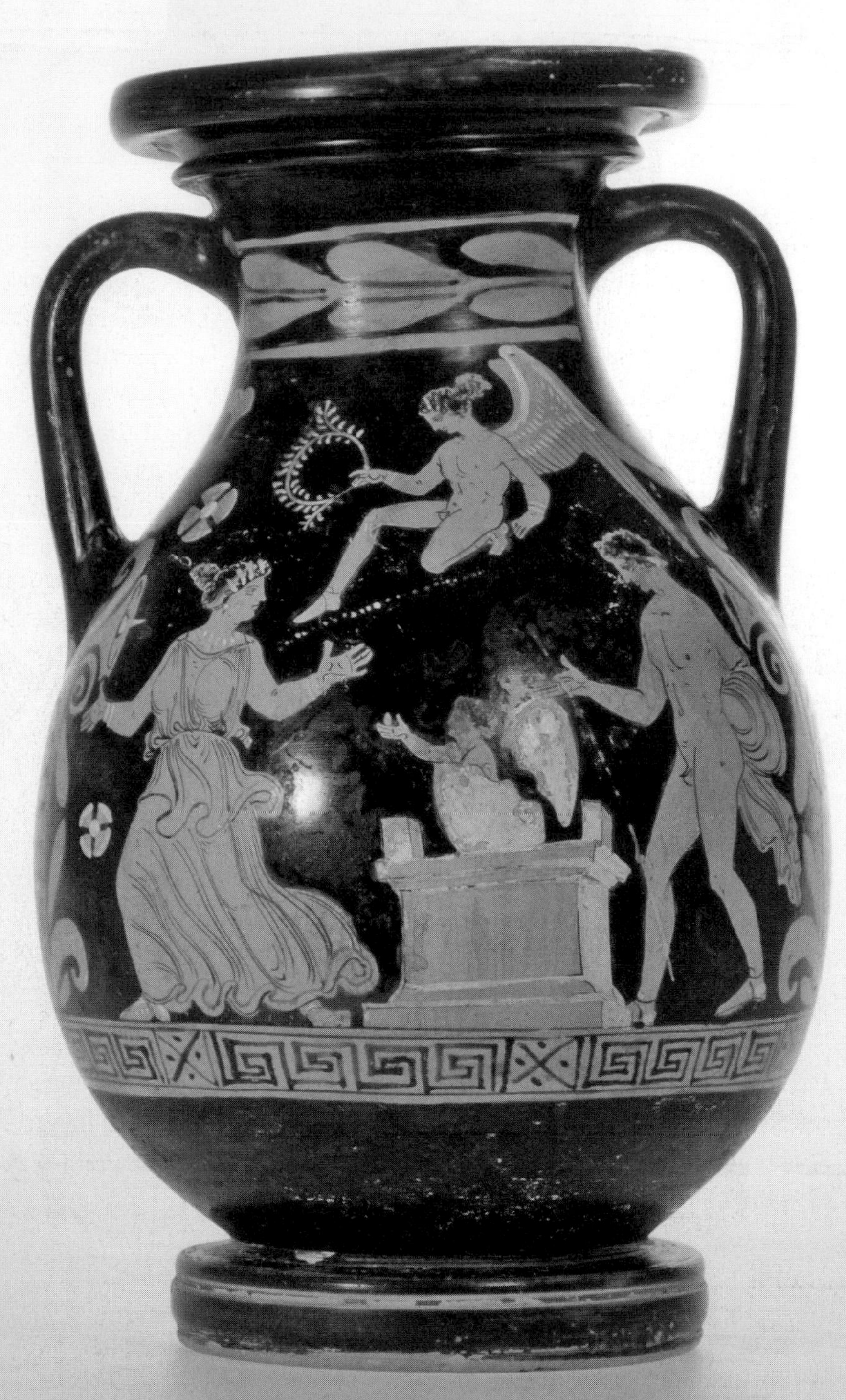

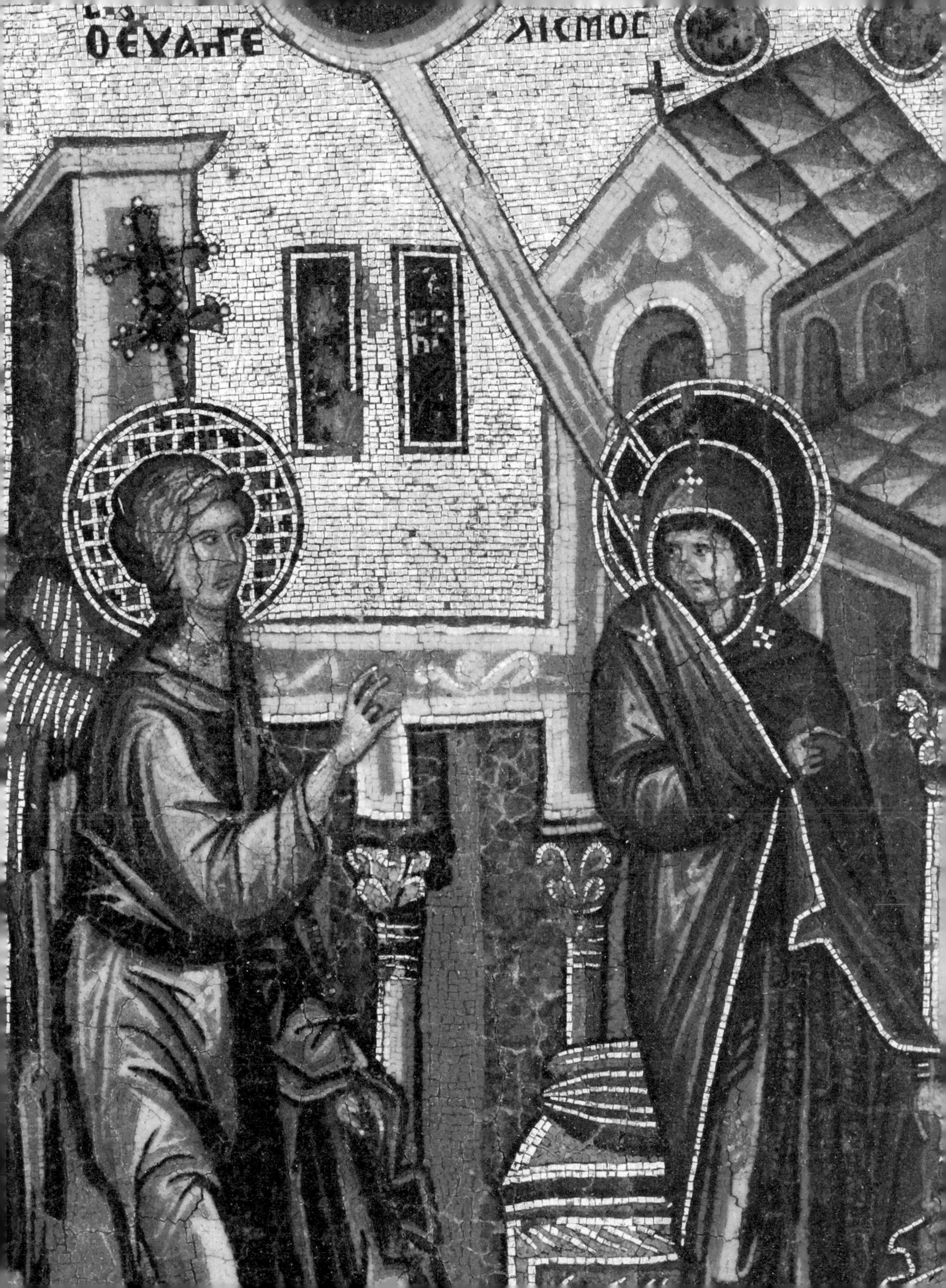

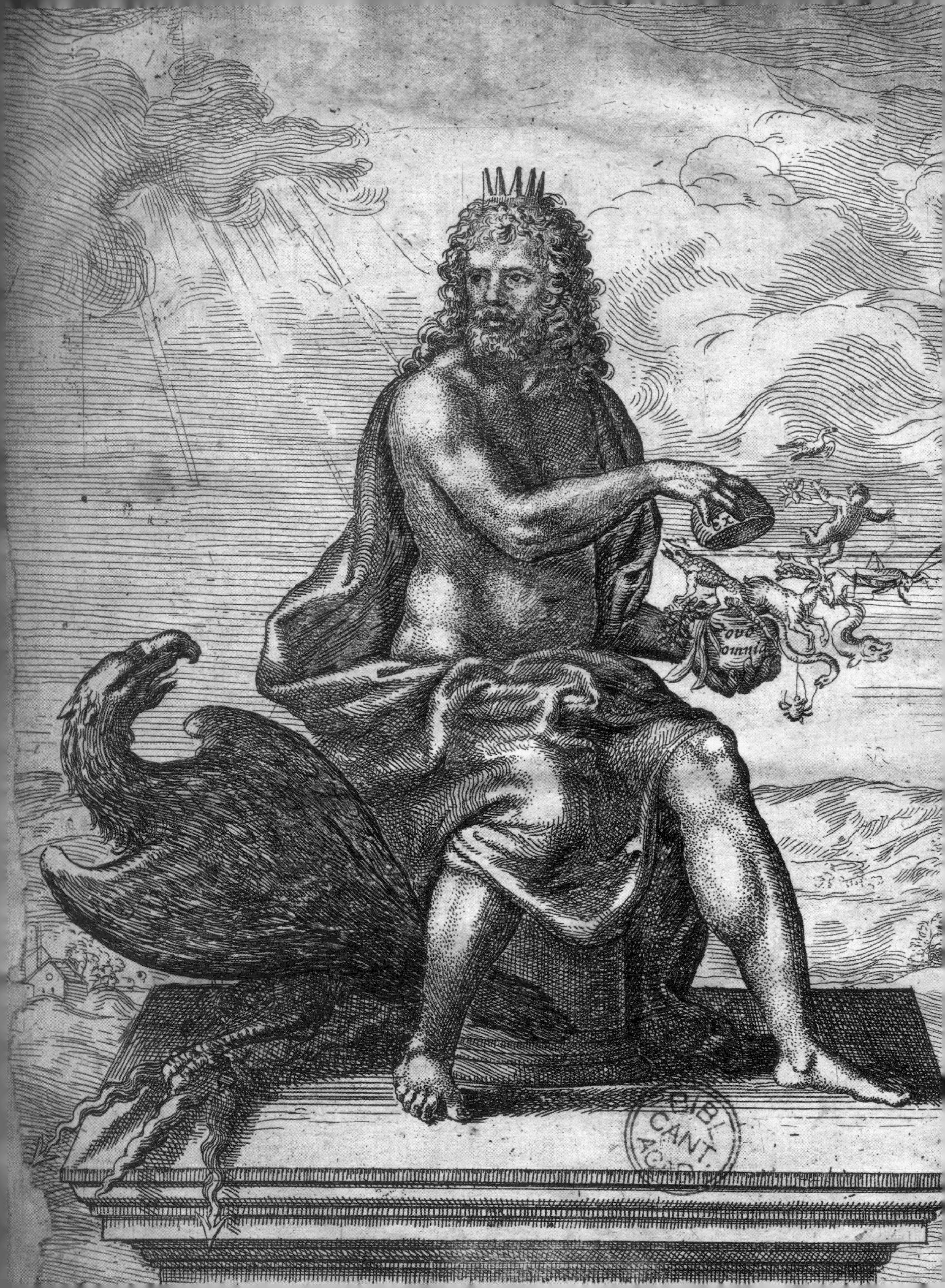
Jove
omnia

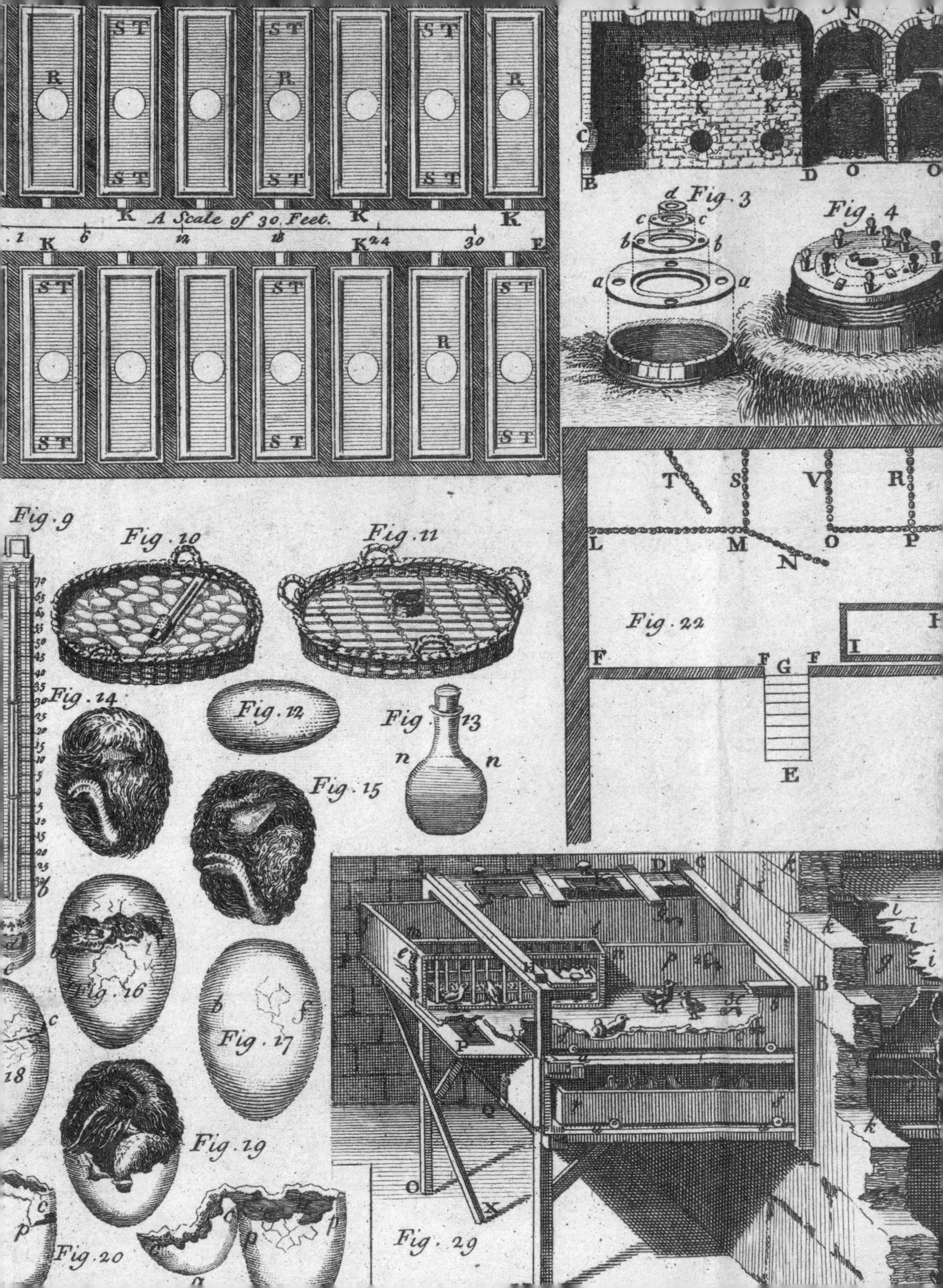

A Scale of 30 Feet.
Fig. 3
Fig. 4
Fig. 9
Fig. 10
Fig. 11
Fig. 12
Fig. 13
Fig. 14
Fig. 15
Fig. 16
Fig. 17
Fig. 19
Fig. 20
Fig. 22
Fig. 29

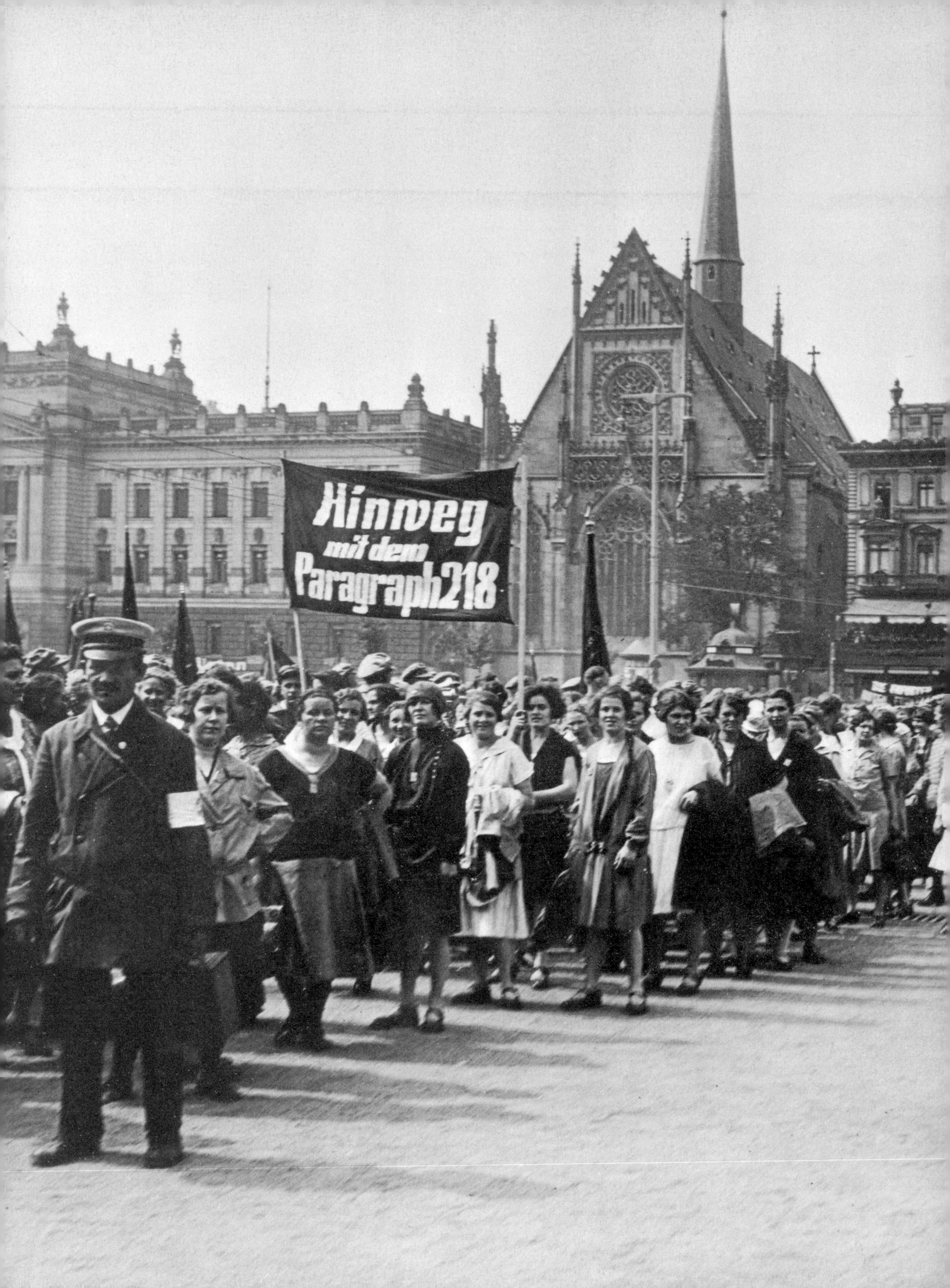
Hinweg
mit dem
Paragraph 218

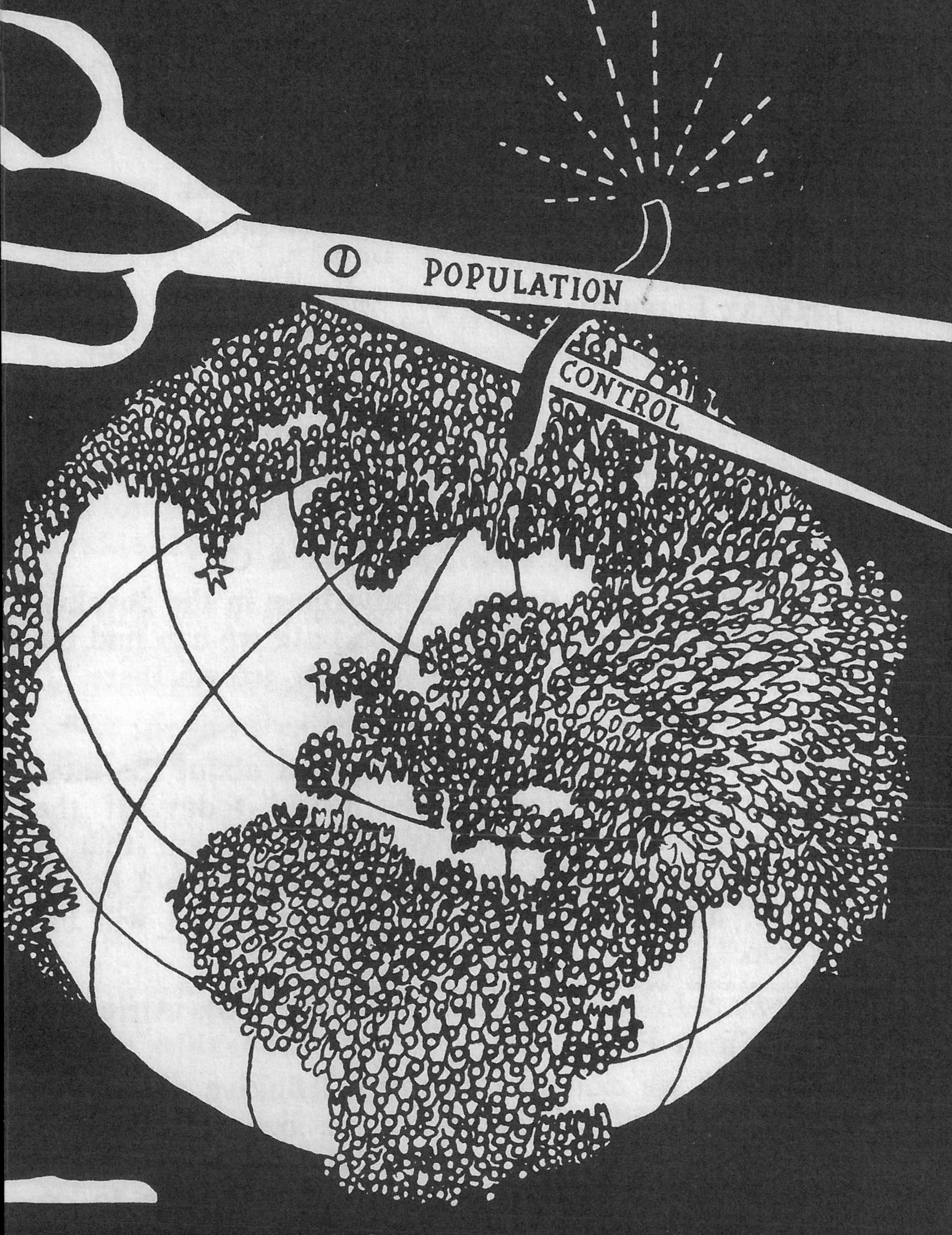
POPULATION
CONTROL

Reproduction

Antiquity to the Present Day

Edited by

Nick Hopwood
University of Cambridge

Rebecca Flemming
University of Cambridge

Lauren Kassell
University of Cambridge

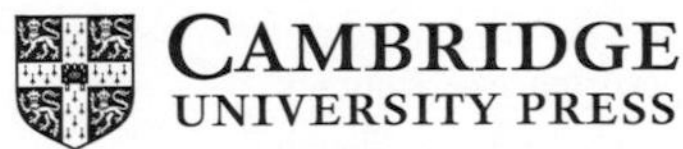

CAMBRIDGE
UNIVERSITY PRESS

University Printing House, Cambridge CB2 8BS, United Kingdom

One Liberty Plaza, 20th Floor, New York, NY 10006, USA

477 Williamstown Road, Port Melbourne, VIC 3207, Australia

314–321, 3rd Floor, Plot 3, Splendor Forum, Jasola District Centre, New Delhi - 110025, India

79 Anson Road, #06-04/06, Singapore 079906

Cambridge University Press is part of the University of Cambridge.

It furthers the University's mission by disseminating knowledge in the pursuit of education, learning and research at the highest international levels of excellence.

www.cambridge.org
Information on this title: www.cambridge.org/9781107068025
DOI: 10.1017/9781107705647

First published 2018
Paperback edition first published 2020

Printed in the United Kingdom by TJ Books Limited, Padstow,. Cornwall

A catalogue record for this publication is available from the British Library

Library of Congress Cataloging-in-Publication data
Names: Hopwood, Nick, editor. | Flemming, Rebecca, editor. | Kassell, Lauren, editor.
Title: Reproduction : antiquity to the present day / edited by Nick Hopwood, Rebecca Flemming, Lauren Kassell.
Other titles: Reproduction (Hopwood)
Description: Cambridge, United Kingdom ; New York, NY : Cambridge University Press, 2019. | Includes bibliographical references and index.
Identifiers: LCCN 2017058265 | ISBN 9781107068025 (hardback)
Subjects: | MESH: Reproductive Health – history | Reproduction | History of Medicine
Classification: LCC RG136 | NLM WQ 11.1 | DDC 613.9/4–dc23
LC record available at https://lccn.loc.gov/2017058265

ISBN 978-1-107-06802-5 Hardback
ISBN 978-1-107-65837-0 Paperback

In memory of John Forrester (1949–2015)

Contents

List of Exhibits — *page* xvii
List of Illustrations — xx
Notes on the Frontispieces — xxvi
List of Contributors — xxviii
Acknowledgements — xxxiii

Introduction — 1

1 Reproduction in History — 3
Nick Hopwood, Rebecca Flemming and Lauren Kassell

Part I Inventing Generation — 19

Introduction to Part I — 20
Rebecca Flemming

2 Phallic Fertility in the Ancient Near East and Egypt — 25
Stephanie Lynn Budin

3 Women and Doctors in Ancient Greece — 39
Helen King

4 Animal and Plant Generation in Classical Antiquity — 53
Laurence M. V. Totelin

5 States and Populations in the Classical World — 67
Rebecca Flemming

6 The Ancient Family and the Law — 81
Tim Parkin

7 Galen's Generations of Seeds — 95
Rebecca Flemming

8 Debating the Soul in Late Antiquity — 109
Marie-Hélène Congourdeau

Part II Generation Reborn and Reformed 123

Introduction to Part II 124
Lauren Kassell

9 Generation in Medieval Islamic Medicine 129
Nahyan Fancy

10 The Multitude in Later Medieval Thought 141
Peter Biller

11 Managing Childbirth and Fertility in Medieval Europe 153
Katharine Park

12 Formed Fetuses and Healthy Children in Scholastic Theology, Medicine and Law 167
Maaike van der Lugt

13 Generation between Script and Print 181
Peter Murray Jones

14 Innate Heat, Radical Moisture and Generation 195
Gianna Pomata

15 Pictures and Analogies in the Anatomy of Generation 209
Karin Ekholm

16 Fruitful Bodies and Astrological Medicine 225
Lauren Kassell

17 Family Resemblance in the Old Regime 241
Silvia De Renzi

18 The Emergence of Population 253
Philip Kreager

19 Generation in the Ottoman World 267
Miri Shefer-Mossensohn and Rebecca Flemming

Part III Inventing Reproduction 281

Introduction to Part III 282
Nick Hopwood

20 The Keywords 'Generation' and 'Reproduction' 287
Nick Hopwood

21 Linnaeus and the Love Lives of Plants 305
Staffan Müller-Wille

22 Man-Midwifery Revisited 319
Mary E. Fissell

23 Biopolitics and the Invention of Population 333
Andrea Rusnock

24 Marriage and Fertility in Different Household Systems 347
Richard M. Smith

25 Colonialism and the Emergence of Racial Theories 361
Renato G. Mazzolini

26 Talking Origins 375
James A. Secord

Part IV Modern Reproduction 391
Introduction to Part IV 392
Nick Hopwood

27 Breeding Farm Animals and Humans 397
Sarah Wilmot

28 Eggs and Sperm as Germ Cells 413
Florence Vienne

29 Movements to Separate Sex and Reproduction 427
Lesley A. Hall

30 Fertility Transitions and Sexually Transmitted Infections 443
Simon Szreter

31 Modern Infertility 457
Christina Benninghaus

32 Modern Ignorance 471
Kate Fisher

33 Imperial Encounters 485
Philippa Levine

Part V Reproduction Centre Stage 499
Introduction to Part V 500
Nick Hopwood

34 World Population from Eugenics to Climate Change 505
Alison Bashford

35 Sex Hormones, Pharmacy and the Reproductive Sciences 521
Jean-Paul Gaudillière

36 Technologies of Contraception and Abortion 535
Jesse Olszynko-Gryn

37 Hospital Birth 553
Salim Al-Gailani

38 Prenatal Diagnosis, Surveillance and Risk 567
Ilana Löwy

39 Artificial Fertilization 581
Nick Hopwood

40 Modern Law and Regulation 597
Martin H. Johnson and Nick Hopwood

41 Sex, Gender and Babies 613
John Forrester

42 Feminism and Reproduction 627
Sarah Franklin

43 Globalization 641
Nick Hopwood

Epilogue 657

44 Concluding Reflections 659
Nick Hopwood, Rebecca Flemming and Lauren Kassell

Select Bibliography 673

Index 701

Exhibits

Exhibits 1–19 are between pages 180 and 181.
Exhibits 20–40 are between pages 612 and 613.

1 An Ancient Egyptian Fertility Figurine
Rune Nyord

2 The Minotaur and Other Hybrids in Ancient Greece
Annetta Alexandridis

3 The Birth Horoscope of a Babylonian Scholar
Eleanor Robson

4 A Swaddled Infant Given to the Gods
Fay Glinister

5 Phallic Fertility in Pompeii
Jessica Hughes

6 A Roman Embryo Hook
Ralph Jackson

7 A Uterine Amulet from the Roman Empire
Véronique Dasen

8 The Tree of Jesse
Margot E. Fassler

9 The Hermaphroditic Hyena
Gabriella Zuccolin

10 Medieval Birth Malpresentations
Lauren Kassell

11 A Medieval Birth Girdle
Lea T. Olsan

12 Renaissance Art, Arousal and Impotence
Patricia Simons

13 Monstrous Births and Diabolical Seed
Jennifer Spinks

14 Jane Dee's Courses in John Dee's Diary
Lauren Kassell

15 A Placenta Painted and Engraved
Karin Ekholm
16 The Generative Parts of Women
Rina Knoeff
17 Pregnant Stones as Wonders of Nature
Sandra Cavallo
18 A Birthing Chair
Lianne McTavish
19 A Painting of a Nursing Mother
Lisa Forman Cody
20 A Microscopical Salon
Mary Terrall
21 A Crystal Womb
Lucia Dacome
22 Man-Midwifery Dissected
Ludmilla Jordanova
23 Images of Human Embryos
Nick Hopwood
24 Population in the South Sea
Rebecca Flemming
25 *Aristotle's Masterpiece*
Mary E. Fissell
26 Spontaneous Generation and the Triumph of Experiment
James A. Secord
27 'Pity the Poor Mother!'
Siân Pooley
28 Condoms
James M. Edmonson
29 Pedigree of a 'Schizophrenic Family'
Paul Weindling
30 Populations, Genetics and Race
Jenny Bangham
31 Menstrual-Cycle Calendars
Martina Schlünder
32 Pregnancy Testing with Frogs
Jesse Olszynko-Gryn
33 Technologies of Adoption Matching
Ellen Herman

34 'Drama of Life before Birth'
Solveig Jülich
35 *Our Bodies, Ourselves*
Wendy Kline
36 *Z.P.G.*
Patrick Ellis
37 Cloned Frogs
Christina Brandt
38 'It's a Girl'
Nick Hopwood
39 Developmental Origins of Health and Disease
Tatjana Buklijas
40 The Room of the Ribbons
Jessica Hughes and Rebecca Flemming

Illustrations

Frontispieces

[1] Birth of Helen of Troy on a fourth-century BC vase
[2] The Annunciation on a mosaic from fourteenth-century Constantinople
[3] Detail from the frontispiece to William Harvey's treatise on generation
[4] 'Method of hatching and bringing up Domestick Fowls' in the *London Magazine*
[5] Photograph of a march against the German anti-abortion law
[6] *Population Bomb* pamphlet published by the Hugh Moore Fund

Part Title Illustrations

Introduction	Babies in hospital, photographed for a *Life* magazine story on 'the baby war'	*page* xxxvi
Part I	Nurse bathing a newborn child, from the side relief of a Roman sarcophagus	18
Part II	'Autumn', one of a series of copper plates of the stages of life	122
Part III	Engraving in which Abraham Trembley teaches the 'reproduction' of the 'polyp'	280
Part IV	Pronatalist poster showing population distribution between age groups	390
Part V	American family planning stamps	498
Epilogue	'Leda and the Swan, after Leonardo da Vinci', print by Vik Muniz	656
Bibliography	Frontispiece to Eucharius Rösslin's *Der Rosengarten*	672

Figures

1.1 Theodore Cianfrani's 'graph showing progress of obstetrics and gynecology' 6
1.2 Barbara Ehrenreich and Deirdre English, *Witches, Midwives, and Nurses* 8
1.3 Staff of Organon celebrate using their millionth litre of mare's urine 12
1.4 José Roy's thirteenth-century spermatozoon in Jules Gérard's *Nouvelles causes de stérilité* 15

2.1 Detail from the *Book of the Dead of Sesu* showing the divine sexual pairing of Geb and Nut 28
2.2 Drawing of a colossal Predynastic statue of the ithyphallic god Min 29
2.3 Detail from the New Kingdom stele of Qeh showing the god Min 29
2.4 Detail from an Assyrian palatial relief featuring the 'tree of life' 31
3.1 Birth of Athena on an Attic red-figure vase 40
3.2 White-ground classical Athenian *lekythos* decorated with a domestic scene 45
3.3 Papyrus fragment of the Hippocratic *Oath* 48
3.4 Index of the Aldine Hippocrates (1526) listing gynaecological works 51
4.1 Attic black-figure vase depicting the olive harvest 55
4.2 Roman mosaic depicting diverse animals and plants 56
4.3 Medieval manuscript of an Arabic translation of Dioscorides containing images of male and female mandrakes 60
4.4 Woodcut from an early printed edition of Virgil, showing Aristaeus's sacrificial generation of bees 64
5.1 Greek manuscript of Plato's *Republic*, belonging to Marsilio Ficino 69
5.2 View of Sparta from a nineteenth-century history of antiquity 75
5.3 Roman census on the relief of Domitius Ahenobarbus 76
5.4 Temple treasury from Republican central Italy 78
6.1 Miniature from a medieval manuscript of Justinian's *Institutes* 82
6.2 Inscribed sarcophagus of Veturia, from Budapest 86
6.3 Gold coin of the Emperor Trajan marking his Italian alimentary programme 90
6.4 Relief from the Emperor Augustus's *Ara Pacis* 92
7.1 Silver coin of the Emperor Marcus Aurelius and his son Commodus 96
7.2 Drawing of a uterus in a medieval manuscript of Muscio's *Gynaecology* 101
7.3 Roman childbirth illustrated on the tomb of Scribonia Attice 104
7.4 Folio of the Syriac Galen Palimpsest 106
8.1 Map of the Roman Empire in the fourth century AD 110
8.2 Miniature illustrating Hildegard of Bingen's vision of ensoulment 117
8.3 Twelfth-century Byzantine icon of the Annunciation 120
9.1 Medieval Arabic commentary by al-Aqsara'i with a discussion of generation 136
9.2 Passage from Jean Fernel's *Physiologia* (1567) 140
11.1 Fifteenth-century birth tray with a boy and pet painted on the bottom 155
11.2 Childbirth scene illuminating Pseudo-Apuleius's *Herbarius* 158
11.3 Lying-in scene on the reverse of the birth tray in Fig. 11.1 159
11.4 Birth of Caesar in a French manuscript of *Li fait des Romains* 161
12.1 Medieval skeleton of a 40-year-old woman, with a fetus in breech position 173
12.2 Miniature in a French chronicle adorning an account of a monstrous birth 175
12.3 Thirteenth-century legal diagram of prohibitions against marrying kin 178

13.1 'Disease woman' from the *Fasciculus medicinae* 186
13.2 Lady Johanna St John's remedy-book, with entries on women under 'W' 192
14.1 The trees of life and of knowledge in the Nuremberg Chronicle 200
14.2 Copulating couple as emblem of the alchemical conjunction of gold and silver 202
15.1 Woodcuts of animal and human uteruses in Andreas Vesalius's *De humani corporis fabrica* 214
15.2 Woodcut of a woman's womb in Vesalius's *Fabrica* 217
15.3 Woman's torso dissected to show the generative organs in Vesalius's *Fabrica* 218
15.4 Non-gravid womb from below in Vesalius's *Fabrica* 219
15.5 Plate from Girolamo Fabrici d'Acquapendente's *De formatione ovi et pulli* 221
16.1 Jan Steen's *Doctor's Visit* 226
16.2 Title engraving from John Sadler, *The Sicke Womans Private Looking-Glasse* 229
16.3 Record of Jane Rolte's consultation with Richard Napier 232
16.4 Seventeenth-century pregnancy calendar in the form of a volvelle 234
16.5 Ballad about a cure for a man afflicted with a scolding wife 236
17.1 Jan Gossaert, *The Children of Christian II, King of Denmark* 242
17.2 Adriaen Thomasz Key, *Family Portrait* 243
18.1 Frontispiece to Thomas Hobbes's *Leviathan* 256
18.2 Title-page of John Graunt's *Natural and Political Observat[i]ons ... upon the Bills of Mortality* 259
19.1 Miniature of a speculum used for extracting a fetus in Sabuncuoğlu's *Imperial Surgery* 273
19.2 Another image of a speculum from Sabuncuoğlu's *Imperial Surgery* 274
19.3 Pair of drawings of women from Itaki's *The Anatomy of the Body* 276
20.1 René-Antoine Ferchault de Réaumur's stages of reproduction of a crayfish leg 293
20.2 Georges-Louis Leclerc de Buffon's 'organic molecules' in seminal fluid of dogs and cows 296
20.3 François Quesnay's 'economic tableau' 297
20.4 Unit opener from *Exploring Biology* by Ella T. Smith 301
20.5 *Chambers's Encyclopaedia* entry on 'Generations, alternation of' 303
21.1 Manuscript diagram of classes in the sexual system by Carl Linnaeus 308
21.2 Manuscript containing botanical drawing by Linnaeus 313
21.3 Plate showing banana flower from Linnaeus's *Musa Cliffortiana* 315
21.4 Drawing that imagines palm planting from Linnaeus's Lapland journal 316
22.1 Engraving showing forceps, from André Levret's *Observations* 322
22.2 Woodcut of a birthing-room scene from Eucharius Rösslin's *Rosengarten* 328
22.3 Engraving from Mme du Coudray's *Abbrégé* showing how midwives could manoeuvre the unborn child 329

23.1 William Heberden's table of maternal and infant deaths 341
23.2 Jacques Tenon's table of live births, stillbirths and maternal deaths 342
24.1 Variations in total fertility rate induced by variations in five proximate determinants of natural fertility 348
24.2 Crude first marriage rates and real wage trends in England, 1541–1850 351
24.3 System of ecological niches showing dynamic feedback linkages capable of maintaining demographic equilibrium 352
24.4 'Natural' age-specific marital fertility rates in East Asian and European populations, 1600–1800 357
25.1 Jean-Baptiste Perronneau, *Portrait of Mapondé* 365
25.2 *Las castas* paintings from the late eighteenth century 370
26.1 Generation of Abraham Trembley's polyp 377
26.2 Frontispiece to *Thérèse philosophe* 379
26.3 Threefold parallel of gestation from *Vestiges of the Natural History of Creation* 384
26.4 Charles Darwin cartoon, 'That troubles our monkey again' 387
27.1 Portrait of T. W. Coke, Esq. with his prize North Devon ox 400
27.2 *Coates' Herd Book* pedigrees for Shorthorn bulls 401
27.3 *Punch* cartoon comparing the breeding of nobles and of cattle 404
27.4 Extract from a bull licence application form 408
27.5 Artificial insemination centre manager demonstrating semen collection 411
28.1 Male sexual organs of the hedgehog by Jean-Louis Prévost and Jean-Baptiste Dumas 416
28.2 Female sexual organs of the frog and tadpole development by Prévost and Dumas 418
28.3 Engraved drawing of frog semen by Gottfried Reinhold Treviranus 420
28.4 'Spermatozoon' penetrating the spiny starfish egg by Hermann Fol 425
29.1 Frontispiece and title-page of Richard Carlile's *What Is Love?* 429
29.2 Interior of Marie Stopes's Mothers' Clinic 435
29.3 Poster for the International Neo-Malthusian Conference 1922 439
29.4 Cover of an Abortion Law Reform Association campaign leaflet 440
30.1 Cinema announcement about venereal diseases, Dundee 447
30.2 T. H. C. Stevenson's diagram of numbers of live births at different ages at, and durations of, marriage 448
30.3 Ansley Coale and Edgar Hoover's graph for India showing projected output per consumer with and without family planning 450
30.4 Graphic accompanying Thomas Parran's campaign against syphilis 455
31.1 Childless couple looking at pictures of children offered for adoption 459
31.2 Caricature of a 'new woman' unwilling to fulfil her partner's 'cry for a child' 465

31.3 Catarrh of the cervix in a plate from Jenny Springer's *Die Ärztin im Hause* 467
31.4 Uterine massage in Anna Fischer-Dueckelmann's *The Wife as the Family Physician* 469
32.1 Lithograph satirizing the publication of obscenity cloaked in medical authority 474
32.2 Article on the Kinsey Report in the men's magazine *Action* 477
32.3 Nurse explains embryology at a maternity welfare centre 479
32.4 Slot machine for 'surgical rubber ware' outside a chemist's shop 482
33.1 Saibai Island woman divining the sex of her unborn child 487
33.2 African delivery scene from George Julius Engelmann's *Labor Among Primitive Peoples* 491
33.3 Postcard of a milk depot in the Belgian Congo 494
33.4 Baby show in Accra 495
34.1 Warren S. Thompson's map of world population density 508
34.2 Participants in world population meetings in 1927 and 1952 510
34.3 Cover of United Nations Population Fund report, *By Choice, Not by Chance* 515
34.4 Population bombs on covers of Moore Fund pamphlet and Paul Ehrlich's book 518
35.1 Three eras of sex-related substances in the twentieth century 523
35.2 The chicken crest test for 'male' potency in a laboratory notebook 524
35.3 Scheme of bio-industrial pathways for deriving sex steroids from cholesterol 526
35.4 Links between keywords in the biomedical literature on endocrine disruption 532
36.1 Advertisement for Dr Patterson's pills, a remedy for female 'irregularities' 537
36.2 *Sunday Pictorial* article about 'X-pills' 540
36.3 Woman's hand displaying IUDs in a *Which?* survey 542
36.4 Cover of *Esquire* about vasectomies 544
36.5 United States patent for the 'Hulka clip' 545
36.6 Spread from a pamphlet by Preterm, a clinic for abortion services 547
37.1 Engraving of the City of London Lying-In Hospital 556
37.2 Oil painting celebrating Ignaz Semmelweis 558
37.3 Flag pins promoting a National Birthday Trust Fund campaign 561
37.4 'Birthrights Rally' on London's Hampstead Heath 565
38.1 Prenatal diagnosis explained in a *Scientific American* article 571
38.2 'Bed-table scanner' for two-dimensional ultrasound 573
38.3 Increased nuchal translucency as a risk marker 575
39.1 José Roy's engravings in Jules Gérard's manual of artificial fecondation 584
39.2 'Test-tube babies' in *John Bull* 585
39.3 *Science* magazine cover, 'Superovulation and embryo transfer in cattle' 589
39.4 An '8-celled egg' developed from a human oocyte fertilized in vitro 591

39.5 Patrick Steptoe with colleagues at Kershaw's Hospital, Oldham 592
40.1 Engraving of Anthony Comstock arresting the abortionist Madame Restell 600
40.2 Abortion opponents march in front of the US Supreme Court 605
40.3 The case of the Relf sisters, reported in an *Ebony* article on sterilization 607
40.4 Human Fertilisation and Embryology Authority website 609
41.1 Sexual response cycles according to William Masters and Virginia Johnson 616
41.2 Fantasy and masturbation in *Women and Their Bodies: A Course* 617
41.3 Dialpak dispenser for oral contraceptives 621
41.4 Photograph of a pregnant Thomas Beatie and his wife Nancy 625
42.1 Photograph of Simone de Beauvoir 632
42.2 Shulamith Firestone's diagram of the achievement of cosmic consciousness 634
43.1 Maternity ward in the Mining Union Hospital for Natives at Elisabethville 644
43.2 'The road to maternal death', a WHO and Ugandan Ministry of Health poster 647
43.3 Indian stamps promoting family planning 648
43.4 Projected IVF devices and consumables market 653

Notes on the Frontispieces

[1] The birth of Helen of Troy on a fourth-century BC vase from southern Italy. In the version of the story illustrated here, Zeus took the shape of a swan to force himself on the goddess Nemesis. A Spartan shepherd picked up the egg she laid and gave it to Leda, his queen. We see the egg hatching on a warm altar. The baby Helen reaches towards a startled Leda (left) as the shepherd (right) looks on. Eros kneels above, signalling that love and desire are key to a tale that, in one form or another, inspires artists to this day (see illustration on p. 656, this book). Apulian red-figure *pelike*, *c.* 360–350 BC. H 33 cm. Kunsthalle zu Kiel, Antikensammlung, inv. no. B501.

[2] The Annunciation depicted on a small luxury mosaic from early fourteenth-century Constantinople, in typical Byzantine style. The archangel Gabriel holds up one hand in the gesture of speech: 'You will conceive in your womb and bear a son, and you will name him Jesus' (Luke 1:31). A beam descends from heaven, the light representing the Holy Spirit touching Mary, who adopts a modest posture as she heeds the angel's words. The theme has endured on devotional objects and altarpieces throughout the Christian world. 15 × 10 cm. © Victoria and Albert Museum, London, no. 7321–1860.

[3] This detail of the frontispiece to William Harvey's celebrated treatise on generation shows Zeus opening an egg labelled 'Everything from an egg'. The release of humans, other animals and plants invoked Pandora's box (originally a jar), from which both all evil and eternal hope flew out into the world. For Harvey, the egg was a product of conception, not the structure we know today; that remained elusive for centuries to come even as the searchers echoed these words. Frontispiece, probably drawn and etched by Richard Gaywood, from William Harvey, *Exercitationes de generatione animalium* (London: Octavian Pulleyn, 1651). Cambridge University Library.

[4] Detail of 'a large and beautiful Copper Plate, representing … the Method of hatching and bringing up Domestick Fowls', to illustrate the work of the Paris academician René-Antoine Ferchault de Réaumur in the *London Magazine; or Gentleman's Monthly Intelligencer*. We see various views of Egyptian ovens, egg baskets and thermometers, stages in the hatching of the chicks and a chicken-house. Réaumur, who wanted there to be a chicken in every peasant's Sunday pot, roused people of varied social station in many countries to experiment with temperature and humidity while raising birds for amusement or profit. From *London Magazine* 19 (July 1750), facing p. 318. Cambridge University Library.

[5] 'Away with Paragraph 218'. Photograph (detail) of a march in Leipzig on 19 August 1928, to protest against the abortion-outlawing paragraph of the German criminal code of 1871. Part of a large campaign, led by the parties of the left and feminist groups, this rally of the Red Women's and Girls' League was organized by the Red Front Fighters' League, a communist paramilitary organization banned the following year. The Nazis made the penalties for abortions harsher in general, while forcing them on 'racial' grounds; significant reform came only in the 1970s, when struggles over reproduction intensified – in the German states and elsewhere. © bpk.

[6] *The Population Bomb*, cover of a pamphlet published by the Hugh Moore Fund in New York in 1954. Moore, the Dixie-Cup millionaire, promoted voluntary sterilization as he extended an interwar programme of Malthusian internationalism into the Cold War. The fund aimed at 'preserving world peace, arresting Communism and improving the lot of people in overpopulated countries'. This image has prompted many variations, most famously Paul R. Ehrlich's bestselling 1968 paperback of the same name (Fig. 34.4, this book). It still shapes debate over the 'carrying capacity' of the Earth today. 15 × 7.5 cm.

Contributors

Annetta Alexandridis
Department of the History of Art and Visual Studies, Cornell University

Salim Al-Gailani
Department of History and Philosophy of Science, University of Cambridge

Jenny Bangham
Department of History and Philosophy of Science, University of Cambridge

Alison Bashford
University of New South Wales, Sydney

Christina Benninghaus
Wadham College, Oxford

Peter Biller
Department of History, University of York

Christina Brandt
Mercator Research Group 'Spaces of Anthropological Knowledge' and Institute of Philosophy I, Ruhr University Bochum

Stephanie Lynn Budin
independent scholar

Tatjana Buklijas
Liggins Institute, University of Auckland

Sandra Cavallo
Department of History, Royal Holloway, University of London

Lisa Forman Cody
Department of History, Claremont McKenna College

Marie-Hélène Congourdeau
Monde byzantin (UMR 8167 Orient-Méditerranée), CNRS, Paris

Lucia Dacome
Institute for the History and Philosophy of Science and Technology, University of Toronto

Véronique Dasen
Faculty of Humanities, University of Fribourg

Silvia De Renzi
Department of History, The Open University

James M. Edmonson
Dittrick Medical History Center, Cleveland

Karin Ekholm
St. John's College, Annapolis

Patrick Ellis
School of Literature, Media and Communication, Georgia Institute of Technology

Nahyan Fancy
History Department, DePauw University

Margot E. Fassler
Department of Theology, University of Notre Dame

Kate Fisher
Department of History, University of Exeter

Mary E. Fissell
Department of the History of Medicine, The Johns Hopkins University

Rebecca Flemming
Faculty of Classics, University of Cambridge

†John Forrester
Department of History and Philosophy of Science, University of Cambridge

Sarah Franklin
Department of Sociology, University of Cambridge

Jean-Paul Gaudillière
Cermes3, Villejuif

Fay Glinister
School of History, Archaeology and Religion, Cardiff University

Lesley A. Hall
Wellcome Library, London

Ellen Herman
Department of History, University of Oregon

Nick Hopwood
Department of History and Philosophy of Science, University of Cambridge

Jessica Hughes
Department of Classical Studies, The Open University

Ralph Jackson
Department of Britain, Europe and Prehistory, British Museum

Martin H. Johnson
Department of Physiology, Development and Neuroscience, University of Cambridge

Peter Murray Jones
King's College, Cambridge

Ludmilla Jordanova
Department of History, University of Durham

Solveig Jülich
Department of History of Science and Ideas, Uppsala University

Lauren Kassell
Department of History and Philosophy of Science, University of Cambridge

Helen King
Department of Classical Studies, The Open University

Wendy Kline
Department of History, Purdue University

Rina Knoeff
Research Centre for Historical Studies, University of Groningen

Philip Kreager
Institute of Human Sciences, University of Oxford

Philippa Levine
Department of History, University of Texas at Austin

Ilana Löwy
Cermes3, Villejuif

Maaike van der Lugt
Department of History, Versailles Saint-Quentin University

Renato G. Mazzolini
Department of Sociology and Social Research, University of Trento

Lianne McTavish
Faculty of Arts, University of Alberta

Staffan Müller-Wille
Department of Sociology, Philosophy and Anthropology, University of Exeter

Rune Nyord
Art History Department, Emory University

Lea T. Olsan
Department of English, University of Louisiana at Monroe

Jesse Olszynko-Gryn
School of Humanities (History), University of Strathclyde

Katharine Park
Department of the History of Science, Harvard University

Tim Parkin
School of Historical and Philosophical Studies, University of Melbourne

Gianna Pomata
Department of the History of Medicine, The Johns Hopkins University

Siân Pooley
Faculty of History, University of Oxford

Eleanor Robson
Department of History, University College London

Andrea Rusnock
Department of History, University of Rhode Island

Martina Schlünder
Max Planck Institute for the History of Science, Berlin

James A. Secord
Department of History and Philosophy of Science, University of Cambridge

Miri Shefer-Mossensohn
Department of Middle Eastern and African History, Tel Aviv University

Patricia Simons
Department of History of Art, University of Michigan

Richard M. Smith
Department of Geography, University of Cambridge

Jennifer Spinks
School of Historical and Philosophical Studies, University of Melbourne

Simon Szreter
Faculty of History, University of Cambridge

Mary Terrall
Department of History, UCLA

Laurence M. V. Totelin
School of History, Archaeology and Religion, Cardiff University

Florence Vienne
Department of the History of Science and Pharmacy, Technical University Braunschweig

Paul Weindling
School of History, Philosophy and Culture, Oxford Brookes University

Sarah Wilmot
John Innes Centre, Norwich

Gabriella Zuccolin
Villa I Tatti, The Harvard University Center for Italian Renaissance Studies, Florence

Acknowledgements

This book owes its birth to one set of parents and three institutional midwives. The parents are the Cambridge 'Generation to Reproduction' Group, in the first place our fellow Principal Investigators, the late John Forrester, Martin H. Johnson, Peter Murray Jones, James A. Secord, Richard Smith and Simon Szreter, with Eleanor Robson as a collaborator in the early stages and Mary Fissell playing an active part, especially in a sabbatical year in Cambridge. During the seminars, reading groups, workshops, conferences, film series, exhibition and other events through which we pooled our knowledge of history of reproduction, we have also learned a great deal from other project members, Salim Al-Gailani, Leah Astbury, Romola Davenport, Karin Ekholm, Fay Glinister, Jesse Olszynko-Gryn and Siân Pooley, as well as those colleagues and visitors who have joined in our discussions, notably Jenny Bangham, Christina Benninghaus, Boyd Brogan, Margaret Carlyle, Sarah Franklin, Vanessa Heggie, Susanne Lettow, Richard McKay, Dmitriy Myelnikov and Gabriella Zuccolin. We are particularly indebted to the people who also took the lead in organizing these events: Francis Neary, Shirlene Badger and Laura Dawes; and we thank Leah Astbury and Sophie Waring for assisting with a workshop that brought the authors of chapters together in a shared endeavour.

Before, during and after that workshop the contributors commented extensively on each other's chapters and 'exhibits' and we are immensely grateful for their generosity. As editors we wish above all to thank Silvia De Renzi, Mary Fissell, Helen King and Katharine Park for showing us how to improve substantially drafts of the first and last chapters and part introductions; and Salim Al-Gailani, Leah Astbury, Alison Bashford, Boyd Brogan, Helen Anne Curry, John Forrester, Sarah Franklin, Martin Johnson, Peter Jones, Ludmilla Jordanova, Elaine Leong, Ilana Löwy, Dániel Margócsy, Jesse Olszynko-Gryn, Simon Schaffer, Jim Secord, Richard Smith, Simon Szreter and Gabriella Zuccolin for many valuable insights and corrections. Editing has been intensely collaborative, too: although one editor took primary responsibility for each part of the book, we all commented on several drafts of every chapter and exhibit. A project as wide-ranging as this one is nevertheless prone to errors and oversimplifications, and we ask readers to look indulgently on those that remain.

Our first institutional debt is to the University of Cambridge, where this project self-organized in the days before strategic research initiatives. It has been based in the

Department of History and Philosophy of Science, a perfect place for cross-disciplinary work, with the support of heads of department John Forrester, Jim Secord and Liba Taub, and the much-appreciated assistance of Tamara Hug, David Thompson, Louisa Russell and Agnieszka Lanucha in the office and Anna Jones, Dawn Moutrey and Clare Matthews in the Whipple Library. We also benefited greatly from interactions in the CRASSH-supported Cambridge Interdisciplinary Reproduction Forum.

We could never have done the work without a second organization, the Wellcome Trust, which made this group possible by funding a strategic award in the history of medicine on the theme 'Generation to Reproduction' [088708] and its predecessor, an enhancement award [074298], as well as other grants that have brought us important collaborators and interlocutors over the years. Anthony Woods and then Daniel O'Connor and their teams have provided a great deal of caring and flexible support, including more than one no-cost extension.

A third institution, Cambridge University Press, let us turn a project into a book. We thank Michael Watson (assisted by Teresa Royle) for commissioning the volume and agreeing to so many pictures, and Lucy Rhymer (assisted by Melissa Shivers and Lisa Carter) for taking over and seeing the project through to completion with imagination and tact. As content manager, Cassi Roberts oversaw the production with great efficiency, and Lindsay Nightingale and Pam Scholefield did sterling work as copy editor and indexer respectively. The Faculty of Classics and the Department of HPS paid for the indexing. For assistance in preparing the manuscript for submission, and especially in sourcing images, we thank Eleri Cousins, Kathryn Schoefert and Tillmann Taape; and for expert photographic work, Ian Bolton and Adrian Newman of the Anatomy Visual Media Group. We further acknowledge the individuals and institutions who have helped with and allowed us to reproduce the pictures that appear on the figures and exhibits; they are credited in the captions. Ronald Ladouceur kindly provided a scan of Hugh Moore's *Population Bomb* pamphlet.

The contributors wish us to record some thanks. For comments on drafts of various chapters, we are very grateful to Keren Abbou-Hershkovits, Leah Astbury, Benedetta Borello, Angela Davis, Sonja Brentjes, Mary Brazelton, Laura Casella, Jo Edge, David Edgerton, Monica Green, Aleka Gürel, Mike Hawkins, Sarah Hodges, Carole Joffe, Natalie Kaoukji, Elaine Leong, Katrina Maydom, Basim Musallam, Caroline Musgrove, Rob Ralley, Leslie Reagan, Susanne Schmidt, Stéphane Schmitt, Sally Sheldon, Emma Spary, Tillmann Taape, John Young and Gabriella Zuccolin. Eleri Cousins translated Chapter 8, and Gabriella Zuccolin provided extensive help with Chapter 14. Nahyan Fancy thanks the Program in Medieval Studies and Center for Historical Analysis at Rutgers University, DePauw University's Fisher sabbatical funds, the Fulton Family Faculty Fellowship and the NEH summer seminar on 'Health and disease in the middle ages' (2012) for supporting the research for Chapter 9. Andrea Rusnock thanks the American Council of Learned Societies for a fellowship that funded the research for Chapter 23. Florence Vienne thanks Kate Sturge for translating first drafts of Chapter 28 and the Deutsche Forschungsgemeinschaft for financial support. Jesse Olszynko-Gryn thanks Elizabeth Watkins for contributing to a draft of Chapter 36 and Michael McGovern for help researching Exhibit 32.

We have some more personal debts. Nick Hopwood thanks Silvia De Renzi for many stimulating conversations about generation and much else, and Janet Westpheling for giving him a copy of François Jacob's *Logic of Life* in 1982. Rebecca Flemming thanks Rachel Aucott for technical and less technical support. Lauren Kassell thanks David Dernie for encouragement, good humour and practical expertise.

Our colleague John Forrester died on 24 November 2015. We think fondly of his brilliant and provocative input into our seminars, reading groups and workshops, and the generosity with which he shared his vast knowledge of the history of sex and many other matters. This book is dedicated to his memory.

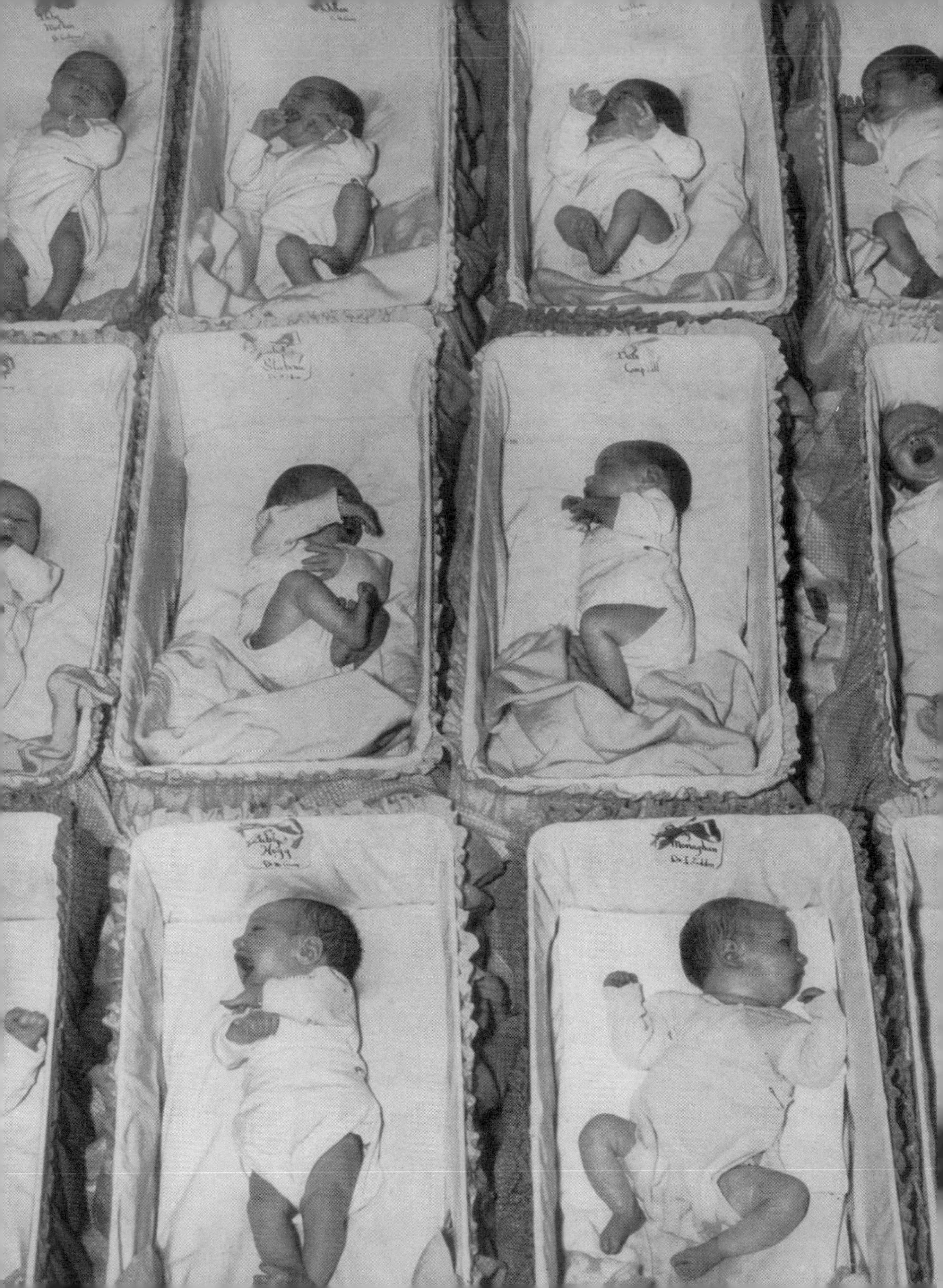

Introduction

Babies at Nazareth Hospital, Philadelphia, photographed for a *Life* magazine story in 1941. *Life* claimed that, in the struggle for fertility with Nazi Germany, America was winning 'the baby war' with a baby boom, a concept that gained traction in demography later. Large-scale hospital birth, which spread rapidly through the mid-twentieth century, became the subject of heated struggles over control and a key issue in what by the 1970s was framed as 'the politics of reproduction'. Detail from photograph by Marty Hyman (*Philadelphia Record*) from 'Boom in babies', *Life* (1 Dec. 1941), 73–4, on 73.

1 Reproduction in History

Nick Hopwood, Rebecca Flemming and Lauren Kassell

Who should reproduce, and how? Is it acceptable to manipulate DNA to make a 'designer baby' or clone a favourite pet? Ought everyone to have smaller families to limit the environmental impacts of population growth? Why do hundreds of thousands of women and millions of babies still die at the time of childbirth every year? Reproduction is in the news because the subject has such wide scope, from the most intimate experiences to planetary policy, and because it raises such large and difficult questions. Innovation fuels controversies over science and technology, economics and politics, ethics and religion, while children keep on being born.

Activists, politicians, scientists and scholars have called on history to celebrate progress or condemn present practices, to understand where we are and how things might take a turn for the better or worse. They have argued that family planning produced prosperity or that fertility control followed social change; that male obstetricians developed techniques to make childbirth safe or increased the danger by edging midwives out. Tales are still told of advance or decline, sudden ruptures or long traditions, but the relevant research has become so vast and diverse that it is hard to see the big picture. Even historians may lose their way in the forests of books and journals.

This volume, the first large-scale history of reproduction, works against this dispersion of scholarship by bringing together and extending some of the best studies. It comes out of conversations between experts in different epochs and approaches, and invites readers to join in the attempt to grasp the whole, to revise old stories and tell new ones. Focusing on the Mediterranean, western Europe, North America and their empires, we span from antiquity to the present day. The book also combines histories of science, technology and medicine with social, cultural and demographic accounts. It aims to set agendas for research, to introduce students and non-specialists to the field and to deepen public debate.

What Was Reproduction?

In the sense of procreation alone, reproduction has had extraordinary reach. Efforts to control fertility and manage births have linked bedrooms to courtrooms, and laboratories to farms and clinics, while involving midwives and embryologists, farmers and anti-abortionists. Explanations have referred to seeds and embryos, eggs and sperm, monsters and clones, sex and the life cycle. Reproduction has been bound up in more general concerns about creation and evolution, race and gender, degeneration and regeneration, not to mention those other meanings of the word: copying and social transmission. The birth of a baby may imply investments in maternity and paternity for families, lineages, even dynasties, and states. The Roman Emperor Augustus legislated to encourage marriage and childbearing, a much-repeated endeavour, while recent Indian governments have run mass sterilization camps, and China launched and eventually loosened a one-child policy. Demands of growing populations for food, and hence land, have propelled migration and been used to justify wars; they have fostered plant and animal breeding, transforming the environment and our diets. Populations that did not reproduce themselves have relied on immigration, with profound effects on economies, politics and cultures.

We can look back like a biologist or demographer and find reproduction in every century, but for historians 'reproduction' also means a set of ideas and practices that are specifically modern. Before the nineteenth century, most educated people wrote not of 'reproduction', but of 'generation', a larger, looser framework for discussing procreation and descent. 'Generation' was an active making, and commentators likened the genesis of new beings to artisanal processes such as brewing, baking and moulding clay. Generation encompassed not just animals and plants, but minerals too, though the human soul received special attention. Only in the mid-eighteenth century did the word 'reproduction', literally 'producing again', begin to gain any currency as the common property of all living organisms (and only them) to beget others of their own kind. Used most influentially in this sense by the director of the King's Garden in Paris, Georges-Louis Leclerc, Comte de Buffon, in 1749, the concept meant a more abstract process of perpetuating species, which were then increasingly defined as 'populations'.

Reproduction, whether as biological universal or time-bound practices, should be central to the writing of history. It has not been, because activities associated with sex, and wrongly perceived as just concerning women, were sidelined for a long time. Since 'reproduction' itself was consolidated as a somewhat unified discourse only in the late nineteenth century, and became prominent only in the mid-twentieth, accounts of the various aspects of its history are scattered.

In the 1970s, some scholars recognized history of reproduction as a broad field comprising individuals and populations. As new social movements fought for women's and gay liberation, and civil as well as workers' rights, people started to talk about 'the politics of reproduction'. Feminists played the leading part. Campaigners for women to take on new social and economic roles demanded the power to choose whether, when and how to conceive, carry, deliver and raise a child. They rediscovered the famous statement about the importance of reproduction by Karl Marx's collaborator Friedrich Engels in 1884: 'the determining factor in history is … the production and reproduction of immediate life … On the one hand, the production of the means of subsistence, of food, clothing and shelter … on the other, the production of human beings themselves, the propagation of the species.'[1] Feminist intellectuals argued that reproductive labour was fundamental to history and social life, and that it should be organized more equitably.

As new methods swept the social sciences and humanities, historians took up topics that their profession had largely ignored: women and gender, the family, the body and sexuality. Reproduction was a magnet for research, but 'history of reproduction' did not acquire an independent identity.[2] Focusing on babies, especially as women's business, risked reinforcing the very assumptions that needed to change, though it might have strengthened ties to the burgeoning studies of procreation in anthropology, sociology and demography.[3] A half-century later, and after much important work, reproduction still invites more concerted historical attention. This book seizes that opportunity.

Frameworks from the 1970s

We begin by going back to the 1970s, when frameworks for the history of reproduction were built in encounters between critical political and intellectual agendas, particularly within feminism, and pre-existing disciplines. Histories of medicine, demography, the family and ideas supplied foundations, component parts and narratives to critique.

Of these, history of medicine was most important. In the 1970s, doctors were at the summit of their power, but denounced for 'medicalization': claiming authority over areas of life that had not been medical at all. The disapproval extended to physicians' and surgeons' dominion over the past through bold, often technology-driven stories of the rise of specialties such as obstetrics and gynaecology. The then largely male practitioners applauded the progress of rationality against female ignorance and incompetence, while obscuring the mutual shaping of technology and society (Fig. 1.1).[4] Activism against hospitalized childbirth, and for improved access to contraception and abortion, spawned histories that decried the denigration of women's contributions to generation and a takeover of childbirth by forceps-wielding men.[5]

The best-known history of reproduction had its origins in 1972 as a talk at a conference on women's health. Barbara Ehrenreich and Deirdre English, teachers at SUNY College at Old Westbury, 'a hotbed of political debate', wrote *Witches, Midwives, and*

1 Friedrich Engels, *The Origin of the Family, Private Property, and the State* (New York, NY, 1972), pp. 25–6.

2 For an early use of the phrase: Mary P. Ryan, 'Reproduction in American history', *Journal of Interdisciplinary History* 10 (1979), 319–32.

3 Faye Ginsburg and Rayna Rapp, 'The politics of reproduction', *Annual Review of Anthropology* 20 (1991), 311–43; Rene Almeling, 'Reproduction', *Annual Review of Sociology* 41 (2015), 423–42.

4 For example, Harold Speert, *Iconographia gyniatrica: A Pictorial History of Gynecology and Obstetrics* (Philadelphia, PA, 1973).

5 Carolyn Merchant, *The Death of Nature: Women, Ecology, and the Scientific Revolution* (San Francisco, CA, 1980); Jean Donnison, *Midwives and Medical Men: A History of Inter-Professional Rivalries and Women's Rights* (New York, NY, 1977).

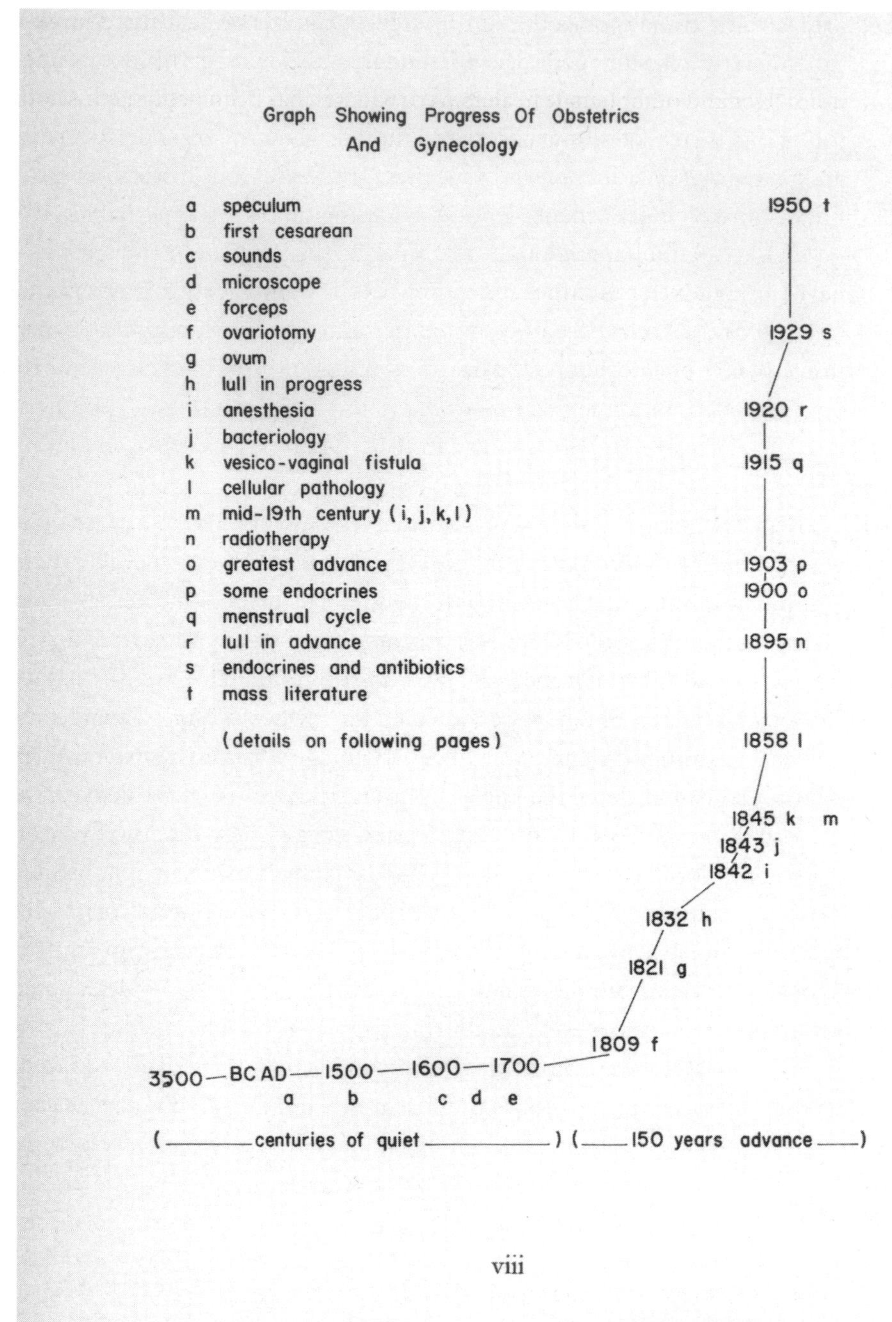

Figure 1.1 'Graph showing progress of obstetrics and gynecology.' The line is 'almost horizontal' until Ephraim McDowell's ovariotomy of 1809 begins 'an abrupt upward trend.' The figure was reproduced for criticism in William Ray Arney's Foucauldian *Power and the Profession of Obstetrics* in 1982. From Theodore Cianfrani, *A Short History of Obstetrics and Gynecology* (Springfield, IL: Thomas, 1960), p. viii. 23 × 15 cm.

Nurses 'in a blaze of anger' (Fig. 1.2).[6] The pamphlet linked the demise of midwives and the rise of male medical professionals, though its premise, that the majority of midwives and other female healers were witches, has been debunked. Another revisionist classic, Linda Gordon's 1976 history of birth control, drew on *A Medical History of Contraception* (1936), which a counterpart of the (American) Birth Control League had funded sociologist Norman Himes to research. Himes contended that for 'half a million years' humans had desired to restrict fertility with 'techniques, now bizarre and pathetically ineffective or injurious, now strangely ingenious, original and workable', but that 'democratized knowledge' of effective methods was 'ultra-modern'. Gordon broadened the scope to encompass politics, from the free-love, socialist and feminist beginnings of the modern movement to states' cooption of contraception to limit the reproduction of the poor and non-white.[7] She horrified conservative historians, but prompted the sympathetic to seek more evidence of how people behaved in the past.

The new politics of reproduction also engaged with population control. Its much-rehearsed history went back to the 'principle of population' articulated by the Reverend Thomas Robert Malthus in 1798: the number of mouths to feed increases geometrically, but resources rise only arithmetically. As nineteenth-century governments re-established the practice of censuses, and instituted civil registration and statistical bureaux, debates over the strength of nations, migration, eugenics and birth control invoked historic trends. After World War II, demographers at the Princeton Office of Population Research offered the European transition to low fertility between 1850 and 1940 as a model for progress in the 'Third World'. 'Demographic transition theory' presented modernization from uncontrolled 'natural' fertility to smaller, planned families as the basis for stable economic growth.[8] Population controllers argued that access to family planning could accelerate this last stage even without social and economic change, but in the 1970s their methods and concepts came under sustained attack from the Left.

Social historians were already giving the history of the family a more distinct identity by going beyond numbers to include sentiments, attitudes and households within their purview.[9] History of the family had started – or so Engels claimed – when *Das Mutterrecht* (Mother right, 1861), by the Basel jurist Johann Jakob Bachofen, disputed the permanence of patriarchy. The American anthropologist Lewis Henry Morgan, drawing on wider research into past kinship, noted the early absence of private property

6 Barbara Ehrenreich and Deirdre English, *Witches, Midwives & Nurses: A History of Women Healers*, 2nd edn (New York, NY, 2000), pp. 7–13.

7 Norman E. Himes, *Medical History of Contraception* (New York, NY, 1970), pp. xiv, 422; Linda Gordon, *Woman's Body, Woman's Right: A Social History of Birth Control in America* (Harmondsworth, 1977), pp. 216–19.

8 Simon Szreter, 'The idea of demographic transition and the study of fertility change: A critical intellectual history', *Population and Development Review* 19 (1993), 659–701.

9 Peter Laslett, *The World We Have Lost* (London, 1965); Louise A. Tilly and Miriam Cohen, 'Does the family have a history? A review of theory and practice in family history', *Social Science History* 6 (1982), 131–79.

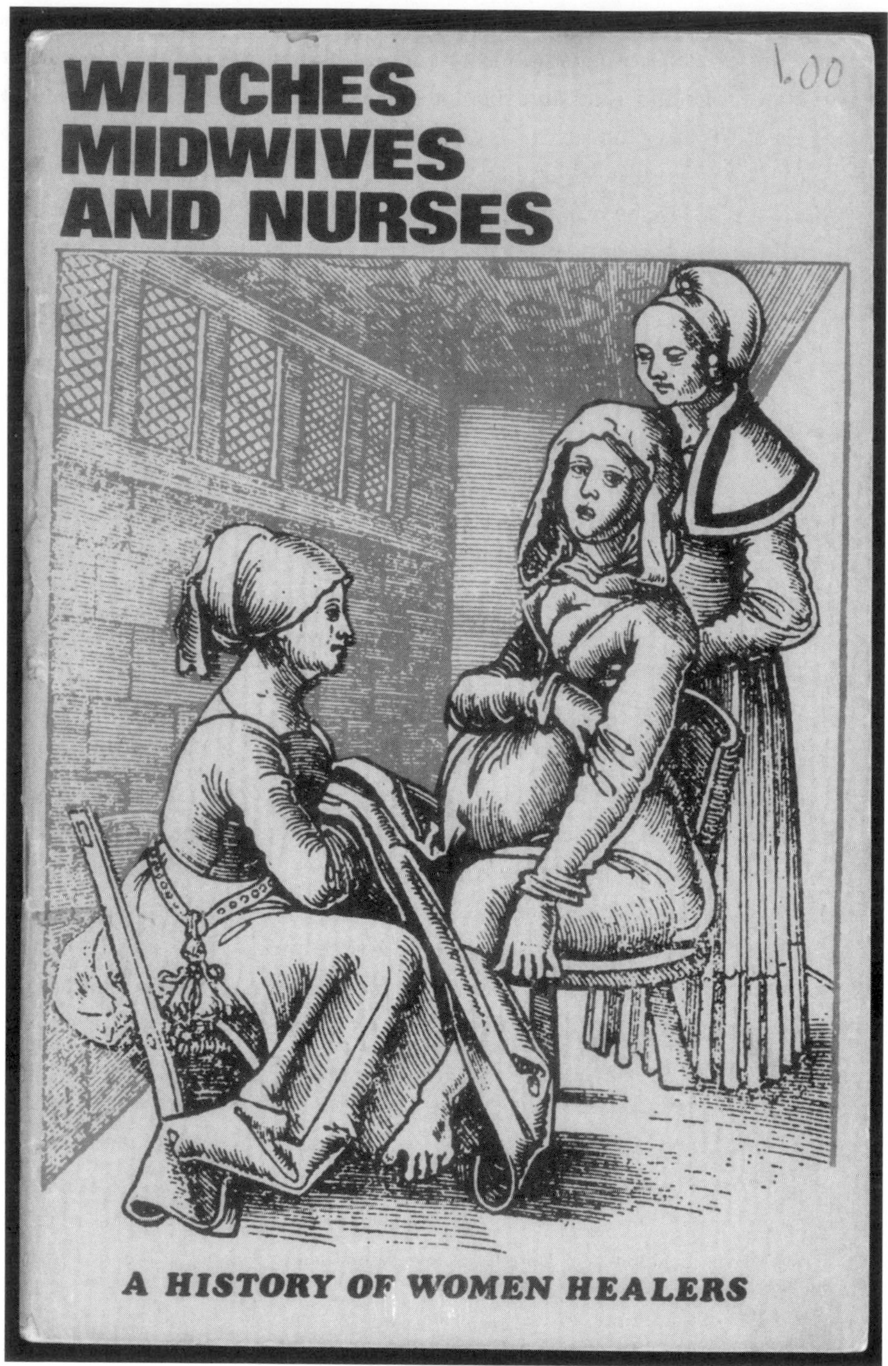

Figure 1.2 Cover of the forty-five-page pamphlet that Ehrenreich and English self-published in 1972 and distributed in old boxes from Pampers nappies; the Feminist Press took it over the following year. The woodcut of a woman in labour, assisted by midwife and birth attendant, is after Eucharius Rösslin's handbook for midwives, first published in 1513. 21 × 14 cm.

and the state, and proposed a universal shift from 'savage' group marriage and maternal clan to 'civilized' monogamy and 'father-family'.[10] Historians were slow to expand their remit, but around 1900 anthropologists classified societies according to practices of family formation and sexual mores, and inquired into understandings of the relations between intercourse, pregnancy and paternity. 'Sexologists' such as Havelock Ellis, author of an early medical textbook on homosexuality, explored human sexual variety past and present.[11] Here were powerful resources for questioning the naturalness of the bourgeois family and its gender roles, a project later developed in feminist philosophy and anthropology.

Fresh approaches enlivened histories of biological and philosophical ideas, in which generation loomed large.[12] By the 1970s, critical scholars were rewriting chronicles of the growth of thought by postulating radical breaks in making the modern world. Most influential has been a French tradition, especially Michel Foucault's notion of 'power-knowledge', the pervasive ways in which power defines thought and the thinkable. Analysing 'apparatuses' rather than intellectual lineages, Foucault had proposed in the 1960s that knowledge could reorganize suddenly, and that a break around 1800 made the medical, life and human sciences possible. In 1976, the introductory volume of his *History of Sexuality* distinguished two forms of 'biopower', a new authority over life that expanded from the seventeenth century. On the one hand, 'anatomo-politics' controlled, trained and shaped individual bodies by disciplines that promoted efficiency and productivity. On the other, a 'biopolitics' of the population, now a phenomenon managed by nation-states, acted through a set of regulations to define peoples, principally workforces, including their racial composition. Anatomo-politics and biopolitics intersected in procreative sex.[13]

Written in the same city, Paris, around the same time, a history of genetics by the molecular biologist François Jacob was the first to locate a break, much like Foucault's, in the late eighteenth-century move from 'generation' to 'reproduction', the framework within which researchers formulated modern concepts of eggs and sperm, genes and populations.[14] Feminist historians of medicine argued further that, between 1750 and

10 Engels, *Origin of the Family*, pp. 28–9, 68, 82–9.

11 Henrika Kuklick, *The Savage Within: The Social History of British Anthropology, 1885–1945* (Cambridge, 1991); Lucy Bland and Laura Doan (eds.), *Sexology in Culture: Labelling Bodies and Desires* (Cambridge, 1998).

12 Still indispensable: Erna Lesky, *Die Zeugungs- und Vererbungslehren der Antike und ihr Nachwirken* (Wiesbaden, 1951); Jacques Roger, *Les sciences de la vie dans la pensée française du XVIIIe siècle: La génération des animaux de Descartes à l'*Encyclopédie (Paris, 1963).

13 Michel Foucault, *The History of Sexuality*, vol. 1: *An Introduction* (New York, NY, 1978); Foucault, *Security, Territory, Population: Lectures at the Collège de France, 1977–1978*, ed. Michel Senellart, trans. Graham Burchell (New York, NY, 2007).

14 François Jacob, *The Logic of Life: A History of Heredity*, trans. Betty E. Spillmann (New York, NY, 1982).

1850, medicine, demography and political economy replaced '*generatio*', or 'fruitfulness', with 'reproduction', which under industrial capitalism became linked to production.[15]

By 1980, then, accounts of loss confronted tales of progress, and claims of sudden ruptures defied assumptions of the smooth advance of knowledge and skill. As histories of medicine and science professionalized, past reproduction stayed unusually politicized. Histories of midwifery fed into battles over high-tech hospital birth,[16] while the Ford Foundation, promoting women's choice about childbearing, supported James Mohr's *Abortion in America* (1978), which was read out during a filibuster in the United States Senate.[17] Histories of eugenics fuelled demands for compensation to people sterilized against their will.[18] Histories of reproductive medicine criticized gender bias and discriminatory provision.[19]

The core insights from the 1970s have enduring value. The feminist attention to the gendered division of labour is fundamental, and now interprets the roles played by men as well as women.[20] It is hard to imagine the field without the idea of 'biopolitics', even if the accumulation of empirical information has qualified Foucault's description of the eighteenth-century rise of 'population' and revealed the limitations of generalizing from France. Jacob named the big shift from generation to reproduction that structures this book, but his history of ideas wants enrichment and re-examination. By pooling expertise, we can reassess these frameworks and ground long views in the latest research.

Challenges of the Long Term

Between the 1980s and the early 2000s, historical practice shifted away from grand narratives while the volume of nuanced studies grew. That has made it harder to draw big pictures, and all too easy to revert to the old ones by default. Instead, we should renew and replace the existing outlines by building on writing that embraced a multiperspectival conception of culture and on histories of science, technology and

15 Barbara Duden, *The Woman beneath the Skin: A Doctor's Patients in Eighteenth-Century Germany*, trans. Thomas Dunlap (Cambridge, MA, 1991), pp. 28–9, 205; Ludmilla Jordanova, 'Interrogating the concept of reproduction in the eighteenth century', in Faye D. Ginsburg and Rayna Rapp (eds.), *Conceiving the New World Order: The Global Politics of Reproduction* (Berkeley, CA, 1995), pp. 369–86.

16 Ann Oakley, *The Captured Womb: A History of the Medical Care of Pregnant Women* (Oxford, 1984).

17 James C. Mohr, *Abortion in America: The Origins and Evolution of National Policy, 1800–1900* (New York, NY, 1978).

18 Daniel J. Kevles, *In the Name of Eugenics: Genetics and the Uses of Human Heredity* (New York, NY, 1985); Gisela Bock, *Zwangssterilisation im Nationalsozialismus. Studien zur Rassenpolitik und Frauenpolitik* (Opladen, 1986).

19 Gena Corea, *The Mother Machine: Reproductive Technologies from Artificial Insemination to Artificial Wombs* (London, 1985).

20 Judith Walzer Leavitt, *Brought to Bed: Childbearing in America, 1750–1950* (New York, NY, 1986); Leavitt, *Make Room for Daddy: The Journey from Waiting Room to Birthing Room* (Chapel Hill, NC, 2009).

medicine that took a 'practical turn'. Historians now pay closer and more integrated attention to everyday activities and experiences, knowledge and technology, as well as empire and globalization. These approaches have inspired the contributors to this book.

In the 1980s, cultural historians rediscovered the body. Norbert Elias's civilizing process, with its internalization of self-restraint, and Mikhail Bakhtin's notion of the grotesque body evoked a rupture between a messy world of sex, excrement, blood and monsters, and the modern bourgeois ideal of order, discipline and hygiene.[21] Enlightenment writers presumed that nature, and bodies, provide a bedrock for society and culture – the assumption that underlay nineteenth-century sexism and racism.[22] Tackling a topic close to reproduction, in 1990 Thomas Laqueur portrayed a concurrent transformation, from a 'one-sex' to a 'two-sex body': men and women, once seen as better and worse versions of the same basic structure, took radically different forms just as anatomy became destiny. Specialists have challenged Laqueur's limited evidence and focus on structure over function and cosmology.[23] These revisions point the way to a fuller appreciation of past experiences of generation and the making of reproductive bodies.

By exploring more scenes of action, historians of medicine again and again brought generation and reproduction to the fore, from the late medieval rise of anatomy and the gendering of early modern English political culture to the 'sexual revolution' since 1960.[24] Historians of science similarly recognized not just universities and hospitals, but also homes and law courts, as places where knowledge was made and generation and reproduction were at stake, for example, in disputes over inheritance and identity.[25] Research more systematically linked industry and agriculture to academic biology (Fig. 1.3).[26]

21 For example, Gail Kern Paster, *The Body Embarrassed: Drama and the Disciplines of Shame in Early Modern England* (Ithaca, NY, 1993).

22 Lorraine Daston, 'The nature of nature in early modern Europe', *Configurations* 6 (1998), 149–72; Susanne Lettow (ed.), *Reproduction, Race, and Gender in Philosophy and the Early Life Sciences* (Albany, NY, 2014); Londa Schiebinger, *The Mind Has No Sex? Women in the Origins of Modern Science* (Cambridge, MA, 1989).

23 Thomas Laqueur, *Making Sex: Body and Gender from the Greeks to Freud* (Cambridge, MA, 1990); Helen King, *The One-Sex Body on Trial: The Classical and Early Modern Evidence* (Farnham, 2013).

24 Katharine Park, *Secrets of Women: Gender, Generation, and the Origins of Human Dissection* (New York, NY, 2006); Mary E. Fissell, *Vernacular Bodies: The Politics of Reproduction in Early Modern England* (Oxford, 2004); Jeffrey Weeks, *Sex, Politics and Society: The Regulation of Sexuality since 1800*, 3rd edn (Harlow, 2012).

25 Silvia De Renzi, 'The risks of childbirth: Physicians, finance, and women's deaths in the law courts of seventeenth-century Rome', *Bulletin of the History of Medicine* 84 (2010), 549–77.

26 Nelly Oudshoorn, *Beyond the Natural Body: An Archeology of Sex Hormones* (New York, NY, 1994); Sarah Wilmot (ed.), 'Between the farm and the clinic: Agriculture and reproductive technology in the twentieth century', special issue, *Studies in History and Philosophy of Biological and Biomedical Sciences* 38 (2007), 303–530. Some earlier studies: Barbara A. Kimmelman, 'The American Breeders' Association: Genetics and eugenics in an agricultural context, 1903–13', *Social Studies of Science* 13 (1983), 163–204; Nicholas Russell, *Like Engend'ring Like: Heredity and Animal Breeding in Early Modern England* (Cambridge, 1986);

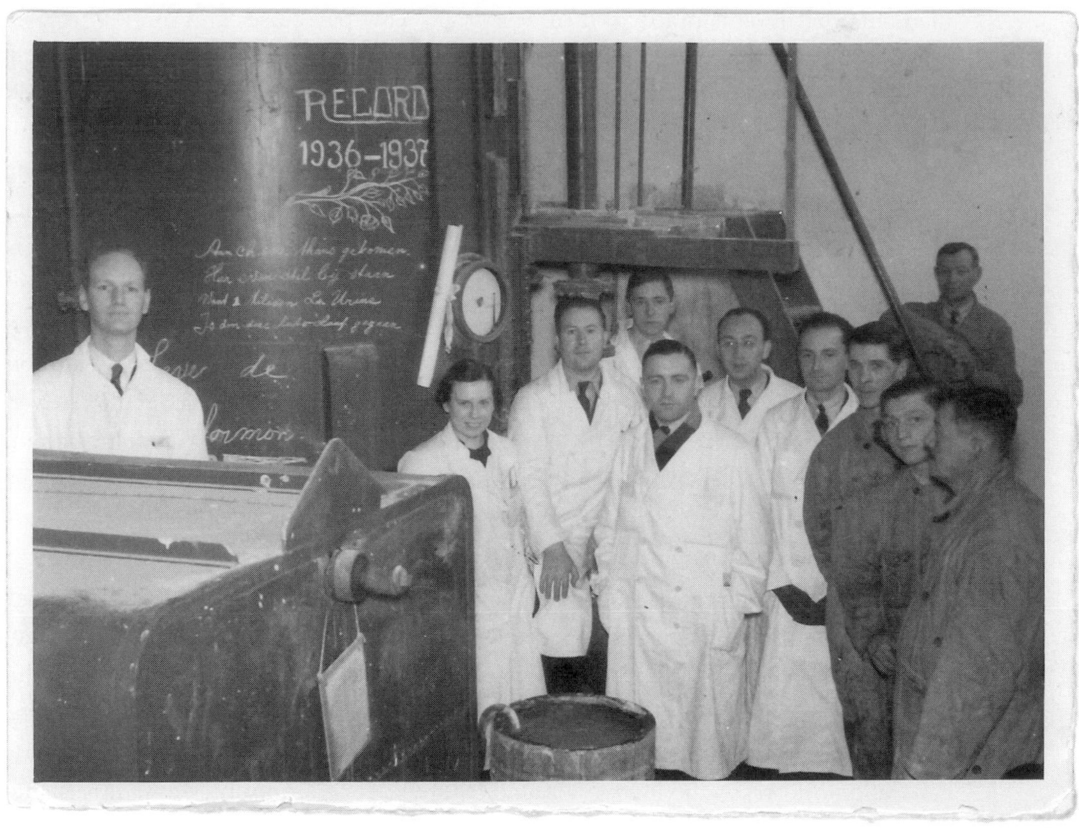

Figure 1.3 Staff of the Dutch pharmaceutical company Organon celebrate their use of the millionth litre of mare's urine in the manufacture of female sex hormone (oestrone, an oestrogen) in the 1936–7 season. This photograph was reproduced in Nelly Oudshoorn's *Beyond the Natural Body* (1994), a pioneering historical sociology of how manufacturing, measuring and marketing made sex hormones effective drugs. Central Archives, MSD, Oss, The Netherlands.

The new cultural history thus included more actors, while approaching their identities more critically. Investigating the making of kinds of practitioner and objects of study has produced guides to their coming into being and passing away. Professional midwives, for instance, seem to have re-emerged only several centuries after the fall of the Roman Empire in the west; the terms 'reproductive sciences' and 'reproductive medicine' were coined very recently.[27] Cultural historians combined this interest in identity formation with a refusal to take seemingly obvious practices for granted, a

Jonathan Liebenau, *Medical Science and Medical Industry: The Formation of the American Pharmaceutical Industry* (Baltimore, MD, 1987).

27 Monica H. Green, *Making Women's Medicine Masculine: The Rise of Male Authority in Pre-Modern Gynaecology* (Oxford, 2008), pp. 34–6, 127–9, 134–40; Adele Clarke, *Disciplining Reproduction: Modernity, American Life Sciences, and 'the Problems of Sex'* (Berkeley, CA, 1998).

sensibility that, with inspiration from the sociology of scientific knowledge, was extended to observation and experiment as well as collecting.[28] Historians of communication reconstructed the authorship, manufacture, distribution, reading and viewing of books and other media, and so embedded ideas in basic routines. Recognizing readers and other audiences as agents of change mirrored the move in history and sociology of technology to appreciate users' power; it put advice books and contraceptives in the same frame.[29]

Sharing the general aim of recovering perspectives from below, scholars sought most importantly to do justice to the agency of colonized groups. They moved subaltern studies to the centre of attention, and brought a more varied set of empires into view together with their medical regimes.[30] Historians of imperialism investigated how colonial enterprises depended on controlling reproduction.[31] Thinking globally highlighted the diversity of reproduction and questioned narratives centred in the metropoles.[32]

In these and other ways, various historical projects converged on generation and reproduction. Yet higher standards of evidence and of contextualization favoured analyses of single topics, periods and places. It is harder to chart long-term transformation while maintaining dialogue with social, political and cultural histories than when the 'Scientific Revolution' was a taken-for-granted break in a long intellectual tradition. But we now have novel strategies for charting continuity and change, for example, by tracking a series of shifts in practices of communication. This volume draws recent work together, presents new research, encourages dialogue and, above all, reconsiders the *longue durée*. We seek to improve the big pictures for their own sake and to allow histories of every century to flourish. A longer view helps studies of short periods to evaluate stability and checks the tendency to overstate change, especially where claims about modern innovations are based on flawed or foreshortened assumptions about the 'pre-modern'.

28 For example, Robert E. Kohler, *Lords of the Fly:* Drosophila *Genetics and the Experimental Life* (Chicago, IL, 1994); Lorraine Daston and Katharine Park, *Wonders and the Order of Nature, 1150–1750* (New York, NY, 1998).

29 Nick Hopwood *et al.* (eds.), 'Communicating reproduction', special issue, *Bulletin of the History of Medicine* 89 (2015), 379–556; Nelly Oudshoorn and Trevor Pinch (eds.), *How Users Matter: The Co-construction of Users and Technology* (Cambridge, MA, 2003); for earlier studies: Roy Porter and Lesley Hall, *The Facts of Life: The Creation of Sexual Knowledge in Britain, 1650–1950* (New Haven, CT, 1995); Patricia Crawford, *Blood, Bodies and Families in Early Modern England* (Harlow, 2004).

30 For the middle ages: Iona McCleery, 'What is "colonial" about *medieval* colonial medicine? Iberian health in global context', *Journal of Medieval Iberian Studies* 7 (2015), 151–75.

31 Nancy Rose Hunt, *A Colonial Lexicon: Of Birth Ritual, Medicalization, and Mobility in the Congo* (Durham, NC, 1999).

32 Alison Bashford and Joyce E. Chaplin, *The New Worlds of Thomas Robert Malthus: Rereading the* Principle of Population (Princeton, NJ, 2016).

Thus, ancient historians and medievalists have disputed that childbirth was ever a matter for women alone.[33] These findings put into perspective arguments about male surgeons' greater involvement in normal births from the eighteenth century. The standard histories are also wrong to imagine that everyone resigned themselves to 'barrenness' until medicine offered treatments for 'sterility' in the nineteenth century and intervened to bypass 'infertility' in the twentieth; learned medical men have targeted female fertility since antiquity.[34] The modern experience is nevertheless distinct in the way in which quests for children became projects in medical consumption on a significant scale.

Long views bring their own temptations, whether to talk up a revolution or claim that nothing changes and everything recurs. Special dangers lurk in tunnel histories. Histories of contraception and abortion rightly stress the antiquity of the desire to regulate fertility – and that all household and kinship systems have limited it somehow[35] – but before the fertility transitions the majority were more interested in promoting than avoiding the birth of children. The false continuities imposed by casual anachronism are most troublesome. Deliberate anachronism may be less problematic (Fig. 1.4). The word 'reproduction', which was rare in its modern senses even in the early nineteenth century, is in our title, but we avoid putting it into the mouths of people who would never have said it. To grasp how the differences between the frameworks mattered, we both revisit the shift from 'reproduction' to 'generation' in the decades around 1800 and trace the longer and overlapping career of 'generation'.[36]

This Book

This book is divided into five chronological parts, each with a short introduction. Part I, 'Inventing Generation', is about ancient Greece and Rome, where fundamental notions of body and soul were articulated, and practitioners in dialogue with philosophy forged a domain of medicine concerned with generation. In the following centuries this framework gained influence across the Mediterranean and was Christianized. Part II,

33 Ann Ellis Hanson, 'A division of labor: Roles for men in Greek and Roman births', *Thamyris* 1 (1994), 157–202; Helen King, *Hippocrates' Woman: Reading the Female Body in Ancient Greece* (London, 1998), pp. 172–87; Green, *Making Women's Medicine Masculine*.

34 Naomi Pfeffer, *The Stork and the Syringe: A Political History of Reproductive Medicine* (Cambridge, 1993); Margaret Marsh and Wanda Ronner, *The Empty Cradle: Infertility in America from Colonial Times to the Present* (Baltimore, MD, 1996); Rebecca Flemming, 'The invention of infertility in the classical Greek world: Medicine, divinity, and gender', *Bulletin of the History of Medicine* 87 (2013), 565–90.

35 Angus McLaren, *A History of Contraception: From Antiquity to the Present Day* (Oxford, 1990); and especially John M. Riddle, *Eve's Herbs: A History of Contraception and Abortion in the West* (Cambridge, MA, 1997); for a critique: King, *Hippocrates' Woman*, pp. 132–56.

36 Ohad Parnes, Ulrike Vedder and Stefan Willer, *Das Konzept der Generation. Eine Wissenschafts- und Kulturgeschichte* (Frankfurt am Main, 2008).

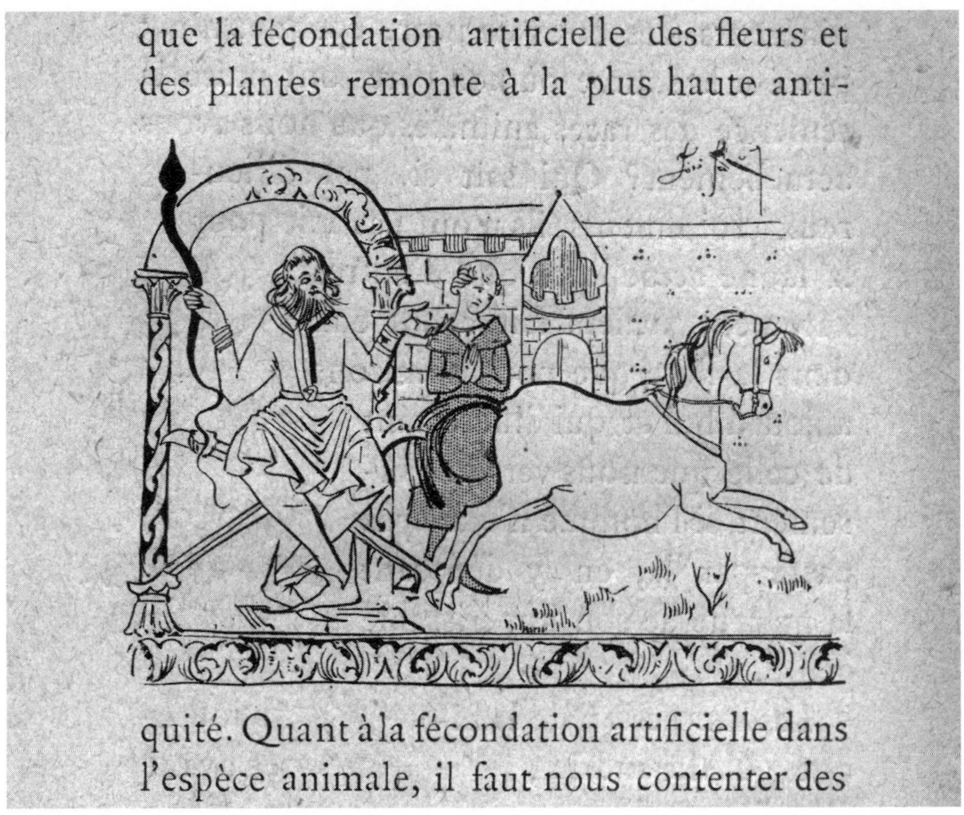
que la fécondation artificielle des fleurs et des plantes remonte à la plus haute anti-

quité. Quant à la fécondation artificielle dans l'espèce animale, il faut nous contenter des

Figure 1.4 A spoof thirteenth-century spermatozoon in a risqué manual of artificial 'fecondation' (insemination) from 1888. The artist, José Roy, represented the semen with which a Darfur man impregnated his mare as a huge sperm within a medieval frame. (See also Fig. 39.1, this book.) Engraving from J. Gérard, *Nouvelles causes de stérilité dans les deux sexes: Fécondation artificielle comme moyen ultime de traitement*, édition définitive (Paris: Marpon & Flammarion, [1888?]), p. 356, width 7 cm.

'Generation Reborn and Reformed', considers the proliferation of discussions about generation in the Islamic and Christian worlds. Involving more laymen and women, debate was invigorated by translations, the foundation of universities and the renaissance of classical learning, the Protestant Reformation of the early sixteenth century and encounters across the Atlantic.

Part III, 'Inventing Reproduction', reassesses the claims that the age of revolutions around 1800 saw the replacement of 'generation' by 'reproduction' and that 'population' was framed as a phenomenon subject to its own laws. Part IV, 'Modern Reproduction', explores the era of capital and empire between 1848 and 1939, when declining birth-rates caused consternation in industrialized countries, and governments, medicine and science increasingly intervened. Part V, 'Reproduction Centre Stage', is about how reproduction became politically prominent and was transformed by science and technology on a large scale. Moving from the high watermark of state power after World War II to neoliberalism, it shows how our reproductive world was made.

We thus track the reworking of an influential body of ideas and practices from Graeco-Roman antiquity onwards, emphasizing those territories for which the most scholarship is available. This is a western regional history, though we spotlight interactions with the rest of the world. Frameworks of generation began in the Mediterranean basin, spread with the Roman Empire and travelled east with the Arab conquests of the seventh century AD and the expansion of domains under Muslim rule. Crossing to the New World with European colonialism, the philosophical tradition of generation acquired global reach even as the paradigm of reproduction began to compete. We review the export and appropriation of western practices, and provide evidence of traffic the other way, from colonial Mexican paintings of racial 'crossings' to the Chinese invention of abortion by vacuum aspiration in the 1950s. We investigate imperial encounters and the discourse of world population, show how an international view decentres the pill, and analyse globalized reproduction today. We cannot do full justice to the spatial dimensions, but sketch connections and comparisons throughout.

The volume foregrounds questions of change and continuity from antiquity to the present, and selects topics that point to a broad history of procreation, without claiming to be comprehensive. Chapters encompass individual medicine and population management, of humans mostly, but also other animals and to a lesser extent plants. We discuss relations of reproduction with sexuality, from love lives in botany to the applicability of Foucault's scheme to sex, gender and baby-making since the 1960s, but concentrate – non-normatively – on procreative sex. For the family and heredity, which overlaps with but came to be framed as distinct from reproduction, we deal with the intersections while referring to the rich histories that already exist.[37] We promote synthesis by grouping topics that are too often separated, for example eugenics and animal breeding, and the various techniques of assisting conception; this lets us uncover the similarities, contrasts and transfers between methods and discourses for humans and livestock, women and men.

Each chapter situates generation or reproduction within a period and develops a theme that offers a path between the parts. Balancing the crowd scenes and long takes, the illustrations present evidence in close-up. Focusing on striking artefacts, the 'exhibits' in the colour sections display some vivid pictures and objects. They hint at the wealth of the archive, raise questions about the kinds of analysis needed to interrogate its contents and showcase topics that deserve more research. The items range from an

37 Elizabeth Foyster and James Marten (eds.), *A Cultural History of Childhood and Family*, 6 vols. (London, 2010); Alison Bashford and Philippa Levine (eds.), *The Oxford Handbook of the History of Eugenics* (Oxford, 2010); Staffan Müller-Wille and Hans-Jörg Rheinberger, *A Cultural History of Heredity* (Chicago, IL, 2012).

ancient Egyptian fertility figurine to a poster for a film about population control, from a phallic wall-painting at Pompeii to a photograph of cloned frogs. A select bibliography of secondary literature represents still more of the field.

One set of questions runs through the book: when and where did 'generation' and 'reproduction' begin and end, what have people meant when they talked in these terms, and how and why were their beliefs and actions like or unlike those that went before and came after? The answers begin to show how different history looks when we highlight generation and reproduction.

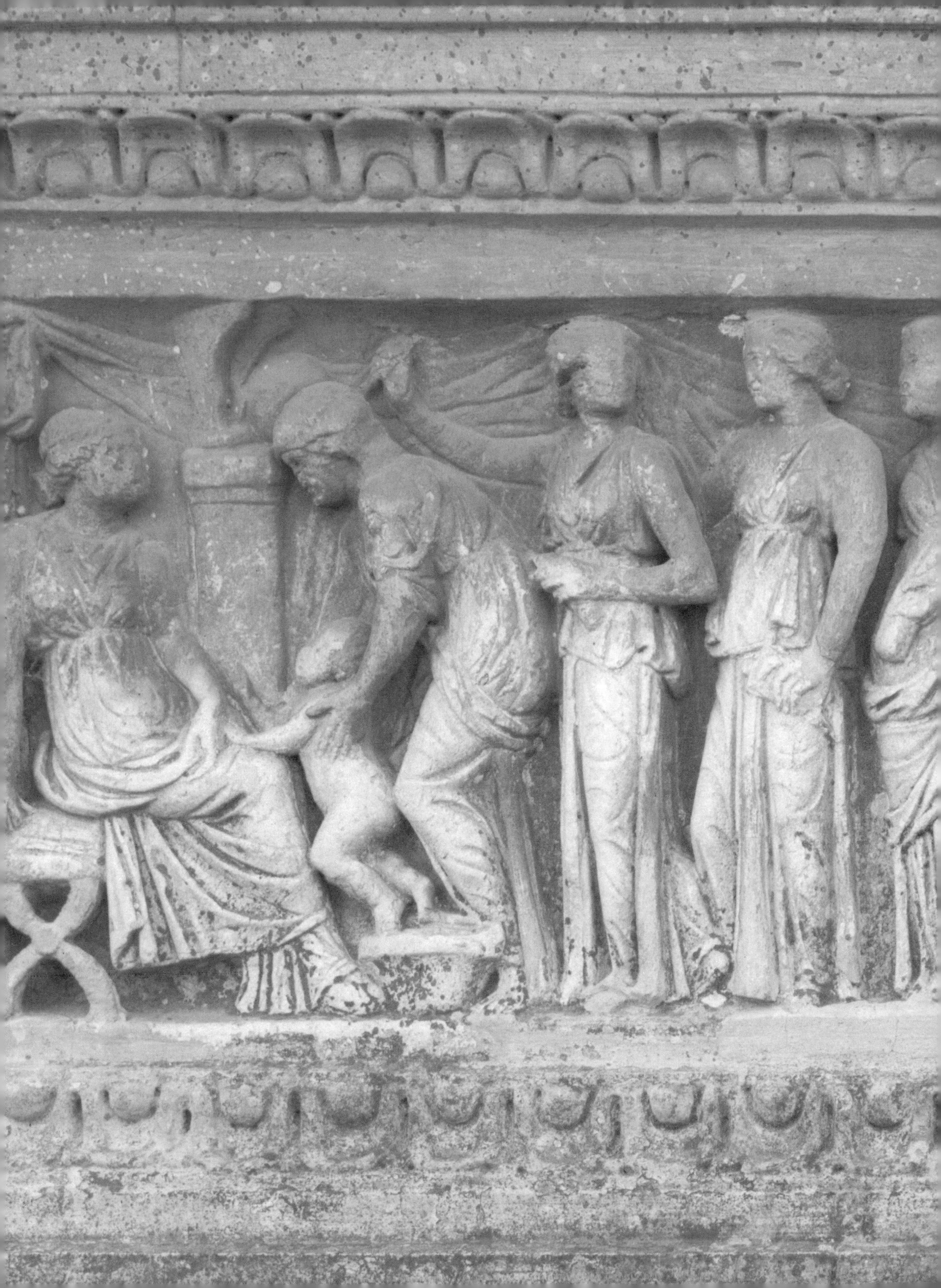

Part I

Inventing Generation

Detail of a side relief from a late second-century AD Roman sarcophagus. A nurse lifts the newborn infant from the bath, and he reaches towards a seated matronal figure, presumably his mother. Behind the nurse the fates look on, the first marking out the course of the child's life on the celestial globe. Often depicted on biographical sarcophagi, bathing was a key stage in the movement towards full humanity after birth. Doria Pamphili sarcophagus: Faraglia, Neg. D-DAI-ROM 8332.

THE STORY OF GENERATION BEGINS IN THE ANCIENT MEDITERRANEAN. Classical Greek poets, philosophers and physicians asked key questions about how humans and others produce more of themselves. Fundamental terms and concepts were established over the late fifth and early fourth centuries BC, most importantly the notion of seed as the crucial substance of generation. The earliest surviving literature on population, about how many and what kind of people the ideal community should contain, and how to achieve that quantity and quality, dates from this same revolutionary moment. Growing wealth and connectivity, and burgeoning cities and politics, enabled an explosion of new and creative activities, of critical inquiry and debate, in writing as well as speech and artefacts. Ways of knowing expanded, becoming more professionally organized and complex in the Hellenistic period, when Greek kingdoms were forged in the territories of the Persian Empire conquered by Alexander the Great and divided up between warring generals after his death in 323 BC.

It may be conventional to claim that classical Greece was so innovative in the form and content of discussions and practices around generation, like so much else, as to make it the right place to begin this account. It is widely recognized, for example, that Greek medical texts gained an explicitly theoretical dimension, adapted from philosophical discourse, which the earlier medical literatures of Egypt and Mesopotamia lacked, within a broader set of divergences between these traditions. Yet the following chapters offer fresh interpretations, and more specific analysis, of both continuity in concerns about human procreation and some clear changes across the ancient Mediterranean world (Rune Nyord, 'An Ancient Egyptian Fertility Figurine', Exhibit 1).

Contrary to standard assumptions, this part of the book argues that the framework of generation produced in classical Greece gave important roles to both women and men. This model contrasts with the one-sided, masculine approach previously dominant in understandings of cosmic and human creation across the eastern Mediterranean (Stephanie Lynn Budin, 'Phallic Fertility in the Ancient Near East and Egypt', Chapter 2). Some ancient Greek poetry still proposed a male monopoly over the power to create life, and the phallus retained its symbolic fecundity in a range of representational forms, even as these larger shifts took firmer hold in the Roman world (Jessica Hughes, 'Phallic Fertility in Pompeii', Exhibit 5). Similarly, hints of a more even-handed approach to procreation can be found in some Neo-Assyrian and late Babylonian medical texts. Persian rule, particularly that of Darius towards the end of the sixth and into the early fifth century BC, instigated a wider set of changes in Mesopotamian intellectual culture, across an array of disciplines, including medicine and celestial divination. The first birth horoscopes joined other readings of the heavens around 400 BC (Eleanor Robson, 'The Birth Horoscope of a Babylonian Scholar', Exhibit 3). Different areas of the Mediterranean world continued to interact, and increasingly converged, contributing to the 'invention of generation'.

The next chapters sketch, probe and position this new model of generation. Hippocratic gynaecology initially takes centre stage: women and procreation became an integral part of the thriving learned, literate Greek medicine of the fifth and fourth centuries BC (Helen King, 'Women and Doctors in Ancient Greece', Chapter 3). Methodological considerations were crucial: writers drew on observation and assumption, theory and experience, while more traditional discourses and practices persisted alongside the new. Asking divinities for help in having and keeping children, for example, remained standard (Fay Glinister, 'A Swaddled Infant Given to the Gods', Exhibit 4), while mythology and art prominently thematized anomalous births and hybrids: the products of mortal and divine unions, or part-human, part-animal creatures, such as centaurs and satyrs (Annetta Alexandridis, 'The Minotaur and Other Hybrids in Ancient Greece', Exhibit 2). Laurence M. V. Totelin moves, more systematically, beyond humans and gods ('Animal and Plant Generation in Classical Antiquity', Chapter 4). The fertility of land and crops and the breeding of livestock were crucial concerns in classical antiquity, which, for all its vaunted urbanization, technical prowess and elaborate trade, was always essentially agricultural. While philosophers such as Aristotle grappled with the more abstract questions posed by the phenomenon of 'coming to be' in all its manifestations, agricultural authors treated practical matters, with much exchange between the two. All were interested in exploring how generation worked and in probing the structure and limits of the framework it offered.

The tradition of agricultural writing flourished in the Roman world as one facet of the general augmentation, adaptation and reorganization of Greek knowledge that followed equivalent processes of expansion and reconfiguration in the political domain. Over the last three centuries BC, Rome rose rapidly from central Italian city-state to international domination, building on victories over Carthage and the Hellenistic kingdoms to forge a vast empire encircling the Mediterranean. That empire was extended and strengthened in the first two centuries AD, incorporating a massive hinterland from Britain to Arabia, the Atlas Mountains to the Carpathians. Rome's practices of population management contributed to this rise. They are discussed in Chapter 5, against the background of Greek population thinking and alongside the policies of other ancient states in relation to their human resources (Rebecca Flemming, 'States and Populations in the Classical World'). The family did much of the practical work for ancient polities in these respects. People pursued the shared goals of continuity and prosperity in conditions of high infant mortality, and within certain social structures and legal rules – of marriage, divorce and the transmission of property. Tim Parkin analyses these issues for the Roman world, with its flexible heirship strategies, active state encouragement of generation and long legal reach ('The Ancient Family and the Law', Chapter 6). The imperial metropolis of the second century AD was also where Galen put seeds, womb and menstrual blood into their most lastingly influential medical arrangement, as outlined in Chapter 7 (Rebecca Flemming, 'Galen's Generations of Seeds'). Physicians were present across the cities and military bases of the empire at around the same time; we have rich archaeological finds of surgical instruments, including some specifically designed for intervention in procreation (Ralph Jackson, 'A Roman Embryo Hook', Exhibit 6). The large scale of the empire shaped and spread this potent mix of knowledge and practice.

Facing heightened military threats from the mid-third century AD onwards, the Roman Empire adapted to changing geopolitical conditions. Whether these had any impact on its transformation into a Christian polity following the conversion of the Emperor Constantine in the fourth century AD is disputed. They certainly contributed to its fracture, to the fall of the Western Empire in AD 476 and its reconfigurations in the East. The successor kingdoms in North Africa and western Europe, like the later Roman (or Byzantine) Empire centred on Constantinople in the east, were Christian, though of different kinds. These plural Christianities moulded the late antique world in diverse and uneven ways. Christian writers entered and came increasingly to dominate philosophical discussion about human generation; church teachings on sex, marriage, abortion and infant exposure called forth various responses from laypeople and state authorities. Part I ends with an exploration of both the common ground among participants in these debates and the divergent fashions in which the Christian emphasis on the soul played out. Marie-Hélène Congourdeau stresses the gaps between theoretical and practical change ('Debating the Soul in Late Antiquity', Chapter 8). The Christian 'procreationist' project that hardened during the middle ages – the insistence that sex is permissible only in marriage and for procreation – was driven by a different set of political and theological concerns from those that drove discussions of ensoulment and fetal life.

Further continuities are evident in the range of divine resources that might be brought to bear on the generative body (Véronique Dasen, 'A Uterine Amulet from the Roman Empire', Exhibit 7), and in the classical medical tradition, which proved impressively robust, implicitly in much of the West, more explicitly in the East. Alexandria was deeply Christian by the sixth century AD, for example, while the curriculum of its prominent medical school was Hippocratic and Galenic, and stayed that way after the city fell to Arab forces in AD 641. Egypt, like much of the territory around it, whether once or never Roman, was then absorbed into the largest and greatest of the states that succeeded Rome, the Islamic empire of the Caliphate. The systematic translation of Greek medical and philosophical texts into Syriac and then Arabic, primarily in ninth-century Baghdad, enabled Avicenna's innovative synthesis of Galenic and Aristotelian approaches to generation, amongst an array of other developments in the Islamicate world (Nahyan Fancy, 'Generation in Medieval Islamic Medicine', Chapter 9).

An earlier translation project had the most ramifications for the topics and themes covered in this volume, however. For it was the making of a Latin Bible, a process consolidated at the end of the fourth century AD, which put '*generatio*' on the path to terminological domination. Previously a rare equivalent of the Greek abstract noun '*genesis*' – birth, engendering or coming-to-be – surrounded by more diverse and frequently used Latin expressions for the same ideas, '*generatio*' attained a virtual monopoly in the Vulgate and among those who worked with it. The word even swallowed up the age-cohort meaning of the Greek '*genea*', which also denotes offspring, tribe or people, and pushed aside equivalent Latin vocabulary, such as '*saeculum*' or '*aetas*', which has a temporal emphasis, signifying a lifespan or generation as an age, period or epoch. The terminological variety integral to the invention of this discursive and practical field in classical Greece and Rome would thus be lost as 'generation' prevailed and came to name that field – part of a homogenizing trajectory both intended and accidental.

REBECCA FLEMMING

2 Phallic Fertility in the Ancient Near East and Egypt

Stephanie Lynn Budin

In the modern west, reproductive fertility is a women's issue. The critical processes of conception, pregnancy and parturition all involve women far more than men. The debate about abortion is fought on (and in) the female body; fertility treatment targets the potential mother's reproductive system; surrogate motherhood invades another woman's reproductive system; and most birth control is aimed at women.

The relentless emphasis on the feminine nature of fertility has caused modern scholars and others to cast this understanding onto the study and reconstruction of the past. Female statuettes from the ancient world, naked and clothed, have been interpreted as 'fertility figurines', while every goddess in the ancient pantheons – be she mother or virgin or both – tends to be described as a 'fertility goddess'. Various and sundry 'mother goddesses' were discovered throughout the ancient world in nineteenth- and twentieth-century scholarship. Today, many reconstructed neopagan religions are devoted to a monotheistic 'Great Goddess' who is understood to have survived the spread across Eurasia of the Indo-Europeans with their patriarchal sky god which ended the peaceful reign of the 'Great Mother'.[1]

The pendulum is now swinging the other way concerning the 'female = fertility' equation, especially in the ancient Mediterranean and Near Eastern territories once most susceptible to its lures. In 1989, Jo Ann Hackett pointed out the innately sexist implications of the theory that females are nothing but wombs.[2] There is also growing interest in the fecund male, as shown by recent publications on the masculine role in fertility in both Egyptian iconography and Sumerian literature.[3] This chapter develops, for the early literate cultures of the eastern Mediterranean, the new emphasis on the understanding of fertility as a masculine attribute, in which it is the life-giving fluids of the penis, rather than what goes on in the womb, that creates new life.

1 Gary Beckman, 'Goddess worship – ancient and modern', in Saul M. Olyan and Robert C. Culley (eds.), *'A Wise and Discerning Mind': Essays in Honour of Burke O. Long* (Providence, RI, 2000), pp. 11–23.

2 Jo Ann Hackett, 'Can a sexist model liberate us? Ancient Near Eastern "fertility" goddesses', *Journal of Feminist Studies in Religion* 5, no. 1 (1989), 65–76.

3 John Baines, *Fecundity Figures: Egyptian Personification and the Iconology of a Genre* (Chicago, IL, 1985); Jerry Cooper, 'Enki's member: Eros and irrigation in Sumerian literature', in Hermann Behrens, Darlene Loding and Martha T. Roth (eds.), *DUMU-E2-DUB-BA-A: Studies in Honor of Åke W. Sjöberg* (Philadelphia, PA, 1989), pp. 87–9.

I focus on mythology – a rich surviving resource – from a swathe of territory from Egypt through the Levant and Mesopotamia into Anatolia, over a period stretching from around the end of the fourth to the early first millennium BC, although the bulk of the material comes from the second millennium. It was in their tales of creation and generation that the residents of the ancient Near East and Egypt were most explicit about their notions of gender vis-à-vis fertility, for both deities and humans. Sources pertaining to historical humans are more scattered and restricted, appearing primarily when productive processes were not functioning as they should, that is, in instances of male impotence and female infertility.[4]

It is convenient to study the phenomenon of male fertility in three separate if overlapping categories. The first is cosmogony, whereby divine action brought reality itself or aspects of the natural world into existence. Here males functioned entirely alone, without any female contribution or assistance. The second is male pregnancy, where male deities were so fecund as to take on the female role of incubator, bringing forth divine progeny. The third is 'child production', which involved the bringing forth of either divine or human offspring, including the creation of humanity itself. In this last category a female contribution was recognized – not as creating new life, but as moulding and nourishing what a male had engendered.

Cosmogony

Male sexuality is the dominant force for fertility in ancient Near Eastern and Egyptian mythologies; it is associated with baseline creation, either of reality itself or of the natural phenomena that make up the world. Typically, this creativity is expressed in phallic and fluid-based imagery, whereby male orgasm brings forth a fluid that either engenders reality *in toto* or 'fertilizes' (that is, waters, feeds or perhaps 'activates') a pre-existing world. The primary example of creation emerging from ejaculation is contained in the Heliopolitan cosmogony of ancient Egypt. The Old Kingdom (*c.* 2700–2250 BC) Pyramid Texts relate how the primordial god Atum emerged upon the *benben* stone from the watery chaos called 'Nun'. In a moment of either loneliness or arousal, he masturbated and ejaculated the deities Shu (air) and Tefnut (moisture): 'Atum evolved growing ithyphallic, in Heliopolis. He put his penis in his grasp that he might make orgasm with it, and the two siblings were born – Shu and Tefnut.'[5]

4 Stephanie Lynn Budin, 'Fertility and gender in the Ancient Near East', in Mark Masterson, Nancy Sorkin Rabinowitz and James Robson (eds.), *Sex in Antiquity: Exploring Gender and Sexuality in the Ancient World* (New York, NY, 2015), pp. 30–49.

5 J. P. Allen, 'From Pyramid Texts Spell 527 (1.3)', in William W. Hallo and K. Lawson Younger, Jr (eds.), *The Context of Scripture: Canonical Compositions, Monumental Inscriptions, and Archival Documents from the Biblical World*, vol. 1: *Canonical Compositions from the Biblical World* (Leiden, 2003), p. 7.

This narrative is repeated in a papyrus from the New Kingdom (*c.* 1550–1100 BC), where it is additionally noted that rather than emerging from Atum's penis, the twins were born from his mouth, possibly suggesting a kind of auto-fellatio.[6] This aspect of the story is also stressed in the Coffin Texts of the Middle Kingdom (*c.* 2000–1650 BC), where the god Shu claims, 'I am this soul of Shu which is in the flame of the fiery blast which Atum kindled with his own hand. He created orgasm and fluid fell from his mouth. He spat me out as Shu together with Tefnut, who came forth after me.'[7] Upon their 'birth', the male and female Shu and Tefnut begin the process of sexual generation, creating the deities Nut (Sky) and Geb (Earth). These grandchildren of Atum themselves engage in such intensive sexual intercourse that their father Shu must eventually separate their bodies so that their children can be born.

Phallic fertility is also emphasized in Egyptian iconography. Several male deities are represented as ithyphallic – with large erect phalluses – as a manifestation of their role in creation, self-regeneration and resurrection.[8] This form of presentation is evident, for instance, in a portrayal of the familial unit of Shu, Nut and Geb on a fragmentary papyrus, the *Book of the Dead of Sesu*, dating from the beginning of the first millennium BC (Fig. 2.1). Here Geb holds his erect phallus, in a manner reminiscent of the earlier description of Atum, while gazing upwards at his sexual partner Nut. Another common image is that of the ithyphallic god Min, whose cult originated in Coptos back in the second half of the fourth millennium BC, and developed during the Early Dynastic period (*c.* 3100–2700 BC). Originally portrayed alone and, once again, masturbating (Fig. 2.2), he also appeared in New Kingdom iconography gazing upon the foreign goddess Qedešet (Fig. 2.3). Qedešet bears a strong resemblance to Egyptian potency or fertility figurines, small terracotta items used to enhance physical or magical potency in Middle and New Kingdom Egypt.[9] The pairing of Min with Qedešet may thus be related to her ability to spark or intensify the god's erection.

Two other deities often depicted with erect penis were Amun and Osiris. Amun appears to have acquired his ithyphallic tendencies through syncretism with both Min and Atum. Osiris is specifically shown with erect penis when in the *duat*, the

6 Lynn M. Meskell and Rosemary A. Joyce, *Embodied Lives: Figuring Ancient Maya and Egyptian Experience* (London, 2003), p. 95.

7 R. O. Faulkner, *The Ancient Egyptian Coffin Texts*, vol. 1: *Spells 1–354* (Warminster, 1973), p. 80 (Spell 77).

8 Ann Macy Roth, 'Father earth, mother sky: Ancient Egyptian beliefs about conception and fertility', in Alison E. Rautman (ed.), *Reading the Body: Representations and Remains in the Archaeological Record* (Philadelphia, PA, 2000), pp. 187–201, on p. 198.

9 Stephanie Lynn Budin, *Images of Woman and Child from the Bronze Age: Reconsidering Fertility, Maternity, and Gender in the Ancient World* (Cambridge, 2011), pp. 126–35; Rune Nyord, 'An Ancient Egyptian Fertility Figurine', Exhibit 1, this book.

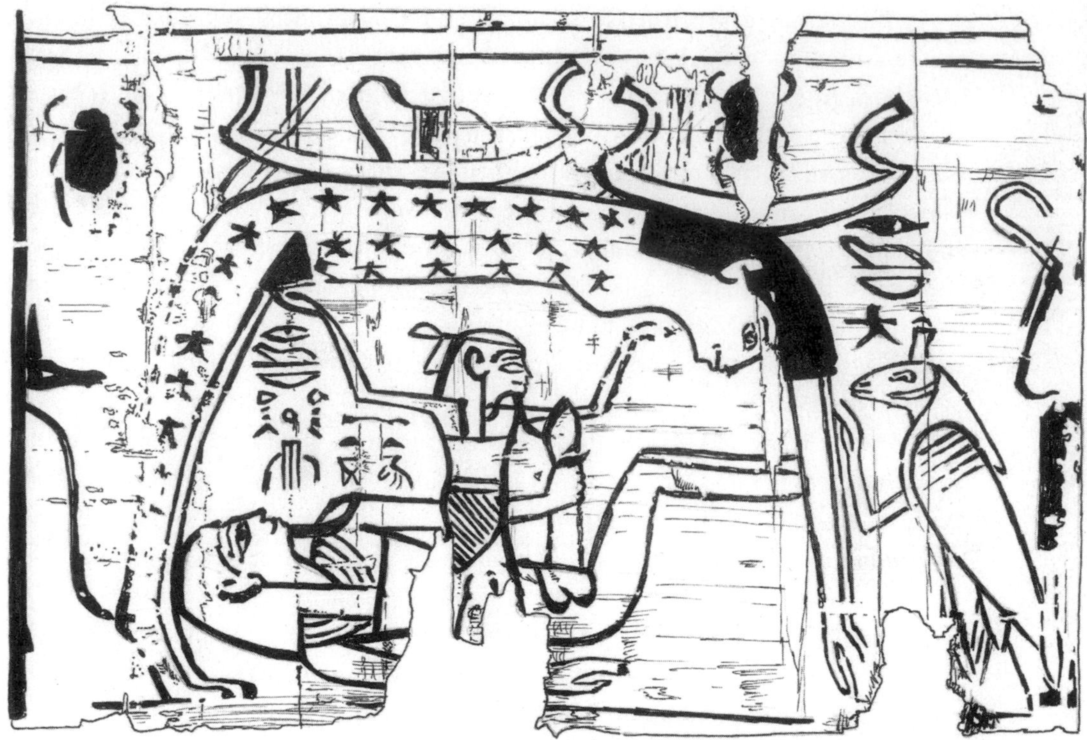

Figure 2.1 Detail from the *Book of the Dead of Sesu*. This fragmentary papyrus roll, excavated from a tomb in Thebes (modern Luxor) in Egypt, contains a richly illustrated collection of spells designed to enable Sesu to navigate the afterlife. Nut (Sky) arches over Geb (Earth). Roll 20.5 cm high: British Museum, EA 9941.1. Drawing by Paul C. Butler, used with kind permission.

underworld, where his ithyphallic rendering represents his resurrection. The erect penis is a sign not only of life, but specifically of new life.[10]

In Mesopotamia, the masculine nature of fertility is expressed in the exploits of some exceptionally creative deities, most notably the god of fresh water Enki. Enki was remarkable for his phallic fertility, giving rise to rivers and with them vegetal, animal and human or divine abundance. This is most explicitly presented in the Sumerian hymn, *Enki and the World Order*, dating to around 2000 BC.[11]

> After he had turned his gaze from there, after father Enki had lifted his eyes across the Euphrates, he stood up full of lust like a rampant bull, lifted his penis, ejaculated and filled the Euphrates with flowing water … By lifting his penis, he brought a

10 Gay Robins, 'Male bodies and the construction of masculinity in New Kingdom Egyptian art', in Sue H. D'Auria (ed.), *Servant of Mut: Studies in Honor of Richard A. Fazzini* (Leiden, 2008), pp. 208–15.

11 Sumerian is an early Mesopotamian language; its central 'classical' corpus of surviving literature dates from *c.* 2150–1650 BC. This hymn is usually placed at the beginning of this period.

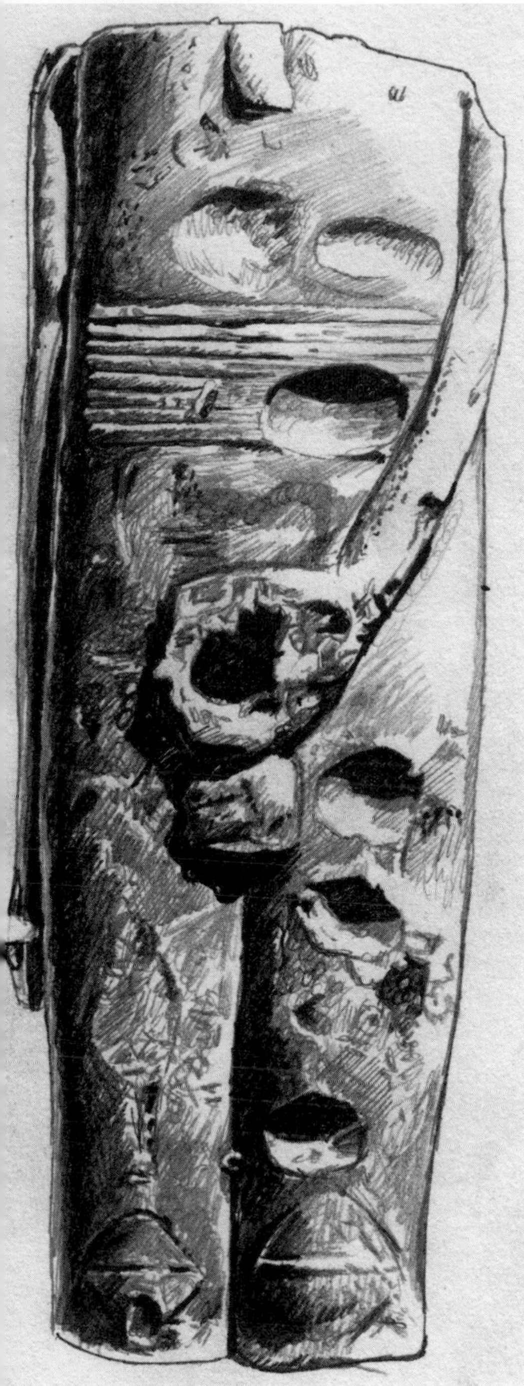

gure 2.2 Surviving segment of one of three colossal
nestone statues of the god Min excavated from his key
nple site at Coptos (modern Qift) in Egypt. Dating from
ound 3300 BC, the whole statue would have stood about 4 m
l. Ashmolean Museum, AN 1894.105e. Drawing by Paul C.
tler, used with kind permission.

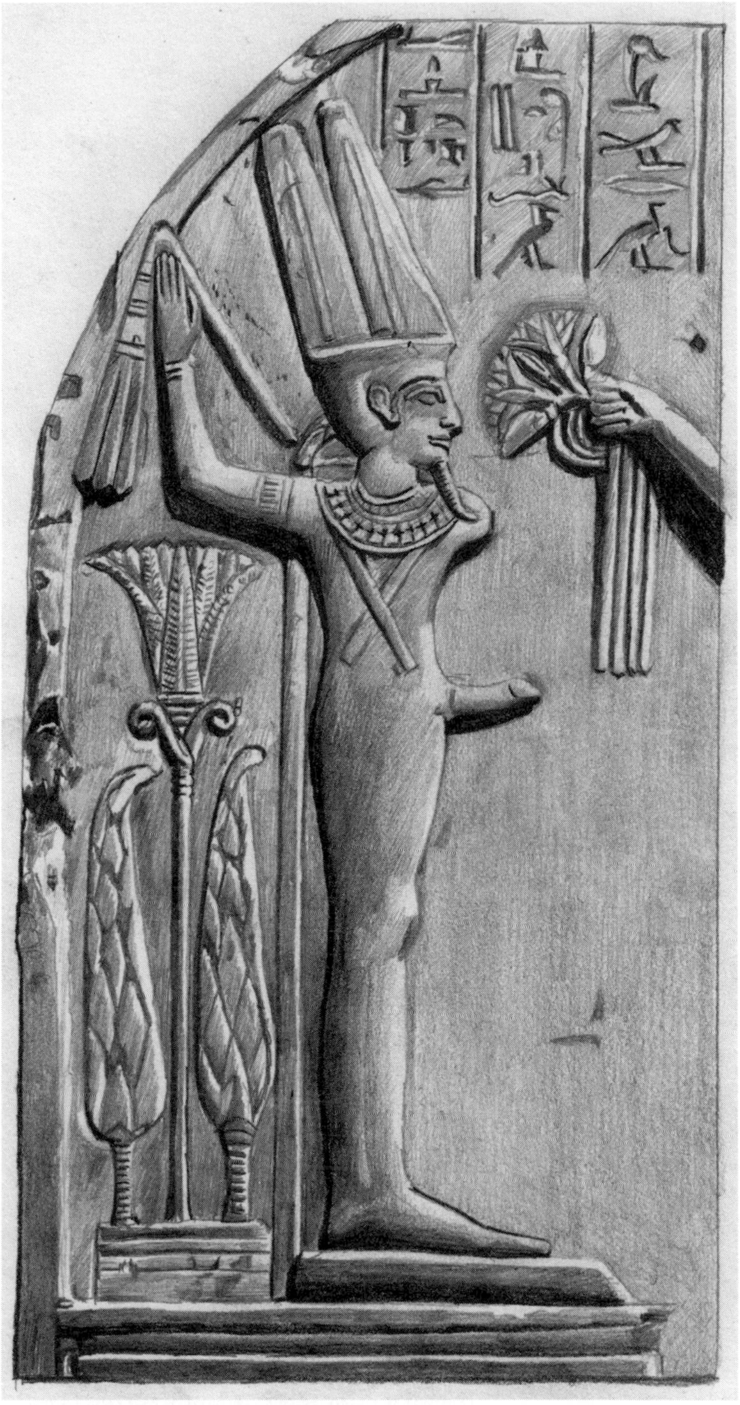

Figure 2.3 Detail from the stele of the chief craftsman Qeh. Min gazes upon Qedešet (to his left, and in the centre of the whole stele, holding flowers in her right hand). Found in Deir el-Medina, across the river from the Valley of the Kings. Figure *c.* 30 cm high. British Museum, EA 191. Drawing by Paul C. Butler, used with kind permission.

> bridal gift. The Tigris rejoiced in its heart like a great wild bull, when it was born … It brought water, flowing water indeed: its wine will be sweet. It brought barley, mottled barley indeed: the people will eat it. It filled the E-kur, the house of Enlil, with all sorts of things.[12]

The fertility theme continues through the hymn, although with less phallic language. The god's mastery of vegetal fruitfulness is noted, for example, and that he makes young men and women sexually appealing and amorous; he can spark fertility in herd animals and field crops, and is even credited with responsibility for the birth of mortal kings.[13]

Earthly fertility is also the domain of other male deities in the Mesopotamian pantheon. In the second-millennium Akkadian tale of *Atrahasis*, the Mesopotamian Noah, when the gods wish to destroy all humans they attempt to starve them to death by withholding the powers of the rain god Adad, once again linking notions of fluid fertility and earthly abundance with a male deity.[14] This association between masculinity and earthly bounty also appears in the high god Enlil. At the end of the Sumerian tale *Enlil and Ninlil*, the poet calls Enlil, 'Lord who makes flax grow, lord who makes barley grow, you are lord of heaven, Lord Plenty, lord of the earth!'[15]

In contrast to Egyptian iconography, Mesopotamian images rarely portray the erect penis. When they do, it is in scenes of mortal sexual revelry that are conceptually divorced from notions of fertility. Instead, the Mesopotamian iconography of fertility typically involved winged male genii impregnating the 'tree of life', as on a wall relief from the throne room of Aššurnaṣirpal II (reigned *c.* 883–859 BC) in Nimrud (Fig. 2.4).

The cosmogony presented in the Hebrew Bible's book of Genesis is distinct in so far as the deity conceptualized by the biblical redactors was transcendent, and thus, although decidedly male, could not be discussed as having a penis or creating the world in any embodied fashion. Nevertheless, elements of both creation accounts (Genesis 1 and 2, composed probably in the fifth and sixth centuries BC respectively) reflect aspects of the Egyptian and Mesopotamian narratives.[16] In addition to the male-as-creator paradigm, the first portrays a primordial state of watery chaos that is equivalent

12 J. A. Black *et al.*, *The Electronic Text Corpus of Sumerian Literature [ETCSL]* (http://etcsl.orinst.ox.ac.uk/, Oxford, 1998–2006), t.1.1.3, ll. 250–65.

13 Ibid., ll. 18–30, 32–7, 52–60 and 326–34, 193–205.

14 Stephanie Dalley, *Myths from Mesopotamia: Creation, the Flood, Gilgamesh, and Others* (Oxford, 1989), pp. 9–35. Over the course of the second millennium, Akkadian increasingly superseded Sumerian as the main literary language of Mesopotamia.

15 *ETCSL*, t. 1.2.1, ll. 144–5.

16 For a summary of issues of biblical composition see John Van Seters, 'Historiography in ancient Israel', in Andrew Feldherr and Grant Hardy (eds.), *The Oxford History of Historical Writing*, vol. 1: *Beginnings to AD 600* (Oxford, 2011), pp. 76–96.

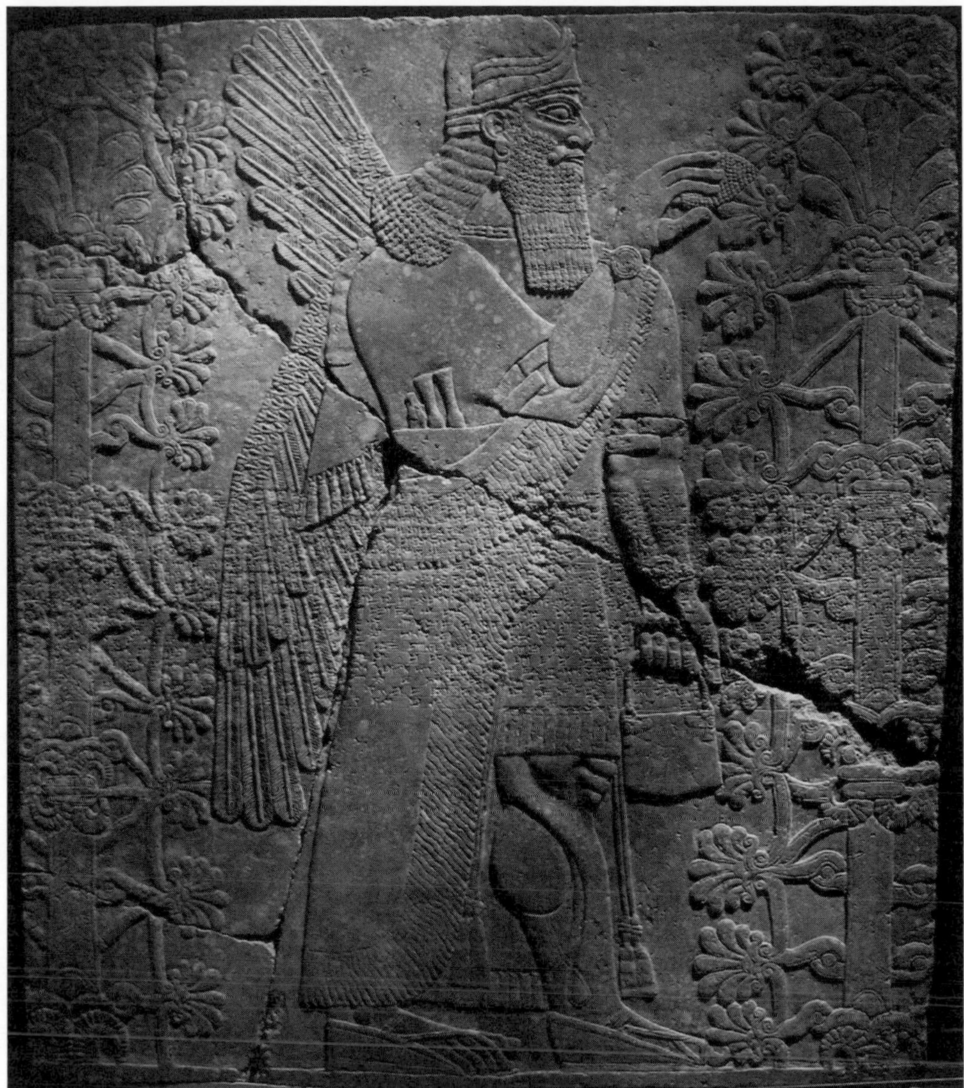

Figure 2.4 Detail from a vast alabaster relief from the Assyrian palace at Nimrud, *c*. 883–859 BC. A winged genie holds a small pail in his left hand, and a cone in his right, through which he 'fertilizes' the 'tree of life' – a prominent symbol of prosperity and fecundity – before him. 230 × 201 cm. Brooklyn Museum, purchased with funds given by Hagop Kevorkian and the Kevorkian Foundation, 55.151.

to the Egyptian Nun. Just as Atum emerged from Nun upon the *benben* stone, so too did Elôhîm command: 'Let there be a dome in the midst of the waters, and let it separate the waters from the waters.'[17] In properly disembodied fashion, then, Elôhîm calls reality into being through the force of his word, rather than of his phallus. The second

17 Genesis 1:6: all translations New Revised Standard Version (NRSV).

account more closely corresponds to the model of creation and male fertility we see in the Mesopotamian myths:

> In that day the Lord God made the earth and the heavens, when no plant of the field was yet in the earth and no herb of the field had yet sprung up – for the Lord God had not caused it to rain upon the earth, and there was no one to till the ground; but a stream would rise from the earth, and water the whole face of the ground ...[18]

Here, earth already exists, but is lifeless. The process of making a living, useful earth is tied to the presence of a stream rising, comparable to the life-giving waters ejaculated by Enki, and the eventual fall of fertile rains, comparable to those of Adad in *Atrahasis*. Creation is still predicated upon male fluids.

Not all of the surviving ancient Near Eastern literary corpora preserve creation accounts; there are, for instance, none amongst the extant Anatolian and Ugaritic or Canaanite texts, which also largely date to the second millennium BC. Nevertheless, even these mythic cycles present evidence of the 'male-as-fertilizer' paradigm, notably in tales of what happens when the relevant deity is absent, as Adad was. When the Hittite rain or storm god Telipinu disappeared:

> Telipinu too went away and removed grain, animal fecundity, luxuriance, growth and abundance to the steppe, to the meadow ... Therefore barley and wheat no longer ripen. Cattle, sheep and humans no longer become pregnant. And those already pregnant cannot give birth. The mountains and the trees dried up, so that the shoots do not come forth. The pastures and springs dried up, so that famine broke out in the land. Humans and gods are dying of hunger.[19]

A similar situation emerges when Baal, the Ugaritic rain or storm god, is vanquished by Mot ('Death') in the Ugaritic *Baal Cycle*: the lands dry up and crops fail until his abundant return.[20]

Male Pregnancy

Perhaps the ultimate representation of male fertility comes from those narratives in which male deities become pregnant, as occurs in second-millennium myths from Egypt, Mesopotamia and Anatolia. The New Kingdom Egyptian tale *The Contendings of Horus and Seth* relates how Seth's attempts to rape Horus are reversed by Isis, leading to Seth's impregnation:

18 Genesis 2:4–76.

19 Harry A. Hoffner, Jr, *Hittite Myths*, 2nd edn (Atlanta, GA, 1998), p. 15 (A i 10–18).

20 Simon B. Parker (ed.), *Ugaritic Narrative Poetry* (Atlanta, GA, 1997), pp. 157–9.

> At evening time, bed was prepared for them, and together they lay down. During the night Seth caused his phallus to become stiff and inserted it between Horus's thighs. Horus then placed his hands between his thighs and caught Seth's semen. Then Horus went to tell his mother Isis: 'Help me, Isis, my mother, come and see what Seth has done to me.' And he opened his hand and let her see Seth's semen. She let out a loud cry, took up her knife, and cut off his hands … Then she fetched some fragrant ointment and applied it to Horus's phallus. She caused it to become stiff and inserted it into a pot, and he caused his semen to flow down into it.[21]

Isis then takes the pot of Horus's semen to the garden of Seth and, discovering from the gardener that Seth is partial to lettuce, pours the semen of Horus onto that vegetable. Seth returns to the garden, and, as usual, ate the lettuce; 'thereupon he became pregnant with Horus's semen'. Seth becomes aware of his pregnancy in court, where he is attempting to wrest kingship from Horus in part based on his perceived 'domination' of the younger god. Upon the discovery of Horus's semen in his uncle, the judge Re causes the semen to emerge from Seth's head in the form of a solar disc, which Re then takes for himself.

Similarly, in the Sumerian tale *Enki and Ninhursag*, Enki eats a large quantity of his own semen which the mother goddess Ninhursag had placed in a variety of plants.[22] Enki becomes sick, as he has thus been impregnated with plant deities which he cannot remove from his body. The deities call for Ninhursag, who functions as a surrogate birth canal for Enki:

> Ninhursaĝa laid Enki in her vulva
> [placed cool hands …]
> 'My brother, what part of you hurts you?'
> 'My brainpan hurts me!'
> She gave birth to Abu out of it.
> 'My brother, what part of you hurts you?'
> 'The top of my hair hurts me!'
> She gave birth to Ninsikila out of it …[23]

In the Anatolian *Song of Kumarbi*, the eponymous deity becomes pregnant after biting off the genitals of the sky-god Anu, whom he is attempting to overthrow.

21 William Kelly Simpson (ed.), *The Literature of Ancient Egypt: An Anthology of Stories, Instructions, Stelae, Autobiographies, and Poetry*, 3rd edn (New Haven, CT, 2003), p. 99.

22 The Sumerian word is 'A', which means 'semen' and 'water', as well as 'urine': Gwendolyn Leick, *Sex and Eroticism in Mesopotamian Literature* (London, 1994), p. 25.

23 Thorkild Jacobsen, *The Harps that Once …: Sumerian Poetry in Translation* (New Haven, CT, 1987), pp. 202–3, with several more lines of aches, pains and births.

> Kumarbi bit his [Anu's] loins, and his 'manhood' united with Kumarbi's insides like bronze. When Kumarbi had swallowed the 'manhood' of Anu, he rejoiced and laughed out loud. Anu turned around and spoke to Kumarbi: 'Are you rejoicing within yourself because you have swallowed my manhood? Stop rejoicing within yourself! I have placed inside you a burden.'[24]

Indeed, several burdens: Anu has impregnated his fellow deity with a number of rivers and divinities of which he must rid himself.

In contrast to the unproblematic, even enjoyable, fertilizing activities performed by gods in the process of creation, these more generative fertility stories place their male deities in difficulty. The gods discover they lack the equipment necessary to give birth. The discomfort of the Egyptian Seth arises more from the fact that he was at least symbolically raped by Horus; but both Enki and Kumarbi realize that once pregnant they are incapable of getting their offspring out of their bodies. Kumarbi needs the support and assistance of an ultra-feminine *harnau* birthing-stool, while Enki must enlist the help of the mother goddess Ninhursag to remove his multiple progeny.[25]

Child Production

These myths illustrate the point that, unlike cosmogonic fertility, producing children required feminine assistance. The male created new life and passed it on to the female, who incubated, moulded and nourished it within her body and through breast-feeding.[26] As a late second-millennium BC Babylonian incantation expressed it, 'My father begot me, my mother bore me'.[27]

We already encountered this uneven, heterosexual aspect of divine child production in the Heliopolitan cosmogony discussed above. After the emergence of Atum from the watery Nun and his engendering of the deities Shu and Tefnut, they and their own offspring begin the process of sexual generation that is henceforth standard. The paradigmatic union is that between Osiris and his sister and spouse Isis, as recounted in a Pyramid Text:

> Your sister Isis comes to you rejoicing for love of you. You have placed her on your phallus and your seed issues into her, she being ready as Sothis, and Ḥar-Sopd has come forth from you as Horus who is in Sothis. It is well with you through him in his name of 'Spirit who is in the *Ḏndrw*-bark'; and he protects you in his name of Horus, the son who protects his father.[28]

24 Hoffner, *Hittite Myths*, pp. 42–3.

25 Jaan Puhvel, '*Genus* and *sexus* in Hittite', in S. Parpola and R. M. Whiting (eds.), *Sex and Gender in the Ancient Near East* (Helsinki, 2002), pp. 547–50.

26 Leick, *Sex and Eroticism*, p. 48.

27 Benjamin R. Foster, *Before the Muses: An Anthology of Akkadian Literature*, 3rd edn (Bethesda, MD, 2005), p. 645.

28 R. O. Faulkner, *The Ancient Egyptian Pyramid Texts* (Stilwell, KS, 2007), pp. 120–1 (§§632–3).

A similar model held for human child production. Nevertheless, when humans are created by a divinity, the male potter deity Khnum is responsible, often moistening his clay with waters from the Nile, represented by the male god Hapi. Thus in the New Kingdom *Tale of Two Brothers*, 'Pre-Harakhti said to Khnum: "Fashion a wife for Bata, that he not live alone!" Then Khnum made a companion for him who was more beautiful in body than any woman in the whole land, for (the fluid of) every god was in her.'[29]

In Mesopotamia, the creation of humans is recorded in the *Atrahasis* narrative. Here, Enki summons Nintu the womb goddess to create humanity, but the goddess counters that Enki must first provide her with purified clay. In this act, Enki infuses his 'water' (or 'semen') into the matter of creation. Furthermore, the god Geštu-e is slaughtered and his blood mixed with the clay, also infusing it with life. Male liquids thus animate the inert matter. However, once the clay is properly invigorated, Nintu, either by herself or with the help of birth goddesses, moulds it into human females and males who henceforth will generate sexually amongst themselves:

She pinched off fourteen pieces of clay
And set seven pieces on the right, seven on the left,
Between them she put down a mud brick.[30]
She made use of a reed, opened it (?) to cut the umbilical cord,
Called up the wise and knowledgeable
Womb-goddesses, seven and seven
Seven created males,
Seven created females,
For the womb-goddess is creator of fate.[31]

The creation accounts in Genesis echo these themes. 'Male and female he created them', after all, with Eve's role as female assistant clearest in the following sequence, where she comes after Adam, with the pair formed to produce offspring themselves.[32] The creation of Eve as an afterthought strongly reflects the male-only monotheism of biblical theology. The Earth and everything necessary for life is created by the male god and cared for by the male human. Human child production is inherently unnecessary but invented to punish Eve. The female role in fertility is functionally accidental.

The Canaanite or Ugaritic repertoire offers a similar understanding of the heterosexual paradigm. In the *Birth of the Gracious Gods*, the focus is on the father god El, whose phallic activities give rise to a pair of voracious deities who suckle at the breasts

29 Miriam Lichtheim, *Ancient Egyptian Literature: A Book of Readings*, vol. 2: *The New Kingdom*, 2nd edn (Berkeley, CA, 2006), p. 207.

30 A reference to the mud bricks upon which women kneeled or crouched during parturition in Mesopotamia and Egypt: M. Stol, *Birth in Babylonia and the Bible: Its Mediterranean Setting* (Groningen, 2000), pp. 117–22.

31 Dalley, *Myths from Mesopotamia*, pp. 16–17.

32 Genesis 1:27 and 2:18–24.

of Athirat, the Canaanite mother goddess. In a more human venue, the *Tale of Aqhat* presents the story of Danel, a wise man who is bereft of heirs. The narrative begins with Danel performing a seven-day ritual to invoke the gods El and Baal so that they might provide him with a son. Baal intercedes with El on Danel's behalf, and El provides his blessing to the man, saying:

> Let him go up to his bed:
> As he kisses his wife, she'll become pregnant,
> As he embraces her, she'll conceive;
> And there will be a son in his house.[33]

Thus we see a man calling on male deities of fertility for a son, who is given to him, incidentally through impregnating his wife.

The need for a female in the process of child production (but not creation) is clear in the ideologies of the ancient Near East. As noted in the earlier discussion, pregnant males cannot bear their offspring themselves, and mortal males must have a female to engender heirs. The idea that the female moulds new life comes across most clearly in the Sumerian tale of *Enki and Ninmah*. Having created humankind, these two deities get drunk and bet that no matter how bad a human the one can create, the other will find a place for it in society. Ninmah, a mother-goddess, begins, creating humans who are blind, incontinent, paralysed or stupid. In each case, Enki can find an employment for the disabled individual, even if it is merely 'standing by the king'. But when Enki must form a human himself, he creates

> Umul (= 'My day is far off'): its head was afflicted, its place of … was afflicted, its eyes were afflicted, its neck was afflicted. It could hardly breathe, its ribs were shaky, its lungs were afflicted, its heart was afflicted, its bowels were afflicted. With its hand and its lolling head it could not put bread into its mouth; its spine and head were dislocated. The weak hips and the shaky feet could not carry (?) it on the field.[34]

Enki created not an adult human, but something like a fetus, for which no occupation could be found. He could provide the start for the being, but only a female could fully form a human.

Conclusion: It's All about the Penis

The female contributions to child production notwithstanding, the credit for creativity – for new life – rested with the male. The male created new life which he then 'gave' to the female. The point comes through clearly in the series of recent studies of ancient Egypt

33 Michael D. Coogan and Mark S. Smith, *Stories from Ancient Canaan*, 2nd edn (Louisville, KY, 2013), p. 36.
34 *ETCSL*, t. 1.1.2, ll. 88–91.

and the Near East that I have synthesized and developed here, although there are also differences in emphasis between the different cultures.

Egypt provides perhaps the most completely masculine approach, in which, as Ann Macy Roth comments, 'the creative role is attached exclusively to the male sex.'[35] This association can be seen clearly in the language. In Egyptian, the verb that we translate as 'to conceive a child' also means 'to receive' or 'to take'; and the hieroglyphic writing system also emphasized phallic pre-eminence in fertility and generation. The image of an erect or ejaculating penis was used as a determinative not only for words such as 'man', 'husband' and 'semen', but also for the nouns 'fetus', 'offspring' and even 'mother', as well as the verbs 'to become erect', 'to beget' and 'to impregnate'.[36]

The womb does receive a little more attention in the Hebrew Bible, providing the same nourishment to the fetus as the mother earth does to vegetation that grows in it. 'There is, however,' as Baruch Levine says, 'no indication … as far as we can ascertain, that the female contributes a life essence … to the embryo: the role of the female is entirely that of nurturer.'[37] The seed, the life essence, is provided by the male, and that grows inside the womb. A rather different kind of imagery emerges from the Sumerian texts of ancient Mesopotamia. Fertility, here, is water-based, and it is this fluid 'irrigation' which the phallus, and male ejaculation, crucially supplies.[38]

In their mythologies as in their daily lives, the inhabitants of the ancient Near East and Egypt privileged the role of the male in matters of fertility and generation. The man was viewed as the creator of new life, and it is not surprising that in these consistently patriarchal and patrilineal societies children were seen as belonging to their fathers and their fathers' families, and that men received the benefits of a prodigious brood. In the Sumerian tale of *Gilgamesh and the Netherworld* we read:

> 'Did you see the man with seven sons?'
> 'I saw him.'
> 'How does he fare?'
> 'Among the junior deities he sits on a throne and listens to the proceedings.'[39]

Amongst the Sumerian proverbs, in contrast, we note that 'A mother who has given birth to eight sons lies down in weakness.'[40]

35 Roth, 'Father earth, mother sky', p. 189.

36 Tom Hare, *ReMembering Osiris: Number, Gender, and the Word in Ancient Egyptian Representational Systems* (Stanford, CA, 1999), pp. 108–9.

37 Baruch A. Levine, '"Seed" versus "womb": Expressions of male dominance in biblical Israel', in Parpola and Whiting, *Sex and Gender*, pp. 337–43, on p. 341.

38 Leick, *Sex and Eroticism*, pp. 53–4.

39 Andrew George, *The Epic of Gilgamesh: A New Translation* (Harmondsworth, 1999), pp. 187–8.

40 Bendt Alster, *Proverbs of Ancient Sumer: The World's Earliest Proverb Collection*, vol. 1 (Bethesda, MD, 1997), p. 72 (2.141).

The male right to rule and dominate was predicated at least in part on this idea of creation and 'ownership'. As males gave rise to reality and offspring, so they had authority over that creation. In the familial context, the father ruled alongside a less authoritative (if not wholly disempowered) mother whose contributions to the continuation of the family could not ultimately be denied. In the realms of mythological, cosmogonic creativity, nothing forced the recognition of the practical feminine contribution to generation. Ideologically speaking, it was the penis that gave rise to all that was, and was good, in the ancient Egyptian and Near Eastern worlds: life came from the male.

3 Women and Doctors in Ancient Greece

Helen King

Discussions of human generation took a new turn in the Greek world of the late fifth and early fourth centuries BC, an increasingly wealthy and interconnected world, where inquiry and argument flourished, in oral and, especially, written forms. The Presocratic philosophers had already started the debate, putting the wider principles of generation, of how things 'come-to-be', into textual question over the previous century. A more particular focus on human bodies and generation emerged when a set of healers started to put their medicine – their ideas and practices around health and disease – into writing, in texts which would later be collected in the 'Hippocratic Corpus'.

These male doctors had general interests in the whole procreative process, as it might fit into their broader physiological discussions, and specific interests in fertility issues which might affect their patients, especially their female patients. In bringing theory and practice together in this way, these men established a new form of written medical discourse, in contrast with the earlier literate traditions of the Near East and Egypt, which lacked an explicit theoretical dimension.[1] The nature of female flesh and somatic fluids became matters of debate, for instance, as they related, on the one hand, to global notions of sexual order and difference, to what might underlie all the perceived somatic divergences between men and women, and on the other hand, to pragmatic matters of treatment, to what might underlie moves to maintain healthy and fertile female bodies.

There was continuity as well as change. As in the ancient Near East, questions surrounding generation continued to be explored in myth. The birth of Athena from Zeus's head after he consumed her mother, Metis, for example, illustrates the mythical thematization of anomalous forms of generation, as does Hera's conception of the god Hephaestus by eating lettuce rather than having intercourse with her husband, Zeus (Fig. 3.1). Significantly, this latter story hinted that the absence of male input would result in a deformed child, as Hephaestus was born lame.[2]

1 On earlier literary medical traditions see, for example, M. Stol, *Birth in Babylonia and the Bible: Its Mediterranean Setting* (Groningen, 2000); Markham J. Geller, *Ancient Babylonian Medicine* (Oxford, 2010); and John F. Nunn, *Ancient Egyptian Medicine* (London, 1996).

2 Marcel Detienne, 'Potagerie de femme, ou comment engendrer seule', *Traverses* 5–6 (1976), 75–81; see further Stephanie Lynn Budin, 'Phallic Fertility in the Ancient Near East and Egypt', Chapter 2, this book.

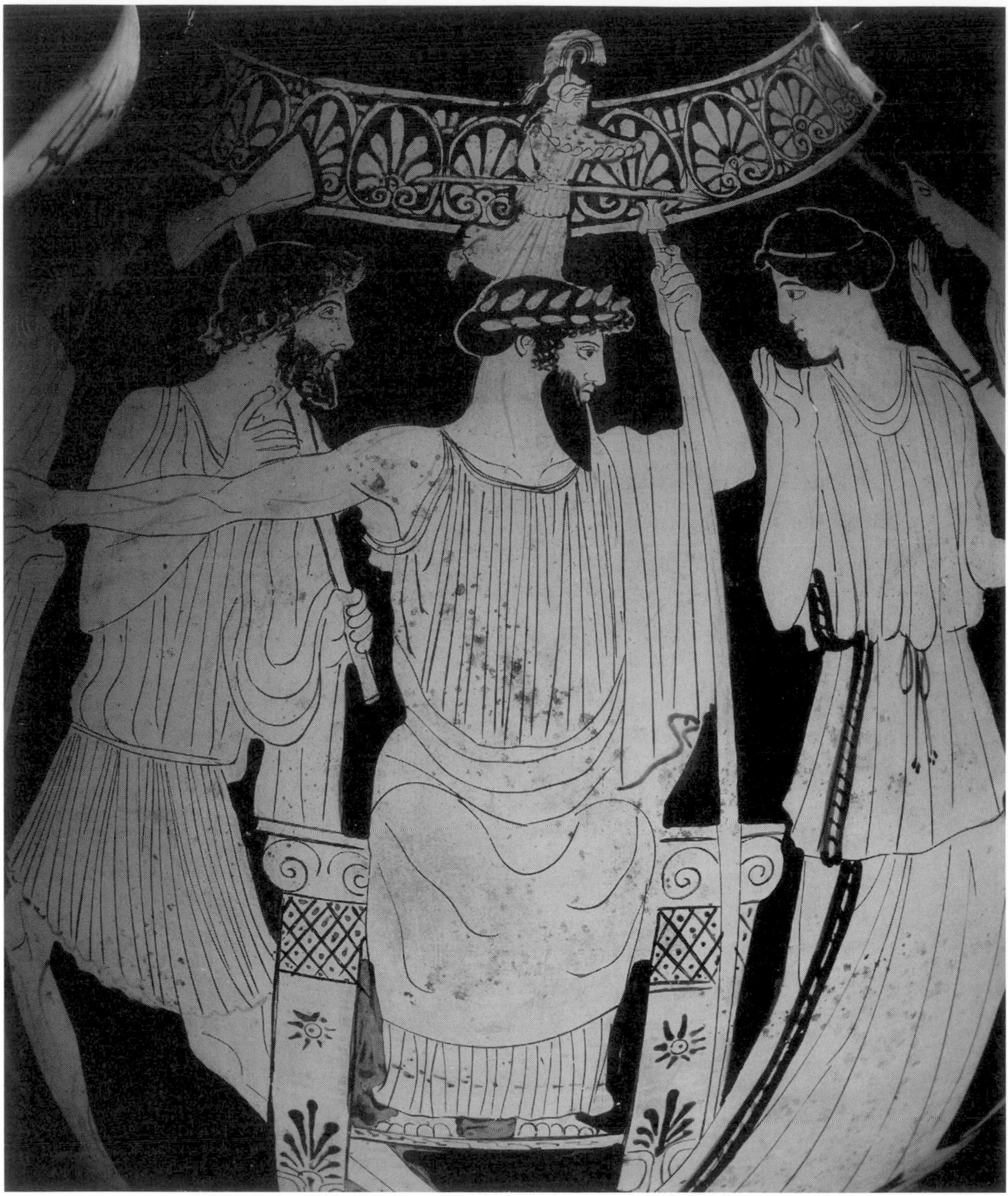

Figure 3.1 Detail of a vase showing the enthroned Zeus giving birth to Athena, flanked by Hephaestus (left) and Eileithyia, the goddess of childbirth (right), and surrounded by other Olympian deities. Depictions of this myth were popular on earlier black-figure Attic pottery, as well as red-figure vases from the classical period, such as this mid-fifth-century BC *pelike*. 41.5 × 31 cm. E 410. © Trustees of the British Museum.

People also continued to bring their desire for children to the gods. The *iamata*, the fourth-century BC inscriptions from the temple of the healing god Asclepius at Epidaurus, include stories such as that about the three-year pregnancy of Ithmonica of Pellene.[3] She 'came to the sanctuary in order to have children', but forgot to ask that the child should in due course be born. She gave birth only after returning to the sanctuary once more. We could rationalize this by suggesting that the early years of this 'pregnancy' were actually some other condition causing amenorrhoea, or that Ithmonica, wanting very much to be pregnant, misread the signs and made a mistake in her dates. These are speculations; a more reliable inference is simply that the beginnings of a child were not automatically assumed to mean that it would eventually be born.[4]

In medical writing, too, the male contribution to offspring continued to be viewed as essential. This did not change, nor did broader notions about gender roles, or the key characteristics associated with male and female, or the assumption of male superiority. The condition known as uterine mole, in which a shapeless mass of flesh rather than a child was produced, could be attributed to the sheer quantity of a woman's blood overwhelming the male seed.[5] The male element in generation was particularly associated with two qualities: strength and speed. When the writer of the Hippocratic treatise *On Generation/Nature of the Child* discussed 'quickening', the point at which the fetus first moves in the womb, he stated that this was generally at three months for a male and four months for a female because the male is 'stronger', formed from seed that is both thicker and stronger.[6]

These two examples from the developing domain of Greek literate medicine also show the burgeoning interest in women's bodies, and as more than simply incubators for men's seed. In this chapter, I shall explore some of the constitutive aspects of these moves: the factors that shaped Hippocratic medicine as a whole, and had a particular impact on its views of women and procreation. There are two main themes in this exploration: the first around the impact of literacy, of writing down what was observed (or claimed as such), and the use of analogy in presenting those observations; the

3 Lynn R. LiDonnici, *The Epidaurian Miracle Inscriptions: Text, Translation, and Commentary* (Atlanta, GA, 1995), pp. 86–7; on appeals for divine assistance, see further Fay Glinister, 'A Swaddled Infant Given to the Gods', Exhibit 4; and Jessica Hughes and Rebecca Flemming, 'The Room of the Ribbons', Exhibit 40, this book.

4 Helen King, 'Illness and other personal crises in Greek and Roman religions', in Sarah Iles Johnston (ed.), *Religions of the Ancient World: A Guide* (Cambridge, MA, 2005), pp. 464–7.

5 Cathy McClive and Helen King, 'When is a foetus not a foetus? Diagnosing false conceptions in early modern France', in Véronique Dasen (ed.), *L'Embryon humain à travers l'histoire: Images, savoirs et rites …* (Gollion, 2008), pp. 223–38.

6 *On Generation/Nature of the Child* (*Genit./Nat. puer.*) 21: retaining the traditional chapter numbers which treat these texts as a single unit, following, most recently, Ann Ellis Hanson, 'A famous handbook and its relevance for science and medicine: Addendum', *Journal of Roman Archaeology* 26 (2013), 738–40. See also, and more generally, Elizabeth Craik, *The 'Hippocratic' Corpus: Content and Context* (London, 2015), pp. 113–18.

second around the interplay of male and female knowledge about women's bodies and their workings in these texts. In both cases I build on existing scholarship in the field of ancient medicine, and look ahead to longer-term debates about the history of medical knowledge more broadly – themes that appear in later chapters in this book.[7] I focus on what is new, and not so new, in learned Greek medicine in these respects, but the stage is also set for thinking about change and continuity in a longer time frame.

Literacy, Observation and the Imagery of Generation

Iain Lonie argued that emerging literacy played a key role in enabling the Greeks of the classical period to focus on different ways of making sense of the body. In various Hippocratic writings, lists of similar symptoms were grouped together, patterns detected and theories constructed to account for them.[8] Descriptions were written of the progress of disease in individual bodies (most famously, the seven books of Hippocratic *Epidemics* use the format of the day-by-day case history). Stages in the progress of human generation could be marked out and described in the same way. They could also be explained through analogy with other natural processes, and by reference to more visible versions of animal production, such as in a chicken's egg.[9]

None of these moves was, however, quite as straightforward as these brief summaries suggest. First, the selection of key events worth noting within the course of a disease or a bodily experience such as conception or birth, or the detection of a pattern, depends very much on what the writer thinks is important; prior theory guides not only what is seen but also what is flagged up as significant in a written description. Second, the relationship between observation and analogy is rarely obvious; the analogy may feel natural, but this may be because it fits with pre-existing ideas. For example, women's flesh was conceptualized as softer and more absorbent than men's: the author of the Hippocratic treatise *Diseases of Women 1* described leaving a closely woven garment and a fleece in a damp place and observing how much more fluid was taken up by the latter. This confirmed that women are 'like' fleece, absorbent, but also

7 For example, Karin Ekholm, 'Pictures and Analogies in the Anatomy of Generation', Chapter 15, this book. See, more generally, Brian Nance, 'Wondrous experience as text: Valleriola and the *Observationes medicinales*', in Elizabeth Jane Furdell (ed.), *Textual Healing: Essays on Medieval and Early Modern Medicine* (Leiden, 2005), pp. 101–17; and Gianna Pomata, 'Observation rising: Birth of an epistemic genre, 1500–1600', in Lorraine Daston and Elizabeth Lunbeck (eds.), *Histories of Scientific Observation* (Chicago, IL, 2011), pp. 45–80.

8 I. M. Lonie, 'Literacy and the development of Hippocratic medicine', in François Lasserre and Philippe Mudry (eds.), *Formes de pensée dans la collection hippocratique: Actes du IVe Colloque hippocratique* (Geneva, 1983), pp. 14–61.

9 Helen King, 'Making a man: Becoming human in early Greek medicine', in G. R. Dunstan (ed.), *The Human Embryo: Aristotle and the Arabic and European Traditions* (Exeter, 1990), pp. 10–19.

closer to nature, unmediated by the cultural process of weaving.[10] Rituals of purification used fleece to absorb impurity, so did this image also include a notion of women's 'difference' that included impurity? As this example suggests, while the need to explain the body in a coherent way was new, the content of the explanations may well be more traditional.

A similar crossover between established motifs and the new literate medicine can be traced in more specifically generative areas. Thus the womb was traditionally presented as a field. In the Athenian betrothal ceremony, for example, the father of the bride gave her 'with a view to the ploughing of legitimate children' and the classical Athenian poet Sophocles had Oedipus refer to his mother and wife Jocasta's womb as 'this field of double sowing whence I sprang, and where I sowed my children'.[11] So, Hippocratic medicine used dung as a form of 'fertilizer' for the womb.[12] Likewise, the Hippocratic image of the womb as a warm place, where a child grows like rising bread dough, can be paralleled with the historian Herodotus's roughly contemporary comment on the necrophilia of the tyrant Periander of Corinth, whose intercourse with his dead wife is summarized by her ghost as 'putting your loaves in a cold oven'.[13] The belief in the womb's transforming heat may thus have been common in ancient Greek culture, taken up by Hippocratic authors and put to particular use in their discussions of generation.

We can find further examples of all these points – selectivity in seeing patterns, the power of analogy in helping people to make sense of what is both seen and unseen, and observation made through the prism of existing theories – in a famous story from *On Generation/Nature of the Child*. When its Hippocratic author observed what he thought was seed 'on the sixth day' after intercourse, expelled from a pregnant slave girl who had taken his advice to jump up and down to remove an unwanted conception, we have no idea what in fact he saw. It looked, he wrote, 'as if someone had removed the outside shell of a raw egg, and the fluid inside was visible within the internal membrane'. In the middle there was something that appeared to the writer to be an umbilical cord, 'and through this the breath moved in and out'.[14] Lonie comments that, other than in the treatise *On Ancient Medicine*, 'Such a systematic and conscious use of observation is unparalleled in the whole Hippocratic Collection'.[15] Some decades later, Aristotle described a detailed examination of a hen's egg on the fourth day in *History of Animals*,

10 *Diseases of Women 1* (*Mul. 1*) 1.

11 Menander, *The Grouch* (*Dyskolos*) 842–3; Sophocles, *Oedipus the King* 1256–7.

12 Ann Ellis Hanson, 'Talking recipes in the gynaecological texts of the *Hippocratic Corpus*', in Maria Wyke (ed.), *Parchments of Gender: Deciphering the Body in Antiquity* (Oxford, 1998), pp. 71–94.

13 Herodotus, 5.92g.2–3; and, for example, on the Hippocratic side, *Genit./Nat. puer.* 12.

14 *Genit./Nat. puer.* 13.

15 Iain M. Lonie, *The Hippocratic Treatises, 'On Generation', 'On the Nature of the Child', 'Diseases IV'* (Berlin, 1981), p. 160.

although he interpreted what the Hippocratic writer saw as an umbilical cord as the heart.[16]

This comparison with Aristotle confirms that, while the Hippocratic writer certainly promoted 'observation' as authoritative, that observation was being interpreted not only according to what he had seen in eggs, but also in terms of his broader beliefs: here that breath, produced when heat meets moisture, is a central factor for life.[17] Later in the same Hippocratic treatise, the umbilicus is linked to the author's statements about the role of 'breath' in forming the fetus. He talks about observing a number of hen's eggs, opening one every day to watch the process of growth, and makes the comprehensive claim that:

> Everything else I have said about the fetus from beginning to end you will discover to be true in the egg of a bird. And indeed, if someone has not seen it before, he will be amazed that there is an umbilicus in a bird's egg. This is how things are, and so have I recounted them.[18]

This individual voice, claiming its authority from personal observation, is something new in the world of medicine and its generative discourses; it simultaneously asserts its own interpretation and appeals to the possibility of shared knowledge.

In the analogical model of what is generated in *On Generation/Nature of the Child*, the shell-less hen's egg is the combined contribution of male and female after six days of development. Both male and female have contributed seed, and the woman has contributed two further things: her womb and her blood. In Hippocratic medicine, blood accumulates in women's flesh from the normal processes of eating and drinking, partly because of the wet and spongy texture of female flesh and partly because women are less active than men, and thus less able to use up any excess blood.[19] Every month, unused blood should flow out, otherwise there is a risk of its over-accumulating, putting pressure on vital organs, or forcing a way out through another orifice. Yet this blood was necessary to nourish a fetus, and thus a key part of generation.

As well as being a container for menstrual blood, the womb was also important for successful conception and formation of the child; if the womb turned around in the body, then male seed would be unable to enter, and if it was the wrong shape then it would deform the baby growing inside. Ancient agricultural writers agreed with the author of *On Generation/Nature of the Child* that, just as cucumbers grow to different sizes and shapes according to the container in which they are placed, so the child's shape

16 Aristotle, *History of Animals* (*HA*) 561a4–21; Ekholm, 'Pictures and Analogies'.

17 Gianna Pomata, 'Innate Heat, Radical Moisture and Generation', Chapter 14, this book.

18 *Genit./Nat. puer.* 29.

19 Helen King, *Hippocrates' Woman: Reading the Female Body in Ancient Greece* (London, 1998), pp. 29–30.

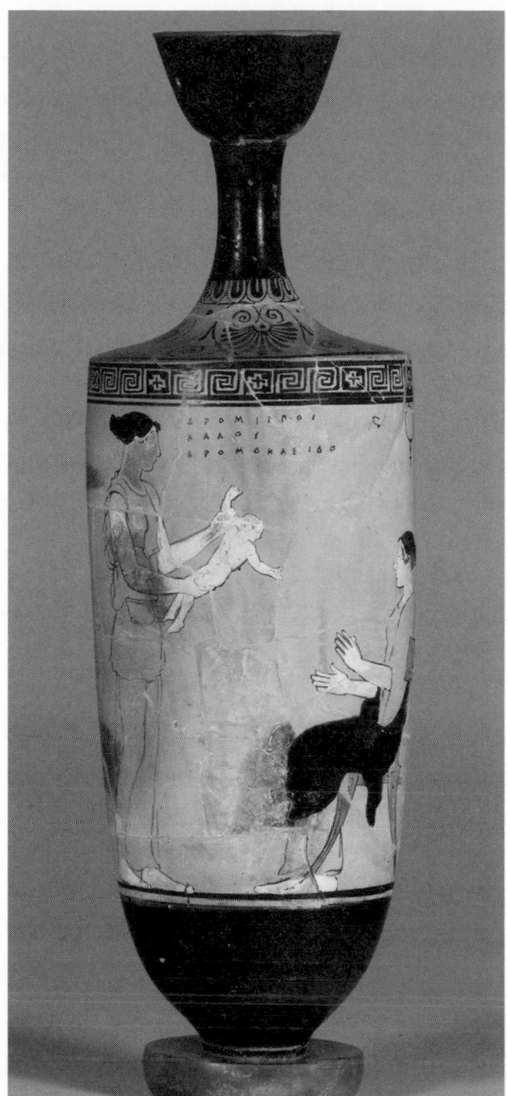

Figure 3.2 This characteristically narrow-mouthed Athenian white ground *lekythos*, from the mid-fifth century BC, shows a small boy, with a cord of protective amulets (*baskania*) across his chest, being passed from a standing to a seated female figure (maybe his mother) in a domestic setting. The inscription reads 'Beautiful Dromippos, son of Dromocleides'. 40 × 11 cm. Berlin Antikenmuseen, F2443. bpk / Antikensammlung, SMB / Johannes Laurentius.

will depend on the womb.[20] Hippocratic texts present the womb as a jar, and a difficult delivery is compared to trying to shake a fruit stone out of a narrow-mouthed jar or *lekythos* (Fig. 3.2).[21]

Thus, in contrast to the belief – most closely associated with Aristotle – that generation resulted from the male seed imposing form on female blood, Hippocratic authors were committed to the idea that women also produce seed, in addition to contributing blood. The idea of two seeds, male and female, proved useful in explaining both the sex

20 Lonie, *Hippocratic Treatises*, p. 5; Hanson, 'Famous handbook', p. 738. 21 *Mul.* 1 33.

of the child and its resemblance to its parents. The Hippocratic treatise *On Generation/Nature of the Child* states that a boy is the result of both partners producing a stronger seed, and a girl the result of both producing weak seed. If one partner produces strong seed, and the other weak, then the child's sex depends on their relative quantities. The author confirms that both men and women can produce both male and female seed, but here again he assumes 'strength' is a male quality.[22]

Women of Experience: Knowledge and Gender

These discussions of blood and seed were theoretical, aimed at explaining the processes of generation, but another important development in ancient Greek medicine was a growing interest in the practicalities of working with women as patients, including as potential mothers. Sick female bodies needed curing, and interventions around fertility covered both specific remedies for procreative failure, and a range of more general measures to support conception, pregnancy and an easy birth.[23]

Treating women was not always easy. They were considered more difficult than men to understand, at least for male practitioners. This was partly phrased in terms of their sheer otherness; the poet Hesiod wrote of 'the race of women'.[24] Hippocratic gynaecology importantly insisted on this radical difference of the sexes, rather than presenting women as inferior versions of men, or as like men but with some different body parts. The claim by the author of *Diseases of Women 1* that 'the treatment of the diseases of women differs greatly from that of those of men' is foundational in this respect.[25]

This writer asserted, in the same passage, that women themselves may not know what is wrong with them, and, even if they do, may not tell their doctor, ashamed by their own inexperience and ignorance; still, 'time and necessity' will eventually teach them.[26] This theme is taken up elsewhere in the Hippocratic Corpus. The 'woman of experience', as Ann Ellis Hanson calls her, does know what is happening to her body.[27] She has menstruated for a long time and been through pregnancy, unlike her younger, less reliable, counterparts. Ithmonica of Pellene, discussed at the start of this chapter, perhaps failed to recognize the signs of pregnancy because she had not felt them before.

22 *Genit./Nat. puer.* 6–7.

23 Rebecca Flemming, 'The invention of infertility in the classical Greek world: Medicine, divinity, and gender', *Bulletin of the History of Medicine* 87 (2013), 565–90.

24 Hesiod, *Theogony* 590; King, *Hippocrates' Woman*, p. 24. 25 *Mul. 1* 62. 26 Ibid.

27 Ann Ellis Hanson, 'The medical writers' woman', in David M. Halperin, John J. Winkler and Froma I. Zeitlin (eds.), *Before Sexuality: The Construction of Erotic Experience in the Ancient Greek World* (London, 1990), pp. 309–38, on p. 310; see also Lesley Dean-Jones, '*Autopsia*, *historia* and what women know: The authority of women in Hippocratic gynaecology', in Don Bates (ed.), *Knowledge and the Scholarly Medical Traditions: A Comparative Study* (Cambridge, 1995), pp. 41–58.

So how did these women know when they had conceived? In a reference to women's shared knowledge, the writer of *On Generation/On the Nature of the Child* mentions that the pregnant slave-girl he saw 'had heard what women say to one another, that when a woman is about to conceive in her belly, the seed does not run out of her, but remains inside'.[28] Similarly, in the Hippocratic treatise *Barrenness* it is noted that a woman knows the seed has been 'taken up' if her husband says he has ejaculated, while she remains dry; if the seed comes out on the same day it will make her wet, so she will know that she cannot be pregnant.[29] The author of the Hippocratic text *Fleshes* mentions that women become aware that they are pregnant through a range of sensations, including chills, heat, shivering and sluggishness.[30] So, doctors certainly asked their female patients – 'Are you pregnant?' – and were willing to trust the answer if the woman was considered to have 'experience'.[31]

But how was it envisaged that these conversations between male physicians and their female patients occurred? Classical Greek society, after all, placed the women of a household under the control of its male head – the *kyrios* – and put a high premium on female chastity, at least for citizen women. The point is reflected in Hippocratic writings. The *Oath* contains a commitment to behave properly, including abstaining from any sexual activity with female or male bodies, free or slave, in any home the physician might enter (Fig. 3.3). The later deontological treatise, *Physician*, concurs: self-control is needed when being given access to the bodies of 'wives, daughters and possessions very precious indeed'.[32] Doctors may prefer not to examine their female patient, but instead to use an intermediary or to ask the patient questions about her self-examination.[33]

Yet, all these texts stress the regularity of physicians' interactions with female patients, and some have clearly implied that at least some women were prepared to talk openly to doctors about their bodies and their sensations. While most of the references mentioned in the previous section are to generic 'women', the writer of *Fleshes* names the *hetairai* ('prostitutes') available for public use as his source of knowledge of the seven-day formation of the fetus, and it was a prostituted slave-girl who produced the six-day seed too.[34] This suggests that a very specific group of women, with their own concerns about their bodies, were being used as evidence for all women. The writer also observes that these women can 'destroy' what is conceived, if they so choose. There are other Hippocratic references to, for example, women pulling away at the moment of ejaculation, or immediately expelling seed, or men practising withdrawal, as contraceptive techniques, but these suggest intervention before there

28 *Genit./Nat. puer.* 13. 29 *Barrenness* 8 (= *Mul.* 3 220). 30 *Fleshes* 19.
31 See also, for example, the Hippocratic *Aphorisms* 5.51; compare Aristotle, *HA* 582b10–12 and 583a35–b3.
32 *Physician* 1. 33 King, *Hippocrates' Woman*, pp. 47–8. 34 *Fleshes* 19.

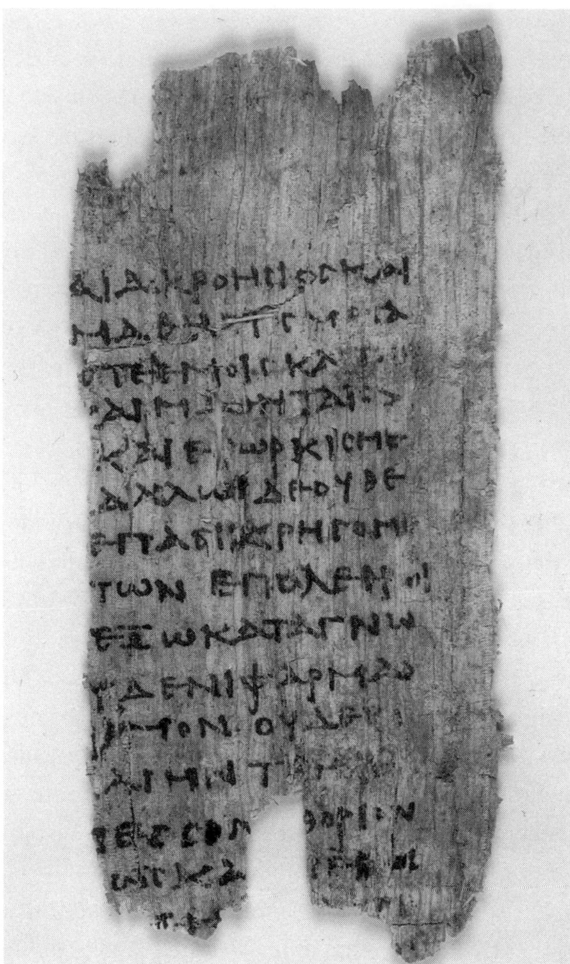

Figure 3.3 A papyrus fragment of the Hippocratic *Oath* from the third century AD, found in Oxyrhynchus (modern El Bahnasa), Egypt. Probably part of a papyrus roll which originally contained a selection of Hippocratic texts, such as standardly circulated in the Roman world. 105 × 52 mm. Wellcome Library, London, MS 5754.

was anything to 'destroy'.[35] Some remedies listed in the Hippocratic gynaecological treatises were 'dislodgers' that could expel retained menses, or perhaps also an embryo. The implication might be, therefore, that these women knew about drugs, as well as possessing a good understanding of their own bodies.

How seriously should we take such statements about women's knowledge? They may be no more than male bluff, with the medical writers creating fictional women to support their beliefs.[36] These beliefs themselves may originate in women's knowledge,

35 Ann Ellis Hanson, '*Paidopoiïa*: Metaphors for conception, abortion, and gestation in the *Hippocratic Corpus*', in Ph. van der Eijk, H. F. J. Horstmanshoff and P. H. Schrijvers (eds.), *Ancient Medicine in Its Socio-Cultural Context*, 2 vols. (Amsterdam, 1995), pp. 297–302.

36 King, *Hippocrates' Woman*, p. 136; Andrea Tone, 'Contraceptive consumers: Gender and the political economy of birth control in the 1930s', *Journal of Social History* 29 (1996), 485–506, on 496.

or in men's attempts to assert control over women's bodies; a third possibility is that they represent the common possession of men and women. The point has been much discussed in the scholarship, with much at stake, in relation to the question about whose understanding of the female body is contained in these particular texts, and to more general questions about the history of fertility control.

The debate began in 1980. For Aline Rousselle, the large number of recipes in the Hippocratic gynaecological texts, many of them to encourage fertility, suggested that these were 'women's remedies', handed down from mother to daughter before a Hippocratic physician eventually committed them to writing; however, she also suggested that women could have been putting together remedies based on recipes given to them by men.[37] In contrast, Paola Manuli regarded the remedies and the theories lying behind them, in which women's bodies were characterized by a womb that moved around the body, as men's creations, imposed on women.[38] This debate was followed up by the more particular, but also more general, arguments of John Riddle about female knowledge of abortifacients and contraceptives. He claimed there was a long tradition of such information being held by women but eventually taken over by men.[39] Nancy Demand then tried to bring these three views together, suggesting that 'the raw material of the gynaecological treatises was information discovered and passed on by women, but doctors perceived that raw material through the conceptual lens of the Greek male and of Hippocratic theory'.[40] Laurence Totelin has, more recently, developed this kind of position further, though more in opposition to Riddle. While folk medicine, she argues, was the shared property of men and women, and what she calls '*haute médecine*' was 'in the hands of male physicians', the two traditions remained in dialogue.[41]

Riddle's assumptions about the ancient world are highly speculative, based on a romantic view of a secret world of powerful women, where 'premodern people knew important things about birth control that we do not'.[42] He regards all remedies labelled 'to expel the menses' as code for abortives, for instance, but the relationship between menstruation and fertility in antiquity was rather different. Because blood was thought to accumulate in women's wet and spongy flesh, there was no concept of 'missing' a period, and, as we have seen, excess blood in the body could be dangerous; hence,

37 Aline Rousselle, 'Observation féminine et idéologie masculine: Le corps de la femme d'après les médecins grecs', *Annales: Économies, Sociétés, Civilisations* 35 (1980), 1089–115.

38 Paola Manuli, 'Fisiologia e patologia del femminile negli scritti dell'antica ginecologia greca', in M. D. Grmek (ed.), *Hippocratica: Actes du Colloque hippocratique de Paris 1978* (Paris, 1980), pp. 393–408.

39 John M. Riddle, *Contraception and Abortion from the Ancient World to the Renaissance* (Cambridge, MA, 1991).

40 Nancy Demand, *Birth, Death, and Motherhood in Classical Greece* (Baltimore, MD, 1994), p. xvi.

41 Laurence M. V. Totelin, *Hippocratic Recipes: Oral and Written Transmission of Pharmacological Knowledge in Fifth- and Fourth-Century Greece* (Leiden, 2009), pp. 127–8.

42 Riddle, *Contraception and Abortion*, p. viii; critiqued in King, *Hippocrates' Woman*, pp. 132–56.

menses needed to be expelled for health. Furthermore, amenorrhoea could be seen as a cause of infertility, not a symptom of pregnancy: no excess blood meant nothing with which to nourish a fetus, and thus no chance of becoming pregnant.

Moreover, whatever we conclude about the reality or otherwise of the women who are supposed to inform Hippocratic beliefs about generation, within an ancient context there was some risk in claiming that knowledge came from women. Passages in which ancient authors mention what women talk about among themselves hint that this is gossip, or knowledge aimed at deceiving men. Male claims of access to women's knowledge may owe more to the complex game of proving that one's sources trump those of one's opponents than to actual processes of knowledge making or other social interactions.[43]

Birthing

At the start of this chapter I suggested that the beginnings of a child did not mean that it would successfully be born, and that Asclepian stories of women becoming pregnant but forgetting to ask for a birth reflected this. Even birth does not ensure parenthood. Exposure of the newborn was always possible, and high infant mortality took its toll.[44] Both the 'raising' and the survival of the child were uncertain. Medical writers not only insisted on the need to prepare for generation by attention to diet and thus to health, but also focused on the difficulty of carrying a child to full term.[45] Birthing itself, the end of the process, was seen as something in which the woman is largely passive. In some Hippocratic texts, birth happened because the child fought its way out of the womb like a chick pecking its way out of a hen's egg.[46] If things went wrong, classical Greek medicine held that, while the seven months' child was at risk, the child born at eight months always died. Hanson has seen this as a strategy which absolved all involved, from the parents to the midwife or physician, of any blame or sense of responsibility, since by recalculating the time of conception any dead baby could be classified as an 'eight months' child'.[47]

Conclusion

The development of learned Greek medicine thus occurred in dialogue with the existing cultural imaginary, and interactions with both philosophy and more traditional

43 Helen King, 'Medical texts as a source for women's history', in A. Powell (ed.), *The Greek World* (London, 1995), pp. 199–218.

44 Cynthia Patterson, '"Not worth the rearing": The causes of infant exposure in ancient Greece', *Transactions of the American Philological Association* 115 (1985), 103–23.

45 *Mul.* 1 2; Hanson, '*Paidopoiïa*', pp. 298 and 294–5.

46 *Genit./Nat. puer.* 30; and *Eight Months' Child* 1.

47 Ann Ellis Hanson, 'The eight months' child and the etiquette of birth: *Obsit omen!*', *Bulletin of the History of Medicine* 61 (1987), 589–602.

ΠΙΝΑΞ ΤΩΝ ΙΠΠΟΚΡΑΤΟΥΣ ΒΙΒΛΙΩΝ.	INDEX LIBRORUM HIPPOCRATIS.
Ὅρκος Ἱπποκράτους.	Iusiurandum Hippocratis.
Περὶ τέχνης.	De arte.
Περὶ ἀρχαίης ἰητρικῆς.	De prisca medicina.
Περὶ ἰητροῦ.	De medico.
Περὶ εὐσχημοσύνης.	De probitate.
Ἱπποκράτους παραγγελίαι.	Hippocratis præcepta.
Νόμος Ἱπποκράτους.	Lex Hippocratis.
Περὶ φύσιος ἀνθρώπου.	De natura hominis.
Περὶ διαίτης ὑγιεινῆς. Πολύβου τοῦ Ἱπποκράτους μαθητοῦ.	De ratione uictus salubris. Polybi discipuli Hippocratis.
Περὶ γονῆς. Πολύβου.	De semine. Polybi.
Περὶ φύσιος παιδίου.	De natura fœtus.
Περὶ σαρκῶν.	De carne.
Περὶ ἑπταμήνου.	De septimestri partu.
Περὶ ὀκταμήνου.	De octomestri partu.
Περὶ ἐπικυήσεως.	De superfœtatione.
Περὶ ἐγκατατομῆς ἐμβρύου.	De extractione fœtus.
Περὶ ὀδοντοφυΐας.	De dentitione.
Περὶ ἀνατομῆς.	De dissectione.
Περὶ καρδίας.	De corde.
Περὶ ἀδένων.	De glandibus.
Περὶ ὀστέων φύσιος.	De natura ossium.
Περὶ τόπων τῶν κατ᾽ ἄνθρωπον.	De locis in homine.
Περὶ ἀέρων, ὑδάτων, τόπων.	De aere, aqua, locis.
Περὶ διαίτης.	Da uictus ratione.
Περὶ ἐνυπνίων.	De insomniis.
Περὶ τροφῆς. ὃ μὴ εἶναι Ἱπποκράτους φησὶ Γαληνός.	De alimento quem esse Hippocratis negat Galenus.
Περὶ ὑγρῶν χρήσιος.	De usu humidorum.
Περὶ χυμῶν.	De humoribus.
Περὶ φυσῶν.	De flatibus.
Περὶ ἱερῆς νούσου. ἀξιολόγου τινός.	De sacro morbo. docti cuiusdam.
Περὶ νούσων.	De morbis.
Περὶ παθῶν. τοῦ Πολύβου.	De affectibus. polybi.
Περὶ τῶν ἐντὸς παθῶν.	De internarum partium affectibus.
Περὶ παρθενίων.	De morbis uirginum.
Περὶ γυναικείης φύσιος.	De matura muliebri.
Περὶ γυναικείων.	De morbis mulierum.
Περὶ ἀφόρων.	De sterilibus.
Νόθα τῇ τελευτῇ τοῦ πρώτου περὶ γυναικείων προσκείμενα.	Supposititia quædam calci primi de morbis mulierum adscripta.
Περὶ ἐπιδημιῶν.	De morbis passim grassantibus.
Περὶ διαίτης ὀξέων.	De ratione uictus acutorum.
Περὶ κρίσεως.	De iuditiis.
Περὶ κρισίμων.	De diebus iudicialibus.
Ἱπποκράτους ἀφορισμοί.	Hippocratis definitæ sententiæ.
Ἱπποκράτους προγνωστικόν.	Hippocratis prænotiones.
Ἱπποκράτους προρρητικόν.	Hippocratis prædictiones.
Κωακαὶ προγνώσεις.	Coacæ præcognitiones.
Περὶ τῶν ἐν κεφαλῇ τρωμάτων.	De uulneribus capitis.

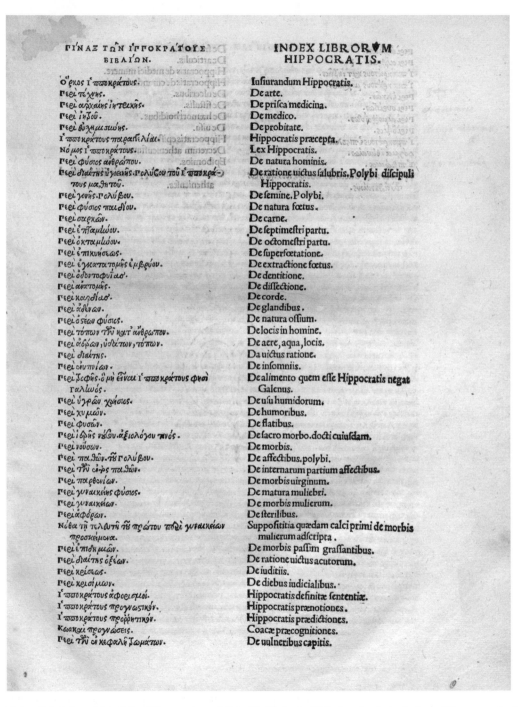

Figure 3.4 Index of the Aldine Hippocrates, published in Venice in 1526, showing its inclusion of the gynaecological treatises. This first printing of the 'complete works' of Hippocrates in Greek followed publication of the collected works in Latin the previous year and further stimulated the study of Hippocratic texts. Published with permission of *ProQuest* as part of Early European Books, 3173/D. Further reproduction is prohibited without permission.

modes of thought continued; but the result was something decisively new in many ways. Human generation was explored as part of a wider trend towards accumulating and ordering knowledge about healthy and sick bodies, trying to understand the general and specific processes involved, and intervening to influence outcomes; all of which was now recorded, described and contested in writing. It might be the focus of attention or dealt with in passing, but the same approaches were taken to generation, the same intellectual resources brought to bear, as to everything else in this emergent medical literature. Observation, experience, conversation, all played their persuasive part, with analogy, shared assumptions and the appeal of comprehensive explanation.

Women were caught up in this new medical project in complex ways. In particular, while the male seed remained crucial, the female contribution to procreation was increasingly recognized, and the female body became the focus of medical activity around fertility; indeed, medical activity around the female body was focused on fertility. *Diseases of Women 1* is, for instance, one of a series of texts which exemplify the principle that female health depends on generation. The womb is the focus of pathological inquiry, and the 'constant refrain' of the therapeutic advice, as Hanson puts it, is to have marital sex, since 'if she becomes pregnant she will be healthy'.[48] This is a key theme of Hippocratic 'gynaecology', of all these treatises dedicated to women's health, diseases and cures. The specific interpretative point will be contested, but the literary genre thus initiated will persist throughout classical antiquity and beyond (Fig. 3.4). Medical texts will continue to be devoted to women, with fertility always a large part of the picture.

48 Hanson, 'Medical writers' woman', p. 318.

4 Animal and Plant Generation in Classical Antiquity

Laurence M. V. Totelin

'Generation' was a particular kind of coming-to-be, which required not just qualitative alteration or quantitative growth, but that a new thing be produced; intimately associated with living beings, it could be extended further. Some minerals, for example, were thought to produce children, or at least re-generate, and more metaphorical generation was widespread across many artistic, artisanal and intellectual realms. Does generation require, or even define, male and female; do both contribute equally? Does the concept have its own typology, or follow external divisions between kinds of things? In what ways, if any, is it valid, for instance, to draw analogies between plant and animal generation? These key questions, with major implications for how any society construes and orders the world, were addressed first sporadically, and then increasingly systematically, in classical antiquity. A range of surviving texts record the early, and very influential, efforts to grapple with these issues.

Despite the significance of generation, the existing scholarship is patchy and incomplete; some areas are much debated, others almost untouched. I attempt here both to provide a general outline of the field, and to explore selected themes within it. The focus is first on some of the earliest philosophical discussions: the systematic efforts of Aristotle in the mid-fourth century BC, especially *Generation of Animals*, and the extensive works on plants by his student and successor as head of the Lyceum, Theophrastus.[1] Together, these texts were conceptually foundational, and though many points, and even principles, were vigorously disputed over the centuries, they also established much shared ground. Most importantly, they developed a theoretical framework around much that was already assumed or taken for granted, and joined many previously disparate pieces into a comprehensive explanatory system, thus setting out a single domain of generation.

This, and much else, can be illustrated by examining the reception, and development, of these discussions in a range of less philosophical textual genres from the Roman world. Particularly important is the tradition of Latin agricultural writing, which begins with Cato in the early second century BC, passes through Varro and Columella

1 Theophrastus also wrote *On Stones*, which mentions the power of some 'to have children'. Information on all authors mentioned in this chapter can be found in Paul T. Keyser and Georgia L. Irby-Massie (eds.), *The Encyclopaedia of Ancient Natural Scientists: The Greek Tradition and Its Many Heirs* (London, 2008).

in the late first centuries BC and AD respectively, and continues to Palladius in the fourth century AD. Ostensibly practical in outlook, concerned with the fertility of the land, crops and livestock, and the particularities of breeding horses and hunting dogs, these texts engage directly and indirectly with many of the same ideas, and ideologies, as their more theoretical predecessors, from the perspective of the Roman landowning elite. Pliny the Elder's first-century AD encyclopaedia, the *Natural History*, does all this and more, in an explicitly encompassing, programmatic and imperial manner. An early-third-century AD Greek work, *On Animals* by the sophist Aelian, also demonstrates the diversity of relevant literary projects that flourished through the Roman Empire. Medieval bestiaries drew on his text, while ancient agricultural writings were multiply excerpted, compiled and translated over the centuries; just as Pliny's authority persisted, albeit subject to increasing criticism, across many disciplines and for a very long time.

Generation in General

Ancient philosophers and technical writers were not alone in puzzling over generation. In his *Eumenides*, the fifth-century BC Athenian tragedian Aeschylus staged a debate, in which the god Apollo famously asserts that the father not the mother is the real parent of any offspring.[2] She 'merely nurses newly-sown seed', caring for what is within her as a host would for a guest, bound by obligations of 'guest-friendship' (*xenia*) not kinship. Poetic engagements with generative themes will continue to be part of this story.

As Aeschylus illustrates, in addition to debating maternal and paternal contributions to generation, ancient writers often applied vegetative metaphors to the processes of human generation: the mother is a field; the father a farmer; the child starts life as a seed.[3] Conversely, the ancients sometimes drew analogies between plant and animal generation. Thus, the Presocratic philosopher Empedocles wrote, in verse: 'So the great trees lay eggs; the olives first' (Fig. 4.1).[4] These comparisons were more than poetic metaphors. The idea of continuity in Nature, common in the ancient world in general and ancient philosophy in particular, implied that the processes were really the same. Aristotle posited that Nature advances continuously, one small step after the other, from the inanimate stone to the most perfect of animals: man.[5] In Aristotle's scheme, soul differentiated inanimate things from animate beings; and the sentient part of the soul differentiated animals from plants – the latter possessing only the nutritive part

2 *Eumenides* 658–61; also Euripides, *Orestes* 544–604.

3 Page DuBois, *Sowing the Body: Psychoanalysis and Ancient Representations of Women* (Chicago, IL, 1988); Helen King, 'Sowing the field: Greek and Roman sexology', in Roy Porter and Mikuláš Teich (eds.), *Sexual Knowledge, Sexual Science: The History of Attitudes to Sexuality* (Cambridge, 1994), pp. 29–46.

4 Quoted by Aristotle, *Generation of Animals* (*GA*) 731a5; and Theophrastus, *Causes of Plants* (*CP*) 1.7.1.

5 *History of Animals* (*HA*) 588b4–589a10.

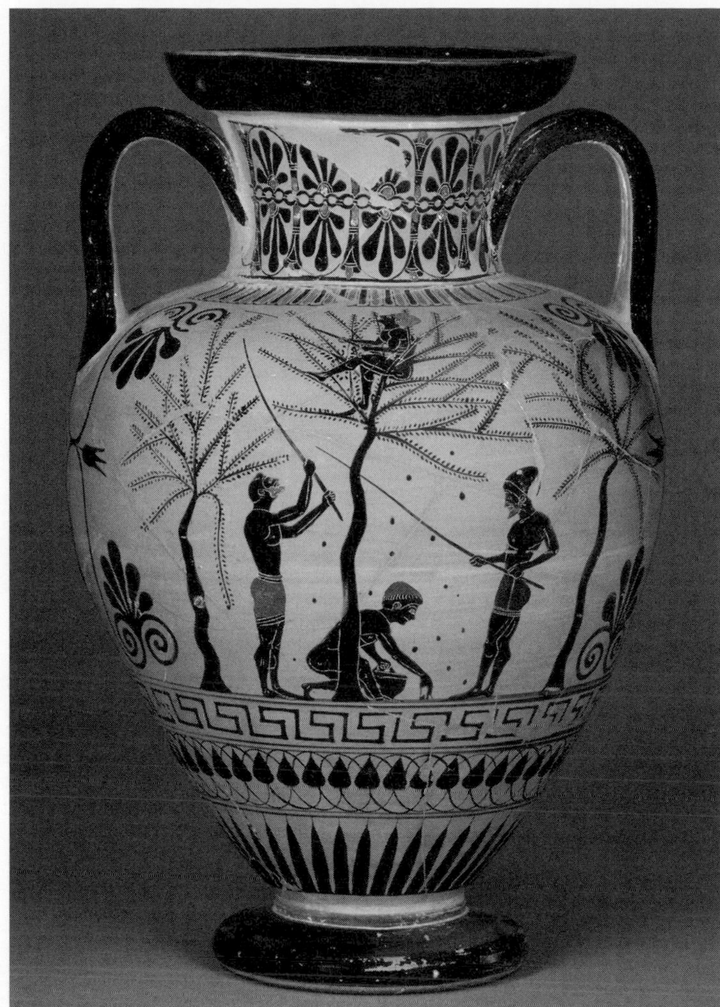

Figure 4.1 The olive harvest representing the bounty of nature on an Attic black-figure vase attributed to the Antimenes painter, *c.* 520 BC. With olives a key crop in the ancient Mediterranean, economically and in terms of lifestyle, metaphors involving them were as abundant as the fruit itself, and easily understood across cultures. H 40 cm: amphora, B 226. © Trustees of the British Museum.

of the soul, responsible for generation and growth. Generation was therefore crucial in defining living beings: it was an activity (*ergon*) common to all living things (*zōnta*), while all animals (*zōa*) also partook in some measure of knowledge, which plants lacked.[6]

Generation, in its variety, also had great classificatory power. Aristotle devised the following hierarchical model in *Generation of Animals*.[7] First are the most perfect blooded animals (hot and wet) that give birth to their young in a perfect

6 *GA* 731a29–30.

7 *GA* 755b29–756a6; G. E. R. Lloyd, 'The development of Aristotle's theory of the classification of animals', *Phronesis* 6 (1961), 59–81; Pierre Pellegrin, *Aristotle's Classification of Animals: Biology and the Conceptual Unity of the Aristotelian Corpus*, trans. Anthony Preus (Berkeley, CA, 1986); Arnaud Zucker, *Aristote et les classifications zoologiques* (Louvain-la-Neuve, 2005).

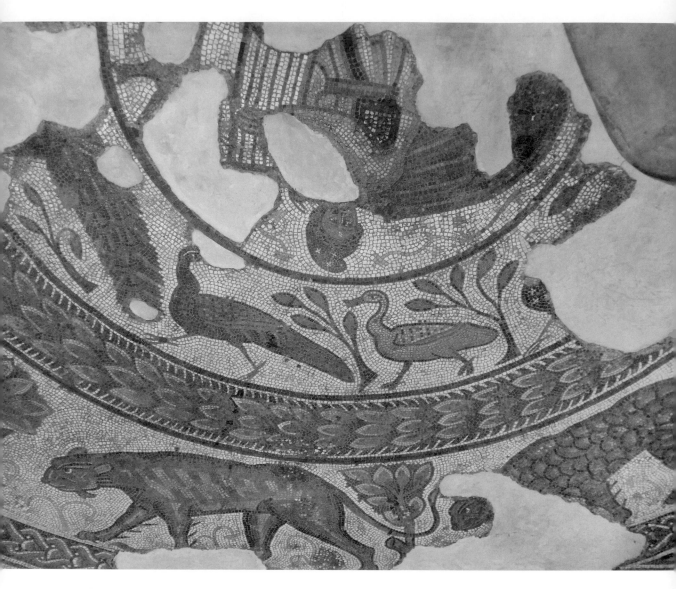

Figure 4.2 Four-footed animals (panthers), birds and plant motifs depicted in a fourth-century AD mosaic from a grand courtyard house in Roman Cirencester. The rich and ordered variety of living things was a favoured subject for mosaics across the Roman Empire. The whole panel, of which this is a section, measures 4.45 m square. Corinium Museum, Cirencester.

state. They are viviparous animals, of which man is the most perfect. The next class are blooded animals (cold and wet), such as cartilaginous fish and vipers, that give birth to living young which had developed in eggs within their mother's body. They are the ovoviviparous animals. Below them are blooded animals (hot and dry), such as birds and scaly reptiles, that lay perfect eggs. The next category of blooded animals (cold and dry) comprises creatures such as scaly fish, crustaceans and cephalopods, which lay imperfect eggs that need impregnation by milt outside the mother's body. The animals in both this and the previous category are oviparous. The final, lowest group is that of insects: bloodless animals that produce larvae. They are the coldest animals of all. In the books on animals in his *Natural History* Pliny also makes extensive use of Aristotle's classifications based on generation (Fig. 4.2).[8]

Other animals fell outside Aristotle's hierarchy. Thus, he argued that shellfish partake of both the animal and the plant and are generated spontaneously.[9] Aristotle also mentioned plant generation on various occasions, stating that it occurred in three different ways: from seeds, from slips or from side-shoots.[10] He did not dwell on the topic, however, leaving it to be developed in a work *On Plants*, which was either never written or has been lost.[11] To learn more about plant generation, one has to turn to the writings of Theophrastus, who listed the following modes of plant generation: 'spontaneous, from the seed, from a root, from a shoot, from a branch, from a twig, from the trunk itself, or even from wood broken into small pieces'.[12] This list calls for comment on several counts. First, it does not mention flowers. Second, it mostly comprises what we would today call 'asexual reproduction' or 'cloning', whereby a part of an existing plant is replanted.[13] Finally, it omits one mode of asexual plant propagation, grafting, of much interest to later Roman writers.

Having defined the basic principles of ancient generation, I will now focus on some of the notions most discussed by ancient authors: male and female, egg and seed, spontaneous generation and hybridity. The first two are at the very core of any debate on generation and, though seemingly very simple, were controversial topics. Spontaneous generation and hybridity were less central to ancient debates, yet they are very illuminating, for they demonstrate the complexity of classical understandings in general, and the fluidity of ancient views of kinds, or 'species', in particular.

Male, Female and Their Union

At the very beginning of *Generation of Animals*, Aristotle noted: 'Now of course some animals occur through the coupling of male and female'.[14] In many cases this statement is straightforward. Most self-moving animals have separate male and female individuals that copulate and are characterized by different generative organs.[15] The male possesses testes (external or internal) and a penis; while the female has a uterus, which is always internal.[16]

8 *Natural History* (*HN*) 11.121–284. 9 *GA* 761a14–19. 10 *GA* 761b26–30.

11 For the complex, multilingual textual history of the *De plantis* (*On Plants*) transmitted in the Aristotelian Corpus: H. J. Drossaart Lulofs and E. L. J. Poortman (eds.), *Nicolaus Damascenus, De Plantis: Five Translations* (Amsterdam, 1989).

12 *History of Plants* (*HP*) 2.1.1.

13 Chr. Gorm Tortzen, 'Male and female in Peripatetic botany', *Classica et mediaevalia* 42 (1991), 81–110, on 88.

14 *GA* 715a18–19. 15 *GA* 730b33–4.

16 *GA* 716b1–2; 719a30–2; also Pliny *HN* 11.209 (uterus) and 263 (testes). Not all the animal organs that Aristotle identifies as 'penis' and 'uterus' would count as such in modern biology; his desire for a single, general pattern is very great.

Aristotle also provided a more theoretical – and universal – formulation of the relationship between male, female and generation: the male is that which 'generates in another' and the female is that which 'generates in itself'.[17] He was, however, aware of exceptions to this rule. Some animals are hermaphrodites; it is not always possible to determine whether an individual is female or male (for instance, the ancients wondered whether to talk of a King or Queen Bee); not all animals were observed to copulate; and some living things, notably shellfish and plants, cannot move and find their partners.[18] Aristotle also acknowledged that, even among copulating animals, male and female were not absolute polar opposites. When castrated, a male animal (or human) became more feminine.[19] Also, while Aristotle claimed that differences in sex lead to differences in character, with females being softer and tamer, he made every effort to note exceptions, such as the courageous she-bear and she-leopard.[20]

Faced with these difficulties, Aristotle concluded that, in the process of generation, a male and a female 'principle' (*archē*) are necessary; these can be provided by two separate individuals or mingled within the same individual. Aristotle's theories were based on numerous observations of animal copulation and on dissections, as well as his wider philosophical commitments. These went a long way to correct popular misconceptions. For instance, the philosopher argued against those who, like the fifth-century BC historian and 'fable-maker' Herodotus, believed that fish do not copulate but conceive by swallowing milt; explaining that fish copulation is very short and difficult for fishermen to observe.[21] He also criticized those who suggested that the hyena had both sets of sexual organs, stating that there is ample opportunity to observe the opposite.[22] Such beliefs, however, continued throughout antiquity and beyond. Aelian's *On Animals*, especially, contains many fabulous accounts, often with a moral conclusion, of strange copulation, hermaphroditism and births in animals.[23]

Aristotle also mixed animal behaviour and human morality. Thus, abhorrence for incest, and to a lesser extent for sexual lust, is reflected in his account of horse breeding: 'After man, the horse, both male and female, is the most lustful of animals … Horses will mount their mothers and their daughters. In fact, a herd of horses is not considered perfect, unless horses copulate with their own offspring.'[24]

17 *GA* 716a14–15.

18 Robert Mayhew, 'King-bees and mother-wasps: A note on ideology and gender in Aristotle's entomology', *Phronesis* 44 (1999), 127–34.

19 *HA* 590a1–2.

20 *HA* 608a25–b4; G. E. R. Lloyd, *Science, Folklore, and Ideology: Studies in the Life Sciences in Ancient Greece* (Cambridge, 1983), pp. 98–9.

21 *GA* 755b7–756b13; against Herodotus 2.93.

22 *GA* 757a3–13; Gabriella Zuccolin, 'The Hermaphroditic Hyena', Exhibit 9, this book.

23 For example, *On Animals* (*NA*) 1.25, 2.46 and 2.55.

24 Aristotle, *HA* 575b31–2 and 576a18–20; and, for example, Aelian, *NA* 4.11.

Throughout antiquity, some creatures, such as the camel and the pigeon, were admired for their monogamy; while others, such as the horse, goat and partridge, were criticized for their sexual incontinence.[25] These anecdotes were entertaining, and morally instructive; but the interest in animal sexual behaviour stemmed primarily from the needs of animal breeding. In that process, horses were particularly troublesome: although salacious, they often refused to mate and required aphrodisiacs or other tricks to make them comply.[26]

There were, then, many opportunities to observe and comment on animal copulation. Plants were more problematic. Theophrastus, and many after him, often referred to 'male' and 'female' plants: for instance, male and female mandrake, male frankincense, male and female cypress (Fig. 4.3).[27] This was not linked to sexual intercourse – 'male' and 'female' plants did not engage in sexual union – but rather reflected cultural assumptions about gender.[28] Thus, 'female' plants carried fruits, whereas males did not; and if both genders carried, the female carried more.[29] Male trees were taller and stronger; female trees easier to work and fatter. Because domesticated plants tend to bear more fruits than wild ones, the former were often considered female and the latter male.

But if 'male' and 'female' plants did not engage in sexual union, how did plants generate? Aristotle suggested that, in plants, male and female principles are mingled together.[30] Theophrastus, for his part, suggested that, in the process of plant generation, the earth was, by analogy, the female principle: it could be compared to a womb, and could be 'in heat'.[31] In doing so, he expressed philosophically a common ancient notion, namely that the earth is female and awaiting 'fertilization'. The Roman agronomists also stressed the fertility of the earth, though Columella noted that some authorities argued it had been exhausted by over-production.[32] A few decades earlier, the philosopher and polymath Nicolaus of Damascus had rejected Aristotle's idea of mixed principles in plants, which he interpreted as an assertion that plants are more perfect than animals. Instead, he argued that the nutritive principle in the generation of plants comes from the earth and their generative power from the sun.[33] Plant generation often involved seeds, but could happen in other ways, by propagation from slips. This raised the question of the function of the seed.

25 Illustrations include: Aristotle, *HA* 630b31–631a7; Aelian, *NA* 3.5, 3.47, 4.11; Pliny, *HN* 10.104; and Columella, 7.6.3.

26 As shown by: Columella, 6.24.2 and 6.27; Varro, *On Agriculture* (*RR*) 2.7.8; Pliny, *HN* 10.180.

27 Lin Foxhall, 'Natural sex: The attribution of sex and gender to plants in ancient Greece', in Foxhall and John Salmon (eds.), *Thinking Men: Masculinity and Its Self-Representation in the Classical Tradition* (London, 1998), pp. 57–70.

28 With one exception, the date-palm: Laura Georgi, 'Pollination ecology of the date palm and fig tree: Herodotus 1.193.4–5', *Classical Philology* 77(1982), 224–8.

29 See especially Theophrastus, *HP* 3.8.1; *CP* 2.10.1.

30 *GA* 730b32–731a29.

31 *CP* 3.2.6 and 4.4.0.

32 Columella, 1.pr.1, 2.1.1.

33 *On Plants* 817a10–26.

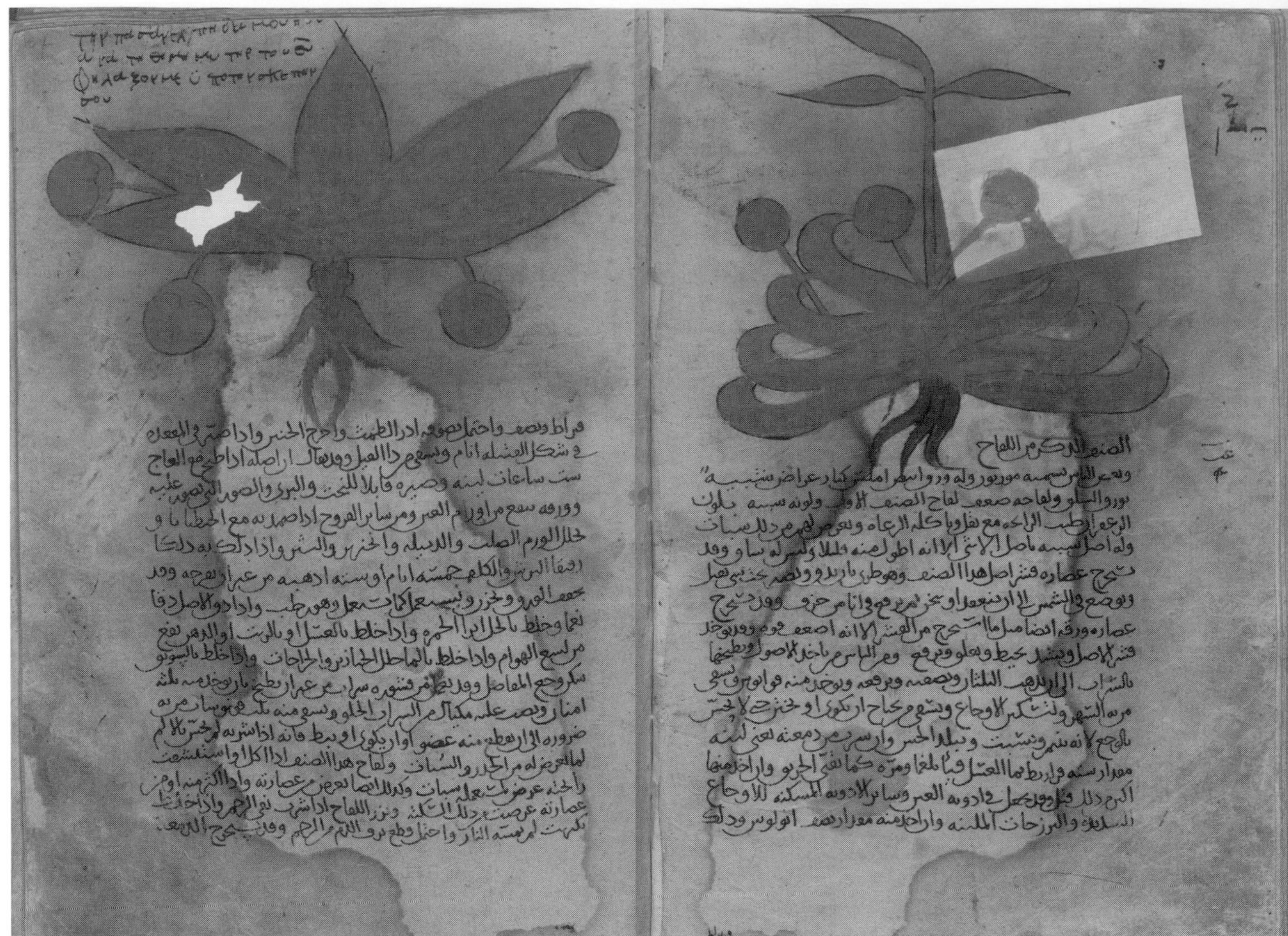

Figure 4.3 Characteristically anthropomorphic mandrakes in a manuscript (dated AD 1083) containing a translation into Arabic of Dioscorides' authoritative Greek herbal. Both male and female plants bear fruit, but the male's (left) are larger, like its roots and its leaves. Bibliotheek der Rijksuniversiteit, Leiden, cod. or. 289, f. 156v–7r.

Seed and Egg

From the very beginnings of Greek literature, the word *sperma* (seed) designated plant seeds and something that has the power to start something else.[34] Greek philosophers took advantage of the metaphorical power of plant seeds, those little things that could easily be observed to grow into a plant. Ironically, this led them to question the application of the notion of seed to plant generation. Thus Aristotle wrote: 'In plants, however, the [male and female] faculties are mingled together; the female is not separate from the male; and that is why they generate out of themselves, and produce not semen

34 Hesiod, *Works and Days* 471; Homer, *Odyssey* 5.490.

(*gonē*) but a fetation (*kuēma*) – what we call their "seeds" (*spermata*)'.[35] He then stated that, as in the case of eggs, plant-fetations contain a part from which the new plant will grow, and a part which will nourish it while it grows, although the earth provides some additional nourishment.[36] Theophrastus too compared plant seeds to eggs: 'This contains in itself innate moisture and heat, and, if these ail, the seeds are sterile, like eggs in the same case'.[37] However, he argued that the analogy between plant seed and egg worked only up to a point. Unlike animals, in which the duration of pregnancy is fixed, plants can take longer to germinate in some places than in others according to the quality of the climate, air and soil: 'for animals have their most important principles in themselves, whereas the seed [of the plant] in general gets them [the starting points] from the air'.[38]

Plant seed, then, is different from animal seed. But what exactly is animal seed? Aristotle devoted a large part of *Generation of Animals* to that question.[39] Discounting the opinion of numerous Presocratic predecessors, he concluded that seed is a useful residue (*perittōma*) of blood.[40] Both male and female produce seed, but the female seed is not as perfect as the male:

> The female is, as it were, a mutilated male; and the menstrual flux is a seed (*sperma*), but not a pure one. For it lacks one constituent, and one only, the principle of soul. For that reason, in the case of the wind-eggs which some animals produce, the egg that takes shape contains the parts of both parents, but it does not have this principle, and therefore does not become ensouled.[41]

This statement has been much debated in modern scholarship, with respect to its meaning and politics. In some readings, Aristotle prejudicially denied women the production of seed.[42] While he was at times certainly biased against women, he did not say that the female role in generation is completely passive.[43] Women do produce a seed: menses are semen, but because women are colder than men, they cannot concoct their seed, which does not contain the sentient part of the soul, and is therefore insufficient in itself for generation.[44] In

35 *GA* 731a1–5. 36 *GA* 740b5–11. 37 *HP* 1.11.1. 38 *CP* 4.11.9.

39 On Presocratic embryology: Erna Lesky, *Die Zeugungs- und Vererbungslehren der Antike und ihr Nachwirken* (Mainz, 1951); Andrew Coles, 'Biomedical models of reproduction in the fifth century BC and Aristotle's *Generation of Animals*', *Phronesis* 40 (1995), 48–88.

40 *GA* 725a11–14. 41 *GA* 737a28–32.

42 Eva C. Keuls, *The Reign of the Phallus: Sexual Politics in Ancient Athens* (Berkeley, CA, 1985), p. 145; Lesley Dean-Jones, *Women's Bodies in Classical Greek Science* (Oxford, 1996), p. 177.

43 For example, *GA* 728a26–7 and b23. See Robert Mayhew, *The Female in Aristotle's Biology: Reason or Rationalization* (Chicago, IL, 2004); and Devin M. Henry, 'How sexist is Aristotle's developmental biology?', *Phronesis* 52 (2007), 251–69; and further Rebecca Flemming, 'Galen's Generations of Seeds', Chapter 7, this book.

44 Mayhew, *Female in Aristotle's Biology*, p. 36.

these circumstances, the main contribution of females in generation is to provide the material (*hulē*) and nourishment (*trophē*) needed for the development of the embryo; and that of males is to transmit the soul, the form (*eidos*) and the principle of movement, but no material whatsoever – that part of the male seed disappears once conception has taken place.[45]

Females on their own can produce wind-eggs (and similar 'products' such as fish eggs in need of 'impregnation'), the formless mass of uterine 'moles' and 'wind-foals' who never live beyond infancy.[46] These 'wind offspring' have the nutritive function of the soul, but nothing else, and in particular they cannot develop the sentient part of the soul. However, while 'wind offspring' are irregular, they still originate from seed (that of the female), and therefore differ from cases of spontaneous generation.

Spontaneous Generation

Starting with the Presocratic thinkers – Theophrastus reported the views of Anaxagoras and Diogenes on the topic – the ancients argued that some animals and plants are generated spontaneously.[47] Aristotle explained the process in *Generation of Animals*:

> Animals and plants occur in the earth and in the wet because, in the earth, there exists water, and in water there exists *pneuma* [that is, a form of warm air], and in all *pneuma* there is soul-heat, so that in a way everything is full of soul. And for that reason they [the animals and plants] are quickly constituted once it [the *pneuma*] has been enclosed. And it gets enclosed when the corporeal liquids are heated, and a foamy bubble, as it were, is formed.[48]

A little before, Aristotle had noted that the seasons provided the heat.[49] When soul-containing *pneuma* becomes trapped in a bubble of liquid and corporeal matter, and is fully heated by the sun, a living being can take shape. Theophrastus's explanation of the phenomenon is similar: 'We need to enquire about spontaneous generation. Simply speaking, it must occur when the earth is thoroughly warmed and the accumulated mixture [that is, of earth and liquid] is altered by the sun, as we also observe in the case of animals'.[50] He provided an example, describing how, in

45 For example, *GA* 729a10–14 and 737a7–15. See further Charlotte Witt, 'Form, reproduction, and inherited characteristics in Aristotle's *Generation of Animals*', *Phronesis* 30 (1985), 46–57.

46 See especially Aristotle, *GA* 750b3–25, 756a15–31, 775b25–776a9 and *HA* 572a13. On wind-foals see also, for example, Aelian, *NA* 4.6; Pliny, *HN* 8.166; and Varro, *RR* 2.1.19.

47 *HP* 3.1.4. Much of the scholarship focuses on Aristotle, and issues of internal doctrinal consistency, but see D. M. Balme, 'Development of biology in Aristotle and Theophrastus: Theory of spontaneous generation', *Phronesis* 7 (1962), 91–104; and Devin M. Henry, 'Themistius and spontaneous generation in Aristotle's *Metaphysics*', *Oxford Studies in Ancient Philosophy* 24 (2003), 183–208.

48 *GA* 762a19–24. 49 *GA* 743a35–6. 50 *CP* 1.5.5.

Paphlagonia, fish are spontaneously generated when warmth and moisture are mixed in the right proportion.[51]

As D. M. Balme noted, Theophrastus expressed scepticism towards theories of spontaneous generation: 'he is always concerned to give a regular physical cause for spontaneity, and he distinguishes it from marvels'.[52] For Theophrastus, the boundary between spontaneous generation and propagation by seed was blurred, and he discussed cases of false spontaneity, when plants grew from imported or unnoticed, very small seeds, as did the cypress tree, the propagation of which was debated throughout antiquity.[53]

But no generation puzzled the ancients more than that of bees. In the words of Aristotle, 'the generation of bees is a great uncertainty (*aporia*)'. Did they copulate; did they obtain seeds from elsewhere; or were they generated spontaneously 'from blossoms or some animal'?[54] It was popularly held that bees came from the rotting carcasses of cows. For instance, Varro repeated the verses of the Greek poet Archelaus:

> They [bees] are the wandering children of a rotting cow
> Wasps are the offspring of horses, and bees of calves.[55]

Nor can the famous verses of the great Roman poet Virgil on the same topic be omitted, with their more political overtones:

> And you shall wonder at this habit that so pleases the bees,
> That they don't indulge in sexual intercourse, or their body lazily
> Release in love, or produce offspring in labour,
> But, from leaves and sweet herbs, their children
> They collect in their mouth, and a ruler and tiny citizens
> They thus elect, and rebuild their palaces and waxen kingdoms.[56]

And they can be regenerated: if an 'entire colony' fails, then the corrupted blood of dead bullocks will bring forth bees; a practice supported by the myth of Aristaeus who raised a new flock of bees from the carcass of a cow he had sacrificed (Fig. 4.4).[57]

There is an ambiguity in these stories about whether this should be seen as a form of spontaneous generation, or whether bees are produced from bovine carcasses in a more direct sense. The fluidity of kinds, the idea that one 'species' might, in the normal

51 Robert W. Sharples, 'Theophrastus: *On Fish*', in William W. Fortenbaugh and Dimitri Gutas (eds.), *Theophrastus: His Psychological, Doxographical, and Scientific Writings* (New Brunswick, NJ, 1992), pp. 347–85, on p. 367.

52 Balme, 'Spontaneous generation', p. 102; also R. W. Sharples, *Theophrastus of Eresus: Sources for His Life, Writings, Thought and Influence. Commentary*, vol. 5: *Sources on Biology (Human Physiology, Living Creatures, Botany: Texts 328–435)* (Leiden, 1995), pp. 122–3.

53 *CP* 1.5.2–4; see also Pliny, *HN* 16.139–43; and Varro, *RR* 1.40.

54 *GA* 759a8–760b28.

55 *RR* 3.16.4.

56 *Georgics* 4.197–202; see also, for example, Columella, 9.14.6.

57 Virgil, *Georgics* 4.281–558.

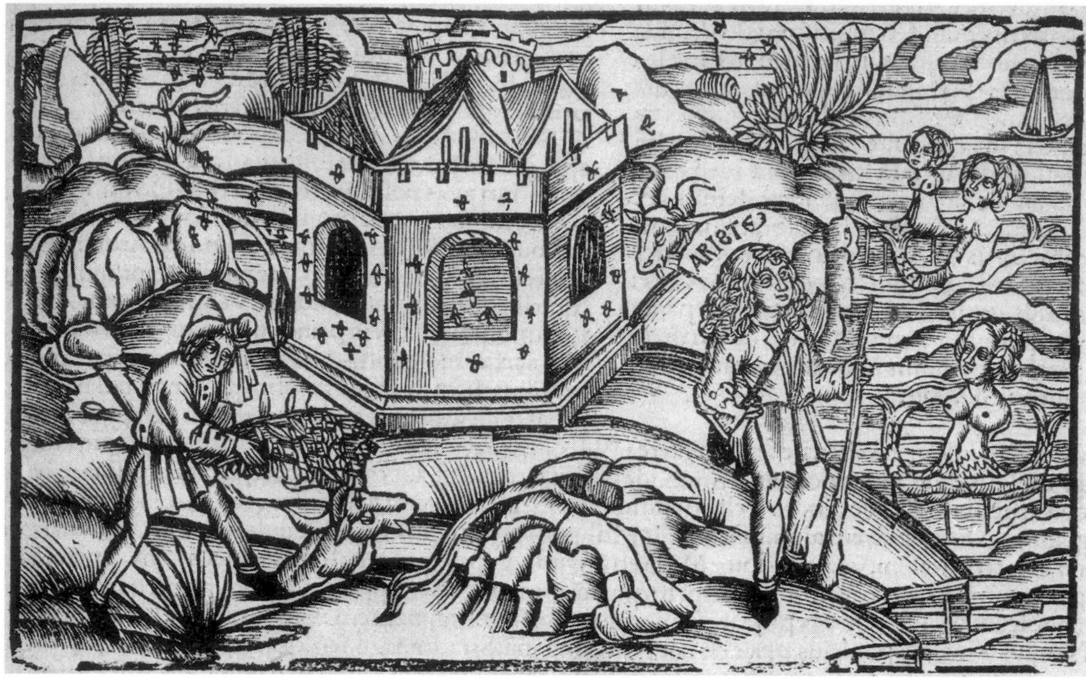

Figure 4.4 A woodcut showing the bees generated through Aristaeus's sacrifice. From the Strasbourg workshop of printer Johann Grüninger, this is part of a series illustrating important early-sixteenth-century printings of Virgil's works. The reimagining of the myth has turned the water nymphs into the more hybrid mermaids. Virgil, *Opera* (Lyon: J. Sacon, 1517). Cambridge University Library.

course of events, generate another quite different one, is, however, further demonstrated in descriptions of hybrid plants and animals.

Hybrids

Aristotle explained that for hybrids to be produced, animals must be close in species:

> Mating occurs naturally between animals of the same kind (*homogeneis*); but beside that, [mating occurs] between animals that have a similar nature, and are not very different in species (*eidos*), if they are of similar size and if their periods of gestation are equal in length. While such unions occur rarely in other animals, it occurs with dogs, foxes, wolves, and jackals.[58]

Exemplifying this principle, the hybrid animal most studied in antiquity was the mule. This useful beast of burden results from the union between an ass and a mare,

58 *GA* 746a29–34.

and is, interestingly, infertile. Aristotle considered mules to be unique among hybrids in their barrenness.[59] Pliny thought the principle a general one: 'It has been observed that the offspring of two different types (*genera*) [of animals] is of a third type (*genus*), and resembles neither parent; and that those thus born, whatever type of animal they may be, cannot generate; therefore mules cannot give birth.'[60] The sterility of mules was a topic of great interest to the ancients, especially since cases of mules giving birth had been recorded, and were seen as omens.[61] Other, even more fabulous, hybrids had been observed in distant parts of the world. According to Pliny, in India, bitches and tigers produced hounds; and a Greek proverb asserted that 'Libya always brings forth something new', as indiscriminate mating there produced all sorts of hybrids.[62]

The Romans (more than the Greeks) were also fascinated by plant grafting, which they saw as a form of hybridization.[63] They constantly experimented in this field; for instance, Columella invented a method to combine trees of different natures:

> But since the ancients denied that any kind (*genus*) of slip can be inserted in any tree, and established as a law that only those slips can unite that are similar in bark, rind and fruit to those trees in which they are inserted, we have thought it useful to destroy this false opinion, and to hand down to posterity this method whereby any type of slip can be inserted into any type of tree.[64]

There follows a long explanation of how to graft olives on figs, a 'graft' that modern horticulture does not consider true. Similarly, Palladius in his short elegiac poem *On Grafting* described thirty grafts, twenty-three of which would be similarly ruled out today. For, despite Columella's claim, it is not possible to graft any slip on any tree.

Most interesting in ancient descriptions of grafting is the constant recourse to sexual and marital vocabulary. Pliny talks of plants' 'desire' for union, with only the earth outdoing them in lust (*libido*), while Palladius is more demurely conjugal.[65] We now consider grafting an asexual mode of plant propagation, but the ancients sexualized it. It is in that process that they saw plants uniting, while they could not usually observe plants mating.

59 *GA* 746b13–16. 60 *HN* 8.173.

61 [Plutarch], *Placita* 5.14 (reporting views of Alcmaeon, Empedocles and Diocles). Reports of fertile mules include: Pliny, *HN* 8.173; Varro, *RR* 2.1.27; Columella, 6.37.3.

62 Pliny, *HN* 8.148; Aristotle, *HA* 606b20 and Pliny, *HN* 8.42. See further Annetta Alexandridis, 'The Minotaur and Other Hybrids in Ancient Greece', Exhibit 2, this book.

63 Modern 'grafting' is distinct from 'plant hybridization'. For antiquity, see Arthur Stanley Pease, 'Notes on ancient grafting', *Transactions and Proceedings of the American Philological Association* 64 (1933), 66–76; and Dunstan Lowe, 'The symbolic value of grafting in ancient Rome', *Transactions of the American Philological Association* 140 (2010), 461–88.

64 Columella, 5.11.12–13. 65 Pliny, *HN* 17.134; Palladius, *On Grafting* 1.1–20.

Conclusion

Ancient Nature – which advanced continuously, without breaks, from the inanimate to man – had generative powers beyond those known in modern biology. Nature herself was often envisaged as essentially fertile and bountiful. The ancient notion of 'generation' (*genesis*) was much broader than the modern notion of 'reproduction' with its focus on the re-production of the species.[66] It included asexual plant propagation, lapidary births and spontaneous generation. By and large, its internal organization followed the general order of beings, but there is a rather different division between the spontaneous and the rest. Male and female principles were necessary for ancient 'generation', but not sexual union, and though mostly 'like begat like', it did not always: two organisms of the same species were not required, and hybrids might be produced. In a sense, then, gender was more central to ancient generation than sex: its relatively simple binarity (male and female, although intersexuality was possible) surpassed more complex generational hierarchies. Spontaneous generation for its part existed mostly outside such hierarchies, though it was grounded in a commitment to natural fecundity.

The encompassing and hierarchical notion of 'generation' thus constructed and elaborated was fundamental for centuries to come. There were plenty of points of contention, but the basic framework, the key categories and concepts, had been solidly established and remained congruent with the main lineaments of the social order. Ancient philosophers, agricultural writers, encyclopaedists and poets all also provided a set of more particular theoretical and practical resources for those trying to understand and intervene in, explain and shape, the generative world around them.[67]

66 For example, Sandra Cavallo, 'Pregnant Stones as Wonders of Nature', Exhibit 17; James A. Secord, 'Spontaneous Generation and the Triumph of Experiment', Exhibit 26, this book.

67 For attempts to intervene with respect to animals and plants, see especially Staffan Müller-Wille, 'Linnaeus and the Love Lives of Plants', Chapter 21; and Sarah Wilmot, 'Breeding Farm Animals and Humans', Chapter 27, this book.

5 States and Populations in the Classical World

Rebecca Flemming

According to Michel Foucault's influential model, ancient states should have had a rather circumscribed, 'essentially negative' notion of their human resources. In this view, 'population' was understood as simply 'the contrary of depopulation' until a new, positive and general version of the concept appeared in the eighteenth century.[1] Old-style sovereigns wanted large, obedient and industrious populations as signs of their power; but ideas about how such an outcome might be achieved, and the efforts which could be invested, were limited.

Peter Biller's magisterial book on the positive complexities of what he calls 'demographic thought' in medieval Europe presents a different picture of pre-modern possibilities.[2] The point is emphasized by Philip Kreager's work on the 'population thinking' of the classical Greek philosopher, Aristotle, particularly as articulated in his *Politics*, also a key text in Biller's account.[3] The crucial contrast between ancient and modern here is one of approach, not invention, as the *Politics* expounds an essentially 'open' form of population thinking, which emerged from a world comprising a multiplicity of autonomous city-states (*poleis*, in Greek) of varying size and constitution, unlike the 'closed' model of the nineteenth-century European nation-state.[4] Fertility and mortality, the two cornerstones of modern demography, play a minor role in Aristotle's considerations because, for him, mobility and shifting patterns of membership were the main shapers of any community. Without stable boundaries there can be no meaningful data-sets from censuses and surveys,

1 The contrast is drawn repeatedly in Foucault's 1978 lectures: *Security, Territory, Population: Lectures at the Collège de France, 1977–1978*, ed. Michel Senellart, trans. Graham Burchell (Basingstoke, 2007), pp. 66–70, 104–6, 351–2. See also Andrea Rusnock, 'Biopolitics and the Invention of Population', Chapter 23, this book. Foucault uses the term 'population' for both old and new forms and so will I.

2 Peter Biller, *The Measure of Multitude: Population in Medieval Thought*, rev. edn (Oxford, 2007); Biller, 'The Multitude in Later Medieval Thought', Chapter 10, this book.

3 Philip Kreager, 'Aristotle and open population thinking', *Population and Development Review* 34 (2008), 599–629; Kreager, 'The Emergence of Population', Chapter 18, this book.

4 On the *polis*, see Mogens Herman Hansen, 'Greek city-states', in Peter Fibiger Bang and Walter Scheidel (eds.), *The Oxford Handbook of the State in the Ancient Near East and Mediterranean* (Oxford, 2013), pp. 250–78; the book provides more generally relevant background for this chapter. On population among nation-states and international institutions: Alison Bashford, 'World Population from Eugenics to Climate Change', Chapter 34, this book.

no 'birth-rate', 'death-rate' or any of the other statistical requirements of Foucault's modern population.[5]

This last point might be considered problematic in a volume dedicated to the history of reproduction. There may have been much more going on around population before the eighteenth century than Foucault alleges, even in the ancient world, but if it did not involve state interest in fertility and mortality then it should presumably be discussed elsewhere. What matter here are the efforts of polities to regulate and intervene in births in order to affect their human resources, actions which depended on, and contributed to, ideas about the role of the state and the wider physical, social, legal and cultural workings of procreation.

This chapter will show that, although the classical world is characterized, broadly speaking, by 'open population thinking', and, indeed, 'open population practice', this was compatible with an interest in fertility, and even in enumeration and censuses. In fact, there was a heavy emphasis on regulating procreation, in theoretical discourse and state action; though not, it should be admitted, of the kind which would qualify as part of a modern, Foucauldian population. The intention here is not to collapse antiquity and modernity, but rather to allow the complex positivities, the alternative coherencies, of the ancient world to emerge more fully. The discussion will proceed in two parts. First, Aristotle's ideas about population will be explored alongside the rather different, but equally extensive, programme of his teacher, the Athenian philosopher Plato. Then the focus will shift to the activities of classical polities in relation to their human resources.

Population Thinking

Though much political thought preceded it, in Greece, Egypt and the Near East, and took a variety of written forms, Plato's *Republic* marks the influential start of a literary tradition dedicated to political philosophy (Fig. 5.1).[6] The ideal community which emerges from this dialogue, composed in the 370s BC, is characterized by a radical approach to marriage and the family: women and children (and property) are to be held in common. The key principles in respect to generation are that: 'Sexual intercourse should occur mostly between the best men and best women, and not between the worst men and women; and the offspring of the first group should be raised, but not

5 Defined most clearly in 'Les mailles du pouvoir', *Dits et écrits, 1954–1988*, ed. Daniel Defert and François Ewald, vol. 4: *1980–1988* (Paris, 1994), pp. 182–94, on p. 193.

6 Kurt A. Raaflaub, 'Poets, lawgivers, and the beginnings of political reflection in archaic Greece', in Christopher Rowe and Malcolm Schofield (eds.), *The Cambridge History of Greek and Roman Political Thought* (Cambridge, 2000), pp. 23–59. The volume also provides further discussions of the texts analysed here.

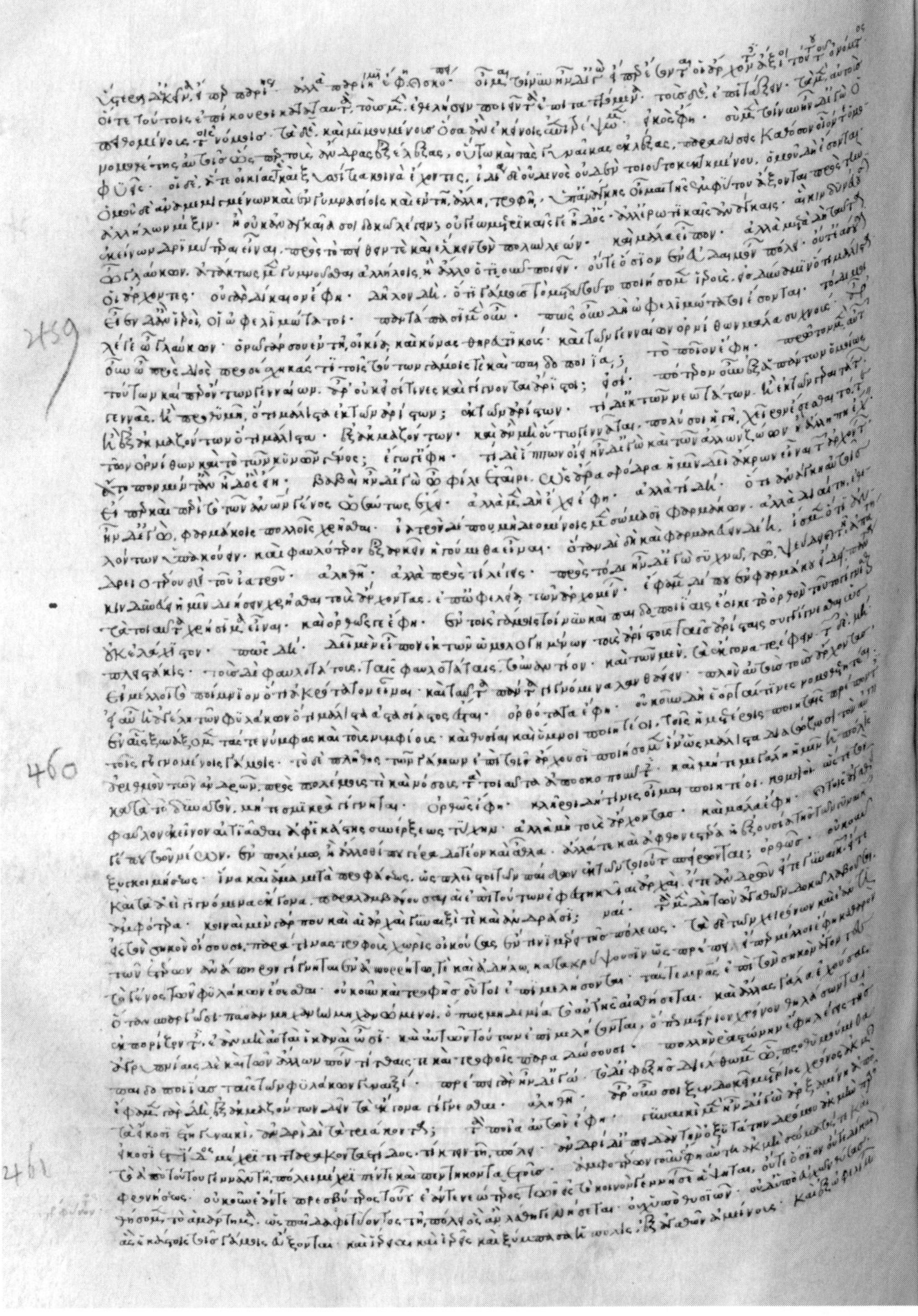

Figure 5.1 Section of Plato's *Republic* from a Greek manuscript which Cosimo de' Medici gave to the leading Renaissance scholar Marsilio Ficino in 1462 to translate into Latin. Ficino's commentary on this text offered a distinctive take on Platonic eugenics. Biblioteca Medicea Laurenziana, Florence, ms. Plut. 85.9, c. 239v. Reproduced with permission of MiBACT. Further reproduction by any means is prohibited.

the second: thus the flock will be improved.'[7] The rulers, however, have to conceal both parts of this practice, in order to preserve unity and order.

A number of 'marriage festivals' will be instituted, when a portion of the right men and women are brought together to have state-approved procreative sex.[8] Selection will operate through some kind of lottery in which all of prime childbearing age are notionally entered, though, in fact, the lots are rigged to favour preferred outcomes without creating resentment amongst the inferior men.[9] The 'quantity' (*plēthos*, in Greek) of 'marriages' will be regulated by the rulers as far as possible to preserve the number of men, despite the depredations of war and disease (women are not mentioned).[10] The city (*polis*) is to become neither larger nor smaller. Appropriate officials then transfer the offspring of good parents to the care of 'nurses' housed in a separate part of the city, while the products of the less good, and the 'deformed' children of those who were expected to do better, are removed to a secret, secluded spot, and presumably exposed there.[11] Mothers with full breasts visit the infant community to provide nourishment, but without knowing which, if any, of the children is theirs.[12] Men who break the rules on state-prescribed sexual activity will be subject to strong social and religious censure; and, though passing the procreative age entails heterosexual freedom for both sexes – only direct descendants and ascendants are off-limits – it is understood that, if pregnancy does occur amongst the more mature, no child will be born or raised.[13]

Plato returned to the project of the *Republic* a few decades later in his final treatise, *Laws*. The precise relationship between the two is much debated, but suffice it to say that though there is strong thematic continuity between them, the later version of the optimal state is more practically detailed and bears a closer resemblance to the historical world of the Greek *polis*. 'Magnesia', the city of *Laws*, will be founded in Crete, roughly along the lines of a traditional Greek colony. It will draw its settlers from several existing states rather than being launched from a single 'mother-city' (*mētropolis*), but will otherwise broadly follow the model of colonization.[14] The settlers and their descendants will be citizens of Magnesia, a community that also explicitly contains

7 *Republic* 459d7–e1. These principles are presented as applying to the 'guardians', the top class in the ideal city's distinctive social hierarchy.

8 *Republic* 459e5–460a2. Though actual marriage is absent from his ideal city, Plato cannot do without marital terminology.

9 *Republic* 460a8–10 and 460d9–461a2. The prime age for women is 20–40, for men 25–55.

10 *Republic* 460a2–6.

11 *Republic* 460c1–5. On what 'deformed' might mean: Martha L. Rose, *The Staff of Oedipus: Transforming Disability in Ancient Greece* (Ann Arbor, MI, 2003), pp. 29–49.

12 *Republic* 460c8–d5.

13 *Republic* 461a3–b7: censure; 461b9–e3: mature freedom. All children born seven or ten months after a 'marriage festival' are considered the offspring of the participants, and thus prohibited, down the generations. Procreative sex with siblings is allowed.

14 John Boardman, *The Greeks Overseas: Their Early Colonies and Trade*, 4th edn (London, 1999).

distinct groups of non-citizens, as Greek *poleis* usually did, that is, slaves and 'metics', the latter group comprising officially resident citizens of other cities plus freed slaves.[15] The question of size – of human number (*arithmos*) or magnitude (*plēthos*) – must be dealt with more concretely in this context, though the basic principle of stability persists, the correlate of a fixed pattern of family landholding.

Thus, Plato decreed that his ideal *polis* should contain 5,040 citizen farmers, male heads of landed households.[16] This number is large enough to defend the city, offer support to neighbouring states in war, and, more importantly, it is highly arithmetically divisible, which is a great organizational advantage.[17] The total will be maintained through a range of measures.[18] A single male heir will be selected to inherit the property, with any additional sons presented for adoption to childless citizens, as also any daughters surplus to the marriage requirements of the state. A high-ranking official will oversee everything, with a set of levers to pull if overall numbers seem too high or too low. Births may be 'checked', or 'encouraged'. No details are provided about how checks are to be achieved, but encouragement operates through the distribution of civic honour and disgrace, together with social admonition. More active and specific measures are demanded in response to larger-scale fluctuations. If the citizenry grows excessively, some will be despatched to found colonies overseas, in the traditional manner.[19] While inserting new adult members into the citizen body to compensate for losses to war and disease is problematic – since they will have been wrongly educated – it is sometimes necessary. How this recruitment should be realized is not specified, but enfranchising 'metics' and relaxing the rules for citizenship – requiring only one, not two, citizen parents, for example, or even including illegitimate children – are both historically attested means to increase local citizen resources.[20] Plato also does not indicate the desired total of Magnesia's inhabitants, including the citizen women and children, as well as metics and slaves.[21]

Laws thus marks a return to marriage and the family, to ideas of household property and inheritance. State control of the citizen population is no longer achieved through the direct regulation of sexual activity and extensive child exposure, but through the

15 Discussed most extensively at *Laws* 776b4–778a5 (slaves); 850a6–d2 (metics); and 914e3–915c7 (freedmen).

16 *Laws* 737e1–4. Most Greek *poleis* were smaller than this, though a few were much larger: Hansen, 'Greek city-states', pp. 260–1. Athens, in Plato's time, had perhaps 30,000 adult male citizens.

17 *Laws* 737d2–5 and 737e4–738b1.

18 *Laws* 740b1–741e5.

19 Traditionally, colonization was about power and trade as well as population.

20 Having once recruited slaves and metics for political purposes (Aristotle, *Politics* 1275b34–6; see also the general discussion at 1278a26–34), Athens apparently also relaxed its strict citizenship laws after plague and defeats in the Peloponnesian War (431–404 BC): Edwin Carawan, 'Pericles the Younger and the citizenship law', *Classical Journal* 103 (2008), 383–406.

21 The model suggests a total of 20,160 citizens (each man has a wife and two children) and perhaps as many slaves, with maybe 2,500 metics (half the number of householders), taking the population towards 45,000.

traditional mediation of the family, by bearing down on births in that setting and then adjusting as necessary. Marriage is compulsory. A man must marry between the ages of thirty and thirty-five or be subject to a hefty annual fine and systematic social dishonour thereafter.[22] The obligation is then for the couple not just to produce children, but to present 'the best and most beautiful children possible to the *polis*'.[23] To this end, female supervisors keep the pair under scrutiny for the first ten years of their marriage. If the decade has been productive, the oversight ends; if not, separation ensues.[24] The attention to quality as well as quantity means that men should not have sex with their wives when drunk, while pregnant women should keep moving; the newborn should be moulded 'like wax' while still 'fluid' and swaddled for two years.[25]

Aristotle's *Politics*, written in the 320s BC, was in part a critical response to his teacher's political works. Amongst the Platonic proposals to which he took exception was the size of Magnesia's population. The territory required to sustain such a multitude of people is impossibly vast, he alleged.[26] But Aristotle's objections to such populousness were not just practical. A key point of his programme is that in measuring the greatness of a *polis*, biggest is not best.[27] Greatness is about happiness and prosperity (*eudaimōnia*), which is produced by effectiveness not numbers. The state which best performs its functions (as a state) is the 'greatest'. This requires a certain minimum citizen-body, so that the city is self-sufficient as a political community in pursuit of the 'good life'; it also creates an upper limit, and not just in relation to territory. If there are too many people then good order breaks down, and the boundary between citizens, metics and foreigners is compromised; governance and justice become impossible, and even military capabilities are undermined, since organization and command become so challenging.

How many is enough and not too much is unclear, nor is anything said here about the ways that quantity might be established and maintained. Yet there generally is, as Kreager argues, more discussion about the (re-)classification of people, their association and movement, than about fertility.[28] Aristotle's ideal state was nevertheless interested in births and he provided extensive explanations of the proposed legislation about marriage, procreation and child-rearing, all intended to optimize the quality of the citizens. The family is a key institution for Aristotle's political theory, and 'child-production' (*teknopoia*) is one of the duties (*leituorgia*) men and women owe the *polis* – a duty the state should encourage and enhance.[29] Most importantly, age at marriage should

22 The point is made twice: *Laws* 720d10–721d6 and 773e5–774e2 (in a longer disquisition on marriage). A female age range (16–20) is also specified (785b2–4) but without legislative context.

23 *Laws* 783e8–19.

24 *Laws* 784a1–b6.

25 *Laws* 775b4–e4 (drinking); 789e1–3 (movement and moulding); Fay Glinister, 'A Swaddled Infant Given to the Gods', Exhibit 4, this book.

26 *Politics* 1265a13–18.

27 *Politics* 1325b34–1326b25.

28 Kreager, 'Aristotle', 620–4.

29 *Politics* 1334b28–1336a2.

be regulated to ensure the best offspring and best succession, amongst other desirable outcomes. 'Mating of the young' is bad for children and parents alike. It generates small, imperfect and often female offspring; while young women are more likely to die in childbirth, and sex when the male seed is still 'growing' impedes bodily development in a young man.[30] Mating of the elderly has similarly deleterious effects on progeny. Parents, in general, must keep themselves healthy and active, and pay attention to the teachings of physicians and natural philosophers about the best season and weather for procreative intercourse. With respect to the exposure or rearing of infants, it will be illegal to raise any 'deformed' child, but otherwise things are more complicated. There must be a numerical limit to procreation, which, if not enacted through exposure, will have to be enforced through early abortion.[31]

There was, then, much more to ancient population thinking than Foucault implied, and plenty of interest in generation. Ideas were, moreover, informed by contemporary notions about human procreation; both Plato and Aristotle articulated their own theories on the subject elsewhere in their oeuvre.[32] The missing piece of the demographic jigsaw is, in fact, mortality, not fertility; that ancient states might intervene around mortality seems to have remained unthought for the time being, at least consciously, or explicitly.[33] Given the utopian mode of the discussions so far, however, questions of practice remain. Greek *poleis* did, on occasion (and for complex reasons), despatch citizens to found colonies, change the criteria for membership, or enrol new groups; but did the recommendations around generation have any purchase on reality?

In providing an answer, the next section looks at classical Greece and its chronological and geographical neighbours. Most important in this respect is Rome, in its formative stages as a central Italian power-broker when Plato and Aristotle were writing, but emerging as the dominant force in the Mediterranean over the following centuries: a rise involving increasing entanglements with Greek culture and in which population policies played a role. Rome, at least in its most *polis*-like period during the Republic, before it abandoned any pretence of being a city-state in the first century BC, makes a good counterpoint to the cities of Greece.[34]

30 *Politics* 1335a11–35. Women should marry around 18, men around 37.

31 *Politics* 1335b19–26. The passage is much discussed because of its reference to abortion: Konstantinos Kapparis, *Abortion in the Ancient World* (London, 2002).

32 Plato, briefly, in *Timaeus*; Aristotle more systematically in *Generation of Animals*: Laurence M. V. Totelin, 'Animal and Plant Generation in Classical Antiquity', Chapter 4, this book.

33 A variety of state actions have an indirect impact on mortality (and fertility), but direct approaches are limited to the latter.

34 For the population policies of a contemporary, non-city state: Willy Clarysse and Dorothy J. Thompson, *Counting the People in Hellenistic Egypt*, 2 vols. (Cambridge, 2006).

Population Practice

In moving on to more pragmatic matters, two general issues must be picked up from the beginning of the chapter. First, the idea of a universal, pre-modern, 'bigger is better' approach to population size has been challenged for the ancient world: by Plato and Aristotle, and through the indications that Greek *poleis* themselves operated with (complex and citizen-focused) notions of 'overpopulation'. So, the objectives of ancient polities with respect to quantities of human resource need to form part of the inquiry. Similarly, a more flexible attitude than is customary should be adopted to these classical states, to their notional and practical reach, their self-conception and operational capabilities in relation to their peoples. Aristotle, and especially Plato, are clearly maximalists in these respects, but the general scholarly consensus is, conversely, too minimalist. It is broadly true that there was little separation between government and the rest of society in ancient Mediterranean states, that they had few ambitions beyond core issues of power and functionality, and developed little administrative capacity; but it does not follow that intervention in individual and family life was unimaginable, inappropriate or impossible.[35] The maintenance of human resources was too important not to be the object of serious state effort.

The institution of the family could be relied on to do most of the work. Family continuity – of property and cult, standing and name – was crucial in Greek and Italian states (and more widely). Family needs and shared values would generally ensure marriage and (as far as possible) the production of offspring. Usually the state simply provided support, through the legal system, to cover cases where things did not work out: enabling and regulating adoption, for instance, as well as divorce and remarriage.[36] In at least two cases, however, polities went further in obligating marriage and children for their citizenry. Sparta and Rome both penalized unmarried men (much as Plato recommended) and rewarded the parents of multiple children.[37] Sparta made efforts to optimize as well as maximize its citizen population. The legendary Spartan lawgiver Lycurgus is reported to have instituted a vigorous gymnastic regime for women as well as men to ensure robust progeny, demanded that men take wives when they were in their physical prime, and allowed a range of extra-marital procreative arrangements for

35 On Greek *poleis* as 'stateless states': Paul Cartledge, 'Greek political thought: The historical context', in Rowe and Schofield, *Greek and Roman Political Thought*, pp. 11–22; on the Roman imperial system as 'government without bureaucracy': Peter Garnsey and Richard Saller, *The Roman Empire: Economy, Society and Culture*, 2nd edn (London, 2014), pp. 35–54.

36 See further Tim Parkin, 'The Ancient Family and the Law', Chapter 6, this book.

37 For Sparta: Plutarch, *Lycurgus* 15.1–2 (penalties) and Aristotle, *Politics* 1270b1–5 (rewards); for Republican Rome: Plutarch, *Camillus* 2.2, with the penalty and reward pattern then reworked by Augustus: Parkin, 'Ancient Family'.

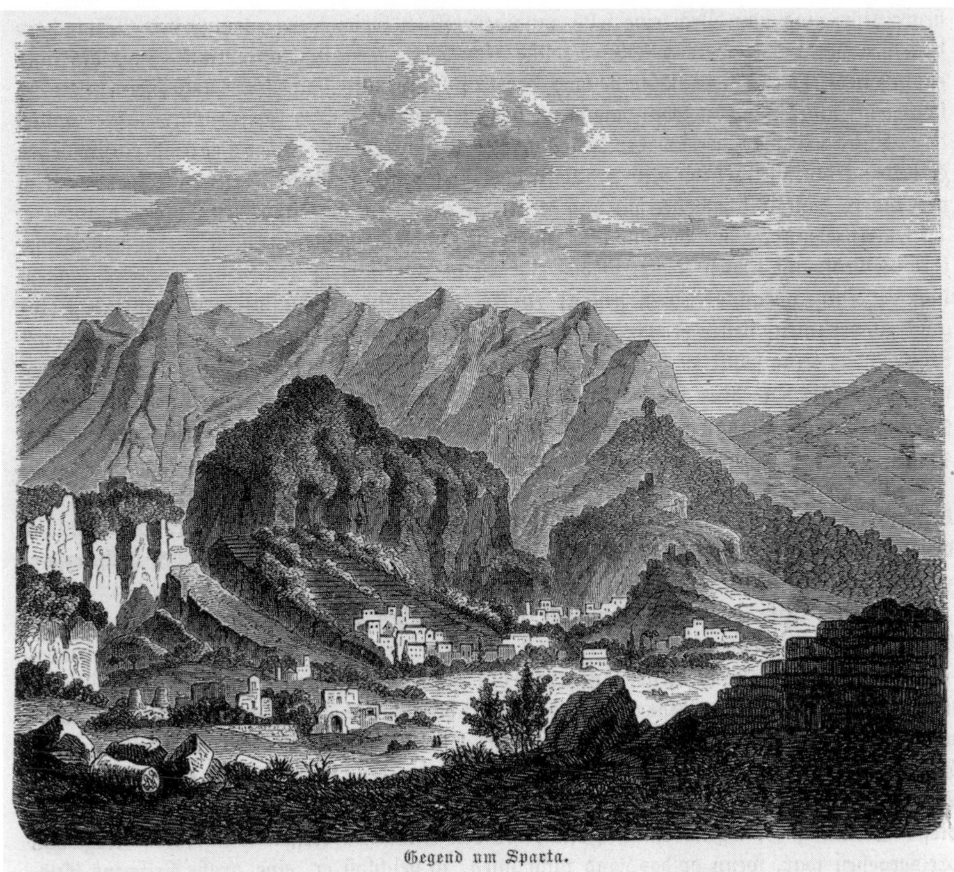

Figure 5.2 A romantic view of Sparta, from a nineteenth-century German history of antiquity. In the background is Mount Taygetus, the site of state-organized infanticide, a practice that evolutionists cited as a case of artificial selection amongst humans. Otto von Corvin, *Illustrirte Geschichte des Alterthums*, 2nd edn, vol. 1 (Leipzig: Spamer, 1880), p. 339. Cambridge University Library.

eugenic purposes.[38] Plutarch, the Greek *littérateur* of the early Roman Empire, asserted in his life of Lycurgus that decisions about the raising (or not) of infants were also taken out of paternal hands (where they usually rested), and given to an official council of elders, with judgements made on the basis of physical fitness (Fig. 5.2).[39]

Rome made no such moves. A situation in which a Roman man who had enough children might be persuaded to divorce his wife and pass her on to a childless colleague could just about be envisaged, but the Spartan idea that he might invite a handsome young man, of proven valour, into the marital home, in the hope of producing offspring

38 Xenophon, *Constitution of the Lacedaemonians* 1.4, 1.6 and 1.7–9 respectively.

39 Plutarch, *Lycurgus* 16.1.

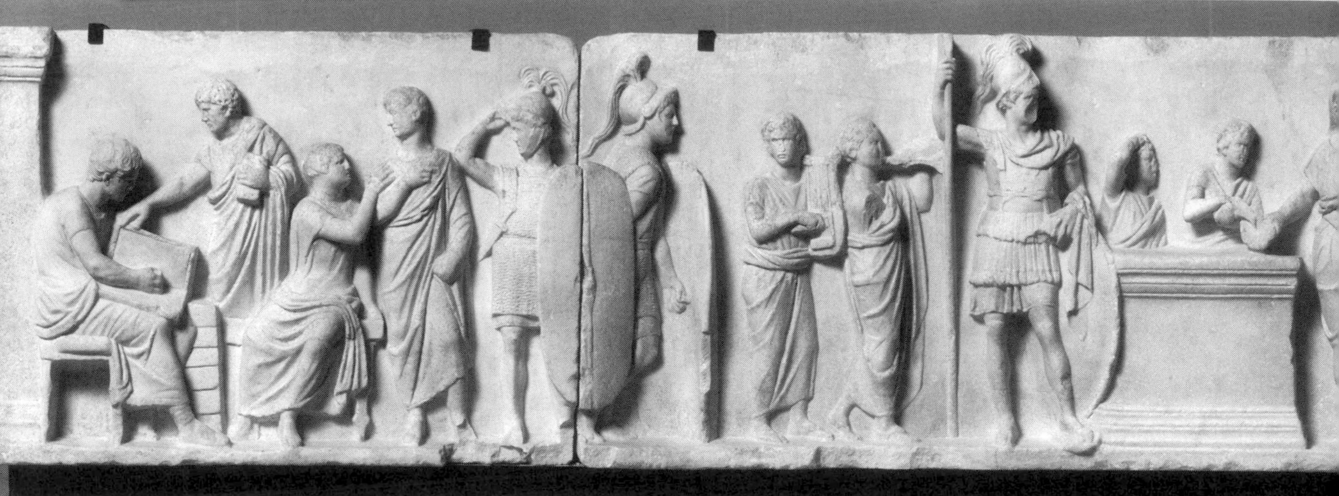

Figure 5.3 Monumental relief from Rome, probably erected by the consul Domitius Ahenobarbus at the end of the second century BC. It shows scenes from the *census* and *lustrum*. On the left, a citizen declares, in public, his name, family, age and property for the official to record. 1.2 × 5.6 m. Musée du Louvre, LL 399/Ma 975. Photo © RMN-Grand Palais / Hervé Lewandowski.

of a similar standard, offended against Roman *mores*.[40] Decisions about raising children, or not, were, with the exception of obviously deformed infants who were to be killed immediately, left up to the family.[41] Indeed, Rome's promotion of citizen fertility forms part of a wider pattern of population maximization through other means, which also stands out. Rome is generally held, by ancient and modern commentators alike, to have taken the notion of an 'open population' further than most classical Greek *poleis*, including Sparta.[42] Roman citizenship was structurally permeable rather than occasionally adjusted. Properly freed slaves became citizens, joining the children of citizen parents, and various Italian migrants might also do so.[43] Additionally, Roman citizenship could be exported, granted to communities, groups and individuals beyond Rome; it was eventually extended to all free inhabitants of the empire.[44]

Territorial expansion enabled Rome's population policies, as did a substantial investment of state effort in the hierarchical organization of the people. Possible problems

40 The only known Roman case: Plutarch, *Cato the Younger* 25. Plutarch, *Comparison of Lycurgus and Numa* 3.1–2 and 4.1–2, compares Roman and Spartan marital practices more generally.

41 Cicero, *Laws* 3.19.

42 Emma Dench, *Romulus' Asylum: Roman Identities from the Age of Alexander to the Age of Hadrian* (Oxford, 2005), pp. 93–151.

43 William Broadhead, 'Rome's migration policy and the so-called *ius migrandi*', *Cahiers Glotz* 12 (2001), 69–89.

44 A. N. Sherwin-White, *The Roman Citizenship*, 2nd edn (Oxford, 1973).

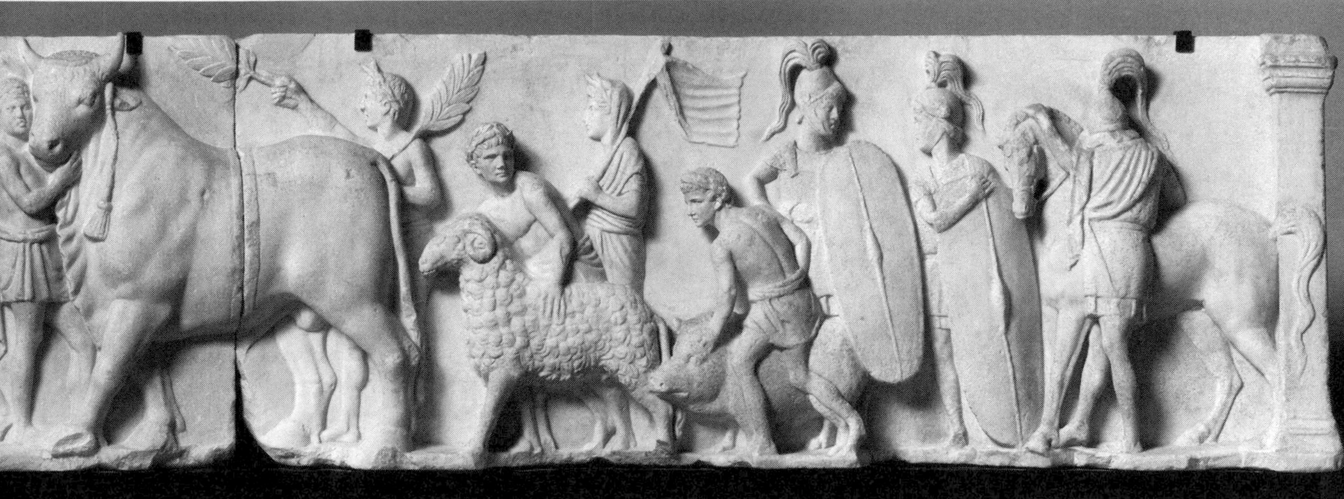

of overpopulation were mitigated, if not avoided, through the former, while the latter ensured that the potential advantages of a large population were realized at minimal political cost to the elite, and largely militarily, thus feeding back into the whole system. The key institution, at least for the Republican period, was the citizen 'census', which occurred on a roughly five-year cycle, overseen by a pair of magistrates, the 'censors'.[45] All citizens were registered, together with their property, and ranked according to wealth (and further subdivided, including by age), for military, tax and political purposes. Men's marital and procreative status came under public scrutiny as part of a wider moral engagement between state and citizenry. The whole process was ritually completed with the *lustrum*, which involved communal sacrifices, censorial prayers and an official announcement of the number of citizens assessed (Fig. 5.3).

More localized processes of recording, classification and enumeration may have operated too. In his Greek history of Rome's foundation and early formation, composed under Augustus, Dionysius of Halicarnassus provides the most expansive surviving account of the ways in which the sixth legendary king of Rome, Servius Tullius (traditionally held to have reigned 578–535 BC), foregrounded and reorganized the Roman population.[46] After reconfiguring the divisions of space and people in the city and its territory (but before instituting the first census), the king established certain

45 The Latin words *census* and *censor* are only poorly represented by the modern English words derived from them. For an overview of the Roman *census* in its ancient context: Rebecca Flemming, 'Identity registration in the ancient Mediterranean world', in Keith Breckenridge and Simon Szreter (eds.), *Registration and Recognition: Documenting the Person in World History* (Oxford, 2012), pp. 169–90.

46 Dionysius of Halicarnassus, *Roman Antiquities* 4.14–24.

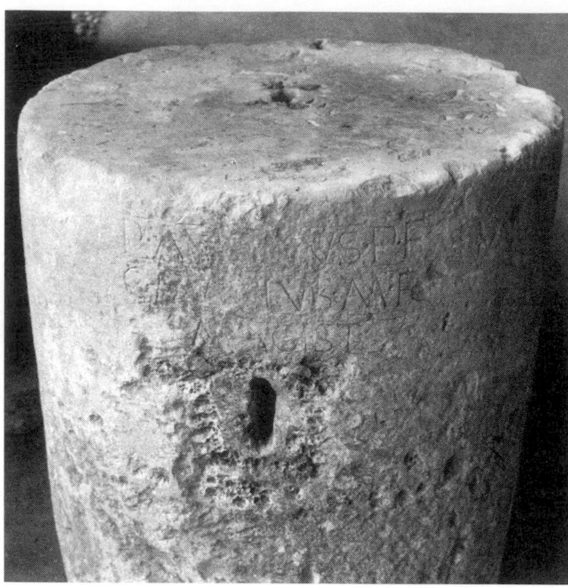

Figure 5.4 Temple *thesaurus*, or treasury, of Republican date, from Hatria (modern Atri) in central Italy, inscribed with the names of the *magistri* responsible. As envisaged by Dionysius of Halicarnassus, coins were paid into such treasuries to keep count of various sections of the population. They were a familiar feature of ancient sanctuaries. 66 × 60 cm. Foto-Archiv CIL, inv. no. PH0001240.

religious obligations for every household, aiming to keep track of the inhabitants. In the countryside, the populace was to pay for an annual local festival – the *paganalia* – with men, women and children each contributing a distinct kind of coin, so that the number in each category would be known.[47] Meanwhile, in the city, specific payments were to be made to the relevant temple treasury for each birth, death and arrival at manhood, a more targeted way of quantifying those (males) of military age (Fig. 5.4).[48] Though there was no real Roman coinage until the third century BC, emphasizing the general point that these foundational stories must be treated with caution, there are elements in the rituals of the Republican *paganalia* and its urban counterpart, the *compitalia*, as reported elsewhere, which might be aligned with this kind of administrative project.[49]

The census was undoubtedly the most important Roman population instrument and, with the censors, had a key role in the ideal city envisaged by the great Roman Republican statesman, Cicero, in his contribution to the tradition of political philosophy launched by Plato. Writing his own *Republic* and *Laws* in the 50s BC, as the Republic unravelled around him, Cicero's optimal state was still conceptually and practically modelled on Rome. It would have a regular census, carried out by a pair of magistrates

47 Ibid., 4.15.3–4.

48 Ibid., 4.15.5, citing the Latin annalist Lucius Piso (*c.* 180–120 BC).

49 Tesse D. Stek, *Cult Places and Cultural Change in Republican Italy: A Contextual Approach to Religious Aspects of Rural Society after the Roman Conquest* (Amsterdam, 2009), pp. 123–212. Like the census, the *paganalia* and other inventions ascribed to Servius certainly existed, but exactly when, how and in what form they came into being is uncertain.

who, as well as recording, assessing, ranking and dividing the citizens, would also 'prevent there from being *caelibes* (unmarried men)', and 'regulate the *mores* (habits) of the people' more broadly.[50] Though all the means of enforcement known to have been used by the censors – variations on Plato's fines and dishonour – had most impact on those of standing and property, that all citizens were included in the censorial compass is also clear. Cicero even claimed that the classifications and terminology of the Servian system emphasized that the poorest were valued for their procreation above all.[51] Servius had called those in the top five 'classes', collectively, the *assidui*, since they contributed money (*aes* or *asses*, in Latin) to the state, while those in the lowest 'class' were the *proletarii*, who contributed nothing but themselves and their offspring (*proles*), that is the *progenies civitatis*, the 'future generations of the community'. Cicero's etymology is dubious, but the basic point about the inclusivity and hierarchy of the census is valid.

Conclusion

There was then population practice, as well as thought, about fertility in the ancient world, and the two are interrelated: as in other areas of political philosophy, actual state institutions, activities and traditions provide resources for theorization. Patterns of colonization, the regulation of citizenship, policies on marriage and childbearing – all informed the writings of Plato, Aristotle and Cicero on population. It is thus likely that Sparta and Rome represent a wider trend, now only really discernible in its most extreme manifestations. Both states were considered, in antiquity, to be particularly interventionist in matters of individual conduct and family life, but there are indications that other polities went at least some way in the same direction.[52]

Classical theory, at least Greek theory, seems to diverge from practice, however, on the question of optimal population size.[53] Both Rome and Sparta had larger citizen numbers than either Plato or Aristotle recommended, and apparently aspired to more; though in neither case was that aspiration unqualified.[54] Everyone accepted Aristotle's argument that the best state is inhabited by the right number of the right kind of people for it to function optimally, but there were different views of what optimal function meant. Thus, Sparta aimed to have as many good citizens as possible, understood that its goals as a state were best served by large numbers of robust, well-formed people, and

50 *Laws* 3.7. 51 *Republic* 2.39–41.

52 Dionysius of Halicarnassus, *Roman Antiquities* 20.13.2–3.

53 The fragmentary remains of Cicero's *Republic* and *Laws* are silent on the question, but he may have taken a more maximizing approach.

54 Reportedly 9,000 Spartiate households constituted the Lycurgan system (Plutarch, *Lycurgus* 8.3–4); the smallest number recorded for Rome's population is 80,000 adult male citizens (counted by Servius: Livy 1.44).

adopted a broadly eugenic approach to the generative part of achieving that objective. Rome aimed to have as many well-organized citizens as possible, brought organization to bear on increasing numbers through generation too, and understood that this was the best way to achieve its aims.

Finally, the relative successes of these projects deserve mention. While Aristotle's explanation for Sparta's catastrophic defeat at the battle of Leuctra in 371 BC – that it was caused by *oligoanthrōpia*', a 'paucity of men' – may be too simple, manpower problems were certainly part of the picture.[55] By contrast, in Rome the number of assessed citizens reportedly rose from 130,000 in the first *lustrum* of the Republic (in 508 BC) to 910,000 in the last (70/69 BC), and Roman territory and power had expanded on a similar scale over the same period.[56] The permeability and extension of the citizenship contributed more to this upward trajectory than procreation did, just as Sparta's failures were not essentially procreative either. Still, Rome never stopped paying attention to citizens' generative duties, and these remained fundamental to continuing imperial success.

55 Aristotle, *Politics* 1270a31–34; Thomas J. Figueira, 'Population patterns in late archaic and classical Sparta', *Transactions of the American Philological Association* 116 (1986), 165–213.

56 Roman census figures are listed in P. A. Brunt, *Italian Manpower: 225 B.C. – A.D. 14* (Oxford, 1971), p. 13. The figures are hotly contested; that there was an increase is not.

6 The Ancient Family and the Law

Tim Parkin

The rules of marriage, inheritance and family formation significantly shape procreative behaviour in various ways, reflecting and reinforcing a wider set of norms and values. If the legal framework for generation is important in any society, that provided by Roman law has been especially crucial. The law of a vast empire had over centuries already begun to influence local traditions before AD 212, when all free inhabitants of imperial territory became Roman citizens, and thus full participants in Rome's juridical community. The fall of the empire in the west in AD 476 fractured, but did not break, this community. Continuity is clearer in the east, with the Emperor Justinian's codification of Roman law in the AD 530s, but the successor kingdoms in the west made use of Roman juristic traditions too, as did the emerging apparatus of canon law, before the more extensive revival of Roman legal scholarship in medieval Europe (Fig. 6.1). Roman jurisprudence remains a resource for a range of legal systems today.[1]

This chapter focuses on the 'formative' and 'classical' periods of Roman law, from the first upheavals of the late Republic in the second century BC to the troubles of the imperial government in the third century AD.[2] I shall refer also to earlier and parallel legal traditions in the ancient Mediterranean, and their approaches to matters of generation and family. Classical Athenian law, for example, demonstrates many of the same concerns as Roman law, though the evidence is more uneven.[3] These were all societies in which marrying and having legitimate children to continue the line was fundamental, legally recognized and elaborated as such; it was the role of the male head of household – the *kyrios* in Greece, the *paterfamilias* in Rome – to ensure the integrity, legitimacy and preservation of his household, in the present and into the future. In Rome, moreover, the *paterfamilias* enjoyed unique power (*potestas*) over his children and descendants in the male line, and greater flexibility in 'constructing kinship', and planning for inheritance and succession, than in most legal systems before and since.[4]

1 Maaike van der Lugt, 'Formed Fetuses and Healthy Children in Scholastic Theology, Medicine and Law', Chapter 12; Silvia De Renzi, 'Family Resemblance in the Old Regime', Chapter 17; Martin H. Johnson and Nick Hopwood, 'Modern Law and Regulation', Chapter 40, this book.

2 For the general history: David Potter, *Ancient Rome: A New History*, 2nd edn (New York, NY, 2014).

3 A. R. W. Harrison, *The Law of Athens*, vol. 1: *Family and Property* (Oxford, 1968); Cheryl Anne Cox, *Household Interests: Property, Marriage Strategies, and Family Dynamics in Ancient Athens* (Princeton, NJ, 1998).

4 Richard P. Saller, *Patriarchy, Property and Death in the Roman Family* (Cambridge, 1994); Mireille Corbier, 'Constructing kinship in Rome: Marriage and divorce, filiation and adoption', in David I. Kertzer and Saller (eds.), *The Family in Italy from Antiquity to the Present* (New Haven, CT, 1991), pp. 127–44.

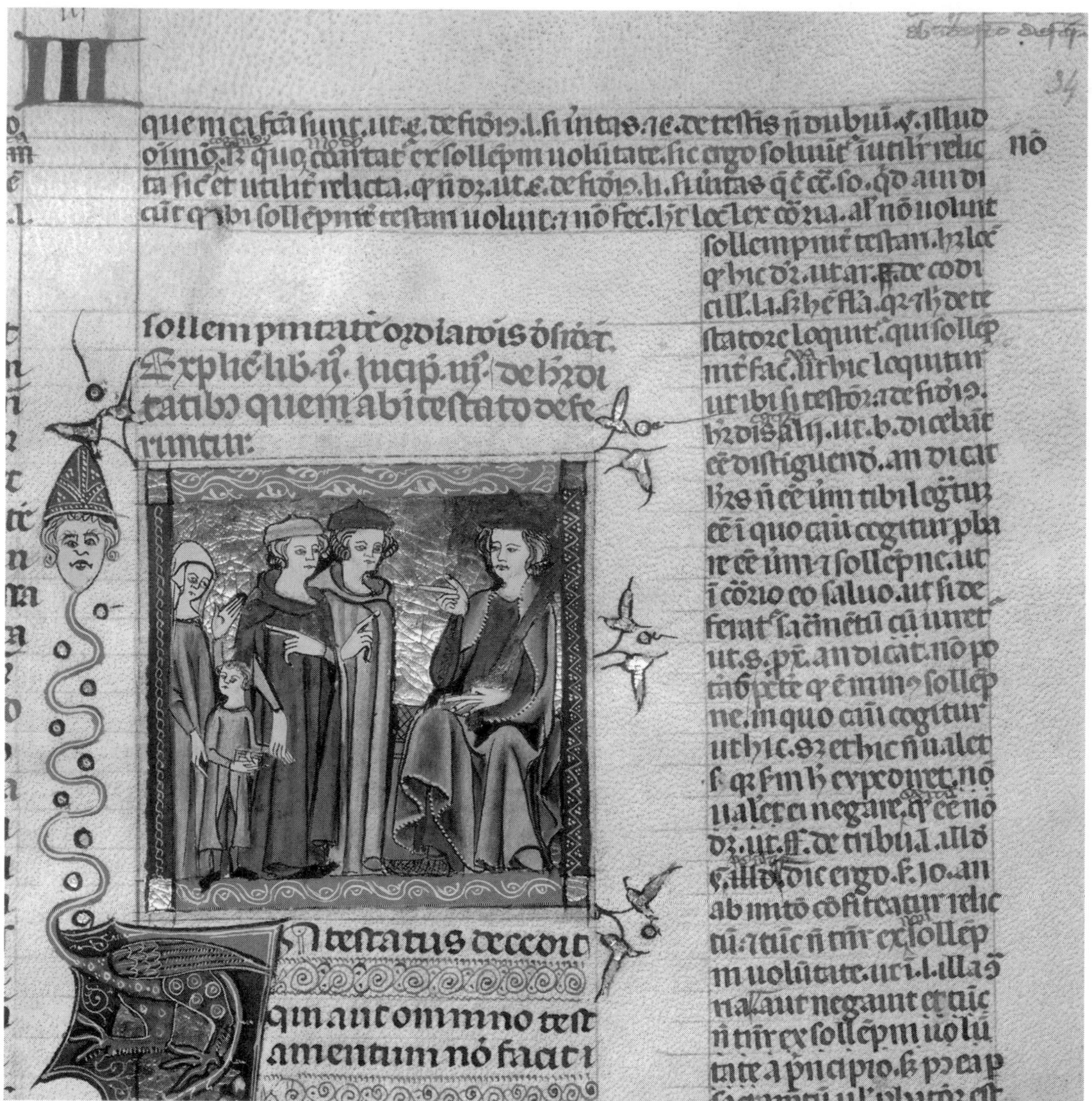

Figure 6.1 A miniature showing a woman and child appearing, with lawyers, before the emperor. It introduces the chapter on intestate succession in Justinian's legal textbook, the *Institutes*, in an early fourteenth-century manuscript of a standard medieval legal compilation. The right-hand column consists of Accursius's twelfth-century glosses on the text. Royal MS 10 E III, f. 34 r. © The British Library Board.

Some of these possibilities began to pull in different and problematic directions as Rome was transformed through the acquisition of empire; and the state increasingly intervened to put things back together and reassert traditional patterns. This intervention has been much debated, in particular those measures directed at promoting marriage and childbearing, and prosecuting adultery, that Augustus, the first Roman emperor, promulgated over the turn of the millennium as part of his broader restoration and reconfiguration of imperial order after civil war.[5] But the Augustan project, and the wider patterns of change and continuity in which it fits, become clearer if the overall shape and key characteristics of relations between generation and the law are set out first.

The Need to Marry and Have Children

The Romans were interested in human generation in many different ways. In his huge first-century AD encyclopaedia – the *Natural History* – Pliny the Elder listed various peculiarities of human compared with animal procreation.[6] Humans, the only bipedal creatures to produce live births, are unique in feeling regret after their sexual debut and, most importantly, in their lack of a fixed mating season. Humans will couple at any time – they alone do not know when enough is enough – a moral failure that Pliny demonstrated most ostentatiously with the example of Messalina, wife of the Emperor Claudius. Apparently, she held a competition with a slave girl (*ancilla*) notorious for her mercenary acts of prostitution, and won, with a tally of twenty-five couplings in one night and day, and then underlined her depravity by celebrating 'a royal triumph'. Pliny completed his diatribe by alleging that, while the males of the human race have devised all kinds of sexual 'crimes against nature', the females have invented 'abortion' (*abortus*).[7] We are worse than animals in these matters, he proclaimed.

Pliny also listed extreme cases of the ideal procreative career for a male of the Roman elite, such as himself. The underlying assumption, stressed again and again in ancient moralizing and legal texts, is that children should be born to parents legitimately married, and that marriage exists first and foremost to produce legitimate children. That was the requirement of citizens. Slaves, such as Messalina's unnamed competitor, could not form a legitimate marriage, and so could not produce legitimate children, though they might be encouraged to procreate nonetheless. Children, for citizens, were the minimum; the ideal was for the man to live to see a long line of descendants, as Pliny's roll of particular honour in this field demonstrates.[8] The Emperor Augustus, though he produced only one legitimate child, exceptionally lived to see a grandson born to his granddaughter (his own great-great-grandson), in the year of his death, that is AD 14. Over a century earlier, Quintus Metellus Macedonicus died leaving six children and eleven grandchildren; counting daughters-in-law and sons-in-law, the total number who greeted him with the title of 'father' was twenty-seven. This scion of an old aristocratic family was, however, outdone by an ordinary freeborn citizen from Fiesole who, in the reign of Augustus, 'went in procession preceded by eight children,

5 Especially debated since P. A. Brunt, *Italian Manpower, 225 B.C. – A.D. 14* (Oxford, 1971), pp. 558–66.

6 *Natural History* 10.171–2.

7 One of Pliny's many idiosyncrasies was his hostility to abortion: Jacqueline Vons, *L'image de la femme dans l'oeuvre de Pline l'Ancien* (Brussels, 2000), pp. 220–42.

8 *Natural History* 7.58–60.

including two daughters, twenty-seven grandchildren, eighteen great-grandchildren, and eight granddaughters by marriage', to the Capitol, where all offered sacrifices.

To marry and have children was a prerequisite to happiness and success in the ancient world, and the male head of household had the duty in turn to provide these opportunities for those in his charge. Daughters had to be dowered: the Roman jurist Papinian emphasized around AD 200 that it is 'absolutely essential for women to have dowries in order to ensure the production of offspring and to replenish the state with children'.[9] Sons might need a different kind of preparation, since misgivings were to be expected; men's duty to marry was imagined to be much more onerous than women's, and not only in satire. The imperial biographer Suetonius, writing in the second century AD, recorded that, in promoting his marriage legislation to the elite, Augustus read out a speech 'urging all men to marry in order to produce children' that Quintus Metellus Macedonicus had delivered as censor in 131 BC.[10] This included the assertion that: 'If, men of Rome, we could live without a wife, we would all avoid that annoyance', but argued that since in general life was not possible without marriage, short-term pleasure must be sacrificed to the requirements of the long term.[11]

Several ancient literary sources provide evidence of the features sought in ideal marriage partners. They emphasized not emotional or sexual compatibility, but birth, background, wealth and family connections. In the first century AD, the Stoic philosopher Musonius Rufus provided a contrasting point of view. Taking Greek philosophical notions and adapting them for a Roman audience, he put forward other ideas about the kind of relationship marriage is, and the part generation plays within it. He also reminds us of the role divorce could play in family strategies; by the late Republic, as in Athenian law, either partner could end a marriage, though with some further complications.[12] Musonius instructed that:

> Husband and wife ought to unite one with the other on these terms: both to live with one another and to produce children; to regard everything as shared and nothing as belonging to the individual, not even their bodies themselves. For while the birth of a human is a great thing and that is the result of this union, it is still not sufficient reason in itself for marrying, since this can also occur without marriage when people simply have intercourse, just as animals too have intercourse with one another. But in a marriage there must be a total union and concern of man and woman for one another, in both health and sickness and at all times: through aiming at this, just as at the production of children as well, they will enter into a marriage.

9 Justinian, *Digest* 24.3.1.
10 *Life of Augustus* 89; Livy, *Summaries* 59.
11 Aulus Gellius, *Attic Nights* 1.6.
12 Louis Cohn-Haft, 'Divorce in classical Athens', *Journal of Hellenic Studies* 115 (1995), 1–14; Susan Treggiari, *Roman Marriage:* Iusti Coniuges *from the Time of Cicero to the Time of Ulpian* (Oxford, 1991), pp. 435–82.

If, however, one partner, or in the worst case both partners, looks out for him- or herself without regard for the other, then the union is doomed, 'and they will either finally be divorced or maintain a union more lonely than solitude'.[13]

Wealth, beauty and nobility add nothing to the success of a marriage, Musonius asserted; basic health, average appearance, self-sufficiency and a suitable soul are all that is required for a productive and harmonious partnership. The prevailing elite perspective would, on the contrary, have valued two of those qualities – resources and lineage – in general and for conjugal purposes specifically. Marriage was evidently not just about children, even if they were usually the primary goal; companionship aside, marriage also provided a tool for securing alliances between families, building political and economic networks and prospects.

Yet whatever political or social advantages a marriage might bring, failure to produce children compromised its success. Sterility was recognized as grounds for divorce, though separation was not inevitable. The point was raised, for example, in a lengthy inscribed funerary speech which survives from first-century BC Rome.[14] The grateful husband praised his deceased wife for giving him everything except children. The issue also came up in Attic court oratory, sometimes just as sympathetically. Almost the entire surviving oeuvre of Isaeus, the noted Athenian speech-writer of the early fourth century BC, deals with inheritance cases. In one speech, an older man offered to divorce his young wife, to free her from a childless marriage so that she could remarry more productively.[15]

Another member of the early imperial Roman elite, Pliny the Younger, provides a personal insight into the powerful need for children; in a letter addressed to Calpurnius Fabatus, his (third) wife's grandfather, he imparted the news of his wife's recent miscarriage.[16] At least to a modern reader, it is a brutal letter, in which the main concern is that this marriage has not yet fulfilled its immediate purpose of producing descendants:

> You are keen to see great-grandsons from us, so you will be that much sadder to hear that your granddaughter has had a miscarriage. In her girlish way she did not know she was pregnant, and so she didn't do what pregnant women are supposed to do to protect the unborn child, and did things which she shouldn't have done. She has learnt some tough lessons, and indeed almost paid for her mistake with her own life. Therefore, although you must find it hard at your advanced age to lose descendants who were already on their way, as it were, you should at least give thanks to the gods that, while they have denied you great-grandchildren for the present, they have saved your granddaughter.

13 Musonius Fr. 13a: Cora E. Lutz, 'Musonius Rufus, "The Roman Socrates"', in Alfred R. Bellinger (ed.), *Yale Classical Studies* 10 (New Haven, CT, 1947), pp. 3–147, on p. 88.

14 Josiah Osgood, *Turia: A Woman's Civil War* (Oxford, 2014).

15 *Orations* 2.6–9.

16 *Letters* 8.10; compare 8.11.

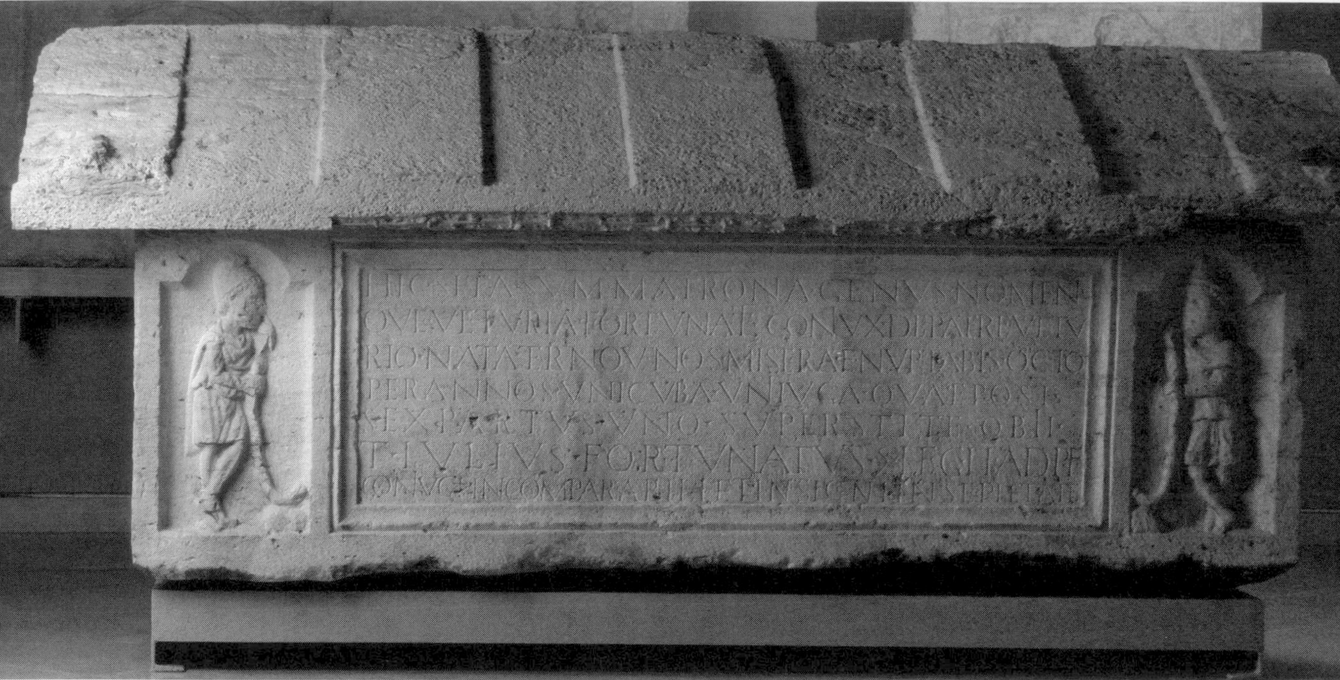

Figure 6.2 Inscribed and decorated limestone sarcophagus of Veturia, commemorated by her husband, a centurion in a Roman legion stationed on the Danube. Many funerary monuments and inscriptions survive from the Roman world, and provide much evidence about families across the empire. 110 × 244 cm. Inv. no. 19.1868.1. © Hungarian National Museum.

Pliny went on to reassure Calpurnius that great-grandchildren would come, and rise to public prominence. That was inevitable, given the lineage on both sides: 'Only let them be born and let them turn this grief of ours into joy.'

Pliny provides a poignant reminder that it was not always easy to do one's duty. The challenges of ensuring family continuity were patent in antiquity, when infant mortality was high. Life's perils, and the challenges of surviving one's children, are epitomized in a second-century AD funerary monument from Budapest (Fig. 6.2). The inscription commemorates Veturia, the loyal and faithful wife of Fortunatus and daughter of Veturius. She lived for 27 years, 16 of them as a married woman, then 'having borne six children, one of whom survives me, I died'.[17]

As we have already seen, the overwhelming requirement or desire was not just for children, but for legitimate children to continue the father's line, the *familia*, in name and property. Two texts from the jurist Ulpian, prominent early in the third century AD, illustrate the absolute necessity for legitimacy and confidence in paternity.[18] They

17 *Corpus Inscriptionum Latinarum* 3.3572. 18 Justinian, *Digest* 25.4.1.pr.–1; and 25.4.1.10.

deal with possible pregnancies in the immediate aftermath of widowing or divorce, a difficult issue and important, since any child thus born would be in the same legal position as if the marriage had persisted: heir to the deceased or former husband. In both cases a very elaborate process of notification, examination and oversight was prescribed, all under the auspices of the urban praetor, the senior magistrate in change of civil affairs in Rome. If there was an eventual birth, for instance, it would take place in the house of 'a very respectable woman', chosen by the praetor, and all the interested parties might send people – men and women – 'to guard the womb'. This involved keeping tabs on all the pregnant woman's movements in the house, and on all visitors, whom the guards had the power to search. Once labour was announced, other women might be sent to be present at the birth, up to five by each party, so that in the birthing chamber, as well as the two midwives, were 'no more than ten freeborn women and no more than six slave women'. All were to be searched, with the room well lit. Interested parties could inspect any child born.

Family strategies were built around the rules and expectations regarding inheritance. As the Roman rules of intestate succession made clear, a dutiful father was expected to pass the family estate on to the children under his *patria potestas* (in his 'power'), generally in equal shares, irrespective of age and gender.[19] A last will and testament that failed to do so could be challenged by aggrieved family members as 'undutiful' (*inofficiosum*). Pliny the Younger told an old friend about a wonderful speech he recently delivered in a dramatic case of this kind, which had excited much public interest.[20] Attia Viriola, a woman of good birth and married into an even more elite, office-holding, family, had been disinherited by her octogenarian father within eleven days of his falling head over heels in love and bringing home a stepmother for her, and she was now suing for her patrimony. The court was not only large, in the number of judges involved and the huge legal teams on both sides, but also crowded with rows of supporters and spectators. 'Great was the suspense among fathers, daughters, even stepmothers.'

There were clear norms and expectations in relation to what those – men and women – making wills should do, but they were also given considerable latitude in how to disperse their property on death. This was particularly the case for women; and, indeed, maternal descendants (as with Calpurnius and his granddaughter), and wider kin, might be included in bequests. Family affection was certainly involved, as were inheritance strategies: there was a range of ways to ensure the continuity of one's *familia* and to secure the future of one's kin. Roman law increasingly recognized the

19 For the Athenian practice regarding the primary rights of sons in succession: Harrison, *Law of Athens*, pp. 122–62; with S. C. Todd, *The Shape of Athenian Law* (Oxford, 1993), pp. 216–21.

20 *Letters* 6.33; and see Justinian, *Digest* 5.2.

rights and importance of non-paternal kin, not least the links between mother and children.[21]

In circumstances of high infant and early childhood mortality, as well as the other vicissitudes of family formation and family life, recourse to adoption of adults appears to have been common, not only to secure succession but also to strategize family ties and allegiances (and ensure that an ageing parent had someone to look after him). The concern in Roman society was not for the adopted person themselves but for the continuity of the paternal line; Isaeus's speeches illustrate the same practice in classical Athenian law.[22] In both contexts these moves were often made within wider kin-groups: Pliny the Younger was adopted by his uncle Pliny the Elder, for instance, while Augustus had been adopted by his great-uncle Julius Caesar; both adopters were childless and the adoptees fatherless. There were risks, however. Valerius Maximus's first-century AD collection of moral *exempla* contains a chapter, 'On parents who have borne the death of children with fortitude', in which the story of Lucius Aemilius Paullus Macedonicus, who made an unlucky gamble with his four sons, is prominent.[23] He gave the older two in adoption, making it easier for the others to advance from his own resources; but the younger pair died early, just days respectively before and after their father's spectacular triumph at Pydna in 168 BC. 'Thus he who had so many children he could afford to give them away found himself suddenly abandoned and childless'.

From Private to Public, Family to State

Concern to produce legitimate children went beyond individual families and their heads of household. The best-known ancient intervention by the state into the bedroom is the legislation passed in the reign of Augustus in an apparent attempt to increase the rate of marriage and legitimate childbearing. Augustus himself claimed that his whole legislative programme was restorative, bringing 'back into use many exemplary practices of our ancestors which were disappearing in our time', just as he 'transmitted exemplary practices to posterity for their imitation'.[24] The specific marriage laws enacted in this larger array were the *lex Iulia de maritandis ordinibus* (Julian

21 Saller, *Patriarchy*; Jane F. Gardner, *Family and* Familia *in Roman Law and Life* (Oxford, 1998), pp. 209–67.

22 Lene Rubenstein, *Adoption in IV. Century Athens* (Copenhagen, 1993); Mireille Corbier, 'Divorce and adoption as Roman familial strategies', in Beryl Rawson (ed.), *Marriage, Divorce, and Children in Ancient Rome* (Oxford, 1991), pp. 47–78; Hugh Lindsay, *Adoption in the Roman World* (Cambridge, 2009). On modern practices: Christina Benninghaus, 'Modern Infertility', Chapter 31; Ellen Herman, 'Technologies of Adoption Matching', Exhibit 33, this book.

23 *Memorable Deeds and Sayings* 5.10.2.

24 *The Achievements of the Divine Augustus* 8.5. For Republican precedents: Brunt, *Italian Manpower*, p. 559; Rebecca Flemming, 'States and Populations in the Classical World', Chapter 5, this book.

Law on the Orders Marrying) of 18 BC and the *lex Papia Poppaea* (the Papian Poppean Law), the latter named after the two (unmarried) consuls of AD 9 who proposed it. Later jurists assimilated the two as the *lex Iulia et Papia*.

The second law remodelled the first, closing some loopholes and softening some of the harshness. In his life of Augustus, Suetonius wrote of a whole sequence of protests and amendments, failures and attempted recuperations.[25] The acerbic historian Tacitus, writing about a century after their passage, simply emphasized the failure of the laws, and the generally corrosive social processes they exacerbated: 'The *[lex] Papia Poppaea* had been passed by Augustus in his later years, after the Julian measures, to increase the penalties for those without children and to enrich the treasury. It did not make marriage and the rearing of children more popular; childlessness held too strong an appeal.'[26] Prosecution was a greater risk as informers took advantage of the new opportunities to target the conjugally and procreatively non-compliant, so that 'whereas before society suffered from its vices, now it suffered from its laws'.

According to Cassius Dio, who composed his Greek history of Rome in the early decades of the third century AD, the laws liberalized marriage between the freeborn and the freed (except for senators and their families).[27] Privileges were granted to those who married, especially if they went on to produce legitimate children; while penalties were incurred by those who did not.[28] These penalties were focused around inheritance: the unmarried (*caelibes*) could inherit nothing from non-kin, the childless (*orbi*) could inherit only half. The rewards were more varied. For elite men, marriage and childrearing brought seniority to a consul, earlier eligibility to hold public office and exemption from onerous civil obligations; freedmen with children were released from duties owed to former masters; special seats in the theatre were on offer too. With three or four children, women gained complete control of their own affairs, and were freed from the oversight of a legal guardian.

One jurist at least, Terentius Clemens in the second century AD, was clear that the laws were enacted 'for the common good, namely, to promote the procreation of children'.[29] But it may not be so simple, and they have had a long and convoluted history of interpretation. They appear not only to have failed but to have been deeply unpopular as well, perhaps because the state was usurping the right of a *paterfamilias* to decide his family's procreative strategies.[30] And yet I wonder if that was really as innovative or shocking as many have assumed: the Republican censor always had

25 *Life of Augustus* 34. 26 *Annals* 3.25. 27 *Roman History* 54.16.2.
28 Summarized in Brunt, *Italian Manpower*, pp. 558–66; and Treggiari, *Roman Marriage*, pp. 60–80.
29 Justinian, *Digest* 35.1.64.1.
30 Dieter Nörr, 'The matrimonal legislation of Augustus: An early instance of social engineering', *Irish Jurist* 16 (1981), 350–64.

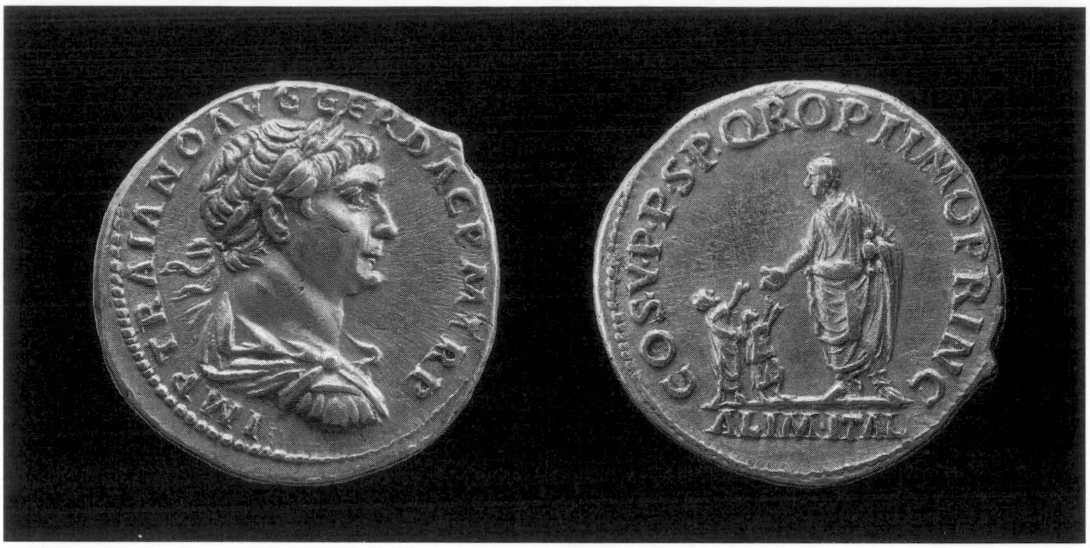

Figure 6.3 Gold coin of the Emperor Trajan, minted in Rome in AD 103–111 to mark his alimentary programme for Italian children. On the reverse, a girl and boy receive money from the emperor over the legend 'ALIM(enta) ITAL(iae)'. The surrounding titles include P(ater) P(atriae): 'father of the fatherland'. Weight 7.11 g. R.7566. © Trustees of the British Museum.

the supervision of laws and morals as his purview. Meddling with wishes expressed in wills may have caused some offence, but the law encroached little on family inheritance patterns, given the exceptions it offered as long as property passed within the traditional kin-group.

If Augustus had wanted to raise the birth-rate, why did he not introduce greater financial rewards? The Emperor Trajan (reigned AD 98–117) took a different approach, as emphasized by Pliny the Younger in a formal speech in praise of his ruler. Generosity is the key:

> Henceforward, reared on your bounty from their earliest days, all should know you as the father of the people; they should grow at your expense while they were growing up to serve you, pass from a child's allowance (*alimenta*) at your hands to a soldier's pay, each owing as much to you as to his own parents.[31]

Spending money on future Romans is the mark of a good, even ideal, ruler; and while 'The rich are encouraged to rear children by huge rewards and comparable penalties', the poor rely entirely on imperial beneficence (Fig. 6.3).

The stakes could not have been higher, Pliny claimed. Unless the emperor looked after the children of the poor, the Roman state and Roman power were under threat.

31 *Panegyric* 26.3–27.1.

Rome's leading men would have no one to lead. Children, still fragile, were now profitable too. In his letters, Pliny also made the point on several occasions that material rewards were required if people were to procreate.[32] Such generosity was expensive, and perhaps that is why Augustus did not go as far to effect a rise in the birth-rate. Or perhaps his motives were not purely demographic. Andrew Wallace-Hadrill argued forcefully, and with some validity, that one key motivation of the laws was to keep property within the family, given that the restrictions on the unmarried and childless inheriting operated only with respect to non-relatives, as has been mentioned, and that these less traditional lines of endowment had been exploited for political purposes in the late Republic.[33]

The literary sources stress the joys of childlessness for elite Romans. The underlying logic was that, in a system of partible inheritance, a *paterfamilias* would limit the size of his family to avoid splitting up his estate among too many children. The risk was that if he had too few children, they might all die at an early age, thus terminating the family line. Relevant here too is the Roman practice of courting the elderly, especially those without living offspring, in the hope of being written into their wills. Inheritance-hunting (*captatio*), a frequent topic in satire and social reality, was alluded to by the philosopher and statesman Seneca the Younger, writing some decades after Augustus's legislative work. In seeking to console the noble Marcia following the death of one of her sons, he lamented: 'In our state childlessness now confers more influence than it snatches away, and loneliness, which used to make old age such a curse, now makes older people so powerful that they actually feign hatred for their sons and disown their children – and thus make themselves childless by their own act.'[34] Many voices made the same complaint throughout the imperial period. If the laws aimed to curtail the practice of leaving substantial inheritances outside the family group, they failed. But that does not invalidate Wallace-Hadrill's argument. The Augustan legislation was a complex body of regulations in a complex social setting, with a complex range of motivations and effects.

This point bears repetition in response to the tendency in modern scholarship to support either the demographic or the moralistic stance. Either Augustus wanted to raise the birth-rate, or he wanted to restore old-fashioned morality and conduct. In fact, the distinction is misleading for antiquity. In 46 BC, as the Republican system was unravelling, its staunch defender Cicero had used a court speech to demand obvious remedial work: 'the law courts have to be reorganized, credit re-established, licentious

32 *Letters* 1.8.10, 4.15.3.

33 Andrew Wallace-Hadrill, 'Family and inheritance in the Augustan marriage laws', *Proceedings of the Cambridge Philological Society* 27 (1981), 58–80.

34 *Consolation to Marcia* 19.2.

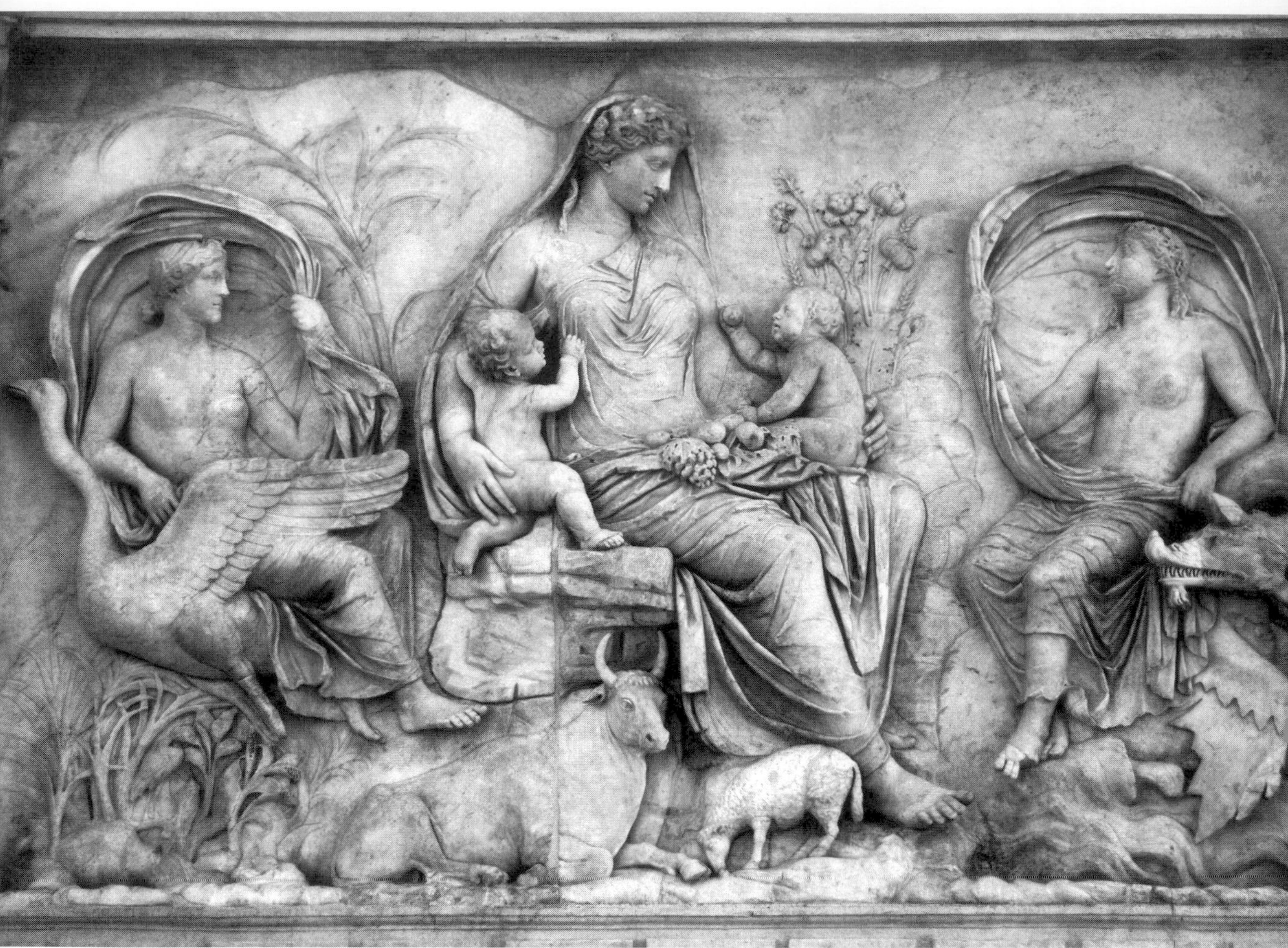

Figure 6.4 Large relief from the *Ara Pacis* ('altar of peace'), a key monument of Augustan Rome. A matronal goddess holds twin children on her lap, amidst a scene of wider fertility, prosperity, peace and order. The figures' identities are debated, but the message is clear, that crops, herds and people, lands and seas, will all now flourish. Photo: akg-images / Album / Prisma.

passions checked and offspring increased [*propaganda suboles*]. Everything that is now in a state of disintegration and collapse needs to be knit together by rigorous laws.'[35] Encouraging procreation and reforming public morals went hand in hand: the restoration of order, peace and prosperity would require both, as Augustus well understood (Fig. 6.4).

Still, it is then all the more remarkable that the laws were unpopular and failed. In 17 BC, the poet Horace praised the *lex Iulia* in his hymn written to help celebrate

35 *For Marcellus* 23.

the new era ushered in by Augustus: 'O goddess, may you produce offspring and make prosperous the decrees of the senators concerning the joining of women in marriage and the marriage law productive of new offspring'.[36] Yet Horace never felt compelled to marry and have children himself. Even Velleius Paterculus, so loyal to Augustus's successor (and step- and adoptive son) Tiberius as both soldier and historian, only went so far as to say that 'old laws were usefully emended and new laws passed for the general good' – not necessarily to everyone's delight or acclamation.[37] Tacitus has Tiberius write to the senate in AD 22 admitting that the Augustan legislation is held in contempt.[38]

Where does this atmosphere of failure and discontent leave the image of Augustus? Or rather is this not a part of the image? In effect, morals are more important than anything. If the laws failed, it was not his fault, but that of Rome's aristocracy. Like sumptuary laws, legislation to encourage childbearing tends not to succeed, but is worth the effort; the effort is the main point. One anonymous panegyrist addressing the Emperors Maximian and Constantine in the early fourth century AD still called these laws, however ineffective, 'the foundations of the state'.[39] Marriage and children are crucial to a community, and one job of any ruler is to emphasize that.

Conclusion

Law determines which sexual relationships can produce legitimate children, and regulates the inheritance of name, status and property that follows legitimacy. This determination, in ancient Greece and Rome, was made from among many legally and socially sanctioned sexual relations (procreative and not). For a respectable citizen woman, sex within marriage was the only option, while men had plenty of others. The process of the production of legitimate children was facilitated by rules enabling divorce and remarriage, and it was supplemented by adult adoption, in these ancient legal systems; while Roman law provided a particularly wide array of heirship strategies and inheritance options in between. Testamentary freedom combined with an expansive notion of kinship to generate great flexibility in making heirs and transmitting property.

Though all about giving male heads of household the tools necessary to ensure family continuity in challenging and unpredictable circumstances, this Roman flexibility allowed the pursuit of other aims, and they were increasingly pursued. Augustus reasserted the point that the production of legitimate children was undertaken on behalf of the state, in support of Roman power, as well as for the *familia*. He provided specific rewards for model behaviour, and penalized those who strayed too far from the ideal;

36 *Secular Hymn* (*Carmen Saeculare*) 17–20. 37 *Roman History* 2.89.4. 38 *Annals* 3.54.
39 *Panegyric to Maximian and Constantine* (*Pan. Lat.* 7) 2.4.

Trajan took the project further practically and ideologically. Means may have changed, but the goals remained much the same throughout, and the various shifts in the laws of inheritance over the same period expanded and finessed an essentially stable structure. The real transformations came later, when this flexibility was progressively curtailed in the Christian and Islamic worlds of the middle ages.

7 Galen's Generations of Seeds

Rebecca Flemming

The most influential understanding of human generation to emerge from classical antiquity belongs to the physician and medical system builder extraordinaire of the Roman Empire, Galen of Pergamum. Born in AD 129, Galen moved from Asia Minor to Alexandria in search of the best medical education, before his ambition led him to the imperial capital, Rome. He largely remained in this vast metropolis, where Greek learning and Roman power mingled and merged, until his death around AD 210: a vaunted practitioner, healer of senators and emperors; a successful, fiercely competitive, rhetorical and anatomical performer; a prolific author and teacher right across the domain of medicine and beyond (Fig. 7.1).[1]

Galen's generative theories come as part of a package which dominated learned medicine across much of the globe into the seventeenth century. He constructed and promoted a holistic, integrated approach to the human being in health and sickness: to the composition, functioning and dysfunctions of the human body and the corresponding modes of cure. He grounded his views epistemologically and cosmologically, and a rigorous ethical outlook pervades almost everything he wrote. His system gained strength from its comprehensiveness and internal cogency along with its synthetic qualities. Galen's ability to integrate key aspects of the medical traditions he inherited was as crucial as the wider congruities of his approach with contemporary political and ideological formations: with imperial ambitions and cosmic hierarchies.[2]

This chapter outlines and analyses the generative parts of Galen's medicine in dialogue with pre-existing medical views and ongoing philosophical debates, on the one hand, and the broader shape and substance of his overall project and Roman imperial society, on the other. It will be argued that the modern focus on Galen's decisive embrace of what has become known as the 'two-seed theory' of generation, in which women as well as men seminate, in contrast to the 'one-seed theory', which has this as a male prerogative, is misleading.[3] It oversimplifies complex debates, and puts the

1 Susan P. Mattern, *The Prince of Medicine: Galen in the Roman Empire* (Oxford, 2013); R. J. Hankinson (ed.), *The Cambridge Companion to Galen* (Cambridge, 2008).

2 Rebecca Flemming, 'Galen's imperial order of knowledge', in Jason König and Tim Whitmarsh (eds.), *Ordering Knowledge in the Roman Empire* (Cambridge, 2007), pp. 241–77.

3 Two classic articles first made the division – Anthony Preus, 'Galen's criticism of Aristotle's conception theory', *Journal of the History of Biology* 10 (1977), 65–85, and Michael Boylan, 'The Galenic and Hippocratic

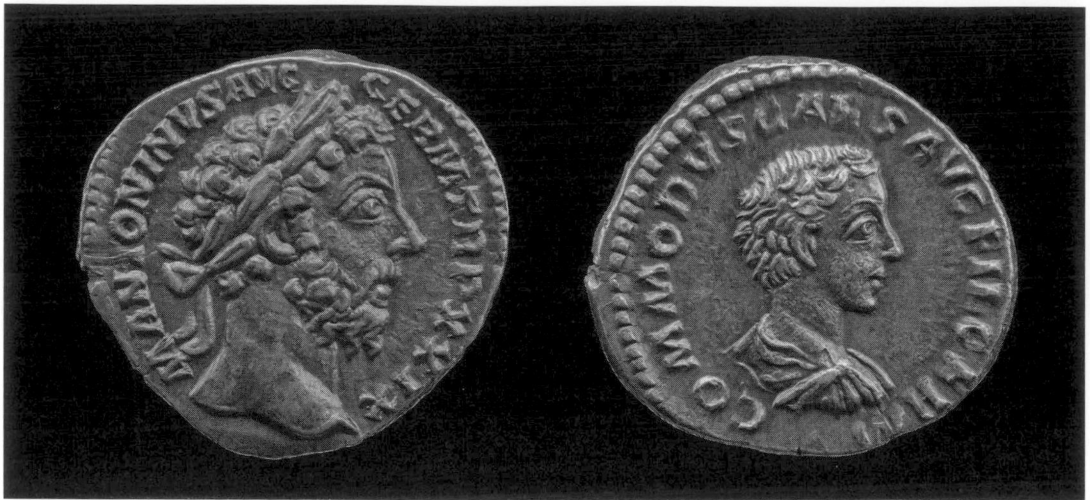

Figure 7.1 Denarius of the Emperor Marcus Aurelius with his son Commodus on the reverse. Commodus was fourteen in AD 175 when this silver coin was issued, but a revolt and deaths in the imperial family accelerated his introduction into public life and made dynastic continuity more of an issue. Galen attended both father and son in the 170s. Weight 3.39 g. 1864.0716.3. © Trustees of the British Museum.

emphasis in the wrong place, problems that are exacerbated if the 'two-seed model' is then labelled 'more egalitarian' (even 'feminist').[4] The approaches current in second-century AD Rome had more in common than divided them, including the crucially shared presumption that females both contribute to their offspring and are inferior. Galen's selections here were thus determined by the internal demands of his system, his authoritative allegiances and competitive environment, rather than any more direct social concerns. All the available options were as patriarchal as the world around them. It will also become clear that anatomical knowledge played only a limited role in shaping ideas. The practice of human dissection elaborated existing understandings, rather than driving conceptual change.

The discussion draws most heavily on the relevant portions of Galen's compendious physiological and anatomical works – *On the Usefulness of the Parts* (*UP*) and *Anatomical Procedures* (*AA*) – and the dedicated treatises *On Seed* (*Sem.*) and *Formation of the Fetus* (*Foet. Form.*), as well as *On the Anatomy of the Uterus* (*Ut. Diss.*), with a little help from elsewhere in his vast surviving oeuvre. These texts addressed specific aims and audiences, at different times in a very long career, but they are broadly consistent in

challenges to Aristotle's conception theory', ibid., 15 (1984), 83–112 – but the now ubiquitous one-/two-seed formula belongs to Thomas Laqueur, *Making Sex: Body and Gender from the Greeks to Freud* (Cambridge, MA, 1990), pp. 35–43.

4 Angus McLaren, *Reproductive Rituals: The Perception of Fertility in England from the Sixteenth to the Nineteenth Century* (London, 1984), pp. 16–17.

approach and content. They also long outlasted their author, and the final section of the chapter will briefly outline their fortunes in the later Roman Empire and its successor states; as Greek ceased to be the dominant language of culture, shared by learned physicians and political elites across the empire, and translation into Latin, in the west, and Syriac (a dialect of Aramaic) and then Arabic, in the east, became crucial.

Beginning with Ends

Galen began with first principles, which, in his teleological universe, were ends.[5] *On the Usefulness of the Parts*, book 14, opens by stating that:

> Nature (*physis*) has three principal aims in the construction of the parts of the animal: she has crafted (*demiourgein*) some of them on account of life itself – such as the brain, heart and liver – some for a better life – such as the eyes, ears and nostrils – and some for the continuation of the kind (*genos*) – such as the genitals, testicles (*orcheis*) and womb (*mētrai*).[6]

These last organs are the focus of that book and some of the next, but before providing any detail, Galen explained that procreation is a compromise. Ideally, nature (or 'the demiurge') would have made her creations immortal, but the material available did not allow that, being innately corruptible, so continuity of kinds, that a new animal always replaces one that has died, was the optimal outcome in the circumstances. To all creatures, therefore, nature has given instruments (*organa*) for conception, the use of which is both innately pleasurable and longed for by the soul.[7] Thus the survival of the kind does not depend on wisdom and learning, but is inevitable; there will be plenty of pleasurable use of those parts, and enough of it generative.

Mortality, and the procreation it necessitates, also explains why there are less-perfect female animals as well as the perfect males; another compromise which would have been avoided if possible, particularly for humans, the most perfect of animals.[8] It would be a grave error, impious even, to think that the demiurge 'would make half of all humanity imperfect, and, as it were, mutilated, unless there was to be some great advantage in such a mutilation'.[9] The advantage is that female 'mutilation' is the best way to ensure that the fetus has the abundant material it needs to form and grow. It can either take this forcibly from the mother or have it provided by a maternal body

5 R. J. Hankinson, 'Galen and the best of all possible worlds', *Classical Quarterly* 39 (1989), 206–27.

6 *UP* 14.1. 7 *UP* 14.2.

8 Rebecca Flemming, *Medicine and the Making of Roman Women: Gender, Nature, and Authority from Celsus to Galen* (Oxford, 2000), pp. 288–358.

9 *UP* 14.6.

which, being inherently excessive, automatically engenders a surplus which the fetus can then obtain without injuring the mother. This requires that the female be colder, so as to be unable to deal effectively with all the nutriment she consumes. She must have an intrinsically unbalanced somatic economy in contrast to the balanced male one, with her surfeit evacuated through menstruation when it is not being more generatively employed.

The necessary female lack of heat has further anatomical and physiological ramifications. It means that women cannot externalize their generative organs, another imperfection, though also highly beneficial to humanity. For what would otherwise become the scrotum stays inside, furnishing the substance of the uterus, an instrument 'well-fitted to receive and retain the seed (*sperma*) and to nourish and perfect the fetus (*to kuoumenon*)'.[10] Indeed, the demiurge has done a marvellous job with the womb, its neck and opening, more generally. Positioning and composition could not be better, with the neck of the uterus the most 'wonderful' aspect of the whole array.[11] Its flexibility and operative precision are astounding. It is also notable that, though the neck is single, nature has made the body of the uterus plural.[12] Double in humans, with left and right 'hollows' (*kolpoi*); much more multiple in pigs, for instance, with the number of cavities matching the number of teats in all animals. Exactly how Galen envisaged this multiplicity taking structural form is unclear, though he claimed that it is revealed in dissection, under the singularity of the two coats which envelop the womb.[13] Still, this internal feature is crucial, and explains, he said, why the uterus is often referred to in the plural.[14]

The basic generative model here was first articulated in the Hippocratic treatises *On Generation* and *On the Nature of the Child* in the late fifth century BC.[15] Galen often quoted from these texts, including the passage most relevant to the understanding just outlined, the foundational statement for the dominant version of Hippocratic embryology: 'If the seed from both remains in the womb (*mētrai*) of the woman, first it is mixed together, since the woman is not still, and it collects and thickens as it is heated.'[16] In *On the Usefulness of the Parts* Galen mentioned this assertion only in passing, and with reference to his fuller engagement in *On Seed*; but he made his general debt to 'the divine Hippocrates' clear nonetheless, in this and other matters.[17]

10 *UP* 14.6. *To kuoumenon* derives from *kueō*, literally meaning 'what is conceived or borne'; Galen also employed *embryon*, from *bryō*, 'to swell or grow', to signify the same thing. Used flexibly and interchangeably, neither seems tied to a specific developmental phase; in English 'fetus' seems to me to come closest to this flexibility.

11 *UP* 14.3. 12 *UP* 14.4. 13 *AA* 12.2; compare *Ut. Diss.* 3.

14 Hippocratic authors, Plato and Aristotle did mostly (not always) use plurals, like *mētrai*.

15 Helen King, 'Women and Doctors in Ancient Greece', Chapter 3, this book; these texts circulated together and separately in antiquity.

16 *On the Nature of the Child* (*Nat. puer.*) 12: Galen contributed to this dominance.

17 *UP* 14.11 (with *Sem.* 2.1.13 and 31); and more generally, for example, *UP* 14.4, 14.7–8 and 15.5.

The two other authorities with whom Galen seriously engaged in this sequence are the fourth-century BC philosopher Aristotle, and the physician Herophilus, active early in the next century. Both are named as contributors to the field, and do more implicit work in shaping and substantiating Galen's generative narrative. Aristotle 'was correct to think that the female is less perfect (*atelesteron*) than the male', but did not follow through on this assertion as he should have.[18] Neither the final cause – the ultimate reason for female imperfection – nor the efficient causes – the material means by which this imperfection is achieved – are fully, even adequately, demonstrated. Galen more than made up for this failing, and in general presented himself as developing and finishing the project Aristotle started.[19]

Herophilus provided Galen with some vital resources for this Aristotelian (and Hippocratic) overhaul. For he and his colleague (and rival) Erasistratus were the key figures in the state-supported programme of human dissection and vivisection in Ptolemaic Alexandria during the first decades of the third century BC.[20] To Galen's regret, this was the first and last time that systematic human dissection was practised in classical antiquity, giving their anatomical writings, including those of Herophilus on the male and female generative organs, huge authority. Herophilus not only described the composition, structure and situation of the womb in detail; he also identified a complex seminal anatomy in both men and women which was significantly (though not totally) shared between the two, with priority given to the former. Both have testicles, which he called '*didymoi*', literally 'twins', as Galen noted in *On the Usefulness of the Parts* (the more modern term is '*orcheis*'), and possess various other vessels involved in the production, storage and transport of seed: most importantly the 'helpers'.[21] Females have only a single pair of these, Herophilus stated, but their seminal ducts, which run from each testicle to the neck of the bladder, follow the male configuration as far as possible.[22] Thus female seed is emitted externally, and does not contribute to the offspring. There are two seeds, therefore, but no 'two-seed theory' of generation. For Herophilus, it seems, the interpretative priority of the male body led him to find testicles and spermatic ducts in women, but not generatively active female seed.

Galen engaged critically, as he had with Aristotle, and took issue with several of these points. Before filling in the details, however, one more name must be added to the roster of Galen's principal authorities. *On the Usefulness of the Parts* does not explicitly

18 *UP* 14.5 (= Aristotle, *Generation of Animals* 728a17–20 and passim).

19 Philip J. van der Eijk, '"Aristotle! What a thing for you to say!" Galen's engagement with Aristotle and Aristotelians', in Christopher Gill, Tim Whitmarsh and John Wilkins (eds.), *Galen and the World of Knowledge* (Cambridge, 2009), pp. 261–81.

20 Philippa Lang, *Medicine and Society in Ptolemaic Egypt* (Leiden, 2013), pp. 243–66; Heinrich von Staden, *Herophilus: The Art of Medicine in Early Alexandria* (Cambridge, 1989).

21 *UP* 14.11.

22 *Sem.* 2.1.15–21.

feature Aristotle's teacher, the philosopher Plato, in its procreative sections, but he was evoked at the outset of the work, and has been a tacit presence throughout.[23] The term 'demiurge' was borrowed from his *Timaeus*, for instance, and the constraint of existing matter on the divine craftsman plays a crucial role in the creation story there too; though women are a result of the moral failure of some of the first, all-male, generation of humans to be made, rather than a material product.[24] Galen's teleology is Platonic as well as Aristotelian.[25]

Beginning with Seeds

A more concrete place to start an exposition of human generation is with the production of the seed itself. Galen asserted that everybody, except his arch-rival Lycus, now agreed that females have testicles (*orcheis*): Herophilus was essentially right.[26] They are, importantly, smaller and flatter than in males, and their associated seminal ducts shorter, narrower and differently configured.[27] Each testicle receives blood and *pneuma* (warm air which has been integrated into the somatic economy) in veins and arteries descending ultimately from the kidney on the relevant side of the torso, and these substances begin to be concocted as the vessels carrying them become increasingly convoluted before attaching to the *orcheis*.[28] This process is less advanced in colder females than males, since heat is the main driver of this kind of transformation in the body, and it will fall further behind in their inferior testicles. The male *orcheis* perfect the seminal fluid, making it ready for generation – thick and white, viscous and full of vital *pneuma* – whereas the female parts cannot fully elaborate their materials in this way, producing 'scanty, cold and watery' seed, which is unable in itself to generate an animal.[29] Long and broad seminal channels then take large quantities of the perfect male *sperma* to the duct through which urine also passes out of the genitals, while the feeble female version requires only a small vessel to transport it the short distance to the 'horns' (*keraia*) of the uterus, from where it passes into the body of the womb (Fig. 7.2).[30]

Still, for Galen, the woman's *sperma* plays a vital role, scanty and thin as it is. It excites sexual desire, and conception, *syllēpsis*, literally 'grasping', occurs when both male and female seed are held by, and within, the womb, then mix together: that is the first step in generating a new being.[31] This mixing comprises both a kind of pneumatic alignment, a combination of the active portions of both seeds in a single pattern of motion, into a single moulding power; and a more material conjunction in which membranes

23 *UP* 1.2 and 8. 24 Plato, *Timaeus* 90e–91a.

25 Rebecca Flemming, 'Demiurge and emperor in Galen's world of knowledge', in Gill, Whitmarsh and Wilkins, *Galen and the World of Knowledge*, pp. 59–84.

26 *AA* 12.1. 27 *UP* 14.6, 10 and 12; *AA* 12.1; *Ut. Diss.* 9. 28 *UP* 14.10.

29 *UP* 14.6 and 9. 30 *UP* 14.10–12. 31 Especially *Sem.* 1.2 and 7; *UP* 14.7 and 11.

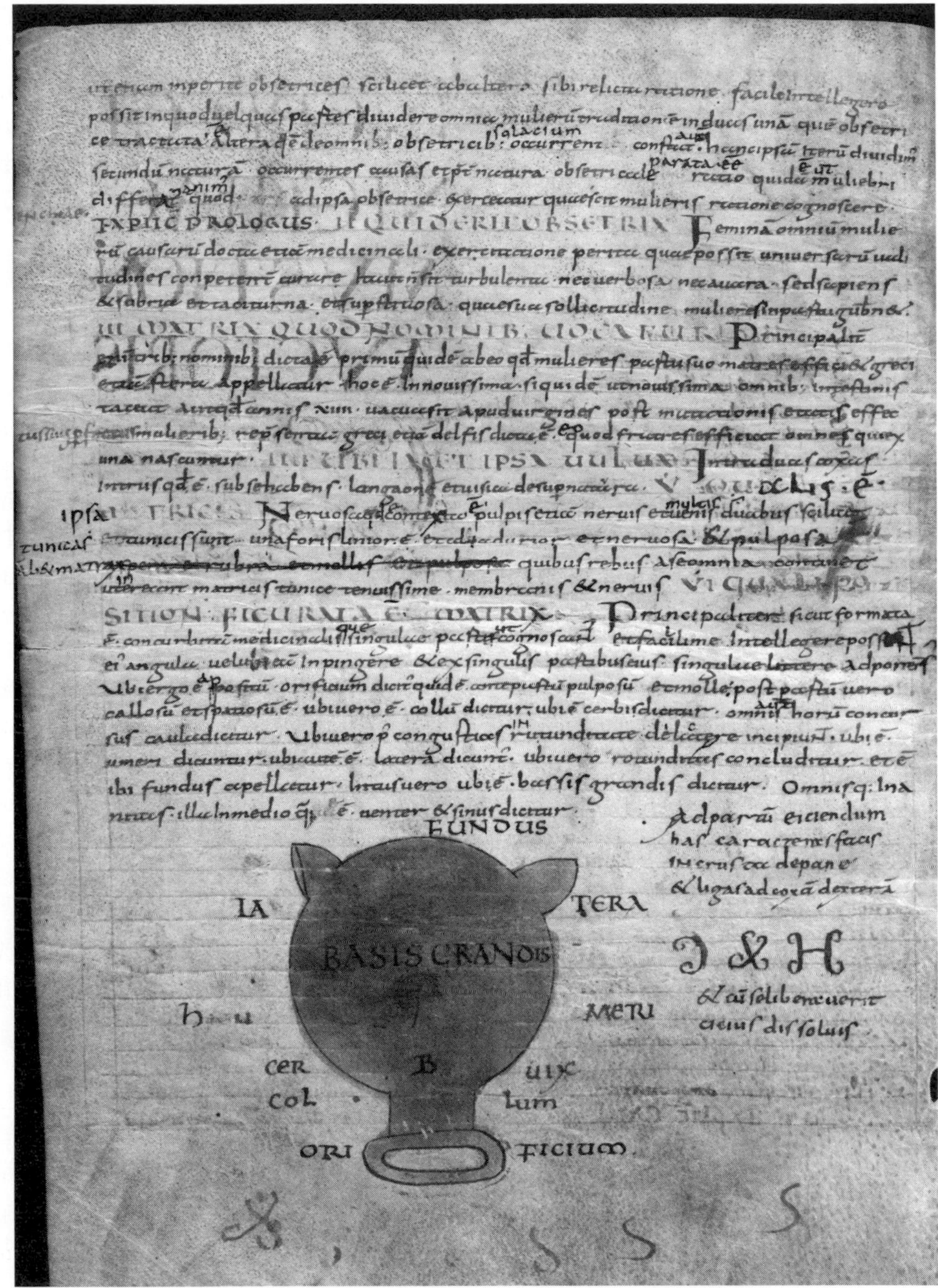

Figure 7.2 Drawing of a characteristically 'horned' uterus from a ninth-century manuscript containing Muscio's late antique Latin adaptation of Soranus's *Gynaecology*. The protuberances are not discussed in the text, which moves (as labelled, from bottom to top of the illustration) from mouth, throat and neck to shoulders, flanks and bottom, with the 'main body' also identified. See further Exhibit 7, this book. Royal Library of Belgium, MS 3701–15, f.16v.

are separately and jointly formed, entwined and arranged, while the female seed also provides initial nourishment for its harder-working male counterpart.[32] For Galen it was crucial that seed, as such, provides both movement and matter, in contrast to Aristotle's argument that it operates only as efficient cause, and contributes nothing of its own substance to the offspring.[33] The Galenic distribution is uneven, with male seed being more active and less material than female seed, but both possess both principles. This latter Galen took to be the Hippocratic position, even if it was not stated as such.

The combined, active force organizes and creates from itself, drawing in further resources – blood and *pneuma* – through vessels descending to the uterus; and a whole supply and removal system is established around what has been conceived.[34] Inside these layers, a four-stage process of fetal development unfolds, though Galen was not entirely consistent in his description of the phases.[35] *On the Formation of the Fetus* sets out his mature position that the liver begins to form in the first stage, followed by the heart and brain, the former probably in the second phase, with all three visible in the third stage (at least in outline), when the other parts also start to emerge.[36] This differentiation is completed in the fourth phase, as all parts are distinguished and strengthened, and growth gets going. Plentiful nourishment extracted from the maternal body enables substantial, but proportionate, expansion. Initially, what is conceived is 'administered' as a plant. It has a nutritive soul from the seed of both parents. Once the heart is formed and pulsation – a form of movement – commences, the fetus is governed not just as a plant, but also an animal, albeit a very lowly one, such as a clam or other shellfish. The rational part of the soul, the 'best' part, distinctive to humans, and located in the brain, develops only after birth.[37] The argument here is mainly with himself, and though there was some wider debate about the order of organic emergence, and the best categorization of fetal existence, the basic framework outlined here was a common holding.[38]

Galen eschewed precise timings in all this, insisting on individual variability. He suggested, however, that the proto-liver is formed within six days, and that the triad of

32 *Sem.* especially 1.7–8; *UP* 14.11.

33 Explicit at *Sem.* 1.1–11; Nahyan Fancy, 'Generation in Medieval Islamic Medicine', Chapter 9; Maaike van der Lugt, 'Formed Fetuses and Healthy Children in Scholastic Theology, Medicine and Law', Chapter 12, this book.

34 *AA* 12.4–6; *UP* 15.5–6.

35 Véronique Boudon-Millot, 'La naissance de la vie dans la théorie médicale et philosophique de Galien', in Luc Brisson, Marie-Hélène Congourdeau and Jean-Luc Solère (eds.), *L'embryon: Formation et animation. Antiquité grècque et latine, traditions hébraïque, chrétienne et islamique* (Paris, 2008), pp. 79–94.

36 *Foet. Form.* 3 (and 6) explicitly amending and overriding *Sem.* 1.9–11 where heart and liver are concurrent (also *UP* 15.6 and *On My Own Opinions* 11).

37 R. J. Hankinson, 'Galen's anatomy of the soul', *Phronesis* 36 (1991), 197–233.

38 Ann Ellis Hanson, 'The gradualist view of fetal development', in Brisson, Congourdeau and Solère, *L'embryon*, pp. 95–108.

principal parts become visible after thirty days.[39] By the completion of the third stage, the generative organs have begun to emerge, perhaps last of all. Still in a rather indeterminate state, they have yet to take up an internal or external location. Whether what has been conceived will be male or female has, however, already been decided, for the two differ 'in their whole body', not just their genitals.[40] This latter divergence is rather inconsequential, effect rather than cause. What matters is whether the seed comes predominantly from the right or left testicle and, more importantly, whether it falls into the right or left uterus. For the blood which sustains and supplies the right side of the abdomen is purer, and so hotter, than the rather thin and murky blood on the left. Seed from the right *orchis* is thus hotter, as is the right womb; and hotter means male (and vice versa). The uterus has most impact, Galen said, since it has longer to work on making what is conceived like itself, thus explaining the Hippocratic aphorism: 'Male fetuses mostly on the right, females on the left.'[41]

The fetus which becomes male has a hotter and drier *krasis* – mixture or temperament – from the outset.[42] This, particularly the heat, drives development faster, as Hippocrates and others claimed.[43] The parts are distinguished more rapidly, bones solidified more quickly and firmly, wider spaces opened up in vessels and the body more generally, everything is stronger and more vigorous. Conversely, a fetus which is colder and wetter in the first stage becomes female. It starts slowly, takes longer, and is too weak, finally, to push its generative parts outside. This weakness is exacerbated after birth.[44]

In *On Seed*, this discussion of fetal sex determination is part of a wider set of arguments for the existence and active role of female seed, combatively articulated.[45] First, Galen refuted Herophilus and unnamed recent physicians who held that, though there is female *sperma*, it is discharged externally, and so does not contribute to the offspring. Amongst these recent rivals should be counted the great 'methodic' physician, Soranus, who asserted this view in his *Gynaecology*, composed around AD 100, though Galen made no direct comment on it.[46] Second, he took on Aristotle and Athenaeus, the first-century BC founder of a medical lineage influenced by Stoic philosophy; both, according to Galen, denied that females produce seed.[47]

39 *Foet. Form.* 1 and 3. 40 *Sem.* 2.5.

41 *UP* 14.7 and 4; Hippocrates, *Aphorisms* 5.48. 42 *Sem.* 2.5.

43 *Nat. puer.* 18 specifies thirty days for male fetal formation, forty-two for the female. Elsewhere in the *Corpus* about forty days covers both.

44 Flemming, *Medicine*, pp. 314–17. 45 *Sem.* 2.1–5.

46 *Gynaecology* 3.12; Ann Ellis Hanson and Monica H. Green, 'Soranus of Ephesus: *Methodicorum princeps*', in Wolfgang Haase and Hildegard Temporini (eds.), *Aufstieg und Niedergang der römischen Welt* II 37.2 (Berlin, 1994), pp. 968–1075; Flemming, *Medicine*, pp. 232–46.

47 The female contribution in Aristotle was more seminal – Laurence M. V. Totelin, 'Animal and Plant Generation in Classical Antiquity', Chapter 4, this book – nor was this the Stoic position.

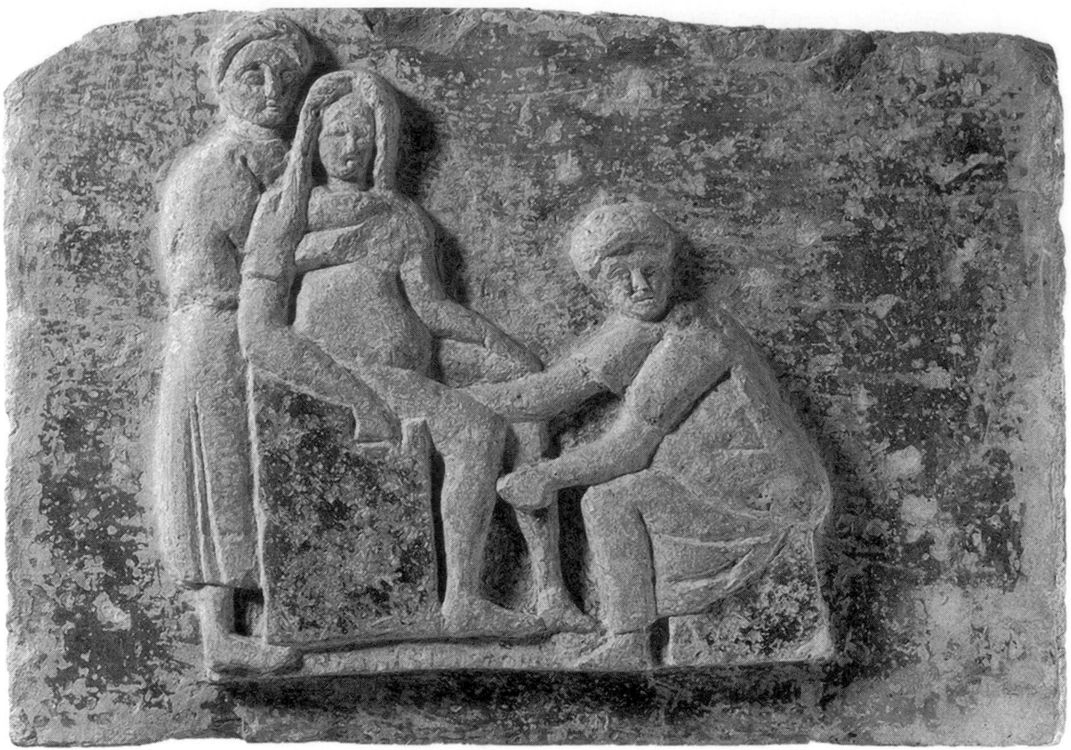

Figure 7.3 A terracotta plaque from the second-century AD tomb of Scribonia Attice (and her family), in the necropolis outside Ostia, Rome's harbour city, showing childbirth as a professional activity. The mother sits in a birthing chair, supported by a female helper behind her, while the midwife assists the emergence of the newborn. See also illustration on p. 18 and Exhibit 18, this book. 28 × 42 cm. Archivio fotografico della Soprintendenza Speciale per il Colosseo, il MNR e l'Area Archeologica di Roma, Sede di Ostia, inv. no. 5203.

Dissection shows that the female testicles and seminal vessels are full of the stuff, Galen countered, and that their spermatic ducts empty, and discharge *sperma*, into the 'horns' of the uterus. General experience, observation and reason also prove that women seminate; it is obvious and makes good sense. Active female seed is the most effective way to account for parental resemblance in all its forms, both general and particular, and that of male and female offspring to both parents. The great advantage is that it allows a single set of causes to operate uniformly across the whole terrain. For, on Galen's model, the similarity to both mother and father (and their respective ancestors) is produced by seed, according to the same principles in both cases and in children of either sex.

Finally, roughly nine months after *syllēpsis*, the fetus is capable of being nourished through its mouth, and so ready to be born (Fig. 7.3).[48] It may bring on birth

48 Ann Ellis Hanson, 'The eight months' child and the etiquette of birth: *Obsit omen!*', *Bulletin of the History of Medicine* 61 (1987), 589–602.

by its own vigorous movements, as Hippocrates said, or the uterus may be stretched to the limit, or over-full of the liquids implicated in fetal support, and so wish to relieve itself of its burden.[49] The wonderful arrangements of nature ensure that the fetus almost always moves towards the exit head first, limbs neatly tucked in; and the neck of the womb, till now closed tight, then opens wide to allow it to pass through.[50] Even more marvellously, at this same moment, milk is ready in the mother's breasts, and the newborn is ready to feed, knowing exactly how to suckle. Milk is another product of female somatic excess. The material which had been nourishing the fetus in the uterus is now diverted upwards, through the key vessels which link womb and breasts, and concocted in the glands around the nipples.[51] Infant understanding of how to feed is a further sign of the wisdom and providence, power and skill of the demiurge.

Afterwards

In the middle of the fourth century AD, the Emperor Julian (the last pagan ruler of the Roman Empire) asked the physician Oribasius to follow his compilation of Galenic medicine with a complete collection of all knowledge useful to the medical art.[52] Oribasius agreed, and composed a vast medical encyclopaedia, in seventy books, around that earlier framework, for, he stated, Galen 'surpasses' all other authorities in the field, in part through his perfect Hippocratism. Whatever exactly had occurred over the 150 years since the death of Galen, this enterprise marks the 'triumph of Galenism', at least in the Greek East of the empire; and over the next few centuries successive Greek medical compendia followed the same Galenic pattern.[53] The curriculum of the medical school of late antique Alexandria, which flourished through the sixth century and survived the Arab conquest of AD 641 in some form, was similarly dominated by Galen and Hippocrates, very much in tandem. *Nature of the Child* was included on the Hippocratic syllabus, for example, because of its subject matter and Galen's favour.[54] An early student of the Alexandrian medical and philosophical schools, Sergius of Resaina, began to translate Galen's works (including *On the Usefulness of the Parts*), and some

49 Galen, *On the Natural Faculties* 3.12.

50 *UP* 15.7. Breech and transverse births occur only once in many thousands, Galen claims; though see Ralph Jackson, 'A Roman Embryo Hook', Exhibit 6, this book.

51 *UP* 14.8.

52 Oribasius, *Medical Compilations* (*Coll. Med.*) 1.pr.; Mark Grant, *Dieting for an Emperor* (Leiden, 1997), pp. 1–17 (and 24–5).

53 Vivian Nutton, *Ancient Medicine*, 2nd edn (London, 2013), pp. 299–317.

54 Surviving lectures on which are in *Corpus Medicorum Graecorum* vol. XI.1,4 (Berlin, 1997), pp. 128–75; with John M. Duffy's introductions, pp. 9–12, 21–3.

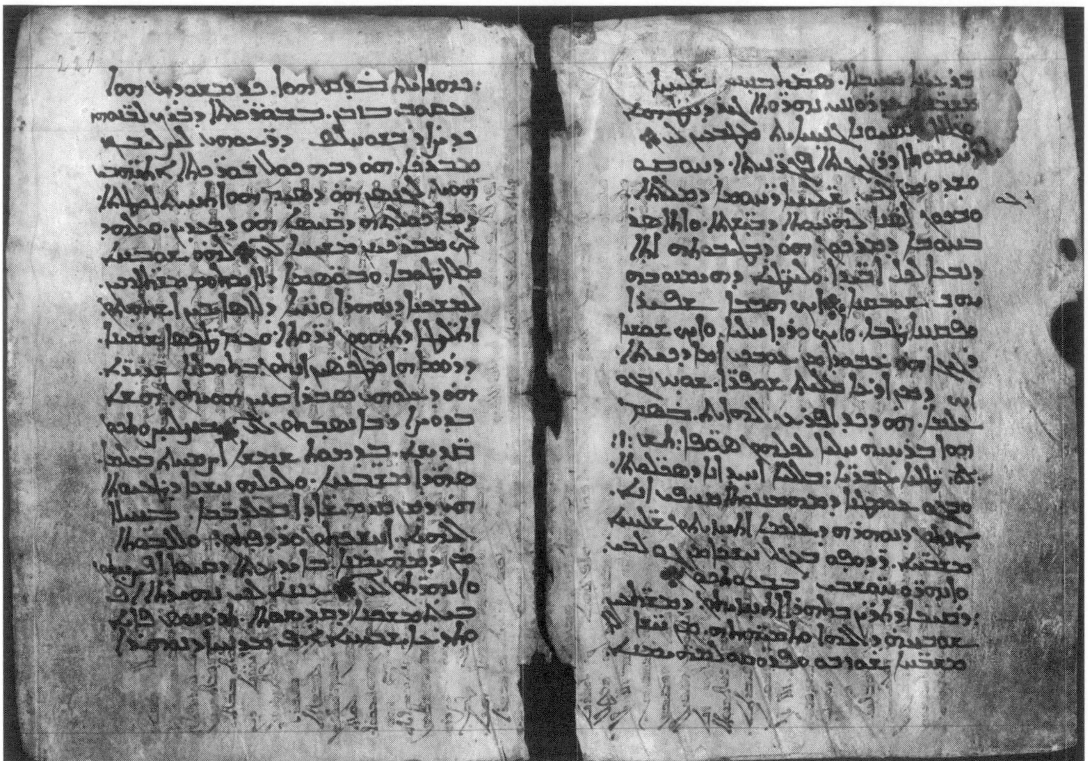

Figure 7.4 Folio of the recently rediscovered Syriac Galen Palimpsest (214v–21r). The earlier undertext – the vertical lines faintly visible beneath this eleventh-century liturgical work – comes from Sergius's translation of Book 8 of Galen's popular treatise *On Simple Drugs*. Books 6–11 contain an alphabetical listing of simples and their powers, many of these generative and gynaecological. © Owner of the Syriac Galen Palimpsest, Creative Commons Attribution 3.0 Unported Access Rights.

Aristotelian texts, into Syriac in the first decades of the sixth century AD, further facilitating the eastern spread of his ideas (Fig. 7.4).[55]

Despite Galen's acknowledged supremacy, Oribasius also incorporated extracts from some of his rivals in his encyclopaedia. Most striking is his inclusion of an abridged description of the female generative organs from Soranus, complete with the denial of the contribution of the female seed to offspring.[56] The Galenic anatomy preceding this passage is not directly contradictory, but subsequent sections on the seed and pregnancy are.[57] The standing of Soranus as a gynaecological authority was even higher in the late antique West, where Galen was less dominant in general. Thus, for example, two 'Latinizations' of Soranus's *Gynaecology* survive, first by Caelius Aurelianus

55 Siam Bhayro, 'Syriac medical terminology: Sergius and Galen's pharmacopia', *Aramaic Studies* 3 (2005), 147–65.

56 Oribasius, *Coll. Med.* 24.31.

57 Ibid., 24.29–30, *lib. inc.* 9–10.

in the early fifth century AD in North Africa, second by Muscio, probably a century later, either in Africa or northern Italy, the other centre of medical learning in the early medieval West.[58] Both describe women's testicles (*testiculi*, in Latin) as 'smaller and softer' than males', and opening into the neck of the bladder; so, Caelius reported, 'it is held that the seed (*semen*) in females is useless in the creation or conception of animals'.[59] The same locations produced Latin versions of some Galenic, and more Hippocratic, treatises from the sixth century onwards, and late antique Ravenna imitated at least parts of the Alexandrian school curriculum, but the focus was on the fundamentals of the medical art, not generation.[60] Still, a range of views were transmitted, both East and West, even as these two halves of a once integrated empire pulled apart, linguistically and politically.

Conclusion

The one-seed or two-seed debate, though not meaningless, was not the most important aspect of the ancient medical conversation about human generation as this took particularly influential form in the Roman Empire of the second century AD. It is not just that the existence of female *sperma* and its contribution to offspring were distinct issues, and that everybody (except Lycus) agreed that females had testicles; but, above all, that this consensus, and its politics, is more representative of the overall picture, despite Galen's studied contentiousness and more modern obsessions. All assumed that the key players in the procreative process are seed, womb and maternal material, and thus that both parents make serious and active contributions to the production of their children. All also assumed that the female is the inferior version of the kind, especially humankind, a principle which their various seminal commitments neither strengthened nor weakened. Galen was, after all, a two-seed man, but his feeble female *sperma* enacts the sexual hierarchy just as clearly as Aristotle's un-concocted female residue. Galen himself argued that it does so more clearly, or, at least, that this forms part of a more complete and cogent account of female imperfection than Aristotle offered.

Other elements of this shared framework should also be summarized here, for they have a long and wide reach: key pieces of the flexible and robust conceptual repertoire of generation as it was developed and flourished in the ancient Mediterranean world. *Syllēpsis* was universally understood as the active closing of the womb around the seminal stuff, whether that was seeds, seed and menstrual fluid, or something else, and of whatever composition and somatic origin. Something special from the parents,

58 Hanson and Green, 'Soranus', pp. 1042–61; Lauren Kassell, 'Medieval Birth Malpresentations', Exhibit 10, this book.

59 Caelius Aurelianus and Muscio, *Gynaecology* 1.16–17.

60 Nutton, *Ancient Medicine*, pp. 305–8.

with generative powers, had to be retained in the uterus. What was conceived then relied on the maternal body for support, formative material and nourishment, drawing on menstrual resources. It first formed, in all its parts, and then grew; operating at rather a low level of existence until birth, a process in which the fetus actively participated. Maternal nourishment continued thereafter. This framework, moreover, stayed in place in the later, Christianizing, Roman Empire and beyond.[61] Debates on details continued and developed in particular directions, while the question of ensoulment came to the fore as other issues faded in importance, but the basic architecture remained secure for centuries.

61 Marie-Hélène Congourdeau, 'Debating the Soul in Late Antiquity', Chapter 8, this book; though see James Wilberding, 'The revolutionary embryology of the Neoplatonists', *Oxford Studies in Ancient Philosophy* 49 (2015), 321–62.

8 Debating the Soul in Late Antiquity

Marie-Hélène Congourdeau

In classical Greek thought, human generation began with the fusion of a male element – the seed – and a female element – seed or menstrual blood – and ended with the emergence of a child. But much rested on what happened in between, and at issue was the formation of not just the body, but also the soul. In the late Roman Empire, as earlier philosophical and medical ideas – of Plato, Aristotle, Hippocrates, Galen and others – were contested and developed, challenged and expanded, the problem of the soul came increasingly to the fore, amongst both pagan and Christian thinkers.[1]

This chapter explores that rise to prominence, and examines in more detail the debates around the 'ensoulment' of the fetus which characterize this period. It emphasizes the flexibility and contingency of much of the discussion, including among Christian theologians, and the relatively loose links between their theoretical discourse and church injunctions about behaviour. Late antiquity saw a basic change in approach to fetal life, as the divinely provided human soul became more important to its constitution. This shift helped to shore up the early Christian use of hostility to abortion, like infant exposure, as a sign of their own higher moral standards, but in a rather vague and diffuse way.[2] These moves, though sharing a direction of travel, seem less connected than might have been expected.

The Parameters of the Debate

The stability of the vast Roman Empire, consolidated and integrated over the first two centuries AD, was disrupted in what is known as the 'Third-Century Crisis'.[3] External military threats (from the resurgent Persian Empire in the east and Germanic groups forced into motion in the north), civil wars and imperial weakness fed political volatility; economic conditions worsened; and Roman civic society and its cultural and religious

1 For these earlier ideas: Helen King, 'Women and Doctors in Ancient Greece', Chapter 3; Laurence M. V. Totelin, 'Animal and Plant Generation in Classical Antiquity', Chapter 4; Rebecca Flemming, 'Galen's Generations of Seeds', Chapter 7, this book.

2 Not that abortion was unproblematic in the classical world, but the Christian view was self-consciously distinctive: Zubin Mistry, *Abortion in the Early Middle Ages*, c. 500–900 (York, 2015), pp. 23–55.

3 For general historical background: Stephen Mitchell, *A History of the Later Roman Empire, AD 284–641*, 2nd edn (Chichester, 2015).

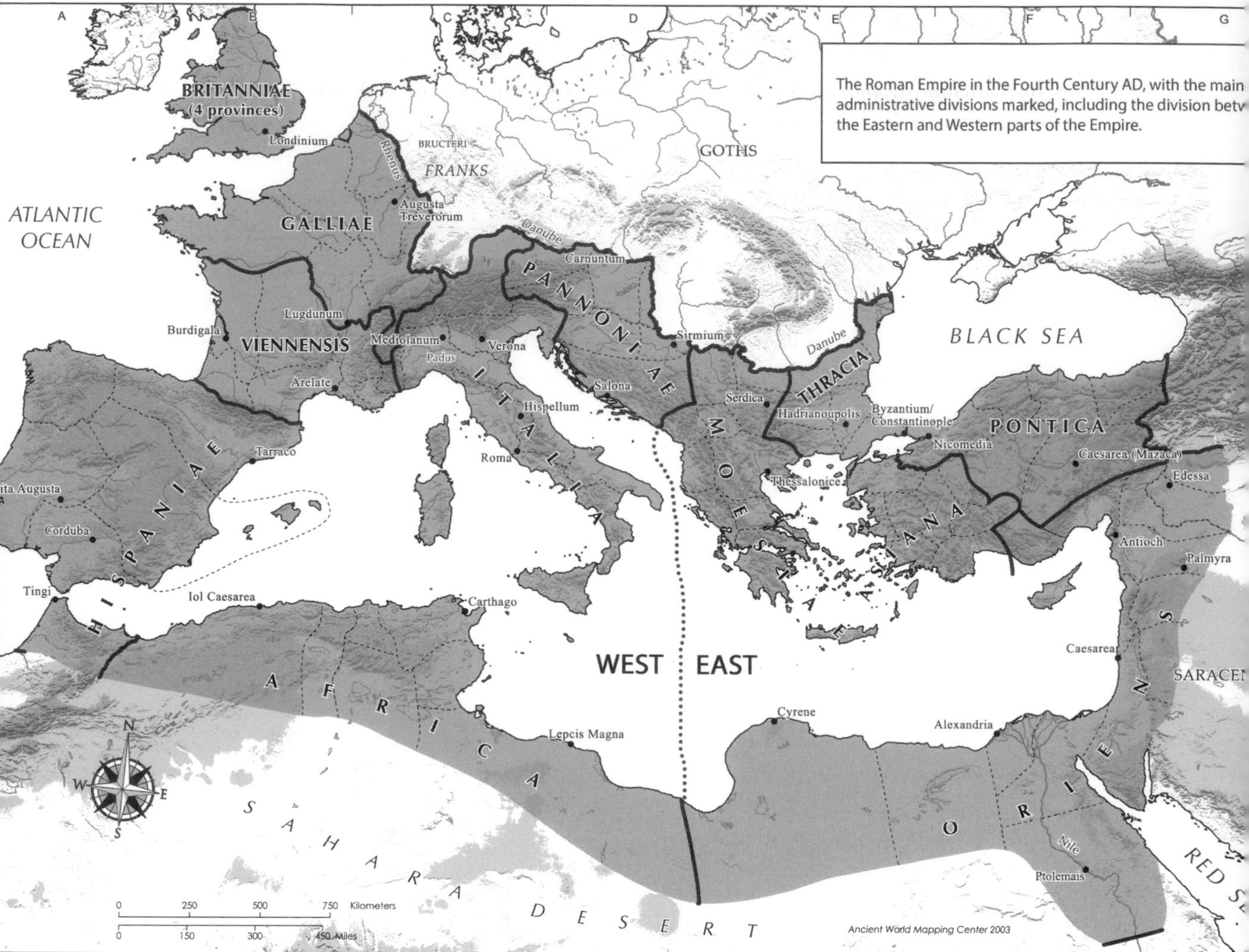

Figure 8.1 Map illustrating the reorganization of the later Roman Empire. Provincial administration was reformed early in the fourth century, then, with effect from his death in AD 395, Theodosius I formally divided the empire between his young sons: Arcadius ruled in the East, Honorius in the West. The two parts enjoyed different fortunes thereafter. Ancient World Mapping Center, adapted by Rachel Aucott.

forms came under pressure. A sense of disquiet born from uncertainty brought philosophy and religion closer together, within a wider set of intellectual and social shifts and realignments. Neoplatonism, which attempted a synthesis between Aristotle and Plato, inflected with revived Pythagorean ideas and informed by the practices of traditional mystery cults, was on the rise. It gradually supplanted Stoicism in the affections of the Roman elite. At the same time, the religions of salvation continued to spread throughout the empire. Despite persecutions, Christianity advanced, church organization grew and Christian discourse expanded.

The resolution of the crisis in the fourth century AD began a process of imperial division between a western part, centred on Rome, and an eastern part, centred on Constantinople, with increasingly divergent cultures (Fig. 8.1). The conversion of the Emperor Constantine in AD 312 set another dynamic in motion, the Christianization of the empire, a project more emphatically pursued by Theodosius I towards the end of the century. With a clearer commitment to a particular orthodox version of the Christian faith than his predecessors, Theodosius famously legislated in AD 380, soon after his accession, that 'all people' under his rule should not only live according to the religion transmitted by the apostle Peter, but also 'believe in the one deity of Father, Son and Holy Spirit with equal majesty and in the Holy Trinity'.[4] His vision thus excluded alternative Christianities, Judaism and traditional pagan religions.

In AD 476, the western empire fell, divided up between various successor states, from the Vandal Kingdom in North Africa, through Ostrogothic Italy and Visigothic Spain to the Frankish and Saxon Kingdoms of more northern Europe; almost all were Christian, though of different stripes. The eastern Roman Empire persisted, and would even reconquer segments of western territory in the sixth century, before losing much ground in Asia and Africa to Persian and then Arab conquests in the seventh. The unravelling political and religious patterns of antiquity were reconstructed differently in East and West.

Many earlier concepts, doctrines and controversies about the soul itself, and its relation to the body, also passed into the later Roman Empire. These were available to philosophers and theologians – the intellectual elite – in the Christianizing world of the fourth century, as they began to focus on how the issues might play out in generation, as part of a wider set of shifting discussions about the nature of human beings. To discern what changed and what was at stake we need to understand the state of the argument going into this period. This is a matter of content and form: what was in dispute and the modes of disputation.

Broadly speaking, from the time of the Presocratics onwards, two basic approaches to the human soul can be identified.[5] According to the first, the soul, whether divine, eternal or created, pre-exists its union with the body. For an undefined reason (punishment, accident or divine plan), it then finds itself in a body, and this event animates the fetus. Death eventually separates the body from the soul, which either migrates into another body or returns to its primitive incorporeal state. This was the view of the Platonists. According to the Atomists, Aristotelians and Stoics, by contrast, the soul is inseparable from the body and emerges from it, and the death of the one signifies the death of the other. These were the two major currents of debate into which Christian theologians introduced alternative, and increasingly dominant, ideas and arguments.

Before examining the late antique debate in more detail, it is important to make one further point about the persuasive resources traditionally deployed to approach

4 *Theodosian Code* 16.1.2.

5 Marie-Hélène Congourdeau, *L'embryon et son âme dans les sources grecques (VIe siècle av. J.-C. – Ve siècle apr. J.-C.)* (Paris, 2007).

these questions. We should not assume that Christian thought relied on revelation, while classical philosophy proceeded through reason alone. The philosophers did use rational arguments; they were interested in coherence and logical demonstration, for instance. Nevertheless, they also referred to an authoritative corpus of texts, especially those of Plato and Aristotle. Moreover, Plato himself had already joined conceptual reasoning and mythical discourse. In the *Republic*, for instance, the Myth of Er helped to explicate the migration of the soul from body to body.[6] This mythic tendency of Platonism was accentuated by leading Neoplatonists such as Plotinus, who began his influential teaching in Rome around AD 250. Amongst the Christians, reference to a revealed body of writings was, however, explicit and emphatic. If reason, on the basis of a shared intellectual heritage, was pre-eminent in philosophical discourse, in the Christian domain it took second place to a textual corpus which, by the late Roman Empire, was made up of two components: the Old and New Testaments of the Bible (the touchstone as the word of God), and the Church Fathers' interpretations of them. This double corpus grounded Christian answers to questions about ensoulment.

The Debate on the Ensoulment of the Fetus

The first question concerned the origin of the soul. For the Stoics, the formation and growth of the fetus necessitated the presence within it, from the beginning, of a material vital breath issuing from the seed. This breath was cooled by the air from the moment of the first inspiration after birth, and this cooling (*psychrōsis*, in Greek) transformed it into a soul (*psychē*). Thus the soul could be considered as coming from the body.[7] The Neoplatonists directly opposed this notion. Porphyry, the key student of Plotinus and influential shaper of the Plotinian tradition into the early fourth century AD, dedicated an entire treatise to the question, *To Gaurus On How Embryos Are Ensouled*, which principally targeted the Stoics.[8] The work concluded by asserting that whatever status one accorded the fetus, the essential point was to affirm that the soul was introduced into it from outside.[9]

Christian theologians explained the origin of the soul more simply: God created the soul and infused it into the fetus. They found this asserted in Genesis: 'Then the Lord God formed man from the dust of the ground, and breathed into his nostrils the breath of life; and the man became a living being' (2:7).[10] Each descendant of Adam received his body and his soul from God in the same way.

6 *Republic* 614b–21d.
7 Plutarch, *On the Principle of Coldness* 2 (*Mor.* 946C).
8 Previously attributed to Galen, this text has now been firmly ascribed to Porphyry, and given sustained scholarly attention: Porphyre, *Sur la manière dont l'embryon reçoit l'âme*, ed. and trans. Luc Brisson *et al.* (Paris, 2012); Porphyry, *To Gaurus On How Embryos Are Ensouled* and *On What Is In Our Power*, trans. James Wilberding (London, 2011).
9 *To Gaurus* (*AG*) 17.1–2.
10 Biblical translations are from the *NRSV* unless otherwise stated.

The question of the moment of ensoulment – when, exactly, the human body and soul are joined – was more difficult and crucial. The answer determined when the fetus should be considered a full human being, which might have consequences for judging behaviour, most obviously with respect to abortion.

Since, for the Stoics, the soul resulted from the cooling of the vital breath by the air, it followed that the final stage of ensoulment occurred at the moment of birth. Porphyry, who summarized various Neoplatonic ideas, was more radical still. *To Gaurus* systematically demonstrated that fetal existence is essentially vegetative – human fetuses are either plants or similar to plants – and moves to a higher level only at birth, when the fetus receives a soul from outside.[11] Porphyry showed, first, that it is not an animal, because none of the characteristic capacities of an animal (sensation, movement, appetite, impulse) is present. He stressed the fact that the fetus is nourished through the umbilical cord, like a plant by its stem, and refuted the idea that the 'cravings' of the mother transfer her appetitive faculty, an animal feature, to the fetus. Then he demonstrated that the fetus is not even potentially an animal – it does not possess the powers of an animal in an unactivated or dormant state – by recalling that, according to Aristotle, all sensation requires organic action, which does not apply to the fetus. Last, Porphyry argued that the soul came from outside, and thus not from the parents.

In contrast, no Christian thinker located ensoulment at birth. The Bible is explicit that the fetus is the object of God's foresight in the mother's womb, and thus is provided with a spiritual soul during this stage.[12] Ensoulment at birth was not the unanimous opinion amongst classical philosophers either. For Aristotle and his followers, since the soul was 'the first actuality of an organized natural body', it could exist only when the body was provided with organs.[13] The human soul was then present once the fetus had a properly human form, which occurred, according to Aristotle, on the fortieth day for boys and the ninetieth for girls.[14]

From the mid-fourth century onwards, Christian exegetes associated with the Antiochene school, such as the bishops Diodorus of Tarsus, John Chrysostom and then Theodoret of Cyrus, arrived at the same conclusion by different routes.[15] They leant on

11 Porphyry preferred the terminology of vegetative 'power' or 'nature', but did not object if others called the organizing and animating principle of this lower, plant-like level of existence the 'vegetative soul' (*AG* 16.1). Vocabulary (and precise conceptions) varied in antiquity, but all posited a hierarchical model of life, ascending from plant via animal to (rational) human forms, each with a corresponding causal force for the relevant functions and activities.

12 Thus, for example, Jeremiah 1:5: 'Even before I formed you in the womb, I knew you.'

13 *On the Soul* 412b5. 14 *History of Animals* 583b2–5.

15 On the two 'schools' of early biblical interpretation, associated with Antioch and Alexandria: Frances M. Young, 'Alexandrian and Antiochene exegesis', in Alan J. Hauser and Duane F. Watson (eds.), *A History of Biblical Interpretation*, vol. 1: *The Ancient Period* (Grand Rapids, MI, 2003), pp. 334–54.

two biblical passages. The first is the verse of Genesis already invoked, which they read to mean that the soul was breathed in, 'after the modelling of the body', that is, after the complete formation of the fetus.[16] The second passage is from Exodus (21:22–3). The Hebrew text reads: 'If men quarrel and jostle a pregnant woman, and her children exit without catastrophe, a fine shall be exacted from the guilty party … If there is a catastrophe, you will give life for life', the catastrophe being the death of the child or the mother. The Greek translation in the Septuagint, produced in Hellenistic Alexandria, is different: 'When two men fight and strike a pregnant woman, if her child comes out but is not configured (*exeikonismenon*), the man shall be punished with a fine … if it is configured, the man will give a life for a life.' The configured, or formed, fetus is that which has a human figure; furthermore, the expression 'a life for a life', which evokes notions of capital punishment, is in the Greek literally 'a soul (*psychē*) for a soul (*psychē*)'. The Antiochene commentators thus concluded that the soul is present in a fetus from the moment of formation.[17]

This interpretation became very popular, particularly in the west. Jerome adopted it, as did Augustine, the two dominant figures of the Latin church in the late fourth and early fifth centuries.[18] In his *Questions on the Heptateuch*, composed around AD 419, Augustine wrote, in relation to the passage in Exodus, that until 'formed' what is carried in the womb is 'not a man'.[19] But he did not come to a final conclusion on the moment of ensoulment: careful as ever in this complex area, he left the question open. His successors were less hesitant. Later in the fifth century AD, the anonymous author of the *Questions and Answers on the Old and New Testament* subsequently ascribed to Augustine influentially asserted ensoulment at formation, relying on these same biblical texts.[20] Eight centuries afterwards and even more authoritatively, Thomas Aquinas would also defend delayed ensoulment, but more for philosophical than exegetical reasons, following Aristotle rather than scripture.[21]

Some philosophers and theologians did place the entry of the soul at conception or even earlier. Porphyry mocked those, such as Numenius and others working in a broadly Pythagorean tradition, who held either that the soul emerges at the same time as the seed or that it is in any case needed for the process of conception to succeed.[22] Various contemporary Christian thinkers concurred, for different reasons.

In early third-century North Africa, Tertullian, writing his most concentrated defence of Christianity, including against charges of 'sacramental infanticide' (and worse),

16 Diodorus, *On Genesis*, Fr. 83: Françoise Petit (ed.), *Catenae graecae in Genesim et in Exodum*, vol. 2: *Collectio Coisliniana in Genesim* (Turnhout, 1986), pp. 86–7.

17 Congourdeau, *L'embryon et son âme*, pp. 169–75 and 303–5.

18 Jerome, *Letters* 121.4.

19 *Questions on the Heptateuch* 2.80.

20 *Questions and Answers on the Old and New Testament* 23.

21 Fabrizio Amerini, *Aquinas on the Beginning and End of Human Life*, trans. Mark Henninger (Cambridge, MA, 2013); Maaike van der Lugt, 'Formed Fetuses and Healthy Children in Scholastic Theology, Medicine and Law', Chapter 12, this book.

22 *AG* 2.2.

underlined its adherents' distinctive, total respect for life, even in the womb, and coined a phrase which would become an adage: 'he is also a man who is going to be one' (*homo est et qui est futurus*).[23] He developed his ideas in the treatise *On the Soul*, asserting that the two substances of the human composite appear at the same time.[24] Just as death is the instantaneous disjunction of soul and body, so conception is their instantaneous joining, therefore the soul appears at the same time as the body, at conception. This insistence on the simultaneous instantiation of body and soul troubled later theologians, such as Augustine. For in this model, the soul appears to issue from the seed, like the body; the simultaneity risks implying a common origin (the Stoic view). This anxiety is well expressed in the anonymous treatise attributed to Augustine, already mentioned, which asserts that the soul 'is not born at the moment of the conception of the body *as if* it was derived from the seed'. In its insistence on the separation of soul from seed, the Latin theological tradition would always worry about ensoulment at conception.

In the East, the theological argument was less with Stoic understandings of the soul as dependent on the body, and more with Alexandrian Christian teachings, especially those associated with their great foundational figure, Origen, which asserted the pre-existence of the soul, and so risked making its embodiment seem to be a moment of decay. Greek theologians thus insisted, in opposition to those in the Latin world, on the union of the composite soul–body – a union desired by God and sanctified by the incarnation and resurrection of Christ. Among the Cappadocian Fathers, Gregory of Nyssa dedicated a chapter of his late fourth-century AD text, *On the Making of Man*, to refuting first those who thought the soul prior to the body (pre-existence) and then those who held that it comes afterwards (delayed ensoulment).[25] Developing philosophical arguments close to those of Tertullian (whom he did not know), Gregory proposed that the elements of a composite necessarily begin to exist simultaneously; neither can exist without nor precede the other. Thus the soul is present from conception, even if its faculties manifest themselves progressively as the body, its instrument, develops.

Almost three centuries later, the most influential Byzantine theologian, Maximus the Confessor, developed this intuition, in his *On Difficulties in the Church Fathers*. He contrasted the 'composite person' (or *hypostasis*) of Christ, whose two parts (divinity and humanity) were each complete in nature, to the 'composite nature' of man whose two parts (soul and body) had no meaning outside of their union.[26] 'Receiving its existence at the moment of conception simultaneously with the body, the soul contributes to the completion of a single human being, whereas the body is created from the underlying matter of another body at the moment of conception, and is joined together with the soul into a single form with it.'[27] The great authority of these two theologians – Gregory of Nyssa and Maximus the Confessor – imposed this opinion on the east.

23 *Apology* 9.8. 24 *On the Soul* 17.2. 25 *On the Making of Man* 28. 26 *On Difficulties* 7.

27 Ibid., 42.10; *Maximos the Confessor, On Difficulties in the Church Fathers: The Ambigua*, vol. 2, ed. and trans. Nicholas Constas (Cambridge, MA, 2014), pp. 138–41.

How the coupling of the soul and the body is accomplished was also debated. For the Stoics, the parents generated the soul and body of their offspring, through the seed.[28] For those who thought that the soul comes from the outside, the issue was more complex, especially if ensoulment was to take place before the fetus left the womb (Fig. 8.2). Many centuries earlier, the Roman Epicurean poet, Lucretius, had mocked those who imagined souls fighting over entrance into the body, or stuck in a body against their will.[29] For Porphyry, everything pointed to full ensoulment at birth: the soul inserts itself naturally into a body entirely formed and ready to receive it, as the child leaves the mother's womb. The congruence between a soul and a body produces a mutual attraction, such as between a magnet and iron filings.[30]

Amongst the Christians, this question was the object of endless debates between those who held that the soul is created and infused directly by God into the fetus, the doctrine which became known as 'creatianism', and those who asserted that it is transmitted through the seed: 'traducianism', from the Latin *traducere*, 'to carry over'.[31] According to this Christian version of Stoicism, God created Adam's soul on the sixth day of creation, and this soul propagates itself and is transmitted to his descendants by means of the seed. Creatianism has two main variants: either God creates each soul at the moment of infusion, or he made all souls on the sixth and last day of his creative activities and draws on this 'treasury of souls' to animate all new human offspring.

The Christian East quickly rejected traducianism, which makes the spiritual soul depend on a corporeal element, seed. Immediate creatianism – God creates each soul at the moment he infuses it into a newly engendered body – was generally preferred. The Antiochenes adopted this view with particular enthusiasm, since it worked well with their model of delayed ensoulment.[32] By contrast, the question inflamed the Christian West for decades. Jerome registered vigorous support for creatianism in an early commentary on Ecclesiastes.[33] He developed a more elaborate creatianist position in arguing against pre-existence of the soul, after many of Origen's works were translated into Latin in the late fourth century, and the debates around them moved west. Augustine also initially averred his preference for this doctrine. But by the end of the fourth century the question of original sin caused him discomfort on this account. Julian of Eclanum, one of the more theologically astute followers of the influential ascetic and teacher, Pelagius, had raised the question of how Augustine's doctrine of original sin

28 A. A. Long, 'Soul and body in Stoicism', *Phronesis* 27 (1982), 34–57.

29 *Nature of Things* 3.778–81.

30 *AG* 11.2: Gwenaëlle Aubry, 'Capacité et convenance: La fonction de la notion d'*epitêdeiotês* dans la théorie porphyrienne de l'embryon', in Luc Brisson, Marie-Hélène Congourdeau and Jean-Luc Solère (eds.), *L'embryon: Formation et animation. Antiquité grècque et latine, traditions hébraïque, chrétienne et islamique* (Paris, 2008), pp. 139–55.

31 The traditional term 'creatianism' is here preferred to the more modern 'creationism', to avoid confusion.

32 Congourdeau, *L'embryon et son âme*, p. 263.

33 *Commentary on Ecclesiastes* 12.6–8.

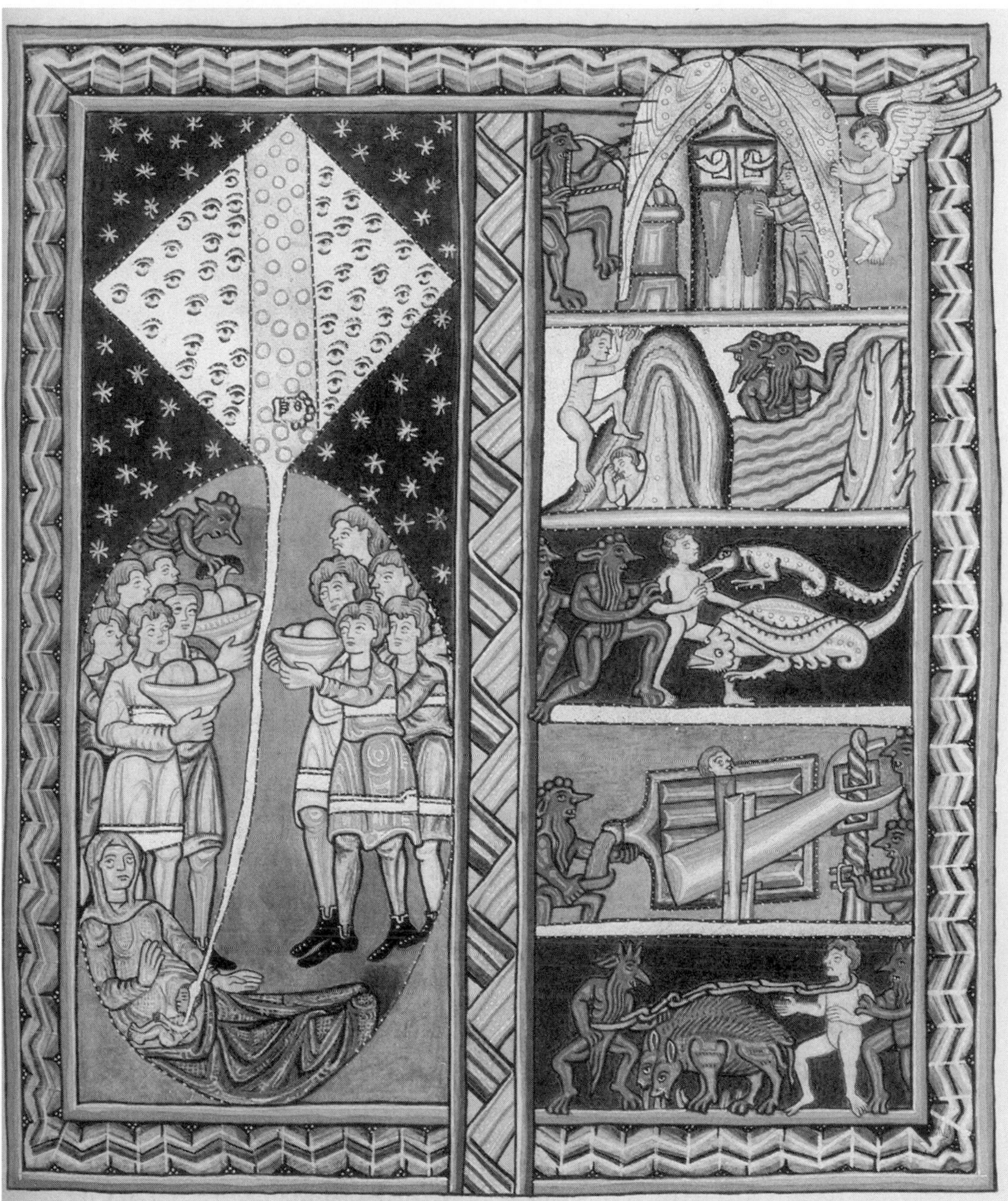

Figure 8.2 Illustrations of the fourth vision of the twelfth-century German nun and mystic, Hildegard of Bingen, as described in her *Scivias*. Though much later than the debates discussed in this chapter, the miniature demonstrates the challenges involved in imagining how the fetus might be infused by an external soul. On the left, the celestial creator animates the perfect human form in the womb through a fiery globe which touches its brain and spreads through all its limbs just before birth. Between creator and womb the production of cheese represents the human part of procreation. The struggles, temptations and possible triumph of the ensouled human are depicted on the right. 22 × 17 cm. Copy of the Rupertsberg manuscript, now lost, St Hildegard's Abbey, Eibingen.

might be squared with the understanding that a good God gives each newborn a newly created soul; and Augustine had turned to a traducian argument in response.[34] If the soul inherits original sin, it is because at the moment of the original fault it was one with the soul of Adam: each soul thus sinned in Adam, which shows that all souls are derived from his.[35]

Jerome was committed to creatianism, but Augustine hesitated, tempted by Adamic traducianism. He would have preferred otherwise, but the transmission of original sin required him to withhold full assent.[36] After many discussions of the origin of the soul, in dedicated treatises and more incidental engagements, he was unable to decide one way or the other. After Augustine's death, however, an anonymous dialogue decided the issue for him.[37] This influential work is composed of quotations from Jerome and Augustine organized so as to demonstrate their agreement on the matter. It does so at the price of distorting Augustine's thought, since it prioritizes his reticence with regards to traducianism and minimizes the worries he may have had with respect to creatianism. At the end of the fifth century, the Bishop of Rome, Anastasius II, cut short the debate by condemning traducianism.[38]

Intersections

Tertullian has already illustrated how Christians laid claim to higher standards than those who surrounded and attacked them, in respect of their protection of life in the womb, and, he added, following the standard apologetic repertoire, in respect to raising all their children too, thus opposing the common (but not Jewish) practice of infant exposure. Similar themes can also be found in early Christian writings in Greek, which include prescriptive as well as more broadly expository texts. The earliest set of surviving community rules, the *Didache*, which perhaps took its transmitted form around the middle of the second century AD, includes amongst its many prohibitions the injunction, 'You shall not murder your child by abortion and you shall not kill it after birth.'[39] The eastern and western traditions diverged as time went on, but shared the same early approach. The question here is to what extent these positions, and their development, intersected with the theoretical debates on ensoulment just outlined.

34 Mathijs Lamberigts, 'Pelagius and Pelagians', in Susan Ashbrook Harvey and David G. Hunter (eds.), *The Oxford Handbook of Early Christian Studies* (Oxford, 2008), pp. 258–79.

35 Congourdeau, *L'embryon et son âme*, pp. 268–74.

36 Augustine, *Letter* 166 (to Jerome).

37 Ralph Hennings, '*Disputatio de origine animae* (CPL 623,37) – or the victory of creatianism in the fifth century', *Studia Patristica* 29 (1997), 260–8.

38 Heinrich Denzinger and Adolf Schönmetzer (eds.), *Enchiridion Symbolorum: Definitionum et Declarationum de Rebus Fidei et Morum*, 32nd edn (Freiburg, 1963), nos. 360–1.

39 *Didache* 2.2.

In the East, the second canon of Basil of Caesarea was fundamental to church teaching. This canon is contained in a letter of Basil to Amphilochus, composed around the same time as the wider debates concerning the key passage of Exodus (21:22–3), and when the *Apostolic Constitutions* were developing the instructions of the *Didache* to construct a more comprehensive set of church regulations. The injunction against abortion and infanticide was glossed and explained: 'because every configured being [*exeikonismenon*] having received from God a soul, if it is killed, will be avenged for having been unjustly put to death.'[40] Basil, significantly, adopted a different line. His canon stipulates: 'A woman who deliberately destroys a fetus is answerable for murder. Fine distinctions about whether it was formed (*ekmemorphōmenon*) or unconfigured (*anexeikoniston*) are not admissible amongst us.'[41] He justified his position by emphasizing the dangers to the woman's life in such cases, and finished by pleading for a mitigation of the punishment. Abortion was considered analogous to murder, whatever the status of the fetus, but the penance was for ten years rather than till death.

In the West, church practice, as attested by penitentials, and later by canon law, did take into account the stage of the pregnancy. The punishment was mitigated if the abortion occurred before the fortieth day, the fetus not being considered to have a human soul prior to this point. This approach, moreover, received canonical confirmation in the twelfth century: the *Decretum* of Gratian stipulates, 'He is not a murderer who provokes an abortion before the soul is infused into the body.'[42] It still took some time for regulation on these matters to pass from canon to state law, but the church was concerned with the issue from the outset.[43]

Other practical matters were at stake. In the Christian empire, the view that the fetus was animated could have had implications in the event of a perilous delivery, for instance, not only for abortion. Who has priority if the woman and the fetus are both ensouled? The question, however, does not seem to have been posed in this period: theologians, like physicians, simply allowed that the child, though endowed at this stage with a rational soul, be sacrificed to save the mother.[44] Such a child would be resurrected, Augustine averred. Indeed he asserted that the promise of resurrection includes formed fetuses which are aborted (and maybe the unformed too), as well as monstrous births, however brief their lives.[45] They will, moreover, be raised in proper human shape.

40 *Apostolic Constitutions* 7.3.2. 41 Basil, *Letters* 188, 2.

42 Gratian, *Decretum*, 2.32.2. 43 Mistry, *Abortion in the Early Middle Ages.*

44 Danielle Gourevitch, 'Chirurgie obstétricale dans le monde romain: Césarienne et embryotomie', in Véronique Dasen (ed.), *Naissance et petite enfance dans l'Antiquité …* (Fribourg, 2004), pp. 239–64.

45 *Enchiridion* 23.85–7.

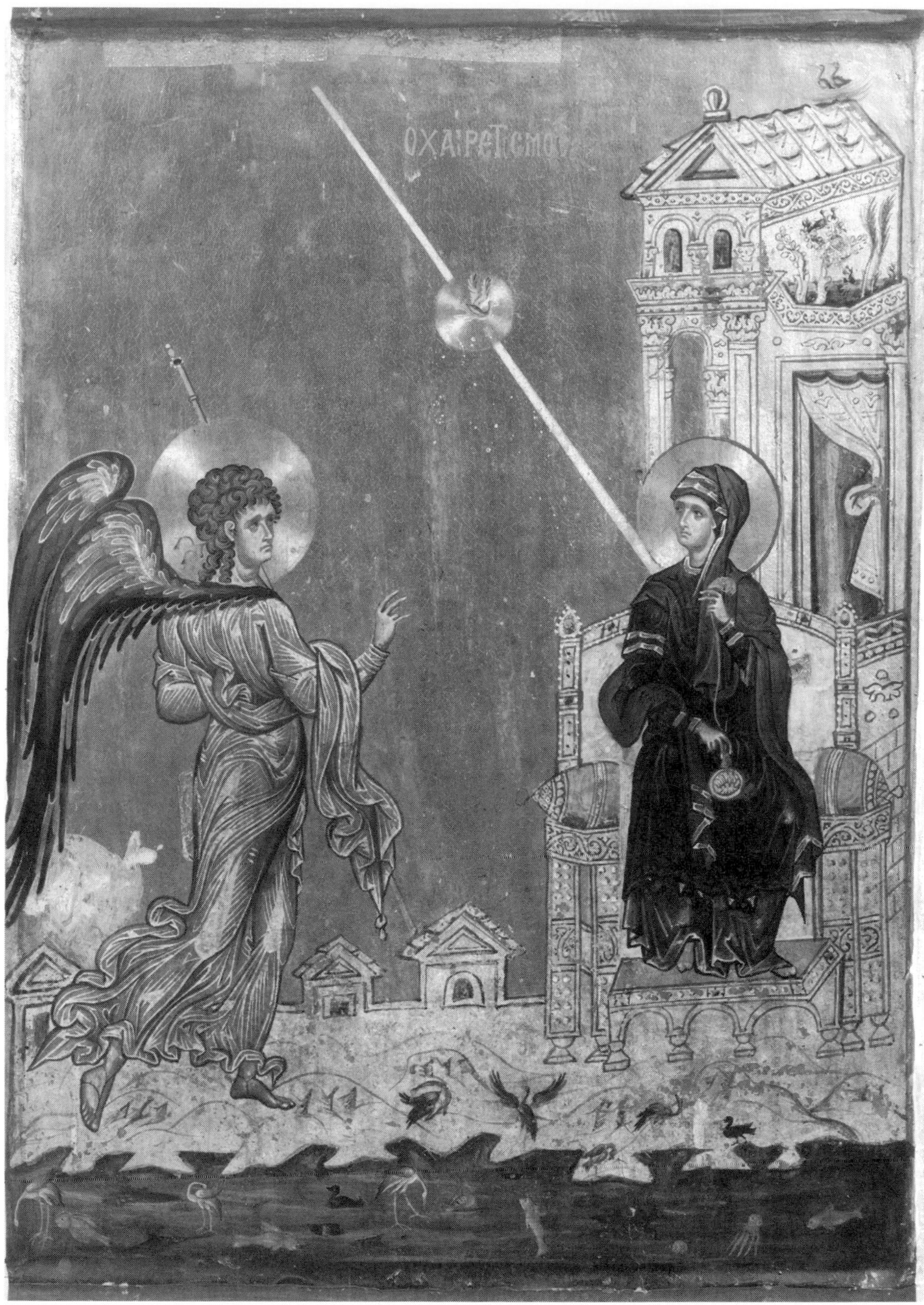

Figure 8.3 Twelfth-century Byzantine icon of the Annunciation. As the angel Gabriel tells Mary she will bear the son of God, the ghostly fetal Jesus, externally engendered by the Holy Spirit, is linked to the Virgin's womb by the (umbilical) thread she holds in her hands; he will be embodied within her. 61 × 42 cm. By permission of St Catherine's Monastery, Sinai, Egypt.

Conclusion

Debates over the soul of the fetus proliferated in the classical world. Neither the Neoplatonists nor the Christians started them; but Porphyry's treatise is the only known philosophical text dedicated to the issue, and Augustine's attention to the matter indicates its ongoing theological importance.[46] Much divided these two currents of thought (and neither was uniform itself), though both externalized the source of the soul to some degree, and both shared a divinely inspired approach to life more generally. Both thus participated in the distinctive discussions about fetal development of late antiquity; but the Christians came to dominate. The emergence and then ascendance of an anthropology marked by the theological concepts of creation and incarnation, built on the authority of scripture, reshaped these and other debates.

All Christian theologians understood the soul as created by God and infused by him into the body during gestation. They introduced a new notion into debates about the soul and its role in human generation, and their views gradually eclipsed those of their philosophical predecessors and interlocutors. But if the discussion became essentially theological, there was still much to discuss. The moments of the soul's creation and of its infusion remained controversial and inherited resources and assumptions played their part. The drama of ensoulment unfolded within a set of physical processes construed much as before – seeds and wombs are crucial, conception is followed by formation (and implicitly growth) – but it had become the overriding centre of attention, because of the relationship with God. Divergences of position within this debate diminished over time, particularly after Anastasius II imposed creatianism, already dominant in the East, on the West. No effort was made to enforce conformity about timing: a general commitment to ensoulment at conception characterized the East, delayed ensoulment the West. Neither perspective was decisive with respect to church rulings on abortion.

These changing concepts and evaluations shaped behaviour, however, because they were tied into a broader cosmological restructuring and helped to sanction certain church teachings about sex, marriage, procreation and the family. Christian imagery also offered new models to, and of, generative women by giving increasing prominence to cycles of motherhood, from conception (the Annunciation) through pregnancy (the Visitation) to birth (the Nativity) (Fig. 8.3).[47] Everything fitted together in the Christian world, however unevenly: conduct and experience shifted, along with attitudes and understandings.

46 See also James Wilberding, 'The revolutionary embryology of the Neoplatonists', *Oxford Studies in Ancient Philosophy* 49 (2015), 321–62.

47 On the early development of this imagery: Leslie Brubaker and Mary C. Cunningham (eds.), *The Cult of the Mother of God in Byzantium: Texts and Images* (Farnham, 2011).

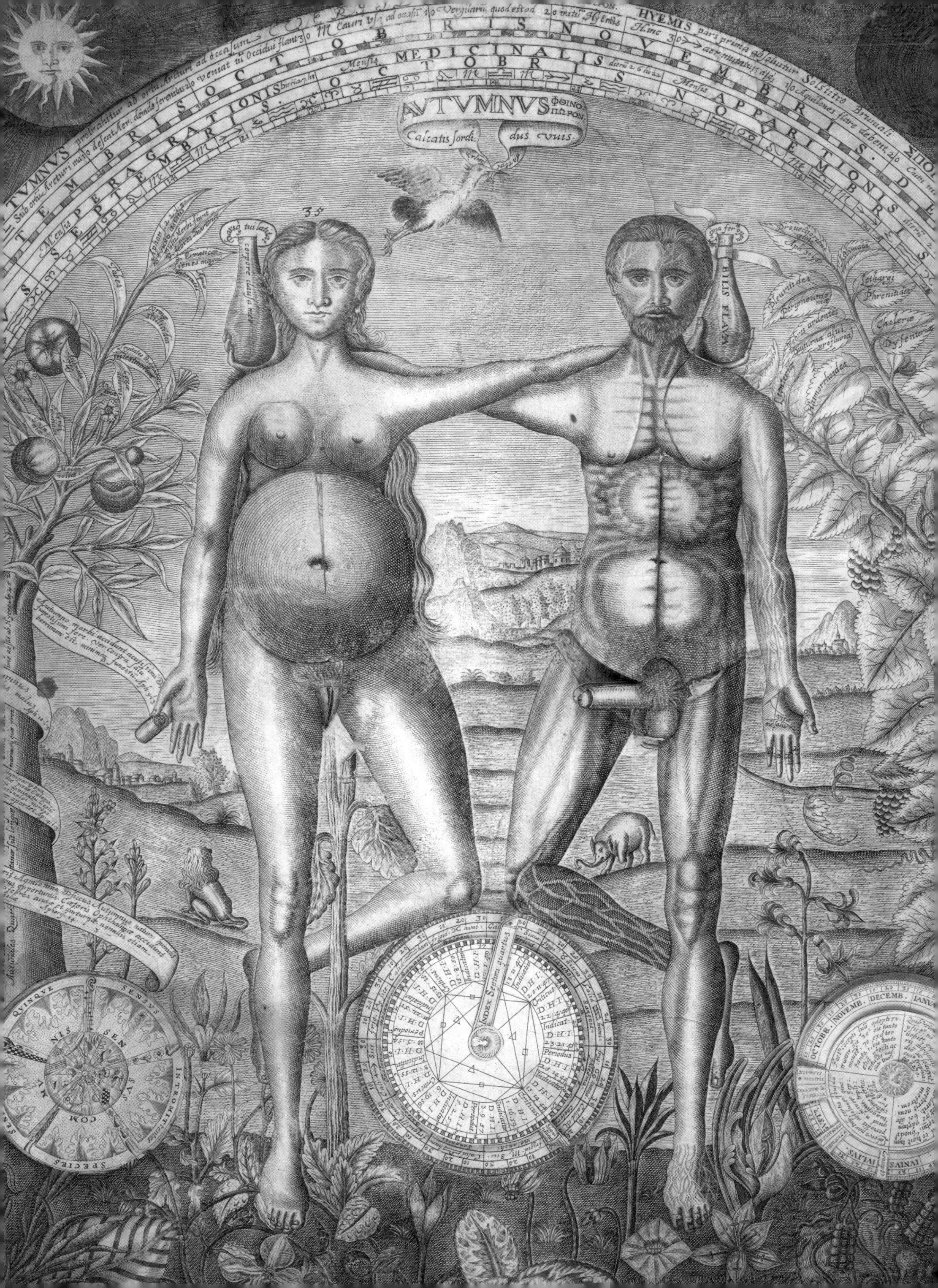

AVTVMNVS
Calcatis sordi- dus uvis
BILIS FLAVA
HYEMIS pars prima
Mensis MEDICINALIS
OCTOBRIS
NOVEMBRIS
SEPTEMBRIS
Lethargi
Phrenitides
Choleræ
Dysenteriæ
Hæmorrhoides
QUINQUE SENSUS
SPECIES
INTROMITTENTIS
OCTOBR.
NOVEMB.
DECEMB.

Part II

Generation Reborn and Reformed

'Autumn', represented by a mature man and pregnant woman, perhaps Adam and Eve, from a series of four copper plates of the stages of life. The work, produced in northern Europe around 1700, was assembled on pasteboard in multiple layers to form flaps and volvelles. Lifting the flaps reveals anatomical details linking the human body, the natural world and the cosmos via astrological, medical and alchemical symbols and imagery. The final flap in the woman's belly uncovers images of birth presentations that go back to late antiquity (Exhibit 10, this book). 51 × 41 cm. History of Medicine Collections, David M. Rubinstein Rare Book & Manuscript Library, Duke University.

Generation became a more pervasive intellectual and cultural framework between the sixth and the seventeenth centuries. Part II treats the millennium as a whole, considering the medieval and early modern periods together to assess long-term changes and continuities. During these eras of social, political and demographic upheaval, scholars brought about the 'rebirth' of ancient ideas and religious reformers sought to restore Christian doctrine to its true form. First refashioned by Arabic and Byzantine scholars, concepts of generation were reformulated within the medieval Christian church and nascent universities, then adapted in response to early modern European encounters with the New World, new methods of inquiry and new modes of communication. Similar changes occurred in the Islamicate Mediterranean, following its political fragmentation and then the rebuilding of the Mamluk and Ottoman Empires.

After the demise of the Western Roman Empire in the decades before 500, the lands ruled by its successor kingdoms became less populated, less urbanized and less connected than they had been for several centuries. A residue of classical medical and philosophical learning, rich with concerns about generation, persisted in writings by scholarly clergymen such as Isidore of Seville. In the Eastern Roman or Byzantine Empire, intellectuals first concentrated on establishing a Christian culture, then on compiling, reordering and retooling classical knowledge, before the more innovative revivals of the thirteenth century. Arab expansion continued after the death of Muhammad in 632 AD, extending the Islamicate world eastwards from Arabia and the Middle East to the borders of China and westwards through North Africa and into the Iberian peninsula. Especially from the eighth century, when numerous Greek works on medicine, philosophy, astrology and other topics began to be translated under the Abbasid Caliphate in Baghdad, classical learning flourished in Arabic. Scholars such as Ibn Sina (Avicenna) in eleventh-century central Asia and Ibn al-Nafis in thirteenth-century Egypt reworked and expanded debates about the importance of the female seed and the formation of the fetus (Nahyan Fancy, 'Generation in Medieval Islamic Medicine', Chapter 9). These ideas circulated in Renaissance Europe as this vital and dynamic engagement continued in the Ottoman Empire.

Ancient Greek and Roman and medieval Arabic views of generation spread through western Europe from the eleventh century. Urban centres grew, trade increased and monarchs aspired to unify Christendom. Where learned men gathered in cathedral schools and then universities, scholastic teachings encompassed questions ranging from how the cosmos was created to how minerals were formed. Efforts to join faith and reason and to reconcile Christian theology and ancient philosophy became foundations of Renaissance learning. Spurred by the mix of wealth, power and creativity in northern Italian courts and city-states in the fourteenth century, concerns about the making of polities and families took on new urgency as scholars studied Greek and

Latin works. Reassessing corrupted manuscripts so classical learning might be reborn, these 'humanists' reconstructed supposedly original texts through reason and empirical evidence. Their collections of observed and reported experiences both endorsed and challenged older authorities, notably Aristotle's ideas about the sequence of fetal formation and Galen's about the importance of female semen.

As commerce reconnected the Mediterranean world to northern Europe, Asia and Africa, it became vulnerable to the spread of disease along the trade routes. When a Mongol army besieged Caffa (modern Feodosia) in the Crimea in 1346, fleeing ships moved plague down the eastern Mediterranean to Constantinople and Alexandria. Starting in the Italian ports of Genoa and Venice in 1347, within a few years the Black Death had cut swathes through populations across Europe, North Africa and the Middle East. It took three centuries of living, working, praying, procreating and policing outbreaks of disease to restore the population to its levels during the boom of the twelfth and thirteenth centuries. Amidst the devastation, church authorities pondered the biblical imperative to increase and multiply, and instructed clergymen to counsel their parishioners about marriage and sex (Peter Biller, 'The Multitude in Later Medieval Thought', Chapter 10). Building on earlier texts about marriage, late medieval scholars argued that unions that produced healthy and beautiful children were essential to the generative success of a state and a family; before the Black Death, theologians had worried more about practices to avoid offspring than to foster fruitful marriages. Throughout the middle ages, parish, civic and state authorities considered notions of the multitude of people that sustained a locale against a number of departures or deaths, without counting total numbers of people, either as a balanced proportion between men and women or in censuses subject to statistical analysis. In the seventeenth century, philosophers and bureaucrats devised methods of political arithmetic that, when developed from the eighteenth century, were used to measure the processes that formed and sustained the groups of people – not breeding individuals – that made up a nation-state (Philip Kreager, 'The Emergence of Population', Chapter 18; Andrea Rusnock, 'Biopolitics and the Invention of Population', Chapter 23).

Medieval experts on church law had encouraged the notion of the marital debt: a binding obligation on spouses to honour one another's desires for sexual gratification. Informed by positive attitudes to sex in Arabic and Galenic texts, this idea was articulated as part of the concerted promotion of responsible procreation and prohibition of fornication (Maaike van der Lugt, 'Formed Fetuses and Healthy Children in Scholastic Theology, Medicine and Law', Chapter 12). Unnatural and unproductive inclinations were symbolized in emblems of sexually ambiguous animals (Gabriella Zuccolin, 'The Hermaphroditic Hyena', Exhibit 9). Families celebrated marriages as promising good, fruitful sex (Patricia Simons, 'Renaissance Art, Arousal and Impotence', Exhibit 12). Some husbands even recorded when their wives menstruated (Lauren Kassell, 'Jane

Dee's Courses in John Dee's Diary', Exhibit 14). Officially the union between husband and wife was sacrosanct, but men might have sex and sire progeny outside marriage, while such behaviour amongst women, even widows, was condemned as threatening the family honour and the strength of the line. Taking a different approach, Islamic law enabled the production of legitimate children with slaves as well as wives, and encompassed a wider set of debates about sexual and marital entitlements, including pleasure, and the avoidance and protection of offspring (Miri Shefer-Mossensohn and Rebecca Flemming, 'Generation in the Ottoman World', Chapter 19).

Lineage was paramount to moral, social and political order. From the arrangement of the household to the state of the nation, the Judaeo-Christian origin myth – the ultimate story of generation – was told and retold in medieval and early modern Europe. Intellectually and ethically dominant, it was adapted to local societies and cultures, and used to justify the political and economic transformations that changed the boundaries of the charted world and the distribution of people within it. Through sacred genealogies, Christians, appropriating Jewish tropes, reinforced patriarchal views of descent of power and property and defined themselves against Muslims and other non-Christians, including Jews. Medieval church windows depicted Christ's pedigree, and royal families linked their genealogies to his (Margot E. Fassler, 'The Tree of Jesse', Exhibit 8). Seventeenth-century paintings of mothers nursing their own infants echoed earlier images of the Virgin and child and idealized domestic and civic order (Lisa Forman Cody, 'A Painting of a Nursing Mother', Exhibit 19). Ancient ideas about how a mother's imagination might affect the appearance of her child persisted at least through the nineteenth century, permitting a lack of resemblance to be explained as the failure of a husband to master the actions or even thoughts of his disobedient wife (Mary E. Fissell, '*Aristotle's Masterpiece*', Exhibit 25). Silvia De Renzi pairs resemblance with dissimilarity to rethink this well-known example of continuity ('Family Resemblance in the Old Regime', Chapter 17). In tracts on the origins of nobility, medical advice for begetting children and paternity disputes, family likeness was a hinge connecting reflections on generation as a natural process and the changing relations between generations.

Much of the history of medieval and early modern pregnancy has been written through the lens of twentieth-century concerns about women's reproductive rights, and thus focuses on contraception, abortion, infanticide and childbirth. Though unwed women in the middle ages feared pregnancy, Katharine Park argues from the evidence of pastoral and legal documents that married people and their medical and moral advisors were more interested in promoting than limiting fertility ('Managing Childbirth and Fertility in Medieval Europe', Chapter 11). Questions about pregnancy, fertility and women's health defined the dynamics of early modern medical encounters (Lauren Kassell, 'Fruitful Bodies and Astrological Medicine', Chapter 16). Across the period and into later centuries, powerful words and objects harnessed natural sympathies and saintly powers to promote (and occasionally prohibit) fertility and birth; whether these methods were superstitious was long debated (Lea T. Olsan, 'A Medieval Birth Girdle', Exhibit 11; Sandra Cavallo, 'Pregnant Stones as Wonders of Nature', Exhibit 17). With a view to aiding births, surgeons and midwives revived and improved ancient knowledge and practice, including the use of taxonomies of fetal positions and birthing chairs (Lauren Kassell, 'Medieval Birth Malpresentations', Exhibit 10; Lianne McTavish, 'A Birthing Chair', Exhibit 18).

The explosions of writing, printing and tools for ordering information that facilitated the proliferation of ecclesiastical, scholarly and civic discourses about sex, procreation and lineage also contributed to increased use of the vernacular. As scholars began systematically to study natural particulars, artisans and women gained audiences alongside clergymen and statesmen, and often contested their authority. Practical knowledge of generation was collected and communicated in recipes and other bundles of information in manuscripts and printed books (Peter Murray Jones, 'Generation between Script and Print', Chapter 13). As householders and artisans assembled practical knowledge, priests encouraged parishioners to engage in devotion focused on Mary and the holy family. Protestant reformers – in the movement later labelled the Reformation – urged their flocks to seek signs of godliness within themselves and in their daily works. Many declared the end of the age of miracles and, for Protestants and Catholics alike, episodes ranging from spontaneous generation to monstrous births became occasions to redefine the explanatory boundaries between divine, demonic and natural causality (Jennifer Spinks, 'Monstrous Births and Diabolical Seed', Exhibit 13).

Over the past fifty years, historians have emphasized the practices of natural knowledge and revised older constructions of the 'Scientific Revolution' as a triumph of rationality and the Enlightenment as a disenchantment of the world. Concentrating on who knew what about generation and how this knowledge was communicated helps to complicate these narratives. Emerging accounts explore collaborations alongside conflicts between different kinds of medical practitioners, and doctors' and patients' shared as well as divergent understandings of health and illness. Vernacular and learned traditions shaped one another, as did knowledge and practice. Within families and households discussions of generation might cross social, gender and generational boundaries. Local habits were often defined against historical traditions or norms dictated by central authorities. The limits of what could and could not be known about the workings of God and nature shifted together with the means to discover them.

The greatest innovations in generation came not in assisting conception or childbirth, baptizing infants, building families or measuring multitudes, but in concerted efforts by people from an increasingly broad social spectrum to understand generation and use it to explain moral, social and political orders. One pressing question was what made a child. Following ancient authorities, there was general agreement that the constituent parts of the fetus were seed, soul and material sustenance (Rebecca Flemming, 'Galen's Generations of Seeds', Chapter 7; Marie-Hélène Congourdeau, 'Debating the Soul in Late Antiquity', Chapter 8), but theologians, natural philosophers and physicians debated what kinds of generative matter each parent contributed. In medieval and early modern legal tribunals from east to west, disputes centred on when the soul entered the fetus, be it at 30, 40, 80 or even 120 days, since this was a necessary premise from which to adjudicate certain cases of inheritance and murder. Seed, moreover, served as a long-running locus for philosophical discussion about vital forces, especially innate heat and radical moisture, from antiquity through the seventeenth century (Gianna Pomata, 'Innate Heat, Radical Moisture and Generation', Chapter 14). Generation posed the decisive challenge for early modern anatomists, and they combined reason, experiment and visual observation – of humans, animals and eggs – in investigations of conception and gestation (Karin Ekholm, 'Pictures and Analogies in the Anatomy of Generation', Chapter 15; Ekholm, 'A Placenta Painted and Engraved', Exhibit 15; Rina Knoeff, 'The Generative Parts of Women', Exhibit 16). Aspects of these processes would remain hidden for at least another century, but by 1700 they were widely debated in relation to sex, race, family and state.

LAUREN KASSELL

9 Generation in Medieval Islamic Medicine

Nahyan Fancy

Any discussion of medicine in the medieval Islamic world, particularly after the Mongol invasions, has to confront at least two assumptions. The first is that Islamic medical texts sanctified 'the Hippocratic and Galenic writings' and 'recycled [their] content'.[1] The second is that medical commentaries restricted themselves to explaining and interpreting 'the tradition' rather than elaborating 'something new'.[2] The combined effect is to depict Arabic texts as mere vehicles for transmitting Greek knowledge to Latin Europe. Though this perception has been challenged for decades, it persists because of resilient disciplinary commitments to the uniformity and universality of science.[3] Scientific developments in the Islamic world are often evaluated using the metric of 'modern science', as if one cannot move beyond Galen without arriving at William Harvey. Once we shed these assumptions, we can understand the Islamic discussions of generation on their own terms and chart their specific trajectories.

Generation is discussed across a wide variety of sources from the medieval Islamic world – the region spanning from the southwestern end of the Mediterranean to the Oxus and Indus rivers during the period between the founding of Baghdad in the eighth century and the conquest of Constantinople in the fifteenth. These sources include medical, philosophical, astrological and religious texts, such as the Quran and its exegeses, hadith (Prophetic traditions) and their commentaries, legal responsa, and even *adab* (belle-lettres) literature, such as advice tracts on conceiving and child-rearing. Consequently, historians have not yet mapped the diversity of views, but have focused on correcting certain western academic misrepresentations. For example, Basim Musallam's *Sex and Society* used a broad range of sources to argue, against western demographers, for the absence of any blanket restrictions on birth control in Islamic societies before 1800. Musallam also examined the religious appropriation of

1 Hormoz Ebrahimnejad, 'Medicine in Islam and Islamic medicine', in Mark Jackson (ed.), *The Oxford Handbook of the History of Medicine* (Oxford, 2011), pp. 169–89, on p. 184.

2 Manfred Ullmann, *Islamic Medicine* (Edinburgh, 1978), p. 71. For a critique: Nahyan Fancy, 'Medical commentaries: A preliminary examination of Ibn al-Nafis's *Shuruh*, the *Mujaz* and commentaries on the *Mujaz*', *Oriens* 41 (2013), 525–45.

3 For a critique of these commitments, see Peter Harrison, '"Science" and "religion": Constructing the boundaries', *Journal of Religion* 86 (2006), 81–106; and Sonja Brentjes with Robert Morrison, 'The sciences in Islamic societies (750–1800)', in Robert Irwin (ed.), *The New Cambridge History of Islam*, vol. 4: *Islamic Cultures and Societies to the End of the Eighteenth Century* (Cambridge, 2010), pp. 564–639.

scientific discussions of generation in order to dispute essentialist claims about Islam's opposition to science.[4] Sherry Gadelrab questioned the relevance of Thomas Laqueur's 'one-sex model' for understanding the establishment of gender hierarchies in Islamic societies, thus adding to the many critiques of this work.[5] Historians have addressed the novelty of some of the objections raised against 'Greek antecedent theories' in respect to generation, thus disrupting standard narratives of medieval Islamic science as a static repository of Greek knowledge in this area too.[6]

An obvious lacuna in the secondary literature is the absence of discussion of medical works composed after 1200.[7] Reflecting a commitment to the 'decline' thesis, the extensive medical commentary tradition of this period, specifically on Ibn Sina's (Avicenna's) *Canon of Medicine* (*c.* 1025), is usually dismissed as uncritical reproductions of earlier knowledge.[8] Yet the commentators advanced new understandings of generation that broke the confines of earlier Graeco-Arabic thought. This chapter highlights these new understandings. The medical commentaries provided the immediate intellectual context for fourteenth-century Islamic religious discussions, as well as medical accounts of generation in the Latin Renaissance – both of which have hitherto been portrayed as depending solely on earlier Hippocratic and Galenic theories. I shall focus on physiological understandings of generation, and not address related issues such as sex differentiation, midwifery, breast-feeding or astrology.[9] I hope nonetheless to offer a model for future examinations of the diversity of discourses on generation across the chronological and geographical expanse of the Islamic world.[10]

4 B. F. Musallam, *Sex and Society in Islam: Birth Control before the Nineteenth Century* (Cambridge, 1983); Musallam, 'The human embryo in Arabic scientific and religious thought', in Peter Pormann (ed.), *Islamic Medical and Scientific Tradition* (London, 2010), vol. 2, pp. 317–31; Julia Bummel, 'Human biological reproduction in the medicine of the Prophet: The question of the provenance and formation of semen', ibid., pp. 332–41.

5 Sherry Sayed Gadelrab, 'Discourses on sex differences in medieval scholarly Islamic thought', *Journal of the History of Medicine and Allied Sciences* 66 (2010), 40–81.

6 Ahmad Dallal, 'Sexualities: Scientific discourses, premodern: Overview', in Suad Joseph (ed.), *Encyclopedia of Women and Islamic Cultures*, vol. 3: *Family, Body, Sexuality and Health* (Leiden, 2005), pp. 401–7, on p. 406; Musallam, 'Human embryo'.

7 Gadelrab, 'Sex differences', briefly examines Ibn al-Nafis's anatomical discussions.

8 For critiques of the view that the commentary tradition stunted scientific development: Asad Ahmed and Margaret Larkin (eds.), 'The *Hashiya* and Islamic intellectual history', special issue, *Oriens* 41 (2013).

9 Paula Sanders, 'Gendering the ungendered body: Hermaphrodites in medieval Islamic law', in Nikki R. Keddie and Beth Baron (eds.), *Women in Middle Eastern History: Shifting Boundaries in Sex and Gender* (New Haven, CT, 1992), pp. 74–95; Avner Giladi, *Infants, Parents and Wet Nurses: Medieval Islamic Views on Breastfeeding and their Social Implications* (Leiden, 1999); Giladi, *Muslim Midwives: The Craft of Birthing in the Premodern Middle East* (Cambridge, 2015); Liana Saif, 'The universe and the womb: Generation, conception, and the stars in Islamic medieval astrological and medical texts', *Journal of Arabic and Islamic Studies* 16 (2016), 181–98.

10 Contrary to Kathryn Kueny's approach in *Conceiving Identities: Maternity in Medieval Muslim Discourse and Practice* (Albany, NY, 2013).

The modern science and religion dichotomy is not useful for understanding the medieval Islamic sources. The Arabic term '*ʿilm*' was used in this period for all forms of organized knowledge, from mathematics to principles of religion (*usul al-din*). Disciplines that we place under the religious category, such as principles of religion, were often categorized under rational sciences, along with medicine and natural science (*al-ʿilm al-tabiʿi*).[11] Moreover, gatherings where intellectual topics were discussed and *ʿilm* acquired – whether in courtly circles, scholars' homes or institutions such as the madrasa – were comprised of scholars and students with varying degrees of expertise across the sciences. Some established jurists and theologians also practised medicine, such as the thirteenth-century Syro-Egyptian physician-jurist, Ibn al-Nafis.[12] My use of 'science/scientific' and 'religion/religious' is thus meant only as a shorthand to refer to works or groups of scholars rather than to posit the existence of sharp dichotomies.

The Avicennan Paradigm

Ibn Sina's works revolutionized medicine, philosophy and the sciences.[13] His *Canon of Medicine* and a philosophical compendium, the *Healing*, became key texts for post-1200 scientific and religious discussions of generation in the Islamic world and, later, Latin Europe. In them, Ibn Sina built upon earlier Hippocratic, Aristotelian and Galenic texts, all of which were translated into Arabic during the ninth century and reworked by tenth-century Persian luminaries such as al-Razi (Rhazes) and al-Majusi (Haly Abbas).[14] Ibn Sina focused on four aspects of the ancient disputes on generation: the nature of the female contribution; the make-up of seminal matter; the precise role played by the male semen; and the identity of the first member formed in the fetus. Ibn Sina's contributions to these disputes were further developed in commentaries on the *Canon* and its abridgements, such as the *Epitome* (*Mujaz*).[15] Medical commentators often incorporated the more philosophical discussions from the *Healing* into their works.

11 Sonja Brentjes, 'On the location of the ancient or "rational" sciences in Muslim educational landscapes (AH 500–1100)', *Bulletin of the Royal Institute of Inter-Faith Studies* 4 (2002), 47–71.

12 Nahyan Fancy, *Science and Religion in Mamluk Egypt: Ibn al-Nafis, Pulmonary Transit and Bodily Resurrection* (London, 2013).

13 Y. Tzvi Langermann (ed.), *Avicenna and His Legacy: A Golden Age of Science and Philosophy* (Turnhout, 2009).

14 Dallal, 'Sexualities', p. 402; on al-Majusi, see also Monica H. Green, 'The transmission of ancient theories of female physiology and disease through the early middle ages', unpublished PhD thesis, Princeton University (1985), pp. 109–17; and on the ancient theories, Helen King, 'Women and Doctors in Ancient Greece', Chapter 3; Laurence M. V. Totelin, 'Animal and Plant Generation in Classical Antiquity', Chapter 4; and Rebecca Flemming, 'Galen's Generations of Seeds', Chapter 7, this book.

15 Fancy, 'Medical commentaries'.

Although the *Healing* provides the necessary proofs for Ibn Sina's complete account of generation, the *Canon* contains most of his final positions. Here Ibn Sina confirmed the existence of female generative organs (*unthayan*) and concluded not only that they produce semen (*mani*), but that women also have to experience orgasm in order to release it.[16] He affirmed that, in both sexes, semen is the residue of the fourth digestion, which is extracted by a species of the generative faculty in the generative organs.[17] The fetus is generated when both semens mix in the womb, where the male semen plays the role of rennet and the female semen that of milk in the fermentation of cheese – an analogy taken from Aristotle's *Generation of Animals*.[18] Ibn Sina also agreed with Aristotle that the first member generated in the fetal body is the heart, though his explanation relied on the changes he instituted in physiology.[19]

Most importantly, Ibn Sina reconceptualized the entire ancient dispute over the process of generation. He asserted that the fetus (*janin*) develops in distinct stages.[20] That is, the fetus relinquishes and receives forms instantaneously from the Giver of Forms (*wahib al-suwar*) during gestation. For example, when the fetus is like a drop of fluid, it grows in its dimensions before 'jumping' to the next stage by adopting the form of a blood-clot. As Ibn Sina explained in the *Canon*, 'The third state is the alteration of the semen into the blood-clot (*'alaqa*), and after that is its alteration into the lump of flesh (*mudgha*) … For each alteration, or two alterations, there is a period of time when [the developing fetus] stays at rest in [that state]'.[21]

Ibn Sina's fits-and-starts model of fetal development mirrored the dominant interpretation of the following quranic verses on generation:

> Indeed, We created humans from an essence of clay.
> Then We placed him as a drop (*nutfa*) in a safe place.
> Then We made the drop into a blood-clot (*'alaqa*); then We made the blood-clot into a lump of flesh (*mudgha*); then We made the lump of flesh into bones; then We clothed the bones with flesh; then We brought him out as another creation. Glory be to God, the best of the creators! (Quran 23.12–14, my translation)

Earlier exegetes had interpreted these verses as implying that God fashions the fetus in distinct stages, thus proving His omnipotence and His ability to resurrect people after

16 Dallal, 'Sexualities', pp. 402–4; Gadelrab, 'Sex differences', pp. 62–5. I have translated '*unthayan*' as generative organs because the term 'testicles' with its Latin root, '*teste*', does not capture the Arabic meaning. The Arabic term is the dual form of '*untha*', which means female and comes from the verb '*anutha*', to become female or feminine. See Edward William Lane, *Arabic-English Lexicon* (London, 1863), s.v. ''-n-th'.

17 Ibn Sina, *al-Qanun fi al-tibb*, notes by Muhammad Amin al-Dinnawi (Beirut, 1999), vol. 1, pp. 95–6 and vol. 2, pp. 726–7.

18 Ibid., vol. 1, p. 39.

19 Ibid., vol. 2, p. 756; Fancy, *Science and Religion*, pp. 84–8.

20 Jon McGinnis, *Avicenna* (Oxford, 2010), pp. 42–8, 238–43.

21 Ibn Sina, *al-Qanun*, vol. 2, p. 757.

death. Many exegetes and legal scholars interpreted the phrase 'We then brought him out as another creation' (Quran 23.14) as marking the point at which the developing fetus became a true human being.[22] Ibn Sina was in accord with scripture, signalled by his use of the quranic terms for two stages, '*ʿalaqa*' and '*mudgha*'. He thus departed from earlier practices of Arabic translators of the Hippocratic treatises and physicians such as al-Majusi.[23] After Ibn Sina, quranic exegetes and medical scholars often co-opted each other's terminology and engaged with each other's accounts of generation.

In the *Healing*, Ibn Sina differentiated between his two-seed theory and Galen's. He argued that since the female semen does not leave the body, properly speaking it is not semen, but rather a type of ripened menstrual blood.[24] Ibn Sina also attacked Galen for maintaining that both male and female semen have the active (*muwallida*) and passive faculties (*mutawallida*) of generation because that would imply that a fetus could be generated from just one of them. As he stated, 'when there is no action, there cannot be a faculty [for that action]'. Ibn Sina thus declared that the female semen cannot possess the active faculty, and the male semen cannot possess the passive faculty (that is, cannot contribute materially to the fetus).[25]

The questions that interested Ibn Sina, and the solutions he proposed, differed from those of the ancients. Ibn Sina's understanding of generation was rooted in his larger philosophical and theological system, and the intellectual contexts of medieval Islamic societies.[26] Later Arabic commentators considered some of these issues to have been definitively resolved, such as the existence of female semen, or the development of the fetus in distinct stages, both of which had very strong precedents in the religious literature.[27] Yet other aspects of his theory, such as how semen is formed or the precise contribution of the male semen, remained contested. Moreover, Ibn Sina's understanding of the faculties of generation and the formative role of male semen raised further

22 al-Tabari, *Tafsir al-Tabari: Jamiʿ al-bayan ʿan taʾwil al-qurʾan*, ed. ʿAbd Allah ibn ʿAbd al-Muhsin al-Turki (Cairo, 2001), vol. 17, pp. 21–5; Marion Katz, 'The problem of abortion in classical Sunni fiqh', in Jonathan Brockopp (ed.), *Islamic Ethics of Life: Abortion, War, and Euthanasia* (Columbia, SC, 2003), pp. 25–50.

23 Hippocrates, *On Embryos (On the Sperm and the Nature of the Child)*, ed. and trans. M. C. Lyons and J. N. Matlock (Cambridge, 1978); *Trois traités d'anatomie arabes par Muhammed ibn Zakariyya al-Razi, ʿAli ibn al-ʿAbbas et ʿAli ibn Sina: Textes inédits de deux traités*, trans. P. De Koning (Leiden, 1903), p. 406. The physician al-Tabari (d. after 855) used *mudgha*, but not *ʿalaqa*; see his *Firdaws al-Hikma fi al-tibb*, ed. M. Z. Siddiqi (Berlin, 1928), p. 32.

24 Ibn Sina, *al-Shifaʾ: al-Tabiʿiyyat, 8. al-Hayawan*, ed. ʿAbd al-Halim Mustansir, Saʿid Zayed and ʿAbdallah Ismaʿil (Cairo, 1970), IX.3, pp. 158–64.

25 Ibid., pp. 161–2.

26 McGinnis, *Avicenna*, pp. 3–4. Compare Marie-Hélène Congourdeau, 'Debating the Soul in Late Antiquity', Chapter 8, this book.

27 The notable exception is the twelfth-century Andalusian philosopher-jurist, Ibn Rushd (Averroes), who reverted to a stricter Aristotelianism and denied any formative role in generation to female semen; Dallal, 'Sexualities', pp. 402–3.

problems. The latter issue resulted from Avicennan physiology, which connected the faculties more directly to a soul-substance.[28] The identification of the soul responsible for governing fetal nutrition and growth, which also had religious ramifications, thus emerged as a central medical concern in the fourteenth century.

Ensoulment in the Medical Commentaries

In the era of the Mamluks that spanned the mid-thirteenth to early sixteenth centuries, the key figure for debates on generation was the aforementioned Ibn al-Nafis, who wrote a lemmatic commentary, following an established form of quoting and expounding one passage at a time, on the entire *Canon of Medicine*. His *Commentary on the Canon* (*c.* 1242), and an abridged *Epitome*, were the fundamental texts of learned medicine in this period. Ibn al-Nafis also had many students who went on to train other physicians in the region.[29] He and his works were extolled by a group of religious scholars, specifically those associated with the fourteenth-century, conservative theologian-jurist, Ibn Taymiyya. They created a new genre of Prophetic medicine wherein they argued for the harmony between medical treatments found in the Quran and hadith and Graeco-Arabic medical theory and practice.[30]

Ibn al-Nafis's critical engagement with the Avicennan account of generation was rooted in the larger debates over reason and revelation prevalent in thirteenth-century Syria and Egypt. The critique centred on two aspects of Ibn Sina's account. The first was Ibn Sina's characterization of the generative organs as the sources of two types of faculties.[31] The second was Ibn Sina's assertion that the male semen possesses active faculties through which it fashions the female semen (and menstrual blood) into a new fetal body.

Ibn al-Nafis rejected the claim that two types of faculties originate in the generative organs: one type to generate semen (generative); the other type to generate the fetus. The latter included two distinct faculties: one to prepare the parts of the semen to receive specific forms of bodily members (first transformative faculty); and another to attach these forms to their respective seminal parts (*musawwira*, meaning formative faculty).[32] He argued that semen is not extracted by the generative faculty, but rather is the residue of the nourishment of the generative organs themselves, just like milk is the residue of

28 Fancy, *Science and Religion*, pp. 69–88.

29 *The Theologus Autodidactus of Ibn al-Nafis*, ed. and trans. Joseph Schacht and Max Meyerhof (Oxford, 1968), pp. 1–19, 75–7.

30 Irmeli Perho, *The Prophet's Medicine: A Creation of the Muslim Traditionalist Scholars* (Helsinki, 1995); Fancy, *Science and Religion*, pp. 23–5.

31 Ibn Sina, *al-Qanun*, vol. 1, pp. 94–5.

32 For Ibn Sina, the formative faculty does not originate in the generative organs but is directly emanated from the Giver of Forms to the prepared seminal matter in the womb.

the nourishment of the breasts.[33] He agreed with Ibn Sina that semen is a residue of the fourth digestion, but clarified that it is the fourth digestion of the generative organs themselves. The material from which the semen is generated, on the other hand, is received by the generative organs from all parts of the body. The secondary fluid, which is found spread across all parts of the body as dew, is vaporized by the heat of each body part and ascends to the brain. There it cools and descends in the veins behind the ears, through the spinal marrow, ultimately joining with the veins proceeding from the kidneys to the generative organs. The natural faculties of the generative organs act upon this mixture, producing semen as a residual excess.[34] With this exposition, Ibn al-Nafis introduced a key component of the Hippocratic theory of seminal formation without adhering to the view that semen was formed by drawing a piece from every part of the body.

As for the first transformative and formative faculties, Ibn al-Nafis accepted their existence but rejected the notion that they emanated from the male generative organs. He wondered, 'how is it possible [for] the semen [to] stay connected to the father's soul' once it is expelled from the father's body, when a hand loses its connection to the soul and degenerates once it is severed?[35] He concluded that neither the male nor the female semen have active faculties. Instead, they both possess specific temperaments (the male is hot and dry, the female cold and moist) that when mixed together in the womb attain a temperament suitable for the emanation of the new human soul from God. Once that soul is connected to this seminal mixture, it emanates these two faculties of generation, along with the remaining natural faculties, to generate the new fetal body.[36]

The immediate impact of Ibn al-Nafis's criticisms is evident in the work of his younger colleague, the famous Christian physician and surgeon Ibn al-Quff. He concurred with Ibn al-Nafis that the male semen cannot possess the two active faculties. Yet, instead of claiming that the rational soul is emanated at conception, he argued that it is emanated to the fetus only after all the vital organs are formed, a process that takes approximately forty days. In the meantime, the soul of the mother (*nafs ummihi*) emanates the transformative and formative faculties and administers the development of the fetus.[37]

Ibn al-Quff's ascription of the active role to the mother in generation is also found in commentaries on the *Epitome* of Ibn al-Nafis by the fourteenth-century Anatolian philosopher-theologian, Jamal al-Din al-Aqsaraʾi, and the fifteenth-century Persian physician, Nafis ibn ʿIwad al-Kirmani. Both commentaries were popular in

33 Ibn al-Nafis, *Sharh al-Qanun*, Wellcome Library, MS Or. 51, ff. 60b3–4, 447b36–448a2.

34 Ibn al-Nafis, *Sharh tashrih al-Qanun*, ed. Salman Qataya and Paul Ghalioungui (Cairo, 1988), pp. 434–5.

35 Ibn al-Nafis, *Sharh al-Qanun*, f. 60b4–7.

36 Ibid., ff. 60b4, 449a1–11. He considered and rejected the possibility that the mother's soul could provide these faculties: f. 448b24 ff.

37 Ibn al-Quff, *Jamiʿ al-gharad fi hifz al-sihha wa-dafʿ al-marad*, ed. Sami Harmaneh (Amman, 1989), pp. 120–1.

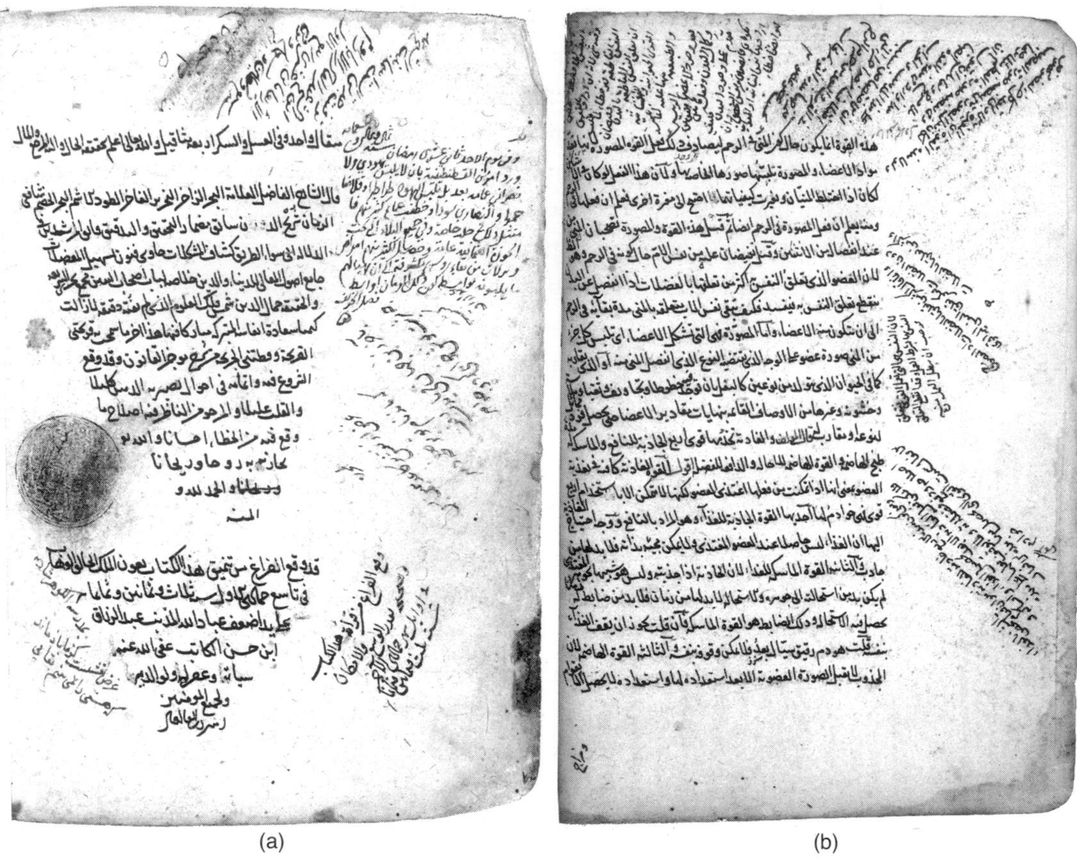

Figure 9.1 Jamal al-Din al-Aqsara'i's manuscript commentary, *Hall al-Mujaz* (The resolution of the epitome). (a) The colophon, which certifies that the copy was completed in 1478 at the Gawhar Shad madrasa, built in Herat, modern-day Afghanistan, about a half-century before. (b) The marginal comment in the top-left-hand corner, which quotes al-Kirmani's *Commentary on the Epitome*, set against the passage in the text on the particular soul responsible for emanating the active faculties of generation to semen. MS Huntington 596, f. 18b, by permission of the Bodleian Libraries, University of Oxford.

Islamic societies until the nineteenth century (Fig. 9.1).[38] Their discussions of generation explicitly combined Ibn al-Nafis's critique of Ibn Sina and Ibn al-Quff's solution: first, by paraphrasing the former ('how is it possible for the soul of the father to stay connected to the semen while it remains in the womb and the parts are generated from it?'); and then, by endorsing Ibn al-Quff's position ('the [first] transformative and formative faculties … are emanated only from the soul of the mother, and their point of origin is the generative organs of the mother').[39]

38 Fancy, 'Medical commentaries', p. 528.

39 Jamal al-Din al-Aqsara'i, *Kitab Hall al-Mujaz*, Wellcome Library, MS Arabic 202, ff. 19b19–20a2; Burhan al-Din Nafis ibn 'Iwad al-Kirmani, *Kulliyat al-Sharh al-Nafisi li-Mujaz al-Qanun* (India, 1904), p. 24.

Thus, Mamluk-era medical commentaries reached a growing consensus over the existence of female semen, the material contribution of the male semen to generation and the development of the fetus in distinct stages. Moreover, the quranic terms for the stages appear freely amidst increasing agreement that the fetus completes its *mudgha* stage forty days after conception. However, debate continued over the timing of fetal ensoulment (conception, forty days or eighty days) and the process of seminal formation. On the last issue, Ibn al-Quff and many other commentators sided with Ibn Sina, though a few, such as al-Kirmani, explicitly defended Ibn al-Nafis's quasi-Hippocratic account, using the analogy of seminal formation to that of milk in the breasts.[40] The religious scholars' explanations of generation built upon these new medical discussions.

Two-Seed Theory and Ensoulment in Traditionalist Circles

Syrian and Egyptian traditionalists associated with Ibn Taymiyya composed new texts on Prophetic medicine starting in the fourteenth century. As part of this project, Ibn Qayyim al-Jawziyya and al-Dhahabi reconciled medical accounts of generation with scriptural depictions. Their writings in turn informed those of their students, such as Ibn Kathir's quranic exegesis, and later were cited explicitly by fifteenth-century Egyptian traditionalists, such as Ibn Hajar al-ʿAsqalani and Jalal al-Din al-Suyuti.

Ibn Qayyim cited contemporaneous medical discussions of generation in his *Commentary on the Oaths of the Quran*: 'Most [physicians] … say that the [fetus] is generated from both semens, and then they are divided into two groups … The second of them says that the members, parts and form are generated from both together, after they mix and temper each other and become one fluid. This is the correct position.'[41] Since a growing majority of Mamluk-era medical commentators agreed, Ibn Qayyim was accurately describing his contemporary medical scene and not relying solely on earlier Hippocratic texts.[42]

Ibn Qayyim's *Oaths* depart even more strikingly from Hippocratic orthodoxy in their refutation of Aristotle's criticism of the Hippocratic account of seminal formation.[43] To Aristotle's objection that if semen was formed by drawing a piece from every

40 al-Kirmani, *Kulliyat al-Sharh*, p. 24.

41 Ibn Qayyim al-Jawziyya, *al-Tibyan fi ayman al-qur'an*, ed. ʿAbdallah ibn Salim al-Batati (Makkah, n.d.), pp. 529–30. See also Cyril Elgood's translation of al-Dhahabi's treatise: 'Tibb-ul-Nabbi or medicine of the Prophet', *Osiris* 14 (1962), 33–192, on 166; and Jalal al-Din al-Suyuti, *al-Minhaj al-sawi wa-l-munhal al-rawi fi al-tibb al-nabawi*, Wellcome Library, MS Arabic 447, ff. 10a–11a.

42 Contrary to Musallam, 'Human embryo', pp. 320–2; and Bummel, 'Human biological reproduction', pp. 335–6.

43 Ibn Qayyim, *al-Tibyan*, pp. 492–502.

part of the body, the semen would in fact be a small animal, Ibn Qayyim responded: 'If you mean by [the semen being a small animal], that it is so actually (*bi-l-fiʿl*), then that is not the case. But if you are implying by this that it is so potentially (*bi-l-quwwa*), then yes. And what prohibits that! [After all,] the semen is a small animal, nay a large one potentially.'[44]

For Ibn Qayyim, the semen is drawn from every part of the body, even if the bit that is drawn is not the body part in miniature. This argument builds upon Ibn al-Nafis's modification of Hippocratic theory: that the material from which semen is generated is drawn from the entire body, albeit as shapeless fluid. Though not the dominant account at the time, some medical commentators accepted Ibn al-Nafis's views on seminal formation.[45] Ibn Qayyim and other religious scholars were thus engaging with contemporary medical disputes, and using scripture to inform and support specific scientific accounts.[46]

On ensoulment, the traditionalists parted from the medical commentators, but continued to engage with them in two ways. First, medical writers contested the timing of fetal ensoulment and the identity of the soul that governs its early development. Ibn Qayyim intervened, claiming that this point can 'only be known through revelation'.[47] He pointed to a Prophetic tradition from the ninth-century collection, Bukhari's *Sahih* (Hadith) – a canonical collection of traditions, which specified that each quranic stage takes forty days to complete.[48] The fetus is a drop of fluid (*nutfa*) for forty days, then a blood-clot (*ʿalaqa*) and a piece of flesh (*mudgha*) for identical periods, only after which (at 120 days) the spirit/soul (*ruh*) is blown into the fetus.[49] Although historians used to cite this tradition as evidence that abortion was legally permissible within the first four months throughout the medieval period, a closer reading suggests that the tradition was more actively invoked after Ibn Sina.[50] Earlier legal scholars, for example, preferred to use criteria such as the dissolution of a blood-clot or the visibility of limbs to determine the 'humanity' of a fetus.[51] Establishing fetal 'humanity' was important for certain civil cases, such as tort and inheritance. Pre-Avicennan quranic exegetes also preferred a different canonical tradition for ensoulment, which refers to its taking place after forty days.[52]

44 Ibid., p. 502. 45 al-Aqsaraʾi, *Hall al-Mujaz*, f. 203a. 46 Elgood, 'Tibb-ul-Nabbi', p. 166.

47 Ibn Qayyim, *al-Tibyan*, p. 507. 48 Ibid., pp. 507–9.

49 '*Ruh*' in the medical literature means spirit, that is, a subtle vapour that acts as the material substrate for the faculties. In the religious literature, '*ruh*' is equated with '*nafs*' (soul), and is the preferred term for a person's soul or identity: Fancy, *Science and Religion*, p. 57 n. 136.

50 Musallam, *Sex and Society*, pp. 57–9; Katz, 'Problem of abortion', pp. 31–2.

51 Katz, 'Problem of abortion'; Miri Shefer-Mossensohn and Rebecca Flemming, 'Generation in the Ottoman World', Chapter 19, this book.

52 al-Tabari, *Jamiʿ*, vol. 16, p. 461.

Second, the traditionalists engaged with medical commentaries in their understanding of what ensoulment entails. Ibn Sina, and many commentators, had followed Hippocratic writings in maintaining that the fetus begins to move around the eightieth day. Ibn Qayyim rejected this standard characterization of movement ('quickening'), stating: 'This is all patently false … The fetus does not possess movement before 120 days, and whatever motion is ascribed to it prior to that is not its own volitional motion, but rather accidental motion'.[53] Medical commentators unanimously accepted that the soul is the source of volitional motion in the fetus. This linking of ensoulment and movement, and the rejection of any wilful movement by the fetus prior to 120 days, seems to be a post-Avicennan development in quranic exegesis.[54]

Conclusion

The discourse on generation in medieval Islamic medicine was rich and diverse. Building upon Greek foundations, Ibn Sina, Ibn al-Nafis and Ibn al-Quff developed new accounts. Moreover, the traditionalists, particularly Ibn Qayyim and his followers, incorporated many of these novelties into their own treatises and so popularized them beyond the limited confines of medical texts. For example, Ibn Hajar's *Commentary on the Sahih of Bukhari* incorporates discussions of seminal formation, ensoulment and fetal growth.[55] This *Commentary* was transmitted orally by Ibn Hajar over the course of many years in live performances, whose audiences included numerous students, powerful patrons and common folk interested in prophetic traditions for pietistic purposes.[56] Since many women learned and taught prophetic traditions at this time, there is a strong possibility that they came to know of the various religious and medical debates on generation through such commentaries on the *Sahih*.[57] This is important since our sources rarely document women's direct participation in learned medical and philosophical circles.

Finally, as with the Islamic discussions, early modern historians have emphasized the Greek foundations of the Renaissance writings on generation.[58] For example, Jean Fernel's views on seminal formation and ensoulment have been explained in terms of

53 Ibn Qayyim, *al-Tibyan*, p. 509.

54 Compare the commentary on the chapter on 'Believers' (*al-Mu'minun*) in al-Tabari, *Jamiʿ* with Ibn Kathir, *Tafsir qur'an al-ʿazim*, ed. Samy ibn Muhammad al-Salama (Riyadh, 1997).

55 Ibn Hajar al-ʿAsqalani, *Fath al-Bari* (Bulaq, 1883), vol. 11, pp. 418–21.

56 Joel Blecher, '*Hadith* commentaries in the presence of students, patrons, and rivals: Ibn Hajar and *Sahih al-Bukhari* in Mamluk Cairo', *Oriens* 41 (2013), 261–87.

57 Asma Sayeed, *Women and the Transmission of Religious Knowledge in Islam* (Cambridge, 2013).

58 Hiro Hirai, *Medical Humanism and Natural Philosophy: Renaissance Debates on Matter, Life and the Soul* (Leiden, 2011), p. 2.

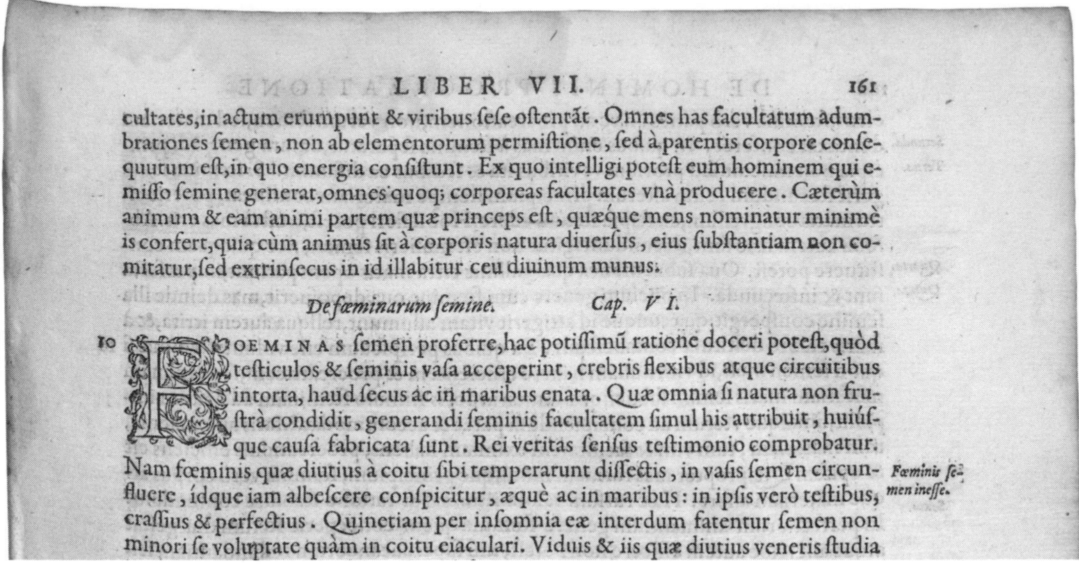

LIBER VII. 161

cultates,in actum erumpunt & viribus ſeſe oſtentăt. Omnes has facultatum adumbrationes ſemen, non ab elementorum permiſtione, ſed à parentis corpore conſequutum eſt,in quo energia conſiſtunt. Ex quo intelligi poteſt eum hominem qui emiſſo ſemine generat,omnes quoq; corporeas facultates vnà producere. Cæterùm animum & eam animi partem quæ princeps eſt, quæque mens nominatur minimè is confert,quia cùm animus ſit à corporis natura diuerſus, eius ſubſtantiam non comitatur,ſed extrinſecus in id illabitur ceu diuinum munus.

De fœminarum ſemine. *Cap. VI.*

FOEMINAS ſemen proferre,hac potiſſimũ ratione doceri poteſt,quòd teſticulos & ſeminis vaſa acceperint, crebris flexibus atque circuitibus intorta, haud ſecus ac in maribus enata. Quæ omnia ſi natura non fruſtrà condidit, generandi ſeminis facultatem ſimul his attribuit, huiúſque cauſa fabricata ſunt. Rei veritas ſenſus teſtimonio comprobatur. Nam fœminis quæ diutius à coitu ſibi temperarunt diſſectis, in vaſis ſemen circunfluere, ídque iam albeſcere conſpicitur, æquè ac in maribus: in ipſis verò teſtibus, craſſius & perfectius. Quinetiam per inſomnia eæ interdum fatentur ſemen non minori ſe voluptate quàm in coitu eiaculari. Viduis & iis quæ diutius veneris ſtudia

Fœminis ſemen ineſſe.

Figure 9.2 Passage on 'The nature, excellence and powers of semen …' from Jean Fernel's *Physiologia*. This conclusion of Book 7, Chapter 5 demonstrates Fernel's debt to Arabic medical commentaries; the next book considers female semen. From the Wellcome Library copy of Fernel's *Universa Medicina* (Paris: A. Wechelum, 1567), p. 161, by permission of ProQuest (www.proquest.com), as part of Early European Books.

the Renaissance Platonism that emerged through humanist engagements with ancient sources.[59] However, many passages in Fernel's *Physiologia* (1567) suggest that the Arabic *Canon* commentaries may have played a significant role in Renaissance discussions. When Fernel wrote that fertile semen receives 'some spirit and faculty' from 'the body as a whole', and that the testicles 'concoct the material of the semen' just as 'the breasts give form to milk', he was reworking the Arabic commentary tradition.[60] Similarly, when he highlighted the fact that the male semen does not 'contribute the soul', which instead comes 'from the outside, a divine gift',[61] he was echoing Ibn al-Nafis and his successors, while framing his own discussion within the terms of Renaissance Platonism (Fig. 9.2).[62] A careful investigation of the contexts of transmission of Arabic medical commentaries into Latin Europe, along the lines of Robert Morrison's recent analysis of astronomical texts, will reveal the full depth of Renaissance engagements with Islamic accounts of generation produced after 1200.[63]

59 Ibid., p. 78.

60 *The Physiologia of Jean Fernel (1567)*, trans. John M. Forrester (Philadelphia, PA, 2003), pp. 543–5.

61 Ibid., p. 552. 62 Hirai, *Medical Humanism*, pp. 47–8.

63 Robert Morrison, 'A scholarly intermediary between the Ottoman Empire and Renaissance Europe', *Isis* 105 (2014), 32–57.

10 The Multitude in Later Medieval Thought

Peter Biller

While the study of medieval population is long-established, the study of medieval thought about population is not. It was brought into existence by *The Measure of Multitude: Population in Medieval Thought* (2000), which looked at European demographic expansion in the twelfth and thirteenth centuries.[1] That book did not go into the later middle ages, and it has not been built upon in early modern scholarship.[2] Nor has it been integrated into general histories of demographic thought.[3] Taking up the story where *The Measure of Multitude* left it, this chapter therefore goes about its business in something of a historiographical void. It asks what followed. How did this body of thought fare after 1300, set against the population decline of the later middle ages? In particular, what interactions were there between demographic decline and thought about population?

The chapter first recapitulates *The Measure of Multitude* to prepare the way for an assessment of what came next. Two points need explaining. First, there is a policy about keywords. To prevent semantic anachronism impeding the history of ideas, where medieval people's thoughts are at issue we use modern English versions of their keywords. 'Population' (*populatio*) is avoided, except in its usual medieval sense, the act of peopling an area. The common medieval word was 'multitude' (*multitudo*), and we therefore talk of 'thought about the multitude'. Only when writing as historians about the population realities of the past do we provide entry permits to 'demography' and other modern keywords associated with it. Second, an account of thought begs the question, who did the thinking? Take as an example a European kingdom around 1300 containing just over four million people, of whom a tiny minority read Latin. Within that tiny minority, an even smaller group wrote works which have come down to us. Within that sub-subgroup, two categories of writers are of interest. The

1 Peter Biller, *The Measure of Multitude: Population in Medieval Thought* (Oxford, 2000; corrected edn, 2003).

2 An exception is Paul Slack, *'Plenty of People': Perceptions of Population Thought in Early Modern England* (Reading, 2011).

3 For example, Yves Charbit, *The Classical Foundations of Population Thought: From Plato to Quesnay* (Dordrecht, 2010). On earlier and later developments: Rebecca Flemming, 'States and Populations in the Classical World', Chapter 5; Philip Kreager, 'The Emergence of Population', Chapter 18; Andrea Rusnock, 'Biopolitics and the Invention of Population', Chapter 23; Alison Bashford, 'World Population from Eugenics to Climate Change', Chapter 34, this book.

first and main category is the lecturers and commentators on university texts and their immediate audience, students. The second category comprises some theologians, where a thread connects university discussions of concrete moral problems, the writers of manuals of instructions for priests and the parish priest. At this point the thread meets a portion of the four million, the multitude inhabiting a particular parish. Leaving no written records, the individuals in that illiterate multitude thought thoughts we cannot access directly. Despite this, on a few very rare occasions we can juxtapose demographic realities and priests' writing or reading, and try to guess their thought about the multitude.

Thought about the Multitude in the High Middle Ages

The earlier construction of thought about the multitude came about through the intellectual revolution of the high middle ages: the translation into Latin of Greek and Arabic philosophy and medicine, the rise of universities, the formation of their curricula through the new translations and textbooks, and thenceforth the production and dissemination into the cities and towns of medieval Europe of graduates whose minds were hardwired with this material. Central to thought about the multitude were two authors, Peter Lombard and Aristotle. Lombard's *Four Books of the Sentences*, a rapid-retrieval source-book of older material from the Church Fathers and councils, was finished in 1157/8 and in the 1220s came to be lectured on in the theology faculty in Paris. Until Luther's time it was the standard classroom text, alongside the Bible. Aristotle's works were translated from Greek into Latin (against a common misconception, only *On Animals* came first via Arabic), and some of these became curriculum texts in the arts faculty, though not always compulsory ones. Significant for our theme is *On the Length and Shortness of Life*, first translated in the first half of the twelfth century, and the *Politics*, translated in the 1260s.

The books of the *Sentences* were divided into sections called distinctions. One distinction in book 2 raised a counterfactual conditional question, 'What would have happened if Adam and Eve had not sinned?' This allowed theologians to speculate about the multitude in perfect natural conditions. Would each sexual act have led to conception? Conception of boy or girl? Ultimately it led to the question, 'Would there have been an equal or unequal number of men and women?' In book 4, distinctions 26 to 42 dealt with the sacrament of marriage. In some distinctions the individual marriage was at issue, especially the purpose of procreation, offspring and the sinfulness of avoiding offspring (*vitatio prolis*) and abortion. But other distinctions envisaged the multitude. A broad theological history of the multitude was implicated, first of all, in the two expansions of the multitude (from two to very many) after Adam and Eve and after the flood. In the beginning, 'Increase and multiply' was a *command*: marriage was a divine precept and virginity was forbidden. Old Testament patriarchs had many wives. Did God allow this, for a time, in order to increase the multitude more rapidly? His dispensations would vary then, according to variations in the multitude. The world is now replete with men (unlike *viri*, the Latin *homines* here covers both men and women), and therefore the binding precept to marry has ceased. But what if the multitude were to be reduced once again, to the point of vanishing?

Aristotle's *On the Length and Shortness of Life* introduced a phrase and disciplined thought about the concept. University lectures and commentaries energetically explored such topics as the different spans of men's and women's lives and of peoples in different parts of the world, including the extremely short lives of Ethiopians. More significant was the *Politics*, the text of which deals with the ideal size of the multitude and marriage ages, and envisages the legislator intervening to encourage people to have more children or taking measures about excess multitude.[4] A rare commentary on book 7, *Libellus de ingenio bone nativitatis* (Tract on the art of good birth), shows the extraordinary stimulus to daring thought that the *Politics* could provide.[5] As discussed in Chapter 12, this work suggests tinkering with marriage ages to achieve perfect babies.[6] But the broader and more lasting significance of the university texts was semantic-conceptual. The Latin Aristotle, the *Sentences* and their commentaries contained phrases articulating the concepts of this genre of thought. These were a 'multitude remaining the same, through the contingencies of births and deaths'; 'inducing parents to have more children'; 'an equal or unequal multitude of men and women'; 'preventing the multitude being excessive'; and 'avoidance of offspring'. They are the dinosaural ancestors of modern demography's 'stable population', 'encourage the birth-rate', 'sex ratio', 'overpopulation' and 'birth control'.

These intellectual developments need to be set alongside experience and observation of contemporary realities within and outside Latin Christendom. These arts and theology masters and students lived at a time of extraordinary increase in population. In 1209, some manors in Taunton, England, contained 509 males; a century later, there were 1,359 males. Increasing local multitudes were accommodated through the multiplication of parishes and the expanding circles of town and city walls; people laboured to clear more and more land for cultivation; and parents were less able to feed their children in the years approaching 1300. At the same time, views of multitudes beyond Latin Christendom changed. The inheritance of Greek geography, travel, the crusader kingdoms and the Mongol incursions expanded notions of the habitable world. The relative size of Latin Christendom diminished: perhaps it was only one-tenth or one-twentieth

4 Flemming, 'States and Populations'. 5 Biller, *Measure of Multitude*, pp. 347–56.
6 Maaike van der Lugt, 'Formed Fetuses and Healthy Children in Scholastic Theology, Medicine and Law', Chapter 12, this book.

of the world? Using a fairly accurate notion of the circumference of the globe, based on ancient Greek calculations, one theologian speculated about the possible multitude of the whole world, given even density. The parts of it that writers knew about expanded to include Mongolia, and there were the first medieval European sightings and descriptions of people from China. The friars who travelled to Mongolia produced ethnographic descriptions *avant la lettre*: one account of the system of Mongol marriage extends to the observation that their women 'never lay in bed for childbirth'.[7] The existence and then fall of the crusader kingdoms entailed intense preoccupation with the multitudes of the eastern Mediterranean. How could the small Christian multitude cope with the military threat of the surrounding hostile and very numerous Arab multitudes? Was the size of these multitudes brought about by Muhammad's permission for a multiplicity of wives? Or was there, as a royal counsellor and bishop of Paris argued, greater 'density' (*numerositas*) of multitude in a Christian kingdom? After the fall of the Holy Land in 1290, if Christians were ever to recapture and populate it, would it be licit to have a multitude of wives, to increase the multitude more quickly?

This juxtaposition of the new locations and opportunities for thought about the multitude in arts and theology, on the one hand, and on the other the experiences of the realities of multitudes within and outside Latin Christendom leads to three observations. First, the emphasis on the fullness of the world in theology and 'medium small is beautiful' in Aristotle coincided with the population conditions of the thirteenth century. It underpins the readiness of understanding and even enthusiasm with which some commentators took up these texts. But it was accidental – and the texts continued into the demographically very different world of the later middle ages. Second, the topic of excess multitude was being articulated at the same time as unprecedented attention was paid to avoidance of offspring in pastoral manuals drawn up for the instruction of those hearing confessions and preaching in parishes; the years around 1300 also saw medical and theological discussions of the licitness of therapeutic abortions.[8]

Third, 'sex ratio' provides an example of thought about the multitude. How did the idea originate, and with whom? The rather contrasting numbers of male and female religious celibates in some kingdoms could have focused some minds. Priests in early thirteenth-century Languedoc were writing down the names of every girl in their parishes above 12 and every boy above 14, in lists which could have stimulated comparison. How did permission for a plurality of wives work, numerically? Some time

7 William of Rubruck, *Itinerarium* vi.5: 'Nunquam cubebant in lecto pro puerperio', ed. Anastaas van den Wyngaert, *Itinera et relationes Fratrum Minorum saeculi XIII et XIV*, Sinica franciscana 1 (Quaracchi, Florence, 1929), p. 183.

8 Peter Biller, 'John of Naples, quodlibets and medieval theological concern with the body', in Biller and Alastair J. Minnis (eds.), *Medieval Theology and the Natural Body* (York, 1997), pp. 3–12, on pp. 8–9; Biller, *Measure of Multitude*, pp. 154, 176–7; van der Lugt, 'Formed Fetuses and Healthy Children'.

after 1218, theological treatises start moving towards the phrase for the ratio, which is commonplace by mid-century. Before 1338, the parish priest at the Baptistry in Florence was placing a white bean in a container for each female baby and a black bean for each male. There was counting, and calculation of the numerical range within which, year by year, the 'male sex was in advance' (*avanzando … il sesso masculine*). Though they are few, the jigsaw pieces suggest the larger picture. Further, they hint at the complex web that contained the thoughts of both the *Sentences* lecturer and the lay woman or man standing around the font and watching the priest count out white and black beans.[9]

The Later Middle Ages I: The Learned

How did *thought about the multitude* fare during the later middle ages? What had been founded in the thirteenth century was consolidated, continued and spread further. The century and a half after the foundation of the University of Prague in 1348 saw new university foundations filling a once-blank map in Germany, central and eastern Europe and the low countries. In theology, masters continued lecturing on the *Sentences* and students continued learning them, and a high proportion of the 1,407 glosses and commentaries on the *Sentences* composed before Luther's time come from this period. Lecturing on the *Politics* was always a smaller affair, but it spread to such new universities as Prague, Vienna, Cologne, Heidelberg, Krakow, Leipzig, Erfurt and Greifswald.[10] William of Moerbeke's translation of the *Politics* continued to be copied; sixty-seven manuscripts are still extant from the mid-fourteenth to the late fifteenth centuries, and notes of ownership and purchase attest use ranging from masters in Erfurt to high humanist circles in fifteenth-century Italy.[11] Moerbeke's Latin was translated into French and glossed by Nicole Oresme around 1371. The 'demographic' words and phrases of the Latin commentaries of the previous century were now in vernacular. And for the first time ever, topics such as 'multitude of children' appeared as headings in alphabetical indices to books. In 1438, Leonardo Bruni made a new translation from Greek, which itself attracted commentaries and was printed in 1478.[12] The matriculation lists from universities including Prague and Vienna begin to provide a telephone-directory

9 Biller, *Measure of Multitude*, pp. 89 (the text), 386, 407, 411–12.

10 Christoph Flüeler, *Rezeption und Interpretation der Aristotelischen* Politica *im späten Mittelalter*, 2 vols. (Amsterdam, 1992), vol. 1, p. 34.

11 The number is from the *Aristoteles Latinus* lists: Georges Lacombe, *Codices, Pars Prior* (Rome, 1939); Georges Lacombe and Lorenzo Minio-Paluello, *Codices, Pars Posterior* (Cambridge, 1955); Lorenzo Minio-Paluello, *Codices, Supplementum Altera* (Bruges, 1961). Humanists were among the owners of nos. 1,444, 1,514 and 1,603; Erfurt masters of nos. 871 and 1,456; and Krakow masters of nos. 1,410, 1,676 and 2,171.

12 Hans Baron, *Leonardo Aretino. Humanistisch-philosophische Schriften* (Berlin and Leipzig, 1928), pp. 70–4, 175–6; Francesco Paolo Luiso, *Studi su l'Epistolario di Leonardo Aretino*, ed. Lucia Gualdo Rosa (Rome, 1980), vi.14, viii.3–4, viii.7, viii.13, ix.2, x.38, pp. 122–3, 138–41, 146, 148–9, 181–2.

solidity to what we already know, the large numbers of literate men going off into the towns and cities of later medieval Europe, their minds stocked with Aristotelian and theological 'demographic' topics and phrases. Courts and rulers were also brought into the picture by dedicatory letters. Oresme's work was for Charles V of France, while Bruni sent a flurry of copies of his Latin translation to the Duke of Gloucester, the Pope, the rulers of Siena and the king of Aragon. His letters construct the *Politics* as important for a ruler – with 'multitude' one of the significant topics mentioned by Bruni in a resumé of the contents.[13]

What can we see beyond continuity and further diffusion? Against the backcloth of the decline and catastrophic mortalities of the fourteenth century, now we will look first at thought discernible in *Politics* commentaries from Paris, and then at a few examples where we can conjecture about grassroots thought about the multitude.

Born around 1322 in Normandy, Nicole Oresme was in his late twenties during the Black Death of 1348–9. In his commentary on the *Politics* he carefully constructs bridges between the classical world and his own. Here he is on childbirth: 'Young pregnant women or their friends went to a temple … to make offerings or vows or prayers to a God or Goddess to help them give birth – Romans had a Goddess called Lucina, the Goddess of childbirth: just as in our faith women call upon St Margaret.'[14] Glossing and first of all explaining Aristotle, he necessarily has to reproduce Aristotle's recommendations, in book 7, of the marriage ages of 18 for girls and 37 for men. But he introduces qualifications – 'one should understand this as applying to temperate places and lands and times, and it is not to be understood that one cannot generate well before the times said above, or perchance after' – which are muffled expressions of his awareness of the gap between Aristotle and the marriage ages of his own world.[15]

Aristotle's Spartan legislator, wanting to increase the number of Spartans, 'calls upon citizens to make more children' (*provocat cives quod plures faciant pueros*).[16] Here is Oresme's version: 'he prods, provokes and prompts the citizens to generate more babies' (*il picquoit et provoquoit et promovoit les citoiens a engendrer pluseurs enfans*).[17] Elsewhere he uses extraordinary historical and classical erudition in what is, essentially, the earliest history of measures to deal with the multitude. The first and longest part concerns measures to keep it down. But he turns in the other direction at the end.

13 'There is, moreover … a long account … of the size of the people' ('Praeterea … de magnitudine populi … longo ordine demonstratur'), *Leonardi Bruni Arretini Epistolarum Libri VIII*, ed. Lorenzo Mehus, 2 vols. (Florence, 1741), vol. 1, p. 105.

14 Nicole Oresme, *Le livre de Politiques d'Aristote*, ed. Albert Douglas Menut (Philadelphia, PA, 1970), p. 332a.

15 Ibid., p. 332b.

16 *Aristotelis Politicorum Libri Octo, cum vetusta translatione Guilelmi de Moerbeka*, ed. Franz Susemihl (Leipzig, 1872), p. 122.

17 Oresme, *Livre*, p. 89.

> Sometimes – going against what has just been said – one applies oneself and strives to multiply generation, in order to populate a region or strengthen a lineage to make it stronger or for some other reason, as our Lord said to Abraham, 'I will multiply thy seed as the stars of heaven etc.' [Gen. 22:17]. But this belongs to another discipline (*science*).

As the subtlest reader of medieval *Politics* commentaries once wrote, when trying to discern intrusions of the realities of the contemporary world, 'One has to develop a nose for the slightest wind of any strange scent'.[18] There is a strong scent in Oresme's multiplying of verbs for the ruler encouraging birth, and his decision to conclude his history of multitude with the attempts to increase it.

Among lecturers on the *Politics* in Paris in the second half of the fourteenth century were Albert of Saxony, Henry Totting of Oyta and Nicholas of Vaudémont; the last was a near contemporary of Oresme. His questions on the *Politics* were written after 1360, and perhaps during the dates when Nicholas was attested in Paris, between 1374 and 1387.[19] Lists of questions raised in other late medieval *Politics* commentaries show in general much repetition and continuity. This highlights one remarkable feature of Nicholas's questions. He borrowed from another discipline, theology, importing three questions from commentaries on the *Sentences*. They were clear signals. 'Whether in a well ruled polity virginity is licit?' (book 4, q. 25); 'Whether virginity, which is a moral virtue, is licit in a well ruled and ordained polity?' (book 5, q. 7); and 'Whether marriage falls under precept?' (book 7, q. 14).[20] As we have seen, a commonplace in the *Sentences* commentaries was the intertwining of the multitude and God's dispensations about marriage and virginity. In extreme necessity, the dispensations would be revoked. As the Augustinian master-general Thomas of Strasbourg wrote, 'such a great mortality of men could happen that those few who were left living would be bound to marry for the preservation of the species'.[21]

Nicholas does not turn 'could' and 'would' into a plain indicative statement: such a great mortality 'has' happened that those people remaining 'are' bound to marry. The orthodoxy of later fourteenth-century Paris probably precluded an outright attack on the infertility of religious celibates or a blunt revival of mandatory marriage. And the maze of logical pros and cons in Nicholas's exploration of the questions, familiar to any

18 Conor Martin, 'Some medieval commentaries on Aristotle's *Politics*', *History* 36 (1951), 29–44, on 38.

19 On Nicholas, see Flüeler, *Rezeption*, vol. 1, pp. 150–5; his questions, once attributed to John Buridan, are listed in vol. 2, pp. 121–40.

20 John Buridan, *Quaestiones in octo libros Politicorum Aristotelis* (Oxford, 1640), ff. 77ra–vb, 79vb–81va, 108ra–vb.

21 *Commentaria in IIII libros sententiarum*, 2 vols. (Venice, 1564; reprint of 2 vols. in 1, Ridgewood, NJ, 1965), vol. 2, f. 146ra.

reader of late medieval scholastic texts, softens the impact of the occasional appearance of these points. Here they are: in certain circumstances through which the whole polity might perish, virginity would be illicit; conjugal chastity (meaning here good marriage and procreation, not abstinence from sex in marriage) is for the common good; and marriage does not fall under precept, such that each person would be obliged to marry: except in the case where there is 'too great scarcity' (*nimia paucitas*) of people. 'The reason why marriage was instituted still remains and perdures.' Together with the extraordinary initial decision to import such provocative questions, these statements will have flagged the drift of Nicholas's thought sufficiently clearly to a late fourteenth-century audience. And perhaps without too much danger to Nicholas himself.

The Later Middle Ages II: Observers on the Ground

Despite the steady vernacularization of the later middle ages and the erosion of the equation between literacy and Latinity, a fundamental division still remained, and the millions were still mainly illiterate. The more than 500 dioceses in Latin Christendom ranged from tiny Italian collections of just a few dozen parishes to large northern European ones, with several hundred. And it was in a parish, 'in the face of a church', that marriages were blessed, in its font that babies were baptized and in the parish cemetery that bodies were buried. The realities of the multitude of the parish loomed largest in the minds of most ordinary people. We come nearer to them when reading those literate men who were closest to them, the parish priests, friars who specialized in preaching and confession, and those pastoral experts who provided instruction manuals for parish priests or legislated for them at the synod of a diocese. While we know virtually nothing about most parishes, we can snatch occasional glimpses or make conjectures about thinking about the multitude in the parish. Let us look at four examples.

First, a phrase in a collection of synodal statutes put together in 1365 for Meaux, a diocese to the northeast of Paris, where the regulation of midwives was detailed. The parish priest was to keep written records of the midwives of the parish, their selection, examination, oath-taking and formal approval. Of all these details one demands our attention. The priest was to ensure adequate provision in each parish. There is to be one sworn midwife *or* two, 'according to the multitude of the parish' (*juxta parochiae multitudinem*).[22] We must always be cautious when interpreting the written legislation

22 *Thesaurus novus anecdotorum*, ed. E. Martène and U. Durand, 5 vols. (Paris, 1717), vol. 4, col. 929; Kathryn Taglia, 'Delivering a Christian identity: Midwives in northern French synodal legislation, *c.* 1200–1500', in Peter Biller and Joseph Ziegler (eds.), *Religion and Medicine in the Middle Ages* (York, 2001), pp. 77–90. For a chronologically conservative view of the re-emergence of the specialized midwife, see Monica H. Green, *Making Women's Medicine Masculine: The Rise of Male Authority in Pre-Modern Gynaecology* (Oxford, 2008), pp. 118–62.

of the high middle ages. What is new may well be not the rule but rather the expression in writing of what is customary, or the use of the opportunity of written legislation to introduce uniformity into existing practice. Either newly introduced, or an existing practice now reduced to writing, this was the rule: every priest running a parish in the diocese of Meaux was to ensure a relationship between the multitude of his particular parish and the number of its sworn midwives.

Second, the *multitude* presented itself in more precise numbers to the parish priests 290 kilometres southeast of Paris, in the Burgundian village of Givry.[23] These priests kept lists of marriages, beginning in 1336. 'Here are contained those who were married after the feast of All Saints', or 'those who were espoused', or 'these are the marriages that took place'. The lists are grouped in relation to Easter, All Saints and the twenty days from Christmas to the feast of Epiphany. The priests also kept lists of deaths, beginning in 1334. 'Here are contained those who died during the time'. Deaths were not grouped, but entered and dated individually. The priests did not note births or baptisms.

The names were not tabulated on a spreadsheet, of course. But the listing of 'those who died during the time' was interleaved with 'those married during the time'. The priest will have had such numbers as fourteen deaths and nineteen marriages in 1336 to hand. As the person who did non-emergency baptisms, he knew that some marriages led to babies, others not. It is inconceivable that the priest did not hold these relatively small numbers in his mind, forming the elementary thought of the contingencies of deaths and marriages, spread over several years, being roughly out of balance or in balance: and that a balance meant the multitude of his parish staying roughly the same. He had in his mind a counterpart of the phrases being learnt by a student at Paris reading the *Politics* and Aristotle's words about a balance between births, 'sterilities' and deaths.

The lists are famous for two sequences of figures.[24] Where deaths had ranged between six and forty-two in any year between 1334 and 1347, 649 died during 1348, the year of plague. Where there were usually between eleven and twenty-nine marriages each year, there were none in 1348. Then they leapt to eighty-six in the following year.

The third example shows how a Carmelite friar living in Paris observed and conceptualized the equivalent of these numbers in 1348 and 1349. 'That same year [1348] and in the following one', he wrote,

23 Pierre Gras, 'Le registre paroissial de Givry (1334–1357) et la peste noire en Bourgogne', *Bibliothèque de l'École des chartes* 100 (1939), 295–308.

24 An asterisk indicates that the figure is incomplete. Deaths: 1334, 6; 1335, 6; 1336, 14; 1337, 25; 1338, 21; 1339, 23; 1340, 18; 1341, 37; 1342, 17*; 1343, 43*; 1344, 26*; 1345, 39; 1346, 25; 1347, 42; 1348, 649*. Marriages: 1336, 19; 1337, 20; 1338, 11; 1339, 29; 1340, 15; 1341, 11; 1342, 1*; 1343, 5*; 1344, 3*; 1345, 2*; 1346, missing; 1347, 19*; 1348, no marriages; 1349, 86.

> in Paris and the kingdom of France and no less, it is reported, in various parts of the world, there was such a mortality of people – of both sexes, and more of the young than the old – that they could hardly be buried … In many places, out of twenty people only two remained alive … When this epidemic, pestilence and mortality stopped, the remaining men and women married each other. The wives who were left in the world conceived beyond the norm. Not one of them was made to be sterile.[25] Rather, the pregnant were to be seen over here, and over there. And also many gave birth to twin children, and some produced [at one birth] three living little babies.[26]

Here there is more than just the sequence of the individual facts of mortality, marriages, pregnancies and births. Even though the friar does not have to hand the generalizing abstract phrases of modern demography, his exaggerations and striving for effect and above all his phrase 'conceived *beyond the norm*' (*ultra modum*) show the distant ancestry of 'marriage and fertility rates'.

The fourth example comes from the instructional literature written by pastoral experts for priests, and from the area where this genre was most highly developed, England. The treatises were based on a dialogue between observation of the facts on the ground and canon law, and they evince continuing concern with the conception and care of babies. A high point was reached in *The Eye of the Priest* (*Oculus sacerdotis*), written in the 1320s by William of Paull near Hull. William knew his stuff, as a former penitentiary, that is, as a diocesan specialist who looked at special sins remitted to him by priests in the diocese because of their enormity or complexity. He shared with another contemporary, John Bromyard, who similarly knew his stuff as penitentiary of the diocese of Hereford, a concern with spilling seed and avoiding conception. Many these days thought this not a sin, he said.[27] This appeared in a long list of things that he instructed parish priests to warn their parishioners against from the pulpit every Sunday. This is one of the many expressions of pastoral experts' concern, in the decades around 1300, with avoidance of conception or procuring abortion, which can be taken as responses to couples' desire and intention to limit children in conditions of excessive multitude.

This text was thoroughly revised by John Burgh between 1380 and 1385. Although renamed *The Eye of the Pupil* (*Pupilla oculi*), it is in many ways a second edition of *The Eye of the Priest*. Here and there the new version accommodates recent events – additional military questions in confession evoke the realities of war with France – and the text continues to evoke a concrete English setting; something is heard in London, and

25 It is possible, but unlikely, that 'nulla efficiebatur sterilis' means 'Not one of them made herself sterile'.

26 *Chronique dite de Jean de Venette*, ed. Colette Beaune (Paris, 2011), pp. 110, 114.

27 Biller, *Measure of Multitude*, p. 213.

later in York.[28] In his very thorough overhaul, John drops the list of things that a parish priest should warn his parishioners about, but he carefully preserves some items from the list, now locating them in various places. These include: pregnant women should avoid heavy work; a mother's milk is best; care should be taken to avoid smothering babies.[29] But he decided not to preserve the coupled injunctions not to spill seed and not to avoid conception. Brevity could have been his motive. It is more likely that his mind, and those of the parish priests who were his intended readers, were full of the realities of their times: conceptualized, as we have seen, in phrases like *too great scarcity* of people, *many marrying*, and *women conceiving beyond the norm*. And that *avoidance of offspring* was no longer at the forefront of the minds of priests and pastoral experts, as it had been during the desperate overcrowding of the years around 1300.

Where about 130 *Sentences* commentaries compiled before the 1340s provided the preliminary dataset for *The Measure of Multitude*, that book's research questions have been put to only a few of the many *Sentences* commentaries compiled after 1348. Ditto for the nineteen late medieval *Politics* commentaries listed by Flüeler. More exhaustive research of these texts might well modify as well as amplify what has been said here. The field beckons.

28 John Burgh, *Pupilla oculi* (Strasbourg, 1518), f. 77va.

29 Ibid., ff. 55va–b, 59ra.

11 Managing Childbirth and Fertility in Medieval Europe

Katharine Park

Procreation lay at the heart of family life in medieval Europe. Unless bound by Christian vows of chastity, men and women defined themselves in large part by their ability to produce the children, especially the male children, on whom the survival of their families depended. Although procreation involved both men and women, it was understood as first and foremost women's work – their 'active and affirmative responsibility', in Joan Cadden's words – and assumptions about gender and sexuality shaped it throughout.[1] In particular, sexual activity and procreation outside marriage were widely accepted for men but strongly stigmatized for women. The fertility and fidelity of wives grounded the continuity of the patrilineal family by assuring that their children, especially their male children, were legitimate descendants of their husbands, while the chastity of its widows and unwed girls guaranteed its honour. These guarantees involved more than sexual chastity, extending to more general taboos concerning women's bodies: for most of the medieval period their genitals were not to be seen or touched by men to whom they were unrelated, even in a medical context. This limited the knowledge available to male practitioners relating to childbirth and sexual health as well as the activities in which those practitioners could engage. It also meant that women were recognized as the principal repository of expertise in the management of birth and, to a lesser extent, fertility.

Nonetheless, as I show in this chapter, the gendering of these functions became more complex during the later middle ages, as men and women increasingly consulted male practitioners in both areas. In childbirth, hands-on male involvement was largely limited to emergency surgical interventions to deliver women or save their fetuses in cases of obstructed birth. Regarding fertility, however, women consulted male practitioners of all sorts, from court physicians to itinerant empirics, in their attempts to conceive or – less often – to avoid conceiving or to rid themselves of unwanted pregnancies. These developments did not reflect the 'marginalization' of female practitioners by male ones. Instead, they reveal a marked increase in the demand for services related to procreation beginning in the early fourteenth century, and a corresponding growth and diversification of the types of practitioners ready to supply those services.

1 Joan Cadden, *Meanings of Sex Difference in the Middle Ages: Medicine, Science and Culture* (Cambridge, 1993), p. 24.

As a result of this growth in demand, one rarely finds direct competition between, say, midwives and surgeons, or female empirics and male physicians, since each group played a different role in the management of procreation.[2] In fact, among and within these groups, practitioners often preferred to work in collaboration on complicated cases, not only to share responsibility for negative outcomes but also because they recognized different types of expertise. Towards the end of the middle ages, some male physicians began directly to assert intellectual authority over midwives in childbirth.[3] In medieval Europe, however, these assertions had little resonance outside courtly or aristocratic circles and no legal or institutional force.

A caveat concerning sources: this chapter focuses on procreation in practice, complementing the discussion of philosophical and theological sources in the next chapter.[4] Because having babies belonged to the spheres of family management and female sociability, procreation was ordinarily not a medical event. The (mostly) women involved in it are poorly represented in the surviving sources, which privilege the authors of medical texts and 'official' practitioners, defined as those explicitly given credentials by local authorities – universities, guilds and municipalities – the vast majority of whom were men. These practitioners worked in the medical marketplace alongside a host of unofficial ones, male and female, who rarely appear in the administrative records of medieval towns. Women practitioners of all sorts thus seldom feature in the written records traditionally used by historians of medicine.[5]

Furthermore, because the vast majority of the interventions and encounters related to procreation involved only oral communication and were spoken, not written, they have left few traces in medical writings, which were oriented towards the transmission of textual information. The best evidence for these encounters appears in non-medical sources, such as witness statements collected in the course of contemporary legal actions regarding, for example, the death of a woman in childbirth that attendants attributed to the negligence of the midwife; an inheritance dispute that turned on whether a fetus excised from the uterus of its dead mother had been born alive; or the prosecution of an unmarried servant girl for suffocating her newborn child.[6] Although constrained

2 On medieval surgeons' obstetric knowledge, see Lauren Kassell, 'Medieval Birth Malpresentations', Exhibit 10, this book.

3 This story is taken up in Mary E. Fissell, 'Man-Midwifery Revisited', Chapter 22; and brought into the present in Salim Al-Gailani, 'Hospital Birth', Chapter 37, this book.

4 Maaike van der Lugt, 'Formed Fetuses and Healthy Children in Scholastic Theology, Medicine and Law', Chapter 12, this book.

5 Monica H. Green, 'Documenting medieval women's medical practice', in Luis Garcia-Ballester *et al.* (eds.), *Practical Medicine from Salerno to the Black Death* (Cambridge, 1994), pp. 322–52.

6 Katharine Park, 'Birth and death', in Linda Kalof (ed.), *A Cultural History of the Human Body in the Medieval Age* (Oxford, 2010), pp. 22–7.

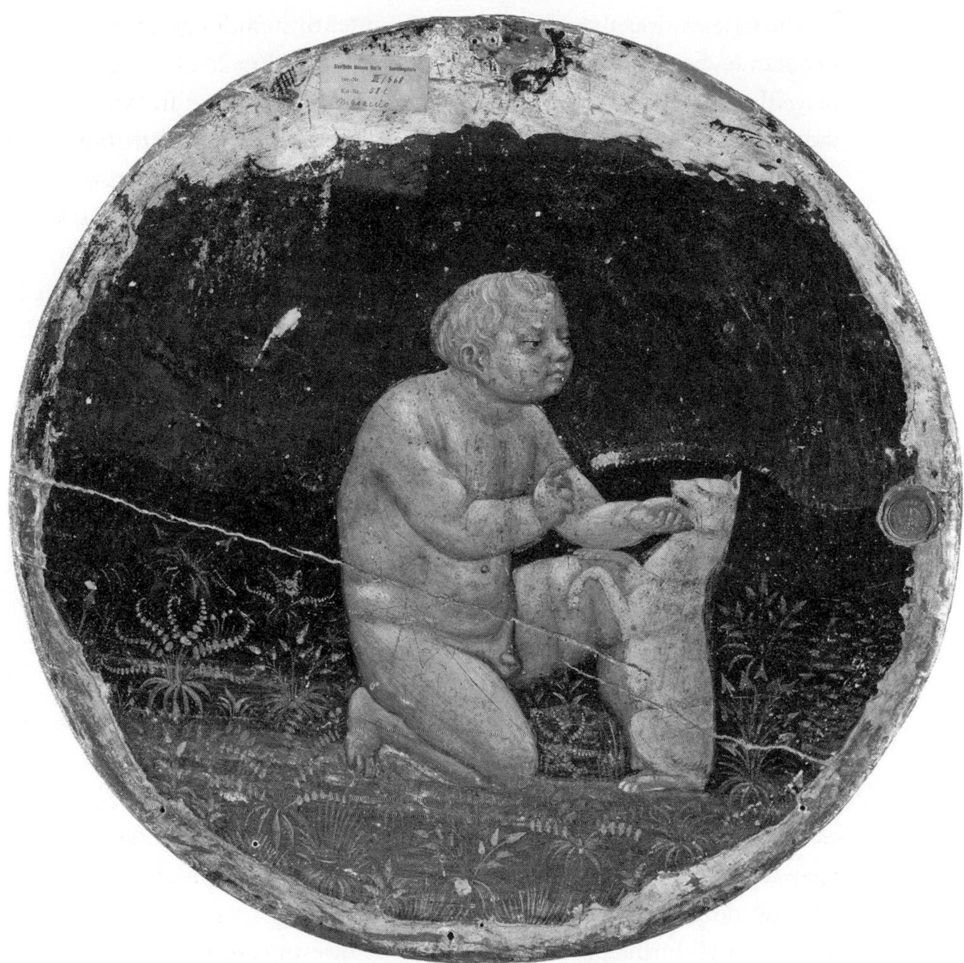

Figure 11.1 Painting by Tommaso Masaccio of a boy with a pet, on the bottom of a birth tray from 1427. A protective lip around the circumference has been lost, and the painting shows signs of wear, reminding us that these trays were utilitarian household objects. Figure 11.3 shows the front of the tray. Oil on wood, 56 cm diameter. © bpk / Gemäldegalerie, SMB / Jörg P. Anders.

and mediated by legal language and procedures as well as an understandable desire to avoid self-incrimination, records like these preserve the voices of the mostly female actors in a way never found in medical texts. Also helpful are miracle lists and private correspondence or account books. Additional sources of information include artworks – tomb sculptures, manuscript illustrations, monumental frescoes of the births of the Virgin Mary or Julius Caesar (thought to have been born by 'caesarean' section) – and remnants of a thriving material culture around fertility and childbirth, such as amulets and decorative objects used to enhance fertility and facilitate the delivery of healthy children. The Florentine 'birth tray' shown in Fig. 11.1 is a good example of the latter: it was thought that looking intently at an image of this sort would help a woman to conceive and bear sons.[7]

In what follows, I use sources of this sort to sketch a history of medieval procreative practices, focusing first on the management of childbirth and then on attempts to enhance or limit fertility. While breast-feeding and infant care were also critical to procreation, I will not deal with them here.[8] For the most part I describe Christian practices. Many had Jewish analogues, for which information is even scarcer; I refer to scholarship on the latter in the footnotes.[9] My goal throughout is to show that these practices and the knowledge they embodied both reflected and shaped the actions of medieval European women and men as they tried – and tried not – to have children.

Managing Childbirth

Through at least the thirteenth century, childbirth normatively took place in domestic spaces and was the province of 'matrons', married kinswomen or family friends, assisted by female servants, if the family could afford them.[10] Matrons' expertise, empirically acquired through giving birth and attending the births of other women, consisted of a mixture of manual technique, moral support and the use of prayers, charms and amulets. These took many forms, including pieces of coral, lodestones and saints' relics.[11] Among the most elaborate were long, thin scrolls of vellum inscribed with the life of St Margaret, the patron saint of childbirth, and intended to be wrapped around the body of the labouring woman.[12] Matrons also helped to wash and swaddle the child.

Not all births proceeded smoothly, however, and additional measures might be required when things went wrong. Glimpses of these appear in *On Treatments for Women*, an influential medical treatise that drew on the work of the twelfth-century female physician Trota of Salerno in southern Italy: a herbal emetic to aid expulsion of

7 Jacqueline Musacchio, *The Art and Ritual of Childbirth in Renaissance Italy* (New Haven, CT, 1999), pp. 125–47; Carole Rawcliffe, 'Women, childbirth, and religion in later medieval England', in Diana Wood (ed.), *Women and Religion in Medieval England* (Oxford, 2003), pp. 91–117.

8 Jütte Gisela Sperling (ed.), *Medieval Lactations: Images, Rhetoric, Practices* (Farnham, 2013).

9 See, in general, Elisheva Baumgarten, *Mothers and Children: Jewish Family Life in Medieval Europe* (Princeton, NJ, 2004).

10 Montserrat Cabré, 'Women or healers? Household practices and the categories of health care in late medieval Iberia', *Bulletin of the History of Medicine* 82 (2011), 18–51.

11 Musacchio, *Art and Ritual*, pp. 139–42; Rawcliffe, 'Women, childbirth, and religion', pp. 103–5; Sandra Cavallo, 'Pregnant Stones as Wonders of Nature', Exhibit 17, this book.

12 Lea T. Olsan, 'A Medieval Birth Girdle', Exhibit 11, this book. Also Wellcome Library, MS 804 (French, *c.* 1465); Musacchio, *Art and Ritual*, pp. 125–47.

the placenta, medicines and poultices to stem postpartum haemorrhages, and a method to aid the delivery of a dead fetus by tossing the pregnant woman in a sheet 'held by four strong men at the four corners'.[13] Trota's own *Practica* confirms that in the twelfth century even difficult childbirth was not managed by midwives – whom its author never mentions – or even by female medical practitioners like herself. Of the sixty-seven short chapters of the *Practica*, only ten relate to fertility, pregnancy and birth, and only one, for 'pain in childbirth', relates to the actual delivery.[14]

The absence of evidence for midwives before the thirteenth century reflects a major historical discontinuity in birth practices between antiquity and the middle ages in the west. Midwifery, an important occupational category in Greek and Roman antiquity, did not survive the dissolution of the Western Roman Empire except in the works of authors parroting ancient texts. The first medieval references to midwives as actual practitioners, rather than literary ghosts, date to the thirteenth century, well after Trota's death. But whereas Roman midwives were a well-defined and often well-educated group with their own occupational title (*obstetrices* in Latin), medieval midwives seem only gradually to have acquired a stable identity separate from matrons, and the titles used to designate them, particularly in the vernacular, overlapped with the words for women performing other domestic functions, such as wet nurses and godmothers.[15]

By the same token, matrons continued to be important presences in the birth room, as supporters, witnesses and sources of advice. Figure 11.2, from a thirteenth-century Italian herbal, offers a schematic portrayal of an uncomplicated delivery and the roles played by the women involved. It shows a labouring woman of apparent wealth and status sitting on a birthing stool, surrounded by four others, two of whom are matrons, married friends or relatives whose social status is indicated by turret hats and veils. The two with simpler turbans are the midwife and the birth attendant in what came to be iconic positions, the latter physically supporting the mother to help her push, and the former attending to what was happening below; here she holds a coriander seed beneath the opening of the woman's vagina, using its fragrance to attract the contents of the uterus downwards.[16] Midwives also used baths and ointments to

13 *On Treatments for Women*, in *The Trotula: A Medieval Compendium of Women's Medicine*, ed. and trans. Monica H. Green (Philadelphia, PA, 2001), p. 92; on other methods of fetal extraction: Ralph Jackson, 'A Roman Embryo Hook', Exhibit 6, this book.

14 *L'inedito opuscolo di pratica terapeutica della medichessa salernitana Trota ...*, ed. and trans. Piero Cantalupo (Salerno, 1995), pp. 22–3, 34–5, 38–45.

15 Cabré, 'Women or healers', 31–5; Monica H. Green, 'Bodies, gender, health, disease: Recent work on medieval women's medicine', *Studies in Medieval and Renaissance History*, 3rd ser., 2 (2005), 13–16. See also Fiona Harris-Stoertz, 'Midwives in the middle ages? Birth attendants, 600–1300', in Wendy J. Turner and Wendy Butler (eds.), *Medicine and Law in the Middle Ages* (Leiden, 2014), pp. 58–87.

16 Musacchio, *Art and Ritual*, pp. 140–1.

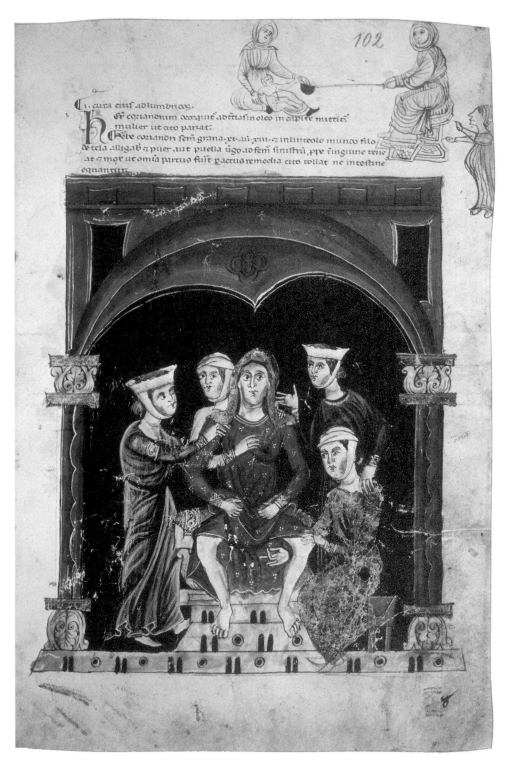

Figure 11.2 Childbirth scene illuminating a thirteenth-century manuscript of the fourth-century *Herbarius* by Pseudo-Apuleius. The text recommends that a virgin boy or girl bind a bag containing eleven or thirteen coriander seeds around a labouring woman's left thigh to hasten birth. This illustration updates the procedure, eliminating the amulet and introducing the expert figure of the midwife. Österreichische Nationalbibliothek Wien, cod. 93, f. 102r.

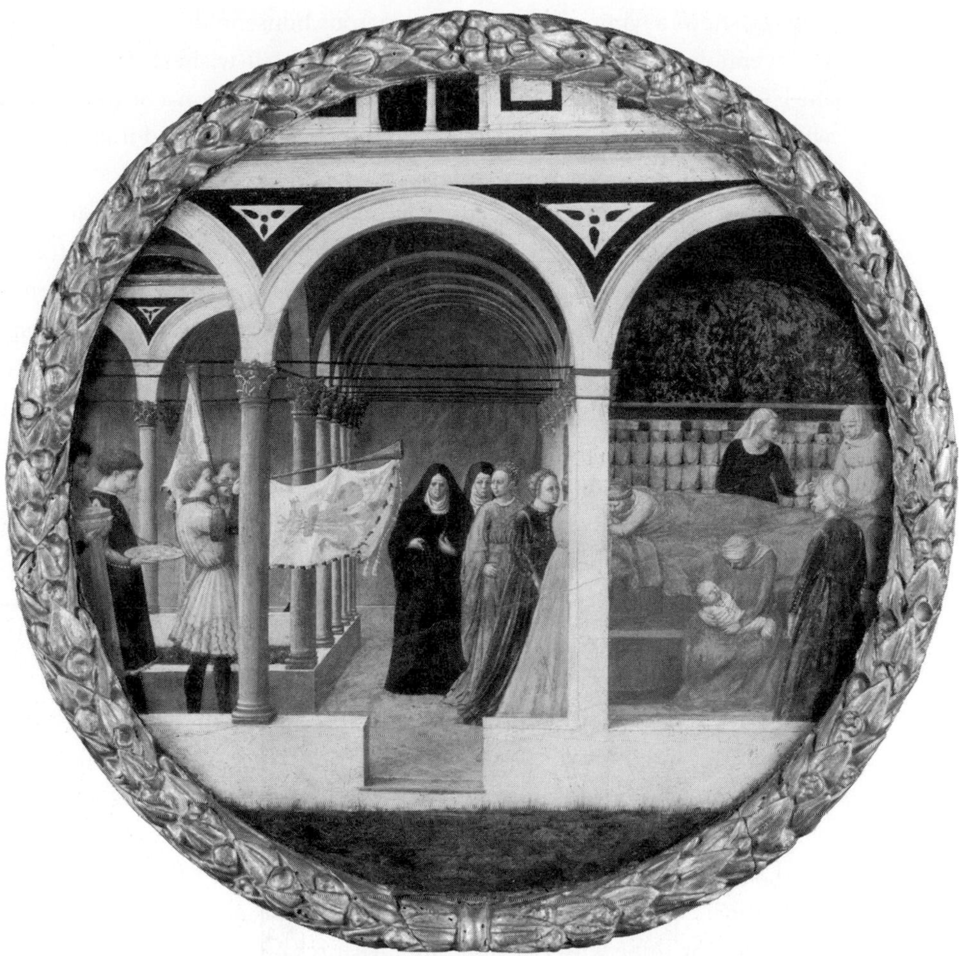

Figure 11.3 Lying-in scene, also painted by Masaccio, on the reverse of the birth tray shown in Fig. 11.1. The servant at the far left carries such a tray. This painting, the 'main view' on the top or interior, is more detailed and skilful than the one on the back. Like Fig. 11.2, it represents childbirth as a ritual enacted by and for women. © bpk / Gemäldegalerie, SMB / Jörg P. Anders.

relax the mother and ease delivery. They turned malpresented fetuses, gave the mother instructions about when to push and assisted the baby's passage through the vagina. They seem also to have performed minor surgeries, such as episiotomy: making a small cut in the perineum to allow the baby to exit the vagina more easily and then suturing the incision after birth. After delivery, they cut the umbilical cord, extracted the placenta, washed and swaddled the child, and presented it to the father. They do not seem to have been responsible for the general medical care of infant or mother, for which families appear to have enlisted the services of medical practitioners. In contrast, the birth assistant might stay on with the family to attend to the needs of mother and baby during the lying-in period. Figure 11.3, the painting on the other side of the birth tray in

Fig. 11.1, shows a lying-in scene in a prosperous household, where the mother, attended by several domestics, greets matrons and female well-wishers. The male attendants on the left bring sweetmeats for the mother and her visitors on a birth tray like the one on which the scene is painted. The woman holding the swaddled infant at her bedside is most likely the birth assistant.[17]

The fourteenth and fifteenth centuries saw a great expansion in midwifery, prompted by families' increasing demand for expert care in childbirth, so that by the fifteenth century it was normative for midwives to attend births of all but the poorest women, including those delivering in some of the larger urban hospitals.[18] Pressure to employ midwives also came from the church, fuelled by ecclesiastical concern for the baptism of dying newborns and salvation of their souls. Preachers campaigned in favour of emergency baptism, and bishops and synods repeatedly decreed that midwives receive instruction in the proper formulae and procedures. One early fourteenth-century Parisian synod required every town to have 'skilled midwives sworn to perform emergency baptism'.[19] To the same end, church authorities encouraged the practice of fetal excision. Sometimes referred to loosely as 'caesarean section', this involved cutting a living fetus from the uterus of a woman who was dying or had just died in childbirth, with hopes that it would survive long enough to be baptized. By the later fourteenth and fifteenth centuries, this procedure had become fairly familiar and was often depicted in illustrated histories of the Roman Empire in connection with the birth of Julius Caesar. These images usually show the incision being performed by a male barber or surgeon, while a midwife extracts or cradles the child. Figure 11.4 provides further detail regarding the caesarean operation: having made the incision, the surgeon holds open the mother's vagina, while a female attendant does the same with her mouth – measures recommended in church legislation to allow the fetus to 'breathe' during the procedure.[20] None of this should be seen as a usurpation of midwives' functions; it was rather a collaborative strategy to deal with a crisis.

17 Louis Haas, *The Renaissance Man and His Children: Childbirth and Early Childhood in Florence, 1300–1600* (New York, NY, 1998), pp. 37–61; Musacchio, *Art and Ritual*, pp. 35–47.

18 Rawcliffe, 'Women, childbirth, and religion', p. 96; Monica H. Green, *Making Women's Medicine Masculine: The Rise of Male Authority in Pre-Modern Gynaecology* (Oxford, 2008), p. 135 n. 49 (Hôtel-Dieu in Paris, 1378) and p. 148. Late medieval hospitals with special wards for parturient women would have employed midwives for deliveries, even if they were not part of the salaried staff.

19 Kathryn Taglia, 'Delivering a Christian identity: Midwives in northern French synodal legislation, *c.* 1200–1500', in Peter Biller and Joseph Ziegler (eds.), *Religion and Medicine in the Middle Ages* (York, 2001), pp. 77–90, on p. 84.

20 Katharine Park, 'The death of Isabella della Volpe: Four eyewitness accounts of a postmortem caesarean section in 1545', *Bulletin of the History of Medicine* 82 (2008), 169–87, on 173.

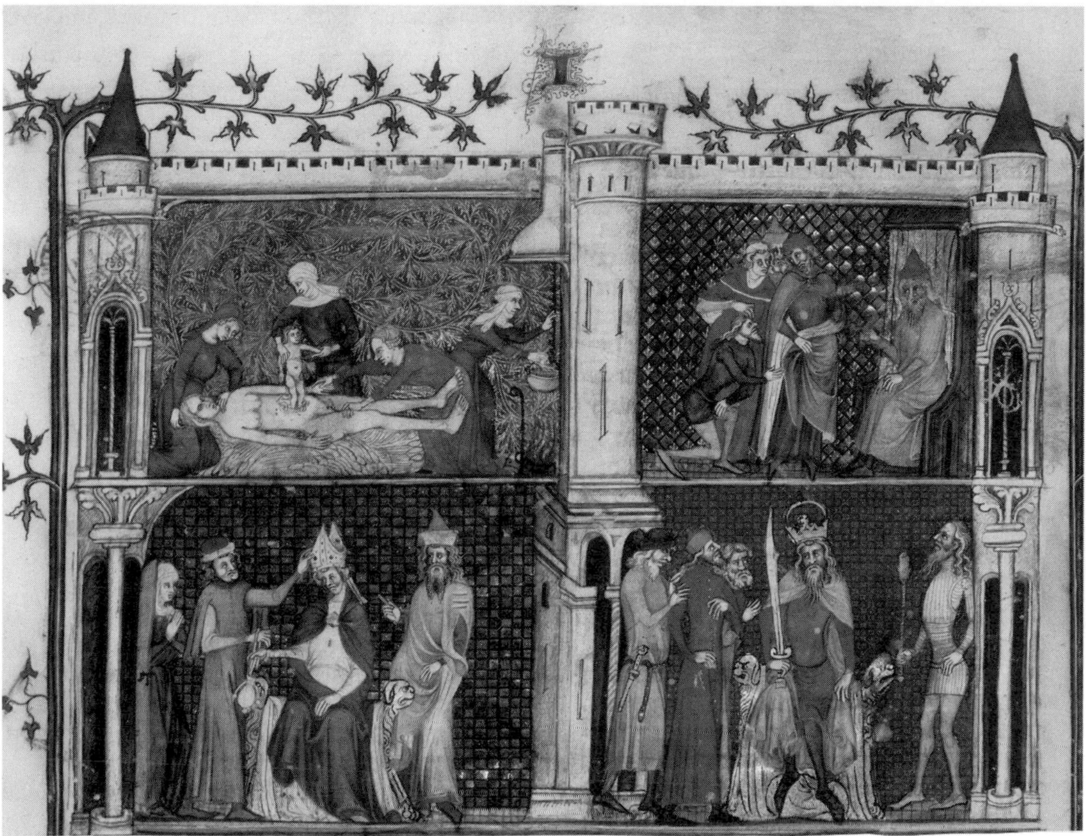

Figure 11.4 The birth of Julius Caesar in a mid-fourteenth-century French manuscript of *Li fait des Romains* (Acts of the Romans). This vernacular history of the Roman Empire, composed *c.* 1213, presents the death of Caesar's mother in childbirth and the extraction of the infant Caesar from her dead body as the originary moment of the empire. Bibliothèque nationale de France, nouv. acq. fr. 3576, f. 197r.

Enhancing Fertility

Because much of the early historical writing on 'women's medicine' grew out of mid-twentieth-century feminist struggles around the legalization of contraception and abortion, it tended to focus on techniques for limiting fertility at the expense of a broader picture of procreative health care. The result was a mythical narrative – often combined with the story of the marginalization of midwives by male practitioners – according to which knowledge concerning the contraceptive and abortive properties of herbal substances was orally transmitted from one generation of women to another, including among midwives, without relying on male medical knowledge or authority. As Monica Green has shown, this contention rested in large part on the conflation of emmenagogues, meant to bring on a woman's period – a function considered essential to women's health and fertility in medieval medicine – and contraceptives or abortifacients, the use of which was advocated by some medical authorities, but only when the mother's life might be endangered by miscarriage or childbirth. There was a demand for abortifacients in medieval society, mostly from unmarried women, but this should not be read into the broad social and medical concern with regular menstruation.[21]

In fact, as might be expected in a period that combined high rates of infant mortality with a strong social and economic investment in procreation, medieval families worried much more about infertility than unwanted pregnancies. This concern was heightened by the advent of plague beginning in 1348, and the subsequent depopulation of late medieval Europe.[22] These factors created a market for the services of practitioners who claimed to be able to facilitate conception and help women carry pregnancies to term. These practitioners were extremely diverse. While women from wealthy families might compete for the services of learned physicians, women on all social levels sought out remedies from official and unofficial practitioners in their communities, typically on the recommendation of other women. Fertility magic, like the love-magic with which it was often associated, often skirted the border between legitimate and illicit procedures.

We can see these processes at work in two sets of documents, one from early fourteenth-century Provence and one from late fourteenth-century Florence. The first records the investigation of a respected local surgeon, Antoni Imberti, accused of having falsely said 'to women that he would make them pregnant and bear children ... and to men who were impotent on account of age or other causes that he would make them capable of intercourse, through the deceptive use of the false and magical art, as well as medicines, baths, potions and other means'.[23] While the judges showed a good deal of interest in Imberti's use of amulets (small bags bound with thread that contained stones and scraps of paper with pious inscriptions), almost certainly seeking evidence of demonic invocation, their main concern seems to have been that his remedies were ineffective and therefore fraudulent.

The other case rests on the correspondence of Margherita Bandini, the wife of a wealthy Tuscan merchant. Still childless in her early thirties, Margherita received much fertility advice from family and friends, including a diagnosis and prescription from the physician Naddino Aldobrandini and a series of recommendations from her sister and brother-in-law that included the pious (charitable donations), the empirical (a ring made by a local woman to be placed inside the vagina during intercourse) and the magical (a belt

21 Monica H. Green, 'Gendering the history of women's healthcare', *Gender & History* 20 (2008), 487–518. For the sixteeth and seventeenth centuries, see Lauren Kassell, 'Fruitful Bodies and Astrological Medicine', Chapter 16, this book.

22 Peter Biller, 'The Multitude in Later Medieval Thought', Chapter 10, this book.

23 Joseph Shatzmiller, *Médecine et justice en Provence médiévale: Documents de Manosque, 1262–1348* (Aix-en-Provence, 1989), pp. 176–83, no. 56.

like the one described in Exhibit 11, to be girded on her by a virgin boy, so that the lettered side touched her skin).[24] This combination of remedies was typical of medieval fertility practices, which also included pilgrimages to the shrines of Christian saints reputed to aid conception, and as a result the material culture of fertility rivals in richness that related to childbirth.[25]

Both cases confirm the intense interest of married women and their extended families in fertility. The available remedies were part of a broad spectrum of health care that included doctors' prescriptions; physicians were regularly consulted about infertility, and their recommendations were in the first instance grounded in their theoretical understanding of the body and its humours.[26] However, if some people explicitly condemned charms as popular 'fables', others included them in their books of practical medicine as part of a well-accepted category of remedies attested by medical experience (*experimenta*), even if their causal mechanism was unclear.[27]

Limiting Fertility

While the enhancement of fertility greatly concerned married men and women, single women faced the opposite problem: how to terminate pregnancies resulting from illicit sexual liaisons, voluntary or involuntary, which might threaten their employment or damage the honour of their families. This problem had theological as well as technical dimensions. Church authorities strictly prohibited terminating pregnancies, in line with the legal and theological doctrine according to which God infused the fetus with a human soul roughly forty days after conception.[28] At least under some circumstances, praying for a miscarriage appears to have been acceptable – witness the miracle granted to the Pisan widow who successfully petitioned the blessed Gérard Cagnoli shortly

24 Ann Crabb, 'Ne pas être mère: L'autodéfense d'une Florentine vers 1400', *Clio: Histoire, femmes et sociétés* 21 (2005), 150–61; Iris Origo, *The Merchant of Prato: Francesco di Marco Datini* (London, 1957), pp. 160–1. Crabb and Origo differ on the nature of the ring recommended by Margherita's sister.

25 Musacchio, *Art and Ritual*, pp. 139–42 (northern Italy); Carol Rawcliffe, 'Women, childbirth, and religion' (England); Gabriela Signori, 'Defensivgemeinschaften. Kreißende, Hebammen und "Mitweiber" im Spiegel spätmittelalterlicher Geburtswunder', *Das Mittelalter* 1 (1996), 113–34 (Germany). See, in general, Katharine Park, 'Magic and medicine: The healing arts', in Judith C. Brown and Robert C. Davis (eds.), *Gender and Society in Renaissance Italy* (London, 1998), pp. 129–49.

26 Green, *Making Women's Medicine Masculine*, pp. 85–91, 249–51. See, in general, Luke Demaitre, *Medieval Medicine: The Art of Healing, from Head to Toe* (Westport, CT, 2013), pp. 153–95.

27 Peter Murray Jones, 'Generation between Script and Print', Chapter 13, this book; Lea T. Olsan, 'Charms and prayers in medieval medical theory and practice', *Social History of Medicine* 16 (2003), 343–66. On pilgrimages related to fertility, see Fiona Harris-Stoerz, 'Fertility', in Larissa Taylor *et al.* (eds.) *Encyclopaedia of Medieval Pilgrimage* (Brill Online, 2012), http://referenceworks.brillonline.com/entries/encyclopaedia-of-medieval-pilgrimage/fertility-SIM_00124, http://dx.doi.org/10.1163/2213-2139_emp_SIM_00124, last accessed 12 June 2018.

28 Rebecca Flemming, 'Galen's Generations of Seeds', Chapter 7; van der Lugt, 'Formed Fetuses and Healthy Children', this book.

after she had been raped.[29] In theory, however, any action that resulted in an intentional miscarriage after the ensoulment of the fetus was classified as homicide in general and infanticide in particular, both capital crimes in large parts of Europe.[30]

While these strictures were in theory universal, in practice denunciations and prosecutions for abortion and neonatal infanticide fell heavily on young single women from humble backgrounds, whose bodies offered an easy target for the enforcement of Christian sexual norms.[31] The judicial records generated by these denunciations and prosecutions reveal a flourishing world of extra-marital sexuality, including a pervasive pattern of sexual exploitation of female servants by their masters and male relatives of their employers, and provide a wealth of information about how young single women, with the aid of their lovers and kinfolk, might attempt to terminate unwanted pregnancies. Among the most revealing sources are the letters of clemency in which the kings of France commuted the death sentences of people convicted of capital crimes. In some cases, the methods described were improvised using materials and techniques at hand, as in the case of the man who tried to provoke a miscarriage by twisting a piece of household linen around the belly of his pregnant maidservant.[32] Pregnant women were also advised to jump from high surfaces or be beaten about the abdomen.

People seeking to terminate pregnancies also turned to practitioners of official medicine under pretexts such as 'constipation', 'uterine illness' or 'abdominal pains', as described in two letters of clemency from 1466. These concerned three individuals living in Clermont l'Hérault, in the south of France: a young woman, Katherine Armant, and the sister and brother-in-law of the man to whom she was engaged. Katherine had become pregnant while her fiancé was abroad, and the letters record a series of attempts by the three to salvage the engagement by provoking a miscarriage; after unsuccessfully pummelling Katherine's abdomen with their fists, they consulted in turn a physician, an apothecary and a barber. The last bled Katherine from the vein in the foot recommended by Galen for terminating pregnancies and prescribed 'potions and powders' to the same end – services that earned him the death penalty as well.[33] It is worth noting

29 Pierre-André Sigal, 'La grossesse, l'accouchement et l'attitude envers l'enfant mort-né a la fin du Moyen Age d'après les récits de miracles', *Actes du 110e Congrès national des sociétés savantes, Montpellier, 1985, Section d'histoire médiévale et de philologie*, vol. 1: *Santé, médecine et assistance au Moyen Âge* (Paris, 1987), pp. 32–41, on p. 26.

30 Wolfgang P. Müller, *The Criminalization of Abortion in the West: Its Origins in Medieval Law* (Ithaca, NY, 2012). In regions still largely governed by customary law, notably Germany, Eastern Europe and England, the legal system was considerably more forgiving (see pp. 12 and 123–48).

31 Laura Gowing, *Common Bodies: Women, Touch, and Power in Seventeenth-Century England* (New Haven, CT, 2003).

32 Cited by Müller, *Criminalization*, p. 166 n. 30.

33 Cited ibid., pp. 163–4, 166. Medieval sources include no known references to surgical abortions; the closest procedure would have been embryotomy, dismembering the fetus in utero in order to extract it piecewise

that the three conspirators did not consult a midwife, nor are midwives ever mentioned in cases of this sort.

Although Katherine's case involved recourse to official practitioners, consultation of unofficial ones, both male and female, was also common, as in the roughly contemporary case of the 18-year-old Jehannette, who obtained a potion from a woman known as Margot of the Large Arms. Two months later she miscarried what was described as an 'apple-sized' fetus, 'whether by illness or otherwise', her letter of clemency noted, and was condemned for suffocating it, since it had achieved human form.[34] Such documents indicate that knowledge regarding abortifacient procedures and preparations – effective or not – circulated widely, and men and women who wished to terminate unwanted pregnancies would have had a good idea whom to consult.[35]

Contraception posed the same religious and ethical problems as abortion, but in less dramatic form. Christian theologians and legal experts classified it as 'quasi-homicide', similar to aborting a fetus in the first forty days after conception, before this had received a human soul; it was punished by penance rather than criminal prosecution.[36] For this reason – and also because it was more difficult to detect – contraception rarely appears in judicial records and other archival sources. Withdrawal (coitus interruptus) was probably the most common method.[37] In addition, as with infertility, lay techniques involved the use of amulets, like the herb worn by Béatrice de Planissoles in early fourteenth-century Montaillou.[38]

Physicians had access to a broad range of information regarding contraception, since, like abortion, it was openly discussed in the Arabic medical encyclopaedias that were the foundation of Latin medical learning; these reflected the more positive attitude to sexuality shared by the ancient Greek and medieval Islamic traditions, which held that regular sexual activity was essential to women's health, and that contraceptives and abortifacients were in order if pregnancy might endanger the woman's life.[39] This matter-of-fact acceptance of fertility limitation posed a dilemma for European

when it had already died or in cases of obstructed birth. There is no evidence that this invasive and dangerous technique was used to terminate unwanted pregnancies; the term Müller translates as 'needle-like instrument' (*Criminalization*, p. 166) in fact refers to a piece of household linen.

34 Ibid., pp. 162–70. 35 On efficacy: Green, 'Gendering the history', 498–500, 505.

36 Müller, *Criminalization*, pp. 51, 53.

37 Peter Biller, 'Birth-control in the west in the thirteenth and early fourteenth centuries', *Past & Present* 94 (1982), 3–26, on 20–4.

38 Emmanuel Le Roy Ladurie, *Montaillou: The Promised Land of Error*, trans. Barbara Bray (New York, NY, 1978), p. 173.

39 Basim Musallam, *Sex and Society in Islam: Birth Control before the Nineteenth Century* (Cambridge, 1983). Jewish law also condemned contraception, though less starkly than Christian law; Carmen Caballero-Navas, 'Medicine and pharmacy for women: The encounter of Jewish thinking and practice with the Arabic and Christian medical traditions', *European Review* 16 (2008), 249–59.

physicians, which is clearly described in a short treatise, 'Whether it is permitted to provoke a miscarriage', written by Gentile da Foligno, professor of medicine at the University of Bologna in the first half of the fourteenth century. In it, Gentile explored (but did not resolve) the tension between the legal prohibition on abortion and the imperative of medicine, 'which is directed toward the well-being of human bodies'.[40] In contrast, Niccolò Falcucci was more lenient, including a long chapter on the 'prohibition of conception' in his influential *Practica* (*c.* 1400), where he stated without reservation that contraceptives should be used if there was any reason to believe that childbirth or a miscarriage might endanger the woman or fetus; counter-indications to pregnancy included uterine conditions, a weak bladder that might rupture during birth, illness and constitutional weakness. Falcucci accordingly detailed a wide range of contraceptive measures, including coitus interruptus, potions and suppositories and amulets.[41] Cautiously, however, he did not include any specific references to his own practice in this connection, as he did in chapters on childbirth.[42]

Conclusion

The comfort of Falcucci and other fifteenth-century Italian physicians in discussing cases of difficult childbirth or the constellation of symptoms known as 'suffocation of the uterus' that they encountered in their own practices signals a new development: the breakdown of the taboo around the inspection of the genitals by male practitioners except in obstetrical emergencies, and physicians' assertion of authority in areas that had previously been restricted to female practitioners. This also took the form of erasing the names of female authorities, such as the mythical Trotula, in treatises on women's medicine.[43] In practice, however, these developments do not seem to have had much impact outside urban elites and princely families, some of whom were already employing physicians to oversee the births of their children as early as the late thirteenth century.[44] Instead of edging midwives out of childbirth or replacing the broad array of people who offered remedies for infertility and unwanted pregnancies, learned physicians simply took their place alongside these other groups in the flourishing field of procreative health care.

40 Müller, *Criminalization*, pp. 160–1, on p. 161.

41 Niccolò Falcucci, *Sermones medicinales septem*, sermo 6, tract. 3, ch. 3 (Venice, 1533), ff. 43v–44r, on f. 43v.

42 Ibid., sermo 6, tract. 3, ch. 10, f. 50r.

43 Green, *Making Women's Medicine Masculine*, pp. 246–324.

44 Michael McVaugh, 'The births of the children of Jaime II', *Medievalia* 6 (1986), 7–16.

12 Formed Fetuses and Healthy Children in Scholastic Theology, Medicine and Law

Maaike van der Lugt

In the medieval west, rules around sexual conduct, marriage and childbearing were largely laid down by the church. Rooted in the pastoral discourse which guided the faithful in everyday life, promising salvation in the next, this moral and legal code gained increasing precision, coherence and dominance from the twelfth century, through the combined efforts of scholastic theologians and canon lawyers, or 'canonists', the experts in ecclesiastical law. Meanwhile, medieval schools and universities also incubated a new learned medicine and natural philosophy. Here, based on fresh interpretations of ancient and Arabic texts, translated into Latin from the late eleventh century, systematic theories of generation took shape.[1]

Historians have shown how this medical and philosophical knowledge acquired new forms and meanings as it became available beyond the university and how pastoral discourse was repackaged in penitentials and handbooks for priests and preachers, relayed to the faithful through sermons and confession, and translated into judicial practice.[2] Yet studies focused solely on the theological, legal or medical frameworks obscure the extent to which procreation pervaded multiple discourses and transcended disciplinary divides. Theologians provided the church with moral and legal norms about sex and marriage, but they also participated actively in debates about the workings of procreation. The primary scholastic treatise on human generation was written by an Augustinian canon who was one of the leading theologians of his time.[3] Moreover, debates over doctrines such as the transmission of original sin or the conception of Christ involved detailed discussion about the physiology of procreation. Scholasticism both stimulated and discouraged

1 Jean Gaudemet, *Le mariage en Occident: Les moeurs et le droit* (Paris, 1987); James Brundage, *Law, Sex and Christian Society in Medieval Europe* (Chicago, IL, 1987); M. Anthony Hewson, *Giles of Rome and the Medieval Theory of Conception* (London, 1975); Romana Martorelli Vico, *Medicina e filosofia: Per una storia dell'embriologia medievale nel XIII e XIV secolo* (Naples, 2002).

2 For example, Monica H. Green, *Making Women's Medicine Masculine: The Rise of Male Authority in Pre-Modern Gynaecology* (Oxford, 2008); Peter Murray Jones, 'Generation between Script and Print', Chapter 13, this book; David d'Avray, *Medieval Marriage Sermons: Mass Communication in a Culture Without Print* (Oxford, 2001); Charles Donahue, *Law, Marriage and Society: Arguments about Marriage in Five Courts* (Cambridge, 2007); Ludwig Schmugge, *Marriage on Trial: Late Medieval German Couples at the Papal Court*, trans. Atria A. Larson (Washington, DC, 2012).

3 Giles of Rome, *De formatione humani corporis in utero*, ed. Romana Martorelli Vico (Florence, 2008).

interdisciplinary cross-fertilization. While every field had its own authorities and commentary traditions, all scholastics shared training in the liberal arts and, from the mid-thirteenth century, Aristotelian natural and moral philosophy. They brought with them a Christian outlook and other common values and beliefs, besides particular, often local, experiences and opinions. This chapter aims to grasp better the extent to which medieval understandings of generation informed legal and religious norms about sex, marriage and childbearing; when and how the different outlooks on procreation converged or conflicted; and how learned debate and explicit rules related to social practices, values and beliefs.

Many medieval discussions of these questions centre on the fetus. Through the Christian doctrine of the immortal soul, the fetus became the focus of intertwining religious, philosophical, legal and social concern. As we shall see, debates about abortion, infant baptism and burial related not only to each other, but also to discussions about the nature of seeds, the formation of the embryo, ensoulment and the body/soul nexus, and to questions about humanity, legal personhood and salvation. Similar questions underlay debates about 'monsters', to use the medieval term. The causality of monstrous births sharply divided opinion, with important implications for their spiritual and legal status.[4] These divergent views lead, finally, to the broader question of whether, why and how norms and rules about marriage, sex and procreation reflected attitudes about physical and mental impairment and the production of healthy and beautiful children. The pastoral ideology promoted procreation and underscored the unity of humankind, combining a concern for survival of offspring and the stability of marriage with indifference about health. However, in the later middle ages new ideas challenged the hegemony of the pastoral view.

Abortion, Burial and Baptism

In moral theology and canon law, abortion was a grave sin. (I use *abortion* in its modern sense, although the medieval *aborsus* also covered spontaneous and accidental miscarriage and efforts to deliver a woman of a dead fetus.) Its prohibition was part of a broader pastoral concern for the offspring's survival, reflected in warnings about the dangers of bed-sharing and heavy penances for women who abandoned their babies, denied them food or killed them.[5] Abortion was not, however, necessarily equated with murder. In the twelfth century, theologians and jurists began to define abortion as a distinct legal category and as a crime, not only a sin or tort. At the same time they qualified abortion as homicide from the moment the fetus was formed. Abortion of unformed

4 Jennifer Spinks, 'Monstrous Births and Diabolical Seed', Exhibit 13, this book.

5 Peter Biller, *The Measure of Multitude: Population in Medieval Thought* (Oxford, 2003), pp. 189–91.

fetuses deserved retribution in the form of penance, whereas abortion of a formed fetus was, like infanticide, also punishable in court.[6]

Fetal form as the criterion for punishment derived from a biblical rule about retribution for accidental miscarriage caused by a third party. Exodus (21:22), in the Septuagint version, stated that 'life must be given for life' when the fetus was fully formed; if still unformed, a fine sufficed to compensate the loss.[7] Physicians placed formation within a range from thirty to ninety days, sometimes differentiating according to sex (females took shape more slowly) and the supposedly variable duration of pregnancy.[8] From a Christian perspective, however, it was not bodily form but the immortal soul that made the embryo a human being. Physicians tended to ignore ensoulment, while most philosophers and theologians agreed that God infused the soul into the fetus once it had acquired its shape. The biblical norm and theories of generation, ensoulment and the acquisition of human status confirmed and reinforced each other.[9]

The fundamental distinction between formed and unformed fetuses applied even to abortions to save the life of the mother, for instance when she was very young. Theologians and canonists conceded that these cases were complicated, but maintained that physicians should not abort formed fetuses.[10] Medical writings were more ambiguous. Recipe collections include explicit prescriptions for contraceptives and abortifacients, but whether the latter served to kill a fetus or drive out one that had died is often unclear. Recipes to 'cleanse the womb' or 'bring back menstruation' are better understood as intended to keep women in good health and prepare them for conception than as disguised contraceptives and abortifacients.[11] In medicine, like in households and families, promoting fertility was the more pressing concern.

While some treatises on generation and medical practice advocated contraceptive measures to avoid dangerous pregnancies as a lesser evil than abortion, they rarely mentioned methods to induce miscarriage, except when the fetus had already died.

6 Wolfgang P. Müller, *The Criminalization of Abortion in the West: Its Origins in Medieval Law* (Ithaca, NY, 2012); Biller, *Measure of Multitude*, pp. 17–112.

7 Müller, *Criminalization*, p. 102; Rebecca Flemming, 'Galen's Generations of Seeds', Chapter 7, this book.

8 Hewson, *Giles of Rome*, pp. 166–78, 214–21.

9 Maaike van der Lugt, 'L'animation de l'embryon humain et le statut de l'enfant à naître dans la pensée médiévale', in Luc Brisson, Marie-Hélène Congourdeau and Jean-Luc Solère (eds.), *L'embryon: Formation et animation. Antiquité grecque et latine, traditions hébraïque, chrétienne et islamique* (Paris, 2008), pp. 233–54; see also Marie-Hélène Congourdeau, 'Debating the Soul in Late Antiquity', Chapter 8, this book.

10 Müller, *Criminalization*, pp. 111–14.

11 Monica H. Green, review of *Eve's Herbs: A History of Contraception and Abortion in the West*, by John M. Riddle, *Bulletin of the History of Medicine* 73 (1999), 308–11; Helen King, 'Women and Doctors in Ancient Greece', Chapter 3; Katharine Park, 'Managing Childbirth and Fertility in Medieval Europe', Chapter 11; Lauren Kassell, 'Fruitful Bodies and Astrological Medicine', Chapter 16, this book.

Around 1300, a leading Montpellier physician warned his readers that teaching the use of abortifacients on living fetuses was a mortal sin.[12] Ancient and Arabic physicians seem to have had fewer qualms. Avicenna (Ibn Sina) matter-of-factly mentioned risks to the mother's health alongside fetal death as indications to expel the fetus. Scholastic physicians, however, did not speak with one voice. One prominent Italian separated medical and pastoral imperatives and claimed that the pregnant woman's health was a doctor's prime responsibility.[13]

Roman law, the basis of medieval civil law, was similarly uninterested in the soul of the embryo. Even though civil law, together with canon law, gradually came to form a common legal system with a claim to universal validity within medieval Christendom, canon and civil law approached the fetus differently. Civil law was concerned with legal status, not salvation. Legal personhood started with the baby's first cry; the fetus was considered a part of the mother's body and only a potential life. Roman law protected the interests of the unborn, most commonly by granting posthumous children inheritance rights; but this was based on a legal fiction, according to which the child had already been born at the time of the father's death or the drafting of his will. Abortion was punished not because of some 'right to life' of the fetus, but on the grounds of other civil or criminal considerations, such as poisoning or depriving someone of an heir. By 1200, however, in a sign of the increasing 'naturalization' of civil law, legal commentators began to treat abortion of formed fetuses as murder.[14]

With the paradoxical exceptions of authorities on English common law and a minority of Italian experts in civil law, later medieval legislation on abortion was based on the distinction between formed and unformed fetuses. This distinction also infiltrated commentaries on Aristotle's *Politics*, which had been translated in the 1260s, giving rise, with his *Ethics*, to yet another normative tradition. Aristotle advocated abortions 'before the emergence of life and sense' to keep numbers down and as more palatable than exposure. Without fully endorsing his views, scholastic commentators agreed that early abortions were not homicides. Legal practice was more lenient than its theory. Since abortion and infanticide were difficult to prove, the authorities were often reluctant to prosecute. Most trials for fetal homicide concerned not abortion, but accidental miscarriage caused by an assault, in which women acted as the claimants.[15]

12 Bernard of Gordon, *Lilium medicinae*, VII.15 (Ferrara, 1486), f. 149r.

13 Biller, *Measure of Multitude*, pp. 153–4; Müller, *Criminalization*, pp. 160–1.

14 On naturalization: Franck Roumy, *L'adoption dans le droit savant du XIIe au XVIe siècle* (Paris, 1998), pp. 136–61.

15 Müller, *Criminalization*, pp. 88–95, 134–48, 233–9; Biller, *Measure of Multitude*, pp. 50–2, 366–78; Rebecca Flemming, 'States and Populations in the Classical World', Chapter 5; Peter Biller, 'The Multitude in Later Medieval Thought', Chapter 10, this book.

The watershed distinctions between formed and unformed fetuses, and crime and sin, converged with theories of ensoulment. Throughout our period, almost everyone who raised the question considered it impossible for ensoulment to occur at conception, in the absence of the structures necessary for the functions of life. The embryo was thought to arise from the mixing of liquids (seed and blood) that gradually solidify. Body and soul had to be adapted to each other, a notion reinforced by the reception of Aristotle's metaphysics and natural philosophy in the early thirteenth century. Philosophers and theologians maintained, with Aristotle, that the embryo possessed a rudimentary soul as soon as it started to attract food, but agreed that it acquired its intellectual soul only when the body was ready. A small minority of scholastics claimed, in the name of the unity of the human soul, that full animation took place at conception.[16]

The majority rejection of immediate ensoulment also had strong religious and social motives. Given the frequency of spontaneous miscarriage, how would a person without a body be resurrected at the end of time?[17] What about all those lost souls? The doctrine of original sin, dating back to Augustine, held that there could be no salvation without baptism. Baptism was seen as a cleansing from sin and a rebirth through which one entered into the Christian faith and community. From the twelfth century, as the western church fostered greater doctrinal precision and stressed pastoral care, it encouraged parents to have their children baptized as soon as possible and instructed midwives in emergency baptisms.[18]

The increasing emphasis on early baptism aggravated the distress of parents of stillborn children. Nameless and without godparents, unbaptized infants could not be buried in consecrated ground. However, the church promoted or allowed several beliefs and practices that mitigated these harsh teachings. Scholastic theologians developed the notion of limbo, a place where unbaptized children did not suffer. By the fourteenth century, the church had begun to tolerate the taking of stillborn babies to special sanctuaries where, when they showed apparent signs of life, they were baptized and buried.[19]

16 Van der Lugt, 'L'animation'; Nahyan Fancy, 'Generation in Medieval Islamic Medicine', Chapter 9, this book.

17 Caroline Walker Bynum, *The Resurrection of the Body in Western Christianity, 200–1336* (New York, NY, 1995).

18 William Maclehose, *A Tender Age: Cultural Anxieties over the Child in the Twelfth and Thirteenth Centuries* (New York, NY, 2006), pp. 53–106; Kathryn Taglia, 'Delivering a Christian identity: Midwives in northern French synodal legislation, *c.* 1200–1500', in Peter Biller and Joseph Ziegler (eds.), *Religion and Medicine in the Middle Ages* (Woodbridge, 2001), pp. 77–90; Tiffany D. Vann Sprecher and Ruth Mazo Karras, 'The midwife and the church: Ecclesiastical regulation of midwives in Brie, 1499–1504', *Bulletin of the History of Medicine* 85 (2011), 171–92; Park, 'Managing Childbirth and Fertility'.

19 Maclehose, *Tender Age*; Jacques Gélis, *Les enfants des limbes: Mort-nés et parents dans l'Europe chrétienne* (Paris, 2006).

From the early eleventh century, church leaders also encouraged the excision of the fetus from its deceased mother, to save the child's life or at least its soul.[20]

In medieval society, fetal excisions could also be motivated by a husband's desire to keep his wife's dowry, which would be returned to her family if she died without issue.[21] Alternatively, the practice reflected beliefs about the impurity of pregnant women and prohibitions of burying them with the fetus inside. The medieval church sometimes endorsed this taboo, but more often rejected or rationalized it by stating that the fetus should be excised if it had already been ensouled or still had a chance of survival.[22] Roman jurists, similarly, had explained an archaic law against burying the mother unless the fetus was removed as a means to produce an heir, and medieval commentators associated this obligation with the ban on executing pregnant women.[23] In both secular and church law, the focus shifted from the woman to the fetus. This neutralized the taboo but exacerbated the moral dilemma: inaction potentially meant killing an innocent human, but if the excised fetus was already dead, it could neither be baptized nor buried in consecrated ground.[24] In canon law the obligation to remove the fetus never became standard; matters were left to the discretion of the local bishop. Excavations of medieval cemeteries have occasionally revealed women's skeletons containing full-term fetuses among the other dead (Fig. 12.1).[25]

Postmortem fetal excisions were not originally considered part of medicine. Evidence for the involvement of barbers and surgeons appears only in the early fourteenth century. By this time, some learned physicians and surgeons had also started to describe the procedure, despite its absence in ancient and Arabic medical sources – a reflection of Christian concerns, new social demands and the growing medicalization of childbirth.[26]

20 Stephen Bednarski and Andrée Courtemanche, 'Sadly and with a bitter heart: What the caesarean section meant in the middle ages', *Florilegium* 28 (2011), 33–69.

21 Ibid.; Osvaldo Cavallar, 'Septimo mense: Periti, medici et partoriente in Baldo degli Ubaldi', in Carla Frova *et al.* (eds.), *VI centenario della morte di Baldo degli Ubaldi, 1400–2000* (Perugia, 2005), pp. 365–460.

22 Van der Lugt, 'L'animation', pp. 251–3; Ludwig Schmugge, 'Im Kindbett gestorben. Ein kanonistisches Problem im Alltag des 15. Jahrhunderts', in Richard H. Helmholz *et al.* (eds.), *Grundlagen des Rechts* (Paderborn, 2000), pp. 467–76, on p. 474.

23 *Corpus iuris civilis*, Digest, 11.8.2 and its standard gloss: Accursius, *Corpus iuris civilis cum Glossis Accursii* (Lyons, 1627), I, col. 1195.

24 Didier Lett, *L'enfant des miracles: Enfance et société au Moyen Âge (XIIe–XIIIe s.)* (Paris, 1997), pp. 207–11; Schmugge, 'Im Kindbett', p. 474.

25 For example, Vilhelm Møller-Christensen, *Æbelholt Kloster* (Copenhagen, 1982), pp. 190–2.

26 Monica H. Green, 'Caring for gendered bodies', in Judith Bennett and Ruth Mazo Karras (eds.), *Oxford Handbook for Medieval Women and Gender* (Oxford, 2013), pp. 345–61, on pp. 353–4; Daniel Schäfer, 'Embryulkie zwischen Mythos, Recht und Medizin. Zur Überlieferungsgeschichte von *Sectio in mortua* und Embryotomie in Spätantike und Mittelalter', *Medizinhistorisches Journal* 31 (1996), 275–97.

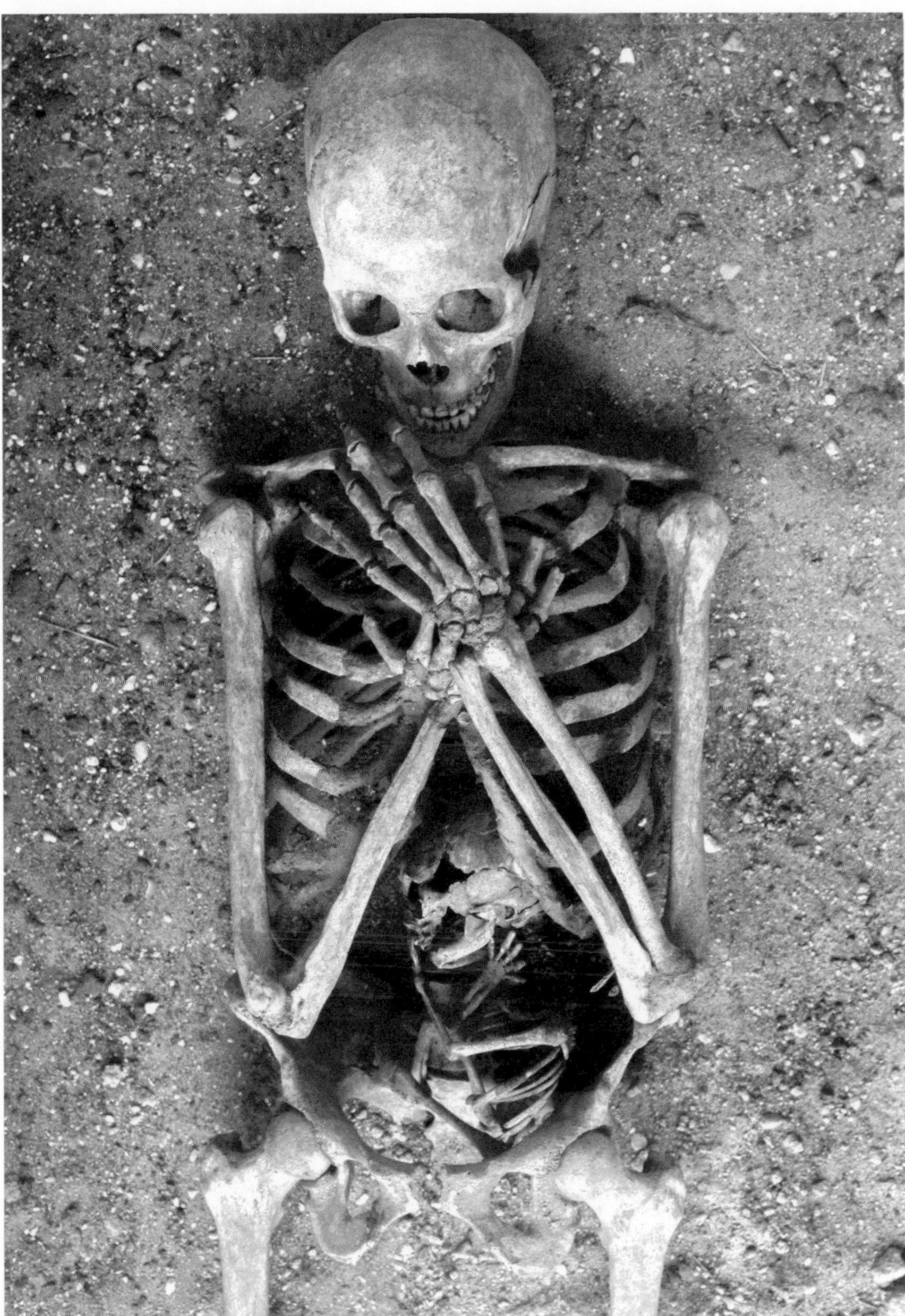

Figure 12.1 This skeleton of a 40-year-old woman, with an eight-month fetus in breech position, was buried at the cemetery of Æbelholt Abbey, Denmark, between 1200 and 1550. It is one of five female skeletons with fetuses, of a total of fifty females of childbearing age, found at this site. Photo: Alwin Göttsche, Museum North Zealand.

The Spiritual and Legal Status of Monstrous Births

The church welcomed all infants as God's creatures; neither an unusual appearance nor limited rational capacities precluded the presence of an immortal soul. Because the soul was associated with reason, medieval canonists and theologians were more concerned with mental than physical impairment, although the latter was more evident in infants than the former. Theologians compared 'half-wits' to children: both could be baptized despite being incapable of professing their faith.[27] Concerning physical deformities, Augustine's inclusive vision of humanity was an enduring influence. In a famous passage of the *City of God* about the 'monstrous races' inhabiting the edges of the known world, Augustine associated these beings of questionable existence with monstrous births, which were, in his view, by definition human.[28] Although medieval theologians, in their sporadic discussions of monstrous races, increasingly echoed the Aristotelian notion of a necessary congruence between body and soul, implying that bodies that did not look human could not have a soul, they continued to suppose the humanity of individual monstrous births.

In theology, canon law and manuals for priests, writers on the access of monsters to the sacraments debated not if they should be baptized, but how. Theologians asked whether hermaphrodites should receive a male or a female name (a minor problem since the sacrament itself was gender neutral) and (more challengingly) whether conjoined twins should be baptized as one person or two (Fig. 12.2).[29] However, a late thirteenth-century question about 'pygmies' reveals the vulnerability of the Augustinian view. To further the argument that a well-proportioned body, but not its size, matters for human status, the author, an anonymous Franciscan, mentioned the undisputed humanity of the 46-day, fully formed embryo. As such, pygmies, though small, are human, but a monstrous child with 'its head on the bottom and its feet on the side' is not, and should not be baptized. The same is true of monsters who are the fruit of bestiality.[30]

This friar's minority position was reminiscent of medieval civil law, where the issue around monsters was not salvation, but succession rights or criminal cases: is it murder to smother a deformed child? Unlike the Laws of the Twelve Tables, classic Roman law did not actively promote the elimination of monsters, but refused to consider

27 Maaike van der Lugt, 'L'humanité des monstres et leur accès aux sacrements', in Anna Caiozzo and Anne-Emmanuelle Demartini (eds.), *Monstre et imaginaire social: Approches historiques* (Paris, 2008), pp. 135–61, with Latin notes at https://halshs.archives-ouvertes.fr/halshs-00175497.

28 Augustine, *De civitate Dei*, 16.8.1–2.

29 Van der Lugt, 'L'humanité'; Irven Resnick, 'Conjoined twins, medieval biology and evolving reflection on individual identity', *Viator* 44 (2013), 343–68.

30 T. W. Köhler, Homo animal nobilissimum. *Konturen des spezifisch Menschlichen in der naturphilosophischen Aristoteleskommentierung des dreizehnten Jahrhunderts* (Leiden, 2008), pp. 419–43.

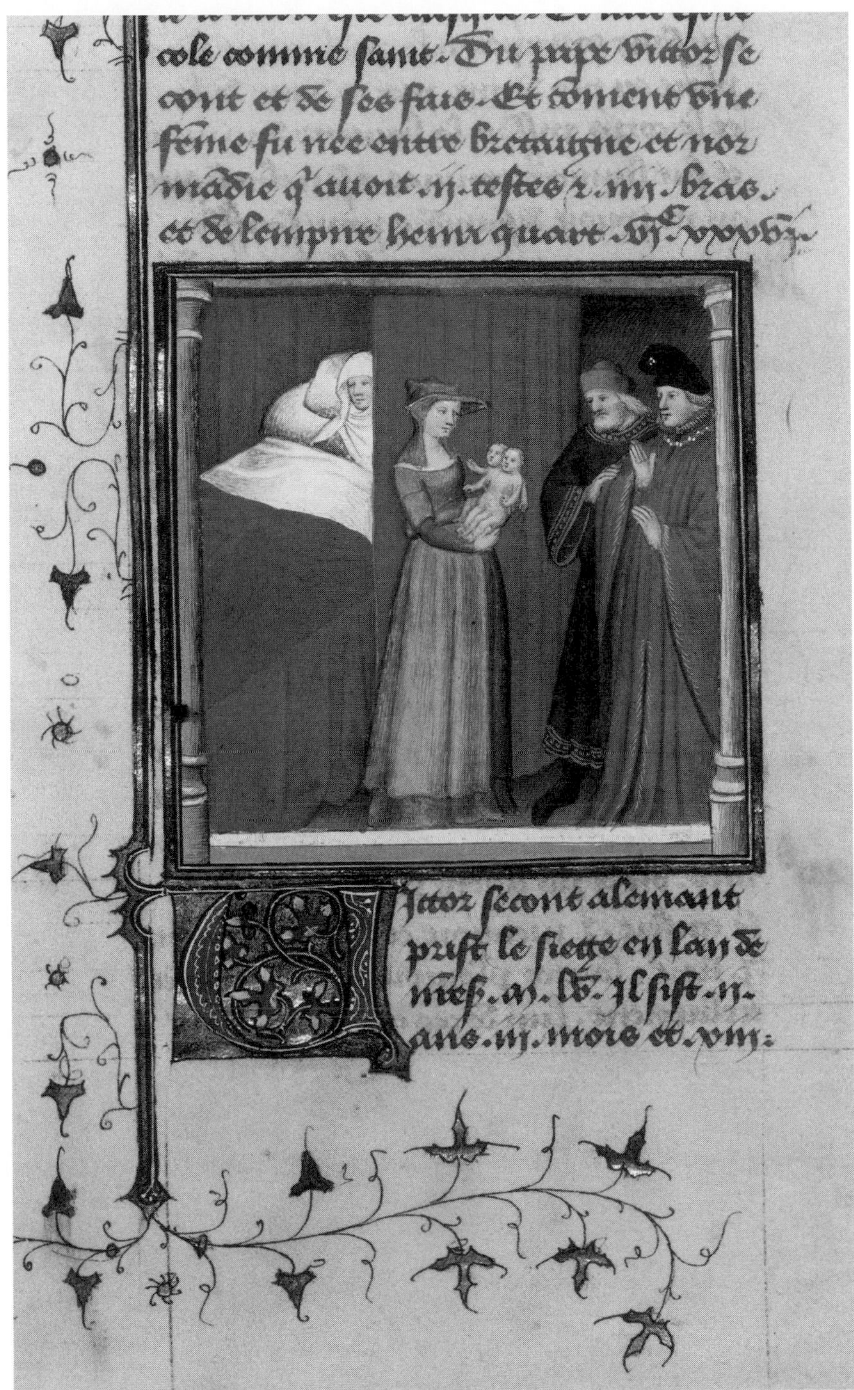

Figure 12.2 This miniature in a French chronicle, copied in 1416, adorns an account of a local monstrous birth. As the mother rests, a midwife or matron shows conjoined twins to two men, one probably the father. The domestic setting implies similar care to other newborns. 'Livre du Tresor des hystoires des plus notables …', Bibliothèque de l'Arsenal, Paris, MS 5077, f. 341r.

them as heirs and deprived them of legal protection. This harsh rule applied only to extreme cases, in which the child was said to lack human form. According to medieval commentators, these births were caused by bestiality, a widespread belief with potentially deadly consequences for the implicated parents, even though most physicians and natural philosophers followed Aristotle in refuting the possibility. They attributed monstrous births to other natural causes: too much or too little matter, corrupted or weak seed, astral influences and the force of the imagination of the father and especially the mother. A late medieval anecdote recounts how Albert the Great once saved a shepherd from execution by convincing the villagers that the stars had caused the birth of a half-human calf. Though fictitious, the story is not implausible: in 1464 the court of Holland sentenced Willem Boudewinsz to die at the stake alongside a cow that had given birth to a deformed calf.

Since external shape was considered decisive for human status, the debate about monsters in civil law centred on defining minimal criteria. At least from the fourteenth century, a well-formed head was believed sufficient. Simultaneously, the religious question of baptism and ensoulment started to infiltrate civil law. In an influential commentary, Baldo degli Ubaldi, a leading Italian jurist in the late fourteenth century, insisted on the necessary congruence of body and soul as a precondition for baptism.[31]

Meanwhile, Aristotle's *Politics* confronted scholastics with the notion that monstrous births were useless to the city and should be eliminated. While commentators agreed that Aristotle's advice was unchristian, the author of a short treatise on the 'art of promoting good births' (*Libellus de ingenio bone nativitatis*), largely based on the *Politics* and written around 1319 for the crown prince of Aragon, proposed to bar monsters from marriage to protect future generations. He also underscored the importance of Aristotle's rules about minimum marital age: children born in marriages that defied this natural norm were weaker, leading their parents to favour quantity over quality and to marry off their own children too young. Poor marriage practices perpetuated poor quality offspring.[32]

Marriage, Sex and the Prevention of Defective Offspring

By contrast, in pastoral discourse about sex and marriage, concerns about defective offspring played a minor role. They also tended to be overridden by the bonds of marriage

31 Van der Lugt, 'L'humanité'; Köhler, Homo, pp. 363–77, 387–411.

32 Biller, *Measure of Multitude*, pp. 347–56, 372–4; Gianfranco Fioravanti, 'Un trattato medievale di eugenetica: Il *Libellus de ingenio bone nativitatis*', *Mediaevalia: Textos e estudos* 21 (2002), 89–111. On marriage, see also Tim Parkin, 'The Ancient Family and the Law', Chapter 6; and Silvia De Renzi, 'Family Resemblance in the Old Regime', Chapter 17, this book.

and the imperatives of the marital debt. Following Paul's stance that it is 'better to marry than to burn', Christian marriage served to keep those who could not stay chaste from fornication. Abstinence was allowed with mutual consent, but intercourse was mandatory if either spouse was tempted to find relief elsewhere, a principle theologians increasingly emphasized from the later twelfth century. The stability of marriage became a priority. The marital debt remained even if one spouse had a disease such as leprosy which, according to common belief and prevalent medical doctrine, endangered the health of the other spouse and future children. Diseases and deformities were neither a reason to abstain from marriage and procreation, nor an excuse for divorce, unless they prevented consummation.[33] By the twelfth century, the notion of marriage as an indissoluble sacrament was firmly established.

By that time, the marital debt tended to trump even some of the sexual prohibitions of the church itself: against intercourse on Sundays and feast-days, before communion, in positions deemed 'unnatural', and during menstruation, pregnancy and lactation. Theologians and canonists increasingly classed these transgressions as venial sins, provided the motivation was avoidance of fornication, despite widespread belief that they could result in deformed offspring. These consequences were sometimes framed not as divine punishment, but as a natural chain of cause and effect backed up by medical knowledge. This was the case, for instance, for the belief that intercourse during menstruation caused leprosy in the child.[34] In high scholastic texts these health warnings were, however, far less present and categorical than in penitentials, sermons and less technical medical and philosophical works.

The danger of defective offspring was even less of an issue in the canonical prohibitions on kin marriage (Fig. 12.3). The *raison d'être* and degree of application of this extensive system are still hotly debated, but historians agree that the motivation was not fear of producing imperfect offspring, a rationalization that arose only in the early modern period.[35] Despite its inclusion in the *Decretum*, the core text of canon law, commentators largely ignored a statement attributed to Gregory the Great (d. 604) that

33 Maaike van der Lugt, 'Les maladies héréditaires dans la pensée scolastique', in van der Lugt and Charles de Miramon (eds.), *L'hérédité entre Moyen Âge et Époque moderne: Perspectives historiques* (Florence, 2008), pp. 272–320, on p. 308; Dylan Eliott, *Spiritual Marriage: Sexual Abstinence in Medieval Wedlock* (Princeton, NJ, 1993).

34 Irina Metzler, *Disability in Medieval Europe: Thinking about Physical Impairment in the High Middle Ages, c. 1100–1400* (London, 2006), pp. 88–9; Eliott, *Spiritual Marriage*, p. 151 n. 62; Luke Demaître, *Leprosy in Premodern Medicine: A Malady of the Whole Body* (Baltimore, MD, 2007), pp. 168–71.

35 Patrick Corbet, *Autour de Burchard de Worms: L'Église allemande et les interdits de parenté: IXème–XIIème siècle* (Frankfurt, 2001); Christof Rolker, 'Two models of incest: Conflict and confusion in high medieval discourse on kinship and marriage', in Per Andersen *et al.* (eds.), *Law and Marriage in Medieval and Early Modern Times* (Copenhagen, 2012), pp. 139–59; Archibald, *Incest*, pp. 21–52.

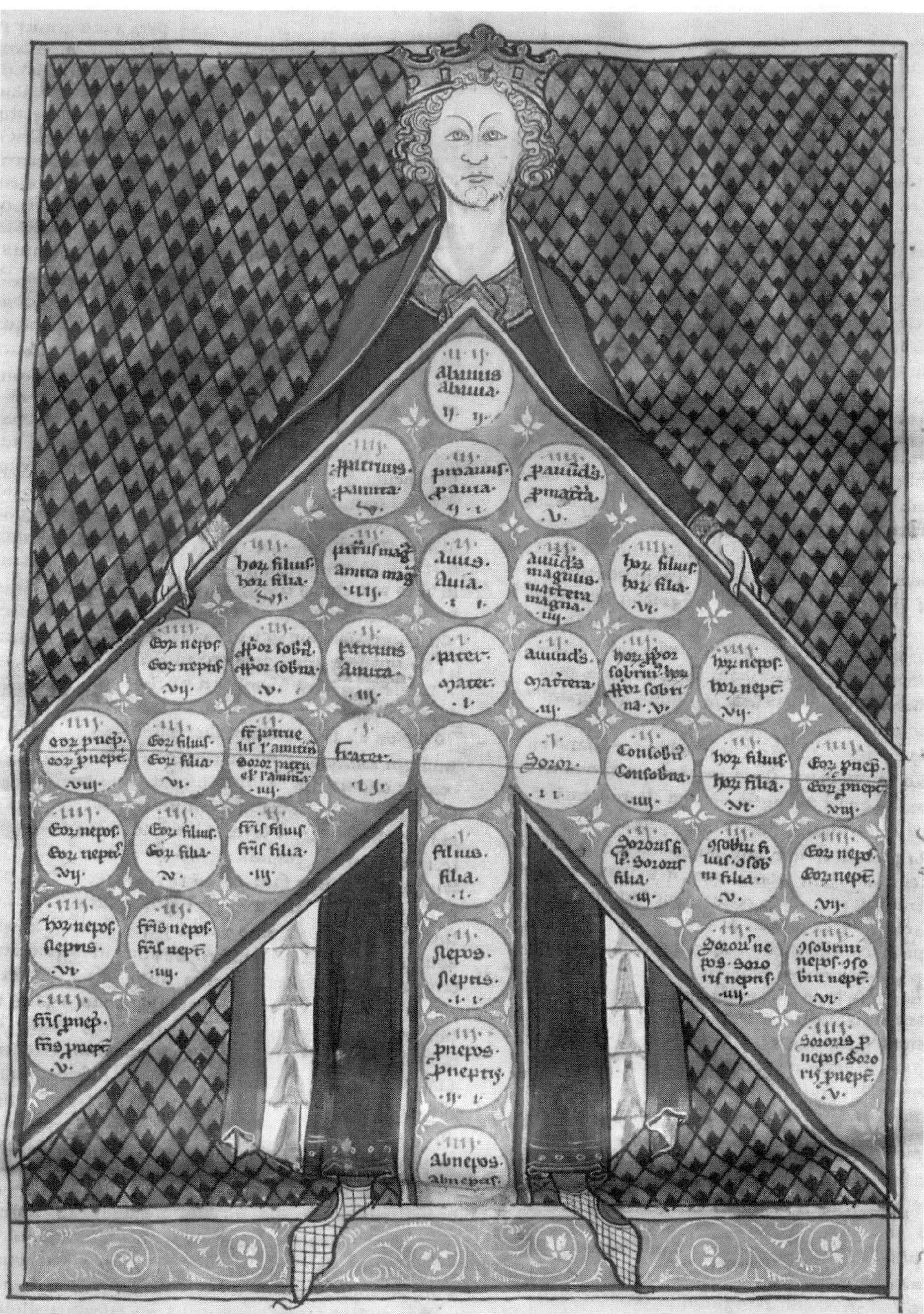

Figure 12.3 Diagram indicating prohibited spouses in a thirteenth-century legal manuscript. In the early church, as in later Roman law, the prohibition of kin marriage extended to first cousins. The interdiction was expanded in *c.* 700–1000 to the seventh degree, and in 1215 reduced to the fourth degree, as represented here. Gregory IX, *Decretales*, Openbare Bibliotheek, Bruges, MS 365, f. 2v.

kin marriage did not produce viable offspring.[36] Instead, medieval sources framed the prohibitions according to two basic models. The first used the biblical language of pollution, conflated kin marriage with incest and framed it as an abomination and a sin against nature. The second interpreted the prohibitions as historically situated legal constructs. Those who adopted the first approach occasionally warned that kin marriage caused defective offspring, a correlation also noted by authors of historical chronicles in their accounts of monstrous births. However, monsters in this view were seen as signs of God's wrath, not a congenital defect. Significantly, incestuous marriages could also lead to collective punishments, such as earthquakes.

The conflation of kin marriage with incest was more common between the eighth and the eleventh centuries, when the prohibitions were expanding. Scholastic theologians and canonists, by contrast, usually adopted the second model. They rated kin marriage a lesser sin than adultery. Like Augustine, they argued that the prohibitions had not always applied; now that the world was full of people, the network of affection should be spread widely. Even in their discussions of incest proper, scholastics did not mention danger to offspring.[37] Contrary to the sexual prohibitions already discussed, prohibitions of incest and kin marriage were not rationalized in medical terms. Scholastic physicians themselves acknowledged hereditary and inborn diseases and sometimes distinguished between the two, but without pointing to consanguinity as a cause.

Conclusion

Questions about the status of the fetus, monstrous births, and the right kinds of marriage and sex reflect the plurality of perspectives about procreation available to scholastic authors. The church presented children as a prime good of marriage and promoted procreation by combining the marital debt with the prohibition of abortion and non-procreative sex. It conveyed an inclusive message about human nature, coupling a concern for the survival of the offspring with indifference to disease and impairment. But in a turning point around 1300, ideas emerged in medicine, natural philosophy, civil law and political thought that challenged the dominant pastoral ideology. Geared towards elite audiences rather than the community of the faithful, these alternative views of marriage, heredity and humanity neither formed a coherent whole nor gained

36 Bede, *Historia ecclesiastica*, I.27; Gratian, *Decretum*, C. XXXV, q. 2, c. 20. Marinus Verbaarschot, 'De iuridica natura impedimenti consanguinitatis in theologia et in iure canonico a S. Petro Damiano usque ad Decretales Gregorii IX (ca. 1063–1234)', *Ephemerides theologicae Lovanienses* 30 (1954), 697–739, on 714–16, 737.

37 Archibald, *Incest*, pp. 50–1; Rolker, 'Two models'; Françoise Héritier, *Les deux sœurs et leur mère: Anthropologie de l'inceste* (Paris, 1994), p. 113.

real momentum. The *Libellus de ingenio bone nativitatis* enjoyed limited circulation and was not translated into actual policies or laws. Hereditary disease never became a central theme of medieval medicine, and even though the fourteenth-century Florentine merchant Paolo da Certaldo advised those seeking marriages to check that such diseases did not run in a prospective bride's family, other lay guides to good living said little about the matter.[38]

The health of offspring was nevertheless an issue for scholastic physicians and philosophers and an increasing worry for lay audiences. There was ample room in theories of procreation for human intervention, with generation, not heredity, as the central concept. The seed or seeds were thought to determine the children's characteristics, yet every child was the fruit of a myriad causes, including the quality of the air and astral influences. Women, especially, were believed to guide generation through many other channels, such as the shape of the womb, level of activity, food intake and imagination.[39] More research is needed, but it seems that in the flourishing later medieval literature on generation, 'women's secrets' and good living, producing healthy children was less a matter of marriage selection than of environment and behaviour before, after and especially during conception.

By concentrating on how couples could produce healthy and beautiful individual babies of the right sex – a great concern – this medieval 'art of generation' is less akin to classic nineteenth- and twentieth-century eugenics, which tended to target groups or populations, than to today's methods of preventing disease through counselling and through prenatal and preimplantation testing. At the same time, the medieval focus on environment and lifestyle, especially of women, resembles the growing tendency, in our times, to subject pregnant women and those trying to conceive to ever more stringent lifestyle advice.[40]

38 Paolo da Certaldo, *Libro di buoni costumi*, ed. Alfredo Schiaffini (Florence, 1945), pp. 83–4; Katharine Park, *Secrets of Women: Gender, Generation, and the Origins of Human Dissection* (New York, NY, 2006), p. 147; Rudolph M. Bell, *How to Do It: Guides to Good Living for Renaissance Italians* (Chicago, IL, 1999).

39 Introduction and articles by van der Lugt and Joseph Ziegler, in van der Lugt and Miramon, *L'hérédité*; Park, *Secrets of Women*.

40 For nineteenth-century eugenic concerns about kin marriage: Sarah Wilmot, 'Breeding Farm Animals and Humans', Chapter 27; for prenatal testing: Ilana Löwy, 'Prenatal Diagnosis, Surveillance and Risk', Chapter 38; for environmental effects on pregnant women: Tatjana Buklijas, 'Developmental Origins of Health and Disease', Exhibit 39, this book.

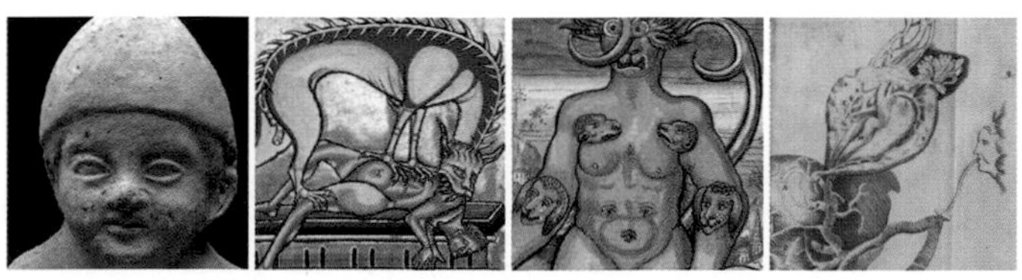

Exhibits 1–19

Exhibit 1

An Ancient Egyptian Fertility Figurine

Rune Nyord

Figurines like this, representing a woman naked but for jewellery and tattoos and carrying a child on her hip, were placed in ancestral tombs during the Egyptian Middle Kingdom (*c.* 2000–1650 BC). The ancient Egyptians, who regarded dead ancestors as a source of fertility and prosperity, treated the tomb as a site of great power that the living could harness. Depositing figurines in the tomb was one way of doing this, and the inscription on the right leg of this statuette asks that 'A birth be granted to your daughter Seh'. The petitioner addresses the deceased father, or other male ancestor, of a living woman, invoking his power over his own offspring's generative capacity.

The exact role of ancestors in the generation of the living was variously understood. One Egyptian spell for use in the ancestor cult, roughly contemporary with this figurine, asks the deceased to petition the gods to allow that children be born to his living descendants, thus ascribing only an intermediary role to the ancestor. By contrast, funerary texts on coffins of the high elite describe the procreative power of the ancestor, his capacity to engender heirs, in explicitly sexual terms. None of these cases mentions the living male sexual partner of the woman wishing to give birth, probably because his contribution was seen as a necessary, but not sufficient, condition for producing a child. Moreover, although ancient Egyptian society was strongly patriarchal, it may be sheer coincidence that all the preserved written petitions for childbirth happen to be addressed to male ancestors, since uninscribed figurines with broadly similar iconography were deposited in the tombs of women as well as men. Nor do we know whether the women desiring offspring presented the figurines themselves, or others acted on their behalf: a man asks his dead father for 'a healthy male child' for himself as well as for his sister (the deceased's daughter) in one votive letter.

The conception of procreative ability as something granted by or transmitted through ancestors is very widespread in societies practising ancestor worship (found as far afield as the Nzema of southern Ghana and the Trobrianders of Melanesia), and has wider ramifications for the construction of kinship in such cultures. The deposition of a figurine bearing the name of a living woman in an ancestor's tomb established a unique bond between the two individuals, and signalled the ancestor's agency in the engendering of the child. Such connections may also be indicated by the common ancient Egyptian practice of naming boys after their grandfathers.

The ties between the living and their deceased ancestors slackened after the Middle Kingdom; religious focus shifted from family tombs to public temples and shrines, and in later periods objects comparable to the figurine shown here were increasingly deposited in temple precincts. The gods gradually became the granters of ancestral fertility in a more general sense, and their role less distinguishable from that of other Mediterranean deities in helping human generation as time went on.

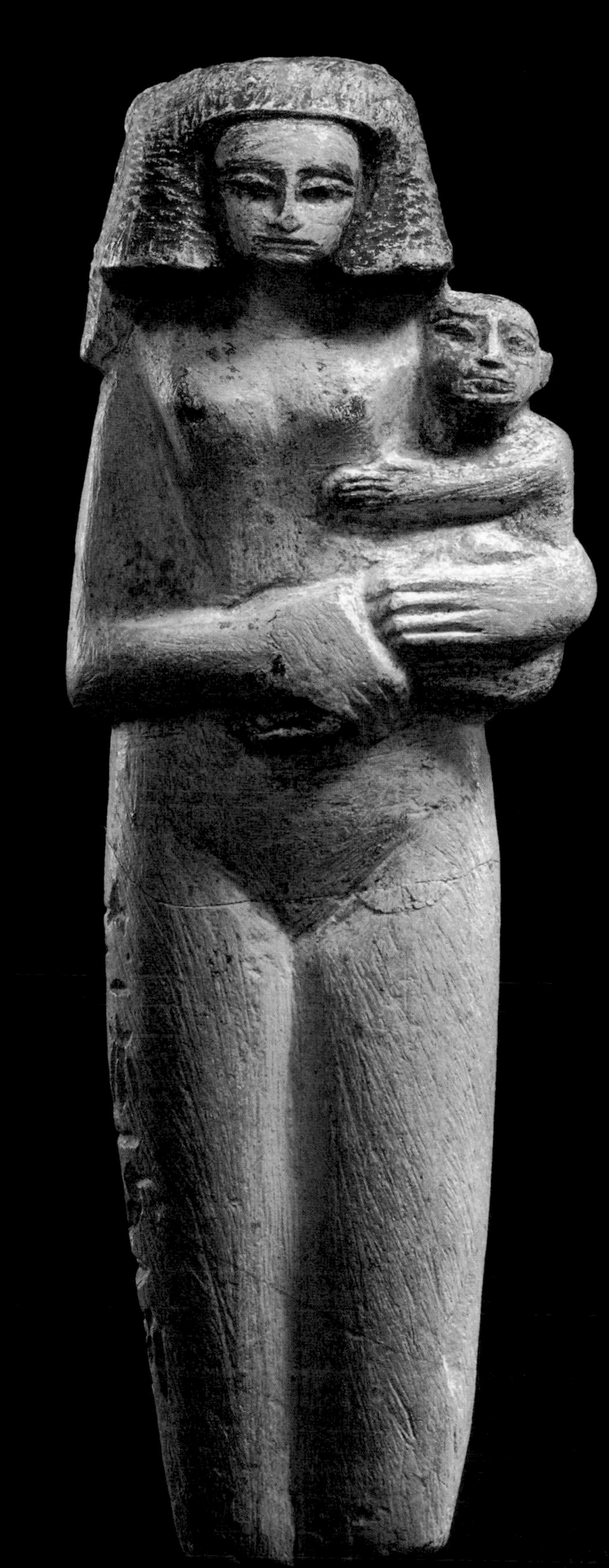

Limestone figurine, *c.* 12 × 4 × 3 cm, bpk / Ägyptisches Museum und Papyrussammlung, inv. no. ÄM 14517, SMB / Sandra Steiß.

FURTHER READING

Chapter 2, this book.

Stephanie Lynn Budin, *Images of Woman and Child from the Bronze Age: Reconsidering Fertility, Maternity, and Gender in the Ancient World* (Cambridge, 2011).

Rune Nyord, '"An image of the owner as he was on earth": Representation and ontology in ancient Egyptian funerary images', in Gianluca Miniaci, Marilina Betrò and Stephen Quirke (eds.), *Company of Images: Modelling the Imaginary World of Middle Kingdom Egypt (2000–1500 BC)* (Leuven, 2017), pp. 337–59.

Geraldine Pinch, *Votive Offerings to Hathor* (Oxford, 1993).

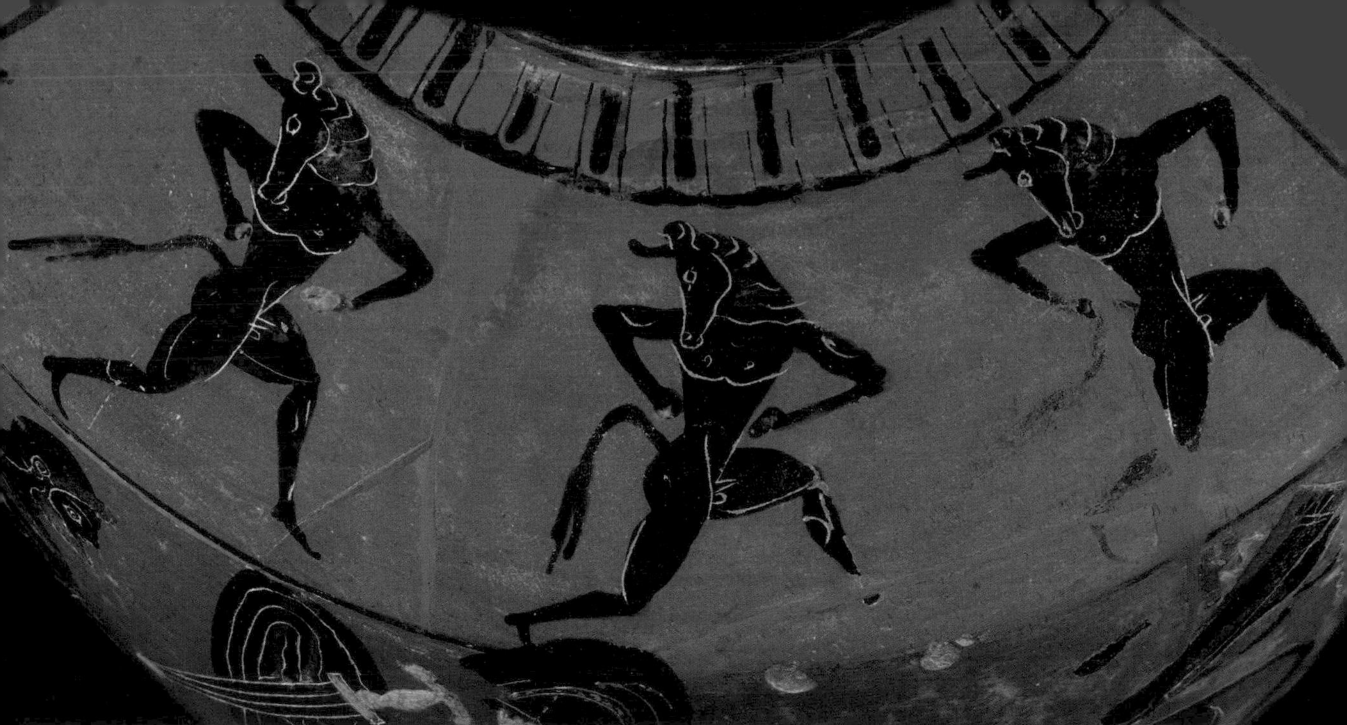

Exhibit 2

The Minotaur and Other Hybrids in Ancient Greece

Annetta Alexandridis

On the shoulder of an archaic Greek *hydria* or water jug, three naked men with bulls' heads and tails are running to the right. Looking backwards, arms akimbo, all three hold small rocks in both hands (the white colour has flaked off). The figures move in almost perfect synchrony, suggesting a choreographed performance. The bulls' heads and stones identify a particular myth: the Minotaur's fatal struggle against the Athenian hero Theseus.

King Minos of Crete owned a beautiful bull, and broke a promise to sacrifice it to the gods. As punishment his wife Pasiphae fell in love with this very bull. She had her court artist Daedalus construct a wooden cow, in which she hid to mate with the animal. The fruit of this perverted relationship was the Minotaur, a mixed creature of bull and man: the monstrous materialization of an abject act of adultery. Able to defend himself only with stones, a primitive form of weapon, he met his death by the sword of Theseus.

Many other mixed creatures populate Greek myth in texts and the visual arts, their pictorial models borrowed from the Near East. There, composites of man, animal and plant form guardian figures or companions of gods and were part of the creation of the cosmos. In the Greek world, specific mythological figures were embodied in this way from the seventh century BC. Living outside human society, as individuals or in groups, mixed creatures often lack clear parentage; they usually share the same sex and do not generate. The satyrs, followers of the god Dionysus, feature a male human body with equine hooves, tail and ears.

Their relentless sexual activity leads to no procreation. Female monsters such as the sphinx and sirens, who combine a human head with feline and/or avian body parts, lure mortals to their doom.

At least of partial human parentage are the centaurs. Born from King Ixion's misbegotten son Centaurus and the wild Magnesian mares, they possess the body and legs of a horse joined to the torso, arms and head of a man. Individual centaurs exhibit additional human traits. A husband and wise teacher, Chiron tutors heroes and demigods such as Achilles and Asclepius.

Hybrids are not necessarily of a lower order, nor do they always look monstrous. The Greek pantheon included composite gods such as Pan, half-human, half-goat, and the river god Acheloos, depicted as a bull with human face. Hybrids may also result from unions between humans and gods, rather than humans and animals, though these distinctions are blurred by the divine transformations that such sexual encounters often involved: Zeus seduced Leda in the guise of a swan to conceive Helen; Achilles' divine mother Thetis changed shape many times before Peleus subdued her. The children of gods and mortals possess appropriately extraordinary qualities, such as Helen's beauty or Achilles' strength. These representations and narratives explore multiple boundaries, ontological, ethical, technological and imaginative, all of which are engaged and enacted in the Minotaur's genesis and death.

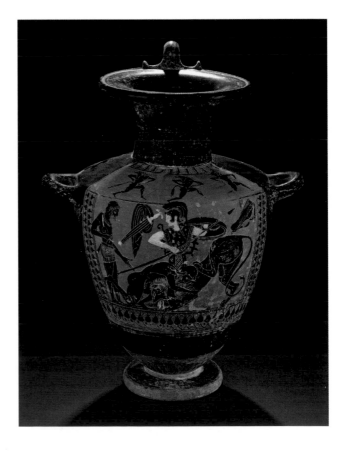

Athenian black-figure *hydria*, with detail, from the last quarter of the sixth century BC. 48 cm high. B 308. © Trustees of the British Museum.

FURTHER READING

Chapters 2, 3, 4 and 12 and Exhibits 9 and 13, this book.

Emma Aston, *Mixanthrōpoi: Animal–Human Hybrid Deities in Greek Religion, Kernos*, suppl. 25 (Liège, 2011).

François Lissarrague, *La cité des satyres: Une anthropologie ludique (Athènes, VIe–Ve siècles avant J.-C.)* (Paris, 2013).

J. Michael Padgett, *The Centaur's Smile: The Human Animal in Early Greek Art* (New Haven, CT, 2003).

Exhibit 3

The Birth Horoscope of a Babylonian Scholar

Eleanor Robson

Year 63, month Ṭebetu, night of day 2 [30 December 249 BC]:

> Anu-belšunu was born.
> That day, the Sun was 9:30° in the Goat.
> The Moon was 12° in the Bucket: his days will be long.
> Jupiter was at the head of the Scorpion: someone will take the prince's hand.
> [The child] was born in the Bucket in the region of Venus: he will have sons.
> Mercury was in the Goat; Saturn was in the Goat;
> Mars was in the Crab.

This unassuming piece of clay is witness to one of the most influential and enduring ideas in the history of generation and reproduction: that one's birth circumstances can shape the course of one's life. This powerful and alluring concept developed in Babylonia (southern Iraq) and eventually spread far across Eurasia thanks to influential proponents such as Ptolemy in the Roman Empire, al-Biruni in the medieval Islamic world and Sacrobosco in the Latin west. It has its appeal even today.

Babylonian scholars began reading the gods' intentions in the night sky in the third millennium BC. For around two thousand years after that, celestial divination was exclusively a method for rulers to check that their actions and intentions met with divine favour; the gods did not concern themselves with the fates of individuals. However, in 484 BC, the Persian king Darius severed royal ties with the Babylonian intelligentsia after a political revolt, and scholars had to find new clients, new sources of income and prestige. Over the next few decades, a radical reconceptualization of the night sky took place that enabled individual destinies to be foretold. The two earliest extant birth horoscopes both date to 410 BC, and by 400 BC, give or take five years, the constellations on the ecliptic – the path of the moon – had become twelve zodiacal signs of exactly equal sizes. They bear essentially the same names today as they did then.

About thirty birth horoscopes from Babylonia survive, all inscribed in cuneiform script on small clay tablets. They typically start, as here, with the date and time of the child's birth, list the locations of the sun, moon and five visible planets as calculated for that time, and some, like this one, include brief predictions. Most seem to have been composed around the time of the subject's birth; though in later traditions they were cast retrospectively. 'The child' was rarely named, but, uniquely, the subject of this horoscope can be identified precisely.

Anu-belšunu was a lamentation priest in the Babylonian city of Uruk in the late third century BC. Celestial observation was an important component of his calling, which also demanded accurate calendrical calculations for the timing of cultic performances, particularly eclipse rituals. He trained three sons in the various aspects of his profession, one of

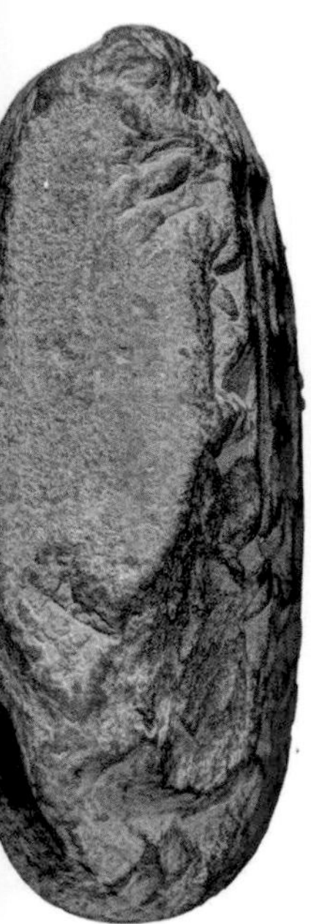
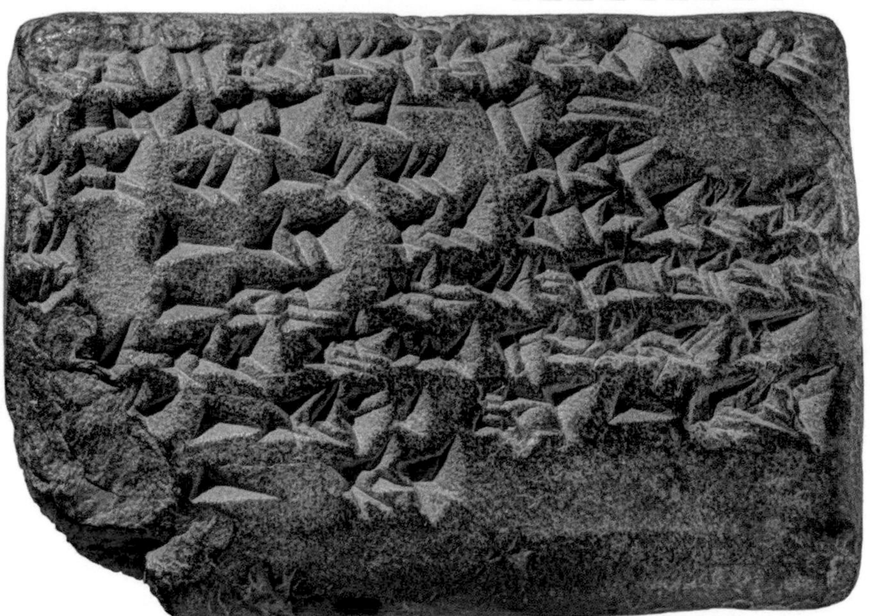
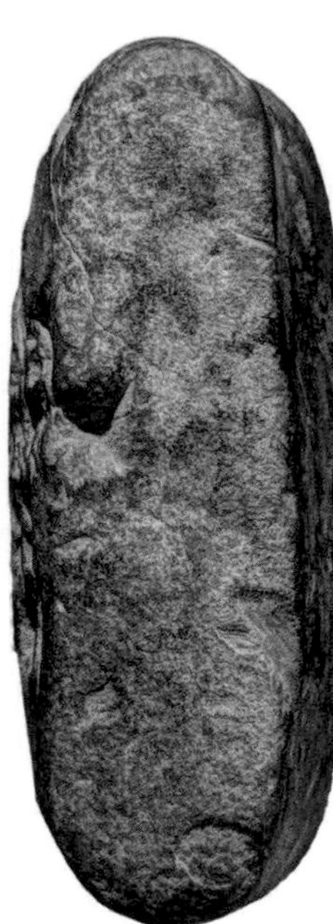

Cuneiform tablet NCBT 1231, Yale Babylonian Collection, New Haven. 32 × 46 × 13 mm. Photograph © Yale Babylonian Collection, 2017. Published with the kind permission of the Associate Curator, Agnete Wiste Lassen.

whom wrote (copied, amended or composed) this horoscope during his apprenticeship. Anu-belšunu is last attested as a wealthy man in his late sixties, witnessing a legal document for a neighbour. The horoscope's predictions, as recorded here, were fulfilled.

FURTHER READING

Chapter 16 and Exhibit 14, this book.

Paul-Alain Beaulieu and Francesca Rochberg, 'The horoscope of Anu-belšunu', *Journal of Cuneiform Studies* 43 (1996), 89–94.

Eleanor Robson, *Mathematics in Ancient Iraq: A Social History* (Princeton, NJ, 2008).

Francesca Rochberg, *The Heavenly Writing: Divination, Horoscopy, and Astronomy in Mesopotamian Culture* (Cambridge, 2004).

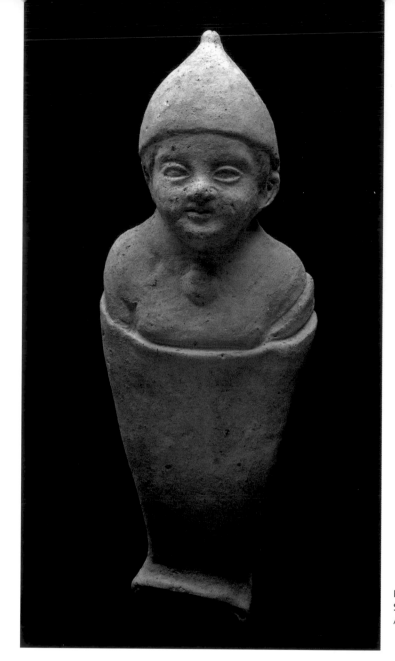

Roughly life-size terracotta figure. Science Museum, London, no. A636026, Wellcome Images.

Exhibit 4

A Swaddled Infant Given to the Gods

Fay Glinister

Mould-made terracotta models of tightly swaddled infants featured in the votive repertoire of central Italy between the fourth and second centuries BC, when Rome extended its control across the peninsula and into the wider Mediterranean world. Part of an expanded array of offerings in which models of diverse human body parts and animal figurines joined and increasingly dominated an existing assortment of votive statuettes, and other miniature objects, mostly metal and ceramic, these terracotta items were dedicated and displayed in their thousands at sites ranging from great urban sanctuaries to remote rural shrines.

The provenance of this example now in the Wellcome Collection is unknown, but with its *bulla* around the neck for safety, bare shoulders, plump features and pointed cap it closely resembles votives found at Capua, near Naples. The cap is restricted to south-central Italy, probably indicating the Greek influences prevalent there; more usually part of the swaddling cloth veils babies' heads. The *bulla* – a protective, apotropaic amulet generally associated with freeborn males – is found in archaeological sites across central Italy, but not all swaddled votives wear one, or its female equivalent, the *lunula*, though they may have originally, if only painted on. Similarly, the wrapping here is smooth, but fabric or painted swaddling bands may once have been present: in some examples the details of the bands were marked out by a modelling tool prior to firing. The faces of some swaddled votives resemble small adults, but this chubby, attentive baby of several months is more typical.

These offerings were vowed to the gods in exchange for the fulfilment of a request, but no ancient author provides details of the process; scholars have only the objects and their archaeological contexts to work with. Some associate swaddled votives with the passage to the afterlife, others with an appeal for divine aid with generation, although more common types, such as votive uteruses, seem more pertinent to that project. Swaddlings are more plausibly viewed as representing a living child in a world of high infant mortality. The child's general well-being or healing was at stake, or perhaps its attainment of a stage on the way to full membership of the community was being marked. Infant swaddling was a formative practice in ancient medical writing. A later text, Soranus's *Gynaecology,* stressed the importance of swaddling to mould the soft and malleable limbs of the newborn into an ideal shape. This suggests that it was a significant part of an infant's development – perfection of the human form – in which the gods might take an interest.

In the broadest sense, swaddled-infant votives were offered to secure divine aid for family success. These terracotta artefacts enact contemporary conceptions of the human body, and symbolize human and divine investment in the status and safety, development and well-being of new citizens of communities across Hellenistic central Italy. A range of votive practices in support of children have persisted, moreover, with simple tin models of swaddled infants still visible in Greek and Italian churches, for instance.

FURTHER READING

Chapter 7 and Exhibit 40, this book.

Rebecca Miller Ammerman, 'Children at risk: Votive terracottas and the welfare of infants at Paestum', in Ada Cohen and Jeremy B. Rutter (eds.), *Constructions of Childhood in Ancient Greece and Italy* (Princeton, NJ, 2007), pp. 131–51.

Fay Glinister, 'Ritual and meaning: Contextualising votive terracotta infants in Hellenistic Italy', in Jane Draycott and Emma-Jayne Graham (eds.), *Bodies of Evidence: Ancient Anatomical Votives Past, Present and Future* (London, 2017), pp. 131–46.

Emma-Jayne Graham, 'Infant votives and swaddling in Hellenistic Italy', in Maureen Carroll and Graham (eds.), *Infant Health and Death in Roman Italy and Beyond* (Portsmouth, RI, 2014), pp. 23–46.

Exhibit 5

Phallic Fertility in Pompeii

Jessica Hughes

A large portion of our surviving Roman wall-painting comes from the ancient town of Pompeii in southern Italy, buried during the eruption of Vesuvius in AD 79. Eighteenth-century excavations brought to light many images of gods, myths and everyday Pompeian life: ancient art 'as it should be'. But some depictions shocked contemporary viewers – scenes of oral sex, satyrs copulating with maenads, and dozens of representations of the human penis, the phallus, shown alone or attached to an owner whose face registered little surprise or embarrassment about the open display of his genitals.

For two centuries after the rediscovery of Pompeii and nearby Herculaneum, these 'obscene' images were often hidden away; their treatment reflecting a squeamishness probably not shared by ancient viewers. In classical Greece, penises had been depicted on a wide range of objects, from vases and statues to 'herms', the marble pillars that often stood at boundaries and crossroads. In Greece the ideal penis size was small enough not to detract from the balance and beauty of the classical body, but during the Roman period penises grew and spread to appear on necklaces, lamps, mosaics, shop signs and paving stones, as well as the walls and floors of public and private buildings. These Roman phalluses were not 'pornographic' in our modern sense of the word, but rather appropriated the imagery of male fertility to indicate abundance and prosperity in other spheres of life, such as business or agriculture.

This is illustrated by the colourful wall-painting shown here, from the Pompeian house believed to belong to two wealthy freedmen brothers, Aulus Vettius Conviva and Aulus Vettius Restitutus. Successful businessmen, the Vettii filled their house with expensive pictures of subjects from Greek mythology. Decorating the vestibule, or entrance hall, this one was among the first an ancient visitor encountered. It shows the god Priapus – an originally Greek deity who became increasingly popular in Roman times – in the act of weighing his enormous penis against a bag of coins. The penis points downwards towards an overflowing basket of fruit, thereby creating (together with the money) a visual triangle of bodily, agricultural and economic fecundity.

The Vettii Priapus uses the productive male body as a symbol for a more general prosperity; we might also argue that it implicitly constructs the world of business as male. But another of this painting's functions is only loosely related to concepts of fertility. Its situation at the entrance of the house suggests it performed an apotropaic role, averting the 'evil eye' and other misfortunes from the house, its inhabitants and contents. That Priapus vigorously guarded crops and gardens was well-documented in Latin poetry, and many other phallic images discovered at Pompeii and around the Roman world, at crossroads and in amulet form, for instance, are thought to have had a protective function. The Roman phallus operated not only in the realm of procreation itself, but also in securing a generally safe and prosperous environment. Earlier themes of male fertility were expanded and materialized in some very particular ways.

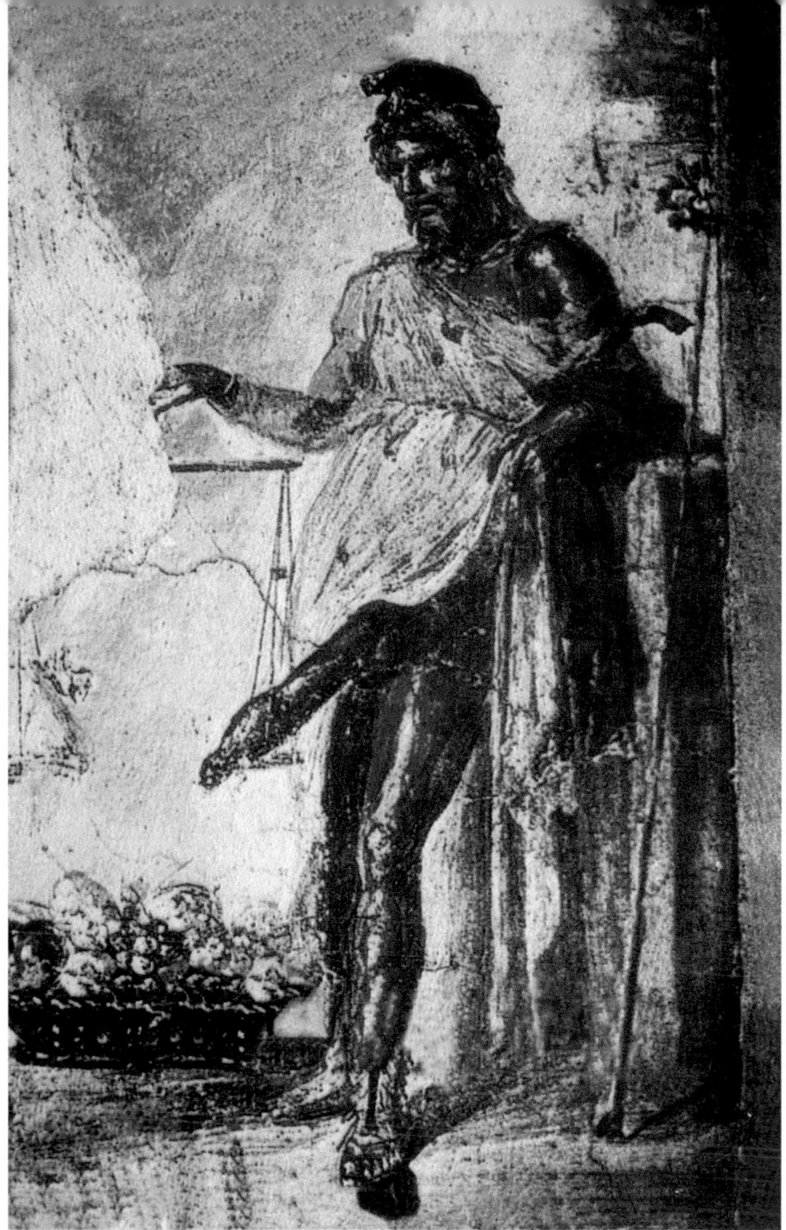

Wall-painting of Priapus from the vestibule of the House of the Vettii in Pompeii, first century AD. The figure and objects are roughly life-size. © Buena Vista Images / Getty Images.

FURTHER READING

Chapter 2, this book.

Mary Beard, 'Dirty little secrets: Changing displays of Pompeian "erotica"', in Victoria C. Gardner Coates, Kenneth Lapatin and Jon L. Seydl (eds.), *The Last Days of Pompeii: Decadence, Apocalypse, Resurrection* (Los Angeles, CA, 2012), pp. 60–9.

Giancarlo Carabelli, *In the Image of Priapus* (London, 1996).

David M. Friedman, *A Mind of Its Own: A Cultural History of the Penis* (London, 2002).

Exhibit 6

A Roman Embryo Hook

Ralph Jackson

In classical medical writing, anything other than a well-aligned, head-first presentation came under the rubric of 'difficult birth' (*dustokia*), and every attempt would be made to manipulate the fetus to the 'natural' position. The fullest discussion of birth procedures appears in Soranus' *Gynaecology*, composed in imperial Rome around AD 100. Soranus advised that, in a normal labour, the woman should remain on her bed until the last stage, when she was to move to a birthing chair for delivery by the midwife and her assistant(s). No mechanical aids were used, just the midwife's voice, giving guidance and encouragement, and her skilled hands.

In a 'difficult birth', the life of the mother took precedence. Thus, in the case of a stuck or dead fetus, if labour was unduly protracted and manual traction ineffective, delivery might have to proceed through what Soranus called 'more forceful methods', employing specific hooks and knives: in Greek, *embruoulkoi* and *embruotoma*, literally embryo- or fetus-pullers and cutters. Similar instruments feature in the operation for extracting an already dead fetus detailed in the surgical book of the Roman encyclopaedist Celsus's influential Latin summary of practical medical knowledge current in the early first century AD. An embryo hook, warmed in olive oil, was introduced and its tip, covered and guided by the practitioner's fingers to avoid injury to the womb, was engaged in an eye socket or other suitable opening. After engaging a second hook to ensure balanced traction, the fetus was to be carefully withdrawn, but if an intact delivery proved impossible, parts were to be amputated as they presented. The finely preserved skeleton of a full-term fetus delivered in this way and carefully buried in a wooden coffin in the fourth century AD was discovered in excavations at the extensive Romano-British cemetery at Poundbury Camp near Dorchester, Dorset.

Based on these ancient descriptions, a handful of items amongst the rich archaeological remains of the Roman medical armamentarium have been identified as 'embryo hooks', with the best examples, such as this one from Pompeii, now in the Naples National Archaeological Museum. When found (probably in the House of the Physician, A. Pumponius Magonianus) it was complete and about 18.5 cm long, as early illustrations indicate, but the corroded iron hook has since become detached. The stout handle is made from solid bronze with terminal mouldings and carefully cut linear ridging to ensure a secure grip. The operative part was of solid iron with a robust sinuous stem terminating in a short curved hook with a round pointed tip. The craftsmanship of the handle is of a very high order, and we can assume a similarly close attention to the finish of the hook's surface, which Celsus stipulated should be 'completely smooth with a short point'.

Such instruments and operations continue to be described in late antique Greek medical encyclopaedias, and feature in the influential surgical books in the great eleventh-century Arabic medical compilation by the Andalusian physician al-Zahrawi (Albucasis); though the archaeological remains of medieval surgery, from either the Byzantine or Islamicate worlds, are sparse.

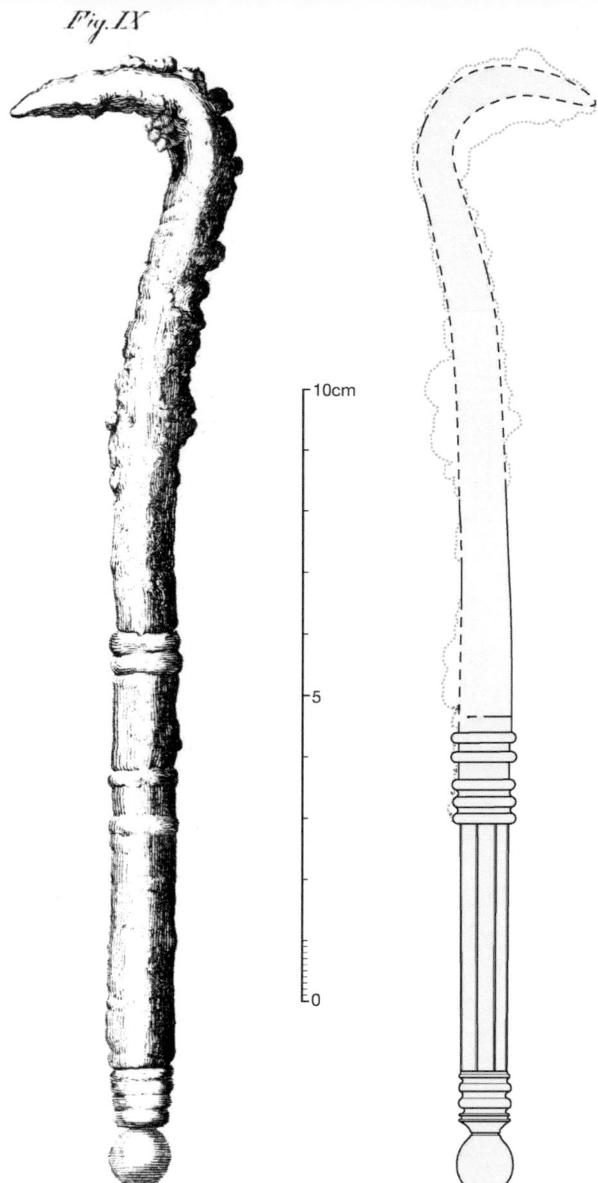

Left: engraving of embryo hook from Pompeii published by Benedetto Vulpes, *Illustrazione di tutti gli strumenti chirurgici scavati in Ercolano e in Pompei e che ora conservansi nel R. Museo Borbonico di Napoli* (Napoli: Stamperia Reale, 1847), plate VII. Right: schematic drawing of the hook based on a 1931 photo and the author's 1981 scale drawing of the handle. © Trustees of the British Museum.

FURTHER READING

Chapters 7, 11, 19, 22 and 37 and Exhibits 10, 18 and 22, this book.

Lawrence J. Bliquez, *Roman Surgical Instruments and Other Minor Objects in the National Archaeological Museum of Naples* (Mainz, 1994).

Innocenzo Mazzini, 'Embriulcia ed embriotomia: Evoluzione e diffusione di due interventi ginecologici dolorosi ed atroci nel mondo antico', in Mario Vegetti and Silvia Gastaldi (eds.), *Studi di storia della medicina antica e medievale in memoria di Paola Manuli* (Florence, 1996), pp. 21–33.

Theya Molleson and Margaret Cox, 'A neonate with cut bones from Poundbury Camp, 4th century AD, England', *Bulletin de la Société Royale Belge d'Anthropologie et de Préhistoire* 99 (1988), 53–9.

Exhibit 7

A Uterine Amulet from the Roman Empire

Véronique Dasen

The rich array of engraved gems surviving from the Roman Empire includes a distinct group of stones aimed at engaging divine forces in the defence, assistance or cure of the human body. These were usually carved on both faces, and sides, with inscriptions in the Greek alphabet, images of animals and deities, and many other motifs. The formulae, letter-like signs and iconography deployed on these items overlap, in their mixture of Graeco-Roman, Egyptian, Jewish and Christian elements, with those contained in the magical papyri from Roman Egypt and displayed on other powerful artefacts, such as curse tablets, from across the empire.

Many of these somatically oriented gems focus on the uterus, and seem to relate to women's main concern: safe and successful generation. The preferred stone, as here, was haematite or bloodstone, a mineral form of iron oxide believed to have the power to control blood flows, among other medical applications. Their engravings typically depict the womb in characteristic 'cupping-vessel' form, borrowing a classical medical metaphor – that consists of a broad main body, narrow neck and wider mouth – with tentacles attached, top and bottom, in conjunction with a door-key. In this example, the key-handle is on the right, and the eight bits engage with the mouth of the uterus. The opening and closing of the womb – most crucially to receive and retain seed (or not), and then allow birth – were the main actions for which divine support was sought through this object.

The three figures carved above the womb and key are Egyptian deities such as were often incorporated to increase the potency of the artefact. Even more typically, the whole scene is encircled by the *ouroboros*, the Egyptian motif of a snake eating its own tail and thus creating a protective space to guard against malevolent forces threatening the womb. A now illegible inscription runs around the outside of the circle, probably words from a formula for opening the womb during delivery, as on other gems in this series.

On the reverse, Greek letters spell out 'Ororiouth', but this is not a standard Greek word. Maybe it is the name of a demon who controls the womb, or a term for the uterus itself, which is more straightforwardly addressed in most examples where there is more text. Much else is uncertain about these gems; their provenance is rarely known and debate continues about their production and the identities of their purchasers and users. Still, as clearly expensive items, their manufacture requiring both technical and ritual skill, 'magical' gems were owned and worn by the elite.

This combination of gems and carving, especially inscription, seems to have been particular to the Hellenistic and Roman period. But it probably developed out of the broadly medicinal use of certain stones, a practice which, like the separate amuletic employment of texts and images, also continued long afterwards. Metal pendants which share motifs and an inscribed *hystera* (womb) formula with these gems also became widespread in the Byzantine world.

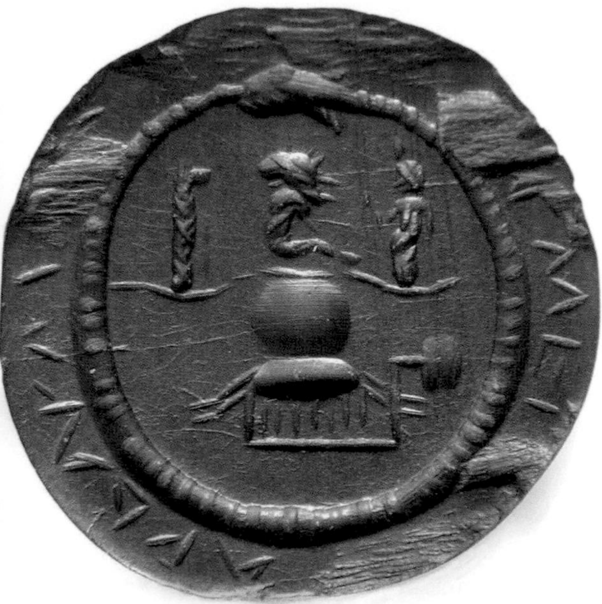

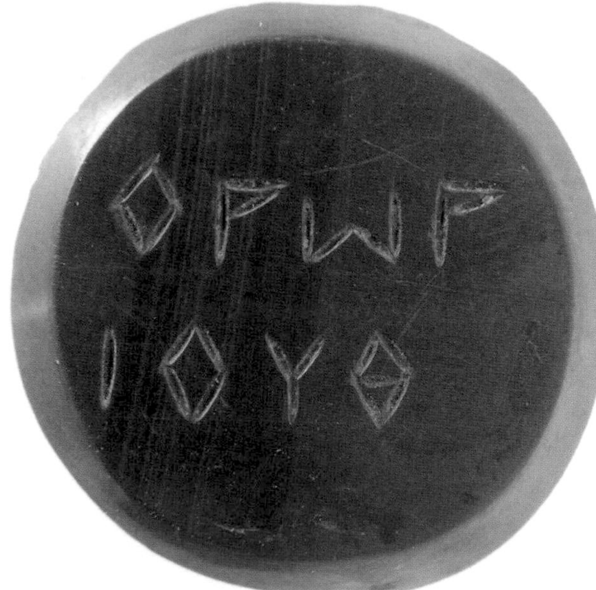

Haematite gem, probably third century AD. Private collection. Front: 1.7 × 1.7 cm, back: 1.5 × 1.5 cm. Photo: Claudia Wagner.

FURTHER READING

Chapters 4 and 7 and Exhibit 17, this book.

Véronique Dasen, *Le sourire d'Omphale: Maternité et petite enfance dans l'Antiquité* (Rennes, 2015).

Katalin Endreffy, Árpad M. Nagy and Jeffrey Spier (eds.), *Magical Gems in Their Context* (Rome, 2017).

Christopher A. Faraone, 'Magical and medical approaches to the wandering womb in the ancient Greek world', *Classical Antiquity* 30 (2011), 1–32.

Exhibit 8

The Tree of Jesse

Margot E. Fassler

One of the most famous Christian images relating to generation and familial relationships developed in late antiquity and the middle ages, when it was first known as the 'stirps Jesse', meaning shoot of Jesse, or, when it took the form of a tree, the 'Jesse tree'. In the Hebrew Bible, Jesse was the father of King David, a key ancestor of Joseph, who was the husband as well as kin of the Virgin Mary and surrogate father of the divinely engendered Christ. Genealogies found in the gospels of Matthew and Luke thus connected Mary, and through her Christ, to the house of David. The 'stirps Jesse' represented the royal pedigree of the messiah and his mother.

In the eleventh century, a liturgical chant on the stirps Jesse was written at Chartres Cathedral for the feast of the Nativity of the Virgin Mary (8 September). It circulated throughout Europe and became a source for the iconography of the Davidic lineage of Mary and Christ: 'The shoot of Jesse produced a rod, and the rod a flower, and over this flower rests the nurturing spirit. The shoot is the Virgin, the female begetter of God, and the flower is her Son.'

The lancet-shaped window shown here, the first in a sequence about the life and death of Christ beneath a rose of the apocalypse in the west façade of the cathedral, represents this chant and the larger meanings of the Davidic heritage of the Virgin and her son. The cathedral canons commissioned these windows as part of a twelfth-century glazing campaign, and they may have been observable from a gallery extant at the time. Enough of the medieval glass of these heavily restored windows remains to attest to their original design. The stirps window shows Jesse, asleep at the bottom, as the root of his ancestral stock. Sprouting from his loins is a lush, flowering plant forming a kind of trunk, with kings, including David and his son Solomon, rising one upon the other. The next-to-last figure is the Virgin Mary, and from her comes Jesus, the culmination of the family tree. The seven doves of the Holy Spirit surround him, proclaiming his identity and connecting him to the chant as well as the messianic prophecy of Isaiah. On both sides of the plant, prophets announce the coming of the Christian messiah.

Images like this served as guides to praying for one's own family, past, present and future. Medieval kings and queens, like parishioners and pilgrims in centuries to come, prayed to the Virgin of Chartres for help. They included her in genealogical trees testifying to their royal pedigrees and procreative powers, and this 'stirps Jesse' may also reflect the lineage of the counts of Chartres/Blois; one daughter married the king of France. Trees continued to represent generation and lineage for centuries. Around 1800, schematic trees began to represent relations in the natural world as well; during the nineteenth century they became the dominant representations of evolutionary pedigrees.

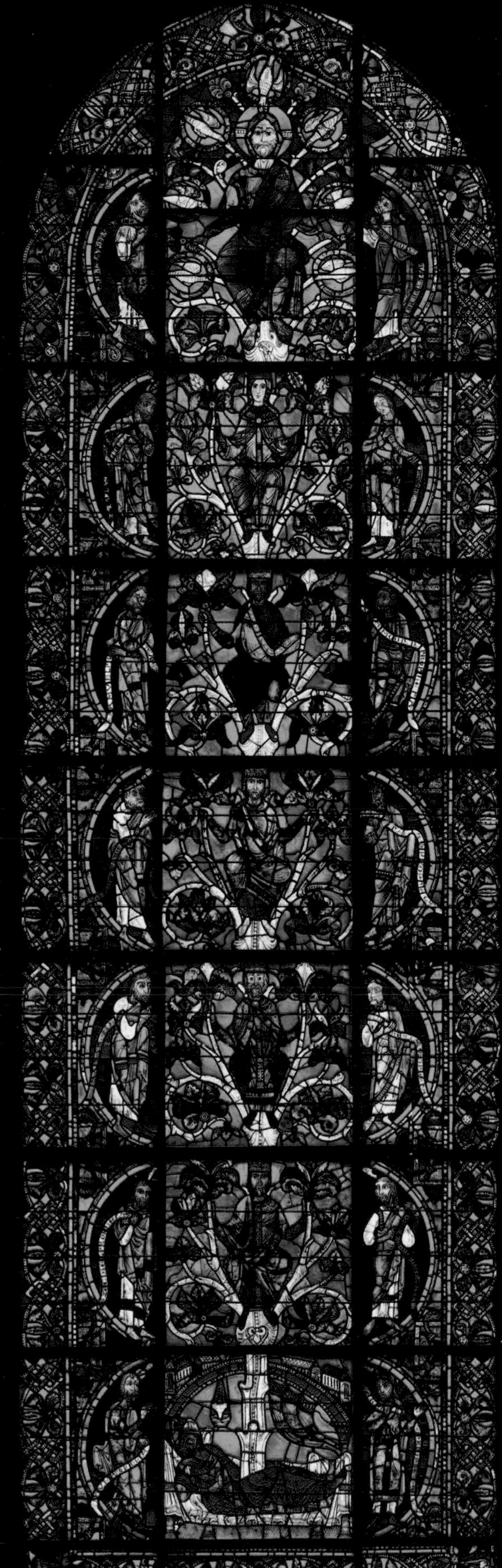

Twelfth-century stained glass window, forming part of the west façade of Chartres Cathedral, 8.4 × 2.6 m. Photograph by Henri Gaud.

FURTHER READING

Chapters 6, 11, 12, 16 and 26 and Exhibits 4, 7, 11, 29 and 40, this book.

J. David Archibald, *Aristotle's Ladder, Darwin's Tree: The Evolution of Visual Metaphors for Biological Order* (New York, NY, 2014).

Margot E. Fassler, *The Virgin of Chartres: Making History Through Liturgy and the Arts* (New Haven, CT, 2010).

James R. Johnson, 'The Tree of Jesse window of Chartres: *Laudes regiae*', *Speculum* 36 (1961), 1–22.

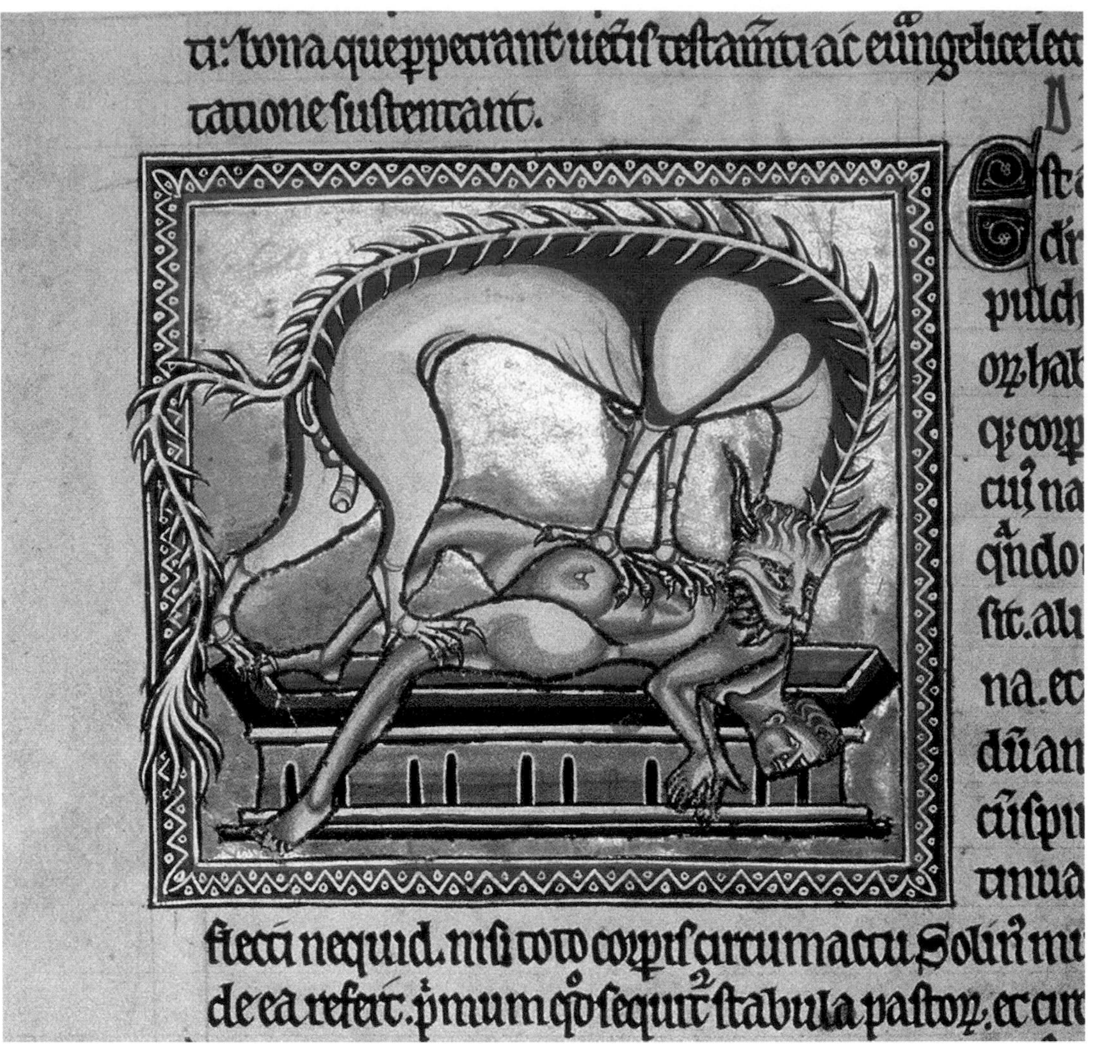

The Aberdeen Bestiary, Aberdeen University Library, MS 24, f. 11v. Detail 10 x 10 cm. © University of Aberdeen.

Exhibit 9

The Hermaphroditic Hyena

Gabriella Zuccolin

From Aristotle's treatises through works of scholastic natural philosophy to early modern natural histories, many learned texts dealt with animals. Bestiaries were distinguished by their allegorical explanations and moralizing frame. They described familiar and exotic creatures, real and legendary, and often foregrounded matters of sex and generation. An example is the hyena, seen here in the Aberdeen Bestiary, probably commissioned for theological exegesis and teaching by a wealthy patron in Lincolnshire or Yorkshire during the golden age of bestiaries around 1200. Little else is known about its provenance except that it was listed in the inventory of the Old Royal Library at Westminster Palace in 1542, and that the son of James I's Royal Librarian had given it to the regent of Marischal College, Aberdeen, by around 1625.

'There is an animal called the hyena', the Latin text begins. 'Its nature is that it is sometimes male, sometimes female, and it is therefore an unclean animal.' A literary tradition, as old as Aesop's fables, assigned alternating sexes to this hermaphroditic creature. The illustration depicts the hyena with both male and female anatomy (a penis and an elongated vagina, not to be mistaken for an anus), together with characteristics typical of the animal in medieval bestiaries: a monstrous spine and tail, demon-like head, fangs and reptilian claws, clasping a corpse. The representation of the hyena's double-sexed genitals is unusual in the bestiary tradition, except, for unknown reasons, in the group which includes the Aberdeen Bestiary, composed in England between the twelfth and fourteenth centuries. Other bestiaries do not represent the hyena's genitals, nor the genitals of other sexually strange animals like elephants, which can only mate once in their life, after eating mandrake; or hares, which can change sex and impregnate themselves.

Despite Aristotle's denial that hyenas were hermaphroditic, this idea persisted in, for instance, ancient and medieval philosophers' discussions of whether hyenas in particular, and hermaphrodites more generally, could self-generate. The hyena was an allegory for human hypocrisy and the devil. Medieval theologians and canonists routinely used hyenas to point to the sins of 'unmanly men' and adulterers; to address fundamental issues about the origins of sex differences; and to think about practical questions such as whether a hermaphrodite infant should be baptized male or female.

To understand why the hyena came to symbolize sexual aberration, it might be useful to recall that their genitalia can easily deceive: the female's enlarged clitoris, through which she urinates, copulates and gives birth, looks like a penis and can develop pseudophallic erections; the labia are shaped much like testicles. Medieval descriptions of hyena anatomy may be strange because, as the ancients taught, its anatomy is strange. But not until Conrad Gessner, the 'Swiss Pliny', published *Historiae animalium* (1551) – a monumental effort to bridge the declining tradition of bestiary lore, ancient zoological knowledge and contemporary observation – was the hyena's hermaphroditism finally dismissed. The animal's strange sex organs became a subject of natural inquiry rather than moral reading.

FURTHER READING

Chapters 4, 14 and 41 and Exhibits 2 and 13, this book.

Jeffrey Jerome Cohen, 'Inventing with animals in the middle ages', in Barbara A. Hanawalt and Lisa J. Kiser (eds.), *Essays on the Natural World in Medieval and Early Modern Europe* (Notre Dame, IN, 2008), pp. 39–62.

Maaike van der Lugt, 'Sex difference in medieval theology and canon law: A tribute to Joan Cadden', *Medieval Feminist Forum* 46, no. 1 (2010), 101–21.

Anna Wilson, 'Sexing the hyena: Intraspecies readings of the female phallus', *Signs* 28 (2003), 755–90.

Exhibit 10

Medieval Birth Malpresentations

Lauren Kassell

Around 500 AD, a North African physician called Muscio or Mustio reworked the influential Greek *Gynaecology* composed by Soranus of Ephesus, the Roman physician, four centuries earlier. Muscio aimed his abbreviated Latin version at midwives who no longer knew the original language; figures illustrated the chapter on difficult births. Just two copies of Muscio's text survive from the early middle ages, and only one with the images. But in the later eleventh century, the figures were reborn when scribes at Monte Cassino, the first abbey of the Benedictine order, recopied Muscio's work. The images long remained the only obstetrical illustrations.

A survey of the twenty-three extant manuscript copies of the Muscian series – including the scroll seen here – shows that the images were not included in collections of works intended for midwives or other women. Instead, in the thirteenth century, they were separated from Muscio's text and circulated with surgical works in Latin, like that by al-Zahrawi (Albucasis), the great Andalusian surgeon, and with vernacular writings on women's medicine aimed at male readers. Then print gave the images a wider audience. They were incorporated into the first printed midwifery book, Eucharius Rösslin's *Rose Garden for Pregnant Women and Midwives*, published in German in 1513, then translated into other European vernaculars and reprinted many times, complete with the figures, over the next century and a half.

This large scroll was produced in England in the 1420s. The two columns of text are mostly extracted from the surgical writings of the fourteenth-century English surgeon, John Arderne; another surgeon may have owned the scroll. In the pictures in the margins, patients display complaints or undergo procedures described in the adjoining text. The centre of the roll shows coloured drawings of human bodily systems from front and rear; stages in Arderne's operation for anal fistula; and the series of fifteen malpresenting infants, each preceded by a caption, of which five are shown in the detail on the left. The sequence of images and their pairings with captions vary across copies.

The Muscio images have sometimes been mistaken for the sort of developmental sequence that anatomists began to depict, first for chicks, in the sixteenth century. In these obstetrical diagrams, however, the only change is in the posture of the fully formed, animated child – or children in the case of twins. The pictures probably provided a surgeon with a handy visual summary of what might go wrong during a birth, such as the hands- or feet-first presentations seen in the detail on the right here, even if he could do little to assist. Like other surgical images, this series was intended to impress a lay clientele with the learned surgeon's expertise. In a similar spirit, Pierre Andrieu, physician to the Count of Foix, included the series in his *Golden Apple*, written around 1450 to help his noble patron produce healthy, legitimate offspring. Images that had begun as instructions for midwives had become instruments of male patronage.

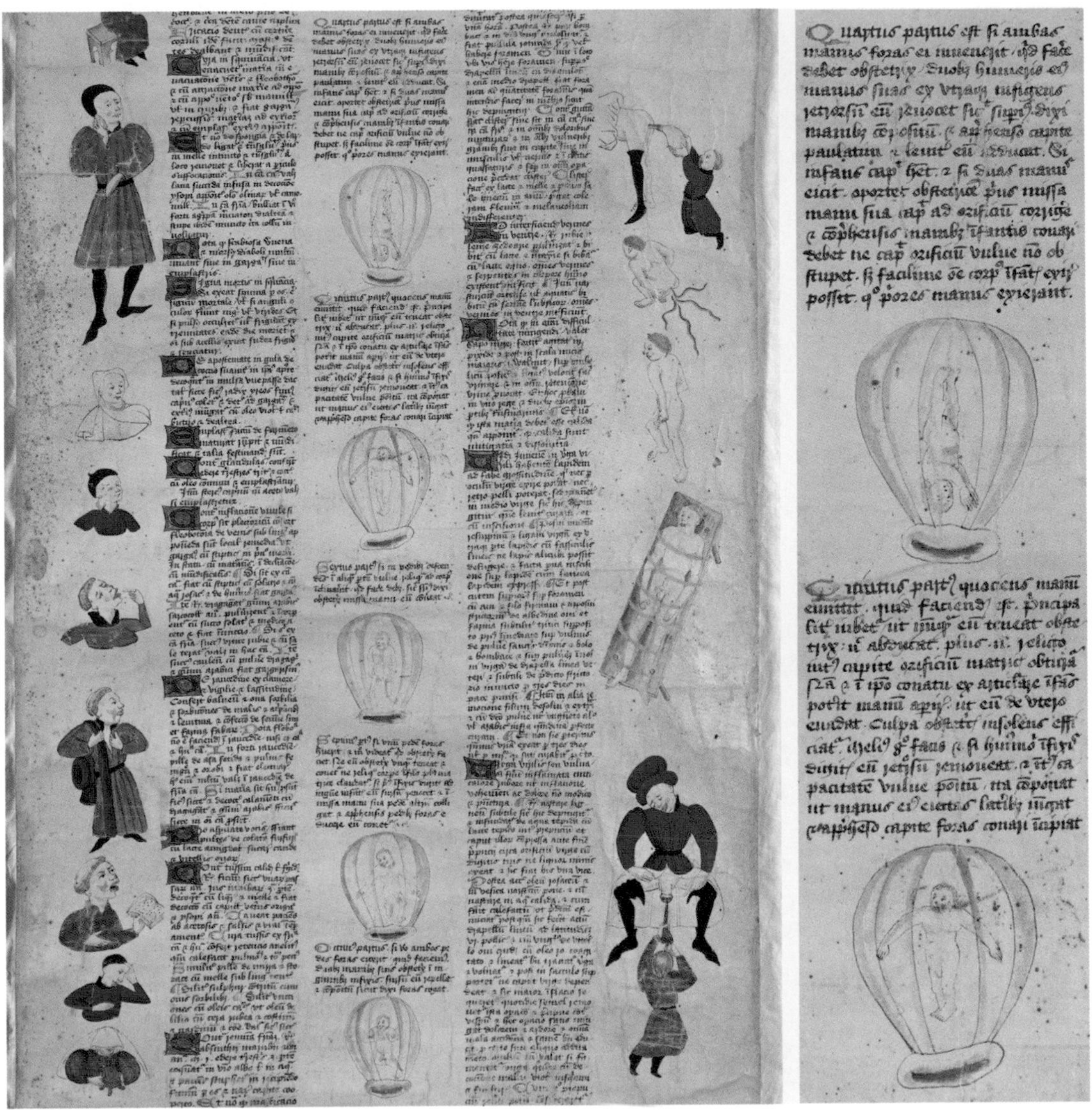

Details of a parchment roll. National Library of Sweden, MS X.118, 542 × 36 cm.

FURTHER READING

Chapters 3, 7, 11, 16, 22 and 37 and Exhibits 6, 18, 22 and 23, this book.

John Arderne, 'Abridged version of "De arte phisicali de cirurgia", "Fistula in ano", including an obstetrical treatise', World Digital Library, www.wdl.org/en/item/11631/.

Monica H. Green, '"Cliff Notes" on the Circulation of the Gynecological Texts of Soranus and Muscio in the Middle Ages' (2017), www.academia.edu/7858536/Monica_H._Green_Cliff_Notes_on_the_Circulation_of_the_Gynecological_Texts_of_Soranus_and_Muscio_in_the_Middle_Ages_2017, accessed 19 July 2017.

Monica H. Green, 'Moving from philology to social history: The circulation and uses of Albucasis's Latin *Surgery* in the middle ages', in Florence Eliza Glaze and Brian K. Nance (eds.), *Between Text and Patient: The Medical Enterprise in Medieval & Early Modern Europe* (Florence, 2011), pp. 331–72.

Exhibit 11

A Medieval Birth Girdle

Lea T. Olsan

From the earliest times, binding and unbinding, opening doors, unlocking locks and reciting magical formulas facilitated childbirth. In fifteenth-century Europe, narrow parchment rolls, or 'birth girdles', inscribed with texts and images and associated with the belt or sash of the Virgin Mary fulfilled this role. Like 'girdles' of other saints, 'Our Lady's Girdle' was lent by churches and abbeys to pregnant women – to contemplate or place on the body. These rolls were brought into the domestic space of a woman's 'lying-in' to protect the lives and souls of mother and child through the dangers of birth. Labouring women and the midwives, other women, and sometimes priests and doctors who helped them used these powerful rolls together with other divine and natural methods to ensure a safe delivery.

The elaborate example seen here, Harley Roll T 11, was produced in the last quarter of the fifteenth century, but that is all we know about its origins. It vividly assembles images of Christ's torments, for contemplation; Latin prayers to saints, particularly the patrons of childbirth Julitta and Quiricus; drawings of amuletic figures authorizing heaven's protection from harms, such as lightning and enemies; and charms to aid childbirth, encourage sleep and staunch bleeding. The two dominant colours, a fresh green and blood red, represent the paradox of the new life that Christ's suffering and death secured for sinners. The text beside the image of the nails is a form of indulgence, stating that Pope Innocent has exempted whoever carries images of the nails on their body, and worships them with a specific number of prayers, from sudden death, death by the sword, poison, pestilence, wicked spirits or fevers, or otherwise dying without the sacraments.

The diamond-shaped side-wound, coloured to show its depth as the 'well' of compassion, acts as a 'measure' of Christ's body authorized in a letter from heaven. The adjacent text promises protection from death and violence. The last promise reads, in Latin, 'if a woman be "travailing of child", on that day that she has seen the aforementioned measure, she shall not die, but the child will have baptism and the mother purification'. Thus, her child's soul will be saved, and the woman herself will live at least until the ceremony at the church door about a month after delivery.

Limited numbers of painted birth girdles have survived. Protestant and Catholic reformers censored charms, devotions to saints and ecclesiastical rituals. Only a few decades after this roll was made, English iconoclasts were retrieving 'birth girdles' from churches and destroying them as products of 'magic' and 'superstition'. Harley Roll T 11 may have survived hidden or forgotten until it acquired new value as an ancient manuscript, rather than a practical talisman, and was then collected by the antiquarians, Robert and Edward Harley. By 1700, women in England placed their hopes for a safe delivery in more mundane objects.

FURTHER READING

Chapters 11, 13, 22 and 37 and Exhibits 6, 10, 17, 18 and 22, this book.

Walter J. Dilling, 'Girdles: Their origin and development, particularly with regard to their use as charms in medicine, marriage, and midwifery', *Caledonian Medical Journal* 9 (1912–14), 337–57 and 403–25.

Joseph J. Gwara and Mary Morse, 'A birth girdle printed by Wynkyn de Worde', *The Library*, 7th ser., 13 (2012), 33–62.

Don C. Skemer, *Binding Words: Textual Amulets in the Middle Ages* (University Park, PA, 2006).

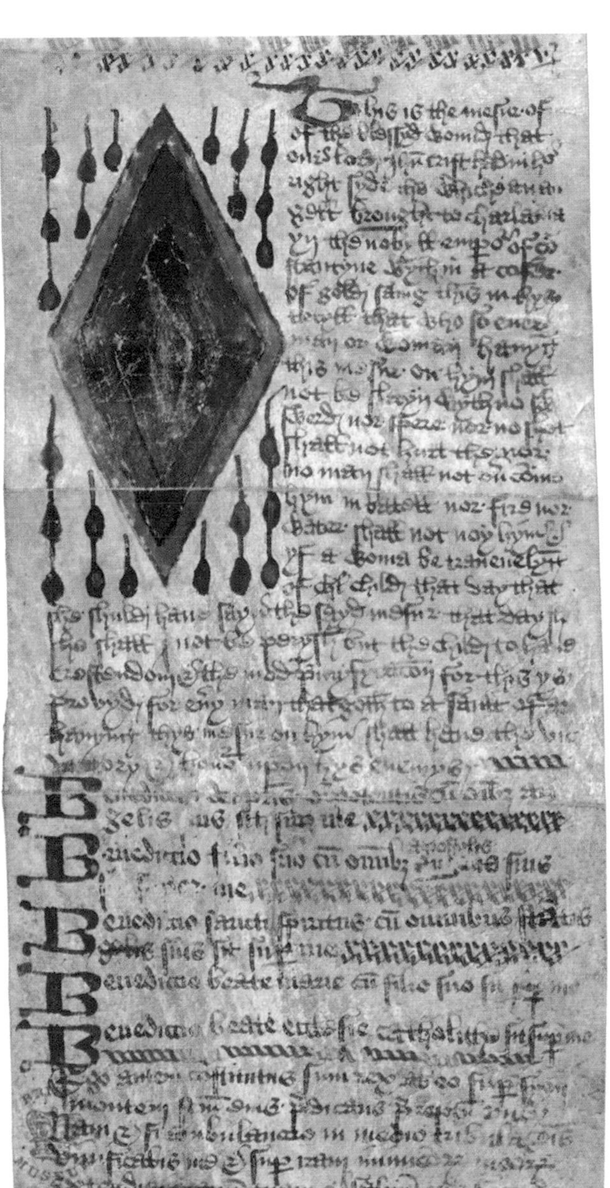

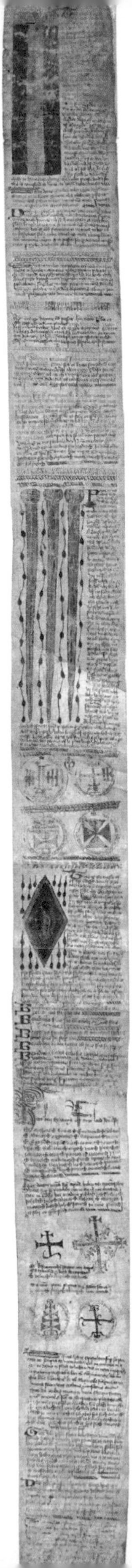

Full girdle made from two parchment membranes, 112.5 x 8.5 cm, and detail. London, British Library, Harley Roll T 11. © The British Library Board.

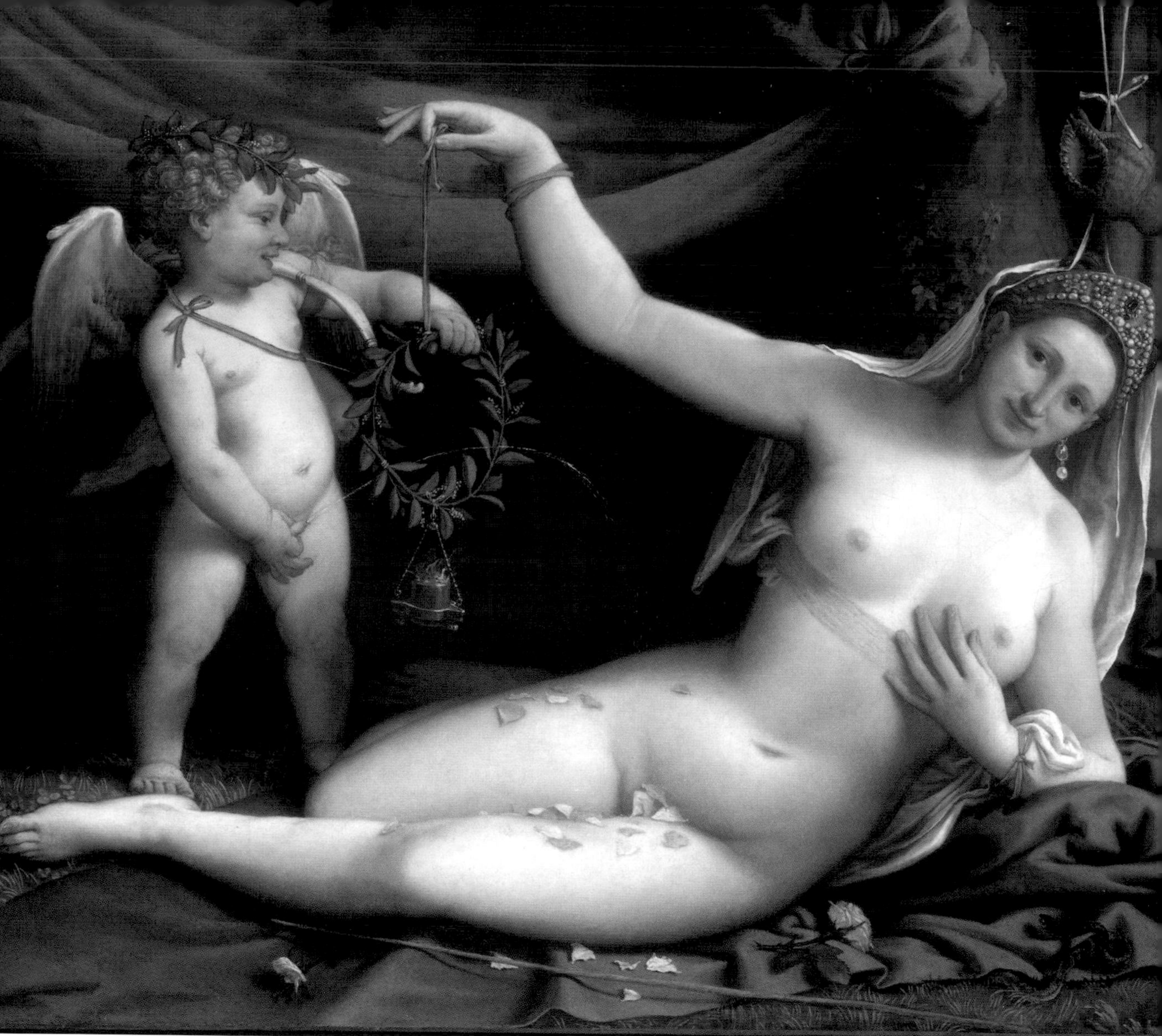

Lorenzo Lotto, *Venus and Cupid*, oil on canvas, 92 × 111 cm, The Metropolitan Museum of Art, Mrs Charles Wrightsman Gift, in honour of Marietta Tree, 1986.

Exhibit 12

Renaissance Art, Arousal and Impotence

Patricia Simons

Renaissance paintings that depict a reclining female nude with nymphs do not always, as some scholars have assumed, celebrate matrimony. Rather, the surviving documentation attests to the non-procreative effects of this imagery, then newly drawn from antiquity, and related items of visual culture. Around 1525, for instance, Pope Clement VII was aghast that the renowned erotic prints, *I modi*, circulated amongst the curia and ordered their destruction. In the 1590s, Pierre de Bourdeille, Lord of Brantôme, wrote of a woman stirred by a picture of bathing women to rush off and have sex with her male lover. Many Venetian noblemen kept their patrimony intact by refraining from marriage, yet Venuses and other amorous images decorated their apartments. Medical texts mention the use of visual materials to promote arousal, couched within advice about fertility, though historians lack records of this practice in use. Most discourse about masculinity and virility focused on pleasure, not the fathering of children; the significance of women's pleasure was joked about and debated in anatomical books. Erotic images could arouse men and women, and were more a part of broad Renaissance sexuality than contributors solely to the production of children within the matrimonial bed.

Lorenzo Lotto's *Venus and Cupid*, probably painted in the mid- or late 1520s, is a likely exception. It displays a masterful and witty combination of imagery about marriage and sexuality, much of it drawn from ancient and popular sources. No information survives about its commission or location, though Lotto's secular patrons were often wealthy merchants or professional men. The imagery suits the poetic and folkloric context of marriage, and the pissing Cupid visualizes the conquest of impotence. Several elements allude to union, including ivy clinging to a tree trunk (amorous in ancient Roman verse). Smiling Venus wears what is probably a bridal veil with crown, and the girdle under her breasts was untied on the wedding night as an augury of children. Other details are sexually witty, especially the red, vulva-like opening of the conch shell and the snake in the grass, a figure used in contemporary literature for male genitals. Rose petals scattered on the goddess's lap and thighs refer to Venus and desire, but also to the seed of chuckling Cupid.

The release of male fluid directed onto the woman's genital region conflates urine with semen, a common joke at the time. Portent of fecundity, Cupid's frothy stream (both piss and ejaculate) jovially demonstrates virility. Reports from sixteenth-century Venice note love-magic overcoming impotence when the husband symbolically pissed through the marriage ring or urinated near a tomb or church door, and these practices were probably commonplace throughout Europe. Lotto's garland and incense-burner more decorously refer to rings and sacred practices. This humour, derived from ancient marriage poems, provided a jubilant release of tension to ward off impotence. Viewers, including the married (and portrayed?) couple for whom the alluring painting was probably produced, are invited to celebrate sexual pleasure. From antiquity through the Renaissance, sex and sexuality were playful as well as productive.

FURTHER READING

Chapters 2, 11, 16 and 24 and Exhibits 5, 19 and 25, this book.

Keith Christiansen, 'Lorenzo Lotto and the tradition of epithalamic paintings', *Apollo*, new ser., 124 (1986), 166–73.

Norberto Massi, 'Lorenzo Lotto's New York Venus', in Lynn Catterson and Mark Zucker (eds.), *Watching Art: Writings in Honor of James Beck. Studi di storia dell'arte in onore di James Beck* (Todi, 2006), pp. 167–70.

Patricia Simons, *The Sex of Men in Premodern Europe: A Cultural History* (Cambridge, 2011).

Exhibit 13

Monstrous Births and Diabolical Seed

Jennifer Spinks

The 'monster of Cracow' (or Krakow) was a human child born in 1543. Of ambiguous sex, it had fiery eyes, webbed claws, a curving tail and animal heads disposed about its body, according to widely circulated contemporary reports. In 1559 the monster, painted by an unknown artist, appeared in a richly illustrated and lavishly bound manuscript about the wonders of the natural world that the French Protestant humanist Pierre Boaistuau prepared as a present for Elizabeth I of England. Over the following decades, French printers reworked the manuscript in multiple, often expanded illustrated editions, which always included a woodcut of the monster of Cracow.

Boaistuau's 'Prodigious Histories' demonstrated a fascination with the generation of 'monstrous births', as children and animals born with physical deformities were typically described. With unnatural extra heads and clawed hands and feet, the monster of Cracow both recalled medieval representations of the devil and prompted new discussions about the manifestations and causes of monstrosity. This image illustrated a chapter discussing whether or not the devil could engender children. Boaistuau listed other births often ascribed to diabolical seed, including the standard example of Merlin, but took a sceptical position. For Boaistuau, it was plausible that devils could have sex with humans – and even fake the process of birth – but, he concluded, 'although evil spirits may copulate, they do not have any seed, and cannot procreate, for there is no division of sex between them'.

One of Boaistuau's sources was a 1554 printed handbook for training midwives. Written by the Swiss surgeon and humanist scholar Jakob Rueff, it was underpinned by a Galenic model of conception in which male and female seed mingled together. In a chapter on monstrous births, Rueff argued that although devils could not generate life, the case of the monster of Cracow demonstrated their power to mingle human and animal seed. The image of the Cracow monster in Boaistuau's work also represented the mixture of human and animal, although his text focused on diabolical causation.

Throughout the sixteenth century, religious explanations were generally given greater weight than theories of natural causation. Particularly after the Lutheran Reformation began in 1517, monstrous births were often interpreted as signs of the imminence of the Last Days. Before Boaistuau many descriptions of the monster of Cracow had been apocalyptic, reporting, for example, that the child cried out, 'Awake, your Lord and God is about to come.' Following Rueff, Boaistuau remained interested in religious causes, but moved his attention away from the Final Judgement and towards an assessment of the devil's actions in the world. Thus his work also reflected rising scholarly concerns about 'preternatural' departures from the norms of nature.

When the eminent French surgeon Ambroise Paré discussed the causes of monsters in the 1570s, he began with the 'glory of God', included both excessive and insufficient seed, and concluded with 'Demons and Devils'. The science of teratology would later dominate discussions of human 'monstrosity'. In the sixteenth century, however, natural causation was often subsidiary to religious explanatory frameworks.

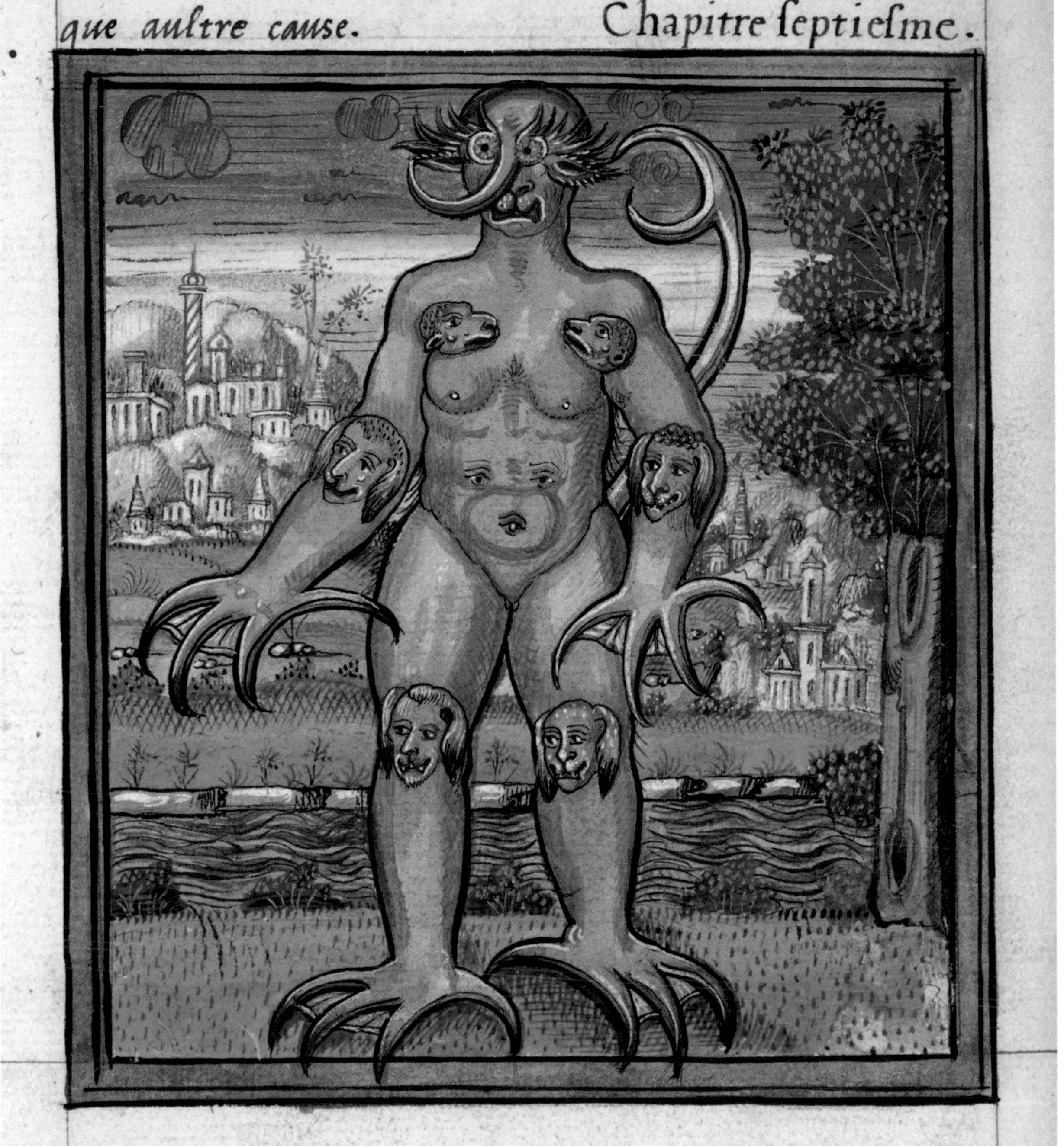

The monster of Cracow, in Pierre Boaistuau, 'Histoires prodigieuses' (1559). Full page, 23 × 16 cm. Wellcome Library, London, MS 136, f. 29v.

FURTHER READING

Chapters 12, 17 and 38 and Exhibits 22, 25 and 38, this book.

Pierre Boaistuau, *Histoires prodigieuses: MS 136 Wellcome Library*, ed. and trans. Stephen Bamforth (Milan, 2000).

Lorraine Daston and Katharine Park, *Wonders and the Order of Nature, 1150–1750* (New York, NY, 1998).

Jennifer Spinks, 'Jakob Rueff's 1554 *Trostbüchle*: A Zurich physician explains and interprets monstrous births', *Intellectual History Review* 18 (2008), 41–59.

Exhibit 14

Jane Dee's Courses in John Dee's Diary

Lauren Kassell

These pages from Johannes Stadius's *Ephemerides*, a table setting out planetary motions day-by-day for five decades, show December 1590. John Dee, a renowned English mathematician and astrologer, used this book as a calendar. Within the grid and in marginal notes keyed to particular dates, he recorded a conversation with Queen Elizabeth, a trip to Chelsea for a disputation with a bishop, payment of debts and when his wife Jane menstruated.

Dee kept 'diaries' from early in his career and more systematically from 1577, when he turned 50: he noted that he had a book published, sought royal patronage and, in 1578, married Jane Fromonds, half his age. Dee's first wife had died in 1575, after a ten-year marriage without issue. Jane was more fruitful. Over the next two decades she bore eight living children, two of whom survived to adulthood. In Stadius's and other printed ephemerides, Dee charted her periods, noting 'Jane had them', a common euphemism, and spelling her name in Greek; other terms included 'courses', 'sickness' and 'flowers'. Dee's system evolved to 'Jane had', sometimes followed by the symbol for Aquarius – perhaps associating water with menstruation – as seen next to 2 December (upper left and detail). Opposite 25 December (lower right), he noted just 'Jane'.

Establishing a family, like publishing books, meeting influential friends and securing royal patronage, marked a gentleman's success. In an era before ovulation was understood or the cessation of menstruation directly linked to pregnancy, Jane's routine bleeding meant health and its interruption was a possible sign of a child. He also noted when they had sex (the symbol Sagittarius, the archer), her miscarriages, childbirths, churchings and the nursing and weaning of the children. It is unclear, however, whether long intervals between entries naming Jane represent her lack of periods or lapses in Dee's diary keeping.

Other early modern men recorded details about women's bodies, and women too might note signs of health or pregnancy. The moment of conception, like of birth, could be astrologically propitious; rulers reputedly postponed consummating marriages until the right time; and travelling husbands recorded dates of conjugal visits. Married noblewomen across Europe mentioned menstruation in letters to family and friends. Women were expected to know their bodily orders, and through the seventeenth century increasingly recorded them, often, like the Swiss aristocrat Angletine Charrière de Sévery, with a simple cross in her diary. Through the eighteenth century, female patients were expected to tell their medical practitioners about the frequency, quantity and quality of their bleeding; paternity, inheritance and sexual misconduct cases invoked evidence of orderly and disorderly menstruation.

The nineteenth century, by contrast, redefined sex and fertility as private, and the twentieth definitively established the link between ovulation and menstruation. Ancient associations between women's blood loss and the phases of the moon, John Dee's records of Jane Dee's flow and twenty-first-century digital menstrual calendars share only the action of charting periods. While debates over its implications continue, the significance of monitoring women's bleeding has changed.

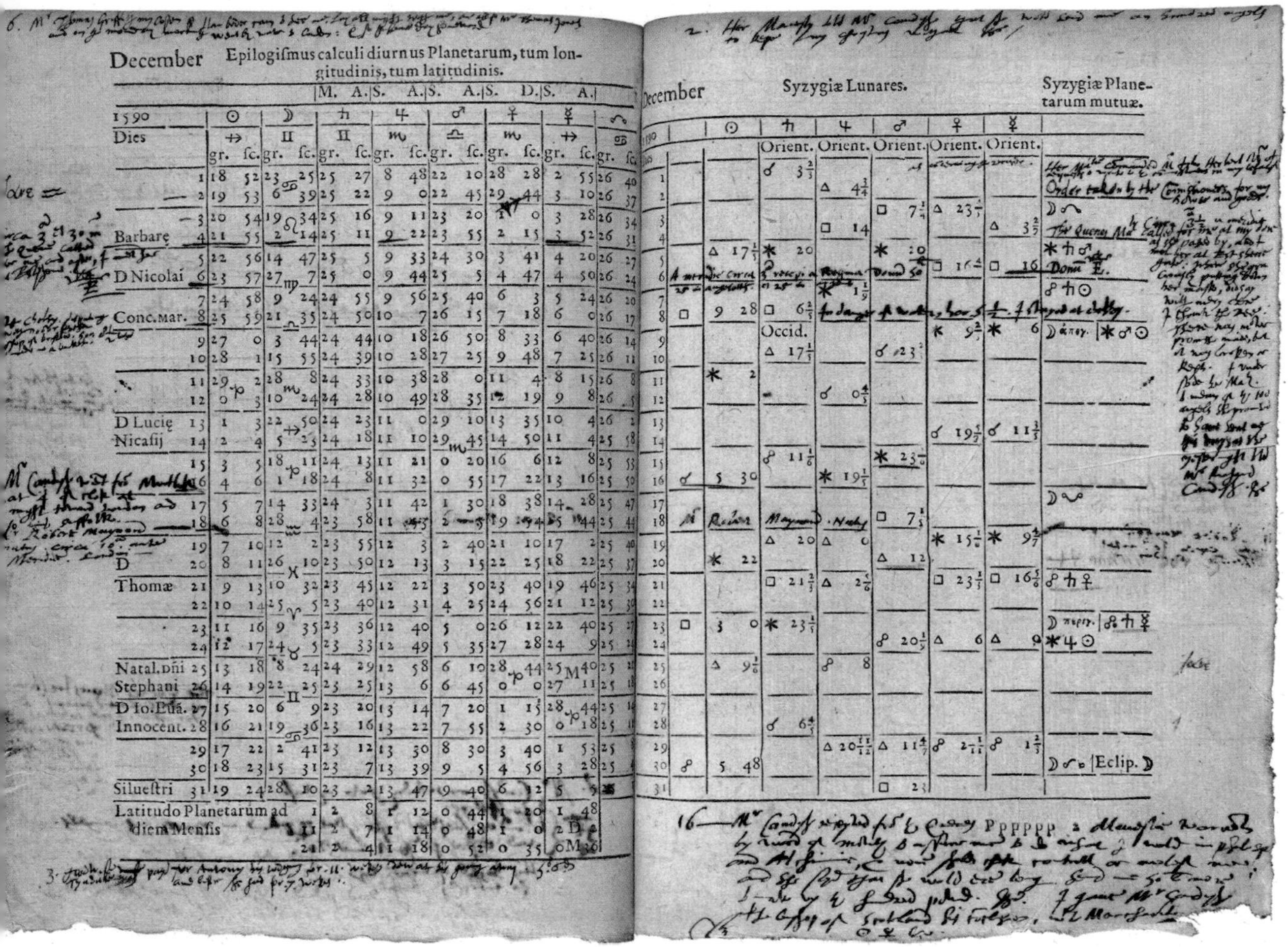

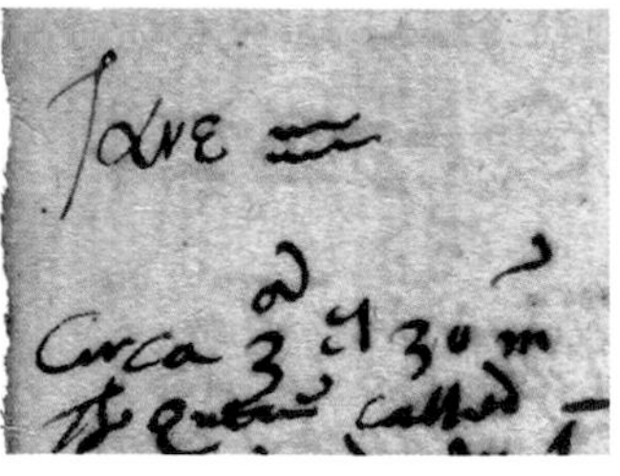

John Dee's 'Diary', recorded in Johannes Stadius, *Ephemerides novae ab anno 1554 usque ad annum 1600* (Cologne: Arnold Birckmann, 1570), Bodleian Library, MS Ashmole 487, Dec. 1590, full opening 21 × 30 cm. By permission of the Bodleian Libraries, University of Oxford.

FURTHER READING

Chapters 3, 11, 16, 31, 32 and 36 and Exhibits 3, 16, 31 and 32, this book.

Deborah Harkness, 'Managing an experimental household: The Dees of Mortlake and the practice of natural philosophy', *Isis* 88 (1994), 247–62.

Lauren Kassell, 'Almanacs and prognostications', in Joad Raymond (ed.), *The Oxford History of Popular Print Culture*, vol. 1: *Cheap Print in Britain and Ireland to 1660* (Oxford, 2011), pp. 431–42.

Cathy McClive, *Menstruation and Procreation in Early Modern France* (London, 2015).

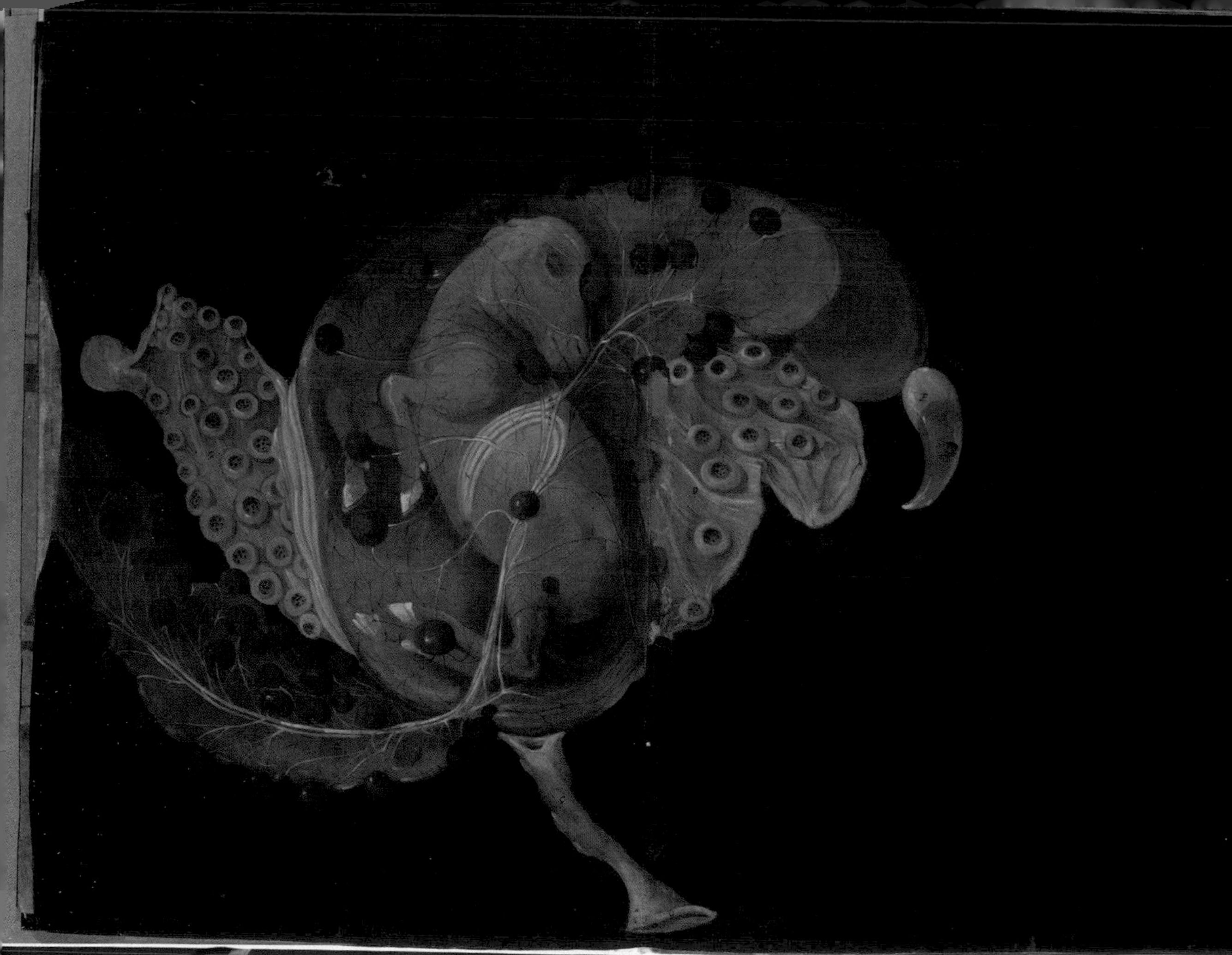

Oil painting of fetal lamb. Cardstock bound with *De formato foetu*. 42.5 × 56 cm. Biblioteca Nazionale Marciana, Venice, Rari 119.10. Reproduced by permission of the library; further reproduction prohibited without written authorization.

Exhibit 15

A Placenta Painted and Engraved

Karin Ekholm

The painting depicts a full-term fetal lamb cut from the amniotic sac and uterus. Girolamo Fabrici d'Acquapendente, who taught anatomy at the University of Padua in the Republic of Venice, commissioned it from unnamed painters as part of a series representing wombs and fetuses. Beside it we see one of the thirty-four copper engravings based on the paintings that then featured in his *De formato foetu* (On the formed fetus, 1604).

Early modern anatomical books commonly included plates, occasionally hand-coloured. Paintings were rare, but Fabrici perhaps took this step because Venice was a great centre

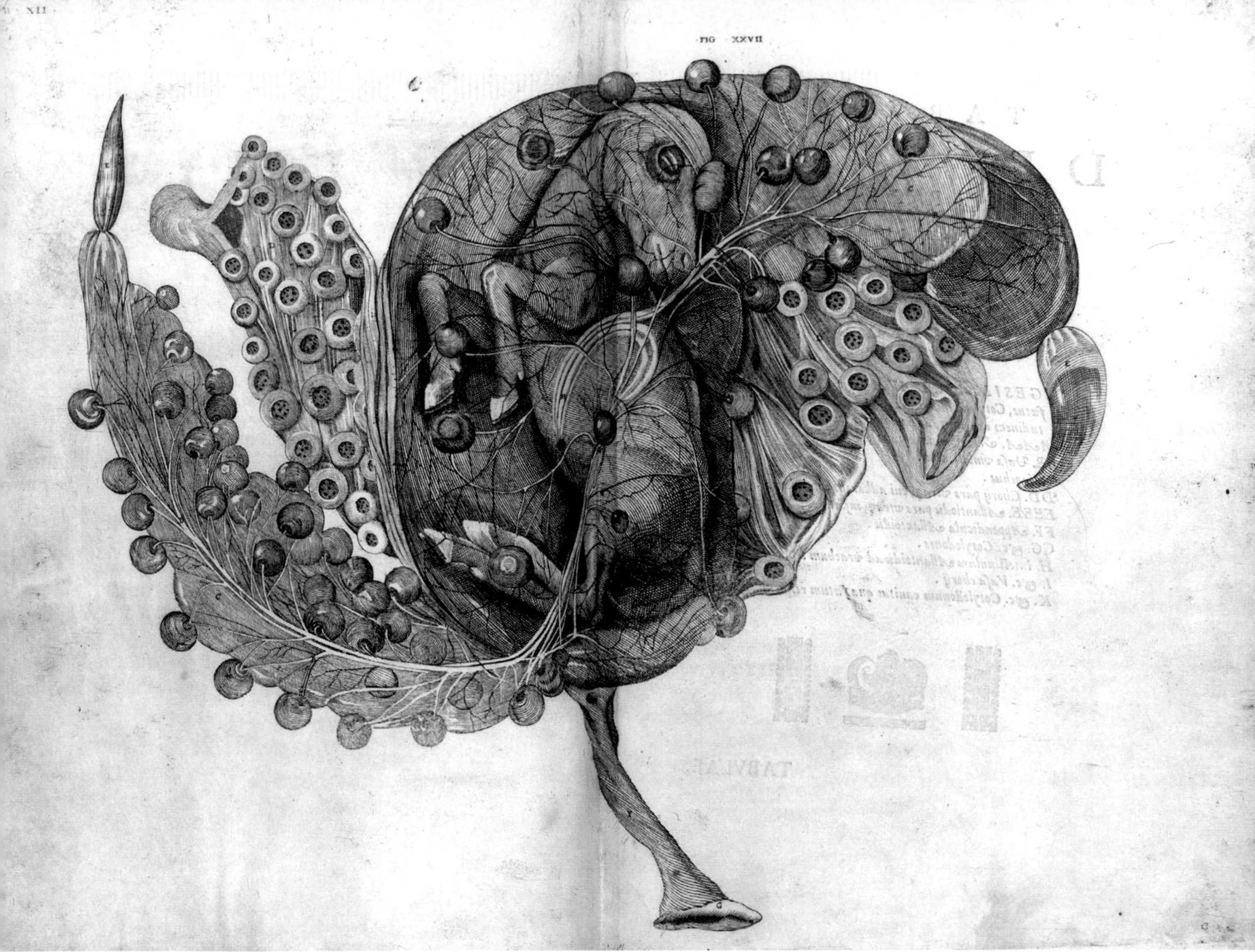

Girolamo Fabrici d'Acquapendente, *De formato foetu* (Padua: Laurentius Pasquatus, 1604, reissued with additional works and a new title page by Roberto Meglietti, 1625), plate XII on pp. 46–7. 42 × 53 cm. Courtesy Lilly Library, Indiana University, Bloomington, Indiana.

of painting, and oils best conveyed the subtle hues and textures on which his arguments depended. The plum-like structures are placentas plucked from the uterus, where they had been attached to the concave knobs resembling buttons (caruncles). Like in still-life paintings of fruit, a tradition newly imported from the Netherlands, the strong tonal contrast makes the placentas appear three-dimensional, an effect lost in the more diagrammatic engraving.

Fabrici's volume contributed to debates about fetal anatomy. Earlier anatomists had disagreed about the fetal membranes, blood vessels and placentas, commonly called the 'fleshy substance', as they tried to make sense of its different shapes, colours, numbers and sizes in different animals. Seeking a resolution, Fabrici presented illustrations with placentas of animals representative of four types: a pancake shape in humans and rodents, a band in dogs, many smaller masses in cows and sheep, and a thin layer covering the amniotic sac in pigs and horses. Though previous anatomists denied the last group a placenta, Fabrici's anatomical investigations, represented in paintings and engravings, led him to claim discovery of equivalent structures in sows and mares.

Fabrici's observations of placentas, moreover, contributed to debates about the connection between fetus and mother. Galen had described placentas as stabilizing the juncture of the uterine and umbilical vessels. In the 1560s, the Bolognese anatomist Giulio Cesare Aranzio challenged this position, arguing that the fetal and maternal blood vessels do not meet. Fabrici sided with Galen. When he separated the small placentas from ewes' wombs, they left black dots – the 'buttonholes' in the painting and engraving – which he identified as broken vessels, thus refuting Aranzio's claim.

Fabrici deposited the paintings, bound with the prints, in the Venetian State Library, for the benefit of posterity. His book was reprinted several times and critiqued by his students, including William Harvey, who owned and annotated the copy shown here. Harvey and other anatomists continued to debate the connection between fetus and mother. Building on the work of another of Fabrici's students, Adriaan van den Spiegel, Harvey suggested that fetuses collect only nutrients from placentas and make blood and vital spirits for themselves. These arguments, like Harvey's discovery of the circulation of the blood, were founded in experiment in addition to anatomical inspection. Though Fabrici's successors rejected many of his views, his classification of four types persisted, and his engravings, which long remained the most accurate representations of animal fetuses and wombs, continue to shape representations of fetal anatomy.

FURTHER READING

Chapters 9, 12, 15 and 38 and Exhibits 10, 16, 23 and 34, this book.

Howard B. Adelmann, *The Embryological Treatises of Hieronymus Fabricius of Aquapendente*, 2 vols. (Ithaca, NY, 1942).

Maurizio Rippa Bonati and José Pardo-Tomás (eds.), *Il teatro dei corpi: Le pitture colorate d'anatomia di Girolamo Fabrici d'Acquapendente* (Milan, 2004).

Karin Ekholm, 'Fabricius's and Harvey's representations of animal generation', *Annals of Science* 67 (2010), 329–52.

Exhibit 16

The Generative Parts of Women

Rina Knoeff

The plate overleaf represents the 'seed-preparing vessels' that feed the female 'balls, trumpets, front part of the womb and vagina'. Drawn and published by Dutch anatomist Reinier de Graaf in his 1672 book on the female organs of generation, it exemplifies his discovery of the follicles that contain the female eggs, as well as the experimental method that led to this find.

The plate and its legend illustrate how de Graaf negotiated between different theories of generation. Although he continued using ancient 'male' terminology such as 'testicles' and 'balls' for female organs, he denounced the idea that these are inverted versions of the male genitalia. De Graaf likewise borrowed ideas about follicles from anatomists including Andreas Vesalius, Gabriele Fallopius and Thomas Bartholin, but in line with William Harvey argued that women contribute only eggs – not seed – to generation. This opposed the Galenic teaching that women produce a weak version of male seed. De Graaf had eggs originate in the ovaries (rather than the womb) and argued that fertilization happens in the 'egg-nests' after they have been sprayed with spirits of the male seed.

Central to de Graaf's work on the male and female generative organs was his invention of syringes to inject fluids and air into vessels and organs and reveal the movement of fluids during life. In this plate, which represents the syringes as blowing faces, de Graaf displayed the course of the 'seed preparing vessels' in support of his argument that the fluids they contain are necessary in the generation of eggs. The vessels branch into tiny arteries that end in bunches of follicles inside the 'egg-nests', where they deliver a substance for the generation of the egg, before returning to the heart. See D and K, and note that the small bump on top of the left 'egg-nest' represents an egg ready to burst from the follicle.

The publication of de Graaf's *De mulierum organis* (1672) caused uproar among his fellow anatomists. Jan Swammerdam, the Dutch anatomist, entomologist and microscopist, claimed that he, together with Leiden professor Jan van Horne, had made the same discoveries much earlier, and that Nicholas Steno, Swammerdam's Danish friend and fellow anatomist, had already written on the ovaries. Much of the debate centred on the production of the plates (who made the first sketches?) and on the trustworthiness of methods of injection (some anatomists argued that vessels, when inflated, push other anatomical structures away). De Graaf retorted that the plates demonstrated that his ideas were based on visible evidence, rather than reason, on which van Horne and Swammerdam had relied.

De Graaf's work was widely known in learned circles and found its way into vernacular medicine; it was posthumously translated into Dutch for audiences of midwives and surgeons. In 1677, Antonie van Leeuwenhoek's discovery of *animalcula* (little animals) in the male seed launched a fierce debate between 'ovists', who championed the egg, and 'animalculists', who revived the opinion that the male seed contains the germ of new life.

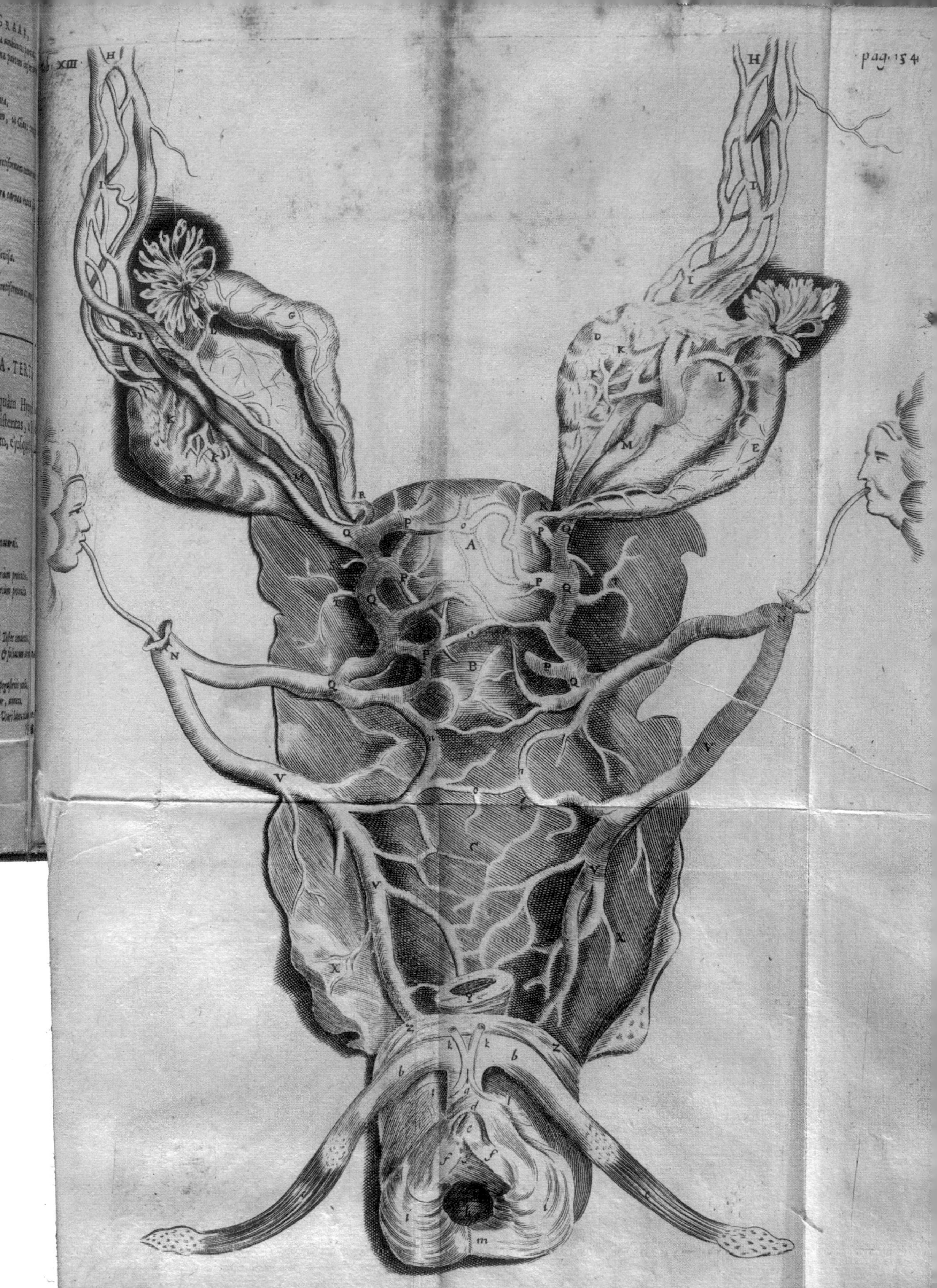
Tab. XIII
pag. 154

FURTHER READING

Chapters 7, 14, 15 and 28 and Exhibits 15 and 20, this book.

Matthew Cobb, *The Egg & Sperm Race: The Seventeenth-Century Scientists Who Unravelled the Secrets of Sex, Life and Growth* (London, 2007).

G. A. Lindeboom, *Reinier de Graaf: Leven en werken, 30–7–1641/17–8–1673* (Delft, 1973).

Evan Ragland, 'Experimenting with chemical bodies: Science, medicine, and philosophy in the long history of Reinier de Graaf's experiments on digestion, from Harvey and Descartes to Claude Bernard', unpublished PhD dissertation, Indiana University (2012).

Reinier de Graaf, *De mulierum organis generationi inservientibus* (Leiden, 1672), published in de Graaf, *Opera Omnia* (1678), p. 154. 30 × 20 cm. Cambridge University Library.

Exhibit 17

Pregnant Stones as Wonders of Nature

Sandra Cavallo

Commonly known as an eagle-stone, because female eagles were thought to use such stones to fortify their nests, the concretion mounted in gold in this picture is an aetites, one of the wonders of nature in the 'Paper Museum' – a visual encyclopaedia of 7,000 images assembled in early seventeenth-century Rome by the scholar and collector Cassiano dal Pozzo. The precious fitting contrasts with the apparently humble stone, which could stand on the small foot or be hung from the loop as a pendant. Rich evidence survives of numerous women who kept such objects as protective amulets during pregnancy, either by the bed or hanging from a long necklace touching the abdomen. Another plate in the 'Paper Museum' and examples surviving in European museums suggest that eagle-stones were also worn unmounted, attached to simple rope strings. These were fastened to the left arm of a pregnant woman to prevent miscarriage or to her thigh during labour to ease delivery.

Various other stones had health-giving properties, some associated with childbirth. From pumice to jaspers and magnets, fossil corals to powdered gemstones and quartz, they prevented sickness during pregnancy, facilitated birth and encouraged lactation if bound on the hip, ingested or applied locally. But belief in their pregnancy-related properties was less widespread and enduring than those of the aetites: references to the powers of this stone are found in natural histories, medical and pharmaceutical texts, Europe-wide and from antiquity to the nineteenth century. The archival evidence also stresses its broad social appeal: letters from Italian and English noblewomen testify to its use during labour in elite circles, and 'a childbirth stone' was listed in the inventory of a modest Florentine household. Price lists published in seventeenth-century German lapidaries present eagle-stones as inexpensive commodities and a staple apothecary ware; in the late nineteenth century, they were still in high demand in French pharmacies.

The popularity of eagle-stones owes much to their material features. As the physician Pietro Andrea Mattioli explained in his expanded edition of Dioscorides' *Materia medica* (first published in 1544), aetites are hollow and contain within them loose pieces which rattle when shaken, 'as if they were pregnant with another stone'. The power of the eagle-stone to aid pregnant women demonstrates the long persistence of analogical reasoning: the stone within a stone was like a child within its mother. Its talismanic power, however, was not an archaic residue, preserved merely through oral transmission and time-honoured domestic rituals. The surge of interest in the marvellous effects of nature in the Renaissance gave new impetus to the exploration of natural phenomena. In an age of commerce, increased communication and print, knowledge of the natural world was pursued by scholars and non-specialists alike, and widely disseminated. Private collections of specimens and images of nature like Cassiano's multiplied while lavishly illustrated vernacular treatises like Mattioli's, of which in Italy alone more than 30,000 copies were sold in twenty years, provided households with user-friendly information about the powers of natural objects. These developments conferred new legitimacy on the prophylactic use of 'pregnant stones'.

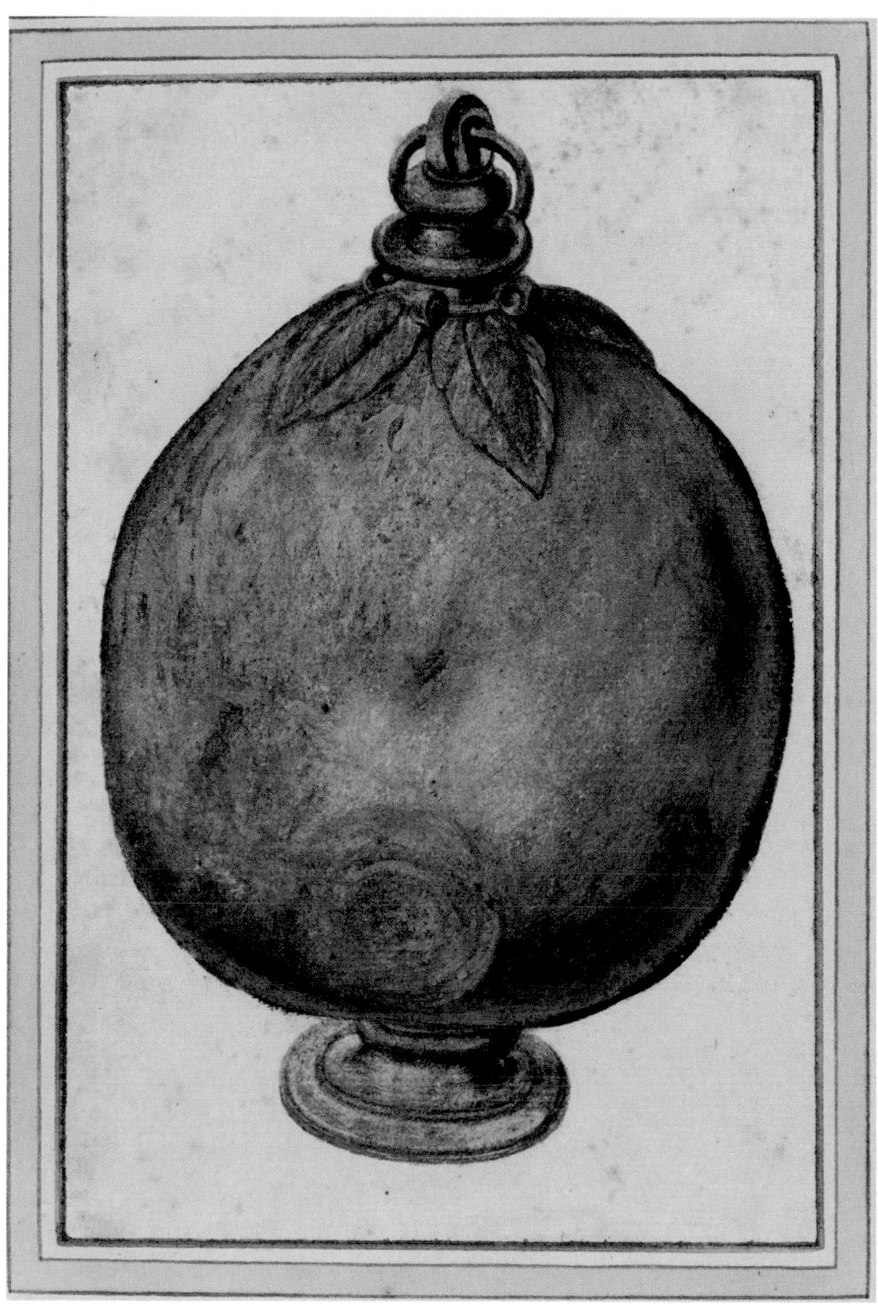

Watercolour of an eagle-stone, or aetites, with gold mounts. Paper, 24.5 × 16 cm, pasted onto album page with wash border drawn around it. Royal Collection Trust, RL 25480.

FURTHER READING

Chapters 4, 11, 13, 16, 22 and 37 and Exhibits 7, 11 and 25, this book.

Lorraine Daston and Katharine Park, *Wonders and the Order of Nature, 1150–1750* (New York, NY, 1998).

C. J. Duffin, R. T. J. Moddy and C. Gardiner-Thorpe (eds.), *A History of Geology and Medicine* (London, 2013).

Jacqueline M. Musacchio, 'Imaginative conceptions in Renaissance Italy', in Geraldine A. Johnson and Sara F. Matthews Grieco (eds.), *Picturing Women in Renaissance and Baroque Italy* (Cambridge, 1997), pp. 42–60.

Exhibit 18

A Birthing Chair

Lianne McTavish

According to the accession records of the Wellcome Trust in London, this wooden birth chair – now on permanent loan to the Science Museum – was owned by three generations of a family of Italian midwives from *c.* 1701 to 1830. When called to assist a woman in labour, a midwife carried this important technology with her, folding the leather-covered seat up, and the arms in, for ease of transportation. It shows signs of wear and has been repainted; hundreds of women may have laboured in it. The semicircular opening in the seat allowed the midwife to monitor the progress of the birth with her expert hands. Chairs like this one enhanced the midwife's authority, and came to symbolize her practice, especially in Italy, where, unlike in many other parts of Europe, childbirth remained a female domain through the eighteenth century.

The design of this chair also enhanced the status of the labouring woman. Seated on a kind of throne with a high back and elaborate arms, she became the centre of attention. Her head overlapped a gilded image of the suffering Christ, signalling the mysteries of childbirth. A child was a divine blessing, and birthing practices included devotional rituals, such as prayers in aid of a safe delivery to Margaret of Antioch, the patron saint of childbirth. At some undocumented point in its history, this chair was called 'miraculous', perhaps because it was associated with successful births, perhaps because the painted image linked it to holy figures with supernatural healing powers. When seated in this chair, the labouring woman was placed in proximity to a sacred body, which supported and blessed her endeavours and drew a symbolic analogy between her pain and Christ's.

Sitting was only one of the positions in which a woman, guided by her midwife, could choose to give birth; other options were resting on all fours, reclining or even sitting on the lap of a female assistant. Yet birthing chairs were an old technology, described in the second-century text of the Greek physician Soranus, and pictured in Roman bas reliefs. A well-known woodcut included in the obstetrical treatise of the German physician Eucharius Rösslin, *The Rose Garden for Pregnant Women and Midwives*, printed in Strasbourg in 1513, shows a parturient woman seated on a simple chair with a curved rather than a straight back. Later chairs could be more complicated, as indicated by the collapsible version featured in a treatise of 1690 by the German midwife Justine Siegemund. Her chair incorporated an open seat, backrest and handles to grip, and had a foot warmer and adjustable footrest. The back of the chair could recline, moving the woman's body towards the horizontal labour position preferred by obstetricians around 1900 – a more passive posture that late twentieth-century activists have associated with birthing women's loss of autonomy. Despite such transformations, birth chairs represent the continuity of obstetrical practices more than their change over time.

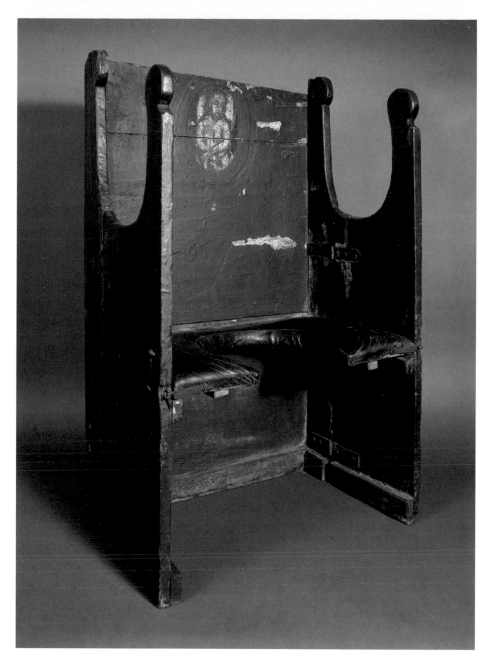

The 'miraculous chair of Palermo', *c.* 1701–1830, possibly crafted in Sicily, Science Museum, London / Science & Society Picture Library, image no. 10284323, inv. no. A602123. 94 × 58 × 38 cm.

FURTHER READING

Chapters 3, 7, 11, 22 and 37 and Exhibits 6, 10, 11, 17, 21, 22 and 25, this book.

Doreen Evenden, *The Midwives of Seventeenth-Century London* (Cambridge, 2000).

Nadia Maria Filippini, 'The church, the state, and childbirth: The midwife in Italy during the eighteenth century', in Hilary Marland (ed.), *The Art of Midwifery: Early Modern Midwives in Europe* (London, 1993), pp. 152–75.

Lianne McTavish, *Childbirth and the Display of Authority in Early Modern France* (Aldershot, 2005).

Exhibit 19

A Painting of a Nursing Mother

Lisa Forman Cody

The family is central to western art, but few works portrayed obviously pregnant women before the twentieth century. Some painters showed the Virgin Mary and other biblical mothers as big with child, but procreation was generally represented through breast-feeding. Hieronymus van der Mij, a minor Netherlands artist, often depicted nursing mothers, including in this small oil painting of 1728. Little more is known about its history: it was acquired by Mary, Countess of Holderness, who avidly collected Dutch works, and soon after her death in 1801 the future George IV purchased it for the Royal Collection where it remains.

Like others of the genre, this painting emphasized breast-feeding as an act of attachment between mother and child, but also used the nursing scene symbolically. Both the pyramidal composition and individual components invoked the Holy Family and Christian values. The dog in the toddler's lap signifies fidelity; the closed birdcage in the upper-left corner suggests the wife's chastity; the torn gold and yellow pincushion with five pins references Christ's crucifixion. The mother's hand over her breast and heart signifies faith, while nursing her child stands for charity.

The original viewers would have recognized these symbols. They might also have been drawn to the interconnected glances between family members. As the husband looks down at his infant at his wife's breast, the child looks upwards at the parents. The mother glances at the toddler, who in turn gazes at the baby. Looking out, the boy's pet spaniel draws us into this intimate scene. The circle of glances and gestures helps the viewer to focus on the painting's main theme: breast-feeding sustains the family and connects its members.

Van der Mij's painting reflects the fact that, throughout the early modern period, most mothers in the Netherlands, Scandinavia and other parts of northern Europe fed their own children. In contrast, the aristocracy and urban elites, especially in London and Paris, often hired wet nurses. Though this image does not explicitly critique wet nursing, it nonetheless underscores the benefits of maternal breast-feeding, a topic that gained political significance during the European Enlightenment.

Within forty years of van der Mij's painting, the Enlightenment philosopher Jean-Jacques Rousseau would argue that women's maternal role, signalled by breast-feeding, naturally suited them for the home rather than the public world of men. The eighteenth-century separation of the sexes is apparent in this painting with mother and infant dressed lightly for the home, but father and son ready for the outdoors. By emphasizing this division between reproduction and production, European images of nursing mothers across the centuries both represented and promoted an idealized view of maternal women. But from the Enlightenment onwards, as wet nursing was increasingly disparaged as unhealthy and unnatural even among elites, imagery of breast-feeding incorporated another layer of meaning: mothers held the family together and naturally ensured the health and strength of the nation by nursing future citizens.

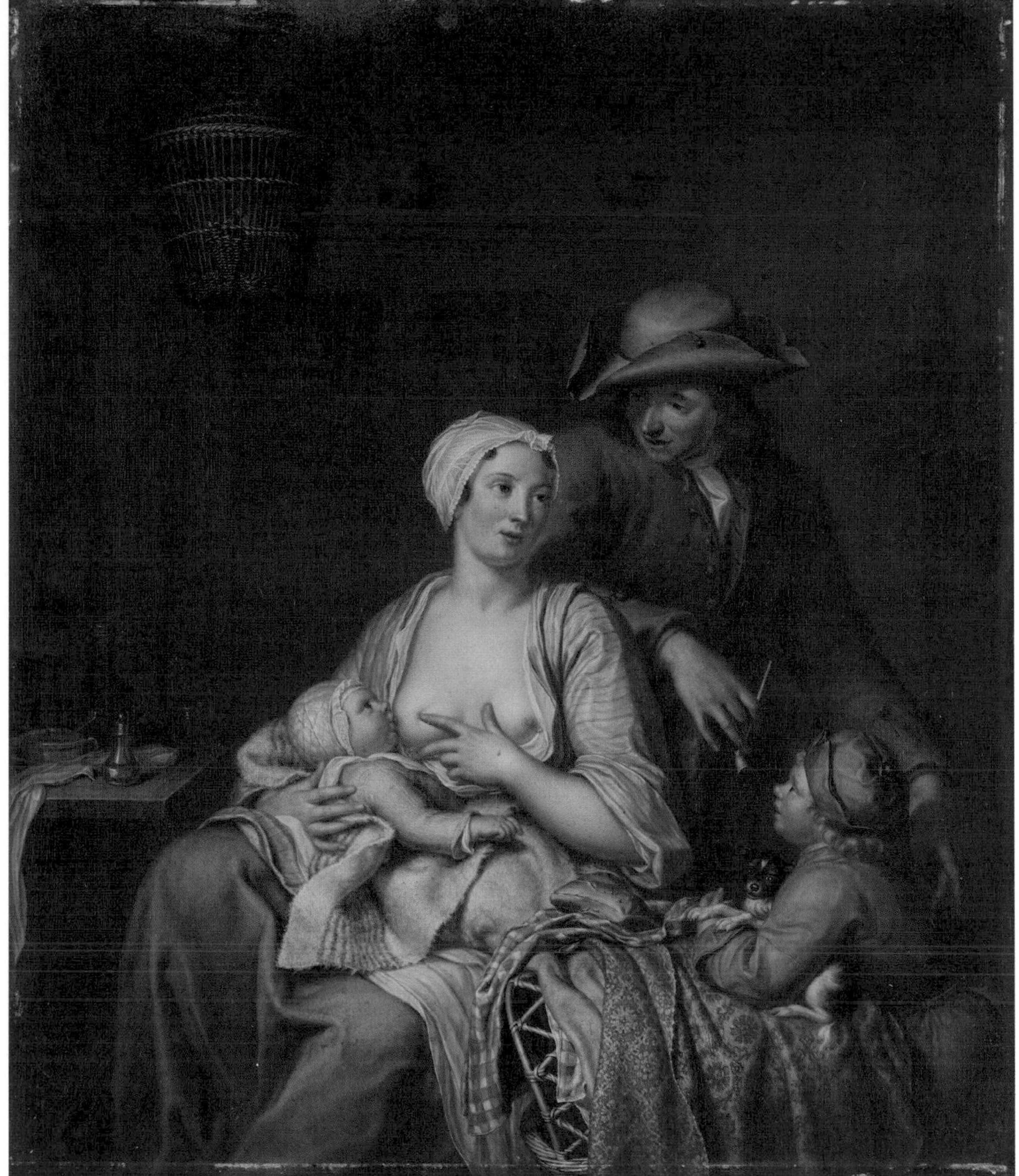

Hieronymus van der Mij, *A Family Group with a Mother Feeding Her Children* (1728). Oil on panel, 34 × 29 cm. Royal Collection Trust.

FURTHER READING

Chapters 6, 17, 24 and 33 and Exhibits 12 and 27, this book.

Jeroen J. H. Dekker, 'Beauty and simplicity: The power of fine art in moral teaching on education in seventeenth-century Holland', *Journal of Family History* 34 (2009), 166–88.

Valerie A. Fildes, *Breasts, Bottles and Babies: A History of Infant Feeding* (Edinburgh, 1986).

Patricia R. Ivinski *et al.*, *Farewell to the Wet Nurse: Etienne Aubry and Images of Breast Feeding in Eighteenth-Century France* (Williamstown, MA, 1998).

13 Generation between Script and Print

Peter Murray Jones

Historians have devoted much attention over the past forty years to the revolution in communication following the emergence of printing by movable type in mid-fifteenth-century Europe. Current scholarship questions whether such a revolution took place, and stresses the coexistence of manuscript and print, the intersection of both media with speech and pictures, and the partialness and gradualness of changes in communication between the fifteenth and eighteenth centuries.[1] In parallel with these general debates, histories of generation have documented the increasing interest of learned men in the workings of women's bodies, and argued that knowledge of generation, even when shared only between women, could be instrumental in upholding the institution of marriage.[2]

This chapter explores what happens when we consider the direct relevance of debates about script and print to understandings of human generation. It focuses on the fortunes of a kind of practical knowledge that is best identified by the medieval Latin term '*experimenta*' (singular '*experimentum*'). Here is an example: if you wish to influence whether you will have a boy or a girl, you should use the herb mercury. It grows in two kinds, male and female, each effective in producing the corresponding kind of children,

> so that the decoction of juice of the Male drank four dayes from the first day of purgation, will give force to the womb to procreate a male Child: but the juice of the Female drank for so many dayes, and in the same manner, will cause a female to be born, especially if the man lye with his wife when the [menstrual] Terms are newly over.[3]

This instruction was first printed in 1559 in the Dutch physician Levinus Lemnius's *Occulta naturae miracula* (Secret miracles of nature), a compendium of wondrous

1 Elizabeth Eisenstein, *The Printing Press as an Agent of Change* (Cambridge, 1979); Adrian Johns, *The Nature of the Book: Print and Knowledge in the Making* (Chicago, IL, 1998); Sabrina Alcorn Baron, Eric N. Lindquist and Eleanor F. Shevlin (eds.), *Agent of Change: Print Culture Studies after Elizabeth L. Eisenstein* (Amherst, MA, 2007); Leslie Howsam (ed.), *The Cambridge Companion to the History of the Book* (Cambridge, 2015).

2 Monica H. Green, *Making Women's Medicine Masculine: The Rise of Male Authority in Pre-Modern Gynaecology* (Oxford, 2008); Laura Gowing, *Common Bodies: Women, Touch and Power in Seventeenth-Century England* (New Haven, CT, 2003); Katharine Park, *Secrets of Women: Gender, Generation, and the Origins of Human Dissection* (New York, NY, 2006).

3 Levinus Lemnius, *The Secret Miracles of Nature: In Four Books …* (London, 1658), p. 27.

phenomena and herbal knowledge proving the presence of God in the workings of nature. Widely translated throughout Europe, it came out in English in 1658. In chapters 3 to 11, Lemnius collected material about generation, beginning with the injunction to remember that procreation was a divine gift, and including information about resemblance, pregnant women's cravings, the roles of female seed and menstrual blood, and the sex of the child.

Experimenta were useful practical techniques for healing, influencing natural processes and foreseeing outcomes; that they had passed the test of experience was their chief recommendation. Written down, *experimenta* were cast as short explanations of techniques of control or prediction. Recipes were a subcategory. Their 'bite-sized' format let them appear as individual items in written collections, embedded within texts or added to the margins of books and documents. Independent and transferable, their value did not derive from their place within a body of knowledge; they represented information.

From an explosion of writing in the fourteenth century to the emergence of printing in the mid-fifteenth century and an increasing vernacularization and commercialization of written and printed works through the seventeenth century, technologies of knowledge changed. So too did the epistemology of generation. As divine creation, generation was increasingly considered knowable through the book of nature as well as that of scripture. As secrets of women, generation shifted from the purview of women to that of men who wished to understand women's knowledge about their bodies. Situating recipes about generation within the broader category of *experimenta* thus draws attention to the gendering of knowledge about the physical operations of natural substances. Men traded in causes, women – often represented as old and illiterate – in experiences.[4] This dichotomy itself became the subject of heated debates from the sixteenth century.[5] Focusing on the communication of *experimenta* instead of learned treatises provides evidence of the transmission of knowledge across scholarly, domestic and commercial spheres as it was shared amongst and between different groups of men and women.[6]

Experimenta concerned with generation fall into three groups: remedies or recipes; prayers or charms; and prognostications. In practice these were often close to each

4 Jole Agrimi and Chiara Crisciani, 'Per una ricerca su "experimentum–experimenta": Riflessione epistemologica e tradizione medica (secoli XIII–XV)', in Pietro Janni and Innocenzo Mazzini (eds.), *Presenza del lessico greco e latino nelle lingue contemporanee: Ciclo di lezioni tenute all'Università di Macerata nell'a.a. 1987/88* (Macerata, 1990), pp. 9–49. See also Alisha Rankin, *Panacea's Daughters: Noblewomen as Healers in Early Modern Germany* (Chicago, IL, 2013), pp. 38–9, 46–8; and Park, *Secrets of Women*, pp. 83–5.

5 Ian Maclean, *The Renaissance Notion of Woman: A Study in the Fortunes of Scholasticism and Medical Science in European Intellectual Life* (Cambridge, 1980).

6 See also Helen King, 'Women and Doctors in Ancient Greece', Chapter 3; Katharine Park, 'Managing Childbirth and Fertility in Medieval Europe', Chapter 11; Lauren Kassell, 'Fruitful Bodies and Astrological Medicine', Chapter 16; James A. Secord, 'Talking Origins', Chapter 26; and Kate Fisher, 'Modern Ignorance', Chapter 32, this book.

other within manuscripts or printed books, and readers or users often flagged their topic, efficacy or noteworthiness in the margins. Such *experimenta* include remedies for infertility or to allay pains in childbirth, performative rituals involving words, actions and objects to achieve the same ends, and predictions of the outcome of a pregnancy, including the sex of a child.[7] They were often written down with brief testimonies to their practical usefulness, statements that they had been proved by experience ('*probatum est*'), or attributions to authority figures ancient or contemporary. Some *experimenta* had deep roots in textual traditions going back to the Hippocratic corpus or Pliny's *Natural History*, and thus invoked the authority of ancient knowledge. Others simply claimed to have worked.

Tracing the different kinds of *experimenta* for generation between script and print, and between Latin and vernacular languages, suggests that while the content of prayers, charms and prognostications was constrained and broadly stable, the producers and consumers of recipes grew in number and variety with innovations in writing, translating and printing.

Experimenta in an Explosion of Writing

The centuries-long continuities in the reappearances of *experimenta* in medieval manuscripts notwithstanding, a major change occurred in western Europe in the fourteenth century, when scribes began to produce so many more copies of manuscripts as to constitute a veritable explosion of writing. This was in part the result of technical novelties. In the twelfth century, parchment made from animal skins began to be replaced by more economical paper made from rags. By the early 1300s, paper was commonly used for administrative documents in cities, cloisters and courts, and by the end of the century also for manuscript books, especially the scientific and utilitarian works that typically contain *experimenta* on generation. Ink was readily available for purchase for the first time, though scribes still usually prepared their own. The introduction of cursive scripts made writing much faster, advantageous for scribes whose business lives required them to draft administrative documents, but who also produced books, professionally or for their own practical purposes. Manuscripts containing texts on cookery, husbandry or medicine were often written quickly in a cursive hand, attesting to the 'private, informal, amateurish, utilitarian, urgent' nature of the occasions when such texts were copied and read.[8]

7 Park, 'Managing Childbirth and Fertility'; Peter Murray Jones and Lea T. Olsan, 'Performative rituals for conception and childbirth in England, 900–1500', *Bulletin of the History of Medicine* 89 (2015), 406–33.

8 Daniel Wakelin, 'Writing the words', in Alexandra Gillespie and Wakelin (eds.), *The Production of Books in England, 1350–1500* (Cambridge, 2011), pp. 34–58, on p. 45.

In the late fourteenth century, when writing in the European vernacular languages also began to compete seriously with Latin, translation of practical and household texts increased. Scientific and medical books often mixed Latin and vernacular languages, and employed a linguistic medley even at sentence level. *Experimenta* on generation might come with vernacular rubrics and instructions for use, with Latin ingredients or words of power. The commissioners and owners of these manuscripts had fewer inhibitions than scholars about this linguistic flexibility. We have only fragmentary evidence about these people, drawn from inscriptions in the manuscripts themselves, but it seems that the interested parties were often secular clergy, mendicant friars or gentry householders, for whom *experimenta* reflected not a vocational commitment to learning, but immediate practical concerns.

Treatise and Remedy-Book

From the late middle ages, *experimenta* began to circulate across a variety of texts, initially in manuscript, then also between script and print. The most famous and widely circulated *experimenta* about generation are in the *Trotula*, a group of gynaecological texts derived in part from the writings of a twelfth-century woman, Trota of Salerno, and in part from the works of medical men. The three texts that made up the *Trotula* complex provided guidance on women's diseases and beautification, and one section, *Liber de sinthomatibus mulierum* (Book on the conditions of women), always dealt with conception, pregnancy and childbirth. From around 1400 this section achieved prominence by juxtaposition with more specialized texts on human generation. It was adapted into new forms in Latin and the vernaculars, and retitled to emphasize women's (procreative) 'secrets' rather than their 'diseases'.[9] Many more versions of these texts were produced in the fourteenth and fifteenth centuries, but all derived from the original *Trotula* complex.[10]

A section on 'impediment to conception' in the *Liber de sinthomatibus mulierum* offered a test to determine whether the man or woman was responsible for infertility; then five recipes followed, sometimes for the woman alone, sometimes for the man and woman together. At least one was explicitly for the generation of males.[11] The 'secrets of women' literature repackaged this material, along with other remedies found in the

9 Monica H. Green, 'From "diseases of women" to "secrets of women": The transformation of gynecological literature in the later middle ages', *Journal of Medieval and Early Modern Studies* 30 (2000), 5–39.

10 Monica H. Green, 'A handlist of the Latin and vernacular manuscripts of the so-called *Trotula* texts. Part II: The vernacular texts and Latin re-writings', *Scriptorium* 51 (1997), 80–104, for translations into Dutch (3), English (5), French (7), German (2), Hebrew (1), Irish (1) and Italian (2).

11 *The Trotula: A Medieval Compendium of Women's Medicine*, ed. and trans. Monica H. Green (Philadelphia, PA, 2001), pp. 34, 77.

same text. The remedies closely resemble those in the section 'Concerning impediments to conception' in *De secretis mulierum* (On the secrets of women), a family of texts composed in the late thirteenth or early fourteenth century by a German admirer of the great Dominican philosopher Albertus Magnus and clearly written for men.[12] An early commentator on *De secretis mulierum* claimed that its author was 'learned in certain experiments [*experimentis*] from women'.[13] Having learned women's secrets, he now made these experiments available to men. But later versions of *De secretis mulierum* disparaged women's own knowledge of generation, reflecting more explicit expressions of patriarchal lineage and inheritance, to elevate the authority of male practitioners and place women in the position of patients dependent on their doctors' knowledge.[14] Like the *Trotula*, *De secretis mulierum* was translated into European vernaculars in the late fourteenth and fifteenth centuries. In one unusually well-documented case from the 1460s, Johann Hartlieb, physician to the dukes of Bavaria-Munich, translated parts of both texts into German for his patron.[15]

The fortunes of the *Trotula* and *De secretis mulierum* diverged between 1475 and 1550, when printing produced multiple copies of books and favoured those texts selected for the press. The *Trotula* languished in manuscript, while *De secretis mulierum* survived and spread in print, probably because it addressed male practitioners and thus promised customers for books. Italian, German, French, Dutch and English presses produced some fifty-four editions of *De secretis mulierum* between 1476 and 1500, and it remained popular for another half-century.[16]

These two texts were also the chief sources of the *experimenta* that accompanied the picture of the 'disease woman' in the most influential example of medical printing before 1501, the *Fasciculus medicinae* (Bundle of medical treatises) of 1491.[17] This book, attributed to the physician Johannes de Ketham, but in fact closely modelled on some anonymous late fifteenth-century manuscripts, keyed the *experimenta* to the image by letters which are connected by indication lines to the womb (Fig. 13.1).

The *Fasciculus medicinae* went into nineteen editions before 1567 (and another in 1668), including translations into Italian, Spanish, German, Dutch and French. It was

12 Helen Rodnite Lemay, *Women's Secrets: A Translation of Pseudo-Albertus Magnus's* De secretis mulierum *with Commentaries* (Albany, NY, 1992).

13 Lynn Thorndike, 'Further consideration of the *experimenta*, *Speculum astronomiae*, and *De secretis mulierum* ascribed to Albertus Magnus', *Speculum* 30 (1955), 413–43, on 430.

14 Park, *Secrets of Women*, pp. 91–103.

15 Kristian Bosselmann-Cyran (ed.), *'Secreta mulierum' mit Glosse in der deutschen Bearbeitung von Johann Hartlieb* (Pattensen, 1985); Margaret Schleissner, 'A fifteenth-century physician's attitude towards sexuality: Dr Johann Hartlieb's *Secreta mulierum* translation', in Joyce E. Salisbury (ed.), *Sex in the Middle Ages: A Book of Essays* (New York, NY, 1991), pp. 110–25.

16 Arnold C. Klebs, *Incunabula scientifica et medica* (Hildesheim, 1963), no. 26.

17 Christoph Ferckel, 'Zur Gynäkologie und Generationslehre im Fasciculus medicinae des Johannes de Ketham', *Archiv für Geschichte der Medizin* 6 (1913), 205–22.

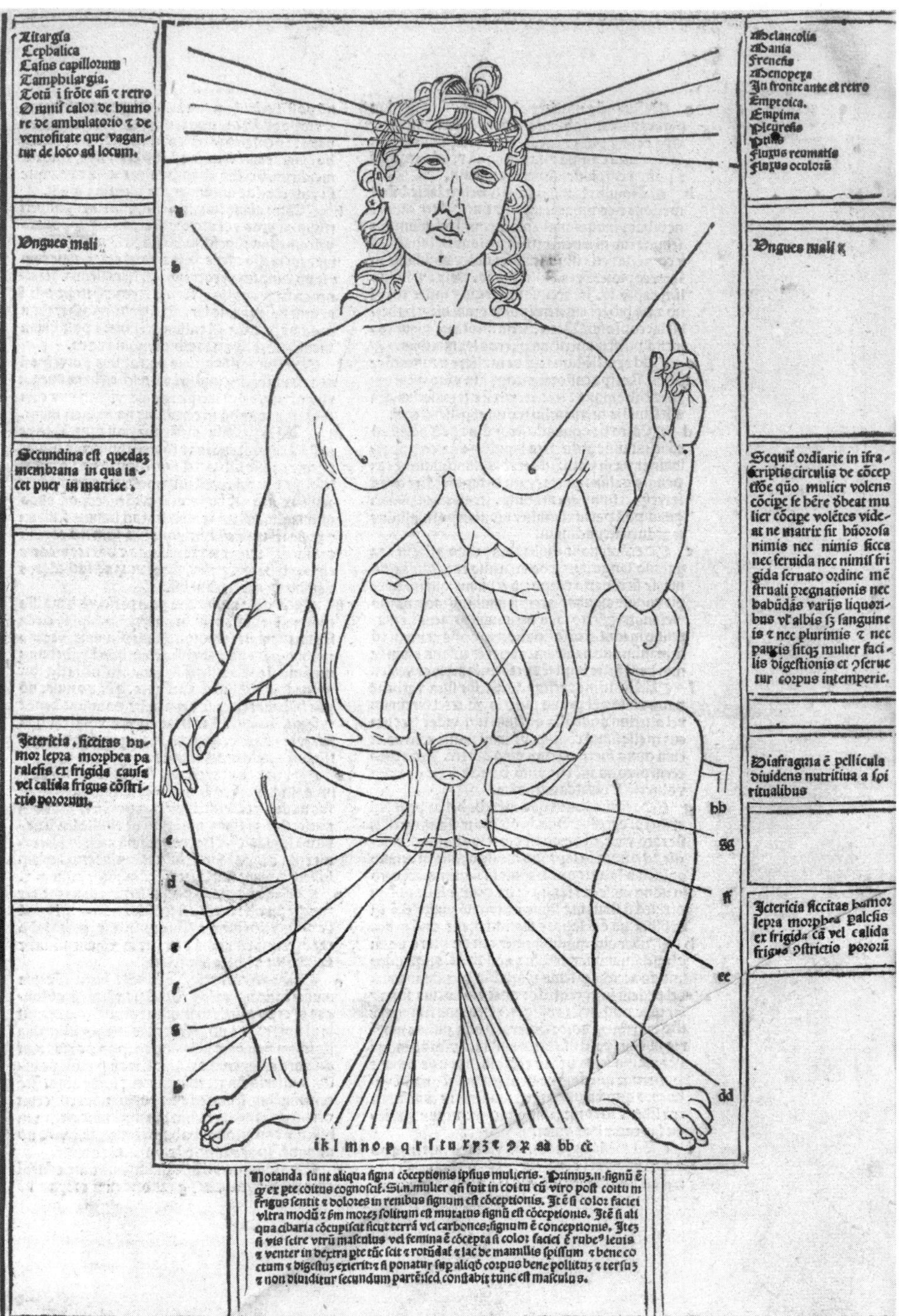

Figure 13.1 Parts of this 'disease woman', a standard mnemonic image in medical compendia, are keyed to *experimenta* borrowed from the *Trotula* and *De secretis mulierum*. For instance, the letter 'o' keys to a treatment for easing childbirth on the following page, noting that 'it is proven'. *Fasciculus medicinae*, attributed to Johannes de Ketham (Venice: de Gregori, 1500), sig. b1r. Cambridge University Library.

recommended to students of medicine by Martin Stainpeis, a stalwart of the University of Vienna, in his *Liber de modo studendi seu legendi in medicina* (Book on the method of studying or reading medicine, 1520), the first reading list for medical students.[18] Together with the pseudo-Aristotelian *Problemata* (Problems), a series of questions and answers on generation, the *experimenta* from the printed *Fasciculus medicinae* then made the transition from print to script as they were copied into manuscripts in Germany, and probably elsewhere.[19] What originated as *experimenta* forming part of longer texts on gynaecology that circulated in scholastic contexts had migrated into short lists of practical information on generation that became popular with householders, medical practitioners and other urban dwellers, as well as medical students.[20]

As part of the explosion of writing in the fourteenth and fifteenth centuries, *experimenta* on generation also circulated in manuscript remedy-books, a newly significant genre of practical medicine. Miscellaneous remedies had been collected for medical practitioners before. The first English 'leechbooks', dating from the ninth through eleventh centuries, preceded those in other vernaculars. But the number of surviving remedy-books from the later middle ages, many combining Latin and vernacular material, shows that these were being compiled and written on a larger scale.[21] While professional scribes, lay or mendicant brothers, were heavily involved in their production, amateur scribes seem to have compiled remedy-books for their own use. The books sometimes contain *experimenta* of all sorts scattered randomly in collections of recipes accumulated over time, and sometimes they give generation a distinct place within an arrangement – for instance, as part of a head-to-toe order of ailments treated.

The compilers' sources are rarely readily identifiable, but they frequently quarried the staple thirteenth-century medical works, such as Gilbertus Anglicus's *Compendium medicinae* (Medical compendium), Peter of Spain's *Thesaurus pauperum* (Treasury of the poor) and Bernard de Gordon's *Lilium medicinae* (Lily of medicine).[22]

As well as compiling remedy-books, scribes copied from each other. In fifteenth-century England, for example, two families of remedy-book texts circulated extensively, one known as the *Liber de diversis medicinis* (Book of diverse medicines), the other as the 'Leechcraft' collection. The first, surviving in sixteen manuscripts, seems to have

18 Christian Coppens, '"For the benefit of ordinary people": The Dutch translation of the *Fasciculus medicinae*, Antwerp 1512', *Quærendo* 39 (2009), 168–205.

19 Britta-Juliane Kruse, *Verborgene Heilkünste. Geschichte der Frauenmedizin im Spätmittelalter* (Berlin, 1996).

20 Margaret Schleissner, 'Sexuality and reproduction in the late medieval "Problemata Aristotelis"', in Josef Domes *et al.* (eds.), *Licht der Natur. Medizin in Fachliteratur und Dichtung. Festschrift für Gundolf Keil zum 60. Geburtstag* (Göppingen, 1994), pp. 383–98; Park, *Secrets of Women*, pp. 77–120, on p. 115.

21 Tony Hunt, *Popular Medicine in Thirteenth-Century England: Introduction and Texts* (Cambridge, 1990) cites many *experimenta* on generation in remedy-books.

22 Britta-Juliane Kruse, *'Die Arznei ist Goldes Wert'. Mittelalterliche Frauenrezepte* (Berlin, 1999) provides a typology of German remedy-books with *experimenta* on generation.

been named by its best-known copyist, Robert Thornton, a gentleman householder from East Newton in the North Riding of Yorkshire.[23] The second, named after one of the titles in the collection, is known in twenty-one manuscripts.[24] Both remedy-book traditions contain *experimenta* on generation consisting of recipes, prognostications and rituals to be performed, and in both, scribe-compilers adapted, added and compressed the remedies and *experimenta*. The same appears true at least of French and German examples.[25] With the rise of print, copying of remedy-books of this type continued but, as we shall see, women began to compile them as well as men; recipes started to outnumber prognostications and prayers or charms; and matters of generation were subsumed under women's health. To understand these changes, we need to consider a novel genre of printed book.

Commodified Secrets

The success in print of the pseudo-Albertus *De secretis mulierum* from 1450 to 1550 made it a forerunner of the new books of secrets. The first such book in Italian, *Opera Nuova intitolata Dificio di ricette* (A new work entitled the house of recipes) of 1527, contained various *experimenta* related to procreation, including one to test for a woman's virginity.[26] The best-known example of the genre, *I Secreti del Reverendo donno Alessio Piemontese* (Secrets of the Reverend Don Alessio Piemontese) by Girolamo Ruscelli, was first published in 1555, amidst a flood of books of secrets. Principally a vernacular genre, the major works were translated between European languages. Alexis of Piedmont, as he was known in England, included artisanal recipes for making all kinds of craft materials, such as dyes and pigments, useful domestic aids, alchemical products and medicinal remedies.[27] Many books advertised products or services that could be bought from the author or his agent. Leonardo Fioravanti's *Capricci medicinali*

23 Susanna Fein and Michael Johnston (eds.), *Robert Thornton and His Books: Essays on the Lincoln and London Thornton Manuscripts* (York, 2014), esp. Julie Orlemanski, 'Thornton's remedies and the practices of medical reading', pp. 235–55.

24 George Keiser, *A Manual of Writings in Middle English, 1050–1500*, vol. 10: *Works of Science and Information* (New Haven, CT, 1998), p. 2840; Keiser, 'Verse introductions to middle English medical treatises', *English Studies* 84 (2003), 301–17; Lea T. Olsan, 'The corpus of charms in the middle English leechcraft remedy books', in Jonathan Roper (ed.), *Charms, Charmers and Charming: International Research on Verbal Magic* (London, 2009), pp. 214–37.

25 Claude de Tovar, 'Contamination, interférences et tentatives de systématisation dans la tradition manuscrite des réceptaires médicaux français: Le réceptaire de Jean Sauvage', *Revue d'histoire des textes* 3 (1973), 115–91 and 4 (1974), 239–88; Kruse, *'Die Arznei'*.

26 *Opera Nuova intitolata Dificio di ricette* (Venice, 1532), [sig. Aiii].

27 William Eamon, *Science and the Secrets of Nature: Books of Secrets in Medieval and Early Modern Culture* (Princeton, NJ, 1994).

(Medical caprices), for instance, advertised remedies for sale at the Bear Pharmacy in Venice.[28] Amongst these secrets, and often mixed up with the other *experimenta*, were those concerned with generation. Information on generation was no longer dependent on a medical context, as it had been through the fourteenth century, but could flourish as easily in books of artisanal recipes and marvels.

The *Italian Books of Secrets Database* contains twelve such books, eight printed between 1532 and 1626 and four manuscript remedy-books from the eighteenth century, chosen because they were compiled in homes, for domestic use, perhaps by women. Of the 3,033 recipes tabulated in total (1,714 from Alessio's four books), forty-four relate directly to fertility, pregnancy and childbirth (twenty-three from Alessio). There are thirty more in the database relating to breasts and lactation, seventeen to menstruation, and twenty-eight to womb disorders. Though these recipes are a small fraction of the total, four features perhaps suggest a decline in the circulation of *experimenta* about generation: there is little repetition of recipes between the different books of secrets and remedy-books sampled; the recipes do not depend closely on the *experimenta* previously circulated in print; no rituals or charms are involved (though the database contains a few of these unrelated to generation); and there are only seven generation recipes in the eighteenth-century manuscripts.[29]

It would be a mistake to rely too closely on the Italian database for general trends. It does not include printed books of secrets marketed as reading for women, which in addition to recipes, chiefly for medical, cookery or cosmetic purposes, contained more sensitive information, carefully framed as suitable for gentlewomen. For instance, a section on 'secret remedies appertaining to women' in some editions of John Partridge's *The Treasurie of Commodious Conceits and Hidden Secrets* published in London between 1573 and 1596 included recipes for encouraging menstruation, limiting bleeding, unblocking the afflictions caused by suffocation of the womb, treating fainting in childbirth and delivering a dead child or placenta. Prognostications of fertility and remedies for barrenness, to speed labour in childbirth and to treat sore lactating breasts were also scattered through the editions.[30]

Learned readers compared and evaluated books of secrets, as is evident in their compilations. Johann Jacob Wecker, the sixteenth-century Swiss physician who had previously translated Alessio from Italian into Latin, assembled *De secretis libri xvii ex variis authoribus collecti* (Seventeen books of secrets collected from various authors).

28 William Eamon, 'How to read a book of secrets', in Elaine Leong and Alisha Rankin (eds.), *Secrets and Knowledge in Medicine and Science, 1500–1800* (Farnham, 2011), pp. 23–46, on pp. 32–4.

29 Tessa Storey, *Italian Books of Secrets Database* (University of Leicester and Wellcome Trust, 2008), http://hdl.handle.net/2381/4335.

30 Allison Kavey, *Books of Secrets: Natural Philosophy in England, 1550–1600* (Urbana, IL, 2007), pp. 110–11.

Book 5 included a section on secrets of generation, some from *De secretis mulierum*, Girolamo Ruscelli's *Secreti nuovi* (New secrets, 1567) and Alessio, alongside others from the philosophical works of the German occult author Heinrich Cornelius Agrippa von Nettesheim, the Italian mathematician, astrologer and physician Girolamo Cardano and the French physician Antoine Mizauld. Wecker's work, with the section on generation intact, was in turn translated into European vernaculars, and acted as a convenient compendium for readers at home.[31]

Many domestic readers annotated their copies or otherwise marked them with underlinings and symbols. Readers also copied sections into personal notebooks or described them in letters to friends and relatives. Fascination with secrets ranged from noblewomen to physicians, courtiers to tooth-drawers.[32] Secrets – occult, natural and generative – passed by word of mouth and by letter as part of an economy of kinship, patronage and gift-exchange.[33] They were also presented to potential patrons by alchemists, like the golden oil that Anna Zieglerin, a minor noble, gave to Duke Julius of Braunschweig-Wolfenbüttel in 1573 in a twenty-page collection of *experimenta*. 'Lion's blood', as she called it, could be used for all kinds of generative activity – to grow summer fruit in winter, create gemstones, cure infertility and nourish infants. She concealed the crucial ingredient, however, thus doing enough to enlist support but stopping the Duke making his own.[34]

Zieglerin walked a tightrope at court to avoid loss of status or accusations of illicit alchemy or witchcraft. Women of lower status ran risks too. In Counter-Reformation Italy, the Inquisition took a hostile interest in women who sold secrets to do with generation or practised rituals that involved Christian liturgical formulae or sacramentals, such as baptismal water, communion wafers and *agnus dei* amulets – wax discs impressed with the figure of a lamb and blessed by the Pope. As the clergy asserted their exclusive right to conduct rituals of the kind found in collections of *experimenta*, these women's ownership of books of secrets was taken as evidence of the practice of magic.[35]

31 Johann Jacob Wecker, *De secretis libri xvii ex variis authoribus collecti* (Basel, 1592), pp. 174–9.

32 'Introduction' to Leong and Rankin, *Secrets and Knowledge*, pp. 1–20.

33 Elaine Leong and Sara Pennell, 'Recipe collections and the currency of medical knowledge in the early modern "medical marketplace"', in Mark Jenner and Patrick Wallis (eds.), *Medicine and the Market in England and Its Colonies,* c. *1450* – c. *1850* (London, 2007), pp. 133–52; Alisha Rankin, 'Becoming an expert practitioner: Court experimentalism and the medical skills of Anna of Saxony (1532–1585)', *Isis* 98 (2007), 23–53.

34 Tara Nummedal, 'Anna Zieglerin's alchemical revelations', in Leong and Rankin, *Secrets and Knowledge*, pp. 125–41.

35 Ottavia Niccoli, *Prophecy and People in Renaissance Italy*, trans. Lydia G. Cochrane (Princeton, NJ, 1990); Silvia De Renzi, 'Secrecy, power and knowledge in early modern Italy', *Studies in History and Philosophy of Science* 27 (1996), 397–407.

Even in Protestant countries, a gulf opened between elites in possession of useful secrets and others whose knowledge was suspected of superstition and witchcraft. Learned authors developed a genre that castigated 'popular errors'; *Erreurs populaires*, by the sixteenth-century French physician Laurent Joubert, was the first and most famous of these books. Although Joubert did not take issue with books of secrets explicitly, in listing and condemning the medical practices of rural folk, midwives and charlatans he targeted the circulation of *experimenta* – recipes, charms and prognostications – through cheap books of secrets and via word of mouth. Ironically, like later works on superstition, Joubert's book was attacked by colleagues who thought that by identifying and listing *experimenta* he was only making the problem worse.[36]

Experimenta in Early Modern Remedy-Books

The extensive circulation of *experimenta* in print did not discourage individuals from writing their own manuscript remedy-books. Rather, owners or borrowers of printed books of secrets dipped into them for promising household remedies, such that manuscript remedy-books frequently cited Alessio and similar authorities. More and more of the many surviving sixteenth- and seventeenth-century manuscript remedy-books were the work of women, while the printed ones were also often issued under aristocratic ladies' names.[37]

Female scribes and authors might have been expected to take a special interest in *experimenta* relating to generation, but in fact these were rarer in manuscript remedy-books than in printed books of secrets. They did not disappear altogether. Lady Johanna St John's mid-seventeenth-century compilation included entries on causing conception, preventing miscarriage and promoting an easy labour (Fig. 13.2).[38] In Lady Ayscough's collection, compiled a few decades later, a liver-cleansing recipe was proven to help a woman, married for four years without a child, to conceive.[39] Women's diseases as a category, and the regulation of the health of the womb in particular, continued to occupy a significant place in remedy-books, but it seems that *experimenta* explicitly to promote generation featured less in the manuscript repertoire. Perhaps the women

36 Natalie Zemon Davis, *Society and Culture in Early Modern France* (Stanford, CA, 1975), pp. 227–67.

37 On manuscripts see, for instance, http://wellcomelibrary.org/collections/digital-collections/recipe-books/; Elaine Leong, *Recipes and Everyday Knowledge: Medicine, Science, and the Household in Early Modern England* (Chicago, IL, 2018); and on print, Elizabeth Grey, Countess of Kent, *A Choice Manual of Rare and Select Secrets in Physick and Chyrurgery* (London, 1653), cited in Mary E. Fissell, 'Introduction: Women, health, and healing in early modern Europe', *Bulletin of the History of Medicine* 82 (2008), 1–17, on 9.

38 Wellcome Library, MS 4338, ff. 213v–14r, cited in Leong, *Treasuries*.

39 Wellcome Library, MS 1026, ff. 104–5, cited in Jennifer Evans, '"Gentle purges corrected with hot spices, whether they work or not, do vehemently provoke venery": Menstrual provocation and procreation in early modern England', *Social History of Medicine* 25 (2012), 2–19, on 11–12.

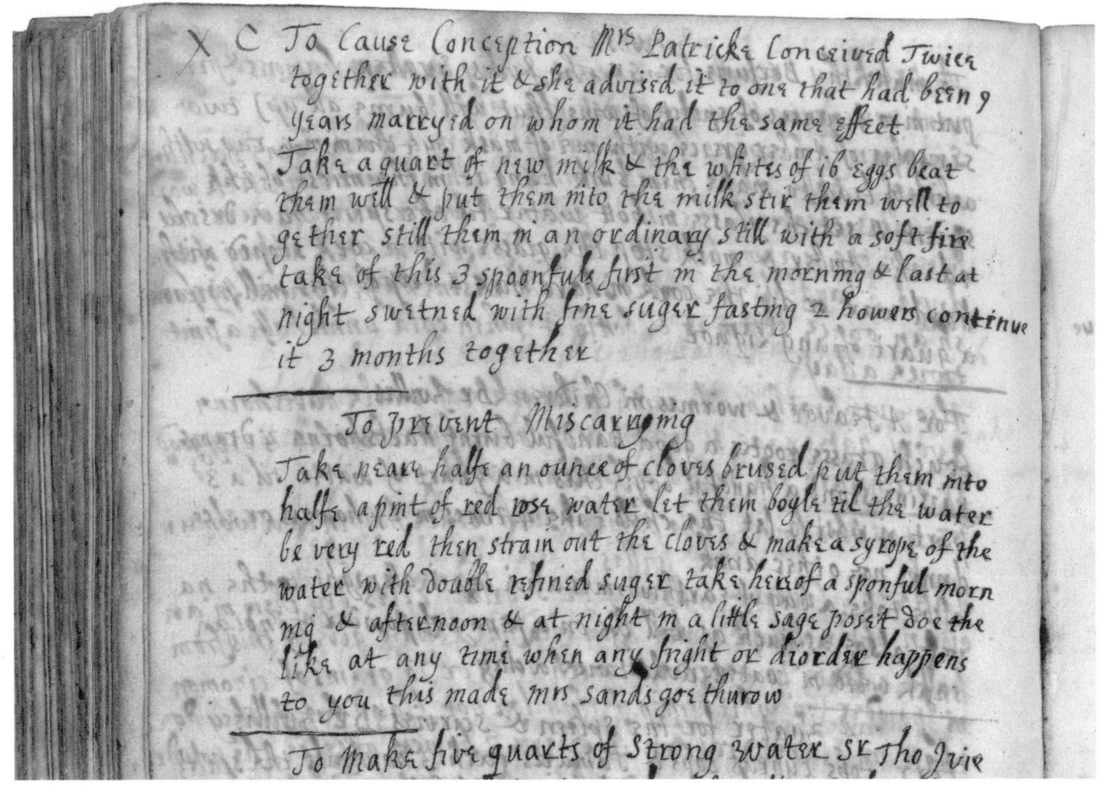
X C To Cause Conception Mrs Patricke Conceived Twice
together with it & she advised it to one that had been 9
years marryed on whom it had the same effect
Take a quart of new milk & the whites of 16 eggs beat
them well & put them into the milk stir them well to
gether still them in an ordinary still with a soft fire
take of this 3 spoonfuls first in the morning & last at
night sweetned with fine suger fasting 2 howers continue
it 3 months together

To prevent Miscarrying
Take neare halfe an ounce of cloves brused put them into
halfe a pint of red rose water let them boyle til the water
be very red then strain out the cloves & make a syrope of the
water with double refined suger take hereof a sponful morn
ing & afternoon & at night in a little sage possett doe the
like at any time when any fright or disorder happens
to you this made mrs Sands goe thurow

To make five quarts of Strong water Sr Tho Ivie

Figure 13.2 A page from Lady Johanna St John's remedy-book, recording proven *experimenta* to promote fertility under 'W', for 'woman'. The first recipe, 'To cause conception', states that 'Mrs Patrick Conceived Twice together with it'. 'X' and 'C' are marked in the margin, probably indicating that it was evaluated or copied into another book. Wellcome Library, London, MS 4338, f. 213v.

who compiled remedy-books found remedies to promote pregnancy indecorous, uninteresting or otherwise dubious.[40]

Whatever the reasons, other inhibitions limited the kinds of generation-related *experimenta* included in manuscript remedy-books. As with the Italian books of secrets, two of the three types of *experimenta* about generation – prayers or charms, and prognostications – disappeared from view in these manuscripts. They suffered the additional penalty of falling foul of the Protestant rejection of the mediation of the Virgin and the saints in childbirth, and of any procedure that smacked of divination or witchcraft.[41] There seem to have been equivalent inhibitions in Catholic Europe after the Council of Trent.

40 Park, 'Managing Childbirth and Fertility'; Kassell, 'Fruitful Bodies'.

41 Lea T. Olsan, 'A Medieval Birth Girdle', Exhibit 11; Sandra Cavallo, 'Pregnant Stones as Wonders of Nature', Exhibit 17, this book.

Despite these worries, the career of printed *experimenta* on generation stretched beyond sixteenth- and seventeenth-century books of secrets. The book by Lemnius with which this chapter began, with its instructions for drinking herbs to produce boys or girls, was widely translated. The English version became the source for the *experimenta* on generation in *Aristotle's Masterpiece*, the sex and midwifery manual that was first printed in London in 1684 and still published in England and the United States in the 1930s.[42]

Conclusion

Experimenta on generation remained popular with producers and consumers of script and print from the fourteenth to the seventeenth centuries through the explosion of writing and translation in the late fourteenth and fifteenth centuries, and the more celebrated coming of print. But the popularity of the different types of *experimenta* changed over time. The advent of a commercial market in printed books of secrets bought mainly by men included *experimenta* in the form of prayers and charms, prognostications and recipes to address matters of generation from conception to nurturing children. As women increasingly wrote remedy-books, by contrast, *experimenta* for generation tended to be cast in terms of women's health more often than the promotion of fertility.

These conclusions are initial impressions drawn from a broad survey of manuscript and printed *experimenta*. Across the period, these bundles of practical techniques were shared by an expanding array of audiences at a crossroads between scholarly, commercial and domestic knowledge of generation. We cannot know whether they became more useful for producing boys and girls, but we do know that a form of knowledge that originated in medieval scholarly writings was transmitted by men and women through the seventeenth century. Whether deemed marvellous, superstitious or wise, they even persisted through the technological innovations of the modern age.

42 Mary E. Fissell, 'Making a masterpiece: The Aristotle texts in vernacular medical culture', in Charles E. Rosenberg (ed.), *Right Living: An Anglo-American Tradition of Self-Help Medicine and Hygiene* (Baltimore, MD, 2003), pp. 59–87; Fissell, '*Aristotle's Masterpiece*', Exhibit 25, this book.

14 Innate Heat, Radical Moisture and Generation

Gianna Pomata

When European literati encountered Chinese medicine in the seventeenth century, they thought they saw a striking commonality in the understanding of vital principles. 'The Chinese, like the Europeans, recognize that human life consists of radical moisture and innate heat', wrote the Jesuit Michael Boym, who in the 1650s conceived a plan to introduce Chinese medical knowledge to Europe.[1] Boym translated the Chinese terms '*yang*' and '*yin*' as '*calidum innatum*' (innate heat) and '*humidum radicale*' (radical moisture), two concepts that had been central to western philosophical and medical traditions since Greek antiquity. Before the early modern period, European philosophers and physicians used 'innate heat' and 'radical moisture' to explain fundamental aspects of life such as ageing, dying, disease, sex difference and generation.[2] This chapter sketches the long-term history of these two fundamental epistemic categories, focusing on their role in the philosophical and medical understanding of generation.

The Primacy of Innate Heat in Ancient Greek Medicine

The conceptualization of heat and moisture as vital principles goes back to the Presocratic philosophers and Hippocratic physicians of the fifth and fourth centuries BC. Hippocratic authors, in particular, made use of paired qualities such as hot and cold, wet and dry, which they saw as materialized in substances such as earth, air, fire and water, blood, phlegm and bile.[3] These paired qualities were also central to their understanding of generation and sexual difference.[4]

The author of the Hippocratic treatise *On Generation/Nature of the Child* described how the movement, pleasure and heat of sexual intercourse produced the seed 'from all of the body, from the hard and the soft parts, and from all its fluid'.[5] In a

1 Michael Boym, *Clavis medica ad Chinarum doctrinam de pulsibus* (Nuremberg, 1686), p. 30. Translations are mine unless otherwise indicated.

2 Classic studies include Everett Mendelsohn, *Heat and Life: The Development of the Theory of Animal Heat* (Cambridge, MA, 1964); Thomas S. Hall, 'Life, death and the radical moisture: A study of thematic pattern in medieval medical theory', *Clio medica* 6 (1971), 3–23.

3 G. E. R. Lloyd, *Polarity and Analogy: Two Types of Argumentation in Early Greek Thought* (Cambridge, 1966), pp. 15–85.

4 Helen King, 'Women and Doctors in Ancient Greece', Chapter 3, this book.

5 *On Generation/Nature of the Child* 3 (compare 1).

process of agitation, liquefaction and frothing, seed was gathered in the spinal marrow, and then transported to the penis and vagina.[6] Both men and women produced seed in this way. While female seed was said to be weak and watery in comparison with its thicker, stronger male counterpart, there was no suggestion that liquidity and weakness were characteristic of women themselves; the heat of the womb, for example, was crucial for fetal formation.[7] By contrast, in the Hippocratic treatise *Regimen*, female and male were aligned with water and fire, respectively: in matters of generation, in composition and in behaviour, the female tended to the wet and cold and the male to the hot and dry.[8] Yet the author of *Diseases of Women 1* described women as hotter and wetter than men because, with soft and spongy flesh, women had more and warmer blood.[9] Hippocratic ideas about heat and moisture did not translate into a hierarchical ranking of the sexes based on their different degrees of heat.

Later in the fourth century BC, Aristotle developed the loose notion of innate heat into a key physiological principle within a coherent philosophical system. He recognized that heat and moisture were associated, but did not give humidity the same theoretical prominence as heat, which he saw as the driving force of many bodily functions and the chief instrument of the soul.[10] In particular, innate heat had a conspicuous role in generation, and in the sexual differentiation required for generation.[11]

Moreover, for Aristotle, innate heat drove the transformation of food into blood, and the further coction of blood into seed. The action of heat on blood engendered *pneuma* – warm air – within it. This contained something hot and 'analogous to the substance of the stars', a kind of 'soul-heat' which was the active principle of generation.[12] Whereas perfected male seed was so endowed, the unfinished, 'impure' female seed or *katamenia* (menstrual fluid) lacked this crucial component.[13] Since coction was driven by heat, the female inability to complete the process of seminal refinement demonstrated that male animals were hotter than females.[14] All of the relevant parts were potentially present in the menstrual fluid, but had to be actualized by the male. The male seed shaped and ensouled the embryo, but did not contribute materially to its body.[15]

What appeared at first to be a quantitative distinction between male and female contributions to generation, with the female seed lagging behind the male in heat and

6 Ibid., 1 and 4. 7 Ibid., 6–7, 18 and 31, 12. 8 *Regimen* 1.27 and 34.

9 *Diseases of Women 1* 1. 10 *Meteorologica* 379b35.

11 Sophia M. Connell, *Aristotle on Female Animals: A Study of the* Generation of Animals (Cambridge, 2015); Robert Mayhew, *The Female in Aristotle's Biology: Reason or Rationalization* (Chicago, IL, 2004); Laurence M. V. Totelin, 'Animal and Plant Generation in Classical Antiquity', Chapter 4, this book.

12 *Generation of Animals* (*GA*) 726a20, 736a1–2, 736b33–8 and 742a15.

13 *GA* 728a26–7, 737a27–30.

14 *GA* 765b9–18; see also Gabriella Zuccolin, 'The Hermaphroditic Hyena', Exhibit 9, this book.

15 *GA* 738b20–8, 741b2–9.

perfection, turned into a radical division. The female was supposed to provide the material, the male the 'form' or 'soul' which fashioned that material into a new being. This was in accordance with the Aristotelian principle that was termed 'hylomorphism' in the nineteenth century: all things were seen as indissoluble compounds of matter and form (in Greek, *hylê* and *morphê*). The male provided no matter, the female no form, and yet both provided heat, which differed in quality and quantity between the sexes.

Five centuries later, in the decades after 150 AD, the great physician Galen formulated his own influential theory of generation. Much has been written about the differences between Aristotelian and Galenic views of procreation, but here their shared assumptions matter more. Both held that the innate heat was fundamental to the making of blood from food and seed from blood, and that males were hotter and therefore more perfect than females. For Galen, however, female seed existed in its own right, though it was colder and more watery than male seed. He further believed that both male and female seed contributed form as well as matter to offspring.[16]

Both Aristotle and Galen associated the substance of the innate heat with the original moisture present in the male semen and the menstrual blood (for Galen, also in the female semen). But although they discussed such 'primigenial' moisture in connection with the issue of ageing,[17] they did not attribute much significance to it in relation to generation. The ancients never granted humidity the kind of theoretical prominence they gave heat. Why was the primacy of the innate heat so deeply entrenched in the ancient understanding of generation? Part of the answer is that the theory served an important social function by explaining and justifying gender hierarchy. Since the female was generally considered colder but moister than the male, humidity could hardly serve the purpose of explaining women's physiological and procreative inferiority, which was an undiscussed premise of philosophical and medical discourse.

The Radical Moisture in Medieval Medicine

Innate heat and radical moisture were reconceptualized in medieval Islamic cultures, when scholars translated the Aristotelian and Galenic texts from Greek into Arabic. As medieval Arabic scholars reformulated Galenic medicine, they turned the concept of radical moisture into an epistemic category comparable in significance to the innate heat.[18] Beginning in the ninth and tenth centuries, this process culminated in the

16 Rebecca Flemming, 'Galen's Generations of Seeds', Chapter 7, this book.

17 Aristotle, *On Youth and Old Age* 469b21–470a19; Galen, *De marasmo* (7 666–704 Kühn).

18 Plinio Prioreschi, *A History of Medicine*, vol. 4: *Byzantine and Islamic Medicine* (Omaha, NE, 2001), pp. 413–22; Philip L. Reynolds, *Food and the Body: Some Peculiar Questions in High Medieval Theology* (Leiden, 1999), pp. 105–19. For Arabic scholarship, see Nahyan Fancy, 'Generation in Medieval Islamic Medicine', Chapter 9, this book.

innovative account of moisture as a vital principle formulated by Avicenna. In his *Canon of Medicine*, he ranked radical moisture with innate heat as a constitutive element of life.[19]

Avicenna rearticulated the Galenic theory of nutrition by stressing the role of moisture. Food was processed into blood and passed through a series of transformations, each producing a specific kind of moisture. Alongside the four primary humours (blood, phlegm, yellow bile and black bile), Avicenna theorized four 'secondary moistures', which he believed were formed in successive stages of the assimilation of food.[20] The fourth of these moistures, however, he saw as derived from semen, and present in the body from the very moment of generation.[21] This fourth humour Avicenna identified as the 'radical moisture' which played a fundamental role in the origin and sustenance of life. He thought that the innate heat could not perform its vivifying function without being nourished by radical moisture, which was indispensable to the innate heat in the same way as fuel is necessary to the flame.[22] He also established a link between radical moisture and his theory of generation by asserting that at the beginning of each new life the radical moisture originated from the seeds of both parents.

Avicenna saw the discrepancies between the Aristotelian and Galenic theories of generation, and used the concept of radical moisture to harmonize them.[23] While accepting Galen's views on the existence of the female semen, Avicenna reinterpreted its function to make it more compatible with Aristotle's hylomorphism. He reaffirmed the Aristotelian view of generation by arguing that the male semen gave form to the embryo, while the female semen and the *menstruum* jointly provided the matter.[24] Along similarly Aristotelian lines, he argued that the female semen was a different substance from the male semen, and should not properly be called 'semen'. And yet, at the same time, in sharp contrast to Aristotle, he insisted on the materiality of semen (male and female) by presenting it as the origin of the radical moisture, which, like the innate heat, he saw as

19 Hall, 'Life', 4–5; Michael McVaugh, 'The "humidum radicale" in thirteenth-century medicine', *Traditio* 30 (1974), 259–83.

20 Avicenna, *Liber Canonis* (facsimile of 1507 Venice edition, Hildesheim, 1964), Lib. 1, fen 1, cap. 1: 'De humoribus', f. 4v.

21 Ibid., Lib. 3, fen 19, cap. 3, f. 351rb.

22 Peter H. Niebyl, 'Old age, fever, and the lamp metaphor', *Journal of the History of Medicine and Allied Sciences* 26 (1971), 351–68.

23 Ursula Weisser, 'Die Harmonisierung antiker Zeugungstheorien im islamischen Kulturkreis und ihr Nachwirken im europäischen Mittelalter', in Albert Zimmermann and Ingrid Craemer-Ruegenberg (eds.), *Orientalische Kultur und europäisches Mittelalter* (Berlin, 1985), pp. 301–26. See also Fancy, 'Generation in Medieval Islamic Medicine'.

24 *Liber Canonis*, Lib. 1, fen 3, doct. 3, ff. 52va–53vb; Michele Nardi, *Problemi d'embriologia umana antica e medioevale* (Florence, 1938), pp. 38, 55, 66 and 76.

the vital core of the new being. Attributing new significance to the materiality of both parents' seed, Avicenna shifted the balance between matter and spirit in generation.[25]

Avicenna saw each person's original endowment of radical moisture as a marker of individuality. At birth, he argued, each person was allotted a specific and fixed amount of radical moisture which determined the upper limit of his or her lifespan. With age, the radical moisture dried out: food provided 'nutrimental humidity', but in insufficient quantities to forestall the exhaustion of the moisture and, ultimately, death.[26] Avicenna's ideas about radical moisture provided not only a reconceptualization of generation, but also a medical theory with which to understand each person's physical individuality and unique, divinely allotted lifespan – a theory that had religious implications.

Avicenna's views became very influential in Europe after his *Canon* was translated into Latin at the end of the twelfth century.[27] His theory of radical moisture, in particular, enjoyed enormous fortune, acquiring great significance especially in theology and alchemy.[28] The physician Arnald of Villanova, active in Montpellier in the last decades of the thirteenth century, devoted the first full Latin treatise to the topic.[29] Christian theologians used the concept to define the 'truth of human nature' (*veritas naturae humanae*), that is, the imperishable core of each person's corporeal identity that would be reconstituted at the resurrection.[30] Radical moisture was seen as the enduring material element of the body, distinct from its transient components that grow and decay. In the Garden of Eden, it was argued, the inevitable drying out of the moisture was counterbalanced by feeding from the tree of life, which constantly replenished it (Fig. 14.1).[31] Therefore Adam and Eve in Eden knew neither disease nor death. After the Fall, by contrast, death is inevitable: the individual can only live, in the best scenario, the number of years corresponding to his or her innate endowment of radical moisture.

But could the consumption of the radical moisture be minimized by proper medical care? Could a humidifying regimen or remedies retard the drying out of the moisture and postpone death? While theologians discussed the radical moisture in relation to identity and resurrection, physicians and alchemists saw it as the key to prolonging

25 Weisser, 'Harmonisierung', p. 323.
26 *Liber Canonis*, Lib. 1, fen 3, doct. 3, f. 53r.
27 Michael Stolberg, 'Die Lehre vom "calor innatus" im lateinischen Canon medicinae des Avicenna', *Sudhoffs Archiv* 77 (1993), 33–53.
28 McVaugh, 'Humidum radicale', 267–8.
29 Arnald of Villanova, *Tractatus de humido radicali* in *Opera Medica Omnia*, vol. 5.2, ed. Michael McVaugh (Barcelona, 2010); see Chiara Crisciani and Giovanna Ferrari's 'Introduzione' to this volume, pp. 319–571, for a thorough review of the intellectual history of radical moisture in the late middle ages.
30 Walter H. Principe, '"De veritate humanae naturae": Theology in conversation with biology, medicine, and philosophy of nature', in Reijo Työrinoja, Anja Inkeri Lehtinen and Dagfinn Føllesdal (eds.), *Knowledge and the Sciences in Medieval Philosophy* (Helsinki, 1990), vol. 3, pp. 486–94.
31 Crisciani and Ferrari, 'Introduzione', pp. 346–59; Joseph Ziegler, 'Medicine and immortality in terrestrial paradise', in Peter Biller and Ziegler (eds.), *Religion and Medicine in the Middle Ages* (Woodbridge, 2001), pp. 201–42.

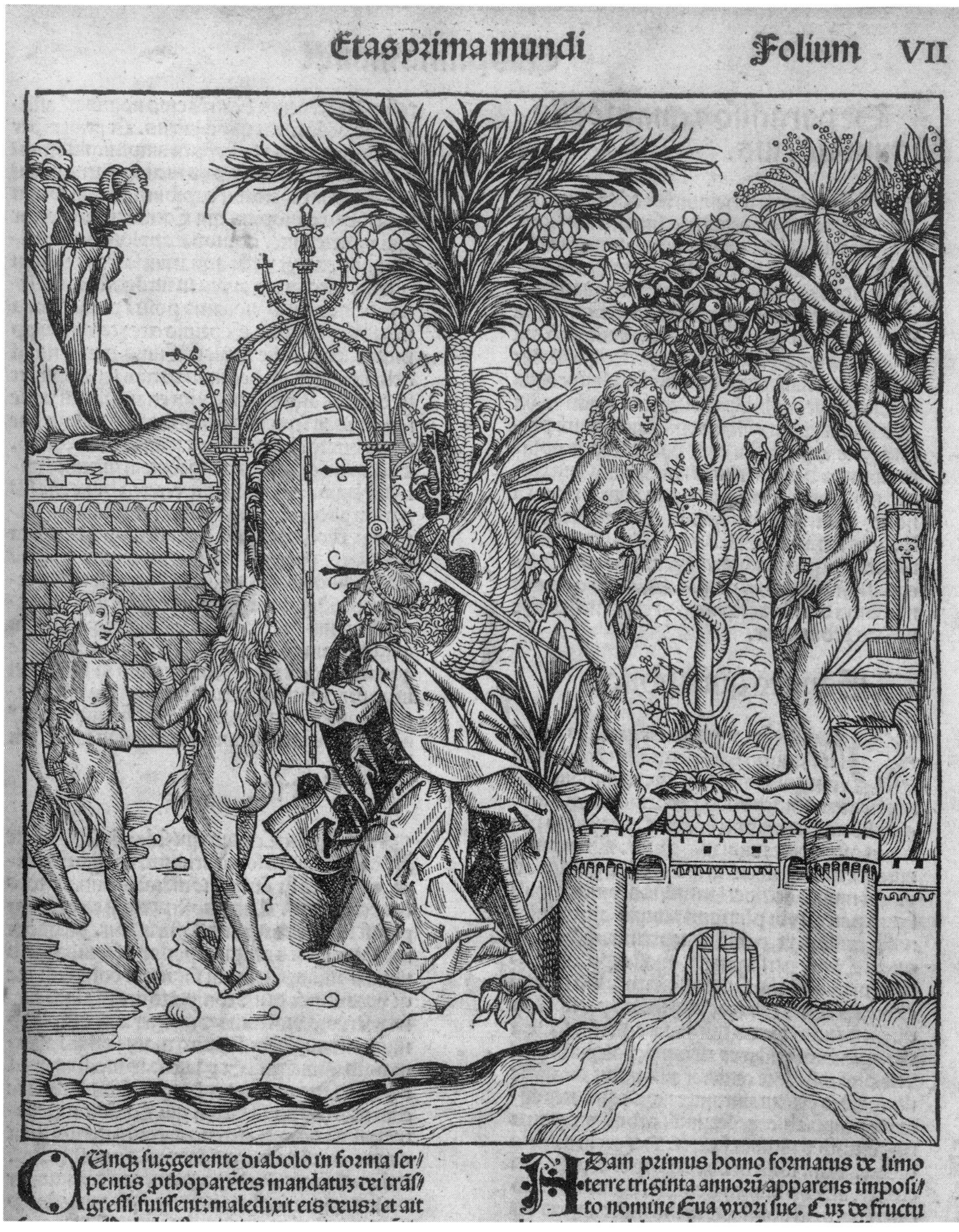
Etas prima mundi
Folium VII
Adam primus homo formatus de limo
terre triginta annorũ apparens imposi/
to nomine Eua vxori sue. Cuz de fructu

Figure 14.1 This woodcut from the Nuremberg Chronicle depicts the tree of life as a dragon-tree (far right), clearly separate from the tree of knowledge and associated with the fountain of life. The text notes that the angel was placed at the gate 'to bar the way to the wood of life'. Hartmann Schedel, *Liber Chronicarum* (Nuremberg: Anton Koberger, 1493), f. 7r. Wellcome Library, London.

life. Most academic physicians recognized that a special regimen and medications could be used to retain the moisture, but were cautious about the possibility of restoring it. Alchemists, by contrast, enthusiastically pursued the goal of prolonging life by means of alchemical preparations, as did Raymond Lull and Roger Bacon.[32] In fourteenth-century alchemy, most interestingly, radical moisture took on a very different meaning from the one it had in theological and philosophical contexts. Theologians understood it as each individual's stable material core, in life and the afterlife. The alchemical notion of radical moisture instead dealt not with issues of stability, continuity and identity but rather with the dynamic transformations of matter, often expressed in terms of generation (Fig. 14.2). In the alchemical texts, radical moisture was seen as a concrete substance that the alchemist could isolate and manipulate – a dynamic aspect of matter that could be captured and used for human purposes. Moisture was still identified with matter, like heat with the spiritual principle of form, but matter was no longer seen as passive and inert; it had become central to a growing interest in natural processes of transformation and change.[33]

How did the debate on radical moisture affect the late medieval theory of generation? Through the teaching of Avicenna's *Canon*, the category of radical moisture was integrated into scholastic medicine in the thirteenth century, at the same time as Aristotle's works on animals were rediscovered and his theories of generation revived. Debates about generation had previously relied on the Galenic theory of two seeds.[34] By contrast, thirteenth-century scholastics drew on the newly accessible Aristotelian works to deny the existence of the female semen as an active principle of generation. Most thirteenth- and fourteenth-century scholastic doctors followed this Aristotelian theory.[35] Yet many of them adopted not the original Aristotelian theory of generation, but Avicenna's subtly modified version. In contrast to Aristotle, who had denied any significance to the material component of the male semen, most representatives of scholastic medicine held that the male semen contributed materially to the formation of the embryo.[36]

Why? The reason is possibly the new significance attributed to the radical moisture as the core of each person's identity. The radical moisture was supposed to be derived from

32 Charles Lohr, 'The Arabic background to Ramon Lull's *Liber Chaos*, ca. 1285', *Traditio* 55 (2000), 159–70; Crisciani and Ferrari, 'Introduzione', pp. 531–5, 580.

33 Crisciani and Ferrari, 'Introduzione', pp. 511, 547, 553. For later developments: Gad Freudenthal, *Aristotle's Theory of Material Substance: Heat and Pneuma, Form and Soul* (London, 1999), pp. 160–91.

34 Joan Cadden, *Meanings of Sex Difference in the Middle Ages: Medicine, Science, and Culture* (Cambridge, 1993), pp. 58–9; Maaike van der Lugt, *Le ver, le démon et la vierge: Les théories médiévales de la génération extraordinaire* (Paris, 2004), pp. 50–3.

35 Cadden, *Meanings*, pp. 58–9; Romana Martorelli Vico, *Medicina e filosofia: Per una storia dell'embriologia medievale nel XIII e XIV secolo* (Naples, 2002), pp. 36–121.

36 Nardi, *Problemi d'embriologia*, p. 58; Maaike van der Lugt, 'Formed Fetuses and Healthy Children in Scholastic Theology, Medicine and Law', Chapter 12; for later arguments: Florence Vienne, 'Eggs and Sperm as Germ Cells', Chapter 28, this book.

ROSARIVM

CONIVNCTIO SIVE
Coitus.

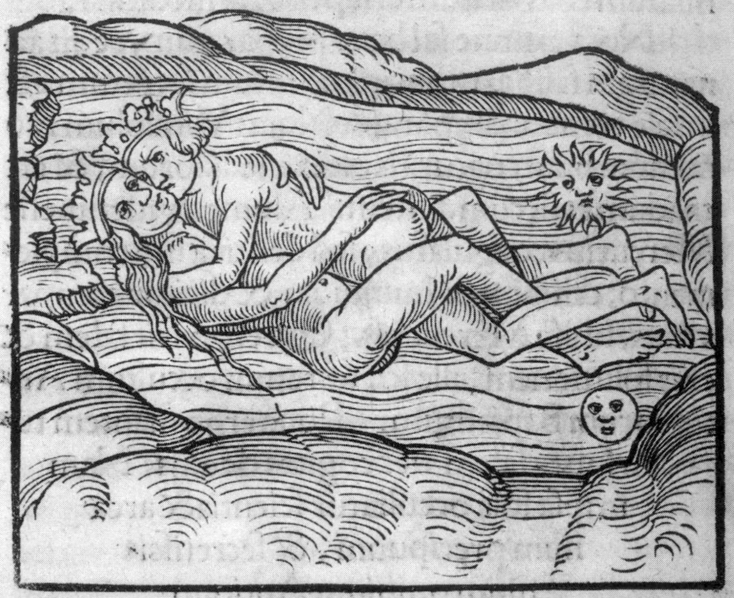

O Luna durch meyn vmbgeben/vnd ſuſſe mynne/
Wirſtu ſchön/ſtarck/vnd gewaltig als ich byn.
O Sol/du biſt vber alle liecht zu erkennen/
So bedarffſtu doch mein als der han der hennen.

ARISLEVS IN VISIONE.

Coniunge ergo filium tuum Gabricum dilectiorem tibi in omnibus filijs tuis cum ſua ſorore Beya

Figure 14.2 Woodcut of a copulating couple as emblem of the alchemical conjunction of gold and silver. In a tradition dating from the middle ages, copulation, generation and death served as allegories for the material transformations necessary to make the philosophers' stone, which could prolong life and turn base metals into gold. *Coniunctio sive coitus* from the *Rosarium philosophorum*, printed in *De alchimia opuscula* (Frankfurt: Cyriacus Jacobus, 1550), sig. F3v. Wellcome Library, London.

the spermatic fluid, that is, the material component of both the father and the mother's semen.[37] While innate heat was seen as wholly spiritual, radical moisture was understood as matter.[38] With respect to the male generative agency, the category of radical moisture was therefore difficult to reconcile with the Aristotelian hylomorphic view of generation, whose cardinal assumption was that the father did not transmit anything material to the embryo. So the scholastics corrected the spiritualist interpretation of the male contribution to generation by adding a material role for the male semen in forming the embryo. The emphasis on radical moisture seems to have led to a new appreciation of the matter of paternal semen.

By the fifteenth century, the radical moisture, as an epistemic category, had mitigated the stark hylomorphism of the Aristotelian view of generation in two ways: by fostering a stronger interest in the material aspect of generation; and by leading to a new emphasis on matter as active – a notion that thrived in the fertile soil of alchemical medicine.

Towards a New Theory of Generation

A novelty of the sixteenth century was the revival of the Galenic two-seed theory. Polarized into Galenist and Aristotelian factions, Renaissance physicians and philosophers battled over theories of generation, hotly debating, in particular, the role of women and the female semen.[39] The Galenist position, which stressed woman's active role, seems to have prevailed. Remarkably, this Galenist victory led to a strong challenge to the Aristotelian view of woman as imperfect male. Though it was still a commonplace that women have a lower degree of innate heat, this was no longer seen as the cause of their inferiority.[40] In the second half of the sixteenth century, the neo-Hippocratic literature on women's diseases combined a two-seed account of generation with the view that men and women were equally perfect in their sex. A neo-Hippocratic or Galenist position on issues of generation often went hand in hand with proto-feminist views – a trend that Ian Maclean described years ago, and that recent research has confirmed.[41]

37 Reynolds, *Food and the Body*, p. 115.

38 Crisciani and Ferrari, 'Introduzione', p. 488.

39 Jacques Roger, *Les sciences de la vie dans la pensée française du XVIIIe siècle: La génération des animaux de Descartes à l'*Encyclopédie, 2nd edn (Paris, 1971), pp. 53–94.

40 Ian Maclean, *The Renaissance Notion of Woman: A Study in the Fortunes of Scholasticism and Medical Science in European Intellectual Life* (Cambridge, 1980), pp. 28–46; Martorelli Vico, *Medicina e filosofia*, pp. 149–95.

41 Maclean, *Renaissance Notion of Woman*, pp. 28–46; Gianna Pomata, 'Was there a *Querelle des femmes* in early modern medicine?', *Arenal* 20 (2013), 313–41; *Pregnancy and Birth in Early Modern France: Treatises by Caring Physicians and Surgeons (1581–1625)*, ed. and trans. Valerie Worth-Stylianou (Toronto, 2013).

If the Galenists seem to have prevailed on the issue of the female semen, the Aristotelians remained strong on the nature of male semen. Was the male semen a purely spiritual substance, it was asked, or does it also act materially, contributing to form the body of the embryo, as do the female semen and the menstrual blood? Despite the ascendancy of the Galenist theory of generation, the 'immaterial' view of male semen, derived from Aristotle, remained widespread in the Renaissance. Nor was it limited to conservative Aristotelians: we find it also in innovative Aristotelians like the anatomists Girolamo Fabrici d'Acquapendente and his pupil William Harvey, the Paracelsian medical reformer Johann Baptist van Helmont, and even those, like Jean Fernel, who affirmed the existence of the female semen.[42]

In contrast with the middle ages, the object of interest among Renaissance physicians shifted once again to the innate heat, at least to judge by the number of works listed under the entries '*calidum innatum*' and '*humidum radicale*' in medical bibliographies.[43] Aristotelian authors were especially inclined to write on the innate heat, sometimes contextually defending the Aristotelian theory of generation against the rival Galenic theory.[44] A survey of medical theses discussed in the sixteenth century also suggests that the primacy of the innate heat was rarely questioned within academic circles.[45]

If this is what we see when we look at academic medicine, a different intellectual landscape emerges when we consider Renaissance alchemy and alchemical medicine. Here the category of moisture remained fundamental to the understanding of natural processes. As a vital principle, moisture was now conceptualized as an oily (not watery) substance, referred to as 'unctuous moisture'. This was seen as the material substrate of heat and spirits, and the principle of material cohesion, in opposition to the Aristotelian view, according to which the soul and innate heat held matter together.[46] Alchemists continued to pursue means for prolonging life, and Paracelsian physicians believed that secret alchemical remedies could achieve this purpose.[47]

At the same time, we can notice the dawning of a new dissatisfaction, if not outright scepticism, about the meaning and value of innate heat and radical moisture. This scepticism would grow considerably in the early seventeenth century, when the two

42 Roger, *Sciences de la vie*, pp. 56, 62–7, 98–103; Gianna Pomata, 'Vollkommen oder verdorben? Der männliche Samen im frühneuzeitlichen Europa', *L'Homme: Zeitschrift für feministische Geschichtswissenschaft* 6, no. 2 (1995), 59–85, esp. 76–81.

43 Martinus Lipenius, *Bibliotheca Realis Medica* (Frankfurt, 1673). Lipenius listed only five texts (two of them medieval) under the entry '*humidum radicale*', and eighteen texts, all from the sixteenth and seventeenth centuries, under '*calidum innatum*'.

44 Cesare Cremonini, *De calido innato et semine pro Aristotele adversus Galenum* (Leiden, 1634). The debate on innate heat was described by Caspar Hofmann, *Syntagma de calido innato et de spiritibus* (Jena, 1686).

45 Roger, *Sciences de la vie*, pp. 56–103.

46 Gad Freudenthal, 'The problem of cohesion between alchemy and natural philosophy: From unctuous moisture to phlogiston', in Z. R. W. M. von Martels (ed.), *Alchemy Revisited* (Leiden, 1990), pp. 107–16.

47 Niebyl, 'Old age', 361–3.

categories were criticized as obsolete and rejected as a symbol of the vacuity of scholastic learning.[48] In his 1623 work on the prolongation of life, Francis Bacon noted: 'These things which the vulgar physicians talk of [namely] radical moisture and natural heat, are but mere fictions'.[49] The alchemical reformer and physician J. B. van Helmont deplored 'the confused traditional notion of [radical] moisture', and attributed ageing and death to the decline of spiritual entities, not the drying of the body.[50] Dissatisfaction with the categories of innate heat and radical moisture did not necessarily lead to their rejection, but sometimes to attempts to rethink them within a new philosophical framework. So for instance Pierre Gassendi, in his 1649 work on Epicureanism, redefined radical moisture and innate heat in corpuscular and mechanical terms.[51]

How did the rethinking of innate heat and radical moisture affect the early modern theory of generation? In the late Renaissance, we see for the first time a challenge to the core idea shared by Aristotelians and Galenists – the derivation of semen from blood. The revival of Hippocratic medicine that took place in this period involved a return of the Hippocratic theory of semen, later called 'pangenesis' and often revised from an atomistic perspective.[52] Most interestingly, a new theory, echoing pre-Aristotelian ideas, argued that semen derived from a hypothetical fluid in the nerves, the '*succus nerveus*' (nervous juice).[53] One of the first formulations of this theory came from an iconoclastic book published in Spain in 1587 under a woman's name, Oliva Sabuco.[54] Sabuco rejected the Aristotelian and Galenic theories of nutrition and generation. She argued that it was not the blood that nourished the body, but a 'white juice' secreted by the brain and distributed through the nerves. Blood, milk, and male and female semen all originated from this 'white juice', the agent not only of nutrition and growth, but also of generation. She stated that the white juice was equivalent to the 'four humidities discovered by Avicenna', but fundamentally reconceptualized Avicenna's theory, arguing that moisture, not heat, was the more fundamental vital principle.[55] After Sabuco, in the seventeenth century the view that semen derived from the 'nervous juice' was championed by a group of English physicians and disciples of William Harvey, which

48 Hofmann, *De calido innato*, p. 49.

49 Francis Bacon, *History Naturall and Experimentall, of Life and Death, or, Of the Prolongation of Life*, in *The Works of Francis Bacon, Lord Chancellor of England*, ed. Basil Montagu (Philadelphia, PA, 1842), vol. 3, pp. 467–518, on p. 468.

50 J. B. van Helmont, *Ortus medicinae, id est Initia physicæ inaudita* (Amsterdam, 1648), p. 722; Niebyl, 'Old age', 365–6.

51 Hall, 'Life', 16.

52 Roger, *Sciences de la vie*, pp. 121–39.

53 Dietlinde Goltz, 'Samenflüssigkeit und Nervensaft. Zur Rolle der antiken Medizin in den Zeugungstheorien des 18. Jahrhunderts', *Medizinhistorisches Journal* 22 (1987), 135–63.

54 Oliva Sabuco, *Nueva filosofia de la naturaleza del hombre* (Madrid, 1587); Sabuco, *The True Medicine*, ed. and trans. Gianna Pomata (Toronto, 2010), pp. 145–6, 206–8.

55 Sabuco, *True Medicine*, pp. 145–6, 206–8; Pomata, 'Introduction', ibid., pp. 45–50.

came to be known as the 'English school' in the European medical discussion of the origin of semen.[56]

The most important rethinking of radical moisture and generation came from Harvey himself, whose *Exercitationes de generatione animalium* (Anatomical exercitations concerning the generation of living creatures) of 1651 advanced a new hypothesis centred on the egg, or ovum, as the product of conception – a theory that would later be appropriated and reconceptualized as 'ovism'.[57] Harvey formulated his theory to explain why, when dissecting animals that had just engaged in coitus, he observed in their wombs neither the mixture of male and female semen supposed by the Galenists nor the menstrual blood posited by the Aristotelians. Consequently, Harvey rejected the Galenic theory of the two seeds and the Aristotelian hylomorphic view that saw the male semen as the only active force in generation.[58] He argued that the conceptus, or ovum, is actively created by male and female together. 'The male is no more to be considered the first principle from which conceptions and the embryo arise … than is the female', he wrote.[59] According to him, the male seed conferred a formative power on the female without direct physical contact, and without contributing any matter to the embryo. Following intercourse, under the fertilizing power of the male semen, the tubes of the uterus opened and released into the uterus 'the first white fluid', out of which the conceptus or ovum was formed.[60] The ovum came from the radical moisture of the mother. 'We call this the radical moisture', he wrote, 'because from it arises the first particle of the embryo, the blood, to wit'. A pulsating speck of blood was formed first, then the heart around it, and then the other organs in epigenetic sequence.[61] Harvey explicitly connected the 'white fluid', or the 'primordium' of the ovum, to Avicenna's theory of the secondary moistures. The fluid that formed the ovum, he wrote, appears to be 'the ultimate aliment, called dew [*ros*] by the Arabians'.[62] Harvey, however, departed from Avicenna's theory in one fundamental detail. He associated the radical moisture with the female contribution to the embryo, and thus put unprecedented emphasis on the female role in generation.

Harvey was aware that his theory was highly speculative – he called it a 'fable'.[63] He also knew that the concepts of innate heat and radical moisture were dubious and

56 Pomata, 'Introduction', ibid., pp. 73–8.

57 William Harvey, *Anatomical Exercises on the Generation of Animals* [1651], in *The Works of William Harvey*, ed. and trans. Robert Willis (London, 1847), pp. 143–571; Karin Ekholm, 'Pictures and Analogies in the Anatomy of Generation', Chapter 15; Nick Hopwood, 'The Keywords "Generation" and "Reproduction"', Chapter 20; Vienne, 'Eggs and Sperm as Germ Cells'; Rina Knoeff, 'The Generative Parts of Women', Exhibit 16, this book.

58 Harvey, *Anatomical Exercises*, pp. 300–1; Ekholm, 'Pictures and Analogies'.

59 Harvey, *Anatomical Exercises*, p. 315.

60 Harvey, 'On conception', in *Works of William Harvey*, pp. 573–86, on p. 577.

61 Harvey, *Anatomical Exercises*, p. 513. 62 Ibid., p. 514. 63 Harvey, 'On conception', p. 580.

puzzling, and he tried to offer a critical reinterpretation. He debunked the category of innate heat: there is no need for this concept, he argued, since the blood as a whole performs the vital roles that heat was assumed to play. Just as the innate heat is nothing but the blood, the radical moisture is nothing but the 'crystalline colliquament' containing the rudiments of an embryo *in potentia*, 'from which the fœtus and its parts primarily and immediately arise'.[64] But since the secondary humidities themselves derived from blood, blood could be said to be 'also the radical moisture, at once the ultimate and the proximate and the primary aliment', 'the immediate instrument and principal seat of the soul'. For the discoverer of the circulation, blood was the only true vital principle, performing those functions that the ancients had attributed to 'fanciful conceits'.[65]

Conclusion

We find a view similar to Harvey's if we look at the entry '*calidum innatum*' in Étienne Chauvin's *Lexicon rationale* (1692), the philosophical dictionary that set out to renew scientific language beyond scholasticism:

> The ancients once imagined the innate heat, which they called the active principle of life; to which they added another passive principle, namely the unctuous radical moisture, used by the heat as nutriment … But the moderns say that this imagined notion [*commentum*] of the Aristotelians and the Galenists is vain and useless.[66]

By the end of the seventeenth century, innate heat and radical moisture were seen as remnants of the outdated scholastic toolkit. In 1686, reviewing Boym's work on Chinese medicine mentioned at the beginning of this chapter, the French philosopher Pierre Bayle remarked ironically:

> We would have much admired … the principles of Chinese medicine if they had been presented to us when we were under the sway of Aristotelian philosophy. Unfortunately, the Chinese theories have reached Europe right at the time when the foundations of mechanical philosophy … have made us adverse to … the *calidum naturale* and the *humidum radicale*, which are the foundational concepts of Chinese medicine as well as of Peripatetic philosophy.[67]

64 Harvey, *Anatomical Exercises*, p. 513.

65 Ibid., pp. 501–18, on pp. 513, 510.

66 Étienne Chauvin, *Lexicon rationale* (Rotterdam, 1692), s.v. *calidum innatum* (cross-referenced with *humidum radicale*).

67 Pierre Bayle in *Nouvelles de la République des Lettres* 6 (July–Dec. 1686), pp. 1005–22, on pp. 1012–13.

The long life of the European *yang* and *yin* – innate heat and radical moisture – was drawing to its close. But we should not be led by Bayle's scepticism to assume that the concept had completely lost significance in early modern scholarly cultures. The attempt to rethink the radical moisture was, in fact, part of the background for the new theory of generation that went under the name of ovism and would be much debated through the eighteenth century.

15 Pictures and Analogies in the Anatomy of Generation

Karin Ekholm

Generation, the creation of new life, posed the ultimate challenge for early modern anatomists. Even when they gained access to women's bodies and fetuses, they had to contend with the ways in which generative organs, more than other body parts, alter with actions and age. Their accounts of these structures focused on variations in shape, size and texture, and on the fluids, eggs and fetuses they contain. Continual changes during intercourse, pregnancy and over a lifetime, together with the small size of nascent creatures, the many clear liquids and the impossibility of watching conception, all complicated efforts to observe, describe and understand generation.

From the sixteenth century, European anatomists prioritized knowledge of bodies acquired through sight over descriptions by ancient authorities, even as they consciously followed Galen and Aristotle.[1] In his monumental *De humani corporis fabrica* (On the fabric of the human body, 1543), Andreas Vesalius exhorted students to refrain from blindly trusting books, to look for themselves and to compare Galen's descriptions with his.[2] '*Autopsia*', seeing with one's own eyes, soon became the watchword. A century later, in *Exercitationes de generatione animalium* (Anatomical exercitations concerning the generation of living creatures, 1651), William Harvey explained his methodology and assured readers that '*per autopsiam*' they would identify errors in Aristotle's and Galen's accounts of how fetuses are conceived and form, and make new discoveries of their own.[3] Seeing was central to anatomists' debates: insisting that Nature's book was open and legible to readers who knew how to look, they criticized others for not seeing and developed their own indirect ways of viewing generative parts and processes. Yet at the same time, echoing long-standing disagreements among natural philosophers, anatomists and physicians, they worried about the practical and epistemological limitations of sight. These worries were especially acute when they tried to explain the workings of the generative organs, parents' contributions and fetal formation.

This chapter examines how anatomists produced pictures, developed figurative language and ventured analogies, and argues that these techniques were central to their

1 Andrew Cunningham, *The Anatomical Renaissance: The Resurrection of the Anatomical Projects of the Ancients* (Aldershot, 1997).

2 Andreas Vesalius, *De humani corporis fabrica libri septem* (Basel, 1543), p. 643.

3 William Harvey, *Exercitationes de generatione animalium* (London, 1651), preface. I quote from the anonymous translation, *Anatomical Exercitations Concerning the Generation of Living Creatures* (London, 1653).

perception, understanding and communication of the things they saw. It takes examples from Vesalius's lavishly illustrated volume and Harvey's plain text, while situating their arguments about observations, analogies and techniques for producing knowledge, as they often did, within older traditions of studying generation and anatomy. Early modern anatomists echoed classical Greek texts that used the word for eyewitness to describe reports on medical and anatomical knowledge and on the geographies and cultures of distant places. They often styled themselves as explorers of unknown lands who mapped the interior of the body.[4] Like cartographers, some anatomists made images, assisted by artists and printers, to persuade readers and guide those who followed in their footsteps. Others warned of the dangers of using either pictorial or verbal maps to form impressions of the interior of the body. In the early sixteenth century, for instance, the military surgeon Alessandro Benedetti – in a book, like Harvey's, without images – urged readers to view dissections, warning that those who rely on written accounts are often deceived, like novices navigating with maps in which geographical features fail to correspond fully to those that 'fall under the eyes'.[5]

Anatomists agreed that direct encounters with bodies should serve as the primary means of learning anatomy, but they diverged in assessing the usefulness and limits of illustrations.[6] Vesalius anticipated that students who lacked opportunities, training or the constitution to open bodies would benefit from his images that 'place a subject before the eyes' more precisely than words, while others, including his teacher at Paris, Jacques Dubois, emphasized the shortcomings of printed images.[7] Dubois urged students to learn by handling specimens, in part because he considered touch the most certain of the five senses, but since physical specimens of generative organs were scarce, he made an exception and displayed 'figures and portraits' when publicly lecturing on these.[8] Through the seventeenth century, anatomists continued to debate the best means to display generative parts and processes. Harvey left images out of his book on animal generation because, he argued, images are always mediated by the imagination. The moment an artist looks away from a face that he is drawing, he forms a mental image that differs from the original.[9] Instead, Harvey recommended that readers learn

4 Harvey, *Anatomical Exercitations*, preface; Caterina Albino, 'Visual bodies: Anatomy and cartography', in Andrew Gordon and Bernhard Klein (eds.), *Literature, Mapping, and the Politics of Space in Early Modern Britain* (Cambridge, 2001), pp. 89–108.

5 Alessandro Benedetti, *Anatomice, sive historia corporis humani* (Paris, 1514), p. 65. Benedetti's book was first published in Venice in 1502.

6 Karin Ekholm, 'Fabricius's and Harvey's representations of animal generation', *Annals of Science* 67 (2010), 329–52.

7 Vesalius, *Fabrica*, preface.

8 Noel du Fail, *Les contes et discours d'Eutapel* (Rennes, 1597), p. 114; Charles Kellett, 'Sylvius and the reform of anatomy', *Medical History* 5 (1961), 101–16.

9 Harvey, *Anatomical Exercitations*, preface.

anatomy from regular dissections, and told them how to see what he saw. Throughout his book, he also detailed the limits to observation and how he negotiated these. Anatomists, physicians and natural philosophers followed his injunction to dissect pregnant animals and eggs, and ironically a Dutch physician supplied pictures of fetal chicks for a digest of Harvey's book.[10]

In examining early modern anatomists' difficulties in seeing generative structures, and how they used words, analogies and images to communicate their findings, I focus on accounts of women's uteruses and birds' eggs, which some considered equivalent to wombs. These organs received the most attention, and representations of them point to important differences in what anatomists sought and saw.

Dissection, Vivisection and the Generative Parts

Historians concur that the sixteenth and seventeenth centuries saw major transformations in how bodies were studied, especially in Italy, France, the Dutch Republic and England, but they differ in their characterizations of these changes. Mid-twentieth-century histories tended to accept Vesalius's rhetoric that he was breaking new ground when he opened bodies and valued his own observations above ancient authorities.[11] Since then, more contextualized accounts have traced medieval traditions of dissection and situated Vesalius in a Galenic revival that informed anatomical practice and understanding. Vesalius's teachers at Paris in the 1530s had been engaged in publishing editions of Galen's work from Greek manuscripts – previously Galen was known from Arab sources – and teaching students his methods.[12] Vesalius aimed to restore anatomy to its ancient splendour by following Galen's approach, informed by his own methods of human dissection, but was led to criticize Galen.

As a physician, Galen's interest was in human anatomy but, limited by cultural prohibitions on dissecting humans, he had deduced descriptions from analogous parts in animals.[13] In the thirteenth century, human dissections began to be demonstrated to medical students, though before then bodies were opened for religious reasons and,

10 Justus Schrader, *Observationes et historiae omnes & singulae e Guilielmi Harvei libello* De generatione animalium *excerptae* (Amsterdam, 1674).

11 Charles O'Malley, *Andreas Vesalius of Brussels, 1514–1564* (Berkeley, CA, 1964), p. 1; Levi Robert Lind, *Studies in Pre-Vesalian Anatomy: Biography, Translations, Documents* (Philadelphia, PA, 1975), pp. 3–9.

12 Jerome Bylebyl, 'The school of Padua: Humanistic medicine in the 16th century', in Charles Webster (ed.), *Health, Medicine and Mortality in the Sixteenth Century* (Cambridge, 1979), pp. 335–70, on pp. 357–8; Bylebyl, 'Medicine, philosophy and humanism in Renaissance Italy', in John W. Shirley and F. David Hoeniger (eds.), *Science and the Arts in the Renaissance* (Washington, DC, 1985), pp. 27–49.

13 Rebecca Flemming, 'Galen's Generations of Seeds', Chapter 7, this book.

for medical and legal purposes, to identify causes of death.[14] The Bologna professor Mondino de Liuzzi codified these practices in the standard dissection manual used in universities from the early 1300s to the 1530s. Mondino incorporated observations from his own dissections and reading, primarily of Arab commentaries on the Hippocratic authors, Aristotle and Galen, who had dissected animals for a variety of reasons.

Aristotle had cut open various animals, including pregnant ones, to identify the essential structure and utility of a given part.[15] He aimed to understand how parts of bodies serve as instruments of the soul: the internal source of motion in a living being, composed of faculties responsible for various actions.[16] Plants, animals and humans shared a vegetative soul responsible for generation, growth and nutrition. Galen and later Arabic authors drew on Aristotle and other philosophical traditions to describe the human body and its activities. By the mid-thirteenth century, a rift had opened between scholastic philosophers, trained in the teachings of Aristotle, and physicians, who followed Galen, in explaining living processes. On generation, Galen disagreed with Aristotle about each parent's contribution, the order in which organs form and how these direct vital functions. The premise, shared by Aristotle and Galen, that living principles govern bodies remained the received view well into the seventeenth century, though anatomists diverged in how they characterized faculties and drew on both sides to formulate eclectic accounts.[17]

Vesalius followed Galen in describing the structures of parts before identifying their action and use. He advised students to begin their training by opening the dead to gain 'accurate knowledge of the number, position, shape, special substance and composition of each part of the body' before cutting into living creatures to understand their function.[18] As the title suggests, the *Fabrica* focused on structure, and in general Vesalius expressed reservations about using animals to understand human bodies. Vivisection would become central to research only later, though Berengario da Carpi, professor of anatomy at Bologna in the early sixteenth century, innovatively used vivisection to understand the function of parts.[19] Yet in the absence of pregnant women

14 Andrea Carlino, *Books of the Body: Anatomical Ritual and Renaissance Learning*, trans. John Tedeschi and Anne Tedeschi (Chicago, IL, 1999); Roger French, *Dissection and Vivisection in the European Renaissance* (Aldershot, 1999); Katharine Park, *Secrets of Women: Gender, Generation, and the Origins of Human Dissection* (New York, NY, 2006).

15 His *Generation of Animals* describes waking sleeping fetuses and refers readers to pictures of how generative parts are situated inside bodies: 779a10–11 and 746a15.

16 Aristotle, *Parts of Animals*, 641a.

17 Nancy Siraisi, *Medieval and Early Renaissance Medicine* (Chicago, IL, 1990), pp. 78–114; Flemming, 'Galen's Generations of Seeds'; Nahyan Fancy, 'Generation in Medieval Islamic Medicine', Chapter 9, this book.

18 Vesalius, *Fabrica*, p. 658.

19 Allen Shotwell, 'The revival of vivisection in the sixteenth century', *Journal of the History of Biology* 46 (2013), 171–97.

to dissect, animals were important in Vesalius's study of generative and fetal anatomy. For Harvey, the use of animals was less problematic. To understand the vegetative soul, one needed to study generation. This meant cutting into living animals, as earlier anatomists had done, to observe actions unobservable in humans. It also involved studying women and fetuses, to which anatomists had less access.

In the decades before Vesalius began work, Berengario lamented that he had difficulty acquiring human fetuses, despite bribing midwives.[20] The state supplied anatomists with cadavers of executed criminals, but since pregnant women were spared until after they gave birth, dissections of the gravid uterus were virtually impossible. Anatomists acquired first-hand experience of the interior of women's bodies mainly through their work as physicians and surgeons, treating gynaecological disorders and diseases, assisting in birth, excising infants from deceased mothers and conducting postmortems.[21] Vesalius, who did not practise medicine, noted that he lacked access to human specimens. He nevertheless included a series of pictures that represent a virtual dissection of a gravid human uterus (Fig. 15.1). As he had scoffed that Galen was deceived by his monkeys, so Vesalius was ridiculed for representing a human fetus with a canine placenta.[22]

Faced with the challenges of studying and communicating generation, sixteenth-century anatomists devised new ways of working. For most parts of the body, they described the typical appearance of organs based on multiple observations, identifying specific donors only for anomalous variations. For female parts, of which anatomists had few examples, they often recorded details about the woman whose body they described. Berengario named patients whose cancerous uteruses he and close relations had removed, and listed the locations and dates of the surgeries; Vesalius noted that he saw the beginnings of umbilical vessels in a woman killed by her husband; and Harvey related the case of a laundress who suffered chronically from a prolapsed uterus.[23] From particular cases, anatomists extrapolated to changes in the uterus and other structures with age, illness and over the course of pregnancy. Yet their ability to draw general conclusions was constrained by the paucity of examples and uncertainties about when conception occurred.

20 Berengario, *Commentaria cum amplissimis additionibus super Anatomia Mundini* (Bologna, 1521), f. 248r.

21 Park, *Secrets of Women*; Renate Blumenfeld-Kosinski, *Not of Woman Born: Representations of Caesarean Birth in Medieval and Renaissance Culture* (Ithaca, NY, 1990).

22 Vesalius corrected the error in 1546 in a published letter, *The China Epistle*, trans. Daniel Garrison (Cambridge, 2015), p. 170, as well as in the 1555 edition of the *Fabrica*, but it was still noted, for example, in Realdo Colombo, *De re anatomica* (Venice, 1559), p. 248.

23 Berengario da Carpi, *Isagoge brevis* (Venice, 1535), p. 21; Andreas Vesalius, *On the Fabric of the Human Body*, trans. William Frank Richardson, vol. 4 (San Francisco, CA, 2008), p. 194; Harvey, *Anatomical Exercitations*, p. 494.

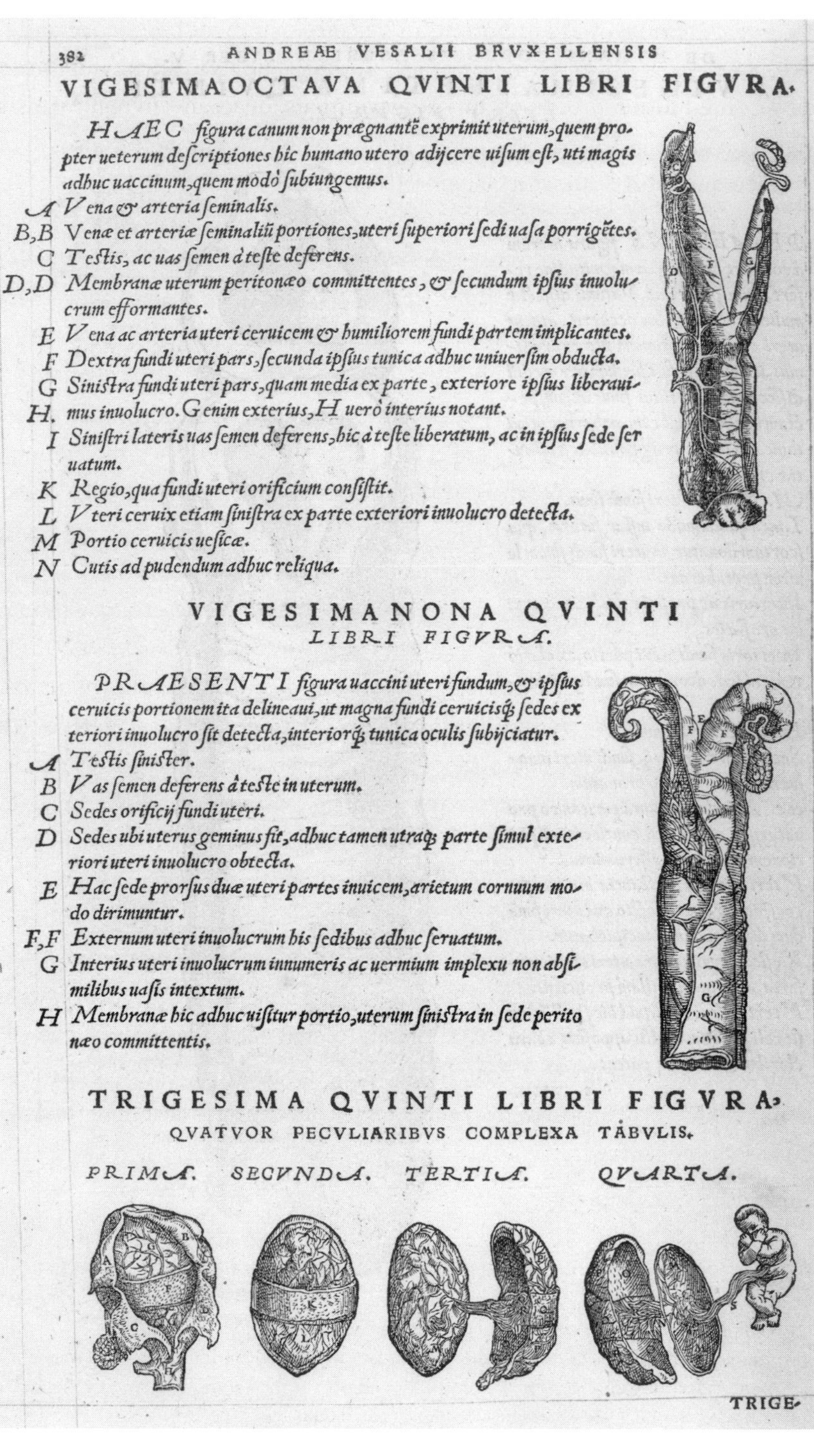

382 ANDREAE VESALII BRVXELLENSIS

VIGESIMAOCTAVA QVINTI LIBRI FIGVRA.

HAEC figura canum non prægnantẽ exprimit uterum, quem propter ueterum deſcriptiones hic humano utero adijcere uiſum eſt, uti magis adhuc uaccinum, quem modò ſubiungemus.

A *Vena & arteria ſeminalis.*
B,B *Venæ et arteriæ ſeminaliũ portiones, uteri ſuperiori ſedi uaſa porrigẽtes.*
C *Teſtis, ac uas ſemen à teſte deferens.*
D,D *Membranæ uterum peritonæo committentes, & ſecundum ipſius inuolucrum efformantes.*
E *Vena ac arteria uteri ceruicem & humiliorem fundi partem implicantes.*
F *Dextra fundi uteri pars, ſecunda ipſius tunica adhuc uniuerſim obducta.*
G *Siniſtra fundi uteri pars, quam media ex parte, exteriore ipſius liberaui-*
H. *mus inuolucro. G enim exterius, H uerò interius notant.*
I *Siniſtri lateris uas ſemen deferens, hic à teſte liberatum, ac in ipſius ſede ſeruatum.*
K *Regio, qua fundi uteri orificium conſiſtit.*
L *Vteri ceruix etiam ſiniſtra ex parte exteriori inuolucro detecta.*
M *Portio ceruicis ueſicæ.*
N *Cutis ad pudendum adhuc reliqua.*

VIGESIMANONA QVINTI
LIBRI FIGVRA.

PRAESENTI figura uaccini uteri fundum, & ipſius ceruicis portionem ita delineaui, ut magna fundi ceruicisq; ſedes exteriori inuolucro ſit detecta, interiorq; tunica oculis ſubijciatur.

A *Teſtis ſiniſter.*
B *Vas ſemen deferens à teſte in uterum.*
C *Sedes orificij fundi uteri.*
D *Sedes ubi uterus geminus fit, adhuc tamen utraq; parte ſimul exteriori uteri inuolucro obtecta.*
E *Hac ſede prorſus duæ uteri partes inuicem, arietum cornuum modo dirimuntur.*
F,F *Externum uteri inuolucrum his ſedibus adhuc ſeruatum.*
G *Interius uteri inuolucrum innumeris ac uermium implexu non abſimilibus uaſis intextum.*
H *Membranæ hic adhuc uiſitur portio, uterum ſiniſtra in ſede peritonæo committentis.*

TRIGESIMA QVINTI LIBRI FIGVRA,
QVATVOR PECVLIARIBVS COMPLEXA TABVLIS.

PRIMA. SECVNDA. TERTIA. QVARTA.

TRIGE-

Figure 15.1 Woodcuts, attributed to Jan van Calcar, in Book V of the *Fabrica*. Figure 28 (top) represents the non-pregnant uterus of a dog, fig. 29 (middle) that of a cow and fig. 30 (bottom) stages in the dissection of a pregnant human uterus. As Vesalius's critics noted, however, the band-shaped placenta in the human series belongs to dogs. Andreas Vesalius, *De humani corporis fabrica libri septem* (Basel: Joannis Oporini, 1543), p. 382. Wellcome Library, London.

To explain what each parent contributed to conception and fetal formation, anatomists, echoing the questions of Aristotle and Galen and borrowing their methods for observing hidden processes, turned to animals, dead and living.[24] This allowed them to control when mating took place and dissect just before and after to track changes resulting from arousal and coition. Using animals also allowed anatomists to observe living fetuses at regular intervals, chart the formation of parts and study their functions. Cutting open living animals, however, raised questions about the representativeness of such inspections. Acknowledging that the animals were distressed, some anatomists questioned whether the observations would reveal how organs appear and function under normal conditions.[25] This was most true for the generative organs, which changed depending on whether animals were sexually aroused or suffering. Further concerns about studying one kind to understand others were raised by variations between different animals in the shape of organs, especially the uterus, fetal structures and placenta. Vesalius complained that persistent confusion about generative parts arose from false assumptions of uniformity and anatomists' failure to disclose which animals they used, and he demonstrated the divergences between Galen's animal-based accounts and his own observations of human structures. Galen described 'horns' of the uterus (Fig. 7.2) and 'cotyledons' on fetal membranes, but, Vesalius noted, these structures are found only in certain animals; generations of anatomists had looked for them in the human body in vain.[26] Once Vesalius had seen what previous anatomists had not, he set out to tell his readers. He also tailored images to show Galen's errors and combined a variety of visual representations to support his own arguments.

Imag(in)ing the Uterus

Representations of animal and human uteruses in the *Fabrica* show how Vesalius used different kinds of images to depict anatomical structures. These include a series of four woodcuts of women's generative organs at successive stages of a dissection that form part of an argument against Galen. The twenty-seventh image in Book V, a 'uterus excised from the body', was often copied into early modern anatomy books and has been replicated widely in histories of the body, especially to illustrate the so-called 'one-sex model' of generative parts (Fig. 15.2).[27] According to this model, these organs in the

24 Cunningham, *Anatomical Renaissance.*

25 Anita Guerrini, 'The ethics of animal experimentation in seventeenth-century England', *Journal of the History of Ideas* 50 (1989), 391–407.

26 Vesalius, *Fabrica* (1555), book V, caption to fig. 32; Flemming, 'Galen's Generations of Seeds'.

27 Examples include Juan Valverde, *Anatomia del corpo humano* (Rome, 1556), book 3, plate V; Caspar Bauhin, *Theatrum anatomicum* (Frankfurt, 1605), book 1, plate XXVI; and Helkiah Crooke, *Microcosmographia* (London, 1615), book 4, plate VII.

two sexes are distinguished by location: in females the passage leading to the uterus is equivalent to an inverted penis, and testes are inside the body, while in males the greater natural heat pushed these parts out. The claim that this was the dominant view of sexual difference from Galen until the eighteenth century, argued most famously by Thomas Laqueur in *Making Sex* (1990), still receives considerable attention. Critics, however, have noted a parallel tradition of texts describing males and females as distinct not only in degree, but also in kind.[28] Helen King has criticized Laqueur for interpreting the illustration as evidence that Vesalius saw vaginas as inside-out penises. One source of confusion, she notes, was that Laqueur reproduced the picture without the title and legend that identify the entire structure as a uterus. For Vesalius, the uterus included not only the 'cavity of the fundus' at the top, but also its 'neck' and 'mound'.[29]

King's argument can be pushed further. Vesalius's images are not self-evident representations of a pristine form of witnessing, but products of how he read texts, sectioned bodies and formulated arguments. He did all this with Galen as his primary interlocutor, testing the ancient doctor's observations against his own dissections. For instance, in discussing the size of non-pregnant uteruses, Vesalius sneered that some – meaning Galen – considered the neck no longer than the fundus (the uterine cavity and tunics).[30] In his experience, the fundus was as long as it was wide, and hardly wider than the uterine neck. Vesalius had artists illustrate this point with fig. 27, created specifically to refute Galen by emphasizing the relative length of the neck (Fig. 15.2). This is the last in the series of prints, each of which calls attention to different characteristics of the uterus. The first displays an opened torso in which the generative organs remain untouched, and in the second figure the bladder is pushed aside to show the positions of the generative organs (Fig. 15.3). Overleaf, a small illustration depicts an excised bladder and the broad ligament, including testes and a womb shown from below (Fig. 15.4). Vesalius never questioned the predominant Galenic view that females produce seed, and he showed vessels joining masculine-looking testicles with the uterus. On the facing page, in fig. 27, the surrounding flesh has been removed to display only the uterus and underscore the proportions between its component parts, which produced its phallic appearance. Considered as a series and within the argument of the work, the reasons for the different renderings of the uterus and adjacent parts become clear. Vesalius presented structures in different ways depending on the questions guiding his observations.

28 Katharine Park and Robert Nye, 'Destiny is anatomy', *New Republic* (18 Feb. 1991), 53–7. See also Gianna Pomata, 'Innate Heat, Radical Moisture and Generation', Chapter 14; and Florence Vienne, 'Eggs and Sperm as Germ Cells', Chapter 28, this book.

29 Helen King, *The One-Sex Body on Trial: The Classical and Early Modern Evidence* (Aldershot, 2013), pp. 53–4.

30 Vesalius, *Fabrica*, pp. 530, 533. The *China Letter*, p. 105, identifies Galen as his opponent.

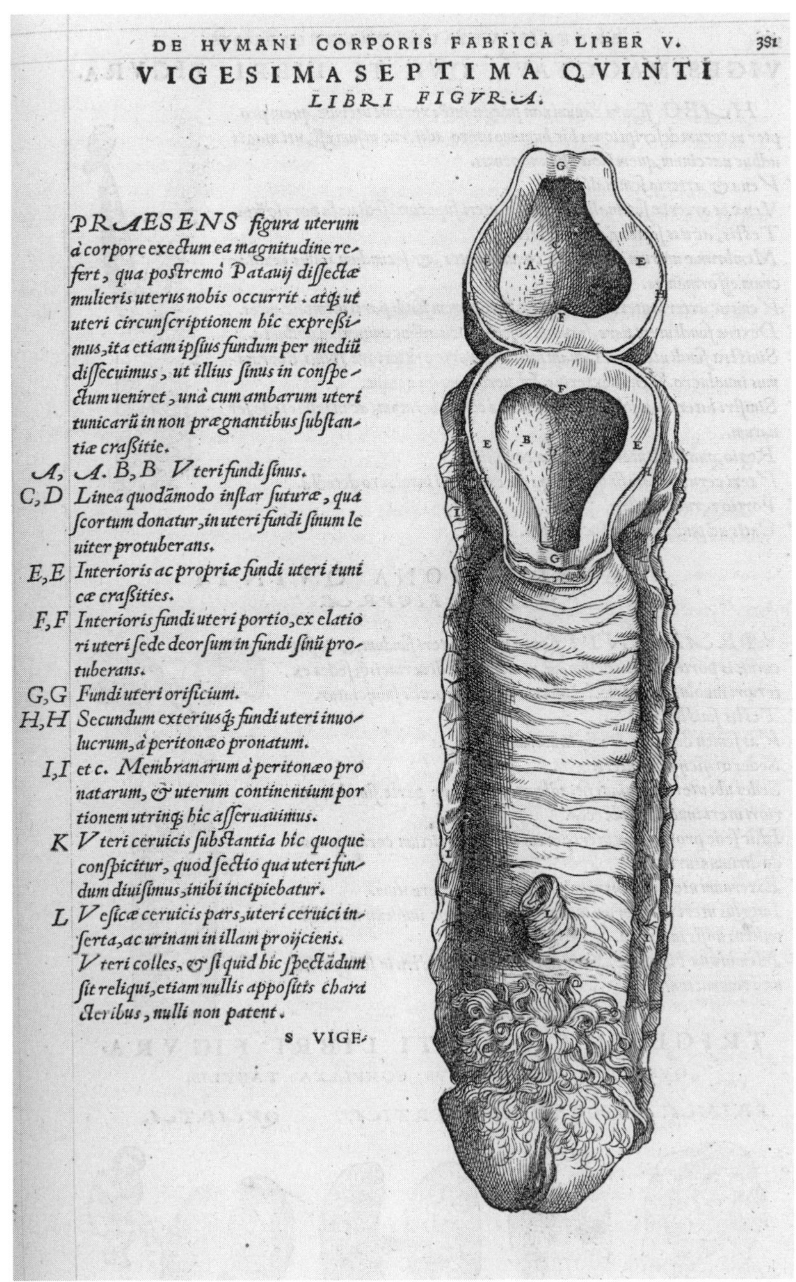

DE HVMANI CORPORIS FABRICA LIBER V. 381

VIGESIMASEPTIMA QVINTI LIBRI FIGVRA.

PRAESENS figura uterum à corpore exectum ea magnitudine refert, qua poſtremò Patauij diſſectæ mulieris uterus nobis occurrit. atq; ut uteri circunſcriptionem hîc expreſsimus, ita etiam ipſius fundum per mediũ diſſecuimus, ut illius ſinus in conſpectum ueniret, unà cum ambarum uteri tunicarũ in non prægnantibus ſubſtantiæ craſsitie.

A, A. B, B *Vteri fundi ſinus.*

C, D *Linea quodãmodo inſtar ſuturæ, qua ſcortum donatur, in uteri fundi ſinum leuiter protuberans.*

E, E *Interioris ac propriæ fundi uteri tunicæ craſsities.*

F, F *Interioris fundi uteri portio, ex elatiori uteri ſede deorſum in fundi ſinũ protuberans.*

G, G *Fundi uteri orificium.*

H, H *Secundum exteriusq; fundi uteri inuolucrum, à peritonæo pronatum.*

I, I et c. *Membranarum à peritonæo pronatarum, & uterum continentium portionem utrinq; hic aſſeruauimus.*

K *Vteri ceruicis ſubſtantia hic quoque conſpicitur, quod ſectio qua uteri fundum diuiſimus, inibi incipiebatur.*

L *Veſicæ ceruicis pars, uteri ceruici inſerta, ac urinam in illam proijciens.*

Vteri colles, & ſi quid hic ſpectãdum ſit reliqui, etiam nullis appoſitis characteribus, nulli non patent.

S VIGE-

Figure 15.2 The concluding woodcut, fig. 27 in Book V of the *Fabrica*, in a series depicting four stages in the dissection of a woman's torso. To a modern eye it looks like a penis, but that was not the original intention. Andreas Vesalius, *De humani corporis fabrica libri septem* (Basel: Joannis Oporini, 1543), p. 381. Wellcome Library, London.

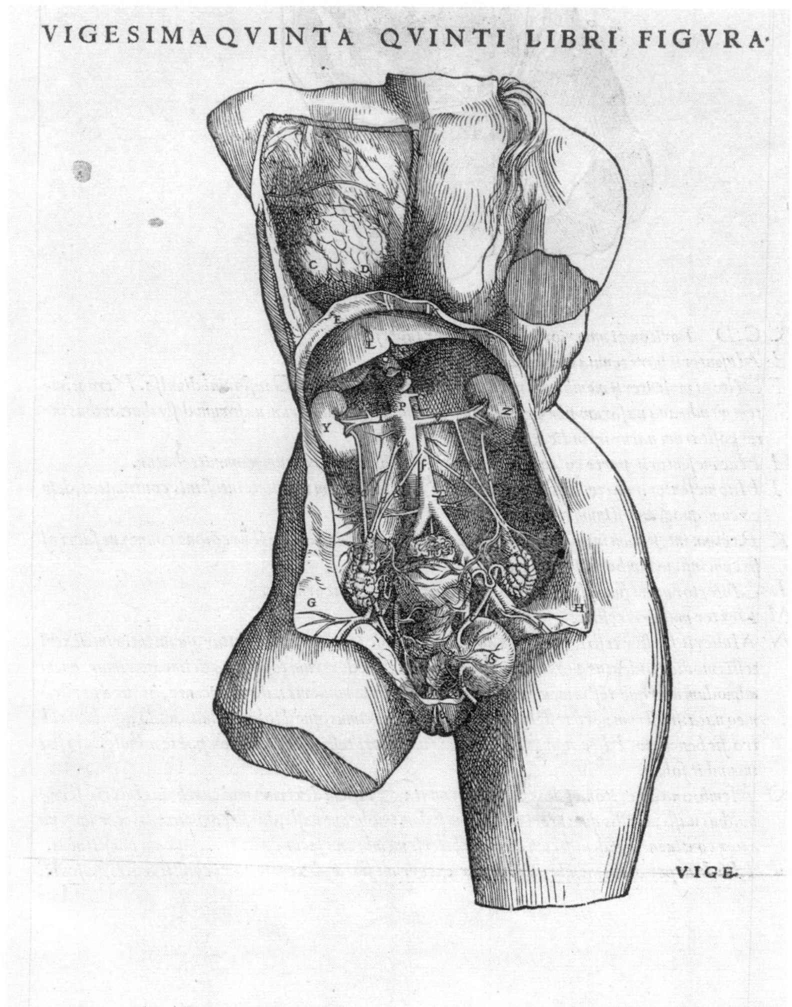

Figure 15.3 Figure 25 in Book V of the *Fabrica*, the second in a series of woodcuts depicting four stages in the dissection of a woman's torso, revealing the generative organs. Andreas Vesalius, *De humani corporis fabrica libri septem* (Basel: Joannis Oporini, 1543), p. 378. Wellcome Library, London.

Histories of sixteenth-century anatomical communication have focused on prints and drawings, but anatomists combined representations of different kinds. To demonstrate that the uterine horns that Galen ascribed to women are found only in certain animals, Vesalius included prints of bovine and canine uteruses; he also appealed to analogies and told readers how to hold their hands to represent their shape (Fig. 15.1). To describe cow wombs, he compared them to ram horns bound at the bottom with a bandage. To picture the same organ in dogs and pigs, he asked readers to spread their

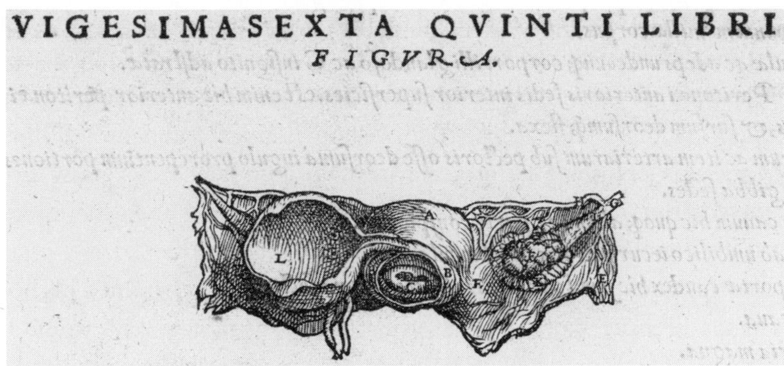

Figure 15.4 The third woodcut (fig. 26) in the series in Book V of the *Fabrica* shows a non-gravid womb from below. The 'broad ligament' holds the uterus in the centre and the female testicles on the right and (covered by the bladder) on the left. Andreas Vesalius, *De humani corporis fabrica libri septem* (Basel: Joannis Oporini, 1543), p. 380. By permission of the CESR Tours and Bibliothèques Virtuelles Humanistes.

index and middle fingers and fold down the remaining digits. The base of the hand represents the fundus, and the fingers are the horns that are usually straight but curve during pregnancy. Hands were used for many early modern practices of signifying, remembering and reckoning, and Vesalius was interested in their structure and what they can do. By engaging readers' hands and making comparisons to common things he helped them to acquire and retain a sense of these unfamiliar objects.[31] He maintained that pictures aided memory once the dissection was over, and these analogies would also have acted as devices for remembering and communicating the various shapes when no books were present.

Eggs as Wombs and Other Analogies

Picture series of another sort were central to the work on generation of Girolamo Fabrici d'Acquapendente, the Padua anatomist who taught Harvey. Fabrici followed Aristotle in studying different manifestations of organs or life processes in various animals. In *De formatione ovi et pulli* (On the formation of the egg and chick, 1621), Fabrici described the generative parts of chickens, explained how eggs form and addressed contested questions about fetal formation. Avian generation, he proposed, involves two wombs. The egg is a uterus where the fetus is formed and fed, after the egg itself is generated in a uterus inside the hen. The 'uterus of the egg' consists of an upper part, the '*ovarium*' – one of the names he coined – where yolks grow like a bunch of grapes

31 For related issues in the training of midwives: Lucia Dacome, 'A Crystal Womb', Exhibit 21, this book.

('*raceme*'), and a lower funnel-shaped section where they are coated in albumen. Fabrici pictured these parts and named them after objects they resembled: the *ovarium* is also nourished like fruit on a tree by a '*pediculus*' (stem) and the lower passage is the '*infundibulum*' (funnel).[32] For Fabrici, like other anatomical and natural historical authors of the time, images formed an integral part of the argument. He oversaw the production of engraved prints and coloured paintings of animal fetuses and generative organs, and paid careful attention to figurative language.[33]

Writing about generation several decades later, Harvey framed his book partly as a response to Fabrici. Worrying that using old words in new ways would lead to confusion, as would minting new ones or adopting metaphors, he postulated that similar concerns had led his teacher to rely on images of animals forming in eggs and wombs.[34] Mistrusting pictures, Harvey instead used analogies to describe the hen uterus. He asked the reader, 'Do you desire an Illustration of this matter? Fashion in your minde a very slender *plant*' and then explained that the knobby roots represent the cluster of yolks and the trunk the funnel. The analogy relates similarities not only in shape, but also in changes with age: just as the stalks of herbs wither in winter, these parts dry up when chickens stop laying eggs (p. 15).[35]

Chick eggs became a central analogy in Harvey's account of generation and shaped his ideas about the formation of fetuses of all kinds. During the 1560s, naturalists at Bologna took up the practice, described by Aristotle and Hippocratic authors, of opening fertilized eggs at intervals. Chick eggs were cheap, available and gave easy access to early transformations (p. 2). At the turn of the seventeenth century, when Harvey studied at Padua, Fabrici demonstrated this procedure privately and commissioned the first series of pictures depicting stages of formation; these were later published in his treatise on chick generation (Fig. 15.5). Harvey, unlike his near-contemporaries, extended the study of eggs to provide a model of formation in all living beings. He explained that since some animals are not available to study and others are tiny, he investigated generation in common creatures like chicks, to whose foundation 'the first originals of all other creatures may be reduced' (preface). He compared the fluids, membranes and nascent bodies contained in fertilized eggs and gravid wombs – of both animals and

32 Fabrici, *De formatione ovi et pulli* (Venice, 1621), pp. 143–5.

33 Sachiko Kusukawa, *Picturing the Book of Nature: Image, Text, and Argument in Sixteenth-Century Human Anatomy and Medical Botany* (Chicago, IL, 2012); Brian Ogilvie, 'Image and text in natural history, 1500–1700', in Wolfgang Lefèvre, Jürgen Renn and Urs Schöpflin (eds.), *The Power of Images in Early Modern Science* (Basel, 2003), pp. 141–66; Karin Ekholm, 'A Placenta Painted and Engraved', Exhibit 15, this book.

34 Harvey, *Anatomical Exercitations*, preface. Further references to this work are given as page numbers in brackets in the text.

35 Helen King, 'Women and Doctors in Ancient Greece', Chapter 3, this book.

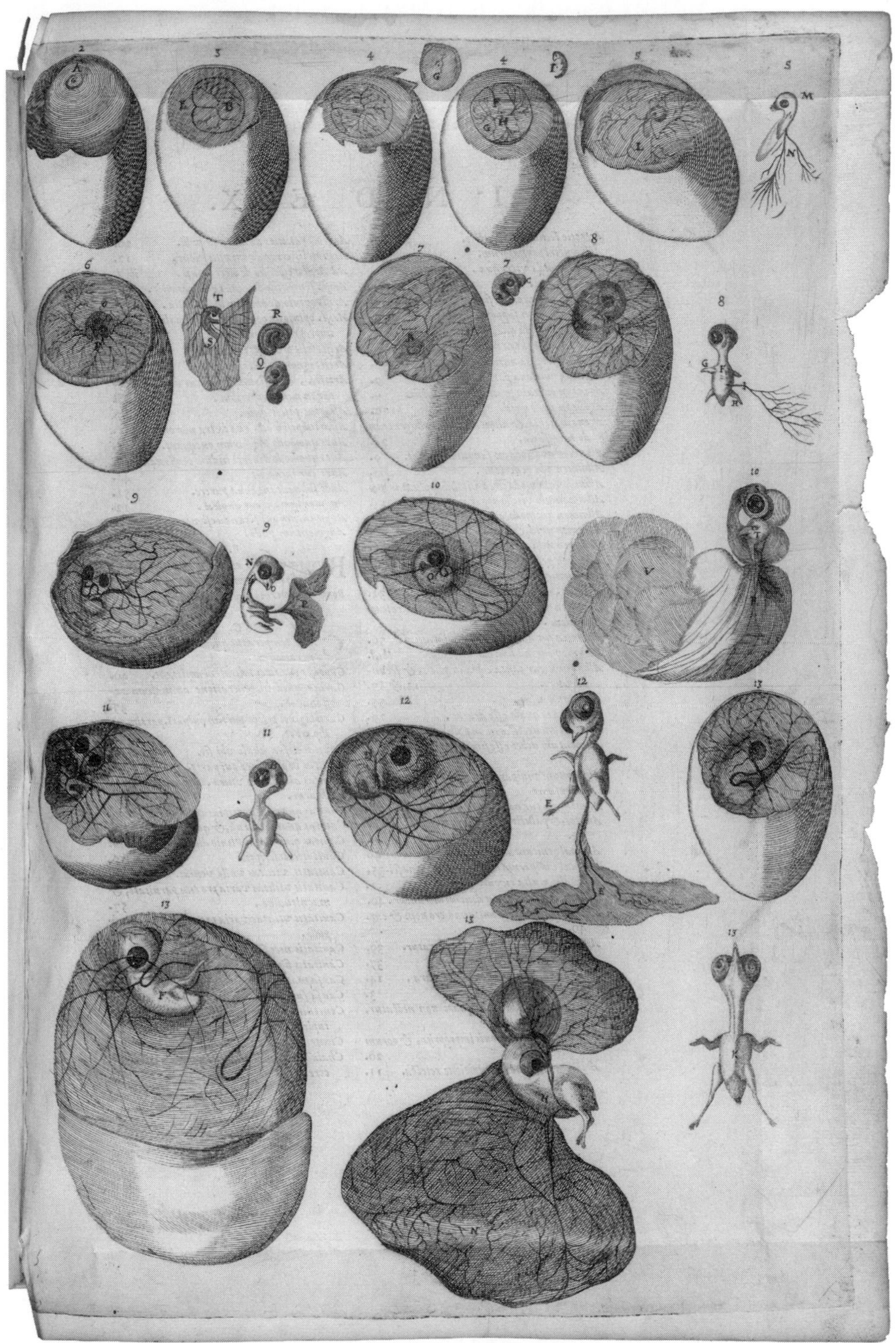

Figure 15.5 The first plate in Girolamo Fabrici d'Acquapendente's series of engravings depicting the changes in fertilized eggs and chicks as they form over the course of twenty-one days. The numbers 1 to 13 indicate the days of incubation, and legends (not shown) identify parts. As formation progresses, the chicks are depicted in various positions. Fabrici, *De formatione ovi et pulli* (Padua: Aloysii Bencii, 1621). Wellcome Library, London.

pregnant patients who had died – and concluded that all animals generate in the same manner (pp. 167, 391–2). Throughout his work, he repeatedly pointed out correspondences between wombs and eggs, often on the basis of similarities he perceived by touch or taste, common means for assessing the qualities of things when nothing could be seen. He also considered plant seeds equivalent to eggs and gravid wombs. An engraved title-page of his book shows beings of all kinds – plant, bird, stag, fish, crocodile, human and various insects – hatching from an egg that Zeus holds with the inscription '*ex ovo omnia*' ('all from the egg') (see frontispiece).

Harvey could observe living fetuses in the eggs for several hours after opening their shells, allowing him to watch the motions of the heart through chests that remained uncovered until relatively late. Another advantage was that changes were recorded from the first day of incubation, which made uncertainties about the time of conception less problematic than in studies of live-bearing creatures. But, like those who had studied eggs before him, Harvey raised questions about the practical challenges of studying eggs and the representativeness of such inspections. He complained that the fetal rudiments were so 'involved in obscurity and deep night, and so perplext with *subtilties*, that they delude the most piercing wit, as well as the sharpest eye' (p. 76). Not only small, the structures changed as the chick 'fetus' was formed within the shell. An anatomist could not watch a single embryo grow and transform; each time he opened a shell, he glimpsed a different individual. Moreover, different eggs developed at different rates and, even if the anatomist worked on eggs fertilized on the same day, he could not account more precisely for variations in the timing of fertilization or his routine of inspections. Harvey mitigated the effects of intruding on the specimen by placing embryonic chicks in silver basins of warm water. They floated freely and lived longer, rendered more visible by the bowl that reflected light. Harvey also augmented visibility by dissecting corresponding organs in larger animals: a dissection of an ostrich revealed features less distinct in chickens (pp. 21–2 and 61).

Anatomists thus developed different methods for dealing with shapes of parts and fetal formation, but conception and the earliest stages of organization hidden within the shell proved particularly difficult to explain on the basis of visual evidence. Harvey failed to find the seminal fluid in the wombs of deer following coitus and concurred with Fabrici that hen uteruses were closed too tightly to admit anything from the male. At a loss to explain this 'dark, obscure business', he appealed to analogies that offered probable explanations of the workings of conception (p. 539). Just as iron acquires magnetic powers and bodies catch contagious diseases through touch, he suggested, momentary contact with male semen changes the uterus in such a way that it gains the capacity to form embryos. Another possibility was that conception was analogous to conceptions of the mind, as was suggested by the similar smoothness and softness of the interior ventricles of the brain and a uterus ready to conceive (pp. 542–3).

To characterize the change effected by the male, Harvey resorted to a further analogy. He related that he grew orange trees in his garden and though the English summer was warm enough to ripen the fruit, the oranges contained no seeds. In the same way, wind-eggs – imperfect eggs, often small and without a yolk – and uteruses prior to conception grow and are nourished, but are made fertile only when the male confers something like the heat of the sun (p. 270). Harvey worked in a tradition that used analogies to communicate sizes, shapes, textures and motions, but here these took on the role of bolstering possible explanations when visual evidence was wanting.

Conclusion

During the second half of the seventeenth century, the dissection of animals of all kinds became widespread not only for teaching, but also for making discoveries. Though concerns about using certain species to understand others persisted, it became common to dissect chick eggs and living animals in efforts to understand how fetuses form and how their changing bodies function. While dissecting the generative organs of a live-bearing dogfish and an egg-laying stingray in the late 1660s, for example, the Danish anatomist Nicholas Steno came to suggest that women's testicles produce eggs.[36] Though microscopes were increasingly used to study living beings, findings pertaining to generation (apart from Leeuwenhoek's discovery of spermatozoa) did not depend on magnification. Anatomists' innovations came instead in how they observed specimens and used images and figurative language in their arguments.[37] Marcello Malpighi, famous as a skilled microscopist, relied on the naked eye and simple magnifying glass to produce ten plates depicting fetal chicks, which he sent in two sets with essays to the Royal Society in 1672. In the second set, he saw more detailed structures not by greater magnification, but by removing chicks from the eggs and spreading them on glass plates that he illuminated from below. The engravings, which remained canonical and unsurpassed for over a century, were organized to depict a given body part at different stages of formation. While Fabrici's plates focused on the formation of the whole animal, Malpighi's pictures called attention to the structure and function of key organs. A century later, when the leading anatomist Albrecht Haller used a microscope to observe embryonic chicks, he referred to Malpighi's drawings to better understand and explain how hearts form.[38] Though new techniques and instruments had allowed early modern

36 Nicholas Steno, *Elementorum myologiae specimen* (Florence, 1668), p. 117.

37 See, for instance, Rina Knoeff, 'The Generative Parts of Women', Exhibit 16, this book.

38 Janina Wellmann, *Die Form des Werdens. Eine Kulturgeschichte der Embryologie 1760–1830* (Göttingen, 2010), pp. 274–80.

anatomists to see structures earlier and more clearly, the challenges of observing generation persisted through the eighteenth century and the making of modern embryology around 1800.[39]

39 Ilana Löwy, 'Prenatal Diagnosis, Surveillance and Risk', Chapter 38; Nick Hopwood, 'Images of Human Embryos', Exhibit 23; Solveig Jülich, '"Drama of Life before Birth"', Exhibit 34, this book.

16 Fruitful Bodies and Astrological Medicine

Lauren Kassell

Am I pregnant? Will we have children? What is my disease? Throughout history, women and their families have formulated these and related questions – Who is the father? Will the child be healthy? Is it a boy or a girl? Do I want it? Will I survive the birth? – according to norms which governed whom to ask and how.[1] This chapter considers how queries about generation were expressed within and shaped by encounters between patients and doctors in early modern Europe. It takes as a premise that medical encounters and women's experiences of their bodies were entwined, and builds on research that allows for long-term continuities without presuming that the encounters have a single, stable structure or that bodily experiences are universal.

Since the 1960s, the 'medical encounter', echoing the earlier 'clinical encounter' and 'doctor–patient relationship', has become shorthand for the dynamics that produced narratives of illness and healing. The phrase is an invitation to interrogate how doctors and patients – terms not intended to imply that doctors were authoritative or patients passive – negotiated power, authority and trust. Medical encounters concerning generation, often focused on women's bodies, mirrored key shifts in women's medicine. Ancient Greek physicians began to include details of women's experience and expertise in their writings. Doctors rekindled an interest in gynaecology in the twelfth century, and from the sixteenth increasingly wrote about women's diseases; accounts of procreation in first-hand narratives, legal cases and medical records burgeoned. From the eighteenth century, medical teachings standardized the female body and devalued women's subjective experiences.[2] Across the period, the ideal persisted of a Hippocratic physician who exercises the authority of reason and experience over a suffering woman (Fig. 16.1). Real medical encounters were shaped by conventions of what could or should be said, observed and recorded. Historians have reconstructed dynamics of

1 Helen King, 'Women and Doctors in Ancient Greece', Chapter 3; Katharine Park, 'Managing Childbirth and Fertility in Medieval Europe', Chapter 11; Christina Benninghaus, 'Modern Infertility', Chapter 31; Kate Fisher, 'Modern Ignorance', Chapter 32; Mary E. Fissell, '*Aristotle's Masterpiece*', Exhibit 25, this book.

2 Lesley Dean-Jones, '*Autopsia*, *historia* and what women know: The authority of women in Hippocratic gynaecology', in Don Bates (ed.), *Knowledge and the Scholarly Medical Traditions* (Cambridge, 1995), pp. 41–59; Helen King, *Hippocrates' Woman: Reading the Female Body in Ancient Greece* (London, 1998), pp. 188–204; Sabine Arnaud, *On Hysteria: The Invention of a Medical Category between 1670 and 1820* (Chicago, IL, 2015).

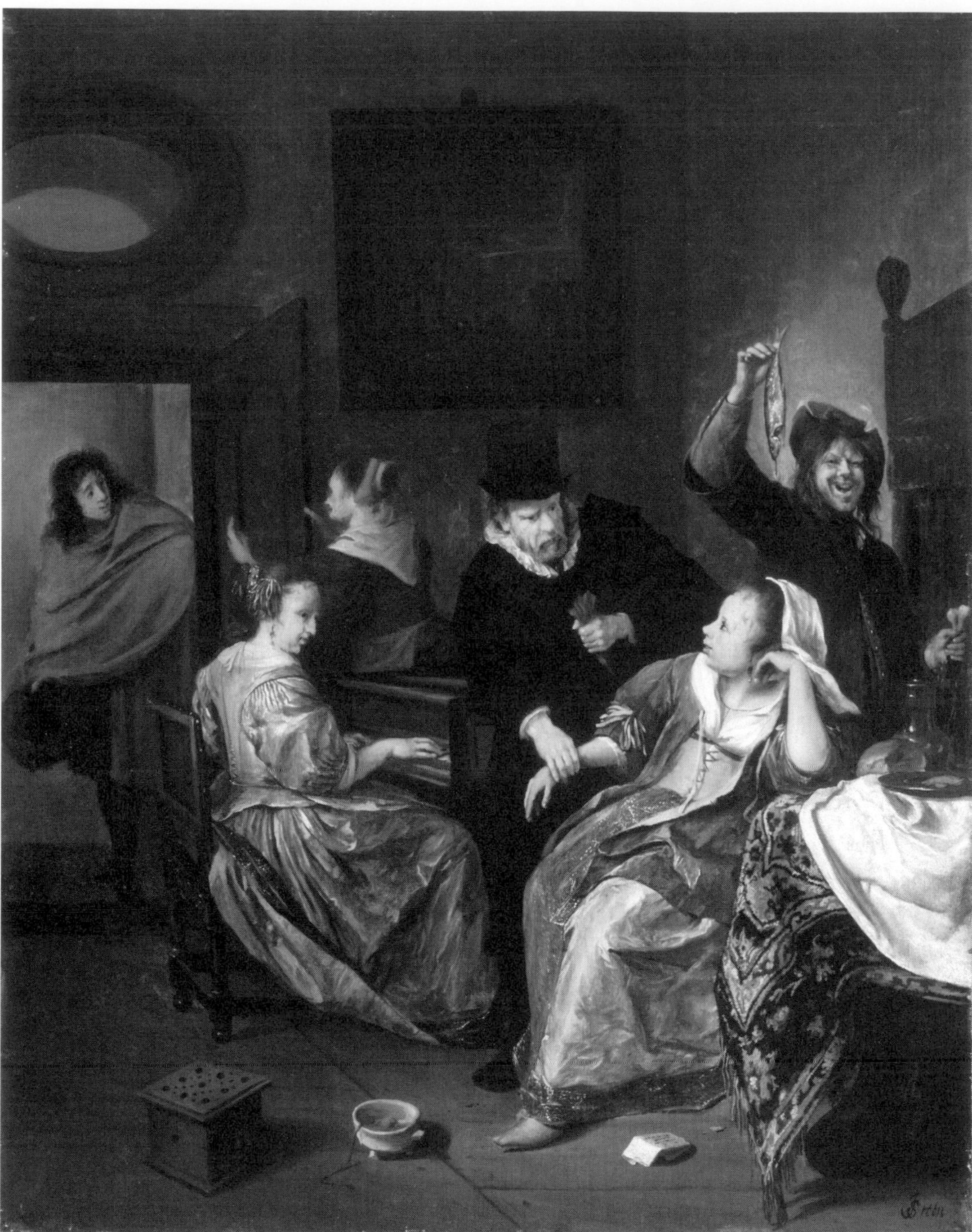

Figure 16.1 Jan Steen's *Doctor's Visit* (*c.* 1663–5). In a play on the gendered dynamic between physician and female patient, he takes her pulse, but fails to note overt hints at pregnancy: the fish, string in a pot and letter on the floor. Oil on panel, 46 × 37 cm, John G. Johnson collection, Cat. 510, Philadelphia Museum of Art.

shared and competing understandings of the body, in some cases through patient writings, but mostly through records of individual doctors, including serial collections of cases labelled diaries, journals, registers, observations and casebooks, the term I shall use for them all.[3] We do not yet have a synthetic history of the medical encounter; the sources are difficult to locate and challenging to interpret.

The earliest surviving European casebooks date from the sixteenth century, when methods of account keeping and an interest in natural particulars converged at bedsides, in consulting rooms and on doctors' desks. While earlier practitioners noted unusual or illustrative cases, early modern records represent ordinary practice, ranging from lists of treatments and payments to narratives of disease and cure, often written from memory or rough notes at the end of the day. Records of around a hundred doctors have been located.[4] Read carefully, they provide evidence about how women, men and their families consulted doctors over generative matters; the norms of gender, status and authority that these encounters rehearsed and reinforced; and how doctors and patients negotiated knowledge of women's bodies, during and beyond the consultation.[5]

Different doctors had different approaches, clients and record-keeping habits. I will focus on the set of consultations recorded by the English self-styled astrologer-physicians, Simon Forman and Richard Napier, day by day from 1596 to 1634.[6] Forman's and Napier's records are remarkable for their extensiveness, totalling around 80,000 cases, and immediacy; unusually, they were written during the consultations. In an era when patients shopped around, three-quarters of them consulted the practitioners only once. Even the cases of regular clients remain dispersed, not consolidated into a narrative. Nonetheless, thousands of cases, brief but vivid, are about pregnancy and fertility.

I group Forman's and Napier's casebooks together because Napier was Forman's student and their records follow the same method. A typical consultation began when a patient asked a question – thus investing the practitioner with the authority to make

3 The best studies remain Barbara Duden, *The Woman beneath the Skin: A Doctor's Patients in Eighteenth-Century Germany*, trans. Thomas Dunlap (Cambridge, MA, 1991); and Michael MacDonald, *Mystical Bedlam: Madness, Anxiety, and Healing in Seventeenth-Century England* (Cambridge, 1981); see also Philip Rieder, *La figure du patient au XVIIIe siècle* (Geneva, 2010). For a survey: Flurin Condrau, 'The patient's view meets the clinical gaze', *Social History of Medicine* 20 (2007), 525–40.

4 Martin Dinges *et al.* (eds.), *Medical Practice, 1600–1900: Physicians and Their Patients* (Leiden, 2015); Lauren Kassell, 'Casebooks in early modern England: Medicine, astrology and written records', *Bulletin of the History of Medicine* 88 (2014), 595–625.

5 Contrast my arguments with Wendy D. Churchill, *Female Patients in Early Modern Britain: Gender, Diagnosis and Treatment* (Farnham, 2012); and Daphna Oren-Magidor, 'Literate laywomen, male medical practitioners and the treatment of fertility problems in early modern England', *Social History of Medicine* 29 (2016), 290–310.

6 Lauren Kassell *et al.* (eds.), *The Casebooks of Simon Forman and Richard Napier, 1596–1634: A Digital Edition*, https://casebooks.lib.cam.ac.uk, last accessed 24 June 2018.

somatic and social judgements – in person, by proxy or in writing. Occasionally the doctors attended wealthy clients at home, in the convention depicted in Fig. 16.1, but patients usually came to their houses or sent messengers, as represented in Fig. 16.2. Forman and Napier asked the patient's name, age and sometimes occupation or address. Where the querent was not the patient, or multiple people were present, the doctor noted their relationships and whether the patient consented to the question. Then he drew a horoscope, also known as a chart or figure, dividing the celestial sphere into twelve zodiac houses or signs, and plotting the locations of the planets within them at the significant moment, usually when the question was asked or the message arrived. This is known as 'horary' astrology.[7] Thereafter the records become less systematic. An entry might contain a judgement based on the horoscope, other sorts of evidence gleaned from the patient's words or appearance, the quality of the urine or the doctor's observations. Unlike most physicians, Forman and Napier did not feel the pulse and seem not to have used touch to examine their patients. Some cases detail remedies and payments, but the account books are lost. The resulting records are rich yet fragmented; they do not narrate a disease or cure and are often ambiguous about whether a patient articulated a complaint or the astrologer discerned it from the stars or other signs. When the doctors added follow-up details, often from third parties, we glimpse communication beyond the encounter.

Forman's and Napier's methods for conducting a consultation were typical of the period. The priority they gave the stars was extreme, but not unusual. Astrology was part of learned medicine, though horary astrology was contested as deterministic or arbitrary. Like other physicians, Forman and Napier also observed signs of a patient's body and listened to her words. In early modern 'bedside medicine', patients and practitioners negotiated narratives of illness and readings of signs, drawing on epistemologies more shared than competing.[8]

Modesty dictated how a doctor or any man who was not her husband saw or touched a woman's body, and constrained what she could say.[9] Some authorities appropriated the trope that ignorance or shame led men and women to suffer rather than acquaint doctors with their symptoms, yet women and men talked between and amongst themselves, and to medical practitioners, about sex, menstruation and pregnancy.[10] These were regular events in the lives of 'breeding' or 'teeming' women, contemporary

7 On natal astrology: Eleanor Robson, 'The Birth Horoscope of a Babylonian Scholar', Exhibit 3, this book.

8 Claudia Stein, 'The meaning of signs: Diagnosing the French pox in early modern Augsburg', *Bulletin of the History of Medicine* 80 (2006), 617–48; Olivia Weisser, 'Boils, pushes and wheals: Reading bumps on the body in early modern England', *Social History of Medicine* 22 (2009), 321–39.

9 Monica H. Green, *Making Women's Medicine Masculine: The Rise of Male Authority in Pre-Modern Gynaecology* (Oxford, 2008), pp. 111–17; Oren-Magidor, 'Literate laywomen', 292, 294–5.

10 Laura Gowing, 'Knowledge and experience, *c.* 1500–1700', in Sarah Toulalan and Kate Fisher (eds.), *The Routledge History of Sex and the Body, 1500 to the Present* (London, 2013), pp. 239–55, on pp. 245–6.

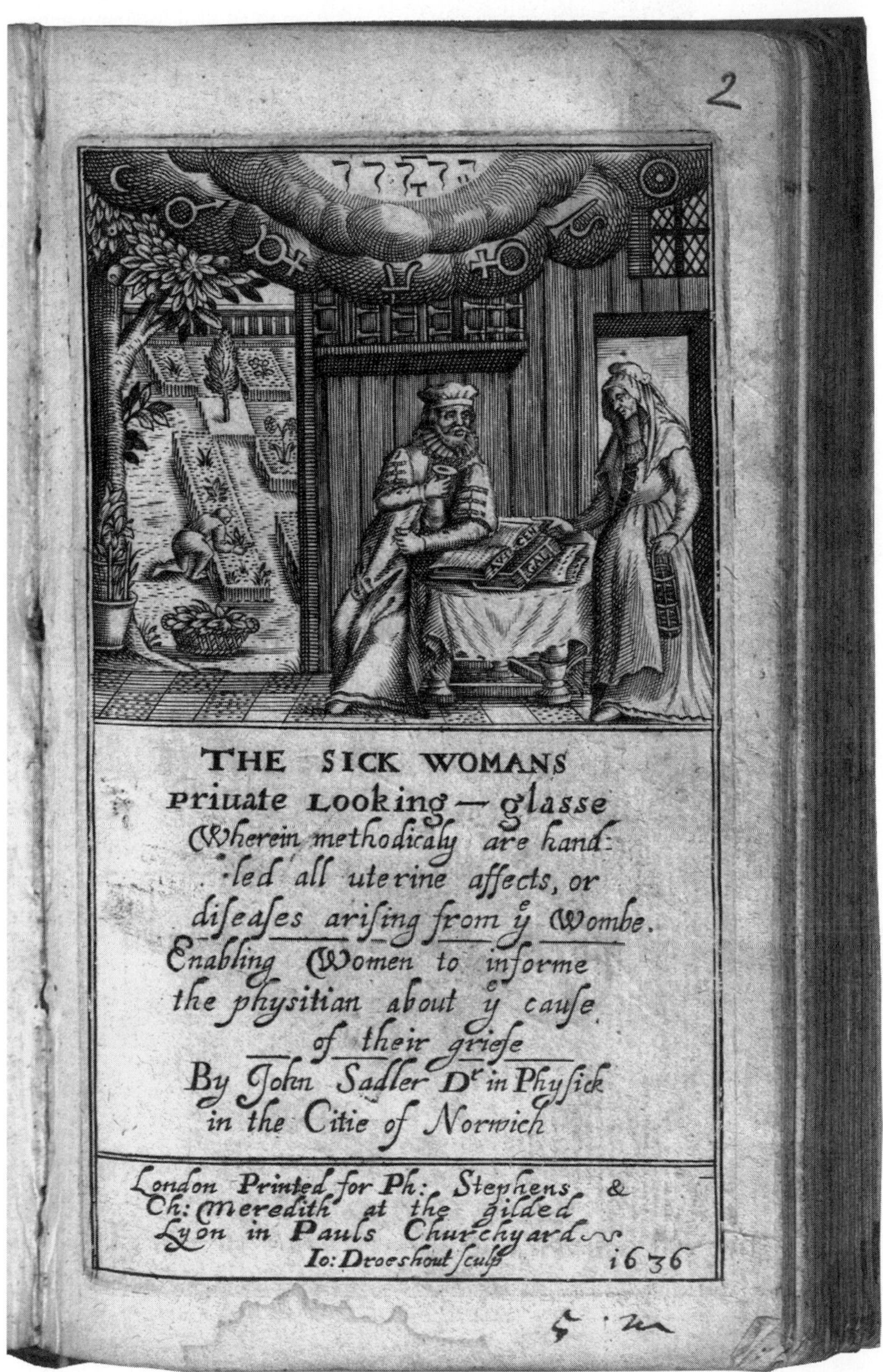

THE SICK WOMANS
priuate Looking—glasse
Wherein methodicaly are hand:
led all uterine affects, or
diseases arising from ye Wombe.
Enabling Women to informe
the physitian about ye cause
of their griefe
By John Sadler Dr in Physick
in the Citie of Norwich

London Printed for Ph: Stephens &
Ch: Meredith at the gilded
Lyon in Pauls Churchyard
Io: Droeshout sculp 1636

Figure 16.2 Title image from a book instructing women how to inform doctors about their diseases. The female patient consulting a physician became a standard motif in depictions of medical encounters. Engraving by John Droeshout in John Sadler, *The Sicke Womans Private Looking-Glasse* (London: by Anne Griffin for Philemon Stephens and Christopher Meridith, 1636), by permission of the Master and Fellows of Trinity College, Cambridge.

terms that capture the defining function of women of childbearing age. During these years, married women were suspended between the potential to bring forth new life and uncertainty about whether they would succeed.

Am I Pregnant?

Early modern married women and their families monitored signs about the state of their bodies and shared these details in letters, diaries and conversations. Recourse to medical practitioners was common, whether a woman was well or experiencing pain, anxiety or illness.[11] Roughly one in twenty women of childbearing age asked Forman and Napier, 'Am I pregnant?' Less often, a husband, family member or employer posed the question, or someone asked the sex of the child or whether mother and infant would survive childbirth, standard topics for fortune-tellers. When a woman asked about pregnancy, she opened a conversation about her experiences of menstruation and other signs, and details about sex and the state of her marriage.

It has often been argued that before the advent of reliable pregnancy tests in the twentieth century, a woman might suspect that she was pregnant if her periods stopped and that her suspicion would be confirmed if she felt the child move, or 'quicken'. She could also use techniques, dismissed by many as superstitious, to divine whether she was pregnant or the sex of the child. Yet for early modern women a lack of menstruation or even quickening were not sure signs. Some knew as soon as they conceived and shared this knowledge in letters to family; others, often in defending themselves against accusations of infanticide, were unaware until the baby was born.[12]

Jane Sharp's *The Midwives Book* (1671), a standard, derivative account designed for midwives and other women, contrasted overlapping but distinct rules of physicians and 'common' people for knowing whether a woman was with child. These rules combined what she felt and others observed. With a medley of details derived from Soranus, Galen and others about the effects of an especially pleasurable sexual encounter, Sharp describes how a woman feels her belly flatten and her 'womb shut close' to retain the

11 Michael MacDonald, 'The career of astrological medicine in England', in Ole Grell and Andrew Cunningham (eds.), *Religio Medici: Religion and Medicine in Seventeenth-Century England* (Aldershot, 1996), pp. 62–90; Michael Stolberg, *Uroscopy in Early Modern Europe*, trans. Logan Kennedy and Leonhard Unglaub (Farnham, 2015), pp. 82–90.

12 Duden, *Woman beneath the Skin*, pp. 157–70; Laura Gowing, 'Secret births and infanticide in seventeenth-century England', *Past & Present* (1997), 87–115; P. Renée Baernstein and John Christopoulos, 'Interpreting the body in early modern Italy: Pregnancy, abortion and adulthood', *Past & Present* (2014), 41–75; Magdalena S. Sánchez, '"I would not feel the pain if I were with you": Catalina Micaela and the cycle of pregnancy at the Court of Turin, 1585–1597', *Social History of Medicine* 28 (2015), 445–64; Leah Astbury, 'Breeding women and lusty infants in early modern England', unpublished PhD thesis, University of Cambridge (2016), p. 60. On hormonal pregnancy tests: Jesse Olszynko-Gryn, 'Pregnancy Testing with Frogs', Exhibit 32, this book.

man's semen rather than belching it forth. As her blood and vital heat run to these parts, she grows cold. She experiences indigestion, cravings, nausea and painful bowel movements; stopped menses; moodiness; and lack of sexual appetite. She might share these signs with others, who could also deduce them from her behaviour, or, depending on access to her body, observe her dark eyes, discoloured complexion and swollen breasts with protruding veins and reddened nipples. Sharp's 'common rules' similarly stressed signs that would be evident to someone living close to the woman – stopped menses and changed complexion – and urine tests, including: leave it to stand for three days, strain it and if it contains worms, the woman is pregnant.[13]

Women who asked Forman and Napier if they were pregnant told the astrologer-physicians their age and how long they had been married. They expected a horoscope to be cast, and often brought their urine. Uroscopy dated from antiquity, had become the principal diagnostic tool of physicians in the middle ages and was practised by various early modern medical practitioners. The colour, consistency and content of urine signalled the state of the bodily humours. Uroscopy began to be discredited around 1600, but some patients still demanded that a skilled practitioner could judge the state of their body from the urine alone.[14] Forman's and Napier's patients were no exception, and in practice, especially in cases of pregnancy, the doctors complied, while questioning its validity. Forman argued that an ability to read the stars allowed him to judge the true cause of a disease.[15] Napier reputedly insisted that the figure was ten times more reliable than the urine, especially 'about women with child'.[16] Diagnosing pregnancy was notoriously hard.

While pots of urine were presented and horoscopes cast, women told the doctors, either outright or with prompting, their assessment of their bodily signs. When Elizabeth Raunfford, aged 40, consulted Napier, he noted, 'thincketh her selfe to be with child for her brestes be very full'.[17] Five years later, she again asked about pregnancy when she thought herself '16 weekes quicke', though the movements were mild, she continued to menstruate and her belly was not very big (Case 46212). Jane Rolte, the wife of a prominent lawyer who began consulting Napier regularly in her twenties, also talked about menstruation, swellings, blockages, heat, discharges, pains and emotions, as part of her history of childbearing (Person 15450) (Fig. 16.3). The uncertainty of the signs allowed

13 Jane Sharp, *The Midwives Book or the Whole Art of Midwifery Discovered*, ed. Elaine Hobby (Oxford, 1999), pp. 81–4.

14 Stolberg, *Uroscopy*.

15 Lauren Kassell, *Medicine and Magic in Elizabethan London: Simon Forman, Astrologer, Alchemist and Physician* (Oxford, 2005).

16 George Atwell, *An Apology, Or, Defence of the Divine Art of Natural Astrologie* (London, 1660), p. 27.

17 Kassell *et al.*, *Casebooks Digital Edition*, https://casebooks.lib.cam.ac.uk/cases/CASE41121. Hereafter individual cases are noted by number in parentheses in the text; a person number refers to a group of cases related to an individual. All references were last checked on 24 June 2018. For full transcriptions of these and related cases, see https://casebooks.wordpress.com/transcribed-cases/pregnancy-and-fertility/.

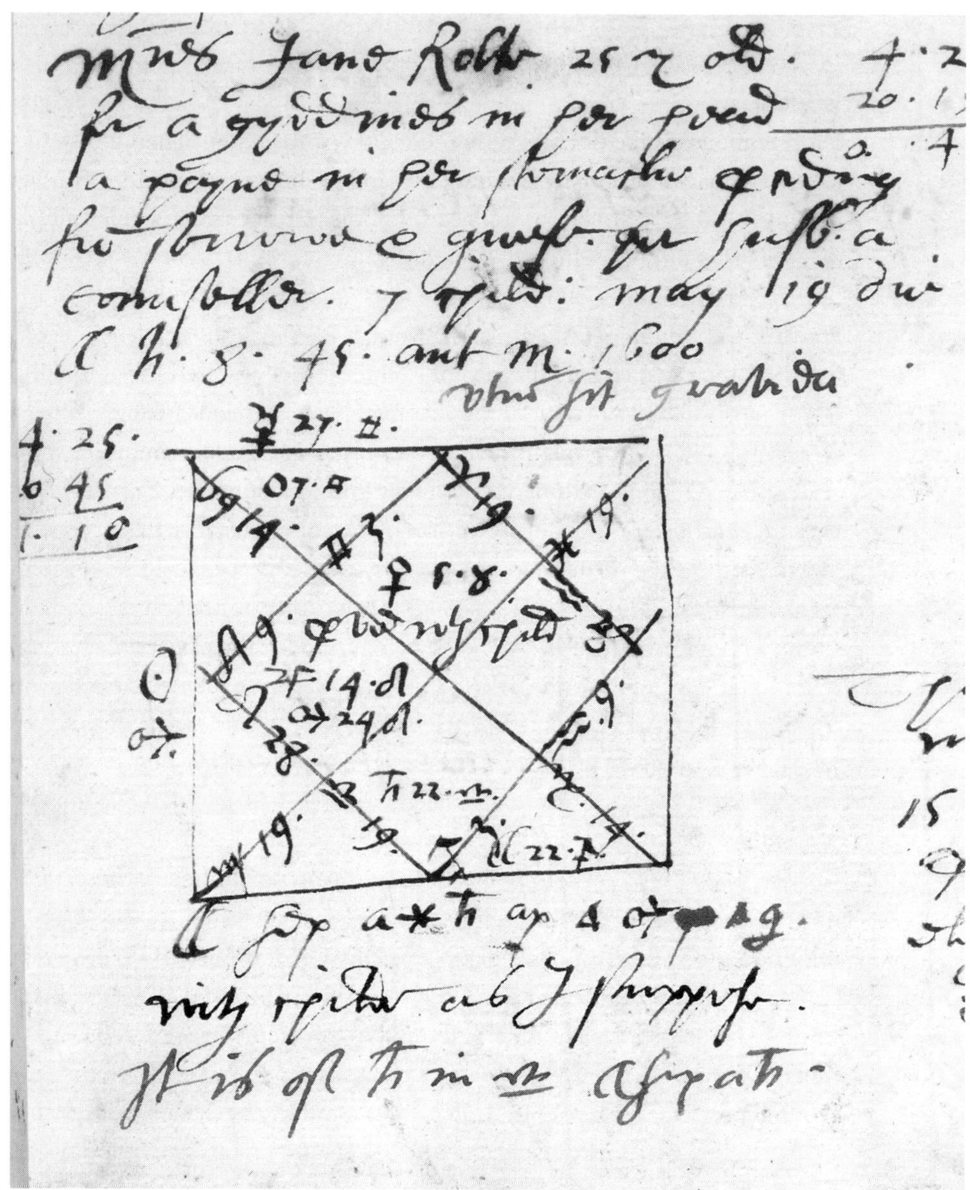

Figure 16.3 Jane Rolte's consultation with Napier on 19 May 1600: 'for a gyddines in her head a payne in her stomacke proceding from sorrowe & greefe. her husb. a counseller. 7 child … utrum sit gravida [whether she is pregnant]'. Napier judged Rolte 'with childe as I suppose', later adding 'p[ro]ved w[i]th child' in the middle of the horoscope. Bodleian Library, MS Ashmole 202, f. 73r (Case 10607), by permission of the Bodleian Libraries, University of Oxford.

the doctors and their clients to disagree. In a typical consultation, Forman noted that Elisabeth Borase, aged 40, 'supposeth her self with child', only to continue, 'but I think yt is not soe' (Case 2294).

Sometimes the doctors were themselves undecided. When Judith Clark, aged 36, asked Forman if she were pregnant, he drew a horoscope and noted 'she should not be with child by her urin', 'but she is with Child by the figur[e]' (Case 513). He had calculated an auspicious conjunction of Venus with Saturn, the ruler of the fifth house, which governed the womb and children.[18] When Agnes Painter, aged 21, asked Forman whether she was pregnant, he looked at her urine and noted contradictory details in the horoscope, which signalled fever and fretfulness, located the cause in her stomach and reins (kidney region), indicated that she did not menstruate, and foretold that she would be unwell and was not with child. '[B]ut yet by judgment of this figure', he noted, 'she seames to be with child'. He concluded, 'she was supposed to be with child. She was very big' (Case 272). While aspiring to provide clear answers, the doctors seem to have communicated their uncertainty to their patients.

Practitioners and patients shared an expectation that they would negotiate the meanings of signs. Precise time intervals featured in these discussions. Just as Forman judged that Clark was with child 'some 6 daies or 6 w[e]cke' – the number six was signalled in the stars – so women, like Raunfford, charted their bodily orders and shared this knowledge with the doctors (Case 193). Healthy women were expected to menstruate regularly and note, in writing or by memory, possible dates of conception. Sharp complained that young wives were especially ignorant and 'not one of twenty almost keeps a just account'.[19] Men might also record when they had sex, and with whom, and when their wives menstruated.[20] Such records documented an interest in the astrological significance of the moment of conception (Fig. 16.4), or, like inscriptions of dates of births, marriages and deaths in the endpapers of Bibles, family history. Whatever the motives, these records were invoked in cases of disputed paternity and inheritance, when physicians and jurists sought to establish dates of conception.[21] In medical encounters, practitioners and their married patients monitored multiple signs to explain the state of a woman's body.

Very few unmarried women asked Forman and Napier about pregnancy. Epistolary consultations could have been discreet, but when a woman asked about pregnancy the doctors sought details about whether she was married, had had previous children

18 Simon Forman, 'The Astrologicalle Judgmentes of phisick and other Questions', ed. Rob Ralley *et al.*, https://casebooks.lib.cam.ac.uk/transcriptions/TEXT5, ¶ 1501–858, last accessed 20 June 2018.

19 Sharp, *Midwives Book*, p. 81.

20 Lauren Kassell, 'Jane Dee's Courses in John Dee's Diary', Exhibit 14; Martina Schlünder, 'Menstrual-Cycle Calendars', Exhibit 31, this book.

21 Cathy McClive, *Menstruation and Procreation in Early Modern France* (Farnham, 2015), pp. 167–94.

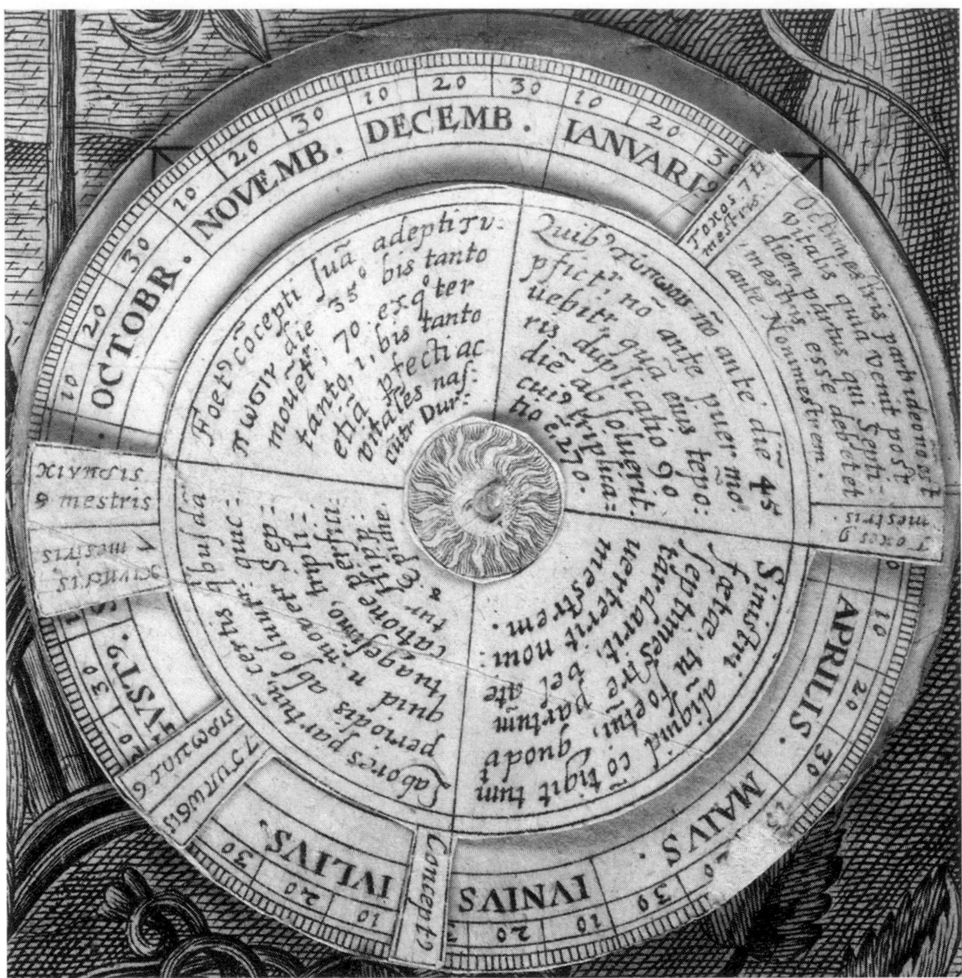

Figure 16.4 Pregnancy calendar in the form of a volvelle. Based on a presumed date of conception, it calculates dates for the completed formation of the fetus, quickening and parturition. These are indicated for 'seven-month' and 'nine-month' children, the two categories that Hippocratic medicine deemed viable. Detail from *Four Seasons of Man*, reproduced in full on p. 122. History of Medicine Collections, David M. Rubenstein Rare Book & Manuscript Library, Duke University.

and, where paternity was uncertain, who was the father, an issue of increasing concern from the early sixteenth century.[22] Perhaps this is why so few unwed women asked. When they did, the doctors took special note. When Elizabeth Key asked Napier whether she was pregnant, he recorded, 'not maryd confesseth that she hath bene naught[y] with on[e]'; the horoscope signalled that she was with child. In consulting Napier, she expressed uncertainty about her bodily state and unburdened herself of her illicit behaviour (Case 38941).

22 Silvia De Renzi, 'Family Resemblance in the Old Regime', Chapter 17, this book.

More often, unwed women asked about disease, and the doctors turned the discussion to pregnancy. Forman insisted, echoing other doctors, that women, especially unwed women, were not to be trusted and that the stars would reveal all.[23] When Alice Sampson, a maid in her mid-twenties, asked Forman the cause of her disease, he judged, 'She should have moch paine in the hed harte & belly but she seames to be with child.' Note his 'should': he was reading the stars. We do not know whether the details about her pains, grief, lack of menstruation and nausea are based on the stars or Sampson's words. We do know that she asked Forman about disease and he brought pregnancy into the conversation. He concluded, 'She saies stoutly she is not with child' (Case 587).

The doctors were on their guard for requests for remedies to effect abortions masked as menstrual regulators, but in practice such cases were rare. Rather, women perceived regular flow to be healthy, and medical theory agreed.[24] Where an illegitimate child was feared, the doctors restored social order by hearing the woman's confession and identifying her paramour. When Dorothy Headlow's mistress asked Forman whether her servant was pregnant, he 'examined' the maid that afternoon 'and she conffessed she was with child' and that one Richard 'Lai with her'. By the time the baby was born ten days later, the couple had been married (Case 491). When things went wrong, women who had attempted to end suspected pregnancies came to the doctors, who tried to discover what had happened. In one case, Forman cautioned himself to 'meddel not thou with her' (Case 6311); in another, Napier noted, 'I gave her nothing' (Case 62118).

Conversations about pregnancy with married and unmarried women might extend beyond the consulting room, prompting the doctors to add follow-up notes. When Forman and Elisabeth Borase disagreed about whether she was pregnant, his judgement was confirmed: 'proved shortly after not to be with child' (Case 2294). Through the medical encounter, the doctors contributed to an idiom in which women and their families and friends expressed hopes and fears about pregnancy.

Will We Have Children?

While a woman typically asked Forman and Napier 'Am I pregnant?' if she expected that she might be, couples asked 'Will we have children?' when they had a history of expectations unfulfilled. This happened rarely, as men and women tended to express concerns about fruitfulness in terms of uncertainty or even optimism about the child to come. But some men and women, whether married for a few months or more than a decade, asked the doctors whether they would have any children or 'for physick & to cause fruictfulnes' (Case 27010).

23 Kassell, *Medicine and Magic*, p. 167.

24 Etienne van de Walle, 'Flowers and fruits: Two thousand years of menstrual regulation', *Journal of Interdisciplinary History* 28 (1997), 182–203.

The New German Doctor:

OR,

An Infallible Cure for a Scolding Wife: Performed by this most Excellent Operator, the like was never known in all Ages.

To the Tune of, Here I love, there I love; or, The English Travellers. Licensed according to Order.

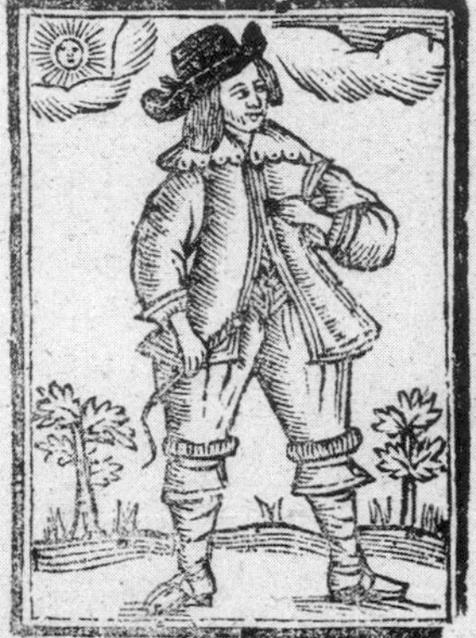

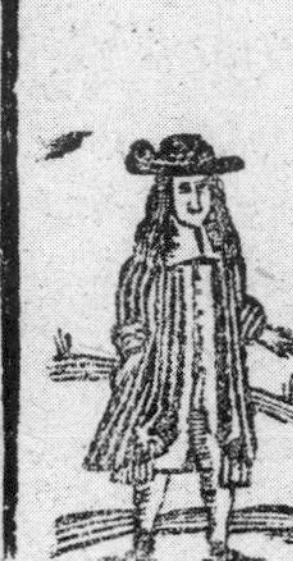

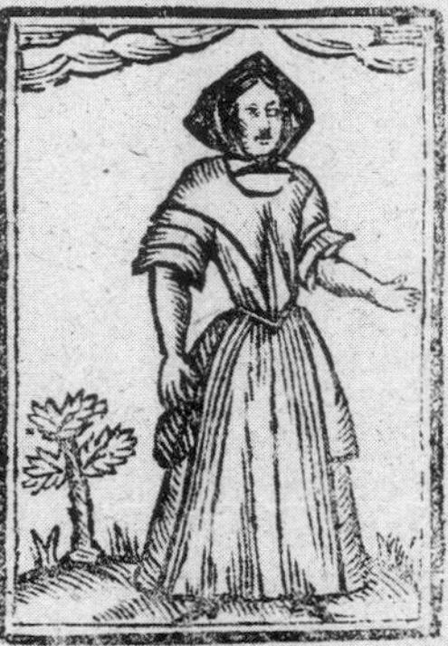

YOu Men that are married, I pray now attend,
Good tydings I bring you, this day as a Friend;
It will be of use to all young Men and old,
Whoever are troubl'd with Women that scold.

A Doctor of late, from the Emperor's Court,
A Person of dextrous Skill by report,
Hath taken a Chamber in London of late,
And cures scolding Wives at a wonderful rate.

This Doctor has travell'd all Poland and Spain,
And now to Great-Britain he crossed the Main:
To one Land and Nation he'll not be confin'd,
But travels the World for the good of mankind.

That Man that is plagu'd with a cross scolding Wife,
Whose railing doth make him quite weary of Life;
Pray what would he give for an absolute cure,
Before such a terrible Life he'd endure?

'Tis like ev'ry Morning when Day-light appears,
She rings him a thundring Peal in his Ears;
And makes him be glad to rouze out of the Bed,
And all by the violent noise of her Head.

Sometimes a good Husband may meet with a Friend,
And happen a penny or two pence to spend;
Then in comes the Wife, who do's thunder and bawl,
And with the Quart-flaggon his Noddle doth maul.

Her Tongue is more keen than a two-edged Sword,
Nay louder than Thunder she Peals will afford;
Instead of fond Pleasures, kind Love and Delight,
She is like a fierce Tygre, both Morning and Night.

It is an unspeakable Torment I know,
You cannot imagine what they undergo:
Who with such cross Women, their Lives now do lead,
But bring them away to the Doctor with speed.

Nay let them be never so aged or young,
This Doctor he takes out the Sting of the Tongue;
Which is the main Cause of that violent noise,
And likewise all modest Behaviour destroys.

A Balsom he has of a moderate price,
Which takes off the frowns of the Face in a trice;
And makes her as mild as the innocent Dove,
And instead of railing, she's all over Love.

He hath been above seven Weeks in the Town,
And yet of young Scolds who was given to frown,
He has cur'd above Seven hundred indeed:
And some full as bad as the Billingsgate-Breed,

There's one I will mention, liv'd near Tower-Hill,
Who would be both fighting and quarrelling still:
From night to next morning, from morning to noon,
Her Pipes I must tell you, was always in tune.

Her Husband he heard of this Doctor of fame,
Without longer tarry, faith thither he came,
With she that was call'd The invincible Shrow,
Fast bound in a Basket, for she would not go.

This Doctor he cur'd her in less than a Week,
And made her as modest, as mild, and as meek,
As any sweet Lady this day in the Land,
And so he do's all, that he e'er takes in hand.

We hear of some Quacks are for curing of Claps,
And some other common Diseases, perhaps;
But when did you hear on our vast British shore,
Of one that cou'd cure this Distemper before!

Whoever is troubl'd this day with a Scold,
Altho' she be youthful, or fourscore years old,
'Tis all one to him, if the Cure he don't do,
He'll not have so much as one penny of you.

Now rather than any that pain shall endure,
The Poor he for little or nothing will cure;
All day at his Chamber he is to be found,
Next Door to the Eel's-foot in Sallengers-Round.

Printed for J. Deacon at the Angel in Gilt-spur-street.

Figure 16.5 A ballad about a cure for a scolding wife. Breaches in marital order are a recurring theme in the few ballads that survive from seventeenth-century England. Other 'quacks cure the clap', but this one takes the sting out of a woman's tongue. *The New German Doctor: or, An Infallible Cure for a Scolding Wife* ([London]: J. Deacon, [1671–1704]), Don. B. 13 (1), by permission of the Bodleian Libraries, University of Oxford.

Children were the main purpose of a Christian marriage. Good sex contributed to a healthy marriage, healthy body and healthy society. Sex was practised outside marriage, often between couples betrothed or otherwise promised but not yet formally married, though transgressions were targeted by the English legal authorities in the early seventeenth century.[25] Sexual fidelity was part of an economy that maintained the social order, but infidelity – and anxiety about it – was rife, with different consequences for rich and poor, men and women. Marital norms were spelled out in conduct literature and sermons, and expressed in writing, pictures and speech, often in terms of inversions (Fig. 16.5). Disorderly behaviour, bodies and society were linked.

25 Faramerz Dabhoiwala, *The Origins of Sex: A History of the First Sexual Revolution* (London, 2012), p. 41.

Married couples took measures to produce healthy, beautiful children, and when they failed, various explanations and actions followed.[26] Everyone knew that fruitfulness was a divine blessing and that disease could prevent a couple from producing issue. Witches, as agents of the devil, were sometimes blamed for generative failures in humans, livestock and crops. Worried couples could use domestic remedies, magical and natural, to promote fruitfulness, counter barrenness and secure a safe delivery.[27] They also appealed to saints, went on pilgrimage to sacred sites and consulted medical practitioners in search of a new regimen or remedies to cleanse the womb and kindle heat.[28]

Aged 38, Alice Woodward told Napier that 'shee had 7 child at full tyme & yet borne still all saving her first'; she 'cannot quiet her mind because shee hath not the l[i]ke fortune that other women have' (Case 21091). By Cicely Coppingford's eighth question, Napier tagged her name, 'that had so many abortus', meaning miscarriages or stillbirths. In her mid-thirties, she had had 'eight child & seven still borne the first livinge'. Her mother-in-law was suspected of using 'evill tongues' against her, but Napier judged her case neither unnatural nor hopeless (Person 10931). Whether couples expressed fruitlessness in terms of ill fortune or vexation, the doctors read its true cause in the horoscope.

When the cause was natural, the doctors prompted women to discuss blockages and flows and, as in cases of pregnancy, they readily shared the details. Orderly menstruation signalled fruitfulness, with the expectation that pregnancy would follow soon after marriage. Married less than a year, Lady Elizabeth Mordaunt, aged 21, asked whether she would have any children. She described 'A rising in her stomacke' and 'disorderly' periods, 'very blacke' and foul smelling (Case 34846). About Judith Honour, aged 45 and married 23 years, Napier noted, 'neaver had any termes at all in her lifetyme & therfore no child' (Case 46577). Yet, Charity Barrowe 'hath her courses well', '8 yeres maryed never had her child'. Napier instilled hope in this couple: ten months later Charity's husband asked for a remedy to make her 'become fruitfull' (Person 9509).

Women's bodies were at the centre of questions about fruitfulness, but the doctors and their patients allowed for a husband's weak seed or an incompatible marriage as factors too. Mary Goddard, aged 28 and married two years, asked Forman 'whe[the]r she shall have Any Child … & whe[the]r the fault be in her or her husband'. He concluded,

26 Linda Pollock, 'Embarking on a rough passage: The experience of pregnancy in early modern society', in Valerie Fildes (ed.), *Women as Mothers in Pre-Industrial England: Essays in Memory of Dorothy McLaren* (London, 1990), pp. 39–67; Ulinka Rublack, 'Pregnancy, childbirth and the female body in early modern Germany', *Past & Present* 150 (1996), 84–110.

27 Lea T. Olsan, 'A Medieval Birth Girdle', Exhibit 11; Sandra Cavallo, 'Pregnant Stones as Wonders of Nature', Exhibit 17, this book.

28 Jacques Gélis, *History of Childbirth*, trans. Rosemary Morris (Cambridge, 1991), pp. 26–33; Park, 'Managing Childbirth and Fertility'; Peter Murray Jones, 'Generation between Script and Print', Chapter 13, this book.

'yt is overmoch drith [dryness] of her matrix is the cause she hath noe children for she hath not her course well & her husband is dry also' (Case 6280). The doctors and their clients shared a model of a healthy, fruitful body that had sufficient moisture to produce seed and nurture a child. Too much or too little heat, whether caused by exertion, emotion or obstruction, dried the body. The astrologers could help set things right. When Anne Tymcok asked Forman whether 'shee shall have anny child or noe', he judged 'her husbandes nature doeth not Agree with her they ar[e] both dry. Let her rectifie her bodie well And her husband alsoe for the gre[a]test faulte is in the man'. We do not know how Forman counselled the woman, nor whether his guidance included his prediction that 'yt seams she shall have a child by som[e] other man and not by her husband' (Case 6494). Talking about fertility could become talking about infidelity.

What Is My Disease?

Most of Forman's and Napier's clients asked, 'What is my disease?' Some of these cases associated a woman's health and generative status. The doctors and their patients shared an understanding of bodies as subject to obstruction and flow, and women's bodies as complicated by the actions of the womb.

Theologians, philosophers and physicians considered the womb a source of wonder and corruption. Church iconography and pastoral guidance told the stories of Eve and original sin, Mary and the annunciation, and the trials and blessings of other biblical and saintly women. In many writings the womb functioned as the sole determinant of a woman's health and disease. In others it was one of many factors, like the liver, that contributed to routine cleansing when it worked properly and caused corruption when it did not. Menstruation, though laden with religious and symbolic significance, was a natural part of a woman's bodily economy.[29] Some, following Galen, even argued that the menstruating female body, with its regular evacuations, was a paragon of health.[30] For the doctors and their patients, healthy women – including unmarried women from their mid-teens, married women who had not been regular since their last child and women around 50, the standard age given for the stopping of the courses – menstruated in an orderly fashion, and a woman with menstrual irregularity was unhealthy.

Forman's short treatise on diseases of women echoed physicians' and midwives' understandings while stressing the value of his experience, gleaned first-hand from

29 Joan Cadden, *Meanings of Sex Difference in the Middle Ages: Medicine, Science and Culture* (Cambridge, 1993).

30 Gianna Pomata, 'Menstruating men: Similarity and difference of the sexes in early modern medicine', in Valeria Finucci and Kevin Brownlee (eds.), *Generation and Degeneration: Tropes of Reproduction in Literature and History from Antiquity through Early Modern Europe* (Durham, NC, 2001), pp. 109–52.

midwives and other women. He explained that women who did not have their courses in due order, quantity or time had blockages that produced lumps and pains. Women with partial stoppages could have children, but a woman who was completely 'stopped' would have none and much pain.[31] In practice, when Jean Winch, in her mid-twenties, asked Forman about disease, he noted that she had pain in her back, felt grief, had never had a child and her womb was full of 'putrefaction' (Person 7960).

Blocked menses were associated with lack of children but also ill health, often manifest in swelling, oozing or bleeding in other places, especially the head or face. When Catherine Kent, aged 30, complained about her 'right eye red waterish' and 'noyse in her hed', Forman detailed the irregular actions of her womb: 'never had them but twice these two yeres from child to child' (Case 24332). Napier noted that Agnes Kent, a servant aged 34 whom a suitor had left in the lurch, had been unwell for six months with various swellings, had a headache and menstruated 'upward at her nose' (Case 11280).[32]

The doctors and their patients shared a view of women's bodies as subject to regular fluxes. Seeking the doctor's help meant entering into a negotiation for judgements and remedies to achieve a fruitful marriage. The doctor was supposed to identify whether a body was obstructed, establish the cause (grief, chill) and take measures to remove the impediments and restore flow. When a woman shared – in person, writing or by messenger – her sense of the state of her body and its order, she was entrusting the doctor with the authority to heal her, even if she might argue with him. When she asked specifically about pregnancy, she was expressing her destiny to breed and potentially opening a conversation about all that was necessary to make her fruitful, from restoring regular menstruation to enjoying sex. These conversations extended beyond what the doctors wrote down.

Conclusion

This reading of Forman's and Napier's rich yet fragmented cases confirms much of the previous scholarship. Early modern married women expected to become pregnant, monitored their bodies for signs of conception, quickening and illness, and discussed their sensations, emotions and experiences with family, friends and doctors.

31 Simon Forman, '"Matrix and the pain thereof": A sixteenth-century gynaecological essay', ed. Barbara Traister, *Medical History* 35 (1991), 436–51.

32 See also Gabriella Zuccolin and Helen King, 'Rethinking nosebleeds: Gendering spontaneous bleedings in medieval and early modern medicine', in Bonnie Lander Johnson and Eleanor Decamp (eds.), *Blood Matters: Theories of Blood in Late Medieval and Early Modern Literature and Culture* (Philadelphia, PA, 2018), pp. 79–92.

With doctors, they negotiated a judgement or treatment that made sense of the uncertainties of their bodies. Unwed women similarly monitored themselves, but were expected to try to conceal any sexual activity from doctors, who in turn reckoned to discover it. This chapter has also reconsidered the dynamics of early modern medical encounters. Forman's and Napier's authority, like that of other doctors, was modelled on their ability to answer questions about pregnancy and fertility by reading observed and reported signs. Diagnosis and divination, during the heyday of astrology and after its decline, were two sides of the same coin. Now we need a more synthetic account of the ways in which gender and generation have shaped medical encounters in other periods and places.

17 Family Resemblance in the Old Regime

Silvia De Renzi

Consider the sixteenth-century portraits of the children of Christian II of Denmark and of an anonymous family (Figs. 17.1 and 17.2). To the modern eye, the royal children share physical traits, while it is unclear whether the others were supposed to look similar. In early modern Europe, family portraits were prominent cultural artefacts, informed by powerful conventions and serving a range of social and political purposes. Showing family resemblance may or may not have been a concern. This ambiguity points to a broader issue. Examining a baby's features to recognize family resemblance is common today and the expression of a broad lay understanding of heredity. But what happened before transmission of characters became a major conceptual frame for relationships across generations? Did early modern people pay any attention to the resemblance or dissimilarity between parents and children or between siblings?

These questions have complex answers. On the one hand, early modern family letters are rich in details about newborns and children, but rarely comment on their physical appearance, except in general terms. Naming, not resemblance, established belonging and family cohesion.[1] On the other hand, physicians and natural philosophers debated the vagaries of resemblance in skin and eye colour and in diseases – discussed for the first time in scholastic medicine – and sought answers in Hippocratic, Aristotelian and Galenic theories of generation. They invoked the power of seeds but disagreed about the maternal contribution. Most argued that the imagination, a faculty held to be stronger in women, could affect children's traits and so explain even the most extreme dissimilarity, monstrosity. Such discussions continued for centuries, but historians of science have recently stressed that these did not coalesce into a 'knowledge regime of heredity' until the nineteenth century. To identify the conditions that allowed this regime to emerge, they have produced a rich account that includes early modern discourses, but emphasizes their weakness and lack of conceptual cohesion.[2] It would

1 Diane Owen Hughes, 'Representing the family: Portraits and purposes in early modern Italy', *Journal of Interdisciplinary History* 17 (1986), 7–38; Gérard Labrot, 'Hantise généalogique, jeux d'alliances, souci esthétique: Le portrait dans les collections de l'aristocratie napolitaine (XVIe–XVIIIe siècles)', *Revue Historique* 284 (1990), 281–304; Christiane Klapisch-Zuber, *Women, Family, and Ritual in Renaissance Italy*, trans. Lydia Cochrane (Chicago, IL, 1985); Benedetta Borello, 'I segni del corpo: Fratelli, sorelle e somiglianze nelle famiglie italiane (XVII–XVIII secolo)', *Quaderni Storici* 145 (2014), 9–40.

2 Staffan Müller-Wille and Hans-Jörg Rheinberger (eds.), *Heredity Produced: At the Crossroads of Biology, Politics, and Culture, 1500–1870* (Cambridge, MA, 2007), p. 15.

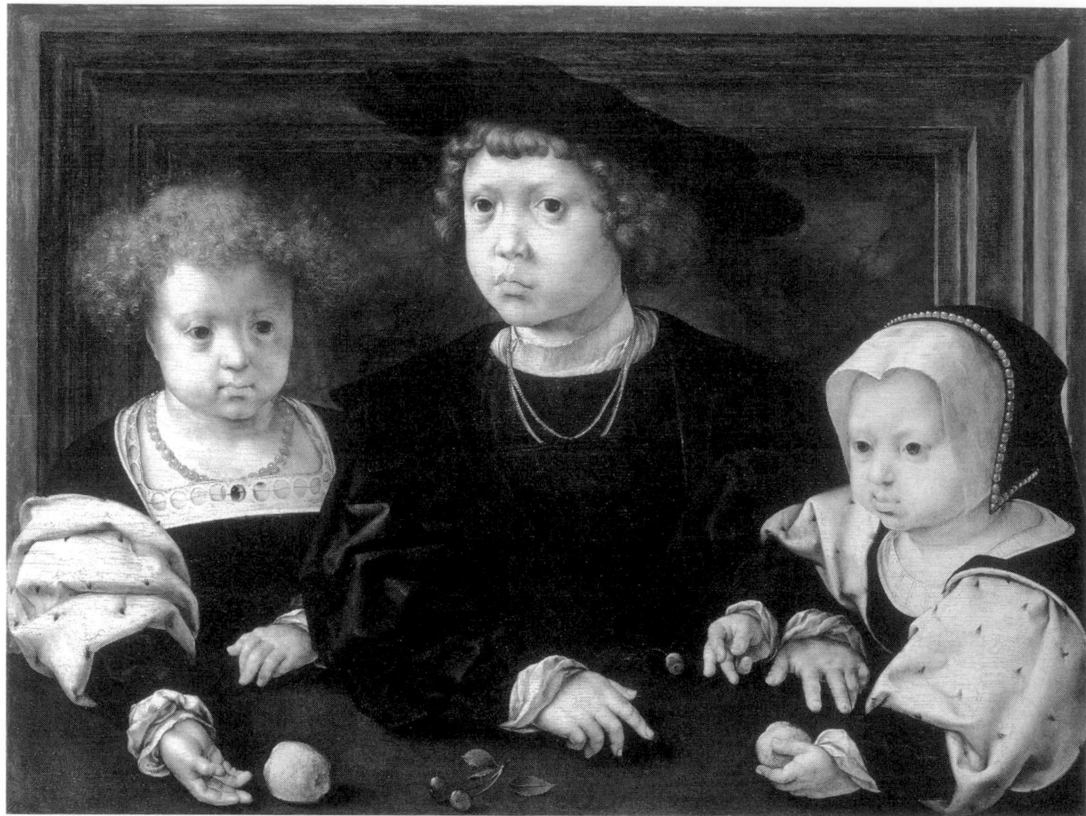

Figure 17.1 Jan Gossaert, *The Children of Christian II, King of Denmark* (*c.* 1526). Strong conventions guided representations of children, but this painting – of children in mourning for their mother – suggests that these could coexist with the perception of, and the intention to express, shared family traits. Oil on oak panel, 34 × 46 cm, Windsor Castle, Bridgeman Images.

be possible to conclude that the early modern history of family resemblance is one of scattered learned debates with little impact on people's experience and negligible epistemological power.

Taking a different tack, this chapter explores how medico-philosophical debates over resemblance were mobilized to respond to deep social and political anxieties. The origins of nobility were of pressing concern in medieval society.[3] In later centuries, apprehension over social taxonomy grew following the expansion of a new aristocracy, the aspiration of professional and mercantile classes to join it, and financial difficulties within the older nobility. At the same time, the stricter discipline imposed on marriage by the church, especially in the decrees of the Council of Trent, had implications in

3 Maaike van der Lugt and Charles de Miramon (eds.), *L'hérédité entre Moyen Âge et Époque moderne: Perspectives historiques* (Florence, 2008).

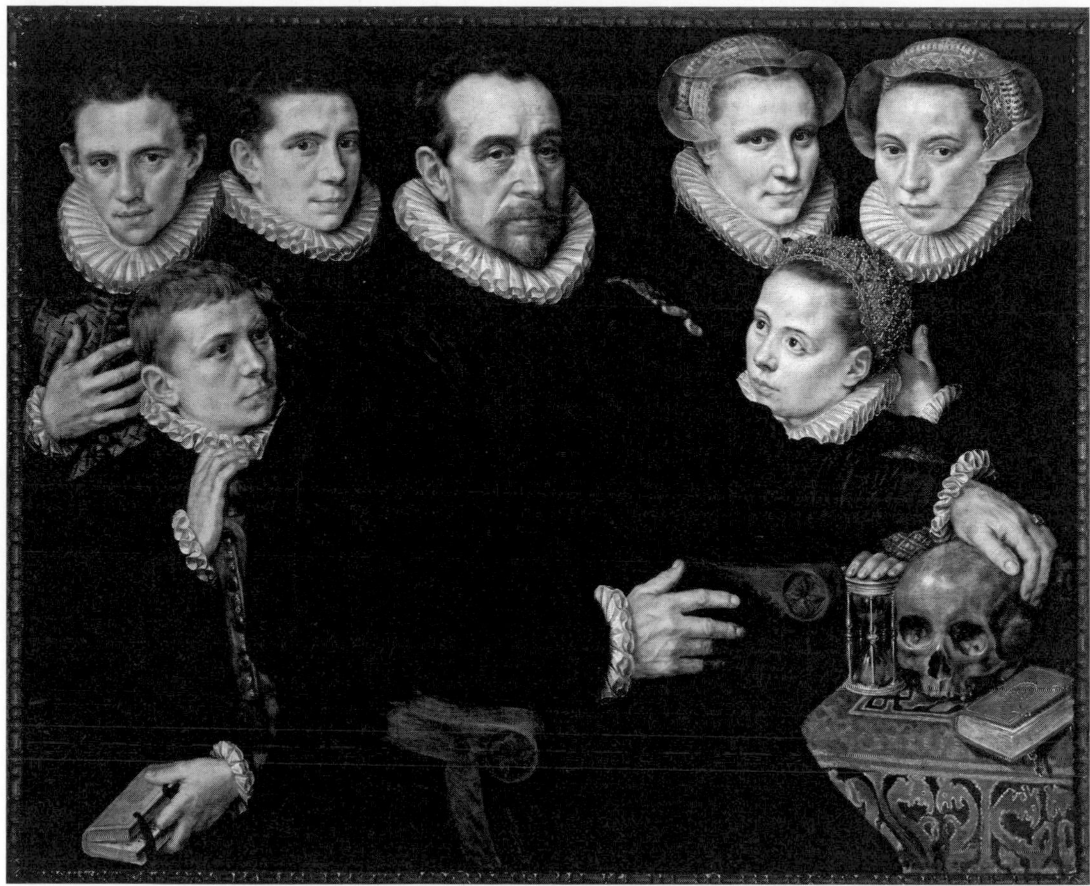

Figure 17.2 Adriaen Thomasz Key, *Family Portrait* (1583). Built around the father's central figure, this family group includes children of different ages and symbols of life's transience. We may perceive shared physical traits, but it is hard to say whether or not representing family resemblance was one of the painter's aims. Oil on panel, 92 × 115 cm, Museo Nacional del Prado, Madrid, akg-images / Erich Lessing.

legal disputes over paternity. Social order in the old regime was bolstered by laws regulating access to family resources, including primogeniture and controversial regulations about illegitimate children. Individuals conceptualized and experienced their relationships to their fathers, ancestors and families within these legal and cultural frameworks; and here, I argue, we gain access to the multifaceted social and political meanings of the dyad of resemblance and dissimilarity. This means bringing into focus the historically specific nexus between 'generation' as a natural process and the socially defined relationships between generations. By the same token, we can ask to what extent late eighteenth-century challenges to the social order transformed perceptions and concepts. While focusing on the continuity between the late sixteenth and the seventeenth centuries, I also sketch areas for research on this later period.

Scholars have discussed the ways in which resemblance shaped Renaissance understandings of nature; but there is no specific literature on the history of family resemblance. Extensive work on the origins of nobility and provision for illegitimate children often advises against generalization. The chapter accordingly takes a case-study approach, focused on the Spanish kingdom and the Italian states. Both were characterized by intense debates about rank and honour and by physicians' long-standing presence in the political arena. If not representative of all Europe, they are ideal sites for an in-depth exploration of the old regime.

Ranking People

Between the mid-sixteenth and the mid-seventeenth century, socially diverse authors wrote extensively on honour and nobility. Arguing for the moral superiority of nobility, some claimed that this was based on blood and the long succession of 'generous' semen. However, since the late middle ages the hegemony of the knightly code had been challenged by the alternative opinion that nobility lay in individual virtue, not lineage; nobility could be an exceptional combination of spiritual or intellectual qualities and achievements that did not belong only to the highest ranks. Over time these disputes became entwined with use of ennoblement by absolutist princes as a financial and political tool. Could nobility be acquired by a legal act ratifying recent success? Did it lie in an innate set of qualities? Or in the venerable past? Pressed to identify ancestry, families across Europe produced family trees and patents of nobility.[4] Ruthless policies of exclusion from power and office also exposed generation as a social and natural process: a college of physicians admitted an apothecary's son only because a jurist had adopted him; his new filiation transcended the limitations of his modest (but not too modest) pedigree.[5] The place of resemblance in these debates and their potential to reach diverse audiences is illustrated by a controversy in print between two Italian literati who lived and wrote in the decades around 1600. Ludovico Zuccolo was an unconventional political writer while Alessandro Tassoni is known for his eclectic literary work. Both stemmed from the provincial nobility and addressed the concerns of educated, but not specialized, readers.[6]

Picking a path amongst competing ideas, Zuccolo argued that nobility resides neither in the possession of wealth nor in noble descent, but in the innate disposition to

4 André Devyver, *Le sang épuré: Les préjugés de race chez les gentilshommes français de l'Ancien Régime (1560–1720)* (Brussels, 1973); Enrique Soria Mesa, *La nobleza en la España moderna: Cambio y continuidad* (Madrid, 2007); Charles de Miramon, 'Aux origines de la noblesse et des princes du sang: France et Angleterre au XIVe siècle', in van der Lugt and de Miramon, *L'hérédité*, pp. 157–210. See also Margot E. Fassler, 'The Tree of Jesse', Exhibit 8, this book.

5 Alessandro Pastore, 'L'onore della corporazione: Il collegio medico di Verona fra il tardo Quattrocento e gli inizi del Seicento', in *Studi di storia per Luigi Ambrosoli* (Verona, 1993), pp. 7–28, on p. 9.

6 On their exchange, Claudio Donati, *L'idea di nobiltà in Italia: Secoli XIV–XVIII* (Bari, 1988).

perform honourable deeds.[7] The appeal to nature commonly justified the link between blood and nobility in aristocratic pedigrees; agreeing that nobility is innate, Zuccolo invoked nature – but to maintain that men with a noble disposition can emerge anew. Nobility is like beauty: although most of the time beautiful parents give birth to handsome offspring, they can bear deformed children. Equally, beautiful children can be born from ugly parents because purer and more delicate spirits, which are not 'poured' from grandparents to parents, can appear in their children; 'poured' (*transfusi*) alerts us to the range of metaphors used to express the passage of traits through generations. The reference to grandparents evoked lineage, but Zuccolo insisted that breaks occur. Showing the vagaries of the process, discontinuity also materializes in moral dissimilarity between fathers and sons: honourable fathers can produce disreputable children. While explaining deterioration in terms of deficiency of matter or accidents to a pregnant woman, Zuccolo did not clarify the mechanism behind improvement – the birth of children with an innately noble disposition to non-noble parents. But this was no gradual purging of bad traits through generations, as often the noble disposition was more robust in the first of a family who possessed it. Nobility, he explained, can be lost through bad habits, but never acquired in the absence of this innate disposition.

While conceding that children generally resemble their parents, it was the opposite phenomenon of children not resembling their parents, in physical beauty or moral disposition, that created the space within which writers like Zuccolo could advocate social mobility. New noble families replace the old, he claimed, like waves upon the shore.

The poet and essayist Alessandro Tassoni deplored the social disorder that would result from Zuccolo's disregard for families' nobility: children of slaves or Jews could claim it.[8] Quoting Aristotle, Tassoni argued that nobility is a quality not of individuals, but primarily of families. When claims to it are vetted, historical and legal evidence, not individual traits, have to be scrutinized. Polemically, Tassoni maintained that otherwise doctors, not noblemen, should be the assessors; but he argued that temperament (a doctor's remit) indicates health not nobility. This social understanding of nobility coexisted with the seemingly contradictory acknowledgement that the noble enjoy 'clarity of blood'.

Tassoni's wrestling with the relationships between nature and history was not exceptional and should alert us to the perceived differences between visible and invisible layers of nature and between kinds of temperament, to which I will return. The question of continuity in generation was also pressing. Tassoni mobilized the well-known anecdote of the white woman who gives birth to a white daughter from a black man. Marrying a white man, the daughter has a black child. This, Tassoni explained, demonstrates that the seed contains the qualities not only of the parents, but also of

7 Ludovico Zuccolo, *Nobiltà commune et heroica, pensier nuovo e curioso* (Venice, 1625).

8 The definitive edition of Tassoni's *Dieci libri di pensieri diversi* came out in 1620; I used the version in *Pensieri e scritti preparatori*, ed. Pietro Puliatti (Modena, 1986), especially pp. 519–22, 705–15.

the lineage: resemblance can be interrupted and then restored. Although this example pivoted on resemblance of skin colour, the implications were broader.

Pervasive concerns over the nature of nobility were discussed in print, manuscript and oral exchanges. Revealing the political relevance of complex theories of generation, they show that key concepts such as temperament and blood were multilayered and contested.[9] Sitting at the heart of these debates, the question of resemblance, or the lack thereof, intersected with ongoing reflections on the sources of individual and family identity.

One question had long bothered male literati – why wise men, such as Cicero, could generate children like his allegedly dim-witted son. To the explanation that men of great intellectual vigour tended to have weak semen and so children who did not resemble them, Tassoni objected that this did not account for why stupid parents sometimes bore bright children. He argued rather that children fail when they are forced into a life that does not suit them. Soldiers' sons may have different dispositions from their fathers and, rather than being chastised, these differences should be cultivated through an appropriate education. The issue was socially charged, as Tassoni knew only too well.

Troubled by his own contested origins, Tassoni was anguished by the failings of the son he had had by a humble woman and legally recognized. Bequeathing a small sum to the boy, Tassoni admitted to doubts, since the child did not resemble him at all, 'at least in his habits'. At a time when poor noblemen were thought to tarnish their blood by marrying down, he was resigned to accepting the product of his demeaning relationship, but keen to stress the lack of moral and social resemblance with his offspring – perhaps despite a physical one. I will come back to proofs of paternity, but Tassoni's appeal to dissimilarity in his mixed paternal feelings is striking. As the son progressed to become a respected army man, Tassoni added him to his will.[10]

Tassoni's comments on education reveal another side of the debate. At a time when professions often ran in families, the management of children's aptitudes within strategies for prosperity shaped experiences of resemblance and dissimilarity. The question intersected with the identification of talents, an issue to which the physician Juan Huarte de San Juan had given careful consideration in his 1575 treatise on the variety of human nature. Among the most widely read texts of Renaissance medicine, Huarte's book was one of Zuccolo's and Tassoni's common sources. Exploring it means moving back in time.[11]

9 Joseph Ziegler, 'Hérédité et physiognomonie', in van der Lugt and de Miramon, *L'hérédité*, pp. 245–71.

10 Antonino Bertolotti, 'I testamenti di Alessandro Tassoni', *Rivista Europea, Rivista Internazionale* 8 (1877), 673–80.

11 Juan Huarte, *Examen de ingenios para las sciencias* (Baez, 1575); references are to the English translation, *The Examination of Mens Wits* (London, 1594); Véronique Duché-Gavet (ed.), *Juan Huarte au XXIe siècle: Actes de colloque* (Anglet, 2003).

Fathers and Sons

A minor noble and town doctor in Andalusia, Huarte promoted medicine as offering answers to growing social and political concerns. In the diverse Spanish monarchy, the preoccupation with purity of race (*limpieza de sangre*) exacerbated tensions between competing sources of rank and identity – traditional privilege and wealth. Endorsing a materialist understanding of the intellectual faculties and the humanist emphasis on education, Huarte offered a simple solution to the vexed question of how young men should choose a career.[12] Children should be directed to the path within the profession – medicine, the law or the church – that requires the combination of faculties in which they naturally excel. For example, within the law, lecturing requires a strong memory while a powerful intellect is necessary for a practising lawyer. Huarte assumed that the material make-up of the individual brain, including degrees of heat, shapes aptitude by determining which of the key faculties prevails – imagination, memory or intellect.

There was no point, Huarte insisted, in forcing a boy with a strong imagination to take up a profession that needed a powerful intellect. We may wonder how his numerous readers across Europe implemented his instruction to assess inclinations. This strong materialist strand coexisted with an emphasis on the ability of individuals to better themselves. Reviewing the controversies over the origins of nobility, Huarte claimed that great achievements by ancestors could lead to a kind of nobility (*hidalguia*) that was then passed down the generations. This was a process of rebirth, as old fathers and identities were shed: 'Yesterday he was called the sonne of Peter, and nephew of Sanchius, and now he is named the sonne of his owne actions.'[13] Complicating his own deterministic approach, this position met the Christian demand to preserve free will: material make-up may define individual fate, but does not preclude initiative. Implicitly building on the notion of habit as second nature, Huarte argued that change can even affect the temperament: manners acquired with social betterment increase humidity which in turn alters behaviour and intellectual faculties.[14]

What place did resemblance have in a medico-political project shaped by the tensions between the determinism of nature and the celebration of change? Huarte examined two main sides of the question: resemblance within what we would now call ethnic groups, and the resemblance of children to parents.[15] Drawing on the recently revitalized

12 Renata Ago, 'Young nobles in the age of absolutism: Paternal authority and freedom of choice in seventeenth-century Italy', in Giovanni Levi and Jean-Claude Schmitt (eds.), *A History of Young People in the West* (Cambridge, MA, 1997), vol. 1, pp. 283–322.

13 Huarte, *Examination*, p. 223.

14 Ibid., p. 60; Maaike van der Lugt, 'L'autorité morale et normative de la nature au Moyen Âge', in van der Lugt (ed.), *La nature comme source de la morale au Moyen Âge* (Florence, 2014), pp. 3–40.

15 On the concept of race: Renato G. Mazzolini, 'Colonialism and the Emergence of Racial Theories', Chapter 25, this book.

Hippocratic tradition, he argued that the former is the product of the environment. Northern people share fair skin and hair because the cold climate preserves a wet temperament. In the received view, this basic mechanism is altered when people move to a new environment. Like plants and animals, Huarte explained, humans respond by taking up new characters. However, overturning the debate on purity of race, Huarte used Jewish history to show that characters can persist for generations, despite relocation. Having lived in the desert and eaten manna for just forty years, the Jews had acquired a choleric temperament that made them brilliant doctors. Hundreds of years later, now living in countries with different climates, they still shone as physicians and were renowned for their wit. The seed is very strong, Huarte claimed, 'when it receiveth thereinto any well rooted qualitie'. Qualities can be acquired and lost, however, and a Hippocratic anecdote helped him explore this reversibility. When the nobles of a country started to prize elongated heads as their distinctive feature, they swaddled newborn babies to achieve the desired shape. Noble children started to be born with elongated heads and 'this artificialnesse grew to such force, as it was converted into nature'. Yet when the practice stopped, heads reverted to the old shape. The story dramatized the complex relationship between natural and acquired traits; readers concerned with the nature and visibility of their families' origins and rank would have appreciated its political relevance.[16]

Discussing the resemblance of children to parents, Huarte challenged the widespread belief that maternal imagination can affect generation. Parental resemblance, he explained, is driven by forces in the seed upon which the imagination has no power.[17] In Galenism, the seed is the final product of concoction and maintains the characteristics of the food ingested. Unlike animals, humans have a varied diet and this is why their offspring do not always resemble their parents. Endowed with various qualities, the seed is responsible for similarity or dissimilarity and, to rephrase Huarte's materialist argument, we are what our parents ate. Because poor people feed on coarse food, they tend to have dull children, wrote Huarte, while implying that they could escape that fate.[18]

To Huarte's socially select readers, the question was how to have the offspring they desired: intellect was at a premium, and patriarchal values meant that sons, not daughters, should be conceived. To achieve this goal, Huarte issued detailed instructions, including dietary advice and basic rules about how, when and with whom to have children. Guidance of this kind had been common since the middle ages, but two

16 Huarte, *Examination*, pp. 199, 195. These tensions are encapsulated in advice to a young aristocrat that to prove himself worthy of his blood he should acquire the taste for literature appropriate to a prince: Roberto Zapperi, 'Odoardo Farnese, principe e cardinale', in *Les Carrache et les décors profanes* (Rome, 1988), pp. 335–58, on p. 337.

17 Huarte, *Examination*, pp. 263–333.

18 For recent twists on such arguments: Tatjana Buklijas, 'Developmental Origins of Health and Disease', Exhibit 39, this book.

aspects of Huarte's advice are worth stressing. First, following the tradition of framing generation as a competition between male and female seed, he explained that physical traits such as nostrils, eyes, mouth and forehead can take the shape of either parent, depending on whose seed is stronger. Yet, if the struggle is unresolved, a child could be born with unmatched pairs of ears or eyes. This shows a sensitivity to physical features that is consistent with the rich taxonomies in books on physiognomy.[19]

Second, to ensure that the father's traits prevail, seed should be produced which, hot and rich with the qualities that secure the desired aptitude, will win out; abstaining from sex for a few days and maintaining the right diet were critical. This emphasis on food and the selection of a suitable partner – a woman's temperament was an indication of proclivity to generate – strengthened the parents' contribution, weakening the power of progenitors' traits. A contemporary tract on midwifery insisted that children resemble their ancestors when during intercourse the mother thinks of them: imagination could disrupt but also ensure resemblance and thus reinforce family relationships.[20] By contrast, denying the role of imagination and focusing on food and sexual hygiene facilitated Huarte's penchant for new beginnings, allowing him almost to discount ancestors.

Perceived as the expression of gender competition, resemblance also revealed the antagonism between natural processes and social conventions. Endorsing time-honoured views, Huarte explained that the illegitimate are more similar to their fathers because they are the product of adulterous, passionate sex, while frequent intercourse in married life weakens the male seed, making children more similar to their mothers. Since the middle ages, 'bastards' had been glamorized, but the laws regulating the status of children born out of wedlock – if not noble – were strict and unforgiving, though concessions were made to ensure basic welfare.[21] Morally castigated, the cohabitation of unmarried people was common in early modern society, as were sexual relationships between servants and masters, and prostitution. Legitimacy could change destiny, but when cases came to court, jurists expected paternity to be extremely hard to prove. Moving from Spain to Rome and the Sacra Rota, one of the most authoritative ecclesiastical tribunals, allows me to discuss resemblance as evidence.

Whose Child?

Over the centuries, a consensus had emerged among jurists that made the following evidence the most reliable in paternity disputes: what most people thought about the

19 Giovanni Ingegneri, *Fisionomia naturale* (Padua, 1626).

20 Scipione Mercurio, *La comare o ricoglitrice* (Venice, 1596), p. 48, refers to physical defects as examples of shared traits passed to children by maternal imagination.

21 Thomas Kuehn, *Illegitimacy in Renaissance Florence* (Ann Arbor, MI, 2002); Matthew Gerber, *Bastards: Politics, Family, and Law in Early Modern France* (Oxford, 2012).

relationship between the alleged parents, the behaviour of the alleged father towards the child, including the name he had chosen, the mother's reputation and, finally, documents such as parish records of the baptism.[22] Jurists had considered the evidentiary weight of resemblance, but, with some exceptions, had mostly expressed reservations on account of the maternal imagination: a child's resemblance to a man could be the effect of the mother thinking of him rather than of his physical presence during the act. By the mid-seventeenth century, judges of the Sacra Rota based their sentences on social rather than natural evidence of paternity. As a few cases show, however, the parties and witnesses sometimes urged judges to consider resemblance.

Claiming that her daughter from an adulterous relationship should be granted rights to the alleged father's wealth, a woman in late sixteenth-century Rome built her case on the man's affection for the girl, including that he called her 'my daughter'. But a witness also testified to a certain resemblance between father and daughter. Whether the witness had been advised that this could count or had projected his assumption, this shows that perception of physical resemblance had currency outside the court and could be mobilized inside. Physical resemblance could be claimed not generically, but, revealing attention to specific traits, on the basis of shared hair colour and shape of mouth, nose, eyes and chin between children and alleged fathers. It was also contested. When the relatives of a cleric challenged a girl's claims that she was his daughter and had a right to a dowry, they objected that the resemblance maintained by three witnesses had no weight because it could have resulted from the mother's imagination. The doctor consulted to resolve the disagreement, Paolo Zacchia, argued, like Huarte, that the imagination, an animal faculty, could not interfere with the activities of the natural faculty responsible for the formation of a child. Resemblance should carry evidentiary weight.

A cautious operator, elsewhere Zacchia qualified his assertion with a theoretical discussion of resemblance, admitting the efficacy of the imagination, but only if repeated: a child born after his or her father's death tended to resemble him because the widow thought of her husband so much.[23] Comparing children's features with those of their late fathers may have been relatively common in grieving families, or a means to assess dubious paternity.

To find reliable evidence for paternity disputes, Zacchia turned deeper into the body to the process by which the heat of the parents' seed determined a child's innate temperament. Resemblance between parents and children could not be modified here; this internal resemblance manifested itself not in physical traits, but in moral disposition and diseases, features unaffected by the imagination. It may seem strange to us that

22 What follows draws on Silvia De Renzi, 'Resemblance, paternity and imagination in early modern courts', in Müller-Wille and Rheinberger, *Heredity Produced*, pp. 61–83.

23 Paolo Zacchia, *Quaestionum medico-legalium tomus prior* (Lyons, 1661), p. 98.

courage or irascibility should provide such strong evidence of paternity, but Zacchia also discussed resemblance in diseases as one of the most genuine expressions of temperaments shared between parents and children. In this he drew on and contributed to the growing interest in hereditary diseases. His view of a deeper level at which resemblance is situated may have been the more technical version of Tassoni's conviction that nobility is an invisible quality of blood rather than of the temperament.[24]

Eighteenth-Century Debates over Generation and the End of the Old Regime

In the late seventeenth century, the debate on generation quickened pace, and soon philosophers and physicians clashed over the competing theories of epigenesis (individuals start as unformed material and forms develop over time) and pre-existence (individuals grow from forms pre-existing in the egg or the male semen). Though resemblance remained hard to explain, it was more easily seen as the result of the mixing of seeds from both parents than in the mere unfolding of an already organized form. But those endorsing pre-existence invoked the role of male semen in initiating the development of the germ, a process during which resemblance could also be imprinted.[25] Scholars have discussed these debates at length, but as I have shown, resemblance had far wider social and political relevance. Exploring how it was explained in a broader range of arenas offers a fresh perspective on the implications of technical discussions.

Endorsing pre-existence, Albrecht von Haller, one of the main protagonists of the epigenesis–pre-existence dispute, challenged the reality of children's resemblance to their parents and, when lecturing on legal medicine at the University of Göttingen in the 1750s, disputed the power of the imagination. Law courts then favoured the stability of families over the establishment of the truth in paternity controversies; Haller's involvement in this field and his family relationship with Friedrich Teichmeyer, a recognized authority, would have made him aware of the complex interactions between knowledge, the law and social expectations in matters of generation.[26]

What remains to be explored is the extent to which the ongoing debates on resemblance and generation interacted with the changes brought about by the erosion of the pillars of the old regime – fathers' authority and privilege by blood. The question

24 Thanks to Maaike van der Lugt for alerting me to this; see further van der Lugt, 'Formed Fetuses and Healthy Children in Scholastic Theology, Medicine and Law', Chapter 12, this book.

25 Mary Terrall, 'Speculation and experiment in Enlightenment life sciences', in Müller-Wille and Rheinberger, *Heredity Produced*, pp. 253–75.

26 Esther Fischer-Homberger, 'On the medical history of the doctrine of imagination', *Psychological Medicine* 9 (1979), 619–28; Sara Paulson Eigen, 'A mother's love, a father's line: Law, medicine and the eighteenth-century fictions of patrilineal genealogy', in Kilian Heck and Bernhard Jahn (eds.), *Genealogie als Denkform in Mittelalter und Früher Neuzeit* (Tübingen, 2000), pp. 87–107.

of hereditary diseases – Zacchia's deepest kind of resemblance – revealed its political sting when in the eighteenth century the focus turned to diseases in noble families.[27] Resemblance to fathers and ancestors became particularly tricky when sons rebelled. How to square fathers' and sons' political opposition with the force of a shared lineage, for instance, troubled the biographer of the Mirabeau family, marked by the clash between revolutionary son Honoré Gabriel and old-regime father Victor.[28]

Conclusion

Early modern families may have forged links with their new members symbolically rather than by perceiving physical resemblance: bearing a name from within the family stock established and signalled belonging, and in law a father's attitude to a natural child counted more than physical traits. Research on ego-documents and visual sources may enrich this picture, but this chapter has explored areas of social practice where the voices of experts more easily mixed with those of interested, though not specialist, parties, from literati to ordinary people seeking justice. Recapturing the distinctive role played by the dyad of resemblance and dissimilarity between parents and children in discourses and practices critical to the old regime opens a new perspective on the cultural history of heredity.

Resemblance and dissimilarity were explained using a cluster of concepts that, contested in medical and philosophical debates, had wide currency: the potency of physical make-up in the identities of individuals and groups; the malleability of nature and the complex relationships between temperament and habit; the ambiguous link between moral and physical traits; the interaction of visible and invisible qualities; and the safeguarding of free will. Ambiguous as it was, resemblance was rooted in these wide-ranging reflections and served different actors' personal, political and social agendas. It may have stood for social order, as when noble parents begot allegedly noble children, and yet everyone knew that generation could be erratic. For many, the challenge was to manage the resulting diversity within family strategies, and unpredictability could also justify social mobility. Advice on good breeding allowed fathers a degree of control, confirming that at the heart of discussions on resemblance lay the multifaceted and complex relationships between generation and generations in the old regime.

27 Carlos López-Beltrán, 'Les *haereditarii morbi* au début de l'Époque moderne', in van der Lugt and de Miramon, *L'hérédité*, pp. 321–51.

28 Laura Casella, '"Comment, en dix ans, ce démon d'une famille est-il devenu le dieu d'une nation? Question profonde!" Storia familiare e storia politica nella storiografia ottocentesca sui Mirabeau', *Cheiron*, no. 49 (2008 [2010]), 137–57; Nick Hopwood, 'The Keywords "Generation" and "Reproduction"', Chapter 20, this book.

18 The Emergence of Population

Philip Kreager

Over the past two centuries, social research on human populations has increasingly focused on the demographics of fertility and mortality. 'Population problems' are now usually assumed to be issues such as whether birth-rates are too high (in stereotyped 'developing' countries) or too low (in 'developed' ones).[1] These concerns are bound up with the priority that modern cultures give to economic growth, and reflect inequalities of supply and demand on which differential rates may have an impact: welfare and health provision, education, ageing, immigration. The usual frame of reference is the nation-state, although states are composed of sub-populations – communities, regions, labour sectors, ethnicities, socio-economic strata – in which the economic rationality of fertility control may play out differently and is often not primary. Local realities are hard to discern from the top-down perspective of national census and survey units, which follow legal and statistical conventions rather than community experience and identities. Indeed, when we adopt the perspective of the latter, the direction of influence usually reverses: differing levels of reproduction and mortality, rather than responding directly to the rationality of supply and demand, become contingent on many compromises that individuals and groups make as members of sub-populations in which they live. Across Europe, different sub-populations respond differently to challenges including the disappearance of regional industries, deficiencies in job creation, obstacles to migration, inadequate housing and changing gender norms.

In the era before the nineteenth-century rise of national statistics, we find a conception of population that was more attentive to the heterogeneity of sub-populations and its importance. Early modern population thinking did not standardize populations, nor pretend to treat them equally. Distinctive histories and political, cultural and religious differences were recognized to shape what numerical information should be collected, on which groups, and its interpretation. From the sixteenth to the early nineteenth century, balancing the heterogeneity of memberships making up the population of a state was a fundamental ground of the form and legitimacy of government, and of arguments for democracy. Population arithmetic and related probabilistic models of population began in the mid-seventeenth century in an attempt to articulate these issues, stimulating wide exploration of different sorts of populations over the next

1 Alison Bashford, 'World Population from Eugenics to Climate Change', Chapter 34, this book.

century and a half. While numbering births and deaths emerged as fundamental to what came to be known as 'political arithmetic', this did not prioritize the narrow focus on fertility and mortality that has become the hallmark of nineteenth- and twentieth-century demography.

Early modern population thinking is thus of interest on two counts. First, it reminds us of a fruitful way of thinking about aggregate properties of societies and states, different from the one we now take for granted. Its open, bottom-up reasoning about human numbers focused on how sub-populations are formed, sustained and compromised in relation to others and to wider forces. This approach to population has again become critical, not only in research on social and environmental adaptation, migration and ethnicity, but also in evolutionary biology and genetics.[2] In this chapter, however, we focus on the earliest systematic and quantitative inquiries into population, asking how these came into being and why. Rooted in classical and humanist ideas of polity and society as composed of diverse but linked memberships, this understanding of human numbers emphasized relative proportion and balance amongst groups. The use of enumeration and calculation to demonstrate such balances began in England, spreading rapidly to the Netherlands and France, and thence to the rest of Europe. For reasons of space, the focus here is on England. In short, classical population thinking created a place for numerical methods and was only displaced by approaches prioritizing fertility from the turn of the eighteenth century. The second interest of early population thinking arises from this contrast, which clarifies the existence of two very different conceptualizations of reproduction and of population in modern European history.

The Generation of a Commonwealth

In *Leviathan* (1651), Thomas Hobbes's now famous defence of kingly rule, he developed a distinction between vital and voluntary human actions: the former, 'begun in generation', are bodily functions like breathing and eating; the latter, characterized by speaking and thinking, are no less natural, but develop as imaginative faculties arising from association with other men.[3] Association begins in families and relations within and between them, expanding with their relations to members of other groups; the 'generation of a commonwealth' is the act by which states are formed as local patterns of association become bound up in the need for peace and security. Because human association leads inevitably to conflict, 'the multitude' can live peaceably only by relying on either 'one Man or [an] Assembly of men, to beare their Person', that is to

2 Philip Kreager *et al.* (eds.), *Population in the Human Sciences: Concepts, Models, Evidence* (Oxford, 2015).
3 Thomas Hobbes, *Leviathan*, ed. Richard Tuck (Cambridge, 1991), pp. 37–8.

co-ordinate and represent the will of the people as a whole.[4] In this 'Generation of the great LEVIATHAN' we have a direct analogy at the level of the state to the classical Greek conception of generation as a process in which parents actively create their offspring. Hobbes provided a concise image of the body politic to demonstrate this (Fig. 18.1). The multitude make up the arms and body of the monarch, their volume constituting his military and civil strength; the sword and sceptre he wields, together with the compartments showing allegorical subjects under each, represent the principal domains of sovereign authority.

Hobbes was following a model of polity laid down in classical sources, especially Aristotle's *Politics*, which continued as the foundation of humanist political discourse and the emerging human sciences well into the eighteenth century.[5] Collective organization arises from families or households, and groups formed by alliances between them. Such groups have their own distinctive character, or *ethos*, consequent on differences produced in the natural and social processes of their association. They can choose alternative forms of government according to a simple numerical logic: Hobbes's government by 'one Man' forming a monarchy; assemblies of 'best' men, or citizens, forming an aristocracy; and participation of the whole multitude, a democracy (not an option Hobbes countenanced). Monarchies and aristocracies are hierarchical, the natural history of association among elite groups in a commonwealth and their habituation in sharing an *ethos* making them not merely distinctive but naturally and politically incommensurable to other groups. This incommensurability exercised a profound influence over the emergence and development of population arithmetic.

'Population' was not a normative term in Hobbes's time, but the processes of group generation laid down in the classical model nonetheless carried implications for how groups could combine to form a state. First, populations are open; association continually leads to the incorporation of outsiders, to the departure of some members, and to collective action uniting (or subjugating) various groups. Second, the analogy to 'generation' in what we would now call the demography of the several sub-populations in a state was not just or even primarily concerned with procreation. To develop and gain influence, polities had to structure and expand their numbers by several sorts of association: by absorbing immigrants; by gaining control of adjacent populations through war, elite marriage or treaty; and by extending influence and capital through trade and colonization. These avenues were of more immediate practical importance than the gradual increment or decline of population due to fertility.[6]

4 Ibid., p. 120; Peter Biller, 'The Multitude in Later Medieval Thought', Chapter 10, this book.

5 Philip Kreager, 'Aristotle and open population thinking', *Population and Development Review* 34 (2008), 599–629; for earlier uses of the *Politics*: Biller, 'Multitude'.

6 Rebecca Flemming, 'States and Populations in the Classical World', Chapter 5, this book.

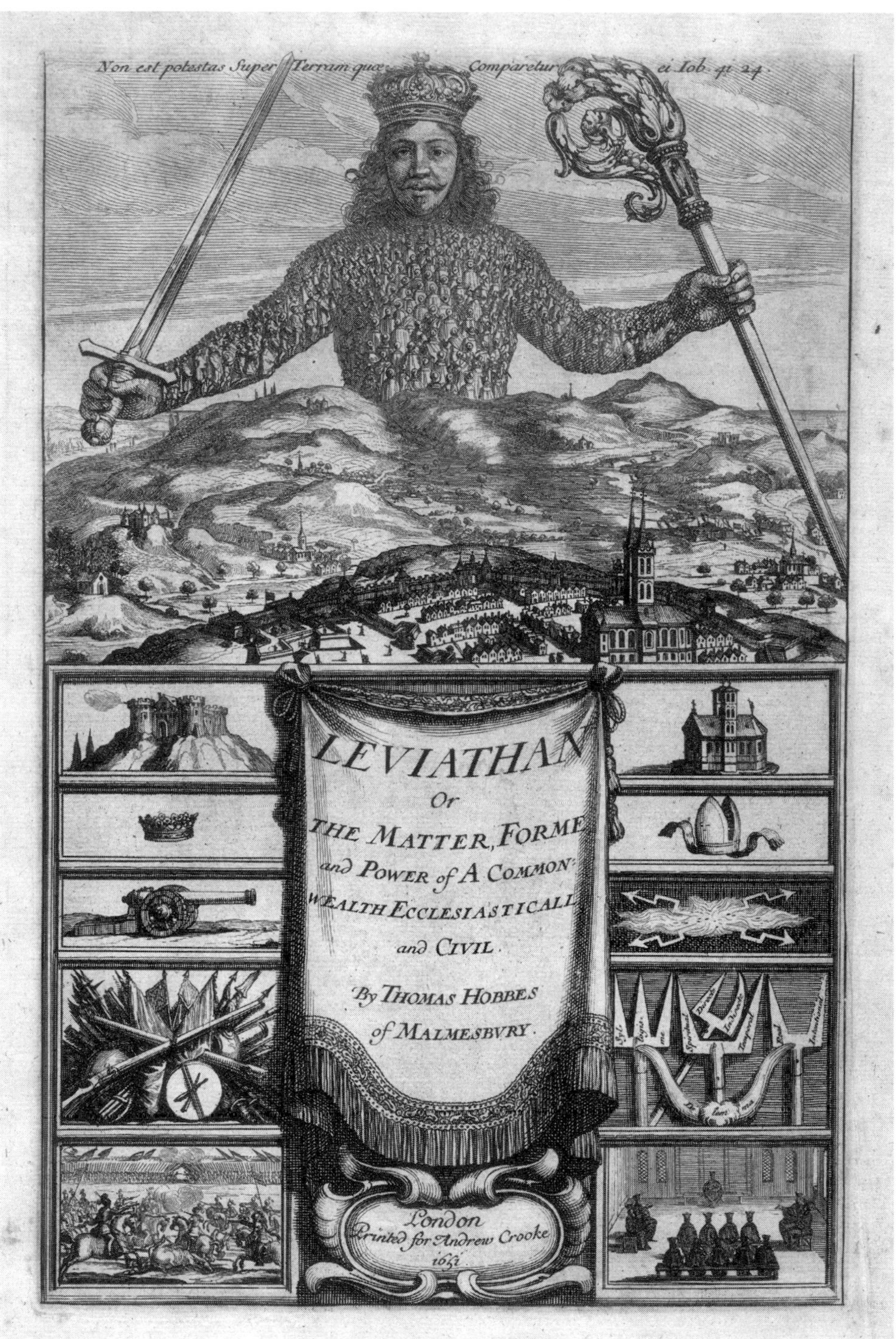

Figure 18.1 Frontispiece to Thomas Hobbes, *Leviathan, or The Matter, Forme, and Power of a Commonwealth Ecclesiasticall and Civil* (London: [by Roger Norton and Richard Cotes] for Andrew Crooke, 1651). Cambridge University Library.

Incommensurability enters here as a third premise because people incorporated into a state rather than born as citizens generally had different rights and statuses. From the Athenian and Roman republics through Renaissance city-states to early modern nations and empires, privileged lineages defined citizen sub-populations (nobility and established families) that were considered superior. The population that mattered was not an aggregate, but a membership built by association through networks of shared *ethos.*

Incommensurability in turn shaped the manner in which population was treated quantitatively. The key issue was not size or strength in numbers, but the strength of ties and reliability of association – the effectiveness and loyalty of networks led by the privileged – that determined the ability of a sub-population or state to develop and secure itself. Censuses were undertaken from time to time, but the modern, statistical assumption that all individuals should be counted regularly and equivalently was not a serious proposition. Mixing up citizens – with their intricate and powerful ties of association through birth, marriage and property – with the multitude of peasants, tradesmen, servants, resident aliens and slaves was natural and political nonsense. Censuses, rather, counted those who counted (propertied household heads, important household members, productive possessions), and only for immediate needs such as taxation and conscription. Counting the unpropertied multitude, who were organized already for practical purposes as retainers of those in power, had little point. Since trade, war and migration frequently displaced people, while conquest and elite alliances between states continually shifted political boundaries, a complete census could represent no continuing reality.

A Natural History of Life and Death

John Graunt's *Observations upon the Bills of Mortality* (1662) is rightly regarded as the key turning point in this story.[7] Graunt wrote fully within the model laid down by Aristotle and other classical sources, his work reflecting the ambiguities and tensions that made the choice between democratic and other forms of association so highly charged. Yet his work also subverted this discourse by initiating the rise of population measurement over the next two centuries, which radically reconfigured the framework of thinking about population and ultimately reproduction.

When Graunt wrote in the mid-seventeenth century, there was no customary vocabulary for describing society quantitatively. He never refers to 'population', employing instead a practical vocabulary in which 'people', 'inhabitants', 'city', 'bills' or

7 *Natural and Political Observations upon the Bills of Mortality* [1662], in *The Economic Writings of Sir William Petty*, ed. Charles Henry Hull, vol. 2 (Cambridge, 1899), pp. 314–436.

'accompts' refer to London's population or sub-populations, to country parishes, or to the country writ large. Nor was there a demographic vocabulary for the several sub-populations that his analysis constructed. When he needed to draw together his findings, he relied on the image of the body politic, calling London 'a head too big for the body, and possibly too strong … it grows three times as fast as the body to which it belongs'.[8] In putting forward a method demonstrating the 'exact symmetry of the several members of the commonwealth', the 'members' Graunt refers to are the sub-populations, those parts of the body politic that generate not just births, but collective life and its values.[9]

Yet Graunt's use of this conventional image strongly opposed that of Hobbes. Graunt belonged to the opposite political camp, having been a captain in the military of the Commonwealth, the mid-century era in which England had violently deposed its king in an attempt to establish parliamentary rule. In writing the *Observations* just after the restoration of the monarchy, Graunt artfully employed the convention of the body politic to affirm his loyalty to the new regime. Yet his method, as we shall see, made the balance of the body politic a natural phenomenon that kings could not control, and he therefore assigned the Royal Society the role of '*Parliament of* Nature': only scientific bodies were fit to represent the conditions of citizens like himself.[10] The frontispiece of the *Observations* accordingly adopts a plain format, merely listing the several domains in which his calculations would inform parliament as to the state of natural and political balances (Fig. 18.2).

The *Observations* quickly became a bestseller, going through four editions in three years and circulating widely. It shaped the principal topics and lines of inquiry in population arithmetic in Europe for the next 150 years, thus providing a convenient focus for understanding this wider development. Graunt's accessibility was owed in part to his directly addressing pressing issues of government and of public and individual health and livelihood. No less important was his synthesis of contemporary method, rhetorical and scientific.[11] In his dedication to the Royal Society, Graunt credited Francis Bacon's *History of Life and Death* for his approach.[12] He followed Bacon's dicta on the conduct of natural observations, and structured his text, step-by-step, according to Bacon's plans for natural histories.[13]

8 Ibid., pp. 320–1. 9 Ibid., p. 401. 10 Ibid., p. 325.

11 Philip Kreager, 'New light on Graunt', *Population Studies* 42 (1988), 129–40; Kreager, 'Death and method: The rhetorical space of seventeenth-century vital measurement', in Eileen Magnello and Anne Hardy (eds.), *The Road to Medical Statistics* (Amsterdam, 2002), pp. 1–35.

12 Graunt, *Observations*, p. 322; Francis Bacon, *History of Life and Death* [1613] in *The Works of Francis Bacon*, ed. James Spedding, Robert Leslie Ellis and Douglas Denon Heath, vol. 5 (London, 1860), pp. 215–335.

13 Francis Bacon, *Natural and Experimental History* [1620], in *Works*, vol. 5, pp. 135–6; *Parasceve* [1620], ibid., vol. 4, pp. 249–71; and *Novum organon* [1620], ibid., vol. 4, pp. 80–1, 94–6, 104–8, 127.

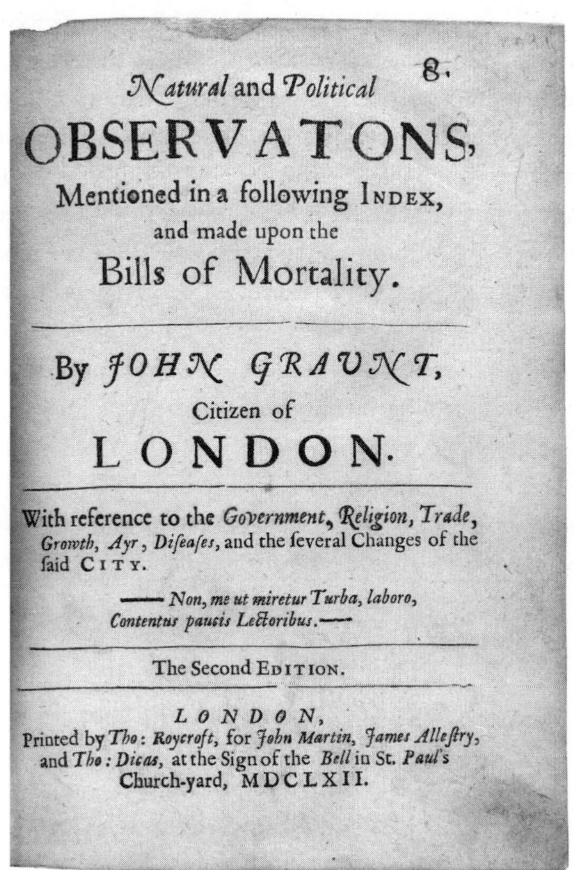

8.

Natural and *Political*

OBSERVATONS,

Mentioned in a following INDEX,

and made upon the

Bills of Mortality.

By *JOHN GRAUNT*,

Citizen of

LONDON.

With reference to the *Government*, *Religion*, *Trade*, *Growth*, *Ayr*, *Diseases*, and the several Changes of the said CITY.

—— *Non, me ut miretur Turba, laboro,*
Contentus paucis Lectoribus.——

The Second EDITION.

LONDON,
Printed by *Tho: Roycroft*, for *John Martin*, *James Alleftry*, and *Tho: Dicas*, at the Sign of the *Bell* in St. *Paul's* Church-yard, MDCLXII.

Figure 18.2 Title-page of John Graunt, *Natural and Political Observat[i]ons, Mentioned in a Following Index, and Made upon the Bills of Mortality*, 2nd edn (London: by Thomas Roycroft for John Martin, James Allestry and Thomas Dicas, 1662). Cambridge University Library.

First, Graunt reviewed the reliability of the mortality bills as evidence based on direct sense impressions, applying Bacon's criteria for classification and compilation. As Bacon proposed that natural histories give a tabular account of evidence enabling readers to assess matters independently, Graunt prefaced his analysis with tables, repeatedly explicating his reasoning so that readers could judge his ratios themselves. Bacon's own natural histories employed a qualitative logic identifying 'simple natures' conceived as proportions or balances; this approach suited Graunt's aims admirably, as the totals he compiled from the bills expressed this logic numerically, showing balances in the political body as natural relationships. His text addressed the central problem of Bacon's *History*, but at a collective level: identification of the causes of differing human longevity. The *Observations* broke down the bills into an extensive set of sub-populations by causes of death, which Graunt then recombined into wider populations reflecting epidemic and endemic causes, and by age, sex, season and location. Arithmetical proportions and balances enabled him, in turn, to separate 'intrinsick' values (natural factors specific to particular environments) from 'extrinsick' ones (those contingent or temporary); on this basis he observed whether the growth or decline of London's and other populations, and the relative healthiness of places, were primary or secondary to the symmetry of the commonwealth. In this way he provided any citizen having even modest arithmetical skills with a method which answered Bacon's questions about why different places and peoples had differing longevity, and indicated whether the policies of king and parliament were consistent with nature, human improvement and, by implication, God's intentions. These were means, in short, to assess the legitimacy and morality of the current polity with regard to procreation, health and strength of the state. We can illustrate this by turning now to how Graunt used his method to evaluate two 'intrinsick' indices of strength as a matter of proportions and balances amongst constituent memberships.

Of 'Teeming Women' and 'Fighting Men'

In the *Generation of Animals*, Aristotle remarked that 'all things that come into being as products of art or nature exist in virtue of a certain ratio'.[14] This natural proportionality, no less indicative of a well-governed body politic, did not until Graunt suggest that mathematics might be applied to numerical evidence to provide independent methods for tracking events and assessing policy. A further century and a half would pass before this possibility became 'statistics', entailing a profound shift in the concept of population and the generation of collective life. As noted, classical and early modern approaches saw groups in nature and society as built primarily by association between individuals and between groups of which they are members. Graunt's method enabled memberships to be viewed simply as aggregates, although his interpretation still located populations in local patterns of association. He accepted, in other words, the classical view of incommensurability in which the 'certain ratio' defining the viability of a population membership places it naturally and politically in a hierarchy of groups, each formed by its own networks of association. In this section, we will consider how he inserted his arithmetical method into the classical model, contrasting this briefly to the modern, statistical conception of populations as ostensibly numerical aggregates. We then take up the different developments of

14 Aristotle, *De generatione animalium*, book IV.2, a17–19, trans. Arthur Platt, in *The Works of Aristotle*, ed. J. A. Smith and W. D. Ross (Oxford, 1949), p. 767.

population and reproduction that the combination of these two approaches made possible.

Graunt's method relied on bookkeeping, and he used 'accompt' to refer to sub-populations.[15] A central instance is his calculation of 'teeming women', those of childbearing age, and 'fighting men', those of age to bear arms. These calculations arose as part of his estimate of London's population size, and of how to interpret the potentially negative implication of its disproportion in the body of England as a whole.[16] First, he shows that country parishes produce more births, and have fewer deaths in infancy and childhood, than the city. London grows through migration, which in the classical model was accepted as a sign of strength. If, however, London is killing off more people than the country produces, and more particularly 'inclines Men and Women more to Barrenness', then its growth would endanger the body politic. Following contemporary accounting practices, Graunt checks proportionalities between several sub-population 'accompts' in order to show that this danger nowhere exists. First, births in the country are so much in surplus that London's mortality does not deplete the country's 'intrinsick' powers of generation. Second, since most migrants are men, the lesser 'prolifickness' of London results from these men having left their wives behind, from rules prohibiting apprentices from marrying and from the frequenting of prostitutes (notoriously 'unhealthful' and 'barren').

Graunt then estimates the proportion of 'teeming women' as double the number giving birth; when births are kept proportional to London's population size, and the same procedure is followed in country parishes, no relative barrenness of London is revealed, even in the most unhealthy parishes. Graunt likewise dispels the possibility that London's 'intrinsick' strength is imperilled by disproportionate mortality of 'fighting men'. Accounting procedure customarily used multipliers to distribute entries uniformly when estimates needed to be made, so Graunt divides male mortality into ten-year age groups, showing that men between 16 and 56 nonetheless make up one-third of the whole, a number more than sufficient for military strength.

Histories of demography and of the early probability calculus often call this kind of exercise 'statistics'.[17] This entails three errors which are important because they obscure both how concepts of reproduction in the state and its several sub-populations evolved in the long era before statistics, and how population thinking subsequently changed in the nineteenth and twentieth centuries. One problem is anachronism: as a

15 Graunt, *Observations*, p. 323; Kreager, 'New light', pp. 133–9.

16 Graunt, *Observations*, pp. 320–1, 369–74, 384–8.

17 For example, Ian Hacking, *The Emergence of Probability: A Philosophical Study of Early Ideas about Probability, Induction and Statistical Inference* (Cambridge, 1991); D. V. Glass, *Numbering the People* (Farnborough, 1973).

term of quantitative reference, 'statistics' emerged later as part of institutional reforms widespread from the end of the eighteenth century. These were based on ideas of polity, nature and society that differed sharply from the classical model. Nineteenth-century statisticians claimed that their quantification established a universal method, compiling all individuals and categories uniformly, exhaustively and purely numerically. This was the exact opposite of incommensurability premised in the classical model.

Second, as noted earlier, the population of a state or society in the classical model was formed through interaction of sub-population memberships, a local history of shifting personal and group associations. In contrast, 'statistics' in common parlance today is programmatic: it takes more or less any numerical compilation as a population. The universalist aims of statistics have made it integral to the rise of modern bureaucracy since the nineteenth century. Calling early modern population arithmetic 'statistics' therefore blurs a historical and conceptual difference between population memberships and populations as constructed in standard datasets. Sub-populations in the latter are aggregates based on individuals' reported characteristics (such as age and occupation) classified in advance by census or survey schedules; while some groups may be numerical outcomes of networks of human association, they are usually compiled without regard to the processes of association which give groups their adaptability. A membership, in short, is not just an aggregate, even if an analyst may treat it as one; population memberships are concerned with how human groups come to be formed, and how they are or are not sustained.

Third, if we take the emergence of sophisticated probabilistic reasoning in the 1660s and 1670s to be 'statistics', we run up against awkward historical evidence. Ian Hacking, for example, has argued that the abstract analysis of probability that emerged in this era can be found not only in the work of brilliant mathematicians, like Blaise Pascal, but among arithmeticians, like Graunt.[18] How this was possible Hacking does not tell us. Scholars familiar with classical literature, however, note that probabilists like Pascal began from ideas of proportional regularity of which Aristotle's 'certain ratio' is an instance.[19] Simple arithmetical proportions were the métier in which Graunt and his fellow merchants used commonplace terms like 'hazard' or 'even lay' to remark an imbalance or risk in a given 'accompt'.[20]

18 Hacking, *Emergence*, p. 103.

19 Daniel Garber and Sandy Zabell, 'On the emergence of probability', *Archives of the History of Experimental Science* 21 (1979), 33–53.

20 Graunt, *Observations*, pp. 350, 384. On the absence of arithmetical concepts and related issues in Hacking's and Michel Foucault's histories, see Kreager, 'Death and method'; and Kreager, 'Histories of demography', *Population Studies* 47 (1993), 519–39. On Foucault's treatment of population: Andrea Rusnock, 'Biopolitics and the Invention of Population', Chapter 23, this book.

The Two Faces of Political Arithmetic

By contrasting statistical population thinking to the older conception in which a state or society consists of diverse sub-populations formed by association, we begin to recognize important differences between 'population' in each. I now turn to how these differences led to a radical transformation in the significance of reproduction, giving rise to the modern concept of fertility. During the long eighteenth century, beginning with Graunt's arithmetic and ending with the rise of institutionalized vital statistics, the idea of the state as essentially quantitative became normative. We see no sweeping away of early modern population arithmetic and the classical model. Rather, approaches that we would now call 'statistical' gradually grew up within the idea of state and society as a hierarchical network of distinctive but interrelated groups.

Our awareness of the tremendous growth of quantitative inquiry into human problems during the eighteenth century has been greatly expanded by Joanna Innes's recent survey.[21] She charts an extensive range of inquiries, addressed not only to stock needs for head counts relating to taxation and war, but also a proliferation of local studies of commercial, criminal, agricultural and other issues relating to the well-being of the multitude. These inquiries, often linked to problems of local government and parliamentary debate, are an index of the developing capacity of civil society. Innes further remarks two principal strands of inquiry, and while she is not concerned with how populations were conceptualized, her distinction captures evolving attitudes to enumeration and the limitations that politics imposed on methods. For simplicity, I will call these the two 'faces' of political arithmetic. One, which remained consistent with the perspective of Graunt and other seventeenth-century pioneers such as Gregory King, Charles Davenant and William Petty, emphasized proportionate supplies of people as the basis of a state's power. The second confined itself to local population characteristics with an eye to moral, bodily and material well-being.

The two approaches fared very differently over the eighteenth century. The first remained substantially hidden from view until nearly the end of the era, because the issues it raised were strongly republican (and hence controversial), and because it required government sources of information that were almost entirely proscribed. There were some safe, if superficial, avenues. It was possible to employ bills of mortality and parish records to contrast population size and strength in different parts of Europe. This was unproblematic if writers simply extolled the 'prolifickness' of native peoples and the benefits of immigration (both implying good government), a

21 Joanna Innes, *Inferior Politics: Social Problems and Social Policies in Eighteenth-Century Britain* (Oxford, 2009), pp. 109–75; Andrea A. Rusnock, *Vital Accounts: Quantifying Health and Population in Eighteenth-Century England and France* (Cambridge, 2002).

pattern only broken by Richard Price in 1780.[22] Consistent with the classical model, however, was recognition that much greater liability and threat lay within the state, owing to internal factionalism and strife amongst constituent population groups. A long line of seventeenth- and eighteenth-century political arithmeticians, including King, Davenant, Petty, John Locke, Benedict Spinoza, David Hume and Price, put forward speculative numerical models of government designed to give due proportional weight to the several incommensurate sub-populations. These analyses effectively questioned memberships then controlling the political status quo. Such work could not be published, or might appear only after the author's death. Even now, King's analysis is the only well-known instance; unusually, he gained access to restricted government records and compiled the first evidence-based political and economic hierarchy of English sub-populations.[23]

The second 'face' meanwhile flourished. Many observers published numerical evidence on local variations in numbers of births and deaths, and speculated about their bearing on health, poverty and trade, without appearing to call established government into question. Few arithmeticians followed Price, who stirred up controversy by arguing that England was experiencing rapid population decline which he linked to loss of national strength, growing poverty, a rising and unchecked public debt and lack of attention to the positive freedoms exemplified in the American and French Revolutions. Price's friend and fellow medic, Thomas Percival, provides a contrasting example of how the majority of arithmeticians proceeded.[24]

Percival drew on the compilations of parish observers around the English north and midlands. While the measures remain Graunt's, and the several localities each constitutes its own 'account', Percival abandoned Bacon's integrative natural historical framework, and the premise that ratios demonstrate an 'intrinsick' structure of the political body. Contrasting household sizes and net surpluses of births over deaths showed that urban locations were less healthy and getting worse. Occasional improvements were attributed to the greater health of rural migrants, whose movement to the towns and cities had increased their size, while inferior urban 'air', child labour, luxury and intemperance were inferred to worsen mortality, births and longevity. There is, as Innes remarks, the implicit suggestion that one could build a picture of the nation from the bottom up by means of such local 'surveys'.[25] Percival and his fellow observers,

22 Richard Price, *An Essay on the Population of England* (London, 1780). An influential instance of the 'safe' approach was Johann Peter Süssmilch, *Die göttliche Ordnung* (Berlin, 1741).

23 Although some excerpts appeared early in the eighteenth century, publication of King's calculations waited until George Chalmers, *An Estimate of the Comparative Strength of Great Britain* (London, 1802).

24 Thomas Percival, 'Observations on the state of population in Manchester, and other adjacent places, concluded', *Philosophical Transactions of the Royal Society of London* 65 (1775), 322–35.

25 Innes, 'Power', p. 143.

however, still viewed this step with caution, and did not directly address Price's contentions. Their sub-populations are mere local aggregates upon which inferences may be made, and Percival was explicit that these were no more than conjectures.

Conclusion

The two faces were thus, in their different ways, circumspect. The first, framed within the older conception of shifting population memberships, was too frankly subversive of the old regime to be widely disseminated. Most practitioners of the second, while greatly extending numerical compilation of populations as local datasets, avoided even the phrase 'political arithmetic'. Four principal consequences of this duality may be noted by way of summary.

First, the profusion of population arithmetic and sometimes more sophisticated applications of probability gradually changed how sub-populations were specified: they came to be aggregates without reference to processes of formation and relation to each other. Populations, in other words, could now be hypostasized as real on the basis of classification and enumeration, and their analysis, interpretation and importance for policy developed without observing processes that form and sustain them.

Second, two fundamental modes of population thinking thus came into coexistence, and were not reconciled.

Third, with the benefit of hindsight, we now know that these first two consequences opened up the possibility of the vast nineteenth-century expansion of institutional statistics, in which quantitative practice was no longer encumbered by the arithmeticians' circumspection, nor by the need to locate the several historical processes that varied population composition. There are elements here of continuity and change. The former is evident in the ideal taken over from early modern population arithmetic that quantification should serve as a basis for assessing the legitimacy and accountability of state policies. As to the latter, while the shift to statistics maintained many specific measurement techniques of the earlier era, population arithmetic was transformed into a universal method, and became a means of articulating new developments in the late eighteenth and early nineteenth centuries, notably political, social and sanitary reforms and the rise of nationalism.[26] States came to be idealized as unitary national populations in which one people shared a common territory, historical experience and culture, in contrast to the several 'estates' or population memberships that had defined political and property hierarchies of the old regime. A complete compilation of the state – its census – thence became necessary to document a nation's population and progress,

26 Philip Kreager, 'Quand une population est-elle une nation? Quand une nation est-elle un état? La démographie et l'émergence d'un dilemme moderne, 1770–1870', *Population* 47 (1992), 1639–55.

while the classificatory procedures employed also served conveniently to marginalize sub-populations not conforming to the national ideal.[27]

Finally, the significance of fertility changed accordingly. Where 'fruitfulness' defined at the level of the state had once contributed to population along with immigration and recurring royal alliances, territorial grabs and military successes, now a national population was supposed to be a self-contained entity, and would have to replenish itself. As fertility became primary, Thomas Robert Malthus was quick to point out the supposed dangers: there could be too many people, as well as too few.[28]

27 Philip Kreager, 'Objectifying demographic identities', in Simon Szreter, Hania Shokalmy and A. Dharmalingam (eds.), *Categories and Contexts: Anthropological and Historical Studies in Critical Demography* (Oxford, 2004), pp. 33–56.

28 [T. R. Malthus], *An Essay on the Principle of Population ...* (London, 1798).

19 Generation in the Ottoman World

Miri Shefer-Mossensohn and Rebecca Flemming

Spreading over three continents – from Arabia to Hungary, from Algeria to Iraq, at its greatest extent – and enduring for six hundred years from the fourteenth to the early twentieth century, the Ottoman Empire was an Islamicate polity blending numerous ethnic, confessional and linguistic communities. It encompassed diverse legal, medical and religious traditions, and an array of established social attitudes and practices that engaged with matters of generation. Islamic theology and jurisprudence dominated, and learned Arabic medicine enjoyed elite prestige – discourses which had been in dialogue for centuries – but the Ottoman world was open and eclectic, recognized multiple sources of authority, and encouraged further translation and exchange.[1]

This chapter tracks generative themes across the Ottoman Empire, from the fifteenth through the seventeenth century. This was the key period of imperial expansion and consolidation: the capture of the Byzantine capital Constantinople in 1453, and its reinvention as the great Ottoman metropolis of Istanbul, was followed by the rapid conquest of the Mamluk Empire in 1516–17. Political and economic evolution continued, with increased challenges posed by the shifting world-order of the seventeenth century, signalled by defeat at the siege of Vienna in 1683, and mixed military fortunes thereafter. How did theorizing, regulating and enacting generation change, or not, over this time: in the move from forging to maintaining a vast empire, and then as the Mediterranean balance of power and wealth began to shift westwards, with the emergence of new colonial trade routes and intellectual projects?

Generation and Empire

Fundamental to the unity of the Ottoman domains was the legal system, essentially Islamic, but flexible across the empire.[2] Non-Muslim religious communities had their own tribunals, in which internal affairs might be settled, but within a larger imperial framework. Town courts operated procedurally according to the rules of sharia, and

1 B. F. Musallam, *Sex and Society in Islam: Birth Control before the Nineteenth Century* (Cambridge, 1983), pp. 40–1; Nahyan Fancy, 'Generation in Medieval Islamic Medicine', Chapter 9, this book.

2 Colin Imber, *Ebu's-su'ud: The Islamic Legal Tradition* (Edinburgh, 1997); Leslie Peirce, *Morality Tales: Law and Gender in the Ottoman Court of Aintab* (Berkeley, CA, 2003).

determined family matters – such as marriage, divorce, paternity and inheritance – on the same terms. They also applied *kanun*, imperial or sultanic law, legislation which was informed, but not bound, by Islamic jurisprudence, as it developed a criminal code and dealt with land and revenue. All Ottoman subjects fell under the jurisdiction of these courts; Christians and Jews used them, including in cases concerning matrimony and generation.

As official appointees, judges (*kadis*) derived their authority directly from the sultan, the figure who unified the imperial domains. His legitimacy depended on descent. In this dynastic state the hereditary rule of the 'sons of Osman', its legendary founder, was justified by appeal to interwoven ideologies of military victory, divine sanction and imperial succession, all vested in the sovereign family. The production of male heirs was thus necessary to perpetuate the state. That this was achieved – thirty-six of its founder's descendants ruled the empire in an unbroken line over six centuries – is 'the central fact about Ottoman history'.[3] Such extraordinary survival was built on making slave concubinage the institution of dynastic generation. Under Islamic law both his wives and his slaves could bear a man legitimate children, with the latter given respectability as a mode of royal procreation by the Abbasids, and embraced by the Ottomans. After the first couple of generations, virtually all sultans were the offspring of concubines.

Centralized systems of provincial administration, revenue raising and military mobilization intersected with each other and the legal structure. Ottoman rule involved large-scale registration for the purposes of taxation – revenue and order, not populousness, were the concerns.[4] As in most other pre-modern states, there was no direct government intervention around fertility – the social and cultural forces ensuring family continuities were largely taken for granted – but energy was invested in the articulation of the different categories of people which made up the overall population, and migration.[5] Bayezid II welcomed the Jews expelled from Spain in 1492, continuing the practices of his predecessors; and sultans claimed the right to settle their subjects wherever they might choose. They transferred loyal groups into newly conquered lands, moved local aristocratic families the other way, and strengthened the human resources in key locations after the depredations of war.

The Ottoman state could thus be interventionist. Sultans attempted universal regulation, through clothing laws, for example, which aimed to distinguish the different

3 Leslie P. Peirce, *The Imperial Harem: Women and Sovereignty in the Ottoman Empire* (New York, NY, 1993), p. 15.

4 Suraiya N. Faroqhi, 'Ottoman population', in Faroqhi and Kate Fleet (eds.), *The Cambridge History of Turkey*, vol. 2: *The Ottoman Empire as a World Power, 1453–1603* (Cambridge, 2012), pp. 346–404.

5 Rebecca Flemming, 'States and Populations in the Classical World', Chapter 5; Peter Biller, 'The Multitude in Later Medieval Thought', Chapter 10; Philip Kreager, 'The Emergence of Population', Chapter 18, this book.

ranks, groups and genders in society.[6] But efforts around generation were minimal, consisting in the provision of courts and laws, and an implicit commitment to family flourishing and ordered imperial multitude.

Generation in Learned Culture

A shared elite culture was forged in the aftermath of the Ottoman defeat of the Mamluks, and the incorporation of the Islamic intellectual and literary heartlands of Syria and Egypt into their empire. Central Asian Turks had long been part of the Islamic world, but rather peripheral to its scholarly traditions. The exercise of their now pre-eminent political power was facilitated in these new territories by acquiring the appropriate learning and cultural fluency; while novel patterns of patronage and influence, anchored in Istanbul, opened up for Arab scholars from those lands. These asymmetries were negotiated in the *majalis*, the intellectual salons of the Ottoman capital and the major cities of Syria and Egypt, which fostered the formation of a learned culture across the empire.[7] Traditional Islamic scholarship – concentrating on quranic exegesis, mastery of the Sunna (the authoritative prophetic traditions or hadith) and jurisprudence (*fiqh*) – was the main currency, and constituted the dominant discursive matrix through which generation was approached in the Ottoman world.

These were also the main subjects studied in the Ottoman *medreses*, or schools, as the education system was expanded and then organized into an integrated hierarchy over the fifteenth and sixteenth centuries.[8] This involved trying to implement a centrally regulated syllabus, at least for the elite schools. Dominated by key texts in the Hanafi tradition, one of the four established legal currents of Sunni Islam, which the Ottoman dynasty promoted as the official school of law – Hanafi jurists wrote all the works of *fiqh* on the curriculum – some classic books of quranic exegesis and hadith commentary from scholars in other schools were also included.[9] Positive law was provided by *al-Hidaya* (The guide), the great synthesis of Burhan al-Din al-Marghinani, composed in twelfth-century central Asia. Massively popular and much commented on, this text

6 Madeline C. Zilfi, 'Whose laws? Gendering the Ottoman sumptuary regime', in Suraiya Faroqhi and Christoph K. Neumann (eds.), *Ottoman Costumes: From Textile to Identity* (Istanbul, 2004), pp. 125–41.

7 Helen Pfeifer, 'Encounter after the conquest: Scholarly gatherings in 16th-century Ottoman Damascus', *International Journal for Middle Eastern Studies* 47 (2015), 219–39; James A. Secord, 'Talking Origins', Chapter 26, this book.

8 Ekmeleddin İhsanoğlu, 'Ottoman educational and scholarly-scientific institutions', in İhsanoğlu (ed.), *History of the Ottoman State, Society & Civilisation*, vol. 2 (Istanbul, 2002), pp. 365–94.

9 Shahab Ahmed and Nenad Filipovic, 'The sultan's syllabus: A curriculum for the Ottoman imperial *medreses* prescribed in a *fermān* of Qānūnī I Süleymān, dated 973 (1565)', *Studia Islamica* 98/99 (2004), 183–218.

remained central to the official curriculum into the eighteenth century, though more specific Ottoman legal compositions were produced from the early sixteenth century onwards and became important teaching texts.

The *Hidaya* covered all the standard topics, including family law. It outlined the two institutions for the production of legitimate children (and for lawful sexual intercourse) – marriage and slave concubinage – in a context in which the Quran prohibited the adoption of heirs, though care for orphans and foundlings was encouraged.[10] While any child born to a wife was presumed to be the husband's, the master could choose whether or not to recognize a child born to a female slave as his. If he did, the slave mother acquired special status, as *umm-walad*: she could not be sold and was freed on the death of her master, and such children were legally indistinguishable from those borne by a man's wife. In contrast to the classical world, slaves could also marry in Islamic law. They could marry each other (with their masters' consent), or a freeman or freewoman could marry a slave. Such a slave had to be owned by someone other than their spouse; concubinage was compatible with ownership, matrimony was not, and this triangulation created complications.

One complication related to the practice of *ʿazl*, withdrawal to avoid procreation, cautiously supported in the Sunna and much discussed in the commentary tradition.[11] Al-Marghinani quoted the eponymous founder of the Hanafi school, Abu Hanifah, who stated that 'If a man marries a slave girl then permission for *ʿazl* belongs to the master', then noted that two of his students asserted the contrary, that permission belongs to her, since intercourse is her right, which is diminished by withdrawal, so her consent is required, as it would be if she were a freewoman.[12] Her status as wife, entitled by marriage to sexual fulfilment (and progeny), conflicts with her status as slave, as her master's property, which gives him a stake in her generative life, since pregnancy and birth may affect her value, and any children will be his slaves. Al-Marghinani prioritized the latter aspect: while a freewoman has rights over her procreative capacity, a slave woman does not, they belong to her master, so it is his consent to *ʿazl* that counts. Other jurists went the other way, or suggested that both must agree, while the Shafiʿi school deemed the question irrelevant. The issue of consent does not arise if wives have a right to sexual intercourse but not ejaculation, as affirmed by the Egyptian exegete Ibn Hajar al-Asqalani in his early fifteenth-century hadith commentary, one of the non-Hanafi works on the imperial curriculum.

10 *Hidaya* book 6 deals with marriage (*nikah*); 9.83 with slave mothers; see also 8.74 on paternity. The quranic prohibition on adoption is 33.4–5. Further: Tim Parkin, 'The Ancient Family and the Law', Chapter 6; Ellen Herman, 'Technologies of Adoption Matching', Exhibit 33, this book.

11 Musallam, *Sex and Society*, pp. 10–38; Abdel Rahim Omran, *Family Planning in the Legacy of Islam* (London, 1992), pp. 113–83.

12 *Hidaya* 6.57.

Seed features as the essential generative substance of human beings in several of the discussions concerning offspring in the *Hidaya*. For example, some combination of male and female seed contributes to determining the status of children borne by slave women in different circumstances, while twins are always the product of one man's seed and thus indivisible in respect to paternity.[13] Seed had appeared in descriptions of human generation in the Quran, and the Sunna elaborated further; both were informed by classical medical concepts embedded in the late antique Mediterranean world. The Arabic medical tradition also developed these concepts following the translation of Greek medical writings into Arabic in ninth-century Baghdad: Ibn Sina's theories emerged as the most authoritative, here as elsewhere. This fed into the rich, ongoing exegetical investments in the Quran and hadith, just as crucial quranic notions and prophetic sayings, about, for instance, the stages of fetal formation or the role of breast-feeding, influenced medicine. It was all one conversation.

Arabic learned medicine was thus integral to elite Ottoman culture. Its ideas about generation informed debates in the *majalis* and were intrinsic to the texts taught in the *medreses* and Islamic law more broadly. Anatolian physicians travelled to Cairo to study and develop their practice in and around its great hospital foundations, especially the Mansuri, before and after the defeat of the Mamluks. Istanbul became a medical centre, notably after 1550, when Suleiman I founded his own hospital complex in the city, with a medical school attached.[14] The office of the chief physician, responsible for the health of the sultan, his family and his realm, took shape earlier, under Bayezid II, though sultans also continued to employ private doctors, and there were other opportunities for court patronage, which attracted physicians from across the Ottoman lands and beyond.[15] In a shared learned medical culture, many were Jews and Christians. Written in diverse languages, Ottoman medical works all drew on Arabic, Persian and Greek sources, recognized the same authorities, and operated with the same key assumptions about disease, cure and the workings of the human body.

Gynaecology and Generation

Ottoman medical writings also shared an integrationist approach to gynaecology and generation, following Galenic models and the Arabic tradition. Some treatises were dedicated to a specific topic, or a single disease, especially plague, but most were synoptic compendia; the first work devoted to pregnancy, birth and child health was not

13 *Hidaya* 9.77 (the reverse seems implied at 9.83) and 8.71.

14 İhsanoğlu, *History of the Ottoman State*, pp. 400–7; Miri Shefer-Mossensohn, *Ottoman Medicine: Healing and Medical Institutions, 1500–1700* (Albany, NY, 2009), pp. 101–44 and 187–91.

15 İhsanoğlu, *History of the Ottoman State*, pp. 396–400.

produced until 1701.[16] Female health, illness and cure and diverse generative matters formed part of general medicine. This is illustrated by three of the best-known medical texts from the Ottoman Empire, spanning the period covered here and demonstrating some of its generic and linguistic variety.[17]

The Anatolian physician Şerefeddin Sabuncuoğlu composed his *Imperial Surgery* (*Cerrahiyetü'l-Haniyye*) in 1465, a Turkish translation of the surgical portion of the Andalusian physician al-Zahrawi's great eleventh-century medical compilation, itself heavily reliant on Greek medical encyclopaedias from the later Roman Empire, especially that of Paul of Aegina.[18] In search of Ottoman patronage to replace that of the local rulers around his home city of Amasya, Sabuncuoğlu dedicated this undertaking to the sultan Mehmet II. He altered al-Zahrawi's text only slightly, amending some techniques and descriptions and occasionally shifting the emphasis, but changed the accompanying illustrations more. In particular, to the existing depictions of surgical instruments he added an extensive array of miniatures displaying many of the operations described.

This surgery was practised on female and male bodies throughout, and there is also a specific gynaecological sequence in the text. Chapters on interventions to the female genitals and uterus were followed by descriptions of procedures for difficult childbirth, what might come after and the instruments required.[19] Sabuncuoğlu followed al-Zahrawi in considering the interior of women's bodies – the womb and any contents – the realm of the midwife (*kabile*), though subordinate to wider male medical expertise. He instructed her in the use of the speculum to open the uterus (Figs. 19.1 and 19.2), in turning an awkwardly presenting fetus, deploying hooks to extract a fetus that had died during labour, and the gentle removal of the afterbirth. A female physician, labelled as such, is depicted performing other operations on female bodies in this sequence in the *Imperial Surgery*, though the text refers to such practitioners only in discussing cutting for kidney and bladder stones in women.[20] There is other evidence, however, of some general female medical practice in the Ottoman Empire, and midwives appear in legal texts, palace archives and court records, attending on the harem and acting as witnesses to birth and related matters.[21]

16 Nükhet Varlik, *Plague and Empire in the Early Modern Mediterranean World: The Ottoman Experience, 1347–1600* (Cambridge, 2015), pp. 207–47; İhsanoğlu, *History of the Ottoman State*, p. 578.

17 Studies remain limited: Miri Shefer-Mossensohn, 'A tale of two discourses: The historiography of Ottoman-Muslim medicine', *Social History of Medicine* 21 (2008), 1–12.

18 See İlter Uzel's (English and Turkish) introduction to his modern Turkish edition, Şerefeddin Sabuncuoğlu, *Cerrahiyyetü'l-Haniyye*, 2 vols. (Ankara, 1992).

19 *Imperial Surgery* 2.70–8; Ralph Jackson, 'A Roman Embryo Hook', Exhibit 6; Lauren Kassell, 'Medieval Birth Malpresentations', Exhibit 10, this book.

20 *Imperial Surgery* 2.61; Bibliothèque nationale de France, suppl. Turc. 693, ff. 110v, 112r–v.

21 Nil Sari, 'Osmanlı sağlık hayatında kadını yeri', *Yeni tıp tarihi araştırmaları* 2/3 (1996/7), 11–64; 'Osmanlı sağlık hayatında kadının yeri (tamamlayıcı belgeler)', ibid., 4 (1998), 247–54.

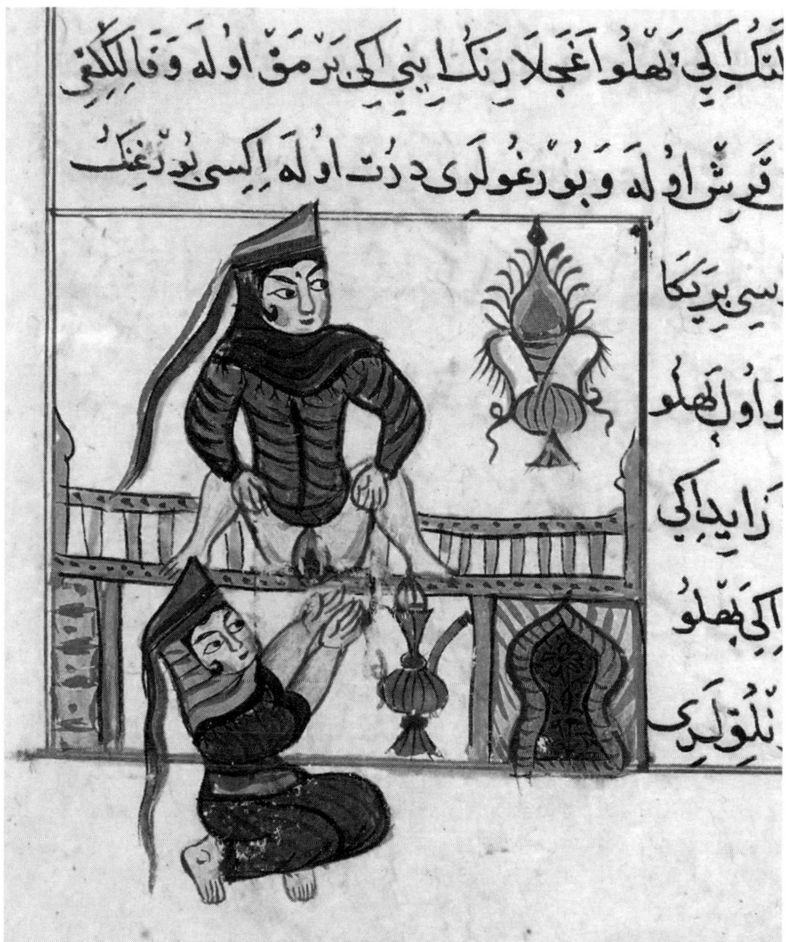

Figure 19.1 Miniature from a 1465 manuscript of Sabuncuoğlu's *Imperial Surgery*, illustrating how to use a speculum (visible only in outline) to extract a fetus that died during labour. The work devotes a whole chapter to instruments used for this purpose. Bibliothèque nationale de France, suppl. Turc. 693, f. 118v.

The *Memorial* (*Tadhkirah*), composed in late sixteenth-century Cairo by the prolific, Syrian-born Dawud al-Antaki, was popular for centuries to come.[22] This major Arabic handbook first broadly introduced the medical art, set out the history of its pharmacological part, mentioning a range of Greek and Arabic authorities, provided a long, detailed list of medical materials and remedies, and concluded with a wider conspectus of disease and cure. Female ailments and therapies featured throughout, and the main sequence of prescriptions included a chapter on contraceptives.[23] Most of the

22 Julia Bray, 'Dawud ibn Umar al-Antaki', in Joseph E. Lowry and Devin J. Stewart (eds.), *Essays in Arabic Literary Biography, 1350–1850* (Wiesbaden, 2009), pp. 41–54.

23 Musallam, *Sex and Society*, pp. 73–5.

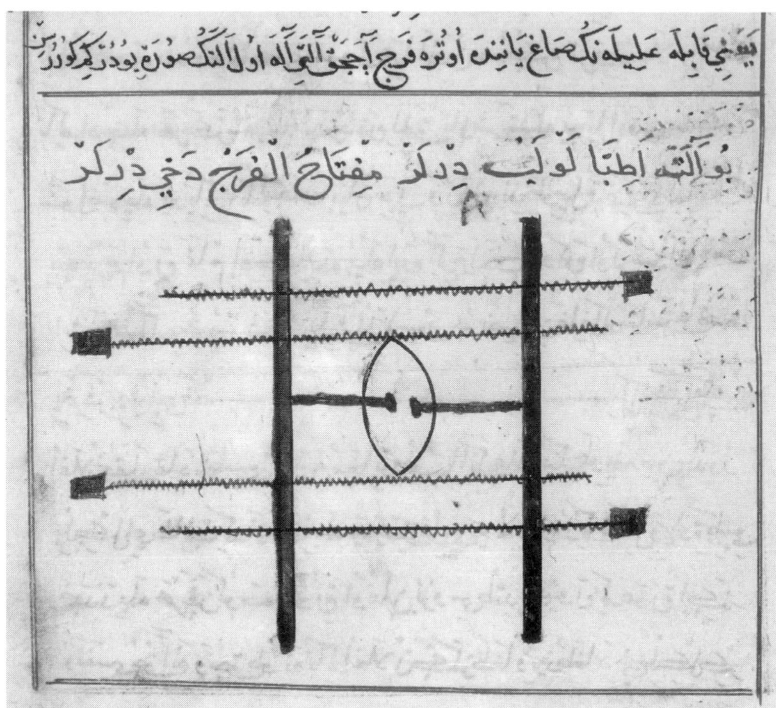

Figure 19.2 Another drawing of a speculum from Sabuncuoğlu's *Imperial Surgery*, this one from the chapter on removing uterine growths and cancers. More schematic, it is a variant on the speculum described and illustrated by al-Zahrawi and diverges from those in classical medical texts or preserved at Pompeii. Bibliothèque nationale de France, suppl. Turc. 693, f. 113r.

recipes – potions, pessaries and a few amulets – were for women to use, but al-Antaki also made a general claim about the kind of substances which, applied to the penis, stopped the woman retaining the seed. He offered two reasons for trying to prevent conception: to ensure that a new pregnancy does not follow too swiftly on the last, and to avoid fathering children with a woman deemed unfit for that purpose. These are social motives in a juristic rather than medical register, and the usually female contraceptive applications of the medical tradition had already been positioned as analogous to *ʿazl* in legal discourse, a point developed further by the noted Egyptian Hanafi jurist Ibn Nujaym soon after the Ottoman conquest.[24] He argued that, by such analogy, a wife needed her husband's agreement to use a pessary to stop his seed entering the womb, a use which he implies was commonplace.

Finally, Şemseddin Itaki, forced from his home in Shirvan by the ongoing conflict between the Ottoman and Safavid dynasties in the 1620s, composed his Turkish

24 Ibid., p. 37.

philosophical-anatomical synthesis, *The Anatomy of the Body* (*Tashrih-i abdan*), to gain recognition and support at the court of Murad IV.[25] An expanded Turkish adaptation of Mansur Ibn Ilyas's fourteenth-century Persian treatise of roughly the same name, though more commonly known as *Mansur's Anatomy* (*Tashrih-i Mansuri*), this work included detailed discussion not only of male and female generative parts, but also of seed, fetal formation and birth, joining authorities such as Hippocrates, Aristotle, Galen, Ibn Sina and Ibn al-Nafis with the Quran and Sunna. In the two-seed world of the hadith, in which the formative stages of the fetus had been clearly set out, there was still much to discuss about, for instance, the male and female contribution and which fetal organ formed first: the heart, asserted Itaki, following Ibn Ilyas and Aristotle, with the brain, liver and navel just behind.

Mansur's Anatomy seems to derive its five illustrations of the main systems or networks in the body from the same source as a set of twelfth-century Latin works.[26] Ibn Ilyas added a sixth, a version of the arterial figure into which a womb containing a fetus has been inserted. An additional set of pictures, borrowed this time from recent western European anatomy, are also incorporated in the surviving manuscripts of Itaki's text, including a drawing of a rather differently embodied uterus, and a disembodied fetus (Fig. 19.3).

Acquisitive engagement with contemporary medical developments in surrounding territories, including the Safavid Empire and western Europe, can also be seen in al-Antaki's oeuvre. His is the first Arabic medical text to discuss the recently arrived and now rapidly spreading 'Frankish chancre', or 'European pox' (*habb ifranji*), usually identified with syphilis. Whether his prescribed treatments – mercury and china-root – are borrowed from west or east, or a combination of the two, is debated.[27] A younger contemporary of Itaki, Ibn Sallum, also travelled to Istanbul in search of court patronage, following a successful medical career in Aleppo, and became chief imperial physician under Mehmet IV in 1656.[28] In this role he encouraged and promoted the Arabic translation of various Paracelsian texts, and synthetic compendia of the new chemical medicine began to circulate in the Ottoman world.

25 Esin Kâhya has produced modern Turkish and English versions with illustrations and facsimiles of the original text: *Şemseddîn-i İtâkî'nin Resimli Anatomi Kitabı* (Ankara, 1996); *The Treatise on Anatomy of the Human Body and Interpretations of Philosophers* (Islamabad, 1990).

26 Andrew J. Newman, '*Tasrih-i Mansuri*: Human anatomy between Galenic and prophetic medical traditions', in Ž. Vesel, H. Beikbaghban and B. Thierry de Crussol des Epesse (eds.), *La science dans le monde iranien à l'époque islamique*, 2nd edn (Tehran, 2004), pp. 253–71.

27 Natalia Bachour, 'Healing with mercury: The uses of mercury in Arabic medical literature', *Asiatische Studien* 69 (2015), 851–7; Anna E. Winterbottom, 'Of the China root: A case study of the early modern circulation of *materia medica*', *Social History of Medicine* 28 (2015), 22–44; further: Simon Szreter, 'Fertility Transitions and Sexually Transmitted Infections', Chapter 30, this book.

28 Bachour, 'Healing with mercury', 857–61.

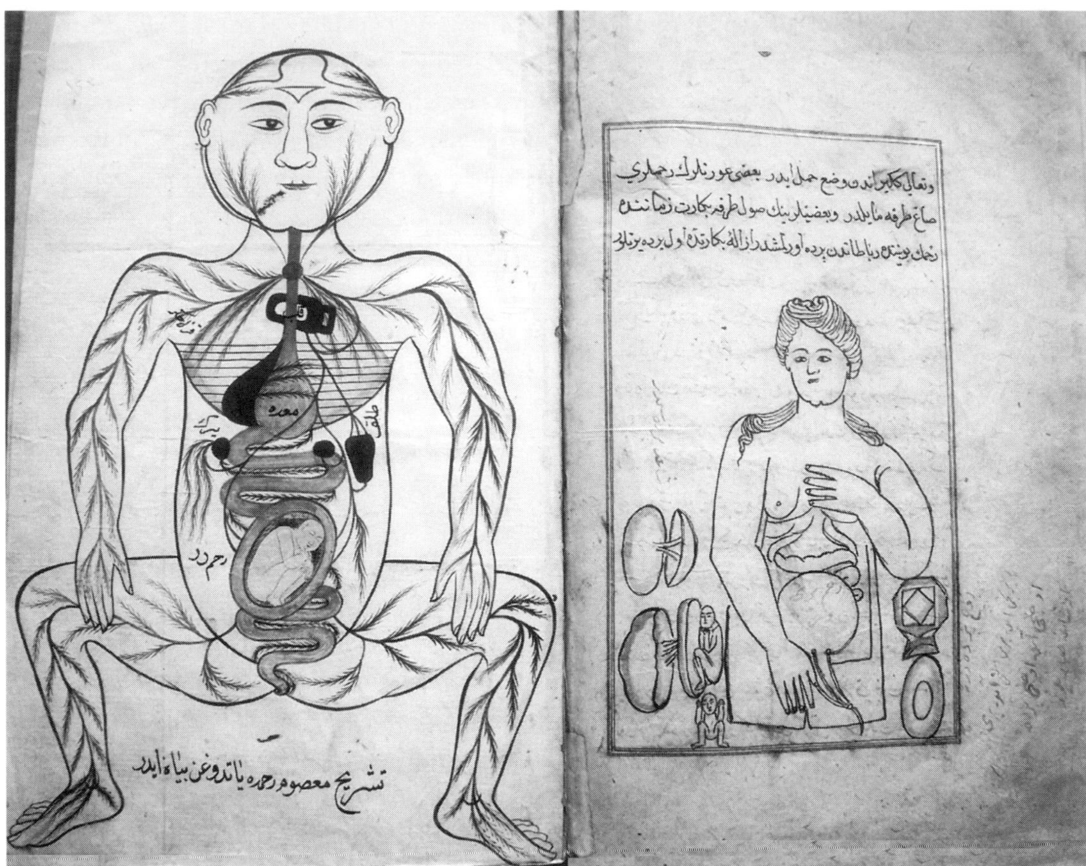

Figure 19.3 A pair of drawings from a 1697 manuscript of Itaki's *The Anatomy of the Body*. A Mansur-style arterial diagram, with axial fetus in the womb, faces a statuesque figure, displaying an empty uterus and flanked by wombs and fetuses, derived from Juan Valverde's *Anatomy of the Human Body* (1560). Istanbul, Suleymaniye Ktp. Bagdatli Vehbi, 1476, pp. 251–2. Reproduced with kind permission.

New perspectives, ideas and materials, from east and west, were thus added to the eclectic mix of Ottoman medicine in the seventeenth century, including some with procreative implications. Juristic discourse, too, was stretched in certain directions by the development of *kanun* and the broader articulation of Ottoman power, but these larger-scale developments made little difference to the intersections of generation and the law.

Courts and Fetuses

Matters of generation are evidenced in the surviving court records of the Ottoman Empire from the sixteenth century onwards, offering glimpses of behaviour as well as its formal regulation. These can be read, moreover, in conjunction with contemporary fatwa collections, that is, compilations of legal opinions issued by noted jurists (muftis) in response to questions posed directly to them, or arising from the ongoing workings of the law. Some muftis were official appointees, and the fatwas of the Grand Mufti of Istanbul often articulated state policy, while others were just locally prestigious, but all, like the *kadis*, operated in the same legal and political framework.

Procreation is less visible in the court records and the muftis' discussions than might be expected.[29] Many family matters were resolved without recourse to the courts, and the injunctions of Islamic law often operated beyond temporal authority. The debate about the permissibility of *ʿazl*, for example, was about how a good Muslim should behave, so the category of the permitted was further ordered from the recommended to the discouraged; but no legal actions resulted.[30] Furthermore, the rules of marriage minimized disputes about paternity, and though divorce and death introduced complications, other aspects of the matrimonial contract proved more conflictual.

The most common generation-related cases in the court records concern claims for *ghurra*, compensation for a lost fetus, an action anchored in prophetic tradition. There was, it is recounted, a fight in which one wife struck her pregnant co-wife with a tent pole, killing both the woman and the fetus; Muhammad demanded that the kin-group of the assailant render blood money (called the *diya*) for the dead woman and a payment (the *ghurra*) of a male or female slave for the fetus.[31] The *ghurra* became a standard topic in legal manuals and commentaries, covered along with other penalties for offences against the person, with the basic ruling of the prophet developed and disputed by the different jurisprudential schools.

The *ghurra* was set at one-twentieth of the *diya*, for instance, about the same as for the loss of half a finger, and jurists often discussed whether this fine should be construed as being paid as compensation for a part of the mother's body or for the person of the fetus itself, or, as the Hanafi school held, a complex combination of the two. In that it was payable within a year, the *ghurra* operated as recompense for a body part, on account of the connection between mother and fetus, but otherwise, in that it was paid by the kin-group (not the assailant), and to the heirs of the fetus, it was for the fetus. In the sixteenth century, the Ottoman Hanafi jurist Qadi Zadeh explicated this hybrid position in detail in his commentary on the *Hidaya*. He explained that, while in the belly, the fetus is a special kind of body part, which has its own life and is in preparation

29 Judith E. Tucker, *In the House of the Law: Gender and Islamic Law in Ottoman Syria and Palestine* (Berkeley, CA, 1998), p. 45; Peirce, *Morality Tales.*

30 Musallam, *Sex and Society*, pp. 30–1.

31 Marion Holmes Katz, 'The problem of abortion in classical Sunni *fiqh*', in Jonathan E. Brockopp (ed.), *Islamic Ethics of Life: Abortion, War, and Euthanasia* (Columbia, SC, 2003), p. 27. Compare Exodus 21:22–3; Marie-Hélène Congourdeau, 'Debating the Soul in Late Antiquity', Chapter 8; and Maaike van der Lugt, 'Formed Fetuses and Healthy Children in Scholastic Theology, Medicine and Law', Chapter 12, this book.

to become a person, so has some rights in relation to others – such as manumission, inheritance, lineage and bequest – but no responsibilities – no liability for damages, for example, or contracts – until the somatic separation of birth. It is 'human in some respects, but not in others'.[32] Birth was a turning-point, also evident in the common view that if an assault on a pregnant woman led to a live birth and then death of the child, full blood money was due.[33]

Demands for *ghurra* were routine in the local Ottoman court records so far studied: from Anatolia, Palestine, Syria and Egypt, and from the sixteenth into the eighteenth century.[34] Claims for compensation were variously pressed by the mother and father jointly or individually, even by a grandparent on occasion, and the alleged assailants include women and men, strangers, acquaintances and family, in diverse scenarios. Many of the Anatolian examples highlight fear as the cause of miscarriage – whether of a husband or of a man on the rampage in a bathhouse – while, in seventeenth-century Ramla, the distinguished mufti Khayr al-Din rejected such expansion of the notion of assault.

The reports sometimes provide further details of the fetus – that it was male, for instance, or six months old – but concentrate on narrating the events, for cause and effect were the key. With high standards of proof, litigants had to mobilize all available resources. In Jerusalem in 1567, the claimant Esther, a Jew, even brought her dead male fetus with her to court, on a tray.[35] The story of her miscarriage was complex, staged over several days, and the accused women admitted some aspects but denied others, leaving the *kadi* unable to reach a verdict. Other cases foundered similarly, since decisive evidence was elusive. Yet claims kept being pressed. The notion of *ghurra*, with its externalization of responsibility, and promise of recompense for the loss of a pregnancy, had traction across the empire.

While such claims were routine in the Ottoman courts, cases in which the woman procured her own miscarriage, though theoretically subject to the same rules, were rare. They are recorded only as incidental to a larger story, attached to a quranic offence or other major matters of social order. For instance, in 1670 an Armenian Christian woman, Sara, was brought to the court of Balikesir in western Anatolia by the police chief, and shockingly confessed to consensual sex with her sister's husband, becoming pregnant, taking drugs to abort the fetus a month before she was due to give birth and burying the evidence with her parents' help.[36] There were general fatwas on the subject, however, with new pronouncements joining established earlier opinions with

32 Katz, 'Problem of abortion', p. 38. 33 *Hidaya* 54; Tucker, *House of the Law*, p. 116.

34 Cases collected, for example, in Ömer Düzbakar, 'Abortion in the Islamic-Ottoman legal systems', *Journal of Islamic Science and History of Medicine* 5 (2006), 28–38; Tucker, *House of the Law*, pp. 122–3.

35 Amnon Cohen and Elisheva Simon-Pikali, *Yehudim be-Veit ha-Mishpat ha-Muslemi: Ḥevrah, Kalkalah ve-Irgun Qehilati bi-Yruhalayim ha-'Othmanit: ha-Me'ah ha-Shesh-'Esreh* (Jerusalem, 1993), p. 164, doc. 167.

36 Düzbakar, 'Abortion', 32.

increasing frequency from the late seventeenth century onwards.[37] If a woman drank a medicament or struck her own belly with the intention of aborting the fetus, then her kin-group had to pay *ghurra*, but if she did so with her husband's agreement, then nothing was owed.

The husband's agreement did not make such conduct right, however. Permissibility was a broader issue, beyond the remit of Islamic penal law, but debated amongst the schools of Sunni *fiqh*. Most interpretations forbade abortion after ensoulment, that is after 120 days, as established by hadith and medically elaborated following Ibn Sina; except in case of danger to the woman's life, which always took precedence. The Hanafi position held that those first four months were a period of uniform permissibility, while the other schools were less liberal.[38] Within the category of the permitted, some Hanafi authorities classified abortion before ensoulment as *mubah* – religiously neutral – while others considered it *makruh* – discouraged but justifiable. The need for a woman to breast-feed was commonly cited as a valid reason for terminating a subsequent pregnancy.

Conclusion

Continuity is more apparent than change in legal and medical approaches to generation in the Ottoman Empire from the fifteenth through the seventeenth century. This continuity was open and flexible, within a dynamic and adaptable imperial system, and not to be mistaken for stagnation or decline: inherited traditions were reworked, amended and expanded, rather than rejected or transfigured. Conception and abortion provide one point of contrast with developments in western and northern Europe over the same period: not just the content of Islamic law remained stable, but also its modes of enforcement in relation to the state.

This would all change, however, as a series of political and economic transformations picked up pace in the late eighteenth and early nineteenth centuries. The Ottoman state and its relationship with its population were radically reconfigured; and western forms of knowledge and technology were explicitly prioritized, with a focus on women, the family and reproduction.[39] The 1830s saw the launch of a revised census, and imperial legislation against abortion, as part of a wider package of reforms; a different set of processes was now under way.

37 Tuba Demirci and Selçuk Akşin Somel, 'Women's bodies, demography, and public health: Abortion policy and perspectives in the Ottoman Empire of the nineteenth century', *Journal of the History of Sexuality* 17 (2008), 377–420, on 384.

38 Katz, 'Problem of abortion', pp. 30–1.

39 Demirci and Somel, 'Women's bodies'; Gülhan Balsoy, *The Politics of Reproduction in Ottoman Society, 1838–1900* (London, 2013); Nick Hopwood, 'Globalization', Chapter 43, this book.

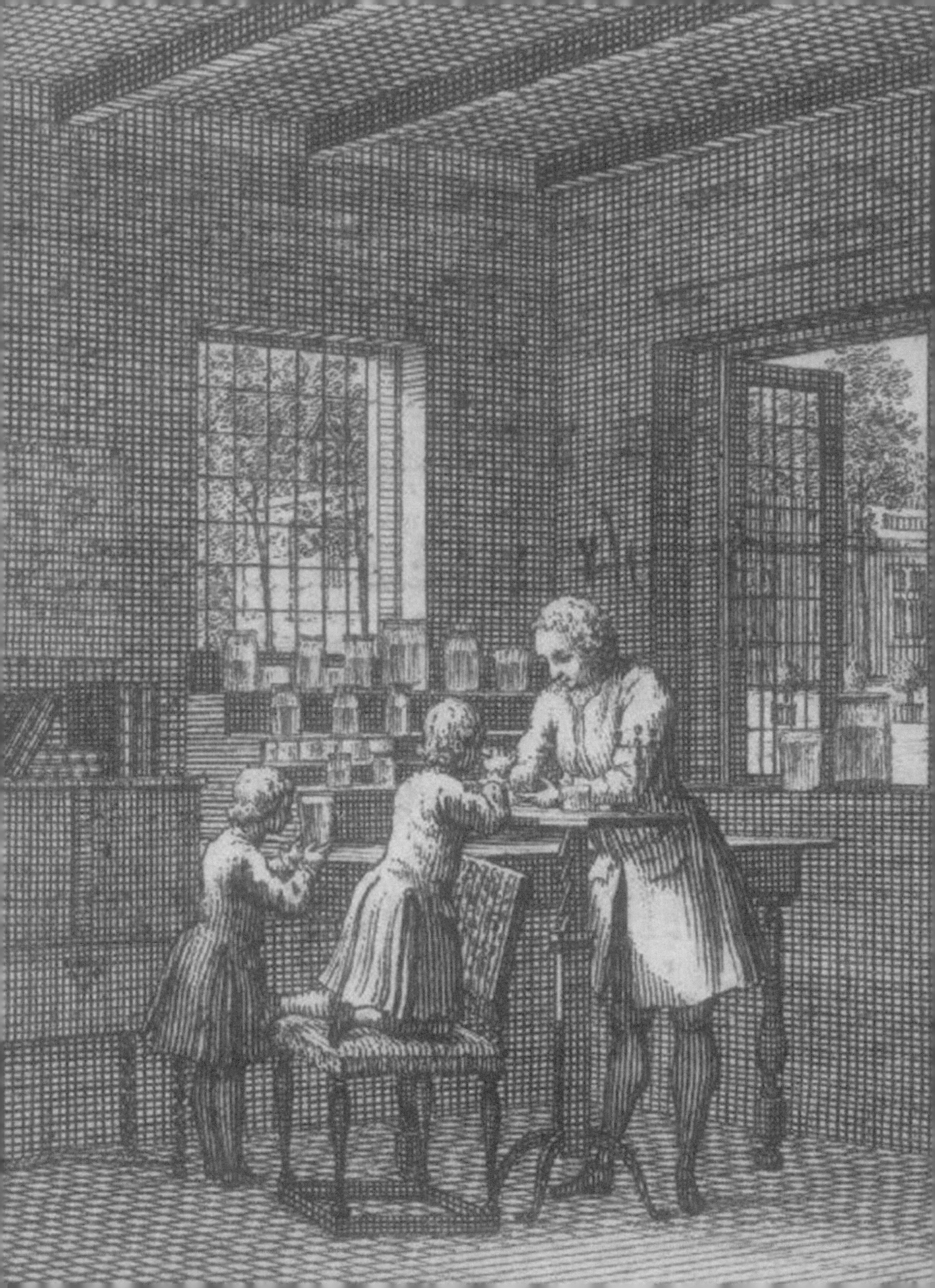

Part III

Inventing Reproduction

Learning about 'polyps' (hydra). Surrounded by jars of the creatures, the Swiss naturalist Abraham Trembley teaches the sons of Count Willem Bentinck, in the laboratory on his estate near The Hague, about their remarkable 'reproduction' (our regeneration). This phenomenon played a significant role in the reconceptualization of 'generation' as 'reproduction'. Detail from header, engraved by Jacobus van der Schley after a drawing by Cornelis Pronk, in Trembley, *Mémoires, pour servir à l'histoire d'un genre de polypes d'eau douce* ... (Leiden: Verbeek, 1744), p. 229. Whipple Library, University of Cambridge.

THE PRESENT CONCEPT OF 'REPRODUCTION' WAS INVENTED in the eighteenth century and gained currency during the transformations between the 1740s and the 1840s that made both the modern world of industrial capitalism and class politics and the vocabulary to describe it. Following the American Revolution of 1776 in the largest colony of the greatest maritime power, the French Revolution of 1789 reorganized the European continent through over two decades of war. The industrial revolution spread, with concomitant urbanization, while steam transport began to circle the globe and facilitated the expansion of empires. The map of knowledge was redrawn. Much changed in this age of revolutions, and rapidly, but as Part III will discuss, the significant novelties, in reproduction as elsewhere, initially had limited reach.

The molecular geneticist François Jacob highlighted the move, beginning in the mid-eighteenth century, from generation, the active, embedded, artisanal view of coming into being that earlier chapters have elucidated, to reproduction, the more abstract approach to the capacity of organisms to beget their like that the rest of this book will explore. Feminist scholars enlarged Jacob's history of ideas by suggesting that, as 'reproduction' replaced 'generation', procreation was both assimilated to the model of capitalist production and marginalized in a separate women's sphere. Histories often invoke this change in terminology, enlisting the shift from generation to reproduction to name a larger transformation in understandings and practices of making plants, animals and people – but it has never been thoroughly studied.

Chapter 20 confirms the semantic innovation, but finds that it took longer and was more complex than is usually assumed (Nick Hopwood, 'The Keywords "Generation" and "Reproduction"'). 'From generation to reproduction' provides a useful shorthand for change between the mid-eighteenth and the late nineteenth centuries, but it is implausible that a conceptual switch set everything in motion. 'Reproduction' was used earlier and in more varied connotations of 'producing again' than has been appreciated, especially in agriculture. In the 1740s, two savants associated with the court at Versailles, Georges-Louis Leclerc, Comte de Buffon, and François Quesnay, developed more abstract meanings in natural history and the analysis of wealth respectively. The regeneration of natural resources interested them both. Yet it took till the mid-nineteenth century for 'reproduction' to capture much territory from 'generation' and build up links to copying, imitation and manufacture, and a few decades more for it to become the subject of a unified discourse. Meanwhile, 'generation' took off, in the sense of a cohort born at the same time or at the same distance from an ancestor, and remained the more common word.

The new 'reproduction' came, in part, out of those investigations into generation in which experimenters had long vied to explain the gradual appearance, over the hours and days of incubation, of the visible structure of the chick embryo in the egg. In the early 1740s, the Republic of Letters buzzed with startling reports that a 'polyp' (hydra) could 'reproduce' (that is, regenerate) itself even when cut in pieces or sieved. The theories of generation that sought to explicate these phenomena had deep philosophical and religious implications in Enlightenment controversy and have been prominent in histories of biological ideas; reworking them set up the very possibility of a science of life. More generally, in the reformed museums, hospitals and professional schools of post-revolutionary Paris, curators and professors carved out fresh roles and practices, audiences and forms of publication for the medical, natural and social sciences. Their analyses were extended especially in the German universities, where microscopists established new objects of study, such as developing embryos and cells (Nick Hopwood, 'Images of Human Embryos', Exhibit 23). But they would not agree on the roles of eggs and sperm in fertilization till the 1870s. Karl Ernst von Baer, the embryologist usually credited with discovering the definitive mammalian egg in 1827, traced the embryo to a 'fetal ovum' that pre-existed the 'maternal ovum' containing it; and though Baer named 'spermatozoa' that same year, he dismissed them as parasites and denied that the semen contributes materially to the offspring (Florence Vienne, 'Eggs and Sperm as Germ Cells', Chapter 28). New disciplines included experimental physiology and a gynaecology now focused on the functions and malfunctions of the ovaries.

Eighteenth-century generation was also bound up in practical projects: classifying and even perfecting human beings, reforming midwifery, acclimatizing and propagating exotic plants, and breeding horses and cattle for improvement (Sarah Wilmot, 'Breeding Farm Animals and Humans', Chapter 27). The classifications of the Swedish botanist Carl Linnaeus depended for material on global networks of exchange; he was obsessed with growing bananas in Scandinavia. His 'sexual system', which ordered plants according to the numbers of male and female parts, is often presented as reinforcing the dominant gender hierarchies and as a static framework that evolutionism would have to overcome. Staffan Müller-Wille shows that his taxonomies were in fact more complex, while his private writings delved into an unruly underworld of sexual forces and desires ('Linnaeus and the Love Lives of Plants', Chapter 21). Late eighteenth-century European savants similarly used encounters with colonized peoples to provide material for the construction of theories of race (Renato G. Mazzolini, 'Colonialism and the Emergence of Racial Theories', Chapter 25).

Attending childbirth was the most important practical task related to generation, and historians have debated how best to explain the advent of man-midwifery: the routine resort to men to deliver babies, especially among elites, combined with increased male surveillance of female midwives. While historians of Britain, where the change was striking, have variously appealed to technology (forceps) and culture (fashion), Mary E. Fissell places the change in the larger Enlightenment concern to improve the lot of mothers and babies ('Man-Midwifery Revisited', Chapter 22). This professional expansion produced fierce quarrels, intriguing models and iconic printed images

(Lucia Dacome, 'A Crystal Womb', Exhibit 21; Ludmilla Jordanova, 'Man-Midwifery Dissected', Exhibit 22). For a long time most women did not use the lying-in hospitals, but these, like so much that originated in this era, announced ambitions that were later realized in altered forms (Salim Al-Gailani, 'Hospital Birth', Chapter 37). The upheavals of revolution and war around 1800, and the corrosive effects of capitalist social relations, fed a sexual revolution, and were countered by the idealization of domesticity, which built on earlier celebrations of motherhood and breast-feeding (Lisa Forman Cody, 'A Painting of a Nursing Mother', Exhibit 19). By presenting female bodies as designed for reproduction, gynaecologists grounded the ideology of separate spheres – the masculine world of work and the feminine hearth and home – and gave women special responsibility for maintaining the population.

With the shift from local and hierarchical associations to modern collectives of equivalent individuals, population was becoming fundamental to thinking about groups of human beings and other organisms. Following on from Chapter 18 (Philip Kreager, 'The Emergence of Population'), Andrea Rusnock approaches this change by reassessing Michel Foucault's remarks on 'biopower' – power exercised in the management of life – and by reconstructing record-keeping about maternal and infant mortality ('Biopolitics and the Invention of Population', Chapter 23). It thus becomes clearer how, through the early nineteenth century, nation-states – now also republics and constitutional monarchies – could once again institute censuses and the civil registration of births, marriages and deaths, and how official bureaux could take an original and mathematical approach to quantifying fertility and mortality. It is also evident that non-governmental institutions, not least charitable hospitals, played a part.

The most influential text is Thomas Robert Malthus's *Essay on the Principle of Population* (1798), still a point of reference in its own right and through Charles Darwin's use of the principle in his theory of natural selection. For Malthus, the problem was not the underpopulation so much discussed in eighteenth-century France, but the geometrical increase of population with which the food supply, expanding only arithmetically, could never keep pace – a gap that dashed Enlightenment optimism as false hope. Writing in the midst of growth in the British population, focused on towns that reproduced themselves without the need for immigration, Malthus was interested in how numbers could be kept low to enhance living standards. He fought the old Poor Laws, England's local welfare system, as supposedly encouraging the birth of children who could not be supported. His attitude to those who found 'no vacant cover' at 'nature's mighty feast' earned him the enmity of romantics and radicals alike. Yet Malthus opposed the illusion that colonialism could provide any lasting solution and pointed to the prior claims to their lands of the aboriginal peoples of the Americas, Australia and the South Sea. In considering populations around the world, he valorized the northwest European household system (or western European marriage pattern) within which couples had first to accumulate the resources for self-sufficiency before they could make a home, over the other ways in which household and kinship systems in Asia and sub-Saharan Africa have suppressed their fertility (Richard M. Smith, 'Marriage and Fertility in Different Household Systems', Chapter 24; Rebecca Flemming, 'Population in the South Sea', Exhibit 24).

Buffon's generalization of the concept of 'reproduction' did not trigger any sharp shift from 'generation' to 'reproduction'. To grasp what did happen, it is crucial to trace the ties between social, political and intellectual changes over many decades. The most convincing accounts take communication seriously, particularly the ways in which debates about origins have been as promiscuous in genre, authorship and audience as they have in transgressing limits of expertise and morality. It matters not just who thought what, but what could be said, written and published. James A. Secord tracks such talk through the circulation of conversation between salon, academy and boudoir, and in medical schools and dining rooms ('Talking Origins', Chapter 26). He explores the potential of close attention to the processes of public discourse and intimate dialogue for understanding the move from generation to reproduction.

In short, several major transformations began in the mid- and late eighteenth century, including the articulation of the modern concepts of 'reproduction' and 'population', the adoption of man-midwifery (and breast-feeding) by high- and some middling-status mothers, and the elite breeding of improved animals and plants. These novelties had limited reach while readerships remained small, few had access to regular medicine, most farmers carried on as before and governments hesitated to become involved. The politics of population, which were established through the first half of the nineteenth century, do not seem initially to have relied much on the keyword 'reproduction'. Yet reformers would importantly draw on, modify and amplify those eighteenth-century innovations as new languages and practices of reproduction gradually moved to the fore.

NICK HOPWOOD

20 The Keywords 'Generation' and 'Reproduction'

Nick Hopwood

The most powerful generalization about the history of reproduction, and the strongest argument for discontinuity, is that there was a shift, starting in the eighteenth century, from a broader, premodern framework, 'generation', to the more abstract, modern notion of 'reproduction'. Much hinges on word usage, and the idea that 'reproduction' gained its modern meaning around that time, while 'generation' in the old sense fell out of use. Raymond Williams's *Keywords: A Vocabulary of Culture and Society* (1983) showed complex and contested terms acting as markers and agents of social change, but did not include 'generation' or 'reproduction'. We still lack a thorough history.

To go beyond schematic generalization, it will be necessary to reconstruct the genesis of 'reproduction'; track its fortunes in new disciplines and among new publics from the eighteenth to the twentieth century; explore what happened to 'generation'; tease out connections, or explain their absence, between domains ranging from the sciences and medicine to economics and manufacturing; and reflect on relations between words, concepts and practices. This chapter cannot do all that. It does review resources for a richer history, while surveying usage to reassess the case for a move from generation to reproduction. I find much truth in that idea, but conclude that the process took longer, and was different as well as more complicated than in the standard account.

From Generation to Reproduction?

Over the last half-century, three groups of scholars have traced the modern concept of reproduction to the mid-eighteenth century: historians of biological ideas, historians of economic thought and feminist historians of medicine. A history of heredity launched the case. In *La logique du vivant* (1970) – translated as *The Logic of Life* (1973) – the molecular biologist François Jacob reacted against gradualist histories of genetics by proposing sharp transitions. Jacob made a series of stages 'integrate' like 'Russian dolls' those that went before, a more progressivist approach than Michel Foucault's in *The Order of Things* (published in French in 1966), but Foucault still applauded 'the most remarkable history of biology that has ever been written'.[1] Like Foucault, Jacob had the analysis of visible structure give way around 1800 to the penetration of hidden

1 François Jacob, *The Logic of Life: A History of Heredity*, trans. Betty E. Spillmann (New York, NY, 1982), p. 16, back cover.

organization and thus usher in a science of life more suddenly than most historians of biology would accept today. Jacob's passage was also from generation to reproduction – for Darwinian molecular biologists the defining 'aim' of life.

'Only towards the end of the eighteenth century did the word and the concept of reproduction make their appearance to describe the formation of living organisms', Jacob announced. Before then, 'living beings did not reproduce; they were engendered'. 'Generation', he exaggerated, 'was always the result of a creation which, at some stage or other, required direct intervention by divine forces.' 'The generation of every plant and animal was, to some degree, a unique, isolated event … rather like the production of a work of art by man.' The doctrine of pre-existent germs had dominated since the late seventeenth century, but a hundred years later, 'facts' supposedly replaced '*a priori* systems'. '[C]ertain facts, such as the regeneration of worms and polyps or the likeness of a child to its father *and* mother, did not fit well with the existence of a preformed being in the germ. The concept of *reproduction* was born of all these observations.' Jacob believed that '[t]he word first appears' in a 1712 memoir about the regeneration of crayfish limbs, but suggested that in 1749 the intendant of the King's Garden, Georges-Louis Leclerc, Comte de Buffon, 'gave a wider meaning to the expression'.[2]

Jacob must have read Jacques Roger's monumental doctoral thesis on 'The generation of animals from Descartes to the *Encyclopédie*', which respected period terms without thematizing the transition.[3] A quarter-century later, Roger's Buffon biography headed a chapter 'From Generation to Reproduction'. '[L]iving beings "reproduce"', Roger explained. 'This very statement excluded creationism and preexistence. It was "reproduction in general", that "power to produce one's likeness", which required study … not … the "generation" of this or that species, but "reproduction" as a universal phenomenon of the living.'[4] The leading specialist endorsed Buffon's heroic role in a grand shift from generation to reproduction.

From the 1980s, feminist historians converged on a similar conclusion, interpreted with an ambition, to link domains and take account of routine usage, that makes Roger's and Jacob's fat histories of biological ideas look thin. While historians of economic thought tended to limit themselves to a rather narrowly defined tradition,[5] feminist scholars stressed the mutual determination of reproduction and production in view of

2 Ibid., pp. 19–20, 71–3.

3 Jacques Roger, *Les sciences de la vie dans la pensée française du XVIIIe siècle: La génération des animaux de Descartes à l'*Encyclopédie (Paris, 1963). The English translation mostly rendered '*génération*' as 'reproduction': *The Life Sciences in Eighteenth-Century French Thought*, ed. Keith R. Benson, trans. Robert Ellrich (Stanford, CA, 1997).

4 Jacques Roger, *Buffon: A Life in Natural History*, ed. L. Pearce Williams, trans. Sarah Lucille Bonnefoi (Ithaca, NY, 1997), p. 127.

5 For a broader view: Margaret Schabas, *The Natural Origins of Economics* (Chicago, IL, 2005).

the dual demands on women of wage labour and childcare.[6] Carolyn Merchant's ecofeminist *Death of Nature* (1980) placed the beginnings of capitalist production and women's loss of control over reproduction in the seventeenth century, but did not discuss terminology. In 1987, in her pioneering study of a doctor and his female patients around 1730, Barbara Duden proposed a later passage from 'generation' to 'reproduction'. Insisting on the otherness of women's preindustrial bodies, understood in terms of *generatio*, or in the vernacular, 'something akin to "fruitfulness"', she argued that between 1750 and 1850 medicine, demography and political economy 'replaced ... *generatio* ... with "reproduction"'. In an endnote on English, French and German dictionaries, the great-great-granddaughter of the lexicographer Konrad Duden located the first uses in economics and about living beings. 'The equipping of women with a reproductive apparatus led to a cultural disembodiment of the processes of *generatio*', Duden concluded, 'analogous to the "disembedding" of the productive economy which accompanied the end of a culture of subsistence and self-sufficiency.' 'Reproduction ... was linked to the context of production as that term moved into the center of political economy around 1850.'[7]

Inspired by Williams's *Keywords*, Ludmilla Jordanova revisited 'reproduction' in 1995, focusing on eighteenth-century Britain and the making of the modern world of busy states, interfering experts and class society. The progenitors of the middle class were 'constructing naturalized categories' through which to manage social relations. Jordanova explored how within discussions of reproduction lurked production, increasingly construed as mechanical, and also imitation and copying, as in 'reproduction furniture' and printing. Around 1800, some represented children as capital. 'Is it coincidental', Jordanova asked, 'that *reproduction*, as the scientific study of generation, was coined at the same time ...?' Yet she stressed the contentiousness and intricacy of such associations.[8]

This programmatic piece has been much cited, sometimes problematically, as a placeholder for the deeper investigation it invited. The change in meaning has too easily anchored the assumption that thinking in terms of capitalist (re)production dehumanized women as baby-producing machines; but women's roles were denigrated earlier.[9] Some historians of the eighteenth century have imposed the modern label or

6 Sarah Franklin, 'Feminism and Reproduction', Chapter 42, this book.

7 Carolyn Merchant, *The Death of Nature: Women, Ecology, and the Scientific Revolution* (San Francisco, CA, 1980); Barbara Duden, *The Woman beneath the Skin: A Doctor's Patients in Eighteenth-Century Germany*, trans. Thomas Dunlap (Cambridge, MA, 1991), pp. 28–9, 205.

8 Ludmilla Jordanova, 'Interrogating the concept of reproduction in the eighteenth century', in Faye D. Ginsburg and Rayna Rapp (eds.), *Conceiving the New World Order: The Global Politics of Reproduction* (Berkeley, CA, 1995), pp. 369–86, on pp. 371 and 378.

9 Allison Muri, 'Imagining reproduction: The politics of reproduction, technology and the woman machine', *Journal of Medical Humanities* 31 (2010), 53–67; Mary Fissell, 'Gender and generation: Representing reproduction in early modern England', *Gender & History* 7 (1995), 433–56.

trivialized the change by treating 'reproduction' as just another name for 'generation'. More legitimately, it has been argued that social and cultural change in the seventeenth and eighteenth centuries preceded the adoption of the new word. Going further, Adele Clarke suggested that association with sex kept reproduction marginal even through the nineteenth century, so that a coherent science was organized only in the mid-twentieth, long after potent discourses had been produced.[10]

A history of keywords can help evaluate these views. In what follows, I begin to outline a more thorough account and raise questions for further research by drawing on recent work and charting usage more systematically.[11] I concentrate on French, English and German because, with the decline of Latin, these vernaculars saw the major modern innovations, but the story begins in antiquity.

Generation as Engendering, Posterity and Cohort

The word 'generation' shares the root *gen**, or 'coming into existence', with Greek and Latin terms also for tribe, family, line of descent and species. *Genesis* (procreation) and *genos* (lineage, family, race) were linked in Aristotle, but historical dictionaries suggest that the Vulgate, a fourth-century Latin translation of the Bible, brought them closer by rendering two Hebrew words as '*generatio*', which thenceforth referred to process and product, the action of engendering and the posterity of a person. In the middle ages there appeared a cluster of meanings closer to the dominant modern one, of a cohort of people of the same age, at the same distance from an ancestor or living around the same time.[12] In Christian theology, the term referred to the begetting of God the Son by God the Father. For natural philosophers and physicians, the most important senses went back to Aristotle's *On Generation and Corruption*, about the basic modes of change, and *On the Generation of Animals*, which established the principal specific application.

Previous chapters of this book have reconstructed medieval and early modern views. By the early eighteenth century, various meanings were current. Ephraim Chambers's *Cyclopaedia* of 1728, the model for the Enlightenment *Encyclopédie*, paid most attention to 'Generation, in Physicks', 'the Act of procreating, or producing a thing,

10 Adele E. Clarke, *Disciplining Reproduction: Modernity, American Life Sciences, and 'the Problems of Sex'* (Berkeley, CA, 1998), pp. 5, 18–21.

11 See especially Ohad Parnes, Ulrike Vedder and Stefan Willer, *Das Konzept der Generation. Eine Wissenschafts- und Kulturgeschichte* (Frankfurt am Main, 2008). Databases consulted include ARTFL (especially FRANTEXT), Deutsches Textarchiv, ECCO, EEB, EEBO, Enzyklothek and Zeno.org. For a complementary approach: James A. Secord, 'Talking Origins', Chapter 26, this book; for another keyword history: Tobias Cheung, 'From the organism of a body to the body of an organism: Occurrence and meaning of the word "organism" from the seventeenth to the nineteenth centuries', *British Journal for the History of Science* 39 (2006), 319–39.

12 Parnes, Vedder and Willer, *Konzept der Generation*, pp. 21–39.

which before was not'. 'Generation is more immediately understood of the production of Animal and Vegetable Bodies, from Seed, or the Coition of others of different *Sexes*, but the same Genus, or *Kind*.' An ancient alternative to 'like begets like', equivocal or spontaneous generation, was dismissed. The main entry concentrated on animals, with special treatment of 'man'; plant generation was discussed separately. Some writers were acknowledged as considering minerals, metals and stones to be products of generation. Gases were generated, and geometry had 'generating lines'.[13] People wrote more generally of 'a chosen generation', 'the present generation' or 'the *n*th generation'.

Chambers stressed the 'Mystery', because animal generation is 'very difficult to be traced. The Parts concurring hereto, are numerous; and their Functions mostly discharg'd in the Dark.' Discussions reviewed competing theories. René Descartes's attempt to apply his purely mechanical philosophy had failed, but gradual formation by 'epigenesis', as the physician William Harvey named the ancient doctrine in 1651, posited matter more active than religious orthodoxy could accept. The pre-existence theory displaced the problem by postulating a single original creation – in the most extreme view the whole human race was preformed in the ovaries of Eve – after which in each generation the embryo had merely to unfold. Most writers placed the embryo in the egg, but some favoured animalcules in the male seed.[14] Theological and philosophical battles were fought in debates over animal generation.

Re-production

'Generation' was the broadest and richest word, though foreign in German till the eighteenth, even nineteenth century; the vernacular '*Zeugung*' and '*zeugen*', '*Erzeugung*' and '*erzeugen*' went back to the middle ages. Meanings included the English 'beget' (more for fathers) and 'engender'. 'Procreation' had long referred to having children and the continuation of the species.[15] The biblical 'multiply' was common too. By contrast, '*Fortpflanzung*', closer to 'propagation' and used since the sixteenth century about faith and sin, was applied in the eighteenth century mainly to plants, though also humans, other animals and things. The French and English 'reproduction' gained some new senses around the same time. Present by the fifteenth century in the Latin '*reproducere*' and '*reproductio*' in theology and the law, it originally meant producing again, with the emphasis on *re*-production: 'the Action whereby a thing is produced a-new, or grows a

13 E. Chambers, *Cyclopaedia* … (London, 1728), vol. 1, pp. 133–6; on spontaneous generation: James A. Secord, 'Spontaneous Generation and the Triumph of Experiment', Exhibit 26, this book.

14 E. Chambers, *Cyclopaedia* … (London, 1728), vol. 1, p. 134; Shirley A. Roe, *Matter, Life, and Generation: Eighteenth-Century Embryology and the Haller–Wolff Debate* (Cambridge, 1981); Justin E. H. Smith (ed.), *The Problem of Animal Generation in Early Modern Philosophy* (Cambridge, 2006).

15 Parnes, Vedder and Willer, *Konzept der Generation*, pp. 21–39.

second time', 'the Restauration of a thing before existing, and since destroyed'.[16] Two uses are most striking.

The first was agricultural, to describe fields annually producing another crop, or cut stems growing again, a meaning close to our 'regeneration'; it appears from 1600 in the key treatise by Olivier de Serres. The academician René-Antoine Ferchault de Réaumur's sensational discovery about crayfish claws became the classical animal example of a phenomenon that remained better evidenced in plants (Fig. 20.1).[17] In the early 1740s, the Genevan naturalist Abraham Trembley announced a still more amazing result: the regrowth of a tiny freshwater 'polyp' (hydra) after bisection or sieving. He distinguished 'this marvellous reproduction' from 'generation', that is, 'the natural manner' in which the polyps 'multiply' by plant-like 'buds'.[18] Well into the nineteenth century regeneration was the main sense in which living beings were 'reproduced'.

A second usage was theological. Defending the reality of Christ's resurrection, the mathematician Blaise Pascal asked in a note first published in 1670, 'Which is more difficult, to produce a man or an animal, or to reproduce (*reproduire*) him [or it]?'[19] The more general problem was the resurrection of the dead at the Last Judgement. Anglican divines held that just rewards and punishments demanded that body and soul be identical in life and afterlife. Immateriality guaranteed the identity of the soul, but how would the decayed body be reproduced, when the dispersed particles could have been incorporated into other living beings?[20]

In the seventeenth and early eighteenth centuries, 'reproduce', '*reproduire*' and '*reproduction*' could already mean procreation. '*Reproduction*' long remained too technical for the dictionary of the French Academy, but in 1690 the main rival included it with the general meaning, 'Action by which a thing is reborn, is produced anew', and the more specific, 'Nature preserves itself by continual *reproductions* of bodies which are engendered & corrupted.' The examples for '*reproduire*' were coppiced trees, one wheat seed producing many, and the regrowth of thistles that had been torn out.[21] In 1713, Archbishop François Fénelon argued that animals could count as mere machines only if one accepted that 'the author of these machines has placed in them what it takes to

16 E. Chambers, *Cyclopaedia* … (London, 1728), vol. 2, p. 996.

17 Charles E. Dinsmore (ed.), *A History of Regeneration Research: Milestones in the Evolution of a Science* (Cambridge, 1991).

18 A. Trembley, *Mémoires, pour servir à l'histoire d'un genre de polypes d'eau douce* … (Leiden, 1744), pp. 15, 149–53; Secord, 'Talking Origins'.

19 Blaise Pascal, *Pensées*, fragment *Fondement*, no. 4, www.penseesdepascal.fr/Fondement/P-R-Fondement4.php.

20 Peter McLaughlin, *What Functions Explain: Functional Explanation and Self-Reproducing Systems* (Cambridge, 2001), pp. 173–9; Udo Thiel, 'Religion and materialist metaphysics: Some aspects of the debate about the resurrection of the body in eighteenth-century Britain', in Ruth Savage (ed.), *Philosophy and Religion in Enlightenment Britain: New Case Studies* (Oxford, 2012), pp. 90–111.

21 Antoine Furetière, *Dictionaire universel* … (The Hague, 1690), vol. 3, p. 388.

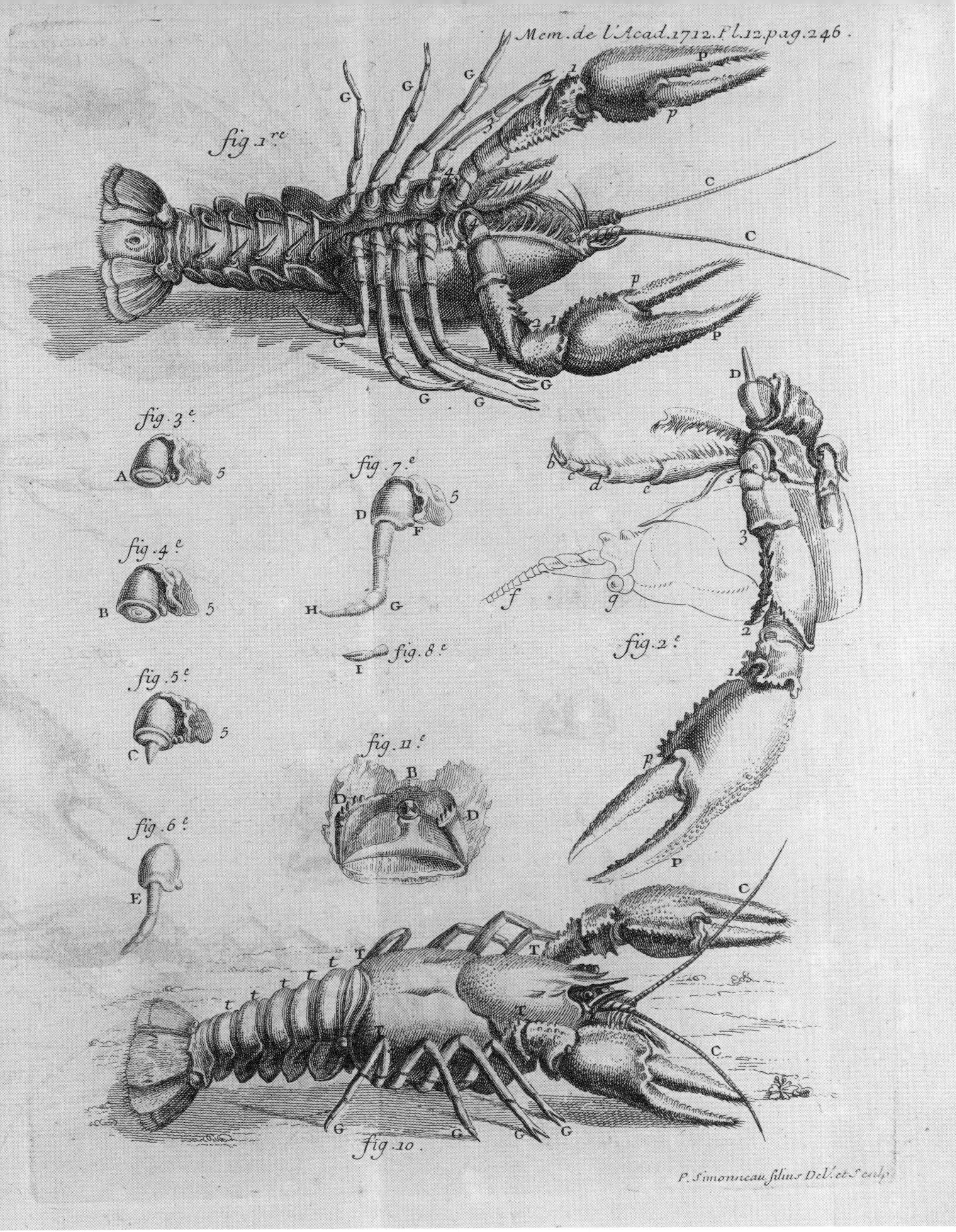

Figure 20.1 Réaumur's stages of reproduction (figs. 3–7) of a crayfish leg broken at *S* in fig. 2, a phenomenon he interpreted in terms of pre-existent germs. Drawing and engraving by Philippe Simonneau from Réaumur, 'Observations sur les diverses reproductions ...', *Histoire de l'Académie royale des sciences* (1712), 223–41, plate 12. 25 × 20 cm. Cambridge University Library.

reproduce themselves (*se reproduire*) endlessly by the joining of the two sexes'. Outside agriculture the word was scarce, however, and this usage rare.[22]

Regenerating Species and Renewing Revenue

Enter Buffon in the company of those academicians, *philosophes*, physicians and improving landlords who form the traditional cast of the French Enlightenment at mid-century. Innovation may have had broader bases, but Buffon himself and the physiocrat François Quesnay are credited for fresh usages of '*reproduction*' in natural history and economics respectively, fields linked by their concern to increase resources.

Buffon's sense is absent from some of his most important sources, including Louis Bourguet's *Lettres philosophiques* (Philosophical letters, 1729), but came out of an intense debate, triggered by dissatisfaction with the mechanical philosophy as much as Jacob's awkward facts, in which savants challenged pre-existence with theories of active matter. Buffon conversed with fellow academician Pierre Louis de Maupertuis, in whose scandalous masterpieces of erotic microscopical materialism of 1744–5 '*génération*' appeared more often, but '*reproduction*' meant regeneration and occasionally species propagation.[23]

Buffon's massive *Histoire naturelle* (Natural history), an instant success with European elites, marked a step-change in prominence. In the second volume (1749), the second chapter, 'Concerning Reproduction in General', begins by defining 'reproduction' and stating what has become the biological species concept: 'Let us examine more closely this property common to animal and plant, this power to produce its likeness, this chain of successive individual existences, which constitutes the real existence of the species; & … let us look in general at the phenomena of reproduction'.[24] Signalling the elevation of the species above the individuals that perish, the term narrowed and widened the scope of 'generation'. On the one hand, it distinguished a defining property of living beings from a process some still allowed for minerals too (and true species reproduction from more transient productions). On the other, that programmatic 'in general' let plants and animals share an activity.[25]

22 Fénelon, *Traité de l'existence et des attributs de Dieu*, ed. Charles Jeannel (Paris, 1872), p. 40; Muri, 'Imagining reproduction', p. 66.

23 Maupertuis, *Vénus physique* (1745); Mary Terrall, *The Man Who Flattened the Earth: Maupertuis and the Sciences in the Enlightenment* (Chicago, IL, 1992), pp. 199–230; Peter Hanns Reill, *Vitalizing Nature in the Enlightenment* (Berkeley, CA, 2005); Secord, 'Talking Origins'.

24 Georges-Louis Leclerc de Buffon, *Œuvres complètes*, vol. 2: *Histoire naturelle, générale et particulière, avec la description du Cabinet du Roy*, vol. 2 (1749), ed. Stéphane Schmitt (Paris, 2008), p. 115.

25 Stéphane Schmitt, 'Introduction à l'*Histoire générale des Animaux*', ibid., pp. 9–58, on p. 32.

The choice of word also signals that, in opposing mechanical creationism, Buffon began with the 'model of the polyp's regeneration' and 'attempted to form a general theory. What had been an incomprehensible exception became … the simplest case of a universal phenomenon.'[26] His theory of sexual reproduction postulated that organic molecules in excess of nutritional requirements were thrown off from every part to accumulate in the semen of both sexes, which formed a fetus in the womb (Fig. 20.2). An 'internal mould' characteristic of the species brought the particles together by means of penetrating forces analogous to gravity. This particular theory was ultimately less successful than the idea of reproduction as overgrowth, but was picked up by writers on natural history and medicine who shared Buffon's interest in acclimatizing exotic plants, breeding nobler animals and perfecting human beings.[27]

A little later, François Quesnay, writer on physiology, physician to Louis XV and Madame de Pompadour at Versailles and a dining companion of Denis Diderot, Jean le Rond d'Alembert and Buffon, ensured 'reproduction' a place in economics. Quesnay's 1747 treatise on the physics of the 'animal economy' had discussed '*génération*', which he presented as driven by an active ether moving something like a worker on a loom. He also referred to 'reproduction of the species', though more often to 'continual reproduction' to replenish the blood and other parts, and once to trees that 'reproduce new branches each time'.[28] When Quesnay engaged with economics, he extended these primarily agricultural usages to the replacement of what consumption had destroyed. His *Tableau économique* (Economic tableau), the physiocrats' founding text, argued that nature (*physis*) – the land and farming – is the source of wealth, while manufacturing and commerce are sterile (Fig. 20.3). In the spirit of *laissez-faire*, the existing mercantilist regulations, designed to promote exports and restrict imports, should be replaced by a single land tax. 'The true riches are the productions which are reborn annually from the land. Without this annual reproduction, the other riches … would soon disappear.' '*Reproduction*' described the renewal of nature in an economy of circulation and replenishment.[29]

26 Roger, *Buffon*, p. 128. *Pace* Staffan Müller-Wille and Hans-Jörg Rheinberger, *A Cultural History of Heredity* (Chicago, IL, 2012), p. 15, I know no evidence that Buffon borrowed from theology. Though the polyp had theological implications, I miss a specific link to the resurrection debate.

27 E. C. Spary, *Utopia's Garden: French Natural History from Old Regime to Revolution* (Chicago, IL, 2000), pp. 99–154; Michael E. Winston, *From Perfectibility to Perversion: Meliorism in Eighteenth-Century France* (New York, NY, 2005); Mary Terrall, 'A Microscopical Salon', Exhibit 20, this book. Carl Linnaeus did not write of 'reproduction': Staffan Müller-Wille, 'Linnaeus and the Love Lives of Plants', Chapter 21, this book.

28 Quesnay, *Essai physique sur l'Œconomie animale*, 2nd edn, vol. 3 (Paris, 1747).

29 Quoted in Jean Cartelier and Marie-France Piguet, '*Produit, production, reproduction* dans le *Tableau économique*: Les concepts et les mots', *Revue économique* 50 (1999), 71–86, on 83–4; see also Paul P. Christensen, 'Fire, motion, and productivity: The proto-energetics of nature and economy in François Quesnay', in Philip Mirowski (ed.), *Natural Images in Economic Thought: 'Markets Read in Tooth and Claw'* (Cambridge, 1994), pp. 249–88; and Andrea Rusnock, 'Biopolitics and the Invention of Population', Chapter 23, this book.

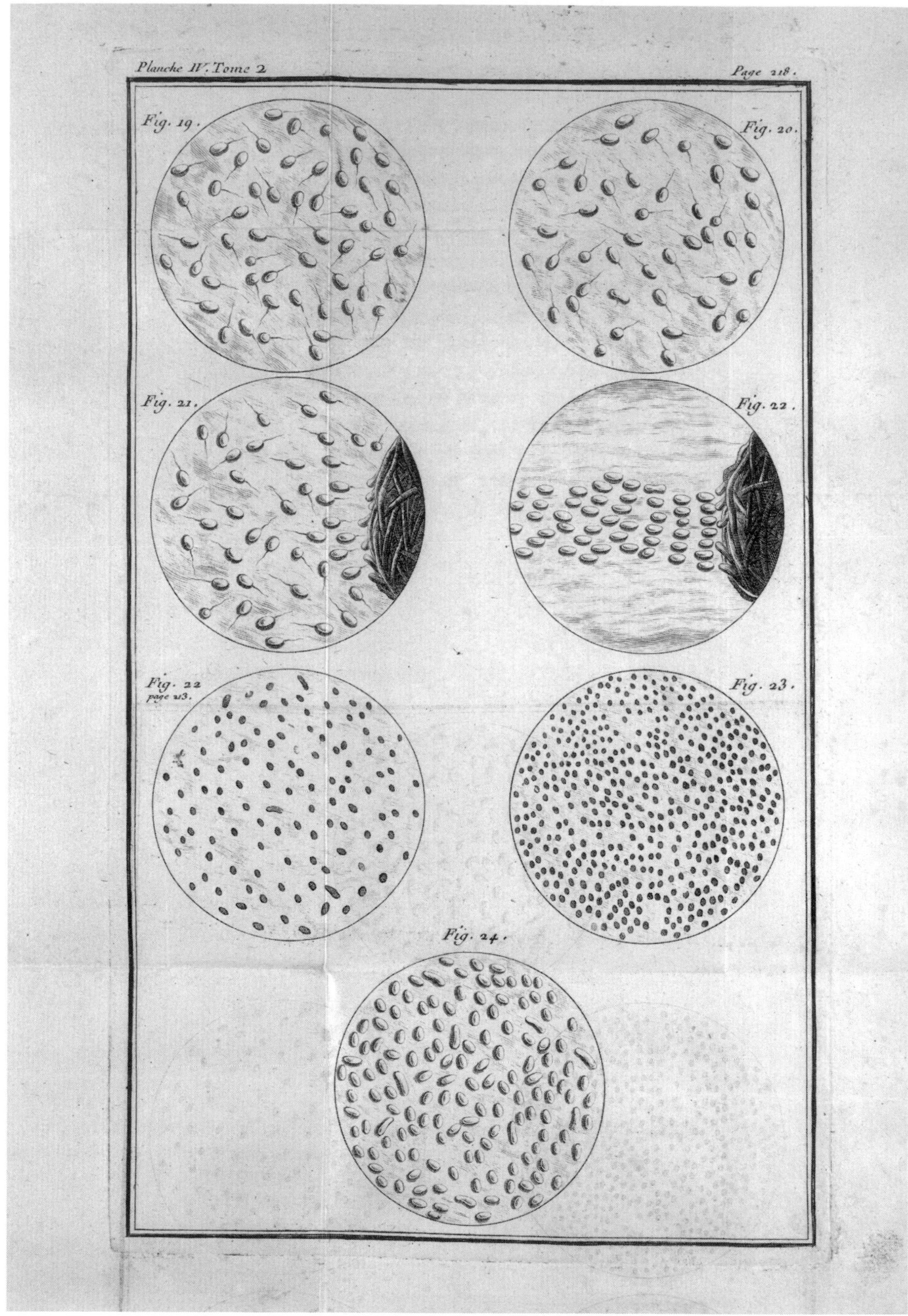

Figure 20.2 Buffon's 'organic molecules' in the semen emitted naturally by a male dog (fig. 19) and fluids extracted from bitches (20–1) and cows (22–4). Exhibit 20, this book, illustrates the performance of these controversial experiments. Engraving after Jacques De Sève's drawing from Buffon, *Histoire naturelle, générale et particulière*, 2nd edn, vol. 2 (Paris: Imprimerie Royale, 1750), plate 4. 30 × 20 cm. Cambridge University Library.

TABLEAU ÉCONOMIQUE.

Objets à considérer, 1°. Trois sortes de dépenses; 2°. leur source; 3°. leurs avances; 4°. leur distribution; 5°. leurs effets; 6°. leur reproduction; 7°. leurs rapports entr'elles; 8°. leurs rapports avec la population; 9°. avec l'Agriculture; 10°. avec l'industrie; 11°. avec le commerce; 12°. avec la masse des richesses d'une Nation.

DÉPENSES PRODUCTIVES relatives à l'agriculture, &c.	DÉPENSES DU REVENU, l'Impôt prélevé, se partagent aux Dépenses productives et aux Dépenses stériles.	DÉPENSES STÉRILES relatives à l'industrie, &c.
Avances annuelles pour produire un revenu de 600 tt sont 600 tt	Revenu annuel de	Avances annuelles pour les Ouvrages des Dépenses Stériles, sont
600 tt produisent net	600 tt	300 tt
Productions, moitié passe icy	moitié passe icy	Ouvrages, &c.
300 tt reproduisent net	300 tt (moitié passe icy)	300 tt (moitié passe icy)
150 reproduisent net	150 (moitié &c.)	150 (moitié &c.)
75 reproduisent net	75	75
37..10 s reproduisent net	37..10	37..10
18..15 reproduisent net	18..15	18..15
9..7..6 d reproduisent net	9..7..6 d	9..7..6 d
4..13..9 reproduisent net	4..13..9	4..13..9
2..6..10 reproduisent net	2..6..10	2..6..10
1..3..5 reproduisent net	1..3..5	1..3..5
0..11..8 reproduisent net	0..11..8	0..11..8
0..5..10 reproduisent net	0..5..10	0..5..10
0..2..11 reproduisent net	0..2..11	0..2..11
0..1..5 reproduisent net	0..1..5	0..1..5
&c.		

REPRODUIT TOTAL .... 600 tt de revenu; de plus, les frais annuels de 600 tt et les interets des avances primitives du Laboureur, de 300 tt que la terre restitue. Ainsi la reproduction est de 1500 tt compris le revenu de 600 tt qui est la base du calcul, abstraction faite de l'impôt prélevé, et des avances qu'exige sa reproduction annuelle, &c. Voyez l'Explication à la page suivante.

Figure 20.3 Quesnay's 'economic tableau' or 'picture'. The zigzag diagram, inspired by hydraulic machines and rolling-ball clocks, shows the flow of money between 'productive' landowners and farmers and 'sterile' trade and industry that took place in the annual reproduction of revenue. It served as a visual calculating machine and rational recreation. From Quesnay, *Tableau économique*, 'third edition' (1759). Hagley Museum and Library.

Diderot and d'Alembert's *Encyclopédie* recognized these usages. Although the brief '*reproduction*' entry referred only to regeneration, the work drew on Maupertuis and Buffon to define animal '*génération*' as 'the faculty of reproducing oneself'. Quesnay's key entries were long unpublished, and physiocracy soon failed, but Adam Smith's *Wealth of Nations* (1776) discussed the physiocrats and used 'reproduction' a handful of times.

Within a few years, then, the same milieu developed more abstract meanings of '*reproduction*' in natural history and the analysis of wealth. Though usage remains to be traced, promises to regenerate (*régénérer*) living beings, including humans, may have been salient alongside a related shift in the concept of population.[30] The disembedding of production and the 'disembodying' of childbearing appear for the moment less relevant. Nor did 'reproduction' yet have much to do with either manufacturing industry or copying, but those connections would strengthen over time.

From 'Requires to Be Explained' to Standard Usage

Encyclopaedias and dictionaries indicate that the new meanings did not settle till the mid-nineteenth century. Differences among Buffon's successors at the Museum of Natural History suggest the potential for conflict: Jean-Baptiste Lamarck accepted his '*reproduction*', while Georges Cuvier reserved '*reproduction*' for regeneration. To add to the complexity, the word was by the 1760s applied to memory as the faculty of recalling sensations.[31] The sense of producing a copy, as of an illustration or previously published work, was present around 1800 and common by the 1830s. Reinforced by new printing techniques and photography, it was reflected in discussions of copying and originality.

Writers in English adopted Buffon's term as a neologism. Oliver Goldsmith borrowed this and more for his *History of the Earth and Animated Nature* (1774), which outsold the three translations of the opening fifteen volumes of the *Histoire naturelle*. In 1780, one translator added a footnote to 'reproduction': 'This word is frequently used by the author, and requires to be explained. It signifies the power of producing or propagating in general, and is equally applicable to plants and to animals. Generation' – in the narrow sense – 'is a species of reproduction peculiar to animated beings.'[32] The note

30 For example, Sean Quinlan, 'Heredity, reproduction, and perfectibility in revolutionary and Napoleonic France, 1789–1815', *Endeavour* 34 (2010), 142–50; on population: Rusnock, 'Biopolitics'.

31 FRANTEXT and *OED* 1d, beginning with Charles Bonnet.

32 Count de Buffon, *Natural History, General and Particular*, trans. William Smellie, 2nd edn, vol. 2 (London, 1785), p. 3; Jeff Loveland, 'Georges-Louis Leclerc de Buffon's *Histoire naturelle* in English, 1775–1815', *Archives of Natural History* 31 (2004), 214–35.

perhaps triggered the objection from Methodist leader John Wesley, fighting Buffon's 'Atheism barefaced', that he 'endeavours to confound the distinction between animals and vegetables' and 'substitutes for the plain word *generation*, a quaint word of his own … in order to level man not only with the beasts that perish, but with nettles or onions'.[33] This comment, in which Wesley expressed a 'fear of levelling' and 'sense of loss' in the face of 'abstract thinking', has become well known through the *OED*.[34]

Thomas Robert Malthus wrote instead of the 'power of population' and 'increase of the human species'.[35] Until mid-century 'reproduction' mostly meant regeneration in physiology and natural history, and encyclopaedias kept 'generation' as the long entry. Then 'reproduction' took over and 'generation' shrank. As a headword in *Chambers* from 1860 and *Britannica* by the 1890s, 'reproduction' referred to sexual and asexual reproduction in animals and plants, but French works of the 1870s acknowledged the wider range. Littré's dictionary gave procreation, regeneration, the action of preserving value in industry and agriculture, and publishing a second time, while Larousse's encyclopaedia concurred before focusing on physiology and especially the rural economy, including how to choose animals to serve as '*reproducteurs*'. Species reproduction was dominant here, although the word was by this time widespread, in these encyclopaedias as elsewhere, in the sense of republishing or copying. In Marxism the concept would be important in the renewal of capital-labour relations, biological life and life in general: 'every social process of production is at the same time a process of reproduction'.[36]

German used '*Reproduktion*' most standardly in the copying sense that Walter Benjamin took for granted in his 1936 essay on the work of art in the age of its '*technischen Reproduzierbarkeit*', or (in the simpler translation) 'mechanical reproduction'. Through the early twentieth century, psychologists commonly referred to reproduction of ideas. But biological and medical usage was distinctive, because while '*Hervorbringung seines Gleichen*' (production of its like) had translated '*reproduction*' in Buffon's title, '*Fortpflanzung*' was the principal successor to '*(Er)zeugung*', and '*Reproduktion*' a minor rival until in vitro fertilization came in around 1980. Like '*reproduction*', '*Fortpflanzung*' emphasized propagation beyond the individual act of '*Zeugung*' and

33 John Wesley, 'Remarks on the Count de Buffon's "Natural History"' (1782), in *Works* …, vol. 7 (New York, NY, 1835), pp. 441–5.

34 Jordanova, 'Interrogating the concept', p. 372.

35 Echoing Wesley, in 1817 the journalist William Cobbett railed against 'Malthus, who considers men as *mere animals*' and complained that 'we now frequently hear the working classes called "the *population*", just as we call the animals upon a farm "*the stock*"': quoted in Robert J. Mayhew, *Malthus: The Life and Legacies of an Untimely Prophet* (Cambridge, MA, 2014), p. 130.

36 Marx, *Capital*, vol. 1, chapter 23.

transferred between domains.[37] But the German situation cautions against ascribing too much significance to the linguistic overlap of biology and economics.

Though Malthus had shown the writer H. G. Wells that 'human life centres about reproduction', and thus pointed the way to eugenics, even around 1900 'reproduction' and '*Fortpflanzung*' had limited reach.[38] During the nineteenth century, 'generation' or '*Zeugung*' had broken down into embryology, the chief successor but itself weakly institutionalized; the study of heredity, later genetics, which overshadowed embryology in the twentieth century; and reproduction, which long lacked an official identity distinct from anatomy, physiology, gynaecology, zoology, botany and other sciences.[39] Historians have accepted Cambridge physiologist Francis Marshall's claim for his *Physiology of Reproduction* (1910) as the founding handbook, but only in retrospect could 'reproductive sciences', rare before the 1980s, serve as a 'generic', 'umbrella-like' term across the twentieth century.[40] A *Journal of Reproduction and Fertility* was founded in Britain in 1960 and a Society for the Study of Reproduction organized in the United States in 1967, by which time 'reproduction' was a regular heading in school biology textbooks and 'reproductive biology' was taking off (Fig. 20.4). With the topic newly central to molecular and evolutionary biology and a site of struggle in medicine, biologists and feminists began to write histories 'from generation to reproduction'.

The Rising Generation

Yet that is only one trajectory. The old meanings lingered, and in embryology and genetics 'generation' had other successors. Above all, it launched a new career from the sense of a cohort of the same age. Represented in 'the rising generation', a standard phrase by the 1750s, this gained a stronger orientation towards the future that expressed a fresh conception of historical time. In the age of revolutions, as mobility loosened ties

37 Editions of *Brockhaus* and *Meyers Konversations-Lexikon*; Jocelyn Holland, '*Zeugung/Fortpflanzung*: Distinctions of medium in the discourse on generation around 1800', in Susanne Lettow (ed.), *Reproduction, Race, and Gender in Philosophy and the Early Life Sciences* (Albany, NY, 2014), pp. 83–103, on pp. 84–5. One indication of further complexities: Karl Friedrich Burdach used '*Reproduction*' for '*Selbstbildung*' (self-formation) in the sense of basal maintenance of the individual organism; by contrast, '*Zeugung*' was concerned with maintenance of the species, when '*Reproduction*' turned into '*Generation*': *Die Physiologie* (Leipzig, 1810), pp. 240–5, 799.

38 Quoted in Mayhew, *Malthus*, p. 155.

39 Nick Hopwood, 'Embryology', in Peter J. Bowler and John V. Pickstone (eds.), *The Cambridge History of Science*, vol. 6: *The Modern Biological and Earth Sciences* (New York, NY, 2009), pp. 285–315; Müller-Wille and Rheinberger, *Cultural History*; Robert A. Nye, 'Love and reproductive biology in *fin-de-siècle* France: A Foucauldian lacuna?', in Jan Goldstein (ed.), *Foucault and the Writing of History* (Cambridge, MA, 1994), pp. 150–64, on p. 153.

40 Clarke, *Disciplining Reproduction*, pp. 69–74, 9; Jean-Paul Gaudillière, 'Sex Hormones, Pharmacy and the Reproductive Sciences', Chapter 35, this book.

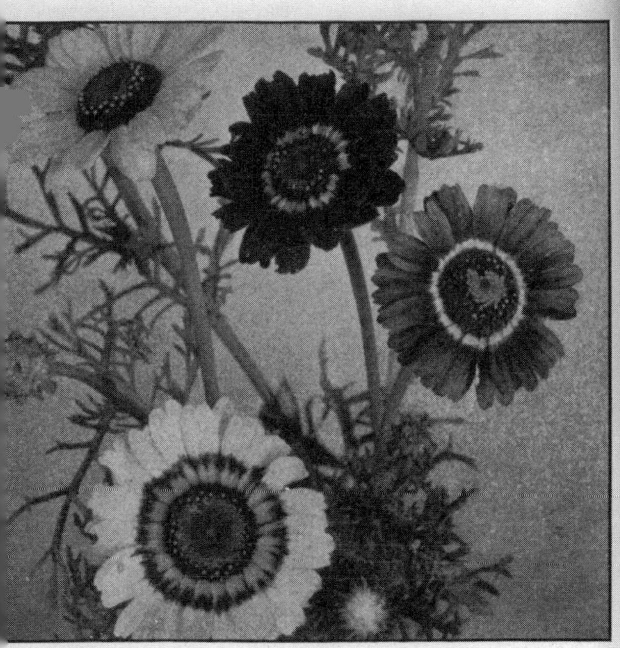

hese chrysanthemums are annuals, grown each year from
eds. Flowers and seeds insure the continued existence of
ese chrysanthemums year after year, just as reproduction
nerally insures the continuity of life. (Courtesy of W.
lee Burpee Company, Philadelphia)

Unit Seven

REPRODUCTION INSURES THE CONTINUITY OF LIFE

PROBLEM 19 *What are the two main methods of reproduction?*

PROBLEM 20 *What part do flowers play in the life of the seed plant?*

PROBLEM 21 *How do the higher animals reproduce?*

PROBLEM 22 *How does an egg grow into an organism?*

SCIENCE DISPROVES ANOTHER SUPERSTITION

It was natural for human beings long ago to wonder where young frogs or mice or rats or other young animals came from. When they found baby mice among a lot of old rags, they jumped to the conclusion that the rags had produced the mice. When they found a nest of bees in the decaying carcass of an ox, they naturally thought the bees had been generated (produced) by the dead body. The famous Latin poet Virgil actually included in one of his books a recipe for getting bees out of an animal's carcass. Even Aristotle, the most scientific of the famous ancient Greek scholars, believed that old rags left in the dark would generate mice and that fleas and mosquitoes were formed in decaying matter.

Thus gradually mankind came to believe that many kinds of young animals

359

Figure 20.4 Unit opener from *Exploring Biology*, Ella T. Smith's successful American high-school textbook. *Reproduction* had figured in chapter and unit titles since around 1920, but was thematized more generally, concertedly and explicitly from the 1960s. This unit began with a 'science *versus* superstition' history of spontaneous generation (see Exhibit 26, this book). From the third edition (New York, NY: Harcourt, Brace, 1949), pp. 358–9, 24 × 31 cm, courtesy of W. Atlee Burpee & Co.

to parents and change devalued their skills, generations became temporary carriers of political sovereignty. Understood as sharing experiences, and thus outlooks, communities of contemporaries served as agents of progress, supposed to pass on the benefits of education, though subject to the constraints of tradition. By the mid-nineteenth century, the sciences, philosophy and political economy, like novels about the modern family, discussed 'generations' with respect to social and natural orders, reproduction, inheritance and transmission.[41]

Ohad Parnes has reconstructed the role of generations in making the modern concept of heredity. In 1826, when the Protestant theologian Friedrich Schleiermacher wrote of the 'alternation of generations' (*Wechsel der Generationen*) in the context of knowledge transmission, a similar term, '*Generationswechsel*', had recently been coined for the phenomenon of a species appearing in two different forms, such that an individual would resemble its grandmother and granddaughters, but not mother or daughters (Fig. 20.5). Inheritance had been understood as maintaining the constancy of the type and individual variations as usually not inherited. By 1860, a new approach, seeking to explain regular changes and patterns of intergenerational 'memory', took the 'seemingly mathematical regularity' of alternating generations as a model. Heredity would be studied as a mechanism for transmitting traits, whether species or individual, between large populations corresponding to generations.[42]

Around 1900, as confidence in progress ebbed, generations came to be seen as separate and crisis-scarred. Karl Mannheim's 'Das Problem der Generationen' (The problem of generations, 1928) put positivist year-counting together with the Romantic-historical insistence on the centrality of consciousness to stress rapid social change as the precondition for a distinctive experience interpreted similarly to produce a shared outlook. Formative crises include the world wars and immigration, which anthropologist Franz Boas identified as producing a 'generation gap'. After the 'baby-boom generation' and 'generation X', use has become inflationary because the term promises attention to numbers and experience. Other applications abound: the 'intergenerational contract', 'generations' of computers. But in English (unlike German), 'generation' and especially 'generate' still also echo the sense of procreation.[43]

Conclusion

Though confirming a shift from generation to reproduction, the words tell a longer story of change that enriches and revises Jacob's and the feminist accounts, and raises questions for research. 'Reproduction' was used earlier and in more various senses of 'producing again' than has been appreciated. The rise of the more abstract modern

41 Parnes, Vedder and Willer, *Konzept der Generation*, pp. 82–119, 150–87; Silvia De Renzi, 'Family Resemblance in the Old Regime', Chapter 17, this book.

42 Ohad S. Parnes, 'On the shoulders of generations: The new epistemology of heredity in the nineteenth century', in Staffan Müller-Wille and Hans-Jörg Rheinberger (eds.), *Heredity Produced: At the Crossroads of Biology, Politics, and Culture, 1500–1870* (Cambridge, MA, 2007), pp. 315–46, quotations on pp. 319, 328, 322.

43 Parnes, Vedder and Willer, *Konzept der Generation*, pp. 218–313.

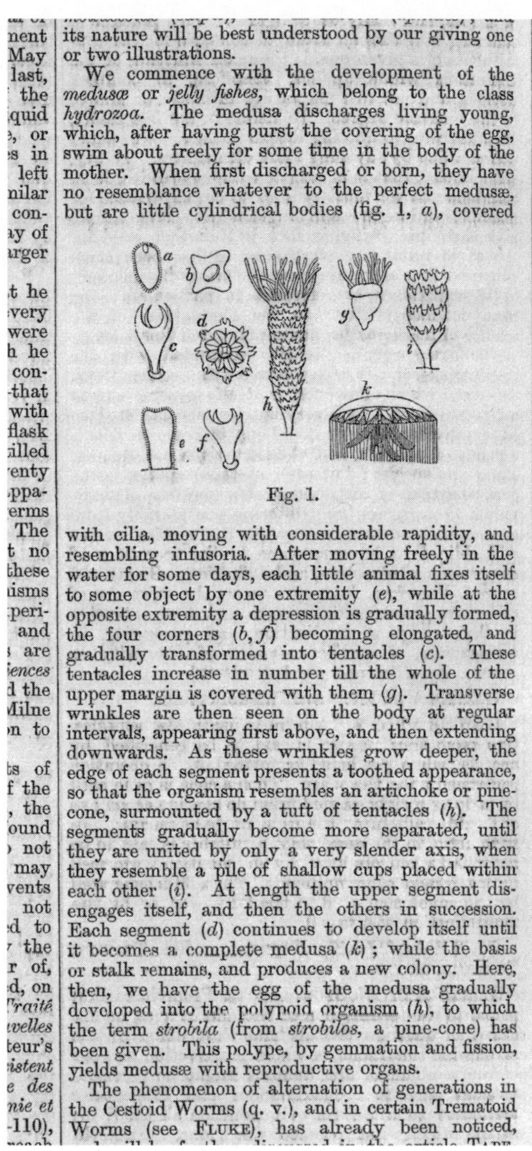
its nature will be best understood by our giving one or two illustrations.

We commence with the development of the *medusæ* or *jelly fishes,* which belong to the class *hydrozoa.* The medusa discharges living young, which, after having burst the covering of the egg, swim about freely for some time in the body of the mother. When first discharged or born, they have no resemblance whatever to the perfect medusæ, but are little cylindrical bodies (fig. 1, *a*), covered

Fig. 1.

with cilia, moving with considerable rapidity, and resembling infusoria. After moving freely in the water for some days, each little animal fixes itself to some object by one extremity (*e*), while at the opposite extremity a depression is gradually formed, the four corners (*b*, *f*) becoming elongated, and gradually transformed into tentacles (*c*). These tentacles increase in number till the whole of the upper margin is covered with them (*g*). Transverse wrinkles are then seen on the body at regular intervals, appearing first above, and then extending downwards. As these wrinkles grow deeper, the edge of each segment presents a toothed appearance, so that the organism resembles an artichoke or pine-cone, surmounted by a tuft of tentacles (*h*). The segments gradually become more separated, until they are united by only a very slender axis, when they resemble a pile of shallow cups placed within each other (*i*). At length the upper segment disengages itself, and then the others in succession. Each segment (*d*) continues to develop itself until it becomes a complete medusa (*k*); while the basis or stalk remains, and produces a new colony. Here, then, we have the egg of the medusa gradually developed into the polypoid organism (*h*), to which the term *strobila* (from *strobilos*, a pine-cone) has been given. This polype, by gemmation and fission, yields medusæ with reproductive organs.

The phenomenon of alternation of generations in the Cestoid Worms (q. v.), and in certain Trematoid Worms (see Fluke), has already been noticed,

Figure 20.5 Part of an encyclopaedia entry on 'Generations, alternation of'. The 'remarkable' phenomenon was illustrated with examples, beginning with '*medusae* or *jelly fishes*'. Spontaneous generation became the other main topic of entries on generation. *Chambers's Encyclopaedia: A Dictionary of Universal Knowledge for the People*, vol. 4 (London: Chambers, 1862), p. 674. 15 × 8 cm. Cambridge University Library.

meanings in natural history and the analysis of wealth was likely bound up with claims about the regeneration of natural resources; arguments directed at rulers rejecting mercantilism might repay further examination. Yet it took 'reproduction' till the mid-nineteenth century to capture a fraction of the old territory – embryology and then also the science of heredity occupied the rest – and by catching a second wind around 1800, 'generation' remained the more common word. References to copying, imitation and manufacture linked 'reproduction' to production in new ways, but the separations of life from economics mattered as much as the connections.

This history of keywords plots a path between and beyond two opposed views which highlight changes around 1800 and 1900 respectively. The first, indebted to Jacob and Foucault, locates the 'conceptual' preconditions for 'the emergence of the political-epistemic regime of reproduction' in a fairly sudden change from generation to reproduction, which it seeks to show was widely potent by the early nineteenth century.[44] But in the present state of knowledge it is unclear to what extent real or imagined interventions were enabled by any simple shift from generation to reproduction or even happened under the banner of reproduction (rather than, for example, population or generation); concepts, not to mention words, may lead, but often follow. The second view accepts these intellectual prerequisites, but stresses the more immediately consequential innovations, not least in eugenics and demography, around 1900. Historians generally assume that by then the topic was obviously reproduction, but Clarke placed this in such a 'hostile' world that it 'coalesced' as a formal object of science only in the twentieth century.[45] Wide resonance did not wait for disciplinary recognition, but that dating still seems right. The crucial question is how reproduction changed as the word was adopted in various arenas and participated in a more unified discourse, and to what extent semantic shifts marked or even drove those changes.

To answer it, we shall need a larger-scale map of practices, concepts and word usage, especially for the long nineteenth century. Caution is in order until that research is done. Contributors to this book have avoided presenting 'reproduction' as an actor's category before about 1750, but mislabelling may be more insidious in and around modern disciplines. For all the exchange, there is no single register for speaking about making babies, breeding animals, planting seeds, making photocopies and socio-economic renewal, and nor has there ever been just one word.

44 Susanne Lettow, 'Population, race and gender: On the genealogy of the modern politics of reproduction', *Distinktion: Scandinavian Journal of Social Theory* 16 (2015), 267–82.

45 Clarke, *Disciplining Reproduction*, p. 5.

21 Linnaeus and the Love Lives of Plants

Staffan Müller-Wille

During the eighteenth century, reproduction and associated processes such as heredity and evolution moved to the centre of a new science of life. The large literature on these intellectual and cultural changes concentrates on the zoological and anthropological writings of scholars including Pierre Louis de Maupertuis, Georges-Louis Leclerc de Buffon, Immanuel Kant, Erasmus Darwin and Jean-Baptiste Lamarck.[1] Yet plants also held a place in eighteenth-century thought, notably the doctrine of physiocracy, which identified agriculture as the source of wealth.[2] Economic historians have demonstrated how the exchange of staple foods such as wheat and potatoes between the New World and the Old facilitated the rise of capitalism.[3] Botanical gardens, in Europe and overseas, served as hubs for this global exchange, and the botanists in charge played a significant role in the propagation of Enlightenment ideas of improvement and progress.[4]

One botanist has been much recognized for his contributions to Enlightenment discourses of generation, propagation and the production of wealth: the Swedish naturalist and physician Carl Linnaeus (1707–78).[5] In 1735, while staying in Holland to complete his medical studies, Linnaeus authored the *Systema naturae* (System of nature), which proposed to classify plants according to the number and arrangement of their 'male' and 'female' generative organs (stamens and pistils). This 'sexual system' made the 28-year-old medical

1 Bentley Glass, Owsei Temkin and William L. Straus, Jr (eds.), *Forerunners of Darwin, 1745–1859* (Baltimore, MD, 1959); Michel Foucault, *The Order of Things: An Archeology of the Human Sciences* (London, 1974); François Jacob, *The Logic of Life: A History of Heredity*, trans. Betty E. Spillmann (New York, NY, 1973); Ernst Mayr, *The Growth of Biological Thought: Diversity, Evolution, and Inheritance* (Cambridge, MA, 1982); Staffan Müller-Wille and Hans-Jörg Rheinberger, *A Cultural History of Heredity* (Chicago, IL, 2012), esp. pp. 15–39.

2 Margaret Schabas, *The Natural Origins of Economics* (Chicago, IL, 2005); Nick Hopwood, 'The Keywords "Generation" and "Reproduction"', Chapter 20; Andrea Rusnock, 'Biopolitics and the Invention of Population', Chapter 23, this book.

3 Nathan Nunn and Nancy Qian, 'The Columbian exchange: A history of disease, food, and ideas', *Journal of Economic Perspectives* 24 (2010), 163–88.

4 Richard Drayton, *Nature's Government: Science, Imperial Britain, and the 'Improvement' of the World* (New Haven, CT, 2000); Emma C. Spary, *Utopia's Garden: French Natural History from Old Regime to Revolution* (Chicago, IL, 2000); Londa L. Schiebinger, *Plants and Empire: Colonial Bioprospecting in the Atlantic World* (Cambridge, MA, 2004); Schiebinger and Claudia Swan (eds.), *Colonial Botany: Science, Commerce, and Politics in the Early Modern World* (Philadelphia, PA, 2005).

5 Pascal Duris, *Linné et la France (1780–1850)* (Geneva, 1995); Lisbet Koerner, *Linnaeus: Nature and Nation* (Cambridge, MA, 1999); Staffan Müller-Wille, *Botanik und weltweiter Handel. Zur Begründung eines natürlichen Systems der Pflanzen durch Carl von Linné (1707–78)* (Berlin, 1999).

student famous and founded a career as Europe's leading botanical authority. According to Londa Schiebinger, the sexual system resonated with eighteenth-century audiences because Linnaeus 'brought traditional notions of gender hierarchy whole cloth into science'. Most importantly, she claims, the sexual system emphasized heterosexual marriage, and thus excluded homosexuality, for example.[6] More recent work has complicated this picture. Ann Shteir found that sexualized botanical representations mattered to eighteenth-century audiences as 'boundaries to be disputed'.[7] This chimes with the observation by earlier historians that the sexual system challenged the long-held conviction that plants did not propagate sexually at all since they lacked the capacity of animals to sense and move.[8]

This chapter uses the case of Linnaeus to reveal some deeper levels of eighteenth-century discourses on sexuality and reproduction. I first take a fresh look at the sexual system, revealing references to behaviours that most eighteenth-century readers perceived as deviant. Sexuality, the subversive message went, was universal and produced a cornucopia of life forms. Then I turn to Linnaeus's writings on dietetics, physiology and the economy of nature, which portray sexuality as a source not only of new life, but also of struggle, dispersion and death. The final section explores Linnaeus's working life, which saw him engaged in propagating plants from all over the world, and his family life, which presented him and his wife with economic and social challenges. In conclusion, I discuss how eighteenth-century botanists projected onto plants their beliefs in a stable natural order that would foster inexhaustible riches, as well as their fears of an unruly underworld of sexual forces and desires.

Perverting the Scale of Nature

Linnaeus designed the sexual system in the summer of 1730 while teaching medical students at the Uppsala botanical garden. To support his course, he arranged the species that were grown there in manuscript catalogues, some of which were probably sold to students, others given as gifts to potential patrons. Five catalogues survive. Two, dating from spring 1730, use Joseph Pitton de Tournefort's classification system,

6 Londa Schiebinger, *Nature's Body: Gender in the Making of Modern Science* (Boston, MA, 1993), pp. 17 (quotation), 4, 25–6.

7 Ann B. Shteir, *Cultivating Women, Cultivating Science: Flora's Daughters and Botany in England, 1760 to 1860* (Baltimore, MD, 1999), p. 274; also Elizabeth Heckendorn Cook, '"Perfect" flowers, monstrous women: Eighteenth-century botany and the modern gendered subject', in Helen Deutsch and Felicity Nussbaum (eds.), '*Defects*': *Engendering the Modern Body* (Ann Arbor, MI, 2000), pp. 252–79.

8 François Delaporte, *Nature's Second Kingdom: Explorations of Vegetality in the Eighteenth Century*, trans. Arthur Goldhammer (Cambridge, MA, 1982); John Farley, *Gametes & Spores: Ideas about Sexual Reproduction, 1750–1914* (Baltimore, MD, 1982); Roger L. Williams, *Botanophilia in Eighteenth-Century France: The Spirit of the Enlightenment* (Dordrecht, 2001).

which was based on flower morphology without any reference to sexual functions. The remaining three, dating from summer 1730 and spring 1731 respectively, present the first versions of the sexual system. One, *Adonis Uplandicus* (Garden of Uppland), does so in the form of a diagram which already contains the basic elements of the version in the *Systema naturae* of 1735 (Fig. 21.1).[9]

The diagram, with its heading 'Classes in our sexual system, named allegorically', can be read in two ways. From left to right, one is led through a series of progressively finer distinctions pertaining to the 'marriages of plants' (*Nuptiae plantarum*). These are either 'private' (leading to the class *Cryptogamia*) or 'public'. The public marriages are conducted in either one or two bedchambers (*Monoclinia*/*Diclinia*), branches that split further according to differences in the social and legal relationships between the partners involved: kin or not (*affinitas*/*diffinitas*), married or adulterous (*conjugium*/*adulterium*) and of equal or unequal social status (*indifferentismus*/*subordinatio*). Only then does the sexual system turn to the number of male partners to distinguish the first thirteen classes (*Monandria*/ … /*Polyandria*). In exploring the metaphor of 'marriage', Linnaeus stressed consummation through sexual union, which explains the inclusion of adultery.

The second reading focuses on the twenty-three classes on the right-hand side of the diagram. These form a vertical series, with *Monandria* (literally 'one-husbanded') at the top, and *Cryptogamia* ('secretly married') at the bottom. The published version in the *Systema naturae*, which accentuated the sexual imagery by adding short explanations, helps us analyse this series. The *Monandria*, that is, plants with one 'husband' only, are placed at the top. Below them is a progressive series of perversions of this ideal. Unions involving more and more partners culminate in the *Polyandria*, with 'twenty or more husbands in the same bed with a woman'. The next two classes involve miscegenation, with females entering relationships with males of different 'potency' (*Didynamia, Tetradynamia*). Then come five classes that exhibit various forms of incest and male homosexuality: the *Monadelphia*, *Diadelphia* and *Polyadelphia*, where women are wed to one, two or more groups of 'cognate' males; the *Syngenesia*, where 'husbands form a union with their genitals'; and the *Gynandria*, with husbands 'monstrously cognate' to the wife. Before arriving at the bottom of the scale – the *Cryptogamia*, which 'celebrate their nuptials secretly' – the series progresses through three more classes, the *Monoecia*, *Dioecia* and *Polygamia*, where adultery takes over, reaching across otherwise separate 'bedchambers' and 'houses'. The 1735 version also adds a division of plants with composite flowers, this time from a population perspective. The *Monogamia* display 'many marriages', while always 'contracting pure conjugals', but 'prostitutes' (*meretrices*)

9 James L. Larson, *Reason and Experience: The Representation of Natural Order in the Work of Carl von Linné* (Berkeley, CA, 1971), pp. 50–8.

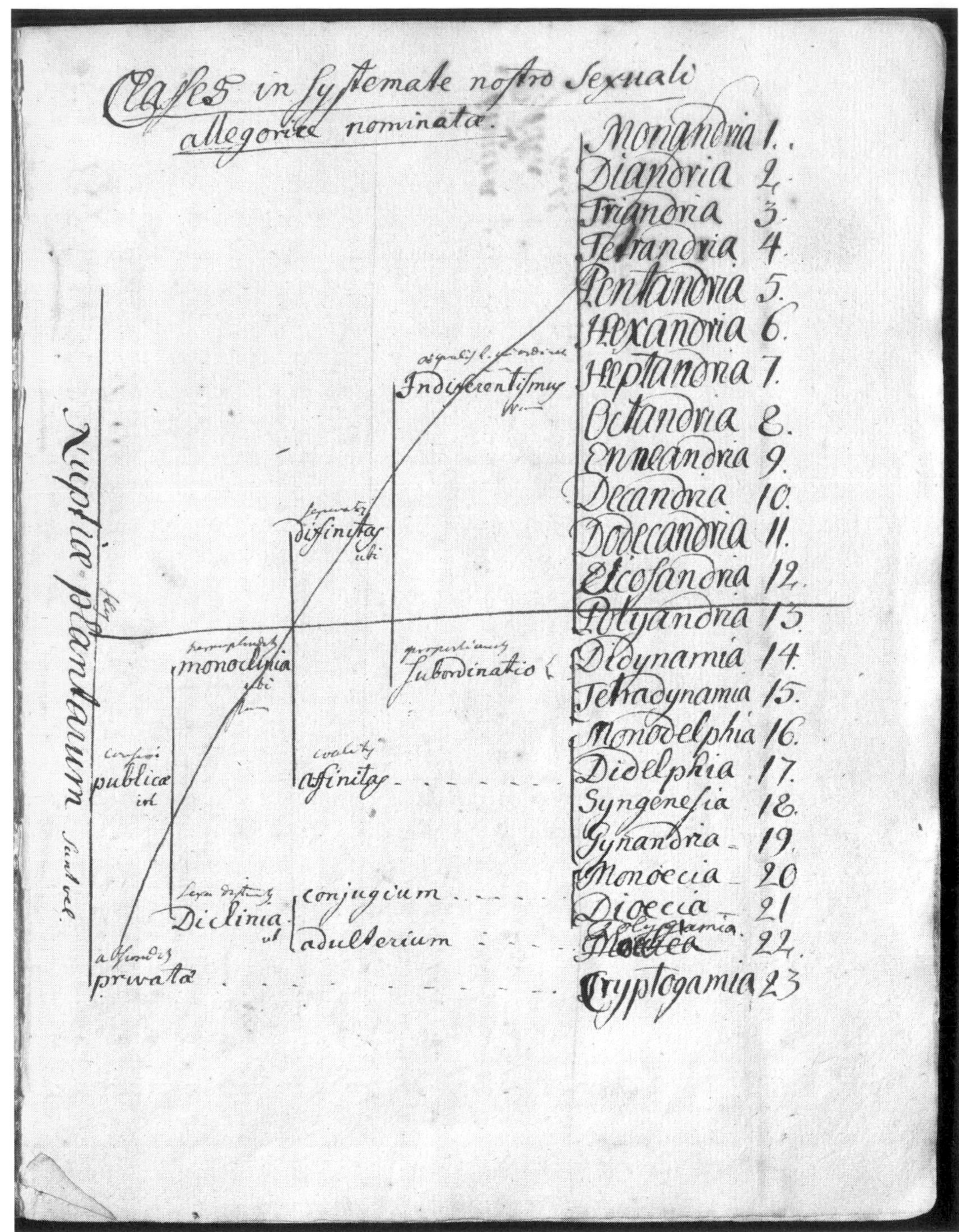

Figure 21.1 'Classes in Systemate nostro Sexuali allegorice nominatae (Classes in our sexual system, named allegorically)', page from Carl Linnaeus, *Adonis Uplandicus*. Ink on paper, 20 × 16 cm. Uppsala University Library, Department of Manuscripts and Music, Leufsta MS 6.

enter the picture in the *Polygamia*. Some of these prostitutes are sterile, while others are fertile and replace sterile wives 'in order to propagate the family'.[10]

Schiebinger noted the rich allusions to eighteenth-century practices – unsanctioned ('secret') marriages, marriage among close kin and prostitution. Yet if one takes into account the full range of practices portrayed, it seems implausible that Linnaeus simply reflected existing custom.[11] The sexual system rather stood in a long tradition of using pornography to entertain medical students.[12] And eighteenth-century audiences understood this, both the many, now infamous critics who denounced the sexual system for its immorality, and those like Jean-Jacques Rousseau, Maupertuis, Julien Offray de La Mettrie and Erasmus Darwin who endorsed its vivid imagery.[13]

The target of the witticisms in the sexual system becomes clear once one realizes its relation to what the historian of ideas Arthur O. Lovejoy called the 'Great Chain of Being', the ancient notion that all beings, from humble mosses to humans, could be arranged on a linear scale of perfection.[14] Only the *Monandria*, the top of the series of twenty-four classes of the sexual system, displays what was deemed a morally acceptable, that is, heterosexual and monogamous, union. From there, one descends into an abyss of deviations and perversions, ending in the unfathomable world of the *Cryptogamia*. Once one reads the sexual system like this, two subversive messages emerge. First, whatever 'rank' plant species may occupy on the scale of perfection, they *all* propagate sexually. This was an affront to conceptions of the scale of nature, since sexual procreation seemed to presuppose the ability to sense and move, which had been considered the prerogative of the more 'noble' animals. Second, the exuberant nuptial arrangements of the sexual system highlighted nature's production of an ostensibly redundant array of variations upon one universal theme. Sexual relations both unified and dispersed plant (and metaphorically human) life. They held these forms together in an apparently stable, 'natural' order of rationally accessible distinctions while at the same time exploding order through illicit transgressions and permutations. This fundamental ambivalence, and the humorous associations it elicited, account for the success of the sexual system.

10 Carl Linnaeus, *Systema naturae, sive Regna tria naturae systematice proposita per classes, ordines, genera, & species* (Leiden, 1735), 'Clavis systema sexualis' (unpaginated).

11 Schiebinger, *Nature's Body*, pp. 25–6.

12 Julie Peakman, *Mighty Lewd Books: The Development of Pornography in Eighteenth-Century England* (New York, NY, 2003), pp. 71–8; Sarah Toulalan, *Imagining Sex: Pornography and Bodies in Seventeenth-Century England* (Oxford, 2007), pp. 21, 53.

13 Schiebinger, *Nature's Body*, pp. 40–74. These debates extended into the nineteenth century: Theresa M. Kelley, *Clandestine Marriage: Botany and Romantic Culture* (Baltimore, MD, 2012).

14 Arthur O. Lovejoy, *The Great Chain of Being: A Study of the History of an Idea* (Cambridge, MA, 1936); also Laurence M. V. Totelin, 'Animal and Plant Generation in Classical Antiquity', Chapter 4, this book.

Sexuality and the Balance of Nature

Does this mean the system was only a joke? Far from it, but to see what concerns lay at its core we need other sources. Linnaeus had a 'hidden philosophy', entangled in the premodern world of symbols and allegories, that idiosyncratically reflected contemporary preoccupations with the roles of the sexes in procreation.[15] This philosophy came to the fore in his writings on medicine and physiology, where sexual relations were a central theme, but in a strikingly different way from the combinatorial logic of the sexual system.

In 1733 Linnaeus prepared a manuscript, *Diaeta naturalis*, on the occasion of private lectures he gave on dietetics, or ways to avoid disease and keep healthy.[16] The lectures followed a conventional Galenic division into 'things natural', that is, the given parts, functions and virtues of the body, and the 'non-naturals', those factors affecting health that regimen can control.[17] Beginning with the former, the manuscript observes that 'all living beings give birth to [beings] similar to them'; conception, pregnancy and birth were seen as the source of bodily constitution and temperament. The rest of the lecture was about the influence on health of the non-naturals: climate, clothes and housing, food and drink, sleep and sexual activity, and the passions.

In the section on things natural, Linnaeus mentions hereditary diseases (*haereditarii morbi*), a topic to which doctors were only beginning to pay attention. Tellingly, he did so in the context of dietetics, since like most contemporaries, Linnaeus blamed the circumstances of conception, rather than dispositions transmitted from generation to generation, for inherited disease. To avoid such diseases, parents should themselves be healthy, neither too old nor too young, and avoid sexual intercourse during menstruation.[18]

15 K. Rob V. Wikman, *Lachesis and Nemesis: Four Chapters on the Human Condition in the Writings of Carl Linnaeus* (Stockholm, 1970); Gunnar Broberg, Homo sapiens *L.: Studier i Carl von Linnés naturuppfattning och människolära* (Stockholm, 1975).

16 Arvid Hj. Uggla (ed.), *Diaeta naturalis, 1733: Linnés tankar om ett naturenligt levnadssätt* (Uppsala, 1958). Further notes served as the basis of eight public lectures at the University of Uppsala, but the manuscripts were never published, probably because of the sexually explicit content; see Axel Otto Lindfors (ed.), *Linnés dietetik på grundvalen af dels hans eget originalutkast till föreläsningar: Lachesis naturalis quae tradit Diætam naturalem och dels lärjungeanteckningar efter dessa hans föreläsningar Collegium diæteticum* (Uppsala, 1907), p. iv.

17 On early modern dietetics, see William Coleman, 'Health and hygiene in the *Encyclopédie*: A medical doctrine for the bourgeoisie', *Journal of the History of Medicine and Allied Sciences* 29 (1974), 399–421; and Steven Shapin, 'Descartes the doctor: Rationalism and its therapies', *British Journal for the History of Science* 33 (2000), 131–54.

18 Uggla, *Diaeta naturalis*, pp. 32–4; in Lindfors, *Linnés dietetik*, p. 31, Linnaeus even used the Latin noun *haeredit[as]*. On heredity in eighteenth-century medicine: Carlos López Beltrán, 'The medical origins of heredity', in Müller-Wille and Rheinberger, *Heredity Produced*, pp. 105–32.

Sexual intercourse was also a theme in the section on the non-naturals, but now with a view to the effect on individuals. Here, Linnaeus stressed that sexual activity was a natural necessity. 'It is certain that the first law was to grow and multiply', and this law, Linnaeus claimed, 'is so ingrained in all bodies, that it is hard to describe … Love is what all wish most, and most enjoy, the most general, necessary, and certain [thing].' Above all, this removed the sexual drive from psychological and moral control. As he told his students:

> Lewdness (*Kåtthet*) is no affect [of the soul], hence nothing foul in girls. No dropsical person will be called drunkard, even if always thirsty. No child greedy and avaricious because it wants to eat. Hence no girl unchaste that wants men, since once the egg (*ovum*) swells she feels desire, and it would be a miracle should she not feel it.[19]

If sexual desire is natural, its suppression will have negative consequences for health, especially mental health. But a balance needed to be struck, Linnaeus warned, since '[s] emen is the flower and quintessence of the blood, hence not to be exhausted'. 'One should not give life to others to such a degree', he continued, 'that one shortens one's own'. Twice per month, or at most twice per week, was his concrete advice, not forgetting to reassure his listeners once more that '[a]ll excellent fellows, enlightened by great reason, … have been lewd'.[20]

This conception of sexuality as a system of regenerative, if potentially exhausting, natural forces also informed Linnaeus's philosophy of nature. Endorsing a 'natural magic' that built on sympathies, antipathies and action at a distance, Linnaeus conceived of organic bodies as composed of two sexualized, dynamically interacting substances, the 'medulla' (pith) and 'cortex' (bark). As he put it in *Generatio ambigena* (Two-sided generation, 1759) with reference to plants:

> Vegetables consist of medullary and cortical substances; the medullary, the chief life of the vegetables, is of a wonderful disposition, which has the power to multiply indefinitely … This medullary [matter] is as it were imprisoned within the cortical substance, which makes every effort to keep it in … But when, owing to height, heat, lack of moisture or nourishment, or disease, it is not strong enough, then the marrow exerts outward pressure, and bursts the cortical substance; and then the plant undergoes a transformation, the fruit-body is perfected, and the marrow is granulated into seeds.[21]

19 Uggla, *Diaeta naturalis*, pp. 111, 109. In mentioning the *ovum*, Linnaeus follows William Harvey and the ancient two-seed model of generation; see Carl Linnaeus, *Sponsalia plantarum* (Stockholm, 1746); and Rebecca Flemming, 'Galen's Generations of Seeds', Chapter 7, this book.

20 Uggla, *Diaeta naturalis*, pp. 111–12.

21 Carl Linnaeus, 'Generatio ambigena', in *Caroli Linnaei Amoenitates academicae, seu Dissertationes variae physicae, medicae, botanicae antehac seorsim editae …*, vol. 6 (Stockholm, 1763), pp. 2–3. I owe the translation to Stephen Freer.

It is striking that these two substances are portrayed as bearing antagonistic forces: one of indiscriminate proliferation, acting from the inside out, which Linnaeus associated with the maternal line, and one of containment and control, which he associated with the male (Fig. 21.2). The constant struggle for balance sustains life. When maternal powers take over, the luscious forms of the flower arise, and if in excess, monstrosities appear, like double flowers. If paternal powers predominate, plant life dwindles. Moreover, it is the male substance that gives plants their specific form, a supposition that Linnaeus exploited to explain the origin of new species from hybridization.[22]

Linnaeus's speculations about medulla and cortex belonged to the genre of 'animal economy', physiological writings that portrayed organic bodies as machines composed of vessels and percolating fluids, or, in more vitalist terms, 'fibres' and 'springs'.[23] Stephen Hales had advocated this model in his *Vegetable Staticks* (1727). Mapping a gendered dualism onto this economy seems to be Linnaeus's addition. There is no evidence that contemporaries adopted it, but the medulla–cortex theory echoed in his far more influential concept of an 'economy of nature' (*oeconomia naturae*) at large.[24] Plant and animal species, he proposed, were interconnected by a web of relationships preserved through a precarious balance between destruction and production. This economy built on a dichotomy of two orthogonal processes: over time, individuals within each species produced more individuals, growing in number from generation to generation; but this process depended on synchronic relationships of consumption and production that curtailed growth so that it remained proportionate to the available means of subsistence.[25] Unlike Buffon, Linnaeus did not use the word 'reproduction', but instead the expression '*generatio continuata*', literally 'continued generation', or generation as a continuous process extending throughout a species and transcending any particular moment – conception, birth or death – in the life of individual beings.[26]

22 P. F. Stevens and S. P. Cullen, 'Linnaeus, the cortex-medulla theory, and the key to his understanding of plant form and natural relationships', *Journal of the Arnold Arboretum* 71 (1990), 179–220.

23 Philippe Huneman, '"Animal economy": Anthropology and the rise of psychiatry from the *Encyclopédie* to the alienists', in Larry Wolff and Marco Cipolloni (eds.), *The Anthropology of the Enlightenment* (Stanford, CA, 2007), pp. 262–76.

24 Trevor Pearce, '"A great complication of circumstances": Darwin and the economy of nature', *Journal of the History of Biology* 43 (2010), 493–528.

25 Camille Limoges, 'Introduction' to Linné, *L'équilibre de la nature*, ed. Limoges, trans. Bernard Jasmin (Paris, 1972), pp. 7–24; Frank N. Egerton, 'Changing concepts of the balance of nature', *Quarterly Review of Biology* 48 (1973), 322–50.

26 Müller-Wille and Rheinberger, *Cultural History*, pp. 31–2; Hopwood, 'Keywords'.

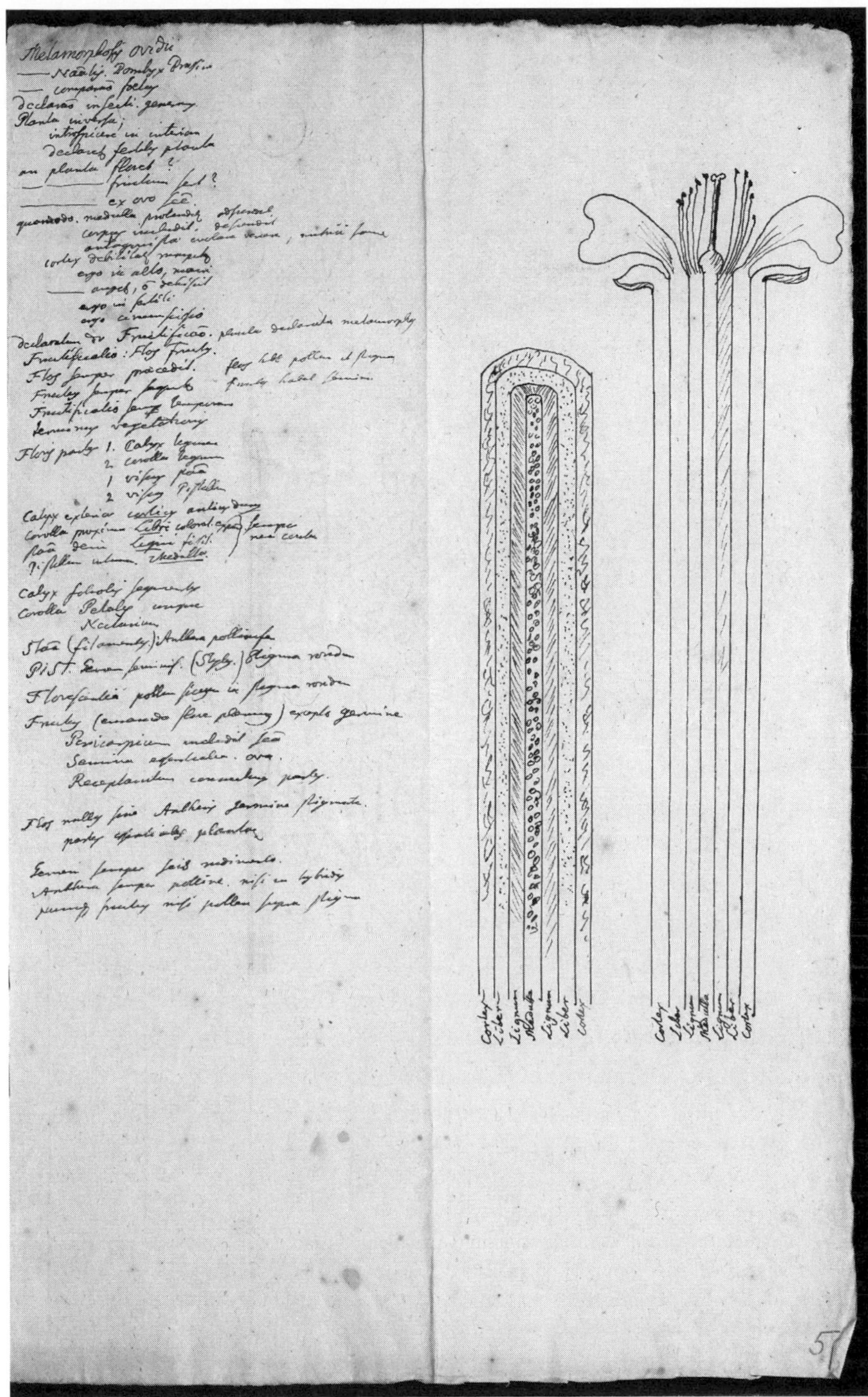

Figure 21.2 Late manuscript containing a drawing by Linnaeus showing the relationship between layers of the plant stem ('cortex' outside, 'medulla' in the centre) and male and female flower parts. Ink on paper, 21 × 8.5 cm. Linnaean Manuscripts, 'Notes on the ontogeny of flowers and leaves' (*c.* 1770), MS GB-110/LM/LP/BOT/6/21, p. 5, reproduced by permission of the Linnean Society of London, Library and Archives, www.linnean.org.

Oeconomia, Work and Family Life

Linnaeus's economy of nature – with species as populations of determinate number and scope engaging in relations of exchange – fits well with his outlook on the human economy.[27] Linnaeus subscribed to the doctrine of cameralism, which aspired to turn territorial states into self-sufficient communities through rational administration of natural resources. In contrast to the economy of nature, however, this ideal had to be enforced through a system of legal 'pulleys and levies' – especially to restrain women's indulgence in imported luxuries.[28] As Linnaeus's philosophy of nature contained a curious antagonism of medulla and cortex, so in his economic views he conceded the potential for imbalance and struggle. To gain a better understanding of this position, one has to turn to the economic projects and practices in which Linnaeus engaged.

A good entry point is *Musa Cliffortiana* (1736), a slim volume to celebrate success in bringing a banana plant to flower and fruit in the hothouse of George Clifford, a merchant banker and botanical amateur, who supported Linnaeus financially during his last two years in Holland. With the help of Clifford's gardener, Dietrich Nietzel, Linnaeus had managed to 'imitate the most productive native locations of Musas [bananas] in every respect, to wit, in temperature, quality of the soil and quantity of water'.[29] Their efforts were rewarded with a flower exhibiting 'a peculiar … sort of polygamy' in which 'one wife, married to useless husbands, embraces the husbands of the other female, while these husbands are united with a sterile and incapable wife' (Fig. 21.3).[30] Linnaeus lured Nietzel to Uppsala several years later, in 1742, when he took over the chair in medicine and botany there and became director of the botanical garden. He eventually served the royal family fresh bananas.

This episode reminds us that Linnaeus cultivated and propagated plants throughout his career, routinely in the botanical garden, but also in trying to acclimatize exotic plants like tea and mulberry to the harsh Swedish conditions in order to turn his home country into a 'miniature mercantile empire' (Fig. 21.4).[31] Many of these attempts failed, however, and Linnaeus's relations with gardeners were fraught.[32] Moreover, success

27 On eighteenth-century conceptions of population: Rusnock, 'Biopolitics'; on Linnaeus's influence on contemporary economic thought: Paul P. Christensen, 'Fire, motion, and productivity: The proto-energetics of nature and economy in François Quesnay', in Philip Mirowski (ed.), *Natural Images in Economic Thought: 'Markets Read in Tooth and Claw'* (Cambridge, 1994), pp. 249–88.

28 Koerner, *Linnaeus*, p. 102; Lisbet Koerner, 'Women and utility in Enlightenment science', *Configurations* 2 (1995), 233–55.

29 Carl Linnaeus, *Musa Cliffortiana: Clifford's Banana Plant*, trans. Stephen Freer (Ruggell, 2007), p. 157.

30 Ibid., p. 167.

31 Koerner, *Linnaeus*, p. 114.

32 Staffan Müller-Wille, 'Introduction' to Linnaeus, *Musa Cliffortiana*, pp. 63–5.

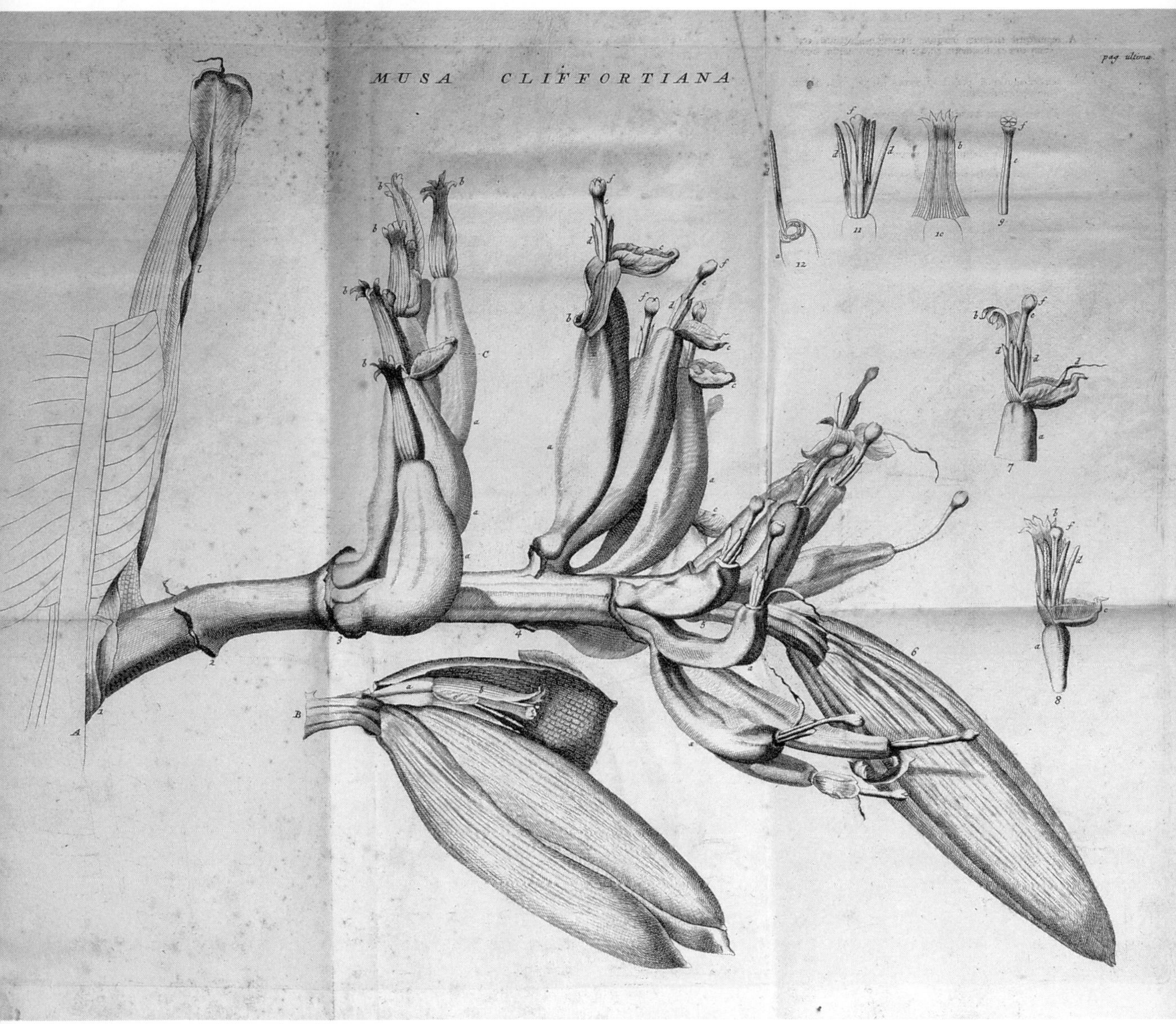

Figure 21.3 Plate showing banana flower with male flower bud at right and female flowers arranged in 'hands' further left. Copper engraving by A. van der Laan produced from a drawing by Martin Hofmann. Foldout from Linnaeus's *Musa Cliffortiana florens Hartecampi 1736 prope Harlemum* (Leiden, 1736), www.BioLib.de. 37 × 52 cm.

often relied on the capacity of plants to reproduce asexually, which was troublesome for someone convinced of the universality of sex. In other cases, which Linnaeus noted with increasing curiosity from the early 1750s, the closeness of species in the beds seemed to foster hybrid unions and the appearance of new 'constant' varieties. Originally destined

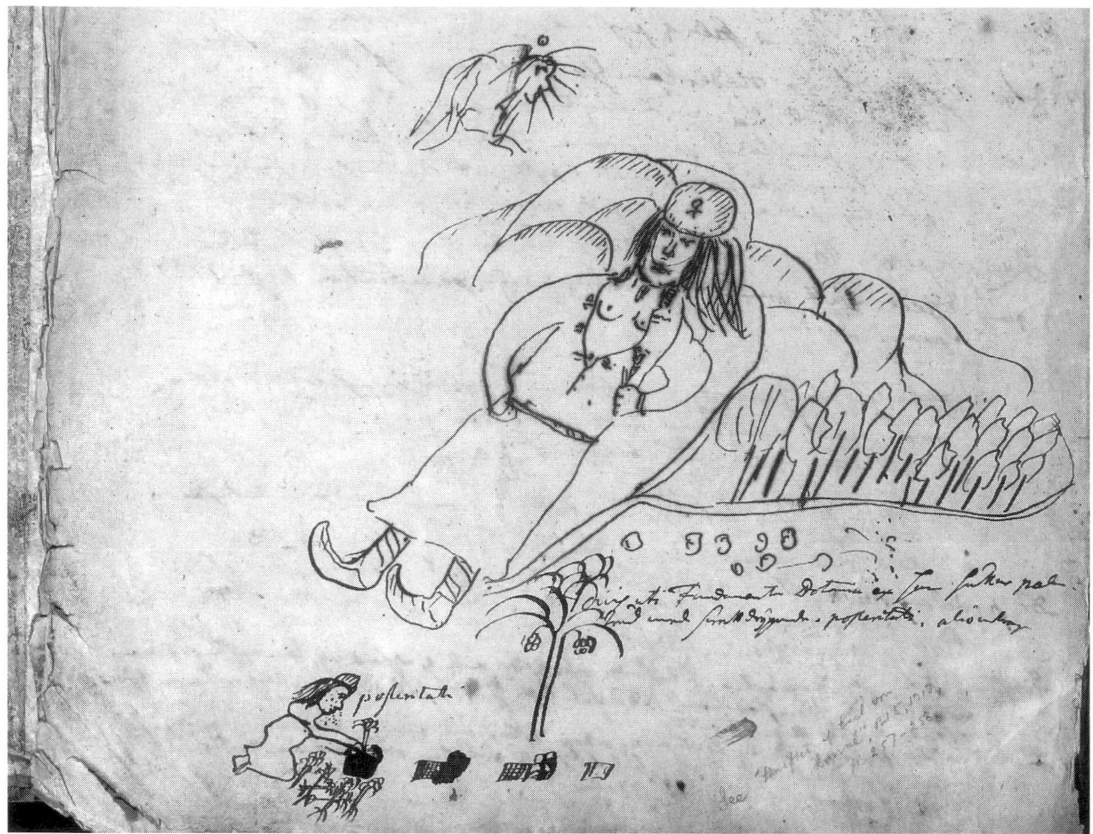

Figure 21.4 Drawing from Linnaeus's Lapland journal, imagining palm planting there. The note by the full-grown palm tree reads, in part, 'one who plants palm trees wet with sweat – For posterity'. The large female figure is dressed in a Sámi costume. Ink on paper, 14 × 18 cm. Linnaean Manuscripts, 'Original cover to Iter Lapponicum', MS GB-110/LM/LP/TRV/1/2/2, by permission of the Linnean Society of London, Library and Archives, www.linnean.org.

to restore the pristine order of Creation, the botanical garden turned into a laboratory of plant reproduction.[33]

If cultivating specimens in the garden was burdensome, so was the associated paperwork. For most of his career, Linnaeus used interleaved copies of *Genera plantarum* (Genera of plants, 1737) to register new species and amend previous descriptions. Other botanists followed, and fed him their own observations in letters, often accompanied by dried specimens or seeds. This collective system of writing natural history proved productive for Linnaeus, including financially. His correspondents' feedback allowed him to prepare updated editions of his major taxonomic publications, each providing a fresh starting

33 Staffan Müller-Wille and Vitezslav Orel, 'From Linnaean species to Mendelian factors: Elements of hybridism, 1751–1870', *Annals of Science* 64 (2007), 171–215.

point for further annotations.[34] There was a drawback, however: Linnaeus received ever more species to describe and assign. Complaints already pepper his correspondence from the late 1740s, when he was working on the manuscript of his opus magnum, the *Species plantarum* (Species of plants, 1753). He confided to a close friend that he was compelled to sit at the desk 'like a broody hen on her eggs, hatching species'. Letters in the late 1760s added an air of doom. 'I am bedridden', Linnaeus wrote in 1769, 'and make observations in my dead science each day'. His last taxonomic works carried the title *Mantissa*, or makeweight, a worthless addition to keep customers happy.[35]

While writing the *Musa Cliffortiana* Linnaeus was already engaged to Sara Lisa Moraea – daughter of the city physician of Falun, a mining town Linnaeus had visited in 1734 – with whom he would experience the pleasures and pressures of reproduction more directly. Posterity has not treated her well. One student, Johan Christian Fabricius, described her as 'a tall, large woman, imperious, egoistic and without any culture'. Sara Lisa brought with her a considerable fortune, and the couple expanded this when they established a household in Stockholm, where Linnaeus set up a practice specializing in the treatment of venereal disease, and then during his years as a university professor, by acquiring no fewer than three large agricultural estates. Sara Lisa, not Carl, managed this small empire of early agricultural capitalism.[36] Linnaeus had this in mind when in a manuscript autobiography he thanked God for having provided him with a wife 'who kept house while I worked'.[37]

Their relationship seems to have been stable, albeit fraught with conflicts over expenses for books and collections, experiments to grow Siberian plants on their estates, and consumption of luxuries like china ware and tea, as well as social events involving dancing and playing cards.[38] It was a productive marriage, however. Sara Lisa bore seven children, five of whom survived into adulthood, four daughters and one son. The daughters were a constant worry, since they needed to be equipped with

34 Staffan Müller-Wille and Isabelle Charmantier, 'Natural history and information overload: The case of Linnaeus', *Studies in History and Philosophy of Biological and Biomedical Sciences* 43 (2012), 4–15; Bettina Dietz, 'Contribution and co-production: The collaborative culture of Linnaean botany', *Annals of Science* 69 (2012), 551–69.

35 Isabelle Charmantier and Staffan Müller-Wille, 'Carl Linnaeus's botanical paper slips (1767–1773)', *Intellectual History Review* 24 (2014), 215–38. The quotations are from *The Linnaean Correspondence*: Carl Linnaeus to Abraham Bäck, 4 Mar. 1752, linnaeus.c18.net/Letter/L1371, and 15 Aug. 1769, linnaeus.c18.net/Letter/L5952, last accessed 18 Sept. 2016.

36 Mariette Manktelow and Petronella Kettunen, *Kvinnorna kring Linné* (Ryd, 2007). Linnaeus and his wife were thus representative of what demographers call the northwest European system of household formation: Richard M. Smith, 'Marriage and Fertility in Different Household Systems', Chapter 24, this book.

37 Carl Linnaeus, *Vita Caroli Linnaei: Carl von Linnés självbiografier*, ed. Elis Malmeström and Arvid Hj. Uggla (Stockholm, 1957), p. 146.

38 Wilfrid Blunt, *Linnaeus: The Compleat Naturalist* (London, 2004), pp. 180–1.

dowries to stand a chance on the marriage market. The son, also Carl, caused concern too. Linnaeus doubted his son's botanical capabilities, and although he inherited the chair, Linnaeus's will excluded Carl the Younger from his botanical collection. The son survived only another five years, during which time he turned his father's stray notes for another *Mantissa* into his own *Supplementum plantarum* (1781).[39]

Conclusion

The static image of nature that *Systema naturae* held up, and its apparent pretension to read the Creator's mind – with respect to plants, a dirty mind, as many contemporaries observed – contrasts markedly with the ideas of obscure vital forces sustaining life that Linnaeus expressed in many other places. The full picture of his life and work challenges previous explanations of his outlook as informed by an outdated, religiously motivated metaphysics of essentialism and species fixism. Linnaeus may have occupied a position at the fringes of the European Enlightenment, but he played a central role in the global networks of exchange through which botanists recruited plants for patriotic and imperial projects of improvement. The sexual system, with its more than 900 genera neatly tabulated under their respective classes and orders, was emblematic of the material riches the plant world offered – foods, medicines, dyestuffs, fibres and timbers – and hinted at the hitherto secret means by which these riches might be multiplied beyond their natural habitats and hence exploited.

Botanists thus engaged in plant reproduction long before they used the term in the modern sense, and Linnaeus was no exception to this rule. Crucially, these practices not only aimed to produce plant specimens that could stand in for their conspecifics all over the world, but were also entwined with botanists' ways of reproducing themselves, of carving out a space to make their own living in the botanical world. Linnaeus serves as a prime example. He was no metropolitan, but the largely self-taught son of a parson from the very poor region of Småland, who came to scientific fame as an outsider. His success depended on developing an acute sense of the social and cultural mechanisms that allowed one to produce, and reproduce, individual standing in the Republic of Letters. In equal measure, however, he developed fears of degeneration and exhaustion over his long career. That the sexual system managed to capture this aspect of reproduction as well, and to portray plant life as an underworld of exuberant sexual drives and desires, may have contributed as much to its long-lasting fame as its more overt messages of order and progress.

39 Charmantier and Müller-Wille, 'Linnaeus's botanical paper slips', 11–13.

22 Man-Midwifery Revisited

Mary E. Fissell

Once upon a time, English women practised a trade, largely in domestic settings. For the middle ages, records of their work are relatively scarce, but by the early modern period we know more. Some women practised more intensively, earning money from their labour and becoming known in their neighbourhoods for their skill. A few opened their homes to their clients, although parish officials intervened quickly if there was any trouble. In the later seventeenth and early eighteenth centuries, however, this occupation was transformed as new technologies developed, clients' expectations changed and men entered the business.

This story might sound like midwifery, but I am describing beer-making. My summary is drawn from Judith Bennett's classic analysis of the gendering of the work involved in making beer versus ale.[1]

The overlap of the two chronologies, however imperfect, is thought-provoking. Women brewed beer and sold it in their homes, or delivered babies in other women's homes. They learned from their mothers or other experienced women. Some made their homes into informal taverns, or took in pregnant women for deliveries. With the development of ale-making, imported from the Low Countries, the scale and gender of brewing changed; some of today's biggest brewers started in the eighteenth century. An immigrant technology also seems to lie at the heart of changes in midwifery: the obstetrical forceps, the carefully managed trade secret of the Chamberlens, a Huguenot family.

This comparison of brewing and midwifery reminds us that both were gendered activities that grew into occupations in the early modern period, and altered their gender associations in the process. At the heart of such change is the puzzle of why and how some practices become gendered, and why and how the gendering changes. Alice Clark, one of the first historians of women's work, used midwifery as a prime example of 'the way in which women have lost their hold upon all branches of skilled responsible work'.[2] My implicit argument in this chapter is that we need to understand midwifery as female work as well as medical practice, and so resituate it as an economic activity shaped by larger shifts in workforces.

Before looking at the time of transition, we should think about midwives themselves, and the longer historiographic traditions that continue to shape our

1 Judith M. Bennett, *Ale, Beer, and Brewsters in England: Women's Work in a Changing World, 1300–1600* (New York, NY, 1996).

2 Alice Clark, *Working Life of Women in the Seventeenth Century* (London, 1919), p. 242.

understanding of their work. 'Midwife' is not a timeless occupational category. In ancient Rome, we know of female midwives from a handful of inscriptions. But then, silence. Not until the high middle ages does the documentary record identify women as midwives.[3] Nor can we assume that women became the sole providers of gynaecologic and obstetric care; most of the medieval and many of the early modern texts on such topics were written by men for men.[4]

Over the past twenty-five years, our understanding of midwives has changed greatly. In the later nineteenth century, as obstetricians created a specialty, they stereotyped midwives in England and America as ignorant, superstitious and dirty. Man-midwives, in this account, used a new technology, the forceps, and saved women and babies from midwives' ministrations. In 1973, that tale was upended in *Witches, Midwives, and Nurses: A History of Women Healers*, a short book by Barbara Ehrenreich and Deirdre English from the Feminist Press.[5] Here, midwives were empirical practitioners envied and feared by men, who branded them as witches to limit their powers. The work inadvertently created a foundational myth; any public lecture on early modern midwives is almost certain to provoke the question 'Weren't they also witches?', no matter how often historians have shown that they were not.[6]

Late twentieth-century women's history, as well as the social history of medicine, prompted detailed scholarship about early modern midwives, which almost completely revised both the 'ignorance' and the 'witch' narratives. The 1993 publication of Hilary Marland's edited volume *The Art of Midwifery* marked the full arrival of the revision. The dust jacket asked 'Were midwives untrained and incompetent?' and the various essays answered 'No!'[7]

Yet even after decades of sustained, rich scholarship, the advent of man-midwives remains perplexing; no one clear answer has emerged. In what follows, I explore three

3 Monica H. Green, 'The possibilities of literacy and the limits of reading: Women and the gendering of medical literacy', in Green, *Women's Healthcare in the Medieval West: Texts and Contexts* (Aldershot, 2000), pp. 1–76. For a different perspective, see Fiona Harris-Stoertz, 'Midwives in the middle ages? Birth attendants, 600–1300', in Wendy J. Turner and Sara M. Butler (eds.), *Medicine and the Law in the Middle Ages* (Leiden, 2014), pp. 58–87.

4 Monica H. Green, *Making Women's Medicine Masculine: The Rise of Male Authority in Pre-Modern Gynaecology* (Oxford, 2008).

5 Barbara Ehrenreich and Deirdre English, *Witches, Midwives, and Nurses: A History of Women Healers* (Old Westbury, NY, 1973).

6 David Harley, 'Historians as demonologists: The myth of the midwife-witch', *Social History of Medicine* (1990), 1–26.

7 Hilary Marland (ed.), *The Art of Midwifery: Early Modern Midwives in Europe* (London, 1993). On the middle ages: Katharine Park, 'Managing Childbirth and Fertility in Medieval Europe', Chapter 11; Lauren Kassell, 'Medieval Birth Malpresentations', Exhibit 10; Lea T. Olsan, 'A Medieval Birth Girdle', Exhibit 11; see also Sandra Cavallo, 'Pregnant Stones as Wonders of Nature', Exhibit 17; and Lianne McTavish, 'A Birthing Chair', Exhibit 18, this book.

central frameworks of the premodern displacement of female by male birth attendants: technologies, fashion and Enlightenment concern for infant life. These should be given context, I argue, by situating the shift to man-midwifery within larger changes in women's work and in childbirth.

Historians have devoted a disproportionate amount of attention to the English case, in part because the advent of man-midwives there was swift, between approximately 1720 and 1770, and accompanied by the novelty of the forceps, changes which generated heated polemic.[8] I argue that the emergent gendered division of labour in the birthing room was variable geographically, but that looking across the Channel at France, at other European countries and at British North America can place England as a special case of a larger phenomenon.

Technology

A nineteenth-century obstetrician, James Aveling, created the 'technology' narrative, in which a new tool remakes social practices.[9] Aveling himself invented a number of obstetric instruments, and advocated for obstetrician-run midwifery training, in part because he thought the new women physicians lacked the *sang-froid* to deal with obstetric emergencies. As Aveling explained, the Chamberlens, who fled from Paris to London in 1576, developed and kept the forceps as a trade secret through four generations. The forceps were designed to exert traction on an infant's head when it was stuck in the birth canal; the instrument has changed but little since its first invention.

Although the Chamberlens preserved their family secret, we know exactly what the forceps looked like. In 1813, a box of their instruments was discovered hidden under floorboards in Woodham Mortimer Hall, where Peter Chamberlen had died a century earlier. The forceps resemble a pair of tongs with long curved loops to grasp the baby's head; usually the two pieces detach so that each can be manoeuvred into the birth canal before being rejoined (Fig. 22.1). But the secret had been out since 1733; Edmund Chapman published the details. Forceps, according to Aveling, prompted a sudden increase in man-midwifery, including lecture courses on obstetrics for male practitioners; lying-in hospitals staffed by men; and men attending routine births. The boom was swiftly met with criticism, often centred on the threat to women's modesty.

Aveling's narrative has obvious appeal, but upon closer examination cannot bear the full weight of the shift from female to male birth attendants. Neither the timing of the advent of man-midwifery nor the uptake of the technology by men fits well with

8 Ludmilla Jordanova, 'Man-Midwifery Dissected', Exhibit 22, this book.

9 J. H. Aveling, *The Chamberlens and the Midwifery Forceps: Memorials of the Family and an Essay on the Invention of the Instrument* (London, 1882).

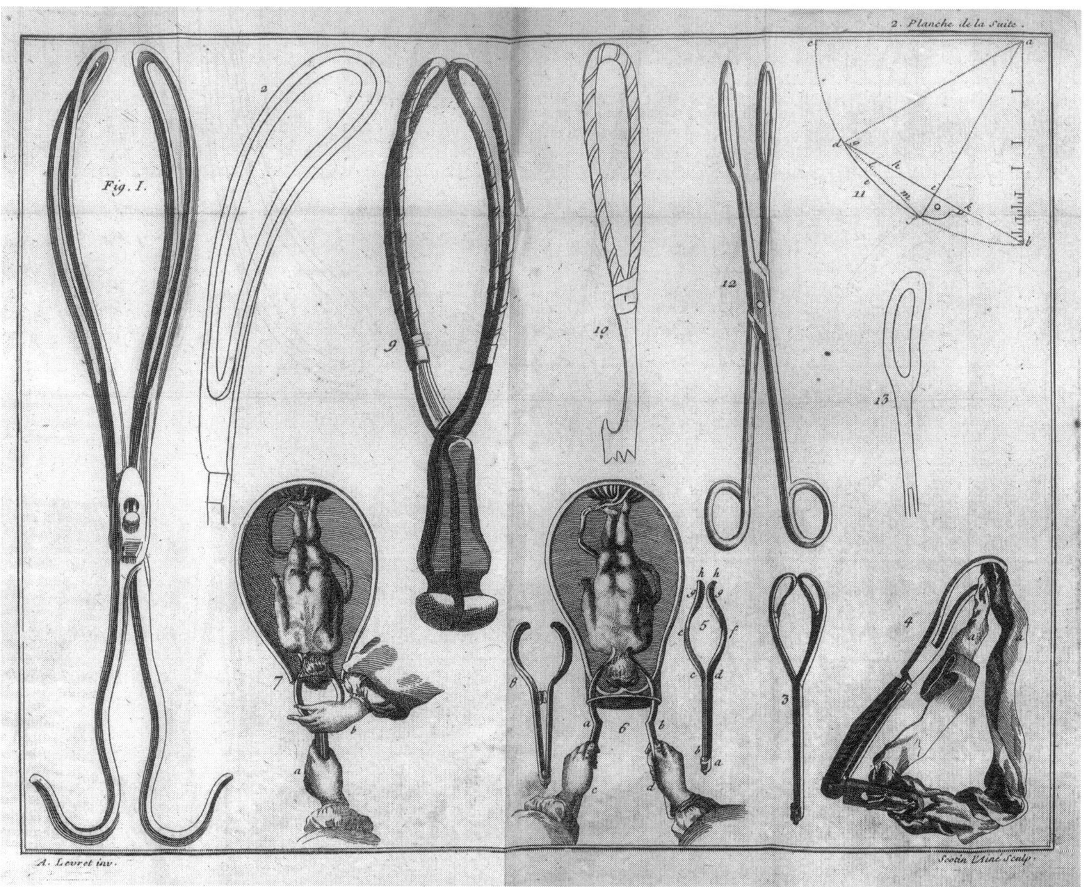

Figure 22.1 Engraving showing various forceps, on the left the standard detachable model, at lower right apparently a combination vectis and fillet. In Fig. 22.3, by contrast, the midwife's hands are the 'tool'. André Levret, *Observations sur les causes et les accidens de plusieurs accouchemens laborieux* (Paris: P. Fr. Didot le jeune, 1770), plate 2. Institute of the History of Medicine, The Johns Hopkins University.

a story of forceps as a game-changer. First, the timing does not match. For example, Sarah Stone, practising in Bristol in the 1720s, complained about all the anatomically trained man-midwives in business, 'For dissecting the Dead, and being just and tender to the Living, are vastly different'.[10] The Chamberlens had no disciples in the city in this period, so forceps were not the reason that Bristol matrons started routinely hiring man-midwives.

Second, man-midwives did not always advocate the new technology. The first London man-midwife to create a successful career for himself was probably James

10 Sarah Stone, *A Complete Practice of Midwifery: Consisting of Upwards of Forty Cases or Observations in that Valuable Art …* (London, 1737), p. xiv.

Douglas, who tried the forceps in 1702; Adrian Wilson surmises that he had received the instrument from Hugh Chamberlen the elder. But Douglas could not make it work properly, and his stellar career as a man-midwife owed nothing to this brief trial. Even William Hunter, the most successful man-midwife of the mid-century, famously remarked of forceps that, 'where they save one, they murder twenty'.[11]

Third, as Wilson has illuminated, the Chamberlen family mobilized not one new technology but three: the vectis, the fillet and the forceps; that box under the floorboards contained them all. All served to deliver obstructed births. The vectis was similar to a one-bladed forceps, somewhat resembling a spoon, the bowl of which could be used to move the baby's head in the birth canal, or even exert traction upon it. The fillet was a ribbon or band that could be placed around the baby's head and similarly used to shift its position (Fig. 22.1). Each instrument has a complex history, with different practitioners adopting one or another.

Wilson suggests that the most fundamental shift was not technological, but mental: the idea that a surgeon had a role in the delivery of a *living* baby. He analyses the cases of Percival Willughby, a seventeenth-century Derbyshire practitioner, unpublished until the nineteenth century. Willughby, like other surgeons, was called to dire cases, when the mother's life was despaired of, and a decision had already been reached that the infant's life would have to be sacrificed. Using a large hook, or crochet, practitioners would 'reduce' the head, a euphemism for cracking the skull, thus killing the fetus if it were still alive. Willughby gives eloquent testimony to the ethical anguish this practice caused him. For Wilson, the real change came when men started routinely delivering live babies, with or without forceps, not when they were called to use the crochet on obstructed births.[12]

The first generation of successful man-midwives in London was not, therefore, much associated with new technologies. The second generation institutionalized the role of men in delivering babies.[13] William Smellie moved from Lanarkshire, in the central lowlands of Scotland, to London in 1739, having specialized in midwifery and sharpened his midwifery skills in Paris. Over the next two decades, Smellie ran lecture courses, teaching over 900 men and an unknown number of women. His 1752 *Treatise on the Theory and Practice of Midwifery* reveals his methods in a series of cases. Smellie and his successors relied upon a detailed knowledge of anatomy to pinpoint how a labour was developing and what might be going wrong. In a 1746 case, in which a poor, starving woman had been in labour for eight days, abandoned by three midwives, he

11 Adrian Wilson, 'William Hunter and the varieties of man-midwifery', in W. F. Bynum and Roy Porter (eds.), *William Hunter and the Eighteenth-Century Medical World* (Cambridge, 1985), pp. 323–43, on p. 343.

12 Adrian Wilson, *The Making of Man-Midwifery: Childbirth in England, 1660–1770* (Cambridge, MA, 1995).

13 Lisa Forman Cody, *Birthing the Nation: Sex, Science, and the Conception of Eighteenth-Century Britons* (Oxford, 2005).

sent for bread and soup from a cookshop and kept the woman quiet and calm. He left her with his senior pupils, telling them that he thought she would be delivered normally if the weak pains strengthened, but that the forceps might be needed if not. Happily, she delivered the baby, and without instruments.[14] Smellie narrates this tale both as critical of ignorant female midwives, who had pushed and pulled the mother into various positions, and as exemplifying Enlightenment sensibility – what starving mother could muster the energy to deliver a child? It was his detailed knowledge of anatomy that enabled him to take an expectant role, rather than rushing in with forceps.

Fashion, Choice and Gender Relations

The second major explanation for how and why men began routinely to deliver babies starts with Smellie's fellow Scot William Hunter. While Smellie retained the mien of Lanarkshire, Hunter remade himself as a London man of fashion, attracting aristocratic patients and even the friendship of the monarch. One detail is telling: Smellie recommended that practitioners diagnose ambiguous cases of pregnancy with a digital anal exam, but that was much too indelicate for Hunter. Wait and see, he advised his pupils, comfort your patient with some meaningless words, and the truth will be revealed soon enough. Hunter became the darling of aristocratic mothers and trained a generation of man-midwives in his genteel ways. As aristocrats came to rely upon man-midwives, the argument goes, so too did their social inferiors, aping their betters in this as in so much else. The problems with this 'fashion' argument are twofold. First, it does not explain why aristocrats employed man-midwives initially. Second, some of the earliest man-midwives made their careers not with ladies, but with the poor.

Take, for example, the clients of William Giffard between 1725 and 1731, many of whom were poor. The practice was largely emergency calls – labours in which something had already gone wrong, long the province of male surgeons. Giffard's book documents the period when he began using forceps and became skilled in their use. These cases call into question the 'fashion' explanation. Whatever else they may have been, the struggling wives and widows of watermen, chair-men and coal-carriers were not the fashionable trend-setters posited as key to man-midwifery by some historians.[15]

Another way of casting the 'fashion' narrative is to think of it as 'patient choice'. Perhaps the best example of this theme is Judith Leavitt's argument that late eighteenth- and early nineteenth-century American women began to employ man-midwives in part because they were more interventionist – including providing bloodletting and

14 William Smellie, *A Treatise on the Theory and Practice of Midwifery*, 3 vols. (London, 1752–64), vol. 2, pp. 337–8.

15 A substantial portion of Giffard's clients are described just as 'a poor woman': William Giffard, *Cases in Midwifry*, rev. Edward Hody (London, 1734).

opium for pain relief. However, those man-midwives were not given complete sway in the birthing room; they had to negotiate with the mothers' friends and families.[16]

In France, surgeons did much the same kind of things as in England, but their roles developed differently. Male surgeons were called in when the delivery had gone wrong, to extract the infant and save the life of the mother. The sixteenth-century French surgeon, Ambroise Paré, devised a technique to deliver a living child in these dire circumstances – but unlike the Chamberlens, his tools were his hands. Paré reinvented the ancient practice of podalic version, that is, turning the baby during delivery so that it could be grasped by the feet and traction applied to effect the birth. However, female midwives also took up the practice; this technology transcended gender. By the later sixteenth century, elite French women were already looking to *chirurgeons-accoucheurs* to deliver their babies. The midwife Louise Bourgeois complained that young women were too much given to the impudence of having male birth attendants. While she 'blushed for them', she acknowledged that in cases of great danger, men might be necessary.[17]

In France, both medical regulation and guilds' regulation of artisanal labour were more developed and complex than in England – and thus the working relations between midwives and surgeons were structured differently.[18] The Hôtel-Dieu in Paris was well-known for its superior training programmes for female midwives; that is where Smellie went to learn. Here, female midwives were at least nominally supervised by male surgeons, although some instructors were female. Late sixteenth-century French male midwives already sniped at their female counterparts, claiming that the women might be able to manage normal deliveries, but their lack of anatomical knowledge made them utterly unfit to handle any difficulties. Different ways of knowing – visual versus haptic – became arrayed in a hierarchy, with a male surgeon's knowledge of anatomy taking primacy over a female midwife's experienced hands.[19]

Gender relations in the birthing room were inflected differently in the French Caribbean colony of Saint-Domingue. As in France, well-to-do women gradually came to select men to deliver their babies, although the change was never absolute. But Saint-Domingue was a slave economy based upon the brutal production of sugar. The Seven Years War of 1756–63 reduced the trade in slaves and put a premium on the health of slave mothers. They were delivered by enslaved midwives, whom their

16 Judith Walzer Leavitt, *Brought to Bed: Childbearing in America, 1750–1950* (New York, NY, 1986), esp. pp. 46–7.

17 *The Compleat Midwife's Practice Enlarged* (London, 1663), p. 29.

18 Laurence Brockliss and Colin Jones, *The Medical World of Early Modern France* (Oxford, 1997); Steven L. Kaplan, *La fin des corporations* (Paris, 2001).

19 Lianne McTavish, 'Reproduction, *c.* 1500–1750', in Sarah Toulalan and Kate Fisher (eds.), *The Routledge History of Sex and the Body, 1500 to the Present* (London, 2013), pp. 351–71.

masters viewed with the deepest suspicion, imagining them to be providing abortifacients, or strangling newborns to save them from a life of slavery. Man-midwives or surgeons were called in not to supervise the actual delivery, but to treat the newborn's cut umbilical cord, because midwives were suspected of causing the ailment known as *mal de mâchoire* by cutting the cord with rusty knives or, as in parts of Africa, tying it with a burnt rag. A few decades later, surgeons began to take a role during delivery, often as supervisors of slave midwives; the Haitian Revolution of 1791 ended these nascent forms of practice.[20]

Farther north, in the new American nation around the same time, some scholarship suggests a relatively easy relationship between female midwives and male doctors. Laurel Thatcher Ulrich's classic study of the Maine midwife Martha Ballard shows us a woman whose midwifery practice was woven into the fabric of her community. Conversely, midwifery was but a part of Ballard's domestic economy; she produced textiles, using the labour of her daughters and others, grew a great deal of her own food and used her own herbs for cookery and healing. She had a cordial relationship with the local male doctors, who on one occasion invited her to join them for an autopsy.[21]

The Italian story reveals another set of working relationships; medical men never came to dominate childbirth. In villages, a midwife was supervised by the parish priest, since she had to summon him for emergency baptisms. However, as we shall see, several Italian states, like those in the rest of Europe, did come to see childbirth as significant to the production of new subjects and as in need of improvement. Italian men intervened in childbirth in an unusual fashion: in *Embriologia sacra* (Sacred embryology, 1745) a Sicilian priest, Francesco Cangiamila, advocated caesarean sections to baptize a dying baby.[22] The argument took a new twist when exported to Peru, where the Peruvian friar Francisco González Laguna argued for fetal baptism within a larger campaign to combat 'superstitious' birthing practices among the Native Americans. These reforms became part of a larger imperial project.[23]

20 Karol K. Weaver, *Medical Revolutionaries: The Enslaved Healers of Eighteenth-Century Saint Domingue* (Urbana, IL, 2006), pp. 55–60; for later legacies of slavery in the Caribbean: Philippa Levine, 'Imperial Encounters', Chapter 33, this book.

21 Laurel Thatcher Ulrich, *A Midwife's Tale: The Life of Martha Ballard, Based on Her Diary, 1785–1812* (New York, NY, 1991).

22 Francesco Emanuele Cangiamila, *Embriologia sacra …* (Palermo, 1745); Nadia Maria Filippini, *La nascita straordinaria: Tra madre e figlio, la rivoluzione del taglio cesareo (sec. XVIII–XIX)* (Milan, 1995); José Pardo-Tomás and Àlvar Martínez-Vidal, 'The ignorance of midwives: The role of clergymen in Spanish Enlightenment debates on birth care', in Ole Peter Grell and Andrew Cunningham (eds.), *Medicine and Religion in Enlightenment Europe* (Aldershot, 2007), pp. 50–62.

23 Adam Warren, 'An operation for evangelization: Francisco González Laguna, the cesarean section, and fetal baptism in late colonial Peru', *Bulletin of the History of Medicine* 83 (2009), 647–75; further: Levine, 'Imperial Encounters'.

Improvement

Working relations between female midwives and their male counterparts varied across Europe and her colonies, shaped by patterns of medical regulation, artisanal work, economic structures and religious attitudes, but there is a common, pan-European emphasis upon the improvement of childbirth outcomes. Such policies were shaped by influences as variable as a mercantilist stress upon population, an Enlightenment revaluation of infant life and a sentimentalization of motherhood, but often coalesced around midwifery education and new institutional provision of maternity care.

Improving midwifery was a constant theme in manuals aimed at midwives. The first to be printed in Europe, Eucharius Rösslin's *Der Rosengarten* (The rose garden), was published in German in 1513 and translated into many European vernaculars (Fig. 22.2). While based upon a manuscript written for men, the printed text is addressed to female midwives and urges them to work competently. Rösslin thundered that men such as Galen, Rhazes and Avicenna had uncovered knowledge of the human body and warned midwives that a (male) god would hold them to account for their work. In other words, Rösslin already posited a hierarchical gender relation between male doctors and female midwives, although interestingly the English translations did not take up this theme. Female authors on midwifery, ranging from Louise Bourgeois in 1609 to Justine Siegemund in 1690 and Teresa Ployant in 1787, also situated their writings within these claims about the need to improve practice.[24]

In the late seventeenth and eighteenth centuries, we see a surge in technical, educational and institutional attempts to improve midwifery all over Europe. For example, in 1701 the Dutch surgeon Hendrik van Deventer published a remarkable book subsequently translated into Latin, German, French and English. It is the first mechanical account of the pelvis and its function in childbirth. Deventer was married to a midwife from whom he learned to manoeuvre the coccyx to facilitate delivery. Significant contexts for his work were his membership in a mystical religious group, the Labadist brethren, and his surgical work on bones, which probably helped him to recognize that mothers who had suffered from rickets often had malformed pelves that obstructed births.[25]

24 Wendy Perkins, *Midwifery and Medicine in Early Modern France: Louise Bourgeois* (Exeter, 1996); Justine Siegemund, *The Court Midwife*, ed. and trans. Lynne Tatlock (Chicago, IL, 2005); Teresa Ployant, *Breve compendio dell'arte ostetricia* (Naples, 1787).

25 Hendrik van Deventer, *Manuale operatien*, part 1: *Zijnde een nieuw ligt voor vroed-meesters en vroed-vrouwen …* ('s Graven-Hage, 1701); on Deventer: M. J. van Lieburg, 'Nieuw licht op Hendrik van Deventer (1651–1724)', *Gewina* 25, no. 5 (2002), 5–120.

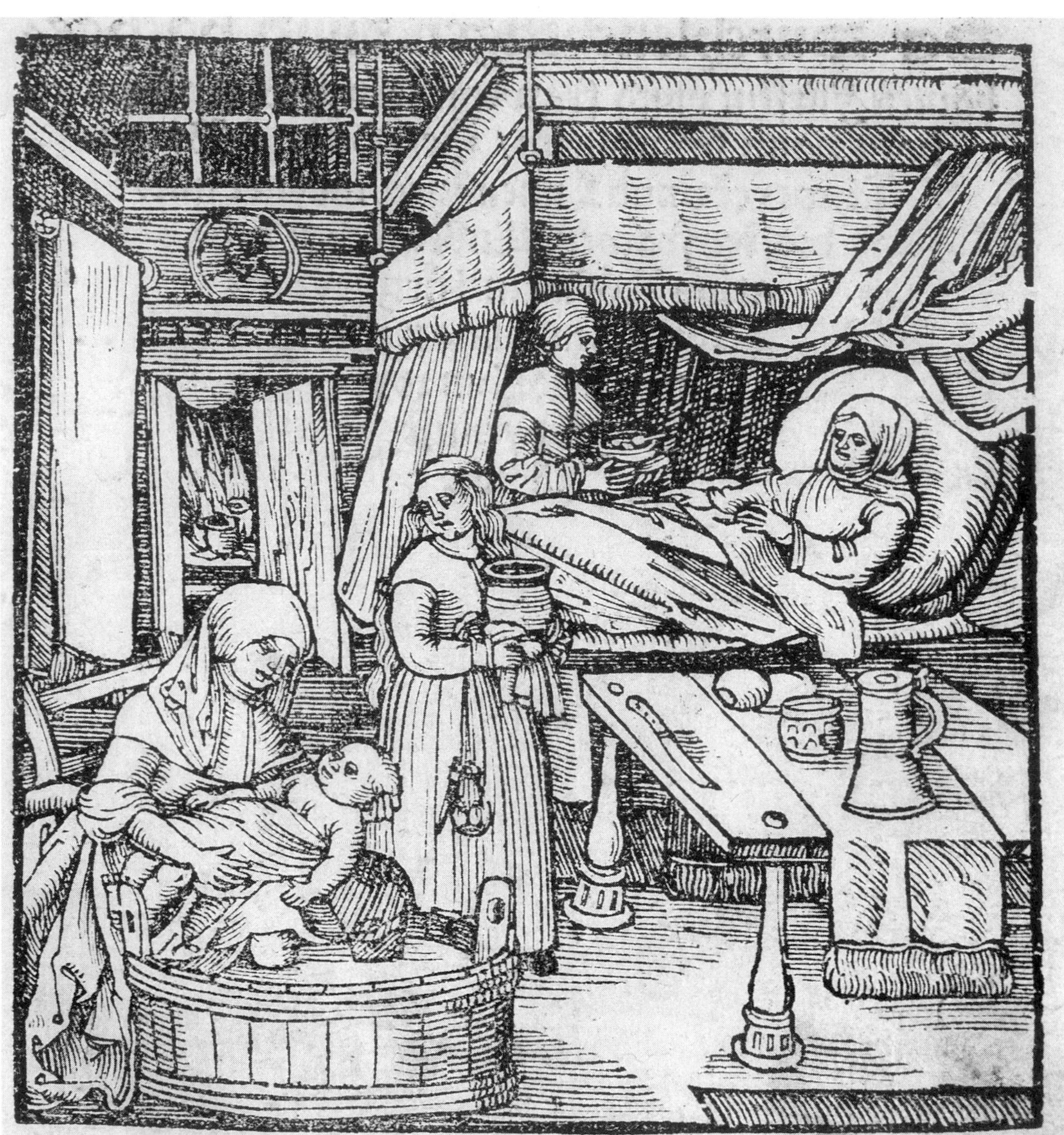

Figure 22.2 This woodcut, from Eucharius Rösslin's *Rosengarten*, depicts a typical early modern birthing-room scene for middle- and upper-class women. As in paintings of the birth of the Virgin Mary, the midwife swaddles the baby while 'gossips' – female friends and relatives – support the mother. Frontispiece to *Der Schwanngeren frawen vnd Hebammen Rosegartten* (Augsburg: Heinrich Steyner, [1528]). National Library of Medicine.

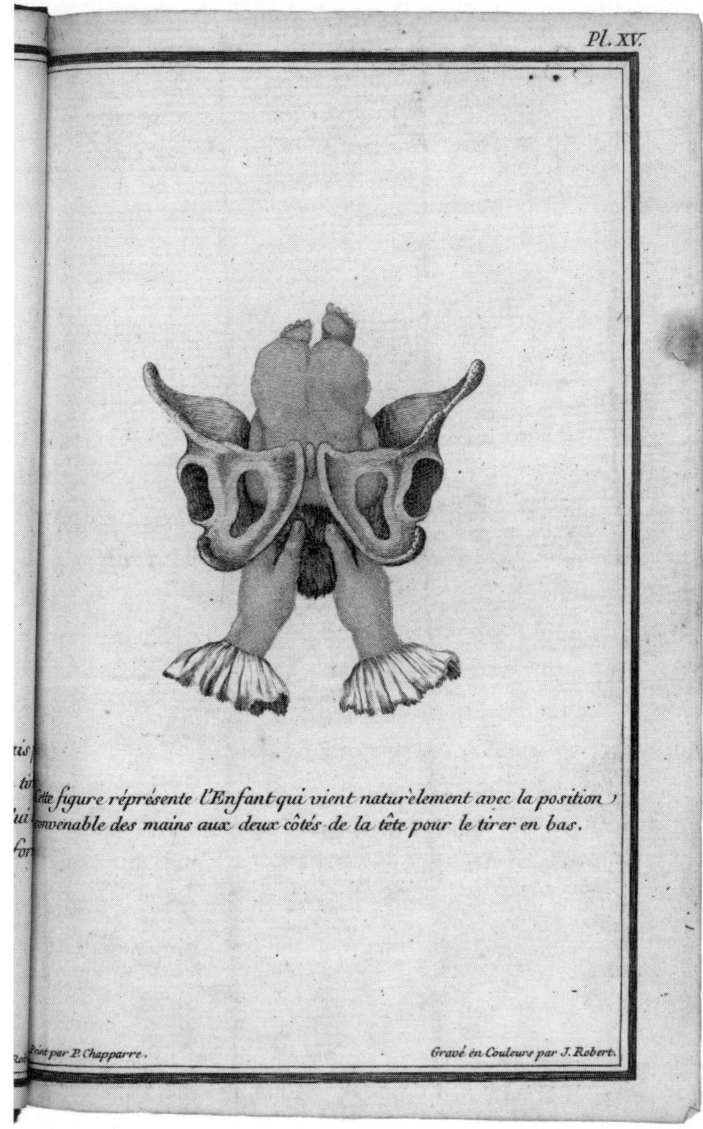

Pl. XV.
ette figure réprésente l'Enfant qui vient naturèlement avec la position
nvenable des mains aux deux côtés de la tête pour le tirer en bas.
Gravé en Couleurs par J. Robert.

Figure 22.3 Plate showing how experienced midwives could manoeuvre the unborn child into a position from which to deliver the baby safely. Skilled hands were tools of the trade. Coloured engraving from Mme du Coudray's masterwork, *Abbrégé de l'art des accouchemens*, new edn (Saintes: Pierre Toussaints, 1769), plate XV. 19 × 12 cm. Cambridge University Library.

Where Deventer sought to improve the practice of midwifery with specific techniques, others did so by means of instruction. In France, Angélique Marguerite Le Boursier du Coudray developed a remarkable educational paradigm for training provincial midwives. Born into a medical family around 1712, she trained as a midwife and became the chief midwife at the Hôtel-Dieu in Paris. She published a manual, *Abrégé de l'art des accouchements* (Summary of the art of delivering children, 1759), and Louis XV commissioned her to teach across the country (Fig. 22.3). She invented what she called her 'machine', ingenious life-sized obstetrical models, which she crafted herself from bone, leather, glass and fabric to enable students to practise a wide range of presentations. From 1760 to 1783 she travelled from town to town, training 4,000 students; her students taught another 6,000.[26]

All over Europe, various institutions sought to improve the standards of midwifery. In Spain in the 1780s and 1790s, the Colleges of Surgery in Madrid and Barcelona made specific provision for instructing female midwives.[27] From 1757, thirteen midwifery schools were founded in and around Venice. As in du Coudray's teaching, instructors used drawings and especially three-dimensional models, sometimes by the famous Bolognese wax-model maker Anna Morandi.[28] Such models were also crucial to the work of Gian Antonio Galli, who taught midwives in Bologna, many of them illiterate. His school began as a private institution, but became part of the state-sponsored Institute of the Sciences; like elsewhere in Europe, safeguarding the health of mothers became part of an enlightened ruler's remit.[29] By the nineteenth century, numerous institutions in the Italian peninsula offered intensive, anatomically grounded education in midwifery to both women and men.

In many European cities, lying-in hospitals began to provide obstetrical care for poor women, even in some cases for unwed mothers, who had usually been deemed morally unfit for charitable help. Rather like Ehrenreich and English, some earlier scholarship portrayed lying-in hospitals as gateways to death with male midwives wielding forceps all too often, but just as in the literature on general hospitals, subsequent work has revealed variation and, for the period before the mid-nineteenth century, a somewhat more optimistic view. The London Lying-In Hospital, for example, had maternal mortality rates equivalent to those of the local population.[30] In the lying-in hospital associated with the University of Göttingen, with births attended by male midwives and their students, about 10 per cent of infants died perinatally in the late eighteenth and early nineteenth centuries, a rate higher than that of home births attended almost entirely by female midwives. However, maternal mortality was about the same as in London, approximately 1 per cent, although also typical in that epidemics caused huge

26 Nina Rattner Gelbart, *The King's Midwife: A History and Mystery of Madame du Coudray* (Berkeley, CA, 1998).

27 Teresa Ortiz, 'Midwives in early modern Spain', in Marland, *Art of Midwifery*, pp. 95–114, esp. pp. 100–1.

28 Nadia Maria Filippini, 'The church, the state and childbirth: The midwife in Italy during the eighteenth century', ibid., pp. 152–75; Rebecca Messbarger, *The Lady Anatomist: The Life and Work of Anna Morandi Manzolini* (Chicago, IL, 2010), pp. 79–83.

29 Lucia Dacome, 'A Crystal Womb', Exhibit 21, this book.

30 Margaret DeLacy, 'Puerperal fever in eighteenth-century Britain', *Bulletin of the History of Medicine* 63 (1989), 521–56; Lisa Forman Cody, 'Living and dying in Georgian London's lying-in hospitals', ibid., 78 (2004), 309–48. For the subsequent history: Salim Al-Gailani, 'Hospital Birth', Chapter 37, this book.

fluctuations from year to year.[31] An institutional alternative – a domestic lying-in service that sent male or female midwives to attend women in their own homes – seems to have reduced mortality.[32] The institutions also present a mixed picture of the gendered division of obstetrical work. Even the German university lying-in hospitals often trained female midwives as well as the male medical students for whom they were primarily designed.

From this pan-European perspective, we see an Enlightenment commitment to improving midwifery, perhaps as a social welfare initiative, or from a mercantilist concern with increasing the population, or due to religious commitments. By the end of the eighteenth century, almost all the variables which have subsequently structured the gender politics of midwifery had appeared: new technologies; arguments about female modesty; hospital births; men as consultants for difficult cases; disparagement of female midwives as superstitious. Even pain relief – usually dated to the mid-nineteenth-century discoveries of ether and chloroform – may already have been in play, albeit in a limited way, if Leavitt is correct that opiates drew Americans to hire male birth attendants. These factors combined and recombined over the next two centuries to structure very different balances between male and female midwives in different places.

Conclusion

First-wave feminism spawned two significant ways to think about the advent of man-midwifery. First is Aveling's narrative of technological determinism, prompted in part by his dislike of the early female physicians, as well as his concerns about midwifery training. Second is Alice Clark's pioneering study of women's history, a declensionist tale about the value of women's work lost. The tension between these two stories explains much of the shape of subsequent historical writing, which we can imagine as something like a figure-ground problem; what is our focus and what mere context? Do we think about female midwives mostly in reference to man-midwives, or in relation to other skilled women workers? If the former, the shift to men seems

31 Jürgen Schlumbohm, 'Saving mothers' and children's lives? The performance of German lying-in hospitals in the late eighteenth and early nineteenth centuries', *Bulletin of the History of Medicine* 87 (2013), 1–31, which is in dialogue with Robert Woods, *Death before Birth: Fetal Health and Mortality in Historical Perspective* (Oxford, 2009).

32 Bronwyn Croxson, 'The foundation and evolution of the Middlesex Hospital's lying-in service, 1745–86', *Social History of Medicine* 14 (2001), 27–57; Mary Lindemann, 'Maternal politics: The principles and practice of maternity care in eighteenth-century Hamburg', *Journal of Family History* 9 (1984), 44–63, esp. 51–5.

remarkable; if the latter, it is just another example of a larger phenomenon. In addition, as this chapter has argued, England is exceptional, but when put in a wider European context, the advent of man-midwives becomes, in part, a somewhat peculiar English version of a bigger project: the Enlightenment attempt to improve the life-chances of mothers and babies.

23 Biopolitics and the Invention of Population

Andrea Rusnock

Population became an object of lively debate in the eighteenth century. In his *Persian Letters* of 1721, the French *philosophe* Charles-Louis de Secondat, Baron de Montesquieu, made the provocative claim that Europe had become greatly depopulated since antiquity. This prompted widespread discussion about the causes and consequences of the decline. Scattered among these philosophical conversations were creative efforts to calculate the size of population, efforts which accelerated in ambition and sophistication after 1750 and indicated that population had not decreased. By the end of the eighteenth century, the English reverend and scholar Thomas Robert Malthus argued that Europe faced overpopulation, a condition as problematic for him as depopulation had been for Montesquieu.[1] Whether too little or too big, population figured prominently in Enlightenment writings, and increasingly it was measured.

The development of quantified and then statistical notions of population coincided with the emergence of modern nation-states comprising more-or-less equal and therefore commensurable individuals. This view replaced an older idea characteristic of hierarchical societies, that populations comprised incommensurable groups of various sizes.[2] In the first decades of the nineteenth century, most states conducted censuses, established civil registration of births, marriages and deaths, and created offices to monitor changes in their populations. In addition, the new social sciences of demography and vital statistics took population as their subject and the mathematics of probability and statistics as their methods. Thus by 1850, population and its quantified attributes, notably fertility and mortality, had become, as they have remained, fundamentally important ways to think about human beings as groups and biologically as a species.

Addressing this transformation, the French philosopher Michel Foucault argued from the 1970s that the notion of population was an eighteenth-century invention and an essential aspect of biopower, a new type of power that takes as its object the management

1 Charles de Secondat, Baron de Montesquieu, *Persian Letters*, trans. John Davidson (London, 1892), Letter CXII; [T. R. Malthus], *An Essay on the Principle of Population, as It Affects the Future Improvement of Society* … (London, 1798).

2 For a helpful comparison of the two ideas: Philip Kreager, 'The Emergence of Population', Chapter 18; see further Rebecca Flemming, 'States and Populations in the Classical World', Chapter 5; and Peter Biller, 'The Multitude in Later Medieval Thought', Chapter 10, this book; and Bruce Curtis, 'Foucault on governmentality and population: The impossible discovery', *Canadian Journal of Sociology* 27 (2002), 505–33, on 507–9.

of life.[3] In Foucault's formulation, biopower operates simultaneously on two levels: on an individual's body (anatomo-politics) and on a population (biopolitics). One of the goals of biopower was (and is) to increase economic productivity by changing the habits and improving the health of individuals, and by encouraging reproduction and the growth of population.[4] Foucault argued that the techniques of biopower were cultivated 'at every level of the social body and utilized by very diverse institutions (the family and the army, schools and the police, individual medicine and the administration of collective bodies)'.[5] This pointed to a fresh way of understanding the emergence of population, a view that puts at its core the connections between new forms of knowledge and the exercise of power. Foucault showed how knowledge, especially scientific knowledge, is central to the operation and maintenance of power in modern societies.

Foucault's writings have proved tremendously fertile, especially in social and political theory. But many historians, wary of adopting his general framework, have challenged his idea that population was invented in the eighteenth century and have offered alternative interpretations of how population was understood and treated by different early modern communities. This chapter provides a reconciliation of Foucault's evocative concept of biopolitics with what we now know about eighteenth-century debates over population. It highlights efforts to quantify particular aspects of population related to reproduction and argues for the importance of understanding the historical roots of biopolitics in Enlightenment writings.

Biopolitics

A variety of theorists have used the term 'biopolitics' in very different ways since the early twentieth century.[6] First coined by Swedish and German scholars who applied biological concepts to understanding nation-states, it also referred to political efforts to preserve life and the natural environment.[7] More recently, reproductive technologies and other biotechnologies that blur the distinctions between natural and artificial have been analysed as biopolitical.[8] Foucault employed 'biopolitics' to represent a new type of knowledge/power that focused on understanding and controlling populations.

3 Foucault addressed the emergence of population most clearly in *Security, Territory, Population: Lectures at the Collège de France, 1977–1978*, ed. Michel Senellart, trans. Graham Burchell (Basingstoke, 2007). See also Foucault, *The History of Sexuality*, vol. 1: *An Introduction* (New York, NY, 1980).

4 Michel Foucault, 'Truth and power', in *Power/Knowledge: Selected Interviews and Other Writings, 1972–1977*, ed. Colin Gordon, trans. Gordon *et al.* (New York, NY, 1980), pp. 109–33, on pp. 124–5.

5 Foucault, *History of Sexuality*, p. 141; also Foucault, *The Birth of Biopolitics: Lectures at the Collège de France, 1978–1979*, ed. Michel Senellart, trans. Graham Burchell (New York, NY, 2008).

6 Thomas Lemke, *Biopolitics: An Advanced Introduction*, trans. Eric Frederick Trump (New York, NY, 2011).

7 Ibid., pp. 9–32.

8 Nikolas Rose, *The Politics of Life Itself: Biomedicine, Power, and Subjectivity in the Twenty-First Century* (Princeton, NJ, 2007).

Over the course of the eighteenth and nineteenth centuries, political economists, doctors, government officials and others developed statistical treatments and understandings of population; by the mid-nineteenth century, these had produced the social sciences of demography and vital statistics. New ideas in political economy – especially the relationship between production and population – helped to shape this quantitative concept of population, which Foucault treated as a new order of knowledge that was intimately linked with new forms of power.

> The great eighteenth-century demographic upswing in Western Europe, the necessity for co-ordinating and integrating it into the apparatus of production and the urgency of controlling it with finer and more adequate power mechanisms cause 'population', with its numerical variables of space and chronology, longevity and health, to emerge not only as a problem but as an object of surveillance, analysis, intervention, modification etc.[9]

Foucault sought to delineate this mechanism of power. Rejecting narratives of progress, he developed what he called an archaeology and genealogy of knowledge: identifying historically specific discursive regimes and practices and showing how these structured knowledge and politics.[10] Foucault did not generally explain how these discursive regimes change or how they were related to one another.

One example that Foucault presented to illustrate structured knowledges concerned smallpox inoculation and vaccination. The introduction of inoculation in the 1720s and vaccination around 1800 provided methods to protect individuals from contracting smallpox. Throughout the eighteenth century, doctors, mathematicians and government officials collected and tabulated information about the number of individuals who had died from natural smallpox, and they calculated the chances of dying from the disease as roughly one in eight. By contrast, the risks of dying from inoculation and later vaccination were far lower. Moreover, the chances of contracting smallpox were very high. To reduce the risk of dying from smallpox, individuals should therefore be inoculated. Foucault labelled the quantitative treatment of the risks of smallpox an 'apparatus' (*dispositif*) in order to signal its novelty and underscore its status as a technique of power. In this 'apparatus of security', the risks of catching smallpox and of dying from it were calculated for a population not an individual, and inoculation was recast as an important security measure for the population.[11]

9 Michel Foucault, 'The politics of health in the eighteenth century', in *Power/Knowledge*, pp. 166–82, on p. 171; also Foucault, *Security, Territory, Population*, p. 79.

10 Lisa Downing, *The Cambridge Introduction to Michel Foucault* (Cambridge, 2008).

11 Foucault, *Security, Territory, Population*, p. 62. The *philosophe* d'Alembert criticized this treatment of risk precisely because it prioritized the population over the individual: Jean le Rond d'Alembert, 'Réflexions sur l'inoculation', in *Oeuvres de d'Alembert* (Paris, 1821), vol. 1, pp. 468–73.

Foucault did not elaborate on his example of inoculation and vaccination; in fact, he wrote very little specifically about biopolitics, and consequently, historians have criticized his work for its lack of empirical evidence, chronological inaccuracies, ahistorical use of concepts and limited applicability to nation-states that differed from the centralized polity of France.[12] Nonetheless, Foucault's work inspired or at least resonated with a growing scholarly interest in population. Sociologists and historians of science and medicine charted the emergence of new disciplines in the social sciences that focused on population,[13] while cultural historians explored how classifying populations contributed to new ideas about the nation-state and its citizens.[14] Historians of mathematics analysed the probabilistic revolution that undergirded the statistical approach to population,[15] and historians of statistics examined the various ways populations were described and quantified.[16] Much of this work demonstrated that the modern statistical concept of population emerged in the nineteenth century with important antecedents in the eighteenth, and that it was not solely a product of state power. Historians continue to explore the broader implications of population, and Foucault's concept of biopolitics remains a fertile framework because it underscores the larger shifts in the way societies value and treat life.[17]

Population Debates in the Eighteenth Century

Montesquieu's claim that Europe in the eighteenth century was far less populated than it had been in antiquity was widely accepted, but the causes of depopulation were a

12 Paul-Erik Korvela, 'Sources of governmentality: Two notes on Foucault's lecture', *History of the Human Sciences* 25, no. 4 (2012), 73–89; Mika Ojakangas, 'Michel Foucault and the enigmatic origins of bio-politics and governmentality', ibid., 25, no. 1 (2012), 1–14; Curtis, 'Foucault on governmentality'.

13 Jacques and Michel Dupâquier, *Histoire de la démographie: La statistique de la population des origines à 1914* (Paris, 1985); Libby Schweber, *Disciplining Statistics: Demography and Vital Statistics in France and England, 1830–1885* (Durham, NC, 2006).

14 Joshua Cole, *The Power of Large Numbers: Population, Politics, and Gender in Nineteenth-Century France* (Ithaca, NY, 2000); Silvana Patriarca, *Numbers and Nationhood: Writing Statistics in Nineteenth-Century Italy* (Cambridge, 1996).

15 Lorraine Daston, *Classical Probability in the Enlightenment* (Princeton, NJ, 1988); Ian Hacking, *The Emergence of Probability: A Philosophical Study of Early Ideas about Probability, Induction and Statistical Inference* (Cambridge, 1991 [1975]); Hacking, *The Taming of Chance* (Cambridge, 1990); Lorenz Krüger, Lorraine J. Daston and Michael Heidelberger (eds.), *The Probabilistic Revolution*, vol. 1: *Ideas in History* (Cambridge, MA, 1987).

16 Éric Brian, *La mesure de l'État: Administrateurs et géomètres au XVIIIe siècle* (Paris, 1994); Alain Desrosières, *The Politics of Large Numbers: A History of Statistical Reasoning*, trans. Camille Naish (Cambridge, MA, 1998); Theodore M. Porter, *The Rise of Statistical Thinking, 1820–1900* (Princeton, NJ, 1986); Andrea A. Rusnock, *Vital Accounts: Quantifying Health and Population in Eighteenth-Century England and France* (Cambridge, 2002).

17 For example, Alison Bashford, 'Global biopolitics and the history of world health', *History of the Human Sciences* 19, no. 1 (2006), 67–88; Roger Cooter with Claudia Stein, *Writing History in the Age of Biomedicine* (New Haven, CT, 2013); Stein, 'The birth of biopower in eighteenth-century Germany', *Medical History* 55 (2011), 331–7.

matter of fierce debate. Historian Carol Blum in her analysis of French writings on depopulation captures the many reasons polemicists advanced to account for the purported decline. The majority focused on births, or more precisely, the failure to multiply. Montesquieu criticized the Catholic church for its practice of clerical celibacy and its ban on divorce. These doctrinal issues were wielded by later authors to bludgeon the church for weakening the nation. Luxury, too, became a target; families that wanted to maintain their wealth were accused of having fewer children by avoiding pregnancy through abstinence and other measures. Many believed that luxury contributed to moral laxity and decreased male virility. Employing too many servants, who often were not allowed to wed and start families, and failing to control prostitution were also regarded as culpable social practices that reduced births.[18] Some writers blamed the prevalence of wet nursing and poorly trained midwives for the deaths of mothers and babies. Overall, the debates focused on increasing the numbers of healthy pregnancies and births by encouraging marriage and making childbirth safer, rather than on creating a larger population through immigration or territorial expansion.[19]

The physiocrats, a group of French political economists writing in the second half of the eighteenth century, explicitly tied population to agricultural production.[20] For François Quesnay, the leading physiocrat, agriculture was the only source of wealth, and when agricultural production became more profitable, more labour would be employed, leading to population growth.[21] Improving general wealth and welfare would thus encourage more and larger families.[22]

Amid the clamour over the causes and repercussions of depopulation came calls to document its existence numerically, or, as Foucault theorized, population became an object of analysis.[23] Political economists, physicians, clergymen and others collected numerical information both private and public from parish registers, bills of mortality, tax records, correspondence networks, hospital records and government inquiries. They developed and debated mathematical techniques that drew on the nascent field of the calculus of probabilities to estimate the sizes of various populations from these sources. They published in books and pamphlets, and in scientific and medical journals such as the *Philosophical Transactions* of the Royal Society of London, and the *Mémoires* of

18 Carol Blum, *Strength in Numbers: Population, Reproduction, and Power in Eighteenth-Century France* (Baltimore, MD, 2002).

19 On childbirth: Mary E. Fissell, 'Man-Midwifery Revisited', Chapter 22, this book.

20 A recent account of pre-Malthusian population ideas: Yves Charbit, *The Classical Foundations of Population Thought: From Plato to Quesnay* (Dordrecht, 2010).

21 *Quesnay's* Tableau Économique, ed. and trans. Marguerite Kuczynski and Ronald L. Meek (London, 1972); see also Nick Hopwood, 'The Keywords "Generation" and "Reproduction"', Chapter 20; and Staffan Müller-Wille, 'Linnaeus and the Love Lives of Plants', Chapter 21, this book.

22 Blum, *Strength in Numbers*, pp. 36–40.

23 Ibid., pp. 44–5.

the Royal Society of Medicine of Paris. Their work fell under the contemporary rubric of political arithmetic (and later medical arithmetic), a branch of mathematics first developed in late seventeenth-century England by the shopkeeper John Graunt and the physician William Petty.[24]

Quantifying Mortality

Two examples related to reproduction – infant mortality and maternal mortality – provide clear examples of how quantification reshaped ideas of population. Using records from general hospitals, foundling hospitals, lying-in hospitals and parish registers, doctors, natural philosophers and government administrators calculated the chances of dying in two distinct populations: infants and pregnant women. The shocking results of these calculations contributed to a growing awareness of and concern about what soon came to be called premature and preventable deaths.[25] These sobering figures were marshalled in efforts to reform conditions in hospitals and to improve the care of children. Better survival chances of children and women would, of course, increase population growth.

Pre-industrial societies experienced high infant and child mortality. Graunt had provided the first numerical estimates of infant mortality in his *Natural and Political Observations Made upon the London Bills of Mortality* (1662). He examined these weekly compilations by parish clerks of the numbers of christenings and burials in each London parish. Initiated in the sixteenth century as a way to track plague epidemics, the bills had been progressively refined so that by 1629 they included lists of the number of burials by cause of death. Graunt grouped causes that primarily affected children, including 'Thrush, Convulsion, Rickets, Teeth, and Worms', and calculated that deaths of infants and children under 4 or 5 constituted about one-third of all burials in London.[26]

Around 1750, as the depopulation controversy proliferated among French and English writers, some returned to Graunt's pioneering calculations and added new sources to investigate and characterize infant and child mortality.[27] English doctors, including Thomas Short, William Heberden the younger and William Black, drew on

24 Kreager, 'Emergence of population'; Andrea A. Rusnock, 'Biopolitics: Political arithmetic in the Enlightenment', in William Clark, Jan Golinski and Simon Schaffer (eds.), *The Sciences in Enlightened Europe* (Chicago, IL, 1999), pp. 49–68; Rusnock, *Vital Accounts*.

25 Zohreh Bayatrizi, *Life Sentences: The Modern Ordering of Mortality* (Toronto, 2008).

26 John Graunt, *Natural and Political Observations Made upon the London Bills of Mortality* (London, 1662), p. 29.

27 Andrea Rusnock, 'Quantifying infant mortality in England and France, 1750–1800', in Gérard Jorland, Annick Opinel and George Weisz (eds.), *Body Counts: Medical Quantification in Historical and Sociological Perspective / La quantification médicale, perspectives historiques et sociologiques* (Montreal and Kingston, 2005), pp. 65–86.

the London bills of mortality as Graunt had done, but they also turned to numbers gathered from hospital and dispensary records, and parish registers. French government officials and academicians, such as Antoine Deparcieux, Antoine Auget de Montyon, Jean-Baptiste Moheau and Jacques-Antoine Mourgue, used parish registers, monastic records and hospital records (including those from foundling hospitals). The French records did not include cause of death, but did provide information about age. All of these authors calculated high rates of infant and child death.

Two books, one English, one French, illustrate how these late eighteenth-century writers quantified infant mortality, developing it as an object of scientific inquiry and a problem to be addressed through reform. In 1778, Jean-Baptiste Moheau, secretary to Montyon, an intendant (royal administrator) of provinces, published *Recherches et considérations sur la population de la France* (Research and considerations on the population of France), which, like Graunt's book, is now considered one of the most important works in early demography.[28] Moheau, perhaps working with Montyon, created tables summarizing the numerical information about christenings and burials from all of France. He arranged many of the tables by age of death. For example, in one table, Moheau created age intervals beginning with the first year of life, and ages 2 to 3. This clearly showed that one in four infants died before their first birthdays.[29]

In England, the physician William Black arrived at the very same figure – 25 per cent of all infants died in their first year of life – in his *Arithmetical and Medical Analysis of the Diseases and Mortality of the Human Species* (1789). Black's calculations, like Graunt's, were based on the London bills of mortality, but for a later period (1701–76). Black's table grouped diseases by categories: acute febrile diseases, stomach and intestinal ailments, and diseases that affected primarily children. It ascribed one in four burials to the conditions that typically affected infants.[30]

Black and Moheau thus found a consistent pattern using very different types of records. Both men sought to identify a universal figure for infant mortality, yet at the same time probed variations due to geography, season, gender and social status. The inclusion of geography and season reflected the continuing use of the Hippocratic *Airs, Waters, Places*, which linked particular localities to patterns of health and disease. Black and Moheau confirmed the widespread beliefs that more children died in cities than in the countryside, and in swampy, low-lying areas than in settlements at higher elevations. The winter months of January, February and March and the autumn months of September and October were the most deadly to children. Both arithmeticians showed that more boys than girls died in every age group, and that poor children died at higher rates

28 Jean-Baptiste Moheau, *Recherches et considérations sur la population de la France* (Paris, 1778).

29 Ibid., p. 213.

30 William Black, *An Arithmetical and Medical Analysis of the Diseases and Mortality of the Human Species* (London, 1789), p. 34.

than children from wealthier families.[31] Reformers noted these enumerated differences and offered suggestions for how to prevent infant mortality and make life longer and more secure.[32] The use of infant mortality figures in policy debates, however, did not become widespread until the second half of the nineteenth century.[33]

Maternal mortality provides another example of the quantification of a particular population in the eighteenth century. As with infant mortality, deaths of women in childbirth were targeted as a cause of depopulation. Unlike the calculations of infant mortality, which drew on a wide range of documents, the risks were compiled almost exclusively from patient records and annual reports of hospitals, which were new sources of numbers. Over the course of the eighteenth century, more and more women gave birth in hospitals largely because of increasing urbanization, the growth of hospital medicine and rising concerns over improving maternity care.[34] Some of the hospitals were old general hospitals such as the Hôtel-Dieu in Paris, while others were new, smaller institutions dedicated to childbirth such as the Lying-In Hospital, soon the British Lying-In Hospital for Married Women, established in London in 1749. Medical arithmeticians gathered information from both types of hospitals in order to calculate the rate of deaths among women giving birth.

William Heberden, for example, a London physician and Fellow of the Royal Society, tabulated numbers taken from the registers of the British Lying-In Hospital in his *Observations on the Increase and Decrease of Different Diseases, and Particularly of the Plague* (1801). He included columns for the numbers of women giving birth, of boys and girls born, of stillborns and of women who died in childbirth (Fig. 23.1). His figures showed that the chances of women dying, while still high, had declined significantly from 1 in 42 for the period 1749–58 to 1 in 288 for 1789–98.[35] Heberden's table both illustrated and contributed to the new concept of population by creating categories of persons to be counted and compared.

A different picture of maternal deaths emerged in France. The Paris surgeon and member of the Academy of Sciences Jacques Tenon, as part of his study of Paris hospitals published just before the Revolution, calculated the chances of dying in childbirth at the Hôtel-Dieu as 1 in 15⅔.[36] Tenon's calculation was based on tables compiled

31 Rusnock, 'Quantifying infant mortality', pp. 74–80.

32 James C. Riley, *The Eighteenth-Century Campaign to Avoid Disease* (New York, NY, 1987).

33 David Armstrong, 'The invention of infant mortality', *Sociology of Health and Illness* 8 (1986), 211–32; Cole, *Power of Large Numbers*; Gretchen A. Condran and Jennifer Murphy, 'Defining and managing infant mortality: A case study of Philadelphia, 1870–1920', *Social Science History* 32 (2008), 473–513; Richard A. Meckel, *Save the Babies: American Public Health Reform and the Prevention of Infant Mortality, 1850–1929* (Ann Arbor, MI, 1998).

34 Fissell, 'Man-Midwifery Revisited'; Salim Al-Gailani, 'Hospital Birth', Chapter 37, this book.

35 William Heberden, *Observations on the Increase and Decrease of Different Diseases, and Particularly of the Plague* (London, 1801), pp. 40–1.

36 Jacques Tenon, *Memoirs on Paris Hospitals*, ed. and trans. Dora B. Weiner (Canton, MA, 1996), p. 226.

(40)

No. of Women Delivered.	Boys Born.	Girls Born.	Total No. of Children Born.	Women had Twins.	Children Still-born.	Children Died.	Women Died.	PROPORTION of DEATHS. Of the Women.	PROPORTION of DEATHS. Of the Children.
3	3		3						
175	93	84	177	2	11	5	3		
337	181	160	341	4	15	9	12		
433	236	201	437	4	22	27	14		
284	141	146	287	3	10	21	10		
321	175	151	326	5	9	66	12	1 in 42	1 in 15.
370	190	185	375	5	8	34	9		
370	188	184	372	2	8	10	3		
478	262	219	481	3	12	22	7		
521	277	254	531	10	6	16	8		
472	253	226	479	7	12	14	6		
427	228	206	434	7	11	58	26		
390	197	198	395	5	20	31	12		
397	199	199	398	1	8	38	7		
414	209	212	421	7	15	32	10	1 in 50	1 in 20.
366	191	178	369	3	15	17	7		
560	311	258	569	9	12	20	9		
588	293	304	597	9	25	17	10		
571	303	272	575	4	7	10	4		
588	301	288	589	1	5	2	3		
561	292	280	572	11	14	13	7		
472	225	249	474	2	13	9	28		
541	266	282	548	7	17	14	4		
596	320	286	606	10	25	17	4		
627	336	298	634	7	19	14	4		
553	292	266	558	5	36	3	18	1 in 53	1 in 42.
570	295	280	575	5	22	13	21		
543	276	275	551	8	26	9	3		
602	312	293	605	3	24	24	6		
572	281	298	579	7	19	18	11		

(41)

A. D.	No. of Women Delivered.	Boys Born.	Girls Born.	Total No. of Children Born.	Women had Twins.	Children Still-born.	Children Died.	Women Died.	PROPORTION of DEATHS. Of the Women.	PROPORTION of DEATHS. Of the Children.
1779	563	310	257	567	4	31	8	3		
1780	566	310	259	569	3	33	4	8		
1781	524	275	255	530	6	26	9	14		
1782	549	298	260	558	9	15	14	13		
1783	587	308	288	596	9	33	17	5	1 in 60	1 in 44.
1784	550	283	272	555	5	24	10	14		
1785	435	231	212	443	8	24	16	6		
1786	597	333	276	609	12	35	19	9		
1787	564	290	283	573	9	36	18	9		
1788	578	296	287	583	5	25	10	10		
1789	599	296	308	604	5	42	12	1		
1790	622	317	313	630	8	34	5	7		
1791	621	325	303	628	7	39	2	1		
1792	610	312	306	618	8	29	4	1		
1793	590	300	297	597	7	24	12	1	1 in 288	1 in 77.
1794	583	286	305	591	8	26	6	2		
1795	612	310	310	620	8	32	13	2		
1796	627	326	305	631	4	24	4	1		
1797	619	332	293	625	6	25	9	3		
1798	566	285	292	577	11	31	12	2		
1799	521	282	248	530	9	21	7	1	1 in 938	1 in 118.
1800	417	211	210	421	4	18	1	0		
Total	26202	13642	12871	26513	311	1073	795	391		

Proportion of Boys to Girls born in the Hoſpital is about 19 to 18.
Children Still-born in ditto, about - - 1 to 25.
Women having had Twins, about - - 1 to 84.

C

Figure 23.1 William Heberden's table of the ratios of maternal deaths to the number of women delivered, and of infant deaths to the number of live births, at the British Lying-In Hospital in London per decade for 1749–1800. The second page reveals remarkable reductions in maternal and infant mortality. Heberden also provided single ratios for male/female births, and incidences of stillbirths and twins. Heberden, *Observations on the Increase and Decrease of Different Diseases, and Particularly of the Plague* (London: T. Payne, 1801), pp. 40–1. Wellcome Library, London.

by gentlemen who had culled the information from the patient registers (Fig. 23.2). The high mortality rate – much greater than those from other French and British hospitals – shocked Tenon, and he called for basic reforms including one woman per bed, isolation of sick women and better ventilation.[37]

37 Ibid., p. 232.

264 MÉMOIRES

ANNÉE 1782.	Enfans nés.	Enfans morts nés.	Accouchées mortes.
Janvier	150.	12.	20.
Février	120.	11.	9.
Mars	150.	12.	8.
Avril	143.	11.	7.
Mai	118.	10.	5.
Juin	102.	6.	1.
Juillet	117.	11.	0.
Août	101.	8.	6.
Septembre	124.	7.	1.
Octobre	115.	5.	6.
Novembre	107.	5.	19.
Décembre	132.	8.	17.
	1479.	106.	99.

ANNÉE 1783.	Enfans nés.	Enfans morts nés.	Accouchées mortes.
Janvier	135.	8.	10.
Février	133.	6.	25.
Mars	112.	11.	30.
Avril	93.	10.	10.
Mai	135.	8.	5.
Juin	105.	10.	4.
Juillet	109.	12.	6.
Août	130.	10.	5.
Septembre	95.	8.	2.
Octobre	124.	12.	9.
Novembre	112.	10.	9.
Décembre	130.	17.	8.
	1413.	122.	123.

ANNÉE

SUR LES HÔPITAUX DE PARIS. 265

ANNÉE 1784.	Enfans nés.	Enfans morts nés.	Accouchées mortes.
Janvier	147.	19.	22.
Février	146.	14.	22.
Mars	146.	15.	8.
Avril	112.	10.	5.
Mai	138.	12.	6.
Juin	106.	7.	1.
Juillet	92.	9.	2.
Août	115.	16.	4.
Septembre	115.	0.	2.
Octobre	81.	10.	4.
Novembre	100.	4.	23.
Décembre	130.	10.	5.
	1428.	126.	104.

ANNÉE 1785.	Enfans nés.	Enfans morts nés.	Accouchées mortes.
Janvier	133.	10.	3.
Février	133.	14.	25.
Mars	144.	14.	13.
Avril	116.	9.	6.
Mai	132.	5.	3.
Juin	120.	8.	2.
Juillet	102.	8.	4.
Août	125.	9.	5.
Septembre	129.	8.	3.
Octobre	115.	15.	5.
Novembre	128.	8.	4.
Décembre	105.	11.	2.
	1482.	119.	75.

Ll

Figure 23.2 Jacques Tenon's table enumerating live births, stillbirths and maternal deaths by month for the period 1782–5 at the Hôtel-Dieu in Paris. Tenon's choice to classify by month reflected his interest in seasonal variation. Tenon, *Mémoires sur les hôpitaux de Paris* (Paris: De l'imprimerie de Ph.-D. Pierres, 1788), pp. 264–5. 26 × 39 cm. Cambridge University Library.

Malthus, Political Economy and Statistics

Taken together, these works cultivated a greater awareness of the loss of human life, a theme Thomas Robert Malthus took up in his *Essay on the Principle of Population*, first published anonymously in 1798. Those 'who have attended to bills of mortality', Malthus noted, have recognized 'that of the number of children who die annually, much too great a proportion belongs to those who may be supposed unable to give their offspring proper food and attention'.[38] For Malthus, like Quesnay and the physiocrats, population size and growth were inextricably linked to the availability of food, which Malthus articulated in his famous law: population increases geometrically, food supply only arithmetically. This law was based on two axioms, that the passion between the sexes is constant, and that food production is limited. Malthus spelled out what he called the positive checks to population – disease, famine, war, infanticide and abortion – forms of 'misery and vice' that raised mortality.

In the first edition, Malthus criticized the optimism of the French *philosophe* the Marquis de Condorcet and the English writer William Godwin about the future progress of humankind. According to Condorcet, Godwin and the physiocrats, greater wealth would inevitably lead to population growth. Malthus, however, contended that population would eventually surpass the means of subsistence, thereby creating a 'redundant population'. According to Malthus, the positive checks to this excess would then sharply reduce the number of persons. In 1803, Malthus authored a completely revised and expanded edition of his *Essay*, adding the idea of preventive checks to overpopulation through delaying marriage and abstaining from sex until married. These moral actions would decrease the production of children in each family. In this view, marriage and the resulting pregnancies were left to individuals, an assumption characteristic of the liberal economic thought of Adam Smith and other political economists of that period.[39]

Malthus fundamentally changed the discussion by identifying overpopulation as the problem, and his idea remains influential even today in debates about poverty, reproduction and food supply.[40] Malthus continued to refine his theories in conversation with other political economists by adding statistical and demographic data to subsequent editions of his *Essay*.[41] In reciprocal fashion, the writings of political economists, including Malthus, stimulated efforts to assess population size. During the first decades of the nineteenth century, nation-states instituted regular censuses and civil registration offices in order to provide more accurate numbers. Sweden, for example, created a national office in 1748 to collect numerical information on births, deaths and marriages from parish registers. The United States established a decennial census as part of its constitution and completed its first national census in 1790. Britain conducted a national census in 1801 and established civil registration in 1837; in France, the Napoleonic government created a national statistical bureau in 1801.[42]

38 [Malthus], *Essay*, chapter 5.

39 Luca Paltrinieri, 'Gouverner le choix procréatif: Biopolitique, libéralisme, normalisation', *Cultures & Conflits* 78 (2010), 55–79.

40 Alison Bashford, 'World Population from Eugenics to Climate Change', Chapter 34, this book.

41 These were published in 1806, 1807, 1817 and 1826; see further Rebecca Flemming, 'Population in the South Sea', Exhibit 24, this book.

42 John Koren (ed.), *The History of Statistics: Their Development and Progress in Many Countries …* (New York, NY, 1918).

These national offices reflected governments' growing interest in quantifying population and its various attributes, such as fertility, mortality, marriage rates and wealth. Non-governmental institutions also contributed to the creation of the concept of population; in hospitals, record-keeping fostered new ways of thinking about groups of patients. In Britain, for example, many new charitable hospitals were created independent of both church and state. They were overseen by lay governors, who required annual reports including numerical accounts of the numbers of patients, treatments and outcomes. More generally, the growth of hospital medicine during the eighteenth and nineteenth centuries, the attendant professionalization of doctors, new scientific and medical societies, and numerous public debates (including those over smallpox inoculation and vaccination), encouraged the turn to quantification to identify and evaluate different populations of patients.[43]

The collection and printing of numbers grew at such a rapid rate between 1820 and 1840 that the philosopher Ian Hacking characterized the output as an 'avalanche of numbers'.[44] Public health officials used population figures to argue for better sanitation, ventilation and other measures that would remediate high mortality rates.[45] Economists debated the impact of poor relief using population statistics, and the new field of insurance utilized mortality tables to put their business on a sounder footing. Physicians compared hospital mortality rates to improve outcomes: the Hungarian doctor Ignaz Semmelweis's work on puerperal fever in the Vienna General Hospital is perhaps the best known. When governments began, regularly, to apportion representatives to national assemblies based on population figures, the modern concept of population had arrived.

Conclusion

Foucault's 'biopolitics' is a useful category of analysis because it underscores the ways in which new forms of knowledge contribute to new types of power that continue to function in the world today. While Foucault himself wrote little about specific individuals, or the motivations and contexts surrounding the development of biopolitics, historians have begun to analyse precisely how the concept of population changed. The modern understanding of population and its features related to reproduction are embedded in these knowledge frameworks, and it is vital to understand their historical constructions.

43 Rusnock, *Vital Accounts*, pp. 109–75.

44 Ian Hacking, 'Biopower and the avalanche of printed numbers', *Humanities in Society* 5 (1982), 279–95.

45 For example, William Coleman, *Death Is a Social Disease: Public Health and Political Economy in Early Industrial France* (Madison, 1982).

During the eighteenth-century debates about depopulation, doctors, clergymen, mathematicians, government bureaucrats and others developed methods which drew on a wide range of public and private records to quantify features of populations. These numerical techniques were part of a general effort to ameliorate suffering and death, and they stimulated comparisons, which in turn contributed to the new statistical idea of population and the role of reproduction in determining its size. At the beginning of the nineteenth century, in the wake of the French Revolution and Malthus's *Essay*, governments began to institute civil registration of births, deaths and marriages, as well as regular censuses, thus providing more uniform and inclusive accounts of the national population. At the same time, the disciplines of probability and statistics, public health, vital statistics and demography developed as both social sciences and tools of governance.

24 Marriage and Fertility in Different Household Systems

Richard M. Smith

Demographers have sometimes distinguished what they term 'natural fertility' from 'family limitation'. The eminent French demographer Louis Henry argued for this distinction most forcefully in research after World War II that encompassed both past and contemporary societies.[1] Henry accepted that under 'natural' conditions fertility might vary considerably for biological and social reasons, but proposed a fundamental difference from societies experiencing or having passed through the Fertility Transition, which began in Europe in the nineteenth century and is still incomplete globally. These post-transitional societies were distinguished by family limitation, in which couples altered their reproductive behaviour with changing numbers of births (parities) as they sought to achieve a desired family size, after which childbearing stopped.[2]

Natural fertility is thus fertility in the absence of parity-specific regulation and can be conceptualized as a product of five proximate determinants which might be supposed in varying degrees to influence the total fertility rate, that is, the number of children a woman would have if she were to experience the fertility rates of the period at each age. The ranges of their relative contributions are plotted in Fig. 24.1. A 'standard' population is shown (vertical line) with a total fertility rate of seven births and the relative potential impact of each of the proximate determinants is displayed by the range of the shaded horizontal bars. It can be seen that the age of marriage and the infecund postpartum period, which is largely caused by maternal breast-feeding, significantly outweigh in importance the impact of intrauterine deaths, coital frequency (influencing waiting time to conception) and the woman's age at last birth. If it can be assumed that the practice of 'stopping' once a particular parity has been achieved is primarily found in post-transitional settings, then demographic research on other societies can focus on behaviour that influences the 'starting' and 'spacing' patterns of fertility. These are largely a function of the ages at which women marry, the proportion doing so and the tempo of births within a reproductive career, which is analysed mainly by investigating the time interval between successive pregnancies.

1 Louis Henry, 'Some data on natural fertility', *Eugenics Quarterly* 8 (1961), 81–91.

2 John Knodel, 'Family limitation and the fertility transition: Evidence from the age patterns of fertility in Europe and Asia', *Population Studies* 31 (1977), 219–49.

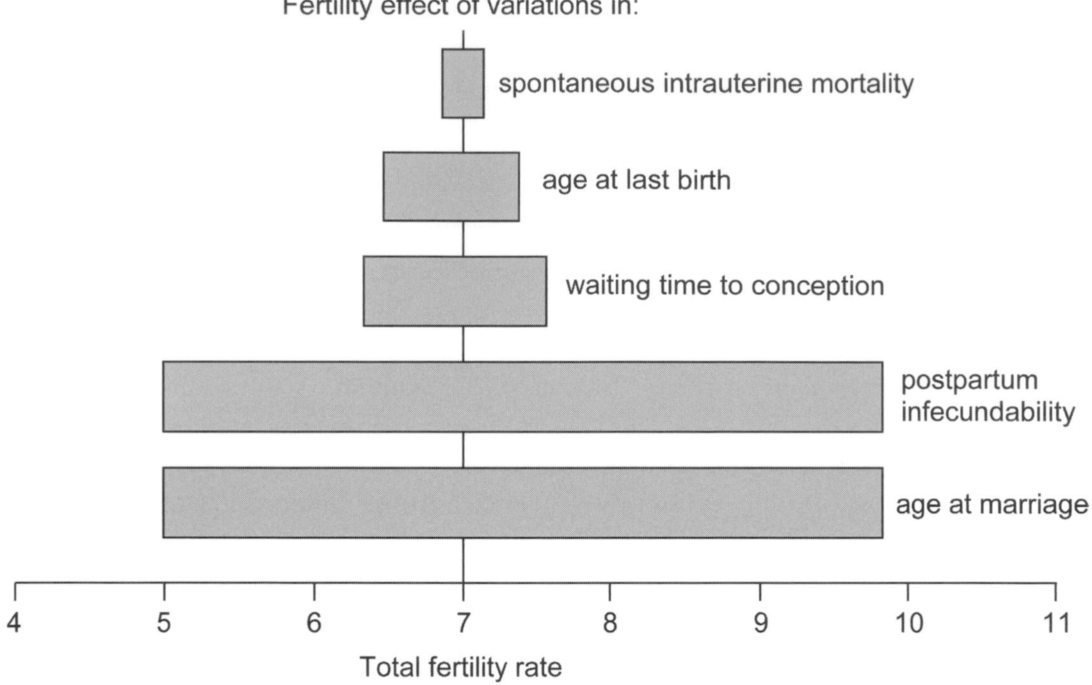

Figure 24.1 Variations in the total fertility rate induced by variations in five proximate determinants of natural fertility. Based on John Bongaarts and Robert G. Potter, *Fertility, Biology and Behavior: An Analysis of the Proximate Determinants* (New York, NY: Academic Press, 1983), p. 45.

This chapter considers the ways in which the starting and spacing patterns of fertility have manifested themselves within various systems of household formation that pre-date the Fertility Transition. It first discusses a framework within which Malthus pondered these issues, particularly with reference to nuclear family households in western Europe, and then proceeds to assess fertility determinants specific to joint household systems in Asia and matrifocal households lodged within lineages in West Africa. The conclusion briefly assesses the extent to which elements of behaviours associated with these patterns have continued to manifest themselves in post-transitional fertility regimes.

The Malthusian Preventive Check and the 'Starting' Patterns of Fertility

In his celebrated *Essay on the Principle of Population* (1798), Thomas Robert Malthus identified two kinds of checks to population growth. Either growth was contained by restricting nuptiality (the age and incidence of marriage), which Malthus termed the 'preventive check'; or, in the absence of this check, population would grow to the point where mortality rose, the 'positive check', and then return to a size more appropriate for the food supply.[3] In the second (1803) edition, Malthus emphasized that he preferred the preventive check, operating through the 'moral restraint' of individuals waiting to marry until they could support a family from their own resources. Such behaviour, Malthus argued, effectively disabled the operation of the positive check. Appealing to history and comparison, he wrote that 'it appears that in modern Europe the positive checks to population prevail less, and the preventive checks more than in past times and in the more uncivilized parts of the world'.[4] Malthus was unambiguously stressing the preventive check of regulating nuptiality, or what would come to be called the starting pattern, as the principal and most effective regulator of fertility.

What features of European marriage in the past do historical demographers regard as particularly supportive of Malthus's ideas about the preventive check as these were formulated in 1803? In a seminal essay, the Hungarian-British demographer John Hajnal identified what he believed was a distinctively European marital attribute.[5] He argued, on the basis of evidence from the seventeenth to the nineteenth centuries, that women in Europe married later than those in other regions (at age 24–27 on average), while a substantial number (between 5 and 15 per cent) never married at all.

In a subsequent article, Hajnal emphasized two other features as characteristic of the core area of what he termed northwest European household formation.[6] First, marriage was for the broad mass of the population 'neolocal': the bride and groom set up their residence apart from those of their respective natal families, and frequently in a different community. Second, a newly married couple would be at least largely economically independent of their kin. In contrasting the household formation systems of northwest Europe and of many other parts of the world, Hajnal highlighted the greater costs borne by the marrying couples in the former area and hence their need to have accumulated the resources for self-sufficiency. They were not absorbed within pre-existing households, but had to carry all of the start-up costs associated with acquiring housing and stocking that household with material possessions.

To obtain these resources, young adults had to spend a long time building up savings. Hajnal noted that in northwest Europe both men and women frequently spent

3 T. R. Malthus, *The Works of Thomas Robert Malthus*, ed. E. A. Wrigley and David Souden, vol. 1: *An Essay on the Principle of Population: The First Edition (1798) with Introduction and Bibliography* (London, 1986).

4 Ibid., vol. 2: *An Essay on the Principle of Population: The Sixth Edition (1826) with Variant Readings from the Second Edition (1803), Part 1* (London, 1986), p. 315; see further Rebecca Flemming, 'Population in the South Sea', Exhibit 24, this book.

5 J. Hajnal, 'European marriage patterns in perspective', in D. V. Glass and D. E. C. Eversley (eds.), *Population in History: Essays in Historical Demography* (London, 1965), pp. 101–43.

6 John Hajnal, 'Two kinds of preindustrial household formation system', *Population and Development Review* 8 (1982), 449–94.

the time between puberty and eventual marriage as unmarried servants or apprentices in households of people to whom they were generally unrelated and from whom they received payment in the form of bed, board and a stipend. Hajnal argued that this institution gave flexibility to marriage timing since, in difficult years, the service 'net' expanded to catch many who had been unable to acquire the resources to embark on marriage. The assumption of household headship by males was thus concentrated in the age range 20 to 35 such that, in England from the sixteenth to the mid-nineteenth centuries, the crude rate of first marriages per thousand persons aged 15 to 34 gives an approximate surrogate measure for the rate of new household creation per thousand persons aged 15 to 34. The incidence of first marriage, the 'nuptiality valve', as Ron Lesthaeghe termed this feature of European reproductive behaviour, determined the long-term shifts in fertility in England before the onset of widespread contraception within marriage.[7] It was closely aligned with a measure of real wages for three centuries from 1541 (Fig. 24.2).[8] Recent research for England on fines paid to lords by peasants to allow their daughters to marry in the thirteenth and fourteenth centuries, and on marriages recorded in parish registers after 1538, shows an even stronger preventive check on marriages and associated births at a manorial or parish level.[9]

The Starting Patterns of Fertility and Demographic Homeostasis in West European Peasant Society

The story of the 'nuptiality valve' in western Europe before 1850 is now familiar, with a sizeable component of women's reproductive capacity under-exploited or unexploited because of the relatively late age of marriage, and a significant number of women never marrying. It has frequently been asserted that this nuptiality pattern acted as a safety valve in the creation of demographic homeostasis, a view that treats fertility as marching to the tune played by mortality (Fig. 24.3). If mortality is assumed to have been unstable, showing no detectable secular trend, nuptiality must be the principal 'driver' of fertility. If mortality fell, then fertility would decline to maintain the same number in the population.[10]

As is well known, France in the period *c.* 1650–1800 exemplifies such an interrelationship. A demographic equilibrium continually re-established itself, despite

7 Ron Lesthaeghe, 'On the social control of human reproduction', *Population and Development Review* 6 (1980), 527–48.

8 E. A. Wrigley, 'British population during the "long" eighteenth century, 1680–1840', in Roderick Floud and Paul Johnson (eds.), *The Cambridge Economic History of Modern Britain*, vol. 1: *Industrialisation, 1700–1860* (Cambridge, 2004), pp. 57–95.

9 Morgan Kelly and Cormac Ó'Gráda, 'The preventive check in medieval and preindustrial England', *Journal of Economic History* 72 (2012), 1015–35.

10 J. Dupâquier, 'De l'animal à l'homme: Le mécanisme autorégulateur des populations traditionelles', *Revue de l'Institut de Sociologie* 45 (1972), 178–211.

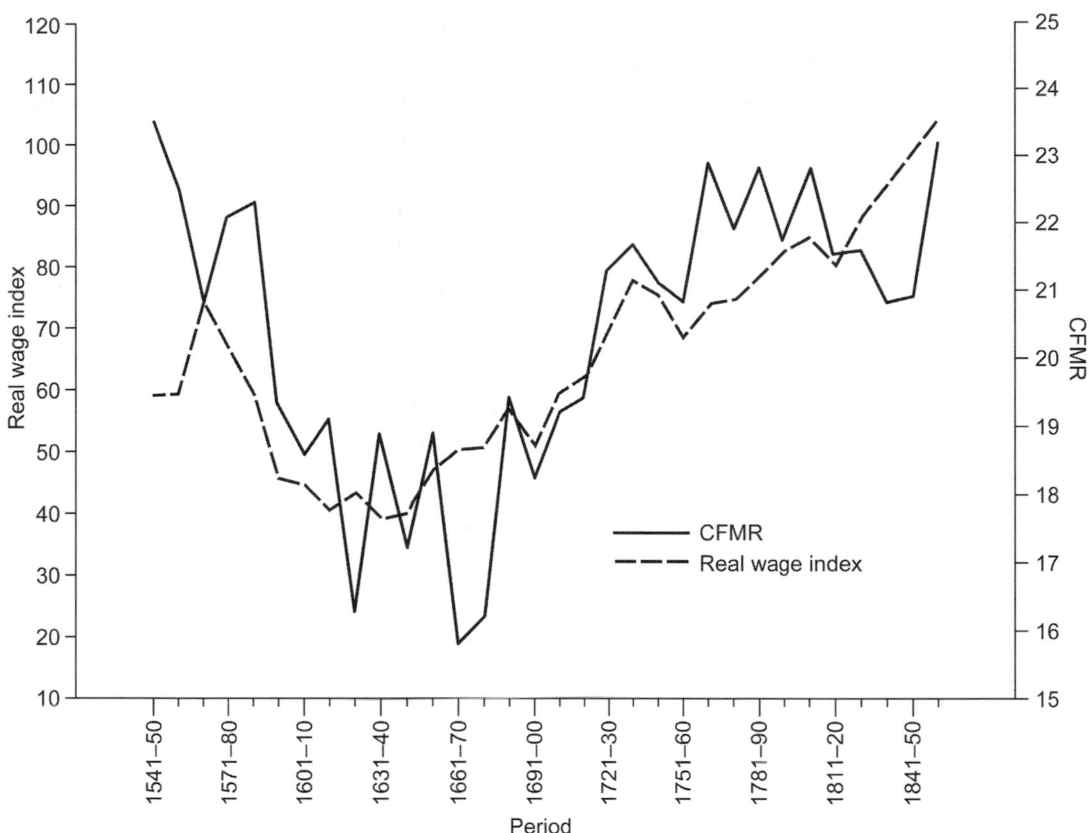

Figure 24.2 Crude first marriage rates (CFMR) and real wage trends in England, 1541–1850. ('Crude' because the birth-rates are ratios of the births occurring in each year to the mid-year total population and make no allowance for age structural variations from year to year.) Based on E. A. Wrigley, 'British population during the "long" eighteenth century, 1680–1840', in Roderick Floud and Paul Johnson (eds.), *The Cambridge Economic History of Modern Britain*, vol. 1: *Industrialisation, 1700–1860* (Cambridge: Cambridge University Press, 2004), pp. 57–95, on p. 78.

disturbances largely initiated by epidemics. The nuptiality valve opened and closed in response to the rises and falls in mortality: marriage age and marital incidence adjusted to reduce fertility as compensation for the losses or savings of lives. For much of the late seventeenth and eighteenth centuries, the number of hearths in the Paris basin barely changed at all. To explain this phenomenon, demographers use the concept of an agricultural holding or craft workshop as fulfilling a function analogous to that of a territory in a bird population in which a new breeding pair is allowed to establish itself only once a nest is vacated, such as when deaths in epidemics provided those in junior positions with opportunities to establish new households.[11]

11 Jacques Dupâquier, *La population rurale du Bassin Parisien à l'époque de Louis XIV* (Paris, 1979).

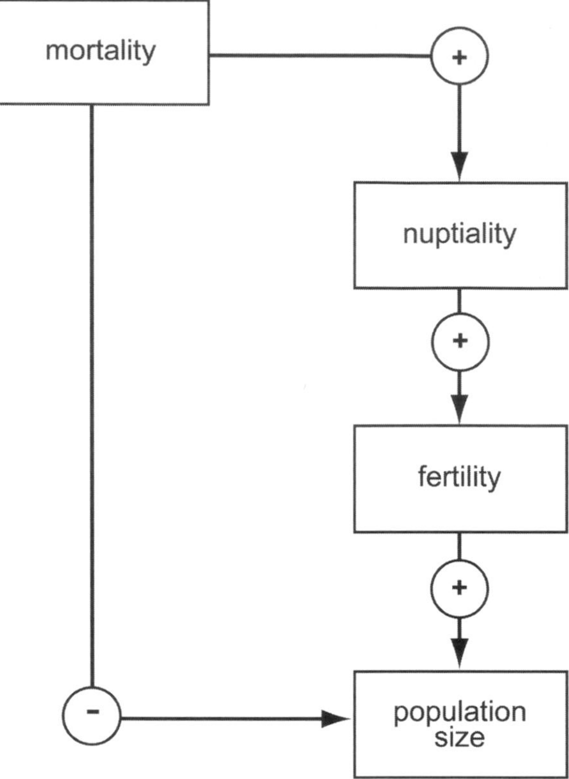

Figure 24.3 A system of ecological niches showing the dynamic feedback linkages capable of maintaining demographic equilibrium. Based on E. A. Wrigley and R. S. Schofield, *The Population History of England, 1541–1871: A Reconstruction* (Cambridge: Cambridge University Press, 1989), p. 461.

There is little doubt that in the eighteenth century the largely peasant agrarian economy of France behaved as a homeostatic regime *par excellence*, with fertility declining as life expectancy increased, especially after 1740.[12] A similar relationship between mortality and fertility may have applied more widely over northern parts of Spain and north-central Italy where marital patterns shifted notably in the eighteenth and nineteenth centuries.[13] In all these regions, mortality fell, and the low nuptiality that prevailed at the end of the eighteenth century was, as Massimo Livi Bacci has noted, 'the culmination of a process initiated in the sixteenth century' after the great late medieval mortalities associated with plague.[14] Some view this nuptiality restraint in response to improving life expectancies as enforced by social superiors rather than self-imposed.[15]

12 E. A. Wrigley and R. S. Schofield, *The Population History of England, 1541–1871: A Reconstruction*, new edn (Cambridge, 1989).

13 Massimo Livi Bacci, *La société italienne devant les crises de mortalité* (Florence, 1978); Vicente Pérez-Moreda, 'Matrimonio y familia: Algunas consideraciones sobre el modelo matrimonial español en la Edad Moderna', *Boletín de la Asociación de Demografía Histórica* 4, no. 1 (1986), 3–51.

14 Massimo Livi Bacci, *The Population of Europe: A History*, trans. Cynthia De Nardi Ipsen and Carl Ipsen (Oxford, 2000).

15 Lesthaeghe, 'On the social control', 530–2.

The Nuptiality Valve and England before the Mid-Nineteenth Century

Yet the concept of a nuptiality valve which took its cue from shifts in mortality to turn fertility on and off is of surprisingly limited value in understanding early modern England. Here, shifts in nuptiality appear not to have operated primarily as a short-term equilibrating force in the wake of mortality surges; rather, shifts in nuptiality and associated fertility were systematically related to changes in real wages through a direct link with the rate of first marriage. Rather than homeostasis, the pattern suggests that fertility behaviour may have been responding systematically to secular changes in society and economy that were in no sense captured by the changing access to a fixed number of niches enabled by mortality shifts.

The economy of early modern England, like the Netherlands, was far more differentiated and urbanized than in the rest of Europe before the nineteenth century. In England, inheritance of land was not the principal means by which an individual secured access to a livelihood, since most of the labour force worked for wages.[16] Children frequently left the parental hearth around the age of 14 or 15, and when later they married, the majority resided in a place in which neither partner had been born. Family was also not a key provider of support during episodes of illness or unemployment or in old age, and the maximization of fertility was hardly prioritized. The most important source of assistance was the community in the form of parish-funded welfare.[17] The family was therefore not the mediating force through which inheritance of a farm or workshop provided a conduit in which mortality and fertility were inversely related. Furthermore, England was an open society with a very mobile population. Emigration from England to the New World and into London in the later seventeenth century disturbed the geographical distribution of the sexes and produced long periods when women were drawn into the labour force as substitutes for men, and so did not marry even when economic conditions might have been favourable.[18]

It is also striking that births out of wedlock did not increase during periods when marriage incidence was very low. Up to 20 per cent of women never married in the later seventeenth century, but births out of wedlock fell too. Similarly, when the incidence of marriage rose and the age of marriage dropped in the late eighteenth and early

16 Richard M. Smith, 'Some issues concerning families and their property in rural England, 1250–1800', in Smith (ed.), *Land, Kinship and Life-Cycle* (Cambridge, 1984), pp. 1–86.

17 Richard M. Smith, 'The structured dependence of the elderly as a recent development: Some sceptical historical thoughts', *Ageing and Society* 4 (1984), 409–28.

18 Richard M. Smith, 'Influences exogènes et endogènes sur le "frein préventif" en Angleterre, 1600–1750: Quelques problèmes de spécification', in Alain Blum, Noël Bonneuil and Didier Blanchet (eds.), *Modèles de la démographie historique* (Paris, 1992), pp. 175–91.

nineteenth centuries, illegitimate births rose sharply too. When nuptiality declined in the seventeenth century, brides were far less likely to be pregnant at marriage than when it rose in the eighteenth century. Such changes suggest that the incidence of sexual relations outside of and in anticipation of marriage increased when marriage rates rose and retracted when they fell.

In France, notwithstanding its presence alongside England within the low incidence and late marriage area of the European marriage pattern, sexual behaviour outside and in anticipation of marriage was strikingly different. As marriage age rose and marital incidence fell with the decline in mortality over the eighteenth century, French women were increasingly likely to become pregnant outside marriage, and more likely to be pregnant when marriage was celebrated. In both cases they did so at older ages than those who were not pregnant at marriage, suggesting some incapacity of the social structure to contain extra-marital sexual activity. In these features we may be observing differences between a French predominantly peasant society for which access to land was an essential prerequisite for marriage and the considerably more differentiated English economy.[19]

Another contrast arises from the fact that births outside marriage in France were much more common in towns, whereas in England they were more likely in the countryside.[20] How far this feature may have reflected differences in the geography of welfare practices deserves more attention. Malthus railed against the English Poor Law as an institution that, he argued, encouraged reckless marriages and childbearing among labouring households which lacked the savings to form households without lowering their own living standards and those of society at large. Such arguments were controversial then and remain a core theme of debate about the fertility-inducing impact of welfare today.[21]

The discussion so far has contrasted the presence and absence of fertility-determined demographic homeostasis in two variants of the west European system of household formation associated with late female marriage, but the differences pale in

19 E. A. Wrigley, 'Marriage, fertility and population growth in eighteenth-century England', in R. B. Outhwaite (ed.), *Marriage and Society: Studies in the Social History of Marriage* (London, 1981), pp. 137–85, on pp. 155–67, Richard M. Smith, 'Marriage processes in the English past: Some continuities', in Lloyd Bonfield, Smith and Keith Wrightson (eds.), *The World We Have Gained: Histories of Population and Social Structure* (Oxford, 1986), pp. 43–99, on pp. 78–98.

20 Richard Adair, *Courtship, Illegitimacy and Marriage in Early Modern England* (Manchester, 1996), pp. 188–223; Richard M. Smith, 'Social security as a developmental institution? The relative efficacy of poor relief provisions under the English Old Poor Law', in C. A. Bayly *et al.* (eds.), *History, Historians and Development Policy: A Necessary Dialogue* (Manchester, 2011), pp. 87–94.

21 Richard M. Smith, 'Welfare of the individual and the group: Malthus and externalities', *Proceedings of the American Philosophical Society* 145 (2001), 402–14.

significance when compared with systems of joint household formation and early female marriage.

Some Fertility Correlates of Joint Household Formation Systems

The most important distinguishing feature of the joint household systems is that newly married couples do not establish separate and independent households, but rather join pre-existing ones.[22]

Such systems are common in South Asia. For instance, in the north Indian joint family system, sons tend to remain with their parents. Daughters marry out, and the groom's parents continue to exercise control over household affairs until death. While daughters marry out at a young age, especially among the landowning castes, the joint family does not extend the opportunity to marry to all sons. In fact, among high-status groups, only one son might marry while his brothers would remain single but share conjugal relations with the in-marrying bride. In such a patrilineal system, the position of those in-marrying women is potentially hazardous. In the north Indian joint household system there are strong inter- and intragenerational bonds between household members related to each other by blood. Women marrying into such households are in a weak position to protect their own and their children's health, resulting in maternal and infant mortality rates higher than those found in systems in which married couples manage their own affairs. Restricted husband–wife communication and the authority vested in the senior household members also have significant implications for fertility behaviour. Sons are strongly preferred because they are so critical to securing the future well-being of the adult women of the household. So mothers develop strong bonds with their sons, and daughters can be subject to discrimination by their mothers and other household members. As a result, mortality rates among girls are significantly higher than among boys but are frequently viewed by commentators as a form of family planning to protect resources.[23]

In south India, female status was and still is significantly higher, and cross-cousin marriage the norm, thereby relieving families of the economic burden of dowry provision. However, like in the north, marital fertility has frequently been lowered by spacing

22 Hajnal, 'Two kinds of preindustrial household formation'.

23 Monica Das Gupta, 'Kinship systems and demographic regimes', in David I. Kertzer and Tom Fricke (eds.), *Anthropological Demography: Toward a New Synthesis* (Chicago, IL, 1997), pp. 36–52; Mead Cain, 'The consequences of reproductive failure: Dependence, mobility, and mortality among the elderly of rural South Asia', *Population Studies* 40 (1986), 375–88; Navtej K. Purewal, *Son Preference: Sex Selection, Gender and Culture in South Asia* (Oxford, 2010).

births by prolonged breast-feeding and various intercourse taboos that older family members controlled. Age gaps between spouses were large and are still notable, with older males marrying younger brides, which probably reduced the frequency of sexual relations, thereby slowing the tempo of conceptions. Traditionally, various forms of stopping behaviour were also present, since it was thought to be damaging to health for men in their forties to engage in sexual relations and for women to become pregnant as grandmothers, a status attained at a relatively young age because of the youthful female marriage regime which in neither north nor south India functioned like the west European nuptiality valve.

In China, another variant of the joint household system prevailed, with universal and early female marriage until very recently.[24] Yet, here again, fertility may not have been higher than in Europe, since reported fertility in marriage seems to have been distinctly low.[25] Birth intervals were longer, as was the interval between marriage and first birth, apparently in part because people exploited the link between long-duration breast-feeding and birth spacing. In addition, infanticide depressed the number of children recorded as having been born to an individual mother. Recent historical investigations suggest that in the eighteenth century approximately 10 per cent of female births resulted in infanticide. Combined with neglect of baby girls, this produced female infant mortality rates frequently between two and three times higher than those in northwest Europe before 1800.[26] Furthermore, because of the depressed fertility and enhanced infant mortality, Chinese parents often resorted to fictive kinship and adoption to overcome the limitations of biology and miscalculation and still preserve family continuity and support in old age.[27]

For eastern Japan in the Tokugawa period, historical demographers have attributed the lack of growth in the population from *c.* 1720 to *c.* 1842 to the ending of every third new life in infanticide. The term *mabiki*, employed to describe such practices, can be translated as 'thinning': children were likened to rice plants, some of which needed to be uprooted as seedlings to give their siblings the space and light to thrive. This was facilitated by societal norms which did not view newborn children as fully formed human beings. Married couples sought to balance the genders of their children and did not consistently discriminate against girls. A dominant stem-household system and a

24 James Z. Lee and Wang Feng, *One Quarter of Humanity: Malthusian Mythology and Chinese Realities* (Cambridge, MA, 2001), pp. 63–82.

25 Zhongwei Zhao, 'Deliberate birth control under a high-fertility regime: Reproductive behavior in China before 1970', *Population and Development Review* 23 (1997), 729–67.

26 Bernice J. Lee, 'Female infanticide in China', in Richard W. Guisso and Stanley Johannesen (eds.), *Women in China: Current Directions in Historical Scholarship* (Lewiston, NY, 1981), pp. 163–77.

27 Arthur P. Wolf and Chieh-shan Huang, *Marriage and Adoption in China, 1845–1945* (Stanford, CA, 1980).

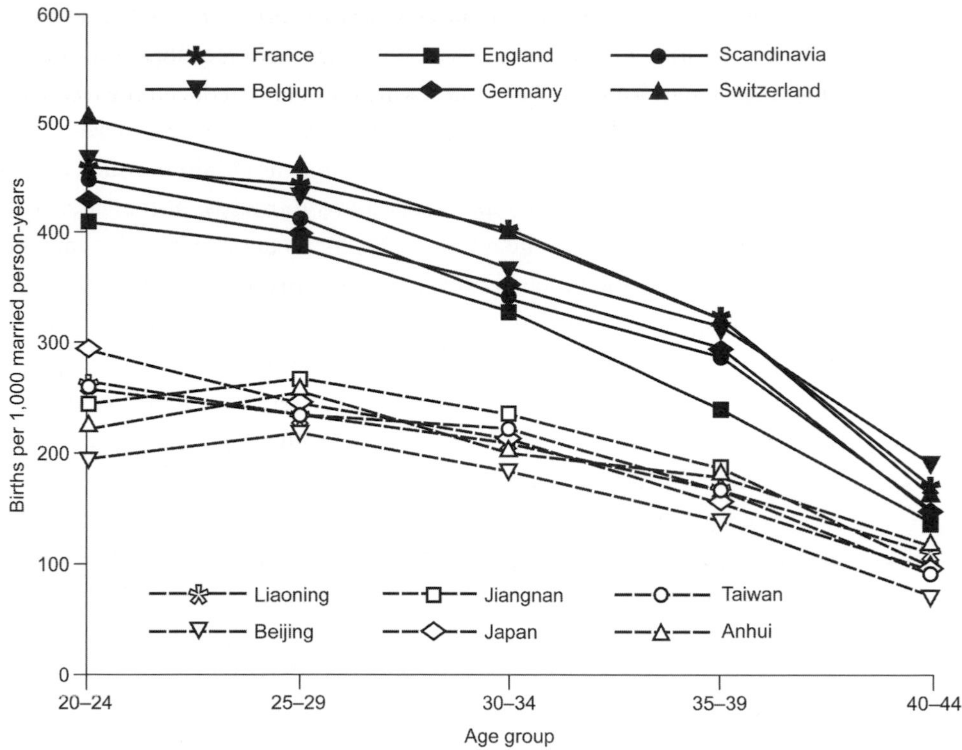

Figure 24.4 'Natural' age-specific marital fertility rates in East Asian and European populations, 1600–1800. Person-years relate to married women. Based on James Z. Lee and Wang Feng, *One Quarter of Humanity: Malthusian Mythology and Chinese Realities* (Cambridge, MA: Harvard University Press, 2001), p. 87.

fear of fragmenting the patrimony, and thus imperilling the household's continuity and undermining the veneration of ancestral spirits, could have motivated this 'thinning', if not strictly 'spacing', behaviour.[28]

Students of these Asian systems have contrasted them with European practices which left the activation of fertility control solely with starting behaviour captured by variations in the age and incidence of female marriage.[29] Asian household formation systems, by contrast, gave rise to a wide array of spacing and stopping choices, some of which included the decision to give away, kill or adopt children. Figure 24.4 compares the much lower Asian marital fertility rates with those found in European populations.

28 Fabian Drixler, *Mabiki: Infanticide and Population Growth in Eastern Japan, 1660–1950* (Berkeley, CA, 2013).
29 Lee and Feng, *One Quarter of Humanity*.

In West Africa, matrifocal households, embedded within lineages to which couples are subordinate, have created another distinctive fertility regime. In this region, marriage is a gradual process and can be easily terminated, thereby increasing the probability of a woman having several partners over her lifetime.[30] Each marital arrangement creates expectations that the woman will bear children, which makes it difficult for her to track their overall number and survival. There is also no assumption that the mother of a child will take the responsibility for its upbringing. This care is just as likely to be provided by other members of the lineage through fostering arrangements. These reduce the likelihood that couples will carry the full costs of their children, leading to relatively high rates of total, if not marital, fertility.[31]

This region is notable for long periods (three to four years) of postpartum taboo on sexual relations with long birth intervals. Such behaviour becomes understandable within the framework of lineage structures in which male elders desire to prevent the formation of close conjugal relationships.[32] Lesthaeghe has argued that the control of those who are reproductively active, and of female and child labour, are only two among many elements of an overall pattern of gerontocratic power exercised over people in lineages. The prevention of close husband–wife solidarity through the long postpartum taboo on sexual intercourse in particular, and through the maintenance of physical and psychological distance in general, also ensures lineage dominance. Hence, married couples do not carry the full cost or indeed responsibilities of their reproductive activities.[33] Of course, one consequence of more recent moves towards a stricter form of monogamous marriage, shorter-duration breast-feeding and the abandonment of the postpartum intercourse taboo was to increase fertility. Furthermore, education weakens gerontocratic authority, especially in the emerging urban areas to which many migrate, thus escaping the control which lineages have traditionally asserted in rural communities. All of these influences may be regarded as the unintended consequence of 'westernization' in diminishing the extent of spacing practices in these societies.[34]

30 Dominique Meekers, 'The process of marriage in African societies: A multiple indicator approach', *Population and Development Review* 18 (1992), 61–78. In some situations, polygyny might be supposed through access to multiple partners and high rates of divorce to spread venereal disease further and lead, as was not uncommon, to high incidences of sterility in substantial areas of sub-Saharan Africa; see further Simon Szreter, 'Fertility Transitions and Sexually Transmitted Infections', Chapter 30, this book.

31 Uche C. Isiugo-Abanihe, 'Child fosterage in West Africa', *Population and Development Review* 11 (1985), 53–73.

32 P. Caldwell and J. C. Caldwell, 'The function of child-spacing in traditional societies and the direction of change', in Hilary J. Page and Ron J. Lesthaeghe (eds.), *Child-Spacing in Tropical Africa: Traditions and Change* (New York, NY, 1981), pp. 73–92.

33 Lesthaeghe, 'On the social control', 530.

34 See also Philippa Levine, 'Imperial Encounters', Chapter 33, this book.

Conclusion: The Shadow of the Past

This chapter began by considering the ways in which demographers in their treatment of 'natural fertility' have given varying importance to starting and spacing patterns. When commenting at the turn of the nineteenth century, Malthus supposed that some parts of Europe had acquired distinctive demographic and economic characteristics, with associated benefits for living standards, because of their unique marriage practices. We have seen that household and kinship systems can influence fertility in various ways through their impact on the starting, spacing and, in certain instances, stopping patterns of fertility. In particular it has been demonstrated that the northwest European system, about which Malthus wrote so approvingly, was not the only one to limit fertility in order to avoid the painful impact of the 'positive check'. The differences between household and kinship systems continue to shape reproductive behaviour into the present.

Malthus argued that the absence of starting practices allowed, for instance, Chinese women to avoid marital restraint through the permission it gave parents to expose their offspring and so limit population growth.[35] He probably would not have denied that Chinese patterns of demographic behaviour rested heavily on collectivist decision-making within the household. This feature of past Chinese family planning has retained a prominent place in more recent practices and policies. Some commentators on the one-child policy of the 1980s stress that this was no fundamental ideological break with the past, but a continuation of collectivist goals in which the control over decision-making relating to family formation shifted from the older generation within the family and household to the commune and the state.[36] It is also perhaps no coincidence that when conscious efforts were made to contain Japanese fertility after World War II, abortion was legalized and served as the principal means by which fertility levels were brought down to western levels in the 1960s.[37] In north India the widespread practice of sex-selective abortion has resulted in exceptional rises in the sex ratio at birth, in effect removing from the death registers infant girls who had previously been killed at birth or neglected thereafter.[38]

Finally, we should note that in England, where for many centuries constraints on marriage shaped secular trends in fertility, the nuptiality valve continued to impact on fertility outcomes well into the twentieth century, notwithstanding the onset of the historic fertility decline. Simon Szreter has shown, by analysing in detail data in the

35 Malthus, *Works*, vol. 2, p. 129. 36 Lee and Feng, *One Quarter of Humanity*, pp. 123–46.

37 Tiana Norgren, *Abortion before Birth Control: The Politics of Reproduction in Postwar Japan* (Princeton, NJ, 2001).

38 Tulsi Patel (ed.), *Sex-Selective Abortion in India: Gender, Society and New Reproductive Technologies* (New Delhi, 2007); Ilana Löwy, 'Prenatal Diagnosis, Surveillance and Risk', Chapter 38; on other aspects of reproduction in modern India: Nick Hopwood, 'Globalization', Chapter 43, this book.

Fertility Census of 1911, that as marital fertility in late Victorian and Edwardian Britain was falling, there was a strong positive relationship between the resort to control of fertility in marriage and marriage age. Later-marrying couples were also lowering the tempo of their childbearing, apparently by resort to sexual abstinence.[39] Here again, the shadow of the past fell strikingly over the present.

39 Simon Szreter, *Fertility, Class and Gender in Britain, 1860–1940* (Cambridge, 1996), pp. 367–439.

25 Colonialism and the Emergence of Racial Theories

Renato G. Mazzolini

From the fifteenth century, increasing numbers of west Europeans either travelled along the coasts of Africa, India and the Far East to explore and trade, or migrated to the new-found lands in the Americas and the Pacific to conquer, colonize and evangelize. These activities involved the exchange of goods and the exploitation of the territories where the Europeans settled. The people they encountered were subjugated and often decimated by wars, epidemics and the destruction of their former ways of life. In their endeavour to render the lands acquired in the Americas economically fruitful, the Spaniards and Portuguese, and later the British, French, Dutch, Danes and Swedes, imported from West Africa a labour force they thought suited to those new environments. From the early sixteenth to the mid-nineteenth centuries, sub-Saharan Africans were subjected to a capitalist trade which produced one of the largest forced migrations in history, as well as a new phenomenon: colour-based slavery, which was unlike previous systems of slavery in the Mediterranean world.[1]

When western European scholars of the sixteenth century learned about the peoples encountered by travellers, they tried to explain their differences in appearance, habits and temperament by appealing not to racial theories, which did not yet exist, but to ancient theories of climate and of constitution.[2] Doubts arose, however, over the explanatory power of those theories when scholars noticed that the skin colours of the inhabitants of Africa and America at the same latitude did not correspond. The climatic theory also could not explain the presence among the people of the Congo of very white individuals who were soon named albinos. More generally, the seventeenth-century development of a mechanistic conception of bodily functions called into question the constitutional theory of the four humours.[3] Even the religious belief in the original

1 Robin Blackburn, *The Making of New World Slavery: From the Baroque to the Modern, 1492–1800* (London, 1997); David Eltis and Stanley L. Engerman (eds.), *The Cambridge World History of Slavery*, vol. 3: *AD 1420–AD 1804* (Cambridge, 2011), pp. 323–475.

2 Valentin Groebner, 'Complexio/complexion: Categorizing individual natures, 1250–1600', in Lorraine Daston and Fernando Vidal (eds.), *The Moral Authority of Nature* (Chicago, IL, 2004), pp. 361–83. Colonial encounters would also inform theories of population: Rebecca Flemming, 'Population in the South Sea', Exhibit 24, this book.

3 Gerhard Klier, *Die drei Geister des Menschen. Die sogenannte Spirituslehre in der Physiologie der Frühen Neuzeit* (Stuttgart, 2002).

unity of the human species, postulated by the book of Genesis, was thrown into doubt, owing to the difficulty of explaining how the inhabitants of America had arrived there. Could they have originated from a different Adam? This speculation led some scholars to reinterpret Genesis and to question the unity of humankind.[4]

In the past fifty years, historians of colonialism and race have studied the dispossession and exploitation of indigenous peoples by west Europeans, and paid attention to colonial sexual relations.[5] The expansion of Europe 'was not only a matter of Christianity and commerce, it was also a matter of copulation and concubinage'.[6] While the policies of the colonial powers generally prevented the intermixture of populations, mixing is well documented for Latin America and colonial Virginia. The low social status to which the offspring of those 'mixtures' were relegated shows the power that their colonizers established over the indigenous people and the imported slaves.

This chapter addresses four major questions rarely discussed by colonial historians, but much debated by European scholars of the period. They concerned human generation, reproduction and descent and were influential both in shaping what was then called the 'natural history of man', our physical anthropology, and in developing the racial theories of the second half of the eighteenth century and the early nineteenth. Special attention will be given to the inheritance of skin pigmentation, since skin colour was the main physical trait of the peoples mentioned by sixteenth- and seventeenth-century travellers. It was used to establish rank as well as legal and religious rights within the colonies, and by natural historians in Europe to classify human groups.

Who Generated the Inhabitants of the Americas?

The doctrine of the unity of the human species, reinforced by the teachings of the late scholastics, was based on Genesis, which all Christians considered to be revealed truth. After the human nature of the inhabitants of the New World had been established in heated controversy among Spanish theologians and jurists, the main challenge was to explain their descent and migration from the Old World, where all men had descended from the second Adam, Noah. According to Spanish friars of the sixteenth century, who saw analogies with Jewish practices in Aztec religion, the Indians descended from the Lost

4 Giuliano Gliozzi, *Adamo e il nuovo mondo: La nascita dell'antropologia come ideologia coloniale, dalle genealogie bibliche alle teorie razziali (1500–1700)* (Florence, 1977).

5 C. R. Boxer, *Race Relations in the Portuguese Colonial Empire, 1415–1825* (Oxford, 1963); Magnus Mörner, *Race Mixture in the History of Latin America* (Boston, MA, 1967); James Hugo Johnston, *Race Relations in Virginia and Miscegenation in the South, 1776–1860* (Amherst, MA, 1970); Werner Sollors (ed.), *Interracialism: Black–White Intermarriage in American History, Literature, and Law* (Oxford, 2000); María Elena Martínez, *Genealogical Fictions: Limpieza de Sangre, Religion, and Gender in Colonial Mexico* (Stanford, CA, 2008); Ronald Hyam, *Understanding the British Empire* (Cambridge, 2010); Damon Ieremia Salesa, *Racial Crossings: Race, Intermarriage, and the Victorian British Empire* (Oxford, 2011).

6 Hyam, *Understanding the British Empire*, p. 364.

Tribe of Israel. However, some scholars had different opinions, and maintained that the inhabitants of the New World must have come 'from a different Adam'. Amerindians were difficult to fit into the framework of biblical revelation. In a devastating analysis of Genesis in 1655, the French theologian Isaac La Peyrère formulated a theory of twofold creation, one of all men, the so-called pre-Adamites, who were unstained by original sin, and one of Adam, the progenitor of the Jewish people alone. He maintained that Amerindians were pre-Adamites who had survived the Great Flood. Notwithstanding harsh criticism by Protestants and Catholics alike, La Peyrère's theory gained support among some scholars, who considered both Amerindians and black Africans to be pre-Adamites.[7] This view of the origin of the human species undermined canonical beliefs and reinforced the idea that there might exist a humankind parallel with, and alien to, the one elected by God and the sole object of sacred history. In everyday colonial life this notion justified subjugation, exploitation and segregation on the grounds of difference in origin and descent.

Why Are the Ethiopians Black?

The question 'Why are the Ethiopians black?' began to be investigated systematically during the seventeenth century. Numerous dissections of the bodies of sub-Saharan Africans were performed, and in 1677 the Dutch physician Johannes Pechlin, following a conjecture put forward in 1665 by his Italian colleague Marcello Malpighi, demonstrated that the 'black pigment' (that is, granules of melanin) was contained in what is now called the Malpighian layer of the epidermis. But what caused this pigment? Some authors distinguished between theological and physical causes. Those who advocated the former identified black people either as descendants of Ham's son, Canaan, who had become black as a consequence of Noah's curse, or as descendants of Cain who had inherited the mark (interpreted as blackness) impressed upon him by God, and had survived the Great Flood. Although no textual evidence supported these interpretations, they were used to legitimize slavery. The physical causes examined were: climate, sperm, bile, blood, the conditioning of the fetus by the mother's imagination, chemical substances purportedly produced by the body and not excreted through respiration, the nervous fluid and the ancient disease leprosy.

Notwithstanding the variety of explanations put forward, most theories agreed that blacks begot blacks, and whites begot whites, and attributed this fact to seminal matter. As the Portuguese traveller Odoardo Lopes put it in the late sixteenth century, the black colour 'did not spring from the heate of the Sunne, but from the nature of the seede'.[8] Several decades later, the English physician Thomas Browne added that if black

7 Richard H. Popkin, *Isaac La Peyrère (1596–1676): His Life, Work, and Influence* (Leiden, 1987).

8 Odoardo Lopes, *A Report of the Kingdom of Congo, a Region of Africa* ..., trans. Abraham Hartwell (London, 1597), p. 19.

people were 'transplanted' to other climates they would still preserve 'their hue both in themselves, and also their generations; except they mixe with different complexions'. He considered 'the tincture of the skin as a spermatical part traduced from father unto son, so that they which are strangers contract it not'.[9] As late as 1768, when arguing against the climatic theory put forward in 1749 by the naturalist Buffon, the *philosophe* Voltaire reiterated that black people 'transplanted' from Africa to the Americas always 'generated blacks like themselves', since their blackness was 'inherent and specific'.[10]

Why Do Black Couples Sometimes Beget White Children?

Travellers and missionaries, however, reported a puzzling phenomenon: cases in the Congo of black couples begetting white children. This also happened on several plantations from which reports were sent to the Académie royale des sciences in Paris and the Royal Society in London. Scholars were incredulous. Some thought that those children had been generated by a mixed white and black couple; others that the children had returned to the original colour of mankind, which was assumed to be white. The perplexity grew when travellers reported the same phenomenon in India, in the Moluccan Islands and among the Cuna Indians of the Panama Isthmus. 'In Spain we call them Albinos', wrote the historian Bartolomé Leonardo de Argensola in 1609, adding that they were as white as Germans and had poor eyesight.[11]

The main discussion of albinos took place in Paris after Mapondé, a 4-year-old child from Cabinda (Angola), was shown in 1744 at the Académie royale and in several Parisian homes (Fig. 25.1).[12] Some of the most influential intellectuals provided descriptions, including the natural philosopher Pierre Louis de Maupertuis in the anonymous *Dissertation physique à l'occasion du nègre blanc* (Physical dissertation occasioned by the white negro). This constituted the first part of his *Vénus physique* (Physical Venus) of 1745, a work which put forward a new theory of generation. He first disputed preformation theories, which held that embryos already existed preformed in either the eggs or the animalcules, by pointing out that mulatto skin was neither black nor white, but a mixture of the two.[13] This suggested that both parents contributed seminal matter to the process of generation. Then, on the basis of information concerning Senegalese families

9 Thomas Browne, *Pseudodoxia Epidemica: or, Enquiries into very many received Tenents, and commonly presumed Truths* (London, 1646), pp. 324, 329.

10 [François-Marie Arouet de Voltaire], *Les singularités de la nature* (Basle [Geneva], 1768), p. 116.

11 Bartolomé Leonardo de Argensola, *Conquista de las Islas Malucas al Rey Felipe III* (Madrid, 1609), p. 71.

12 Renato G. Mazzolini, 'Albinos, Leucoæthiopes, Dondos, Kakerlakken: Sulla storia dell'albinismo dal 1609 al 1812', in Giuseppe Olmi and Giuseppe Papagno (eds.), *La natura e il corpo: Studi in memoria di Attilio Zanca* (Florence, 2006), pp. 161–204.

13 Maupertuis, *Vénus physique* (1745), p. 75; see also Nick Hopwood, 'The Keywords "Generation" and "Reproduction"', Chapter 20; and James A. Secord, 'Talking Origins', Chapter 26, this book.

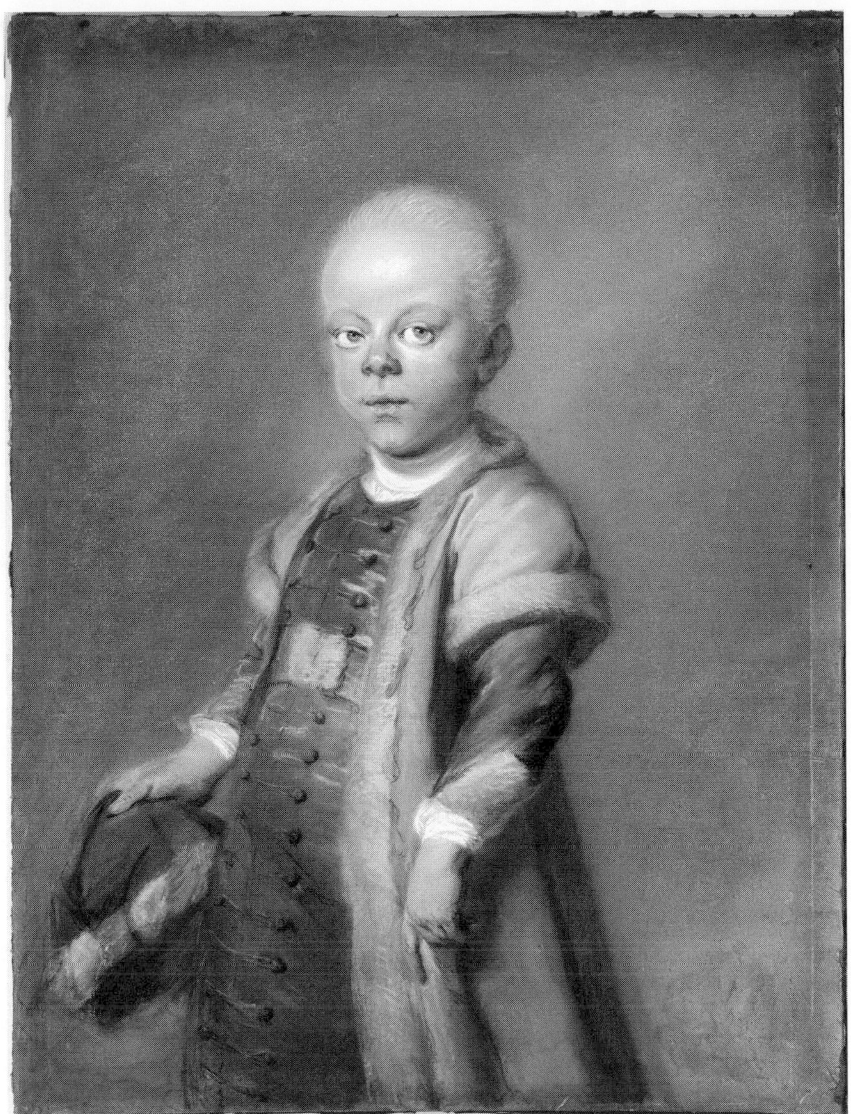

Figure 25.1 Jean-Baptiste Perronneau, *Portrait of Mapondé*, 1745, pastel on paper, 75 × 56 cm. Photo © Nationalmuseum, Stockholm.

into which albino children had been born, Maupertuis suggested that albinism could be inherited even if only one ancestor had been albino. He also endorsed the hypothesis of a certain Monsieur du Mas who had long lived in the Far East and surmised (correctly) that albinism is a disorder of the Malpighian layer of the skin.

In several works, Voltaire maintained that albinos constituted a distinct species, since he could not conceive that blacks might generate whites, while the Swedish naturalist Carl Linnaeus classified them as troglodytes. It was only in 1776 that the Swiss naturalist Marc-Théodore Bourrit acknowledged that albinos existed in Europe as well.

In 1784, by dissecting the eyes and skin of an albino man who had died in Milan's Ospedale Maggiore, the eye surgeon Francesco Buzzi established that albinos did not constitute 'a specific species', and that du Mas had been right. In 1786 the Göttingen professor of medicine and natural history, Johann Friedrich Blumenbach, reached a similar conclusion by a complex induction based on dissection of the eyes of albino rabbits. The only substantial difference between the two authors was that Blumenbach held albinism to be hereditary, while Buzzi did not. In later works Blumenbach insisted that albinos were 'patients', and that albinism was further proof of the unity of the human species since it occurred all over the world.[14] The enormously influential ideas of Voltaire and Linnaeus were thus defeated, and the English surgeon William Lawrence could write in 1819: 'So far is this variety from being peculiar to the Negro, or even to the torrid zone, that there is no race of men, nor any part of the globe, in which it may not occur.'[15]

Classifying Humans by Colour

The classification of human groups by their skin colour characterized the first natural histories of man published during the eighteenth and early nineteenth centuries.[16] But selection of the colours was slow and often controversial. Skin colour was the main physical trait mentioned by travellers. It was also one of the markers used in the Mediterranean by merchants to describe the slaves they intended to sell, and by slave owners as an aid to identification when they ran away. The surprising feature of both kinds of descriptions is that the terminology used to indicate the various nuances of skin pigmentation was extremely rich. It is documented by the collection of travel accounts published in many editions by the Italian geographer Giovanni Battista Ramusio during the second half of the sixteenth century.[17] Note, however, that the term 'yellow' was not used to describe the hue of the Chinese; this was a later invention.[18]

European intellectuals had long grasped that humans exhibit differences in skin pigmentation as, after all, was apparent in Europe itself. They tended to codify such

14 Mazzolini, 'Albinos', pp. 186–9.

15 W. Lawrence, *Lectures on Physiology, Zoology, and the Natural History of Man, Delivered at the Royal College of Surgeons* (London, 1819), p. 287.

16 Nina G. Jablonski, *Living Color: The Biological and Social Meaning of Skin Color* (Berkeley, CA, 2012); Renato G. Mazzolini, 'Skin color and the origin of physical anthropology (1640–1850)', in Susanne Lettow (ed.), *Reproduction, Race, and Gender in Philosophy and the Early Life Sciences* (Albany, NY, 2014), pp. 131–61.

17 Giovanni Battista Ramusio, *Navigazioni e viaggi*, 6 vols., ed. Marica Milanesi (Turin, 1978–8).

18 Walter Demel, 'Wie die Chinesen gelb wurden. Ein Beitrag zur Frühgeschichte der Rassentheorien', *Historische Zeitschrift* 255 (1992), 625–66; Michael Keevak, *Becoming Yellow: A Short History of Racial Thinking* (Princeton, NJ, 2011).

differences in broad chromatic categories. As the Italian philosopher Giordano Bruno wrote in 1590: 'The species of men are of many colours: the black progeny of the Ethiopians, and the red offspring of America'.[19] The description of Amerindians as 'red' was a generalization drawn from selected sources. It became customary only during the second half of the eighteenth century,[20] but was rejected by several scholars who compared the untanned arm of a north American Indian with their own.[21]

During the late seventeenth and early eighteenth centuries, the process of codifying differences into broader chromatic categories, by combining the geographical distributions of populations and their supposed complexions, temperaments and constitutions, took paradigmatic form in the classification drawn up by Linnaeus in the tenth edition of his *Systema naturae* (1758–9), where the varieties of the human species were classified thus:

American	red, choleric, erect.
European	white, sanguine, brawny.
Asiatic	sallow, melancholy, rigid.
African	black, phlegmatic, relaxed.[22]

The German philosopher Immanuel Kant propounded a similar scheme in a text of 1775, revised in 1777. He adopted Buffon's rule to define a species, that is, fertile progeny. Kant postulated that the skin colour of the original human stock was 'white of brunette colour', and that as humans had migrated to different climates they had adapted by developing hereditary characters from predispositions unified in the original stock. Kant thus distinguished four races of men:

First race	Noble blond (northern Europe) from humid cold.
Second race	Copper-red (America) from dry cold.
Third race	Black (Senegambia) from humid heat.
Fourth race	Olive-yellow (Indians) from dry heat.[23]

Classifying Human Mixtures

The notion of 'species of men', 'varieties of men' or 'races of men' emerged mainly from the combination of skin colour with geographical distribution. But what happened

19 Giordano Bruno, *Opere latine*, ed. Carlo Monti (Torino, 1980), pp. 783–4.

20 Nancy Shoemaker, 'How Indians got to be red', *American Historical Review* 102 (1997), 625–44.

21 Constantin-François Volney, *Tableau du climat et du sol des Etats-Unis d'Amérique*, 2 vols. (Paris, 1803), vol. 1, p. 435.

22 Carl Linnaeus, *Systema naturae …*, 10th edn, 2 vols. (Stockholm, 1758–9), vol. 1, pp. 20–2.

23 Immanuel Kant, 'Von den verschiedenen Rassen der Menschen', in *Der Philosoph für die Welt*, ed. J. J. Engel, 22 (1777), 125–64, on 159–60.

when different populations mixed and had offspring? Among European scholars interested in the natural history of man, this question became a topic of investigation only during the second half of the eighteenth century, although it had been an administrative problem for the Spaniards and the Portuguese from the beginning of their conquests.

In 1533 the Spanish Crown ordered that the fathers of the many abandoned natural (illegitimate) children, or 'mestizos', born from intimate relations between Castilians and Indian women, be found and compelled to support their offspring.[24] A scandalized Jesuit, Nicola Lancilotto, wrote to the founder of the society, Ignatius Loyola, in 1550 concerning the licentiousness of Portuguese men in India: 'There are innumerable Portuguese who buy droves of girls and sleep with all of them, and subsequently sell them'.[25] A manuscript census, probably written between 1550 and 1570, shows that the archbishopric of Mexico comprised 9,495 Spaniards, 10,593 black slaves, 2,000 'mestizos' and 1,050 'mulattoes'. The accuracy of the figures may be questioned, but they do show an extraordinary increase in the slave population and in the number of 'hybrids', as they were sometimes called, which is documented in many other sources. The census also shows that the inhabitants of the region were subdivided into categories: Spaniards, black slaves, mestizos and mulattoes.

In 1580 another Italian Jesuit, Alessandro Valignano, classified the inhabitants of Portuguese India in a similar way.[26] For the Portuguese, as for the Spaniards, the question was whether countrymen born abroad, as well as 'half-breeds', could be admitted into religious orders. By the end of the sixteenth century, the general answer was 'no', but the debate continued through the seventeenth century.

The Spanish colonial government in Central and South America and the Catholic church – which was responsible for baptisms and marriages – gradually established an administrative system known as the '*sistema de castas*'.[27] This consisted in the classification of a newborn child on the basis of his or her ancestry. The terminology used by this system had local variations, but this did not alter its importance, for it allowed or precluded access to certain careers and to religious orders depending on membership of a given caste. In his *Politica Indiana*, published in 1647, the jurist Juan de Solórzano Pereira discussed the tensions within the caste system and expressed a much contested view: that the '*criollos*', individuals born in America but of Spanish ancestry, had the same rights as the '*Españoles*' residing in America but born in Spain. They too, he added, could pursue ecclesiastical careers. '*Mestizos*' and '*mulatos*' also had the same right of

24 Antonio de Herrera, *Historia general de los Hechos de los Castellanos en las islas y tierra firme del Mar Oceano*, decada quinta (Madrid, 1615), p. 154.

25 Boxer, *Race Relations*, p. 61.

26 Ibid., p. 62.

27 Max S. Hering Torres, María Elena Martínez and David Nirenberg (eds.), *Race and Blood in the Iberian World* (Vienna, 2012).

access as Spaniards to offices and religious orders provided they were the offspring of a legitimate marriage. But they seldom were. He observed that the number of illegitimate *mestizos* and *mulatos* was steadily increasing, and that they were potentially dangerous because they refused to work in the mines like the poor '*Indios*', thus aggravating the conditions of the latter. Illegitimate *mestizos* and *mulatos* were not to be privileged in any way, because they were the offspring of lust and were themselves vicious: an evaluation that endured for centuries.[28]

The caste system was illustrated, from the late seventeenth century, in numerous cycles of paintings produced in Mexico.[29] They usually began with a Spanish man and an Indian woman, a Spanish man and a black woman, and an Indian man and a black woman, and depicted four successive 'crosses' from each pair, some of which are shown in Fig. 25.2. Other paintings showed more complex crosses, such as that producing a '*coyote*', a person with Indian, African and European blood in his or her veins. These paintings also reveal a parallel between social structure and skin colour: the higher a Spaniard rose in the social hierarchy, the whiter the complexion of his wife had to be. Unfortunately, these Mexican cycles of paintings were unknown to non-Iberian scholars of the eighteenth century, because, with very few exceptions, foreigners were forbidden to travel to Central and South America. But the system was not exclusive to Spanish America, for it was maintained or adopted in a less formalized way also in the British and French West Indies.[30]

Non-Iberian scholars came to know the Spanish caste system mainly through the 1758 French translation of a book by the Jesuit José Gumilla, who provided the following scheme for white–black crosses:

1. European × negra [black] → mulata, 2/4 from each parent;
2. European × mulata → quarterona, 1/4 of mulata;
3. European × quarterona → octavona, 1/8 of mulata;
4. European × octavona → puchuela, completely white.[31]

Gumilla knew that crosses were more complex, but did not elaborate because his purpose was to maintain that, according to the Catholic church, '*quarterones*' and '*octavones*' must be considered '*blancos*' (white), and only the *Indios* and *mestizos* newly converted.

Building on Gumilla, Blumenbach, a strenous supporter of the unity of the human species, described four generations of human mixed breeds when discussing the question of pigmentation in his epoch-making doctoral dissertation *De generis humani*

28 Juan de Solórzano Pereira, *Politica Indiana* (Madrid, 1647), pp. 244–8.

29 Ilona Katzew, *Casta Painting: Images of Race in Eighteenth-Century Mexico* (New Haven, CT, 2004).

30 Jean-Luc Bonniol, 'La couleur des hommes, principe d'organisation sociale: Le cas antillais', *Ethnologie française* 20 (1990), 410–18.

31 José Gumilla, *Histoire naturelle, civile et geographique de l'Orenoque* ... (Avignon and Marseille, 1758), pp. 114–15.

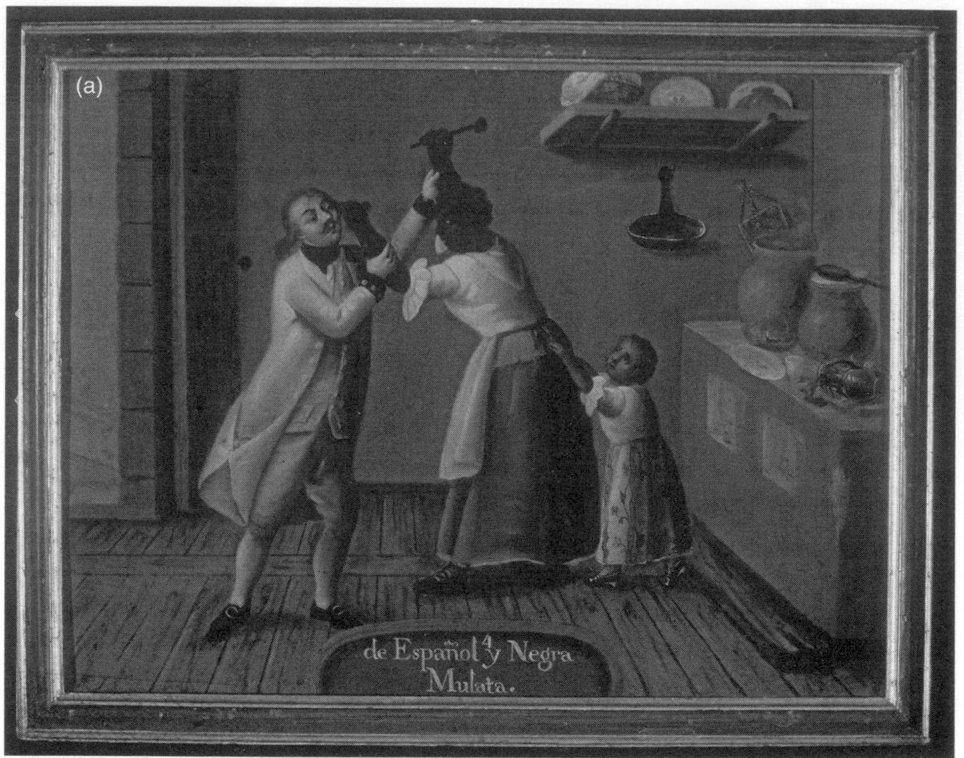
(a)
de Español 4 y Negra
Mulata.

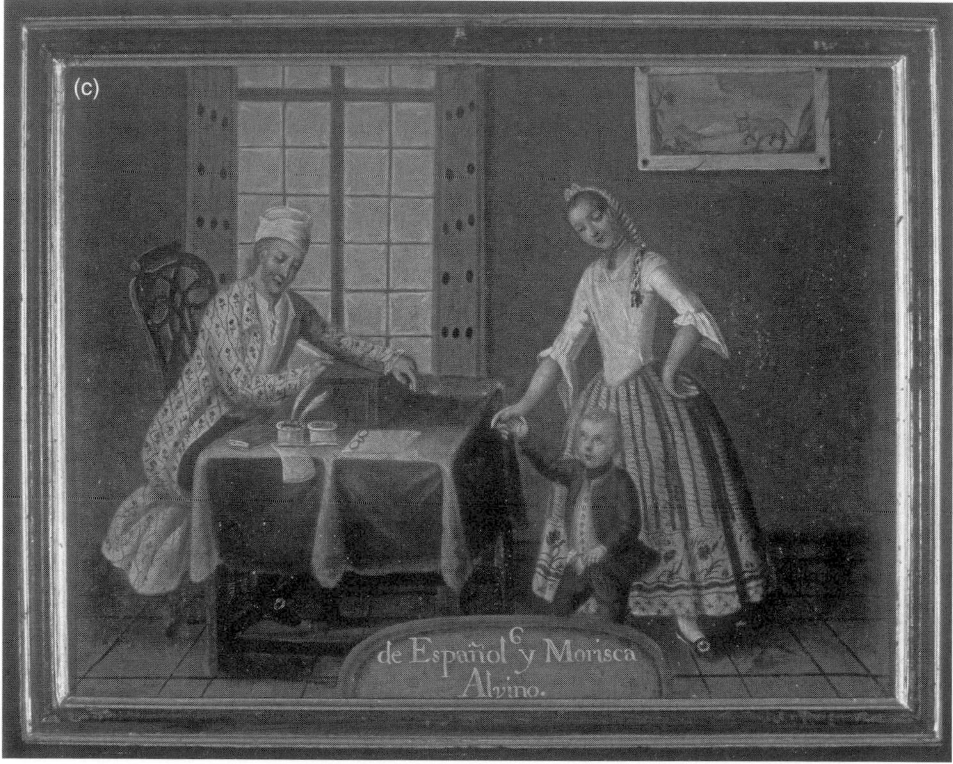
(c)
de Español 6 y Morisca
Alvino.

Figure 25.2 *Las castas*, anonymous late eighteenth-century paintings: (a) *From Spanish Man and Negro Woman a Mulatto Woman*, (b) *From Spanish Man and Mulatto Woman a Morisco*, or *quarteron*, (c) *From Spanish Man and Morisco Woman an Albino*, (d) *From Spanish Man and Albino Woman a Negro Throwback*. Each panel 36 × 48 cm. © Museo de América, Madrid.

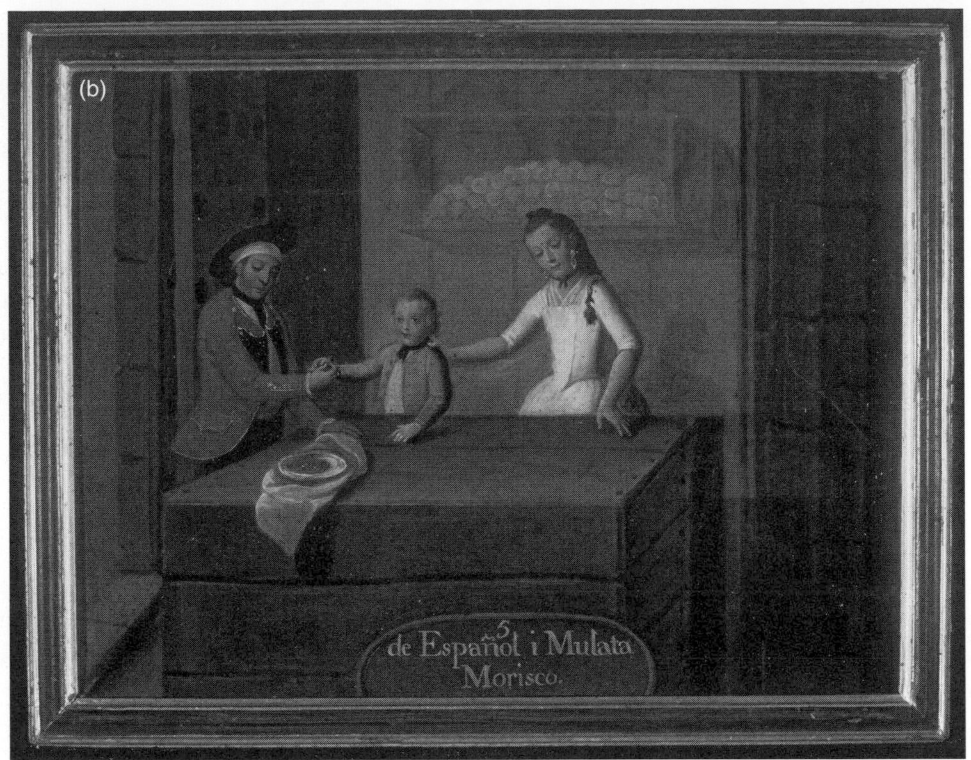

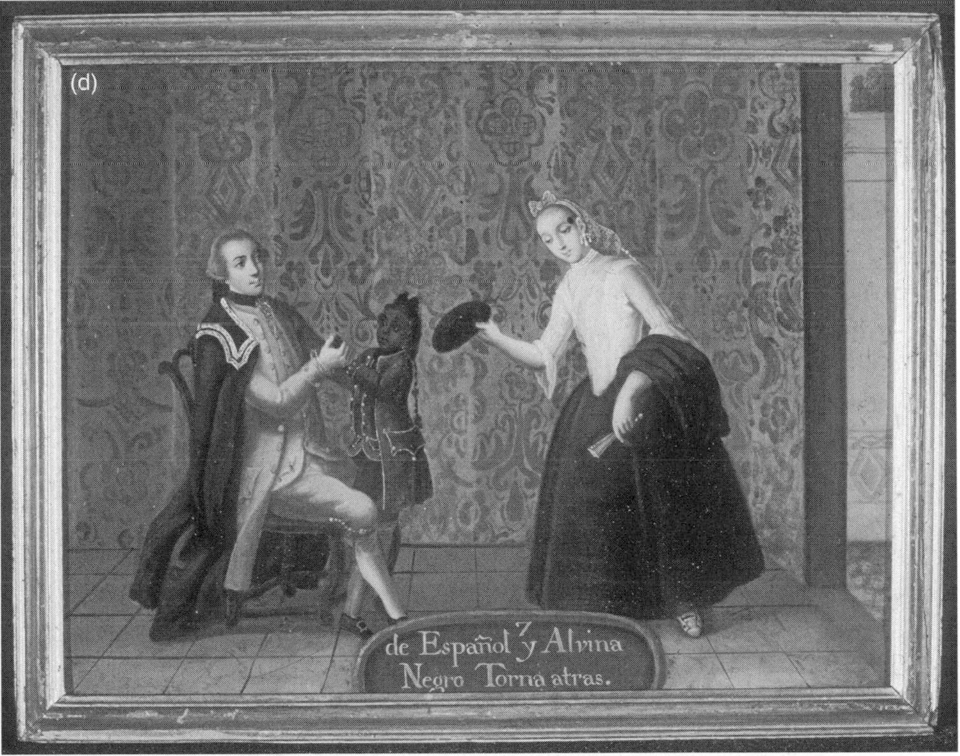

Figure 25.2 (*cont.*)

varietate nativa (On the natural varieties of mankind) of 1775. He drew the conclusion that whatever might be the cause of human skin colour, the intermixture of human varieties demonstrated that colour was changeable and could never be considered a feature constituting a diversity of species.

In an influential essay of 1777, Buffon described four mixed generations of white and black people, mainly in relation to skin colour. This was his simplified scheme of 'four generations mixed in order to make the colour of Negroes disappear':

1. White × black → mulatto, half white, half black;
2. White × mulatto → quarteron, tanned;
3. White × quarteron → octavon, less tanned than the quarteron;
4. White × octavon → a perfectly white boy or girl.

The inverse scheme demonstrated how 'to blacken whites':

1. Black × white → mulatto with long hair;
2. Black × mulatto → quarteron, 3/4 black and 1/4 white;
3. Black × quarteron → octavon, 7/8 black and 1/8 white;
4. Black × octavon → a perfectly black boy or girl.[32]

Yet Kant, in his last attempt to clarify his notion of race, an essay of 1788, argued that Nature seemed 'to permit the melting together' of races, but not 'to favour it, since thereby the creature becomes fit for several climates but not suited to any one of them to the degree achieved by the first adaptation to it'. Races differed from varieties because only their characters were unfailingly hereditary.[33]

Non-Iberian scholars learned about the social system in which this population 'interbreeding' was embedded only in 1811 when Alexander von Humboldt published his *Essai politique sur le royaume de la Nouvelle-Espagne* (Political essay on the Kingdom of New Spain). In Mexico and Cuba, Humboldt studied the social effects of the caste system, describing Mexico as a country where inequality reigned: all economic and political power was in the hands of the whites, and the *Indios* and coloured *castas* did all the hard manual labour. He concluded that they would never progress given the conditions of absolute inequality in which they were forced to live.[34] Much the same could have been concluded of other countries.

32 Georges-Louis Leclerc, comte de Buffon, 'Addition à l'article qui a pour titre, Variétés dans l'espèce humaine', in *Histoire naturelle, générale et particuliére*, supplément, vol. 4 (Paris, 1777), pp. 454–582, on p. 504.

33 Immanuel Kant, 'Über den Gebrauch teleologischer Principien in der Philosophie', *Teutsche Merkur*, Jan. and Feb. 1788, 36–52, 107–36, on 50; English translation in Kant, *Anthropology, History, and Education*, ed. Günter Zöller and Robert B. Louden (Cambridge, 2007), p. 202.

34 Renato G. Mazzolini, 'Physische Anthropologie bei Goethe und Alexander von Humboldt', in Ilse Jahn and Andreas Kleinert (eds.), *Das Allgemeine und das Einzelne – Johann Wolfgang von Goethe und Alexander von Humboldt im Gespräch*, Acta Historica Leopoldina 38 (Halle, 2003), pp. 63–79.

During the early history of colonial Virginia, for instance, marriages of white men and Indian women were not uncommon. Owing to the imbalance of the sexes among Europeans, these were seen at times as a strategy for attaining a peaceful coexistence with the natives and as a means to favour colonialism. White female servants were also known to marry black men. However, after the extermination of even peaceful Indians during the rebellion of 1676, following the example of Barbados, the main labour force in Virginia changed: white indentured servants were replaced by increasing numbers of black slaves. On the grounds of their 'abominable mixture and spurious issue', marriages of whites with blacks, mulattoes or Indians were outlawed in 1691.[35] Children were to take the status of their mother. A white mother giving birth to a mulatto child was severely fined, but the child was free. Since slaves were considered property, the offspring of a black or mulatto slave woman and a white man took the status of the mother and was therefore a slave. Considering the possibility of emancipating a slave, Thomas Jefferson, the former Governor of Virginia, wrote in 1787: 'When freed, he is to be removed beyond the reach of mixture', that is, sent away, lest his blood 'stain' that of his master.[36] In Virginia's plantations, segregationist practices were imposed. But sexual relations still occurred: planters continued to assert their rights to sexual property even over their own offspring.

Conclusion

Racial theories and racial classifications were mainly elaborated not in the colonies, but by west European scholars who seldom left their own shores. Only at the end of the eighteenth century were racial theories imported to flourish in the United States, where the question of colour was pre-eminent in daily life. But the practices of what we now call 'racism' – a twentieth-century coinage – were fully developed in the colonies from the sixteenth century onwards without having a proper name.

Between the end of the eighteenth century and the first decades of the nineteenth, as the movement for abolition of the slave trade and of slavery won its first victories in England, the term 'race' slowly replaced 'variety'. Most authors conceived races as stable natural entities, and the inheritance of skin pigmentation provided the main phenomenon on which their conceptions were based. However, they no longer distinguished races by skin colour alone; they did so also by hair type and Petrus Camper's facial angle, which measured the projection of the upper jaw and teeth, as well as the shapes of skull and pelvis and other canons of European aesthetics, intellectual capacity, moral

35 A. Leon Higginbotham, Jr and Barbara K. Kopytoff, 'Racial purity and interracial sex in the law of colonial and antebellum Virginia', in Sollors, *Interracialism*, pp. 81–139, on p. 107.

36 Thomas Jefferson, *Notes on the State of Virginia* (London, 1787), p. 240. Further on slavery and reproduction: Philippa Levine, 'Imperial Encounters', Chapter 33, this book.

virtues and vices, political practices and level of civilization. By the 1850s, belief in a common origin of all mankind (monogenesis) was giving way to that in the independent origins of human races from several ancestors (polygenesis). Furthermore, during the 1820s, historians used the concepts of race and racial struggle to explain great European historical events; they interpreted the French Revolution as a clash between descendants of the Franks and of the Gauls. Because of its scientific appeal, race replaced religion in creating clear-cut barriers between the populations of an earth dominated by whites. In the preface to his *Races of Men*, the Scottish anatomist Robert Knox declared in 1850: 'Race is everything: literature, science, art, in a word, civilization, depend on it.' A new ideology was born.

But what about the offspring of those now called 'hybrids', 'racial crossings' or 'interracial mixtures'? Lawrence, a declared supporter of the unity of the human species, wrote in 1819: 'the intellectual and moral character of the Europeans is deteriorated by the mixture of black or red blood: while, on the other hand, an infusion of white blood tends in an equal degree to improve and ennoble the qualities of the dark varieties'.[37] In British and French colonies, people of mixed parentage were excluded from higher military and government offices, just as the Spaniards and the Portuguese had excluded them from religious orders at the end of the sixteenth century. Testifying to this continuity of exclusion are the many sources which portray 'half-breeds' as troublemakers and individuals torn between different cultures and loyalties: a threat to order and empire. In the long run, however, and notwithstanding the tragedies they suffered, mixed-race people may well be considered the lasting but unintentional contribution of colonialism to proving the unity of the human species, and a visible refutation of the notion of race as a stable natural entity.

37 Lawrence, *Lectures on Physiology*, p. 300.

26 Talking Origins

James A. Secord

The question of origins has always involved generation in the widest sense; apprehending how individuals come into being is as relevant to planets and stars as to plants, animals and people. Over many centuries, hidden forces of repulsion, attraction and desire have been understood to govern the physical as much as the human world. Since the Renaissance, the association between matter and the passions has been traced to the ancient Roman epic *De rerum natura* (On the nature of things) by the Epicurean poet Lucretius, who invoked Venus as a symbol of the generative power of nature in the opening lines.

Venus has not featured much in histories of origins, and especially of evolution, many of which still follow a narrow agenda set in the 1950s by the founders of the modern evolutionary synthesis. More generally, the history of ideas dominated twentieth-century surveys such as Arthur Lovejoy's *Great Chain of Being* (1936) and Peter Bowler's *Evolution: The History of an Idea* (1983). This tradition, which aimed to unite the advancing flow of time with rational inquiry into the laws of nature, goes back to the universal histories that emerged in late Enlightenment narratives of progress, and was reshaped through late nineteenth-century evolutionism; Lovejoy's book began as lectures at Harvard University named for the evolutionary psychologist William James. If any history were going to be evolutionary and developmental, it would be the history of evolution and development.

Yet the history of thought is an odd approach to adopt for debates about origins, which have been extraordinarily promiscuous in genre, authorship and audience. Conversations in the bedroom, salon and bookshop were continuous with the contributions of scholars and experts in journals and learned societies. Discussions of origins are implicated in mapping social hierarchies and racial stereotypes, defining gender roles, probing the limits of decency, and legitimizing state intervention. These processes of public debate and intimate discourse are not 'context' or 'background', but the story itself. We need to know what could be written, published and said, and under what circumstances – not simply who thought what.[1]

1 For a related approach to medieval advice on generation: Peter Murray Jones, 'Generation between Script and Print', Chapter 13, this book.

Recent studies reinforce the need for a new history of origins, with generation, reproduction, gender and sexuality at its core. Mary Terrall located mid-eighteenth-century French discussions of generation in 'salon, academy, and boudoir'. Gowan Dawson, Angelique Richardson and Evelleen Richards have shown that Victorian evolutionary writings were implicated in controversies about promiscuity and contraception.[2] Focusing on Britain and France from the mid-eighteenth to the late nineteenth century, this chapter sketches what bringing these approaches into a long-term perspective could look like.

Polyps and Flaming Chaos

In 1741, one topic dominated elite conversation in Paris and London: the freshwater polyp, today known as hydra (Fig. 26.1). Take one of these tiny aquatic organisms, cut it in two, wait a few hours, and – astonishingly – it does not die, but instead grows back, walks and even regenerates arms and other missing parts. Cut it into as many pieces as you like, and that number of new individuals will result. The Genevan naturalist Abraham Trembley, who had discovered the powers of the polyp while teaching two boys at a country house on the outskirts of The Hague, found the powers of the polyp so incredible that he sent living specimens throughout Europe so that others could witness what he had seen. Travelling by fast carriages and ships, the creatures arrived in Paris, Rome, Stockholm and London, to be wondered at by the learned, curious and fashionable in the salons.[3] Often led by women, salons encouraged enlightened conversation in many European cities from the sixteenth through the mid-nineteenth century.[4]

The polyp raised questions anyone could understand. A living thing that swung its arms and walked must be an animal. But one that could be divided and 'reproduce' (we would say 'regenerate') was, clearly, a plant. As the philosopher Voltaire remarked on seeing a jar of the organisms on a friend's mantelpiece, 'this production called a

2 Mary Terrall, 'Salon, academy, and boudoir: Generation and desire in Maupertuis's science of life', *Isis* 87 (1996), 217–29; Gowan Dawson, *Darwin, Literature and Victorian Respectability* (Cambridge, 2007); Angelique Richardson, *Love and Eugenics in the Late Nineteenth Century: Rational Reproduction and the New Woman* (Oxford, 2003); Evelleen Richards, *Darwin and the Making of Sexual Selection* (Chicago, IL, 2017). See also Jonathan Hodge, 'Against "revolution" and "evolution"', *Journal of the History of Biology* 38 (2005), 101–21.

3 Marc J. Ratcliff, *The Quest for the Invisible: Microscopy in the Enlightenment* (Farnham, 2009), pp. 103–23; Rebecca Stott, *Darwin's Ghosts: The Secret History of Evolution* (New York, NY, 2012), pp. 86–106.

4 For instance, Dena Goodman, *The Republic of Letters: A Cultural History of the French Enlightenment* (Ithaca, NY, 1994); Steven Kale, *French Salons: High Society and Political Sociability from the Old Regime to the Revolution of 1848* (Baltimore, MD, 2006); and Jon Mee, *Conversable Worlds: Literature, Contention, and Community 1762 to 1830* (Oxford, 2011).

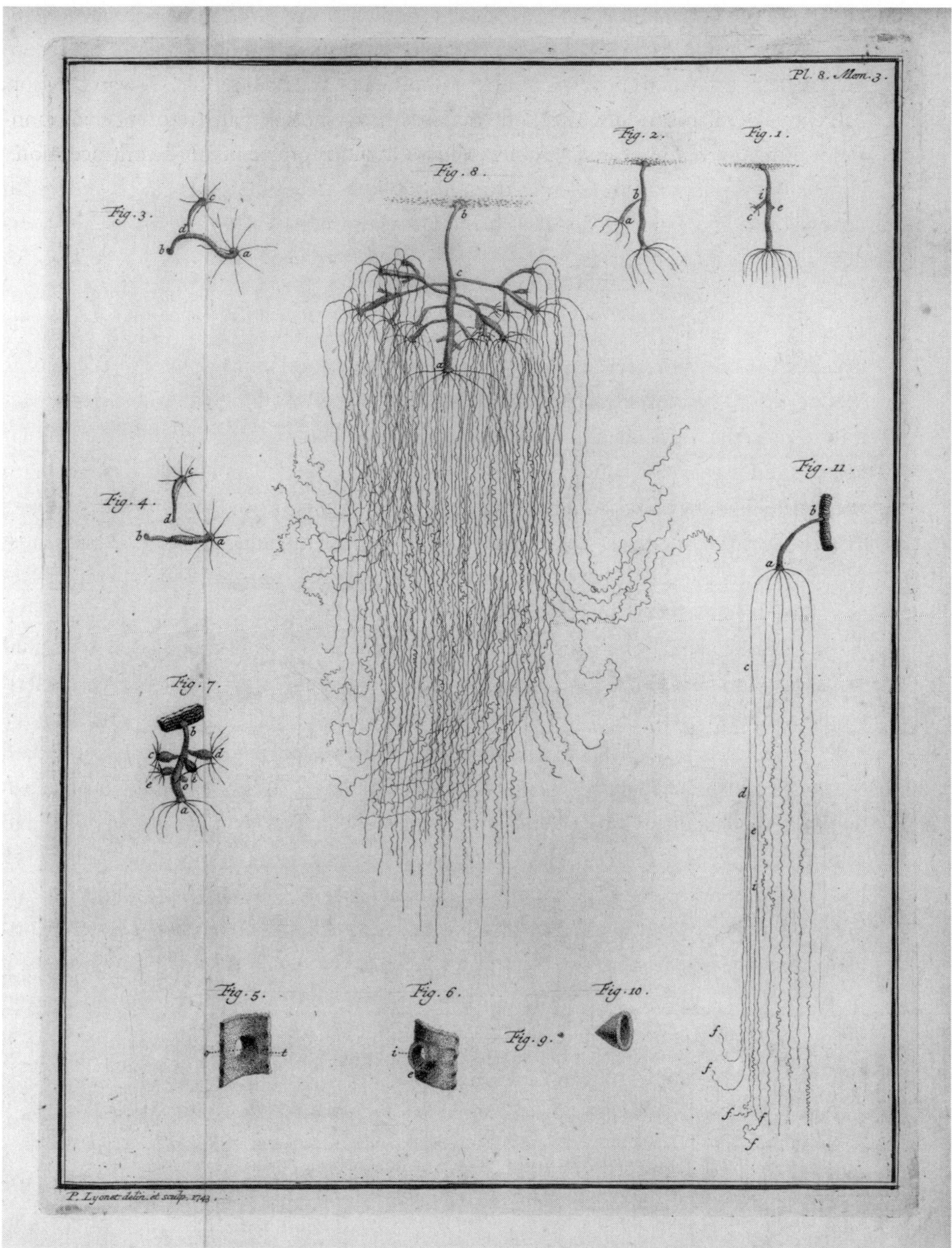

Figure 26.1 Abraham Trembley's polyp. This plate shows 'generation', that is, the 'natural manner in which these animals multiply' by the plant-like growth of 'offshoots'. Other plates illustrate what Trembley called the 'reproduction' of individuals from experimentally isolated parts; vignettes depict the tutor with his pupils (see illustration on p. 280, this book). Trembley, *Mémoires, pour servir à l'histoire d'un genre de polypes d'eau douce* … (Leiden: Verbeek, 1744), plate 8. 22 × 16 cm. Whipple Library, University of Cambridge.

polyp resembled an animal less than a carrot or an asparagus did'.[5] The polyp's ambiguity opened a range of possibilities for understanding how new living beings came into existence.

As central institutions of enlightened discussion, salons revolutionized the significance of the polyps, just as happened earlier with Lucretian atomism and Cartesian mechanical philosophy. Trembley saw himself as a man of knowledge engaged in detailed observations and experiments; the salon elite, by contrast, used the creatures to pose questions about life, matter, sex and the soul. As the Parisian salonnière Madame Geoffrin told the president of the Royal Society of London, at her gatherings the topic was exciting even more attention among 'the ignorant' than the learned.[6] Over the following decades, various books and pamphlets – notably the natural philosopher Pierre Louis de Maupertuis's *Vénus physique* (Physical Venus, 1745) – exploited the polyp's bizarre behaviour to raise the wider issues. These works placed the polyp alongside other wonders involving generation (including an albino African child and the apparently virgin birth of aphids), facilitating conversation and bridging science, fiction and libertine philosophy.[7] The celebrated erotic novel *Thérèse philosophe* (Thérèse the philosopher, 1748) declared, 'Voluptuousness and philosophy produce the happiness of the sensible man. He embraces voluptuousness by taste. He loves philosophy by reason' (Fig. 26.2).

The most widely read account of origins to emerge from these salon conversations was in the *Histoire naturelle* (1749) by the French naturalist Georges-Louis Leclerc, Comte de Buffon. Any theory of the coming into being of new forms, this work argued, had to be as clear as Newtonian explanations for astronomy and cover everything from the genesis of the earth to the sexual union of birds. Towards this end, the crucial chapter posited elementary forms of an organic matter that was 'ever active, ever ready to mould itself, to be assimilated, and to produce beings similar to those that receive it'.[8] Irreducible to brute physical matter, these primal living molecules were subject to the 'internal mould' of the organism. This guaranteed 'reproduction', ensuring the continuity of living beings.

Buffon's work, often identified by historians as a milestone in the transformation of more general theories of generation to a specific focus on reproduction,[9] targeted the

5 Quoted in Jacques Roger, *The Life Sciences in Eighteenth-Century French Thought*, ed. Keith R. Benson, trans. Robert Ellrich (Stanford, CA, 1997), p. 158; also Susannah Gibson, *Animal, Vegetable, or Mineral? How Eighteenth-Century Science Disrupted the Natural Order* (Oxford, 2015).

6 Quoted in Harcourt Brown, 'Madame Geoffrin and Martin Folkes: Six new letters', *Modern Language Quarterly* 1 (1940), 215–41, on 226.

7 Terrall, 'Salon, academy, and boudoir'; Robert Darnton, *The Forbidden Best-Sellers of Pre-Revolutionary France* (New York, NY, 1995); Renato G. Mazzolini, 'Colonialism and the Emergence of Racial Theories', Chapter 25, this book (Fig. 25.1 portrays the child).

8 Quoted in Roger, *Life Sciences*, p. 450.

9 Nick Hopwood, 'The Keywords "Generation" and "Reproduction"', Chapter 20, this book.

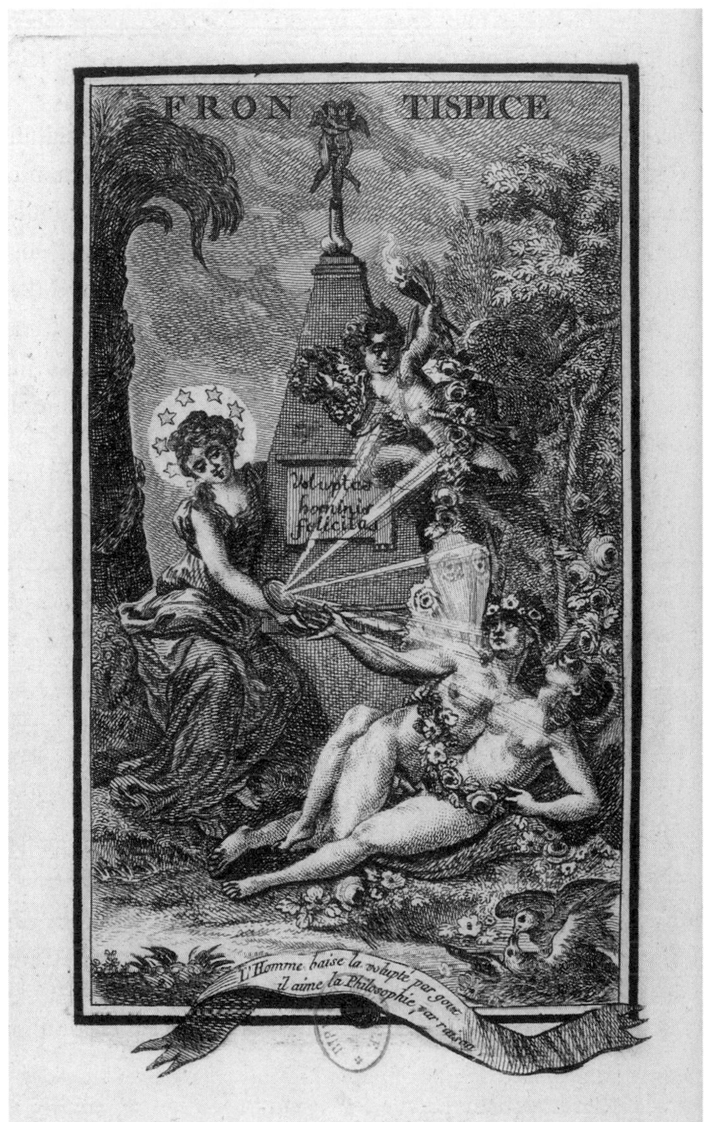
FRON TISPICE
Voluptas
hominis
felicitas
L'Homme baise la volupté par gout
il aime la Philosophie par raison

Figure 26.2 The goddess of Reason enlightens the coupling of Mars and Venus, while Cupid brings to their embrace the fire of passion. Frontispiece to a mid-eighteenth-century edition of *Thérèse philosophe*, usually attributed to Jean-Baptiste de Boyer Argens. From *Thérèse philosophe, ou Mémoires pour servir à l'histoire du P. Dirrag et de mademoiselle Eradice* (n. p., n. d.), Bibliothèque nationale de France, Réserve des livres rares, Enfer-404.

salon elite. Readers were led to appreciate geometrical rigour and naturalists' obsessive attention to observation; but the theory attempted to block the use of such findings in support of materialism, particularly by avoiding spontaneous generation from non-living matter. Although few accepted Buffon's ideas, his volumes became a Europe-wide bestseller.[10] The salons had thus framed naturalists' surprising findings in a sexualized, sublime account of the origins of all things. Buffon was frequently discussed in Britain,

10 Roger, *Life Sciences*, p. 426; Mary Terrall, 'A Microscopical Salon', Exhibit 20, this book.

where the poet Oliver Goldsmith found that French writers tilted too far towards speculation, as in the positing of active matter and 'organic molecules'. He worried less about atheism (a doctrine with few British followers), and more about imaginative excess and over-excitement of the passions.[11]

By the late eighteenth century, concerns about the dangers of active matter were becoming more dominant, especially in Britain, as is evident in responses to the Lichfield physician Erasmus Darwin's posthumous *Temple of Nature* of 1803. This long poem, an encomium to nature's fecundity, argued that organic particles explained the generation of life from matter, as well as providing a mechanism for understanding how the polyp's mutilated fragments could contain the possibility of reproducing the whole.[12] Organic matter was presented as linking processes of generation, the origins of disease and the wider laws governing the formation of the universe. As Darwin put it:

> Ere Time began, from flaming Chaos hurl'd
> Rose the bright spheres, which form the circling world;
> Earths from each sun with quick explosions burst,
> And second planets issued from the first.
> Then, whilst the sea at their coeval birth,
> Surge over surge, involv'd the shoreless earth;
> Nurs'd by warm sun-beams in primeval caves
> Organic Life began beneath the waves.[13]

Darwin's earlier writings, especially the *Botanic Garden*, had been designed to stimulate fashionable repartee, combining scientific discoveries and speculations in erotic verse. The *Temple of Nature* addressed the same audience only a few years later, but flopped. Theories that denied the limits between life and matter were tarred as 'materialism'. Darwin's works were out of favour, victims of the conservative climate after the French Revolution. Readers were told to avoid the *Temple of Nature* as morally tainted. The poem, as the *Monthly Review* noted, was 'in no way adapted to improve either the judgment or the morals of his readers'. Most damningly, it was silly: 'we feel a difficulty in determining whether we ought to be angry, or to laugh'.[14]

11 Oliver Goldsmith, 'Of the generation of animals', in *An History of the Earth and Animated Nature*, vol. 2 (London, 1774), pp. 15–51; Jeff Loveland, 'Georges-Louis Leclerc de Buffon's *Histoire naturelle* in English, 1775–1815', *Archives of Natural History* 31 (2004), 214–35.

12 Erasmus Darwin, *The Temple of Nature; Or, the Origin of Society: A Poem, with Philosophical Notes* (London, 1803), 'Additional notes', pp. 1–11.

13 Ibid., canto I, lines 227–34, pp. 19–20.

14 'Darwin's *Temple of Nature; a Poem*', *Monthly Review* 43 (1804), 113–27, on 124 and 123; Norton Garfinkle, 'Science and religion in England, 1790–1800: The critical response to the work of Erasmus Darwin', *Journal of the History of Ideas* 16 (1955), 376–88.

Politics of Generation

In the decades after the French Revolution, conversation about the generation of individuals, species and the cosmos became increasingly politicized. Unlike Erasmus Darwin's poetic celebrations of sex and generation, technical terminology dominated the subject. From the 1820s, findings tended to be presented in medical journals, anatomical lecture theatres and scientific academies: a specialist domain akin to those that had emerged at the end of the eighteenth century in and around the French professional schools and German universities. Conversation about generation was centred in the masculine world of medicine, particularly London's medical schools. Booksellers' shops, notably that belonging to the publisher John Churchill, were hotbeds of discussion about the emerging genre of specialist books, such as Professor Friedrich Tiedemann's *Systematic Treatise on Comparative Physiology*, a work advocating serial transformism that was translated from the German in 1834. The *Lancet*, a crusading medical weekly, included instalments of works by Étienne Serres, Henri Blainville, Étienne Geoffroy Saint-Hilaire and other French authors on animal morphology. Geoffroy, for example, experimented on embryological monstrosities to explore arrested development; he elaborated a theory of the 'unity of type' that allowed correlations across very different animal groups.[15] In France, these doctrines attracted considerable discussion and support. Geoffroy's transcendental anatomy was the subject of a widely reported public dispute at the Paris Academy of Sciences with the comparative anatomist Georges Cuvier, who denied that such correlations could be made. As the poet Johann Wolfgang von Goethe asked a friend after reading of the debate in a German newspaper, 'Now … what do you think of this great event? The volcano has come to an eruption; everything is in flames, and we no longer have a transaction behind closed doors!'[16] But interest in such matters was becoming unusual: even Goethe's friend thought he was talking about the fall of Charles X from the French throne after the July 1830 revolution.

In Britain, medical men, ultra-radicals and commercial journalists dominated the discussion. Reproductive knowledge was deemed too esoteric for mainstream working-class politics, and attempts to use it there generally failed. Instead, it was free-thinking socialists such as Emma Martin who argued that embryological evidence suggested a material origin for humanity. If humans developed from apes, there was no need for a god. Her lectures, targeted at working and middle-class women, developed the consequences of a materialist philosophy for understanding fetal development, pregnancy and abortion. Like her predecessor Mary Wollstonecraft (who in arguing for women's

15 Adrian Desmond, *The Politics of Evolution: Morphology, Medicine, and Reform in Radical London* (Chicago, IL, 1989).

16 Quoted in Toby A. Appel, *The Cuvier–Geoffroy Debate: French Biology in the Decades before Darwin* (New York, NY, 1987), p. 1.

rights denied any connection between matter and the higher qualities of mind), Martin was condemned for encouraging promiscuity.[17]

Despite this hijacking by radicals, the subject could still be presented to ordinary readers without challenging accepted norms of decency. Such attempts were now identified as 'popular', 'elementary' or 'familiar', with the implication that they had been neutered for a non-expert readership. A key title was the young medical writer Perceval Lord's *Popular Physiology* (1834), published by the Society for Promoting Christian Knowledge. The *British and Foreign Medical Review* praised the book as an inoffensive introduction:

> The great point *here* is to illustrate processes which every child knows to take place, without referring to those which, it is universally agreed, should be kept in the back-ground. What possible evil, we will ask, can result from tracing the development of the chick during incubation, and from showing the curious correspondence between the different stages of the evolution of its organs, and the permanent forms of the same in the lower animals? … or in explaining the process of reproduction in sponges and polypes?

Better to teach such subjects (replacing offensive terms such as 'male and female organs' with their technical equivalents), than to allow readers to linger on 'the undisguised exhibition, in glowing colours, of the passion of love and its effects'. In dry, unemotive language, *Popular Physiology* could present the latest theories, so that even susceptible young women could appreciate Geoffroy, Serres and others. Much better this than French novels, continental philosophy or the poems of Erasmus Darwin.[18]

The delicate position of generation on the margins of respectability is further illustrated by another standard text, the Scottish physician Neil Arnott's *Elements of Physics, or Natural Philosophy, General and Medical* (1829). Here the purchaser had two options for binding. The details of human development and reproductive anatomy, dealt with in the final pages, could be left in; or removed, leaving the book to conclude with an anodyne paean to the creator.

Such gestures were accepted as ways of reconciling embryonic development with divine foresight, but formulating general explanations for the material origin of new species and of the cosmos remained anathema to all but a few. To the end of his life, Charles Darwin remembered his shock as a young man when his teacher Robert Edmond Grant 'burst forth in high admiration' of the transmutation theory of the French

17 James A. Secord, *Victorian Sensation: The Extraordinary Publication, Reception, and Secret Authorship of* Vestiges of the Natural History of Creation (Chicago, IL, 2000), pp. 314–19.

18 'Aitkin, Lord and Hayward on popular physiology', *British and Foreign Medical Review* 7 (1839), 214–17, on 215; further: Kate Fisher, 'Modern Ignorance', Chapter 32, this book.

naturalist Jean-Baptiste Lamarck: 'I listened in silent astonishment'.[19] Darwin's reaction was typical; to engage in such loose speculation about origins, as he later joked to a friend, was 'like confessing a murder'.[20] Even at the most liberal London salon, only after 'the ladies' left the dinner table was the topic broached, with Lord Holland commenting in 1837 that knowledge of the creation of man had not advanced beyond Lucretius.[21] In polite circles, developmental theories, associated with sex, belonged with port and cigars.

Universal Gestation of Nature

A few months after Lord Holland's party, Darwin, living in a bachelor flat in London and preparing his *Beagle* voyage publications, began a clandestine inquiry into generation. Kept in notebooks marked 'private', this initially culminated in a theory in which higher forms emerged through environmental effects on developing embryos. Darwin was committed to explaining all natural phenomena, from the origins of the earth to human thought, as the products of the laws of matter, and his notebooks reveal that he knew where this could lead: 'love of the deity effect of organization. oh you materialist!'[22]

Writing in *Man, in His Physical Structure and Adaptations* (1838), the working-class author and editor Robert Mudie condemned the '*doctrine of developments*' that would create a complete progression from primordial matter, through the nebular system of the origins of the universe, to organic life and human mind. Like readers of Erasmus Darwin's poems, Mudie believed laughter the only response:

> Well, an indefinite number of developments – whirlings – bring us to the sheep, and the sheep eat turnips; a few more develop the dog, and he eats mutton; a few more still develop Man, and he eats both the mutton and the turnips. How many more whirlings may be necessary in order to develop a philosopher capable of inventing or appreciating this theory, we pretend not to know … But in reality it is no laughing matter; for it is from beginning to end the doctrine of materialism in its most malignant and inveterate form …[23]

19 Charles Darwin, 'Recollections of the development of my mind and character', in Darwin, *Evolutionary Writings*, ed. James A. Secord (Oxford, 2008), pp. 355–425, on p. 371.

20 Charles Darwin to Joseph Dalton Hooker, [11 Jan. 1844], in *The Correspondence of Charles Darwin*, vol. 3, ed. Frederick Burkhardt *et al.* (Cambridge, 1987), p. 2.

21 Charles Lyell to Sophia Lyell, 19 Mar. 1837, in *Life, Letters and Journals of Sir Charles Lyell, Bart.*, ed. [Katharine M.] Lyell, vol. 2 (London, 1881), pp. 8–9.

22 Charles Darwin, notebook entry C166, in *Charles Darwin's Notebooks, 1836–1844: Geology, Transmutation of Species, Metaphysical Enquiries*, ed. Paul H. Barrett *et al.* (Cambridge, 1987), p. 291; M. J. S. Hodge, 'Darwin as a lifelong generation theorist', in David Kohn (ed.), *The Darwinian Heritage* (Princeton, NJ, 1985), pp. 207–43.

23 Robert Mudie, *Man, in His Physical Structure and Adaptations* (London, 1838), p. 251.

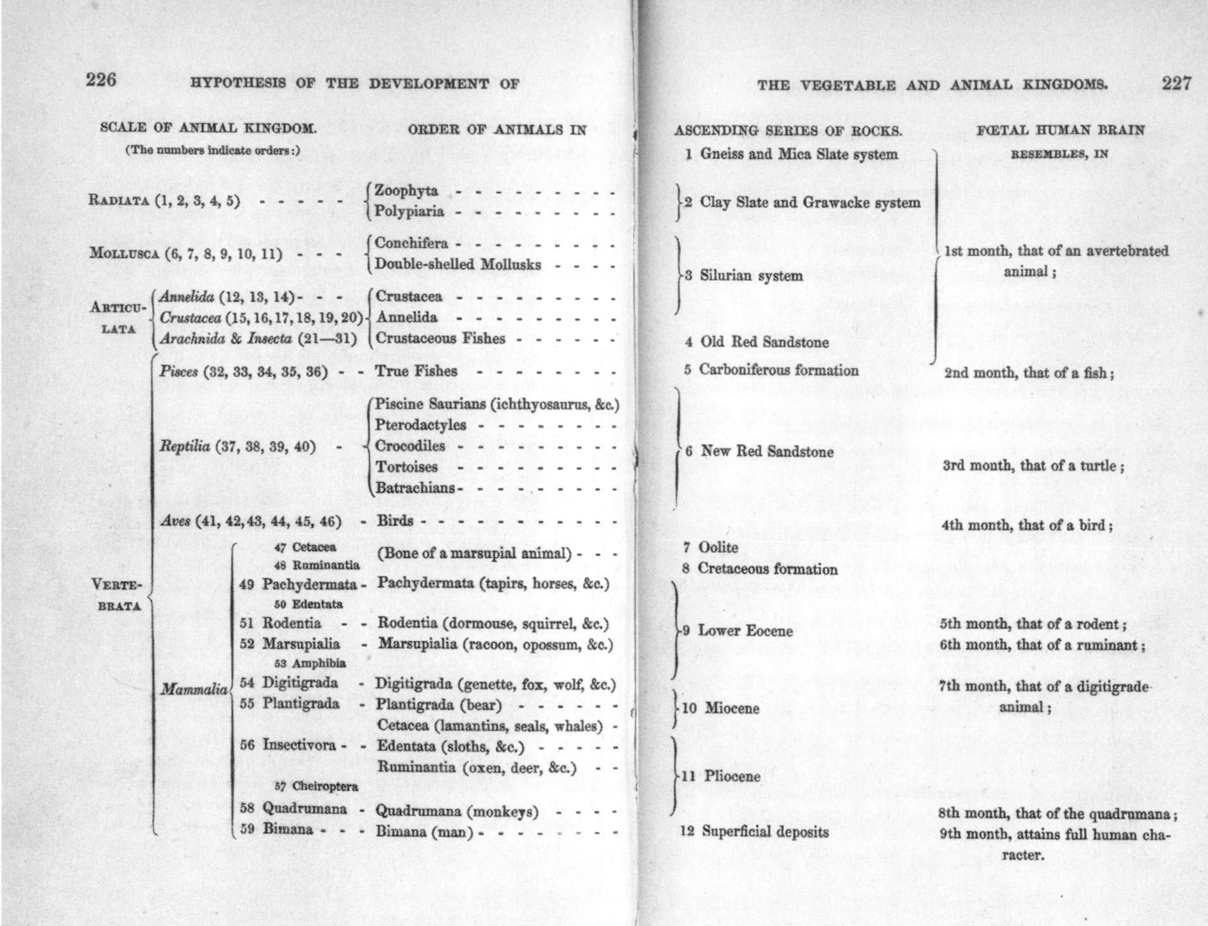

226 HYPOTHESIS OF THE DEVELOPMENT OF | THE VEGETABLE AND ANIMAL KINGDOMS. 227

SCALE OF ANIMAL KINGDOM. (The numbers indicate orders:)		ORDER OF ANIMALS IN	ASCENDING SERIES OF ROCKS.	FŒTAL HUMAN BRAIN RESEMBLES, IN
RADIATA (1, 2, 3, 4, 5)		Zoophyta Polypiaria	1 Gneiss and Mica Slate system 2 Clay Slate and Grawacke system	
MOLLUSCA (6, 7, 8, 9, 10, 11)		Conchifera Double-shelled Mollusks	3 Silurian system	1st month, that of an avertebrated animal;
ARTICULATA	*Annelida* (12, 13, 14) *Crustacea* (15, 16, 17, 18, 19, 20) *Arachnida & Insecta* (21—31)	Crustacea Annelida Crustaceous Fishes	4 Old Red Sandstone	
VERTEBRATA	*Pisces* (32, 33, 34, 35, 36)	True Fishes	5 Carboniferous formation	2nd month, that of a fish;
	Reptilia (37, 38, 39, 40)	Piscine Saurians (ichthyosaurus, &c.) Pterodactyles Crocodiles Tortoises Batrachians	6 New Red Sandstone	3rd month, that of a turtle;
	Aves (41, 42, 43, 44, 45, 46)	Birds		4th month, that of a bird;
	Mammalia: 47 Cetacea 48 Ruminantia	(Bone of a marsupial animal)	7 Oolite	
	49 Pachydermata	Pachydermata (tapirs, horses, &c.)	8 Cretaceous formation	
	50 Edentata 51 Rodentia	Rodentia (dormouse, squirrel, &c.)	9 Lower Eocene	5th month, that of a rodent;
	52 Marsupialia	Marsupialia (racoon, opossum, &c.)		6th month, that of a ruminant;
	53 Amphibia 54 Digitigrada	Digitigrada (genette, fox, wolf, &c.)	10 Miocene	7th month, that of a digitigrade animal;
	55 Plantigrada	Plantigrada (bear) Cetacea (lamantins, seals, whales)		
	56 Insectivora	Edentata (sloths, &c.) Ruminantia (oxen, deer, &c.)	11 Pliocene	
	57 Cheiroptera 58 Quadrumana	Quadrumana (monkeys)		8th month, that of the quadrumana;
	59 Bimana	Bimana (man)	12 Superficial deposits	9th month, attains full human character.

Figure 26.3 The threefold parallel of gestation between the 'scale of animal kingdom', the 'order of animals in ascending series of rocks' and the 'foetal human brain'. [Robert Chambers], *Vestiges of the Natural History of Creation* (London: Churchill, 1844), pp. 226–7. 18 × 23 cm. Cambridge University Library.

A commercial writer, Mudie knew that such ideas were rife in the urban underworld, even if no book had brought them together in an accessible, up-to-date way.

The anonymous *Vestiges of the Natural History of Creation*, published by Churchill in 1844, did just this. Beginning with a blazing fire mist and ending with the destiny of the human race, *Vestiges* combined the progressive narratives of the new sciences of nebular astronomy, geology, physiology and phrenology (Fig. 26.3). Uniting them was a vision in which lower forms gave birth to higher, so that stars, strata, living beings and the human mind were products of a single developmental sequence. Mudie's mock system had been based on digestion; this one was grounded in reproduction, although the term itself was used interchangeably with 'generation'. The moulding of individuals through a repeatable law-like process, which had come to dominate discussion of the origin of living beings, was now applied to the entire physical world. The resemblance between the planets was perceived to be 'a true *family likeness*'.[24] The *Vestiges* author hailed this as 'the universal gestation of Nature'.[25]

Vestiges was fiercely attacked, especially for failings in its treatment of specialist science. In the interests of simplicity, it fudged the distinction between the two main models of embryological development, both imported from continental Europe, where they were better known. In the one, the embryo passed through the stages of a fish, reptile, bird and mammal; in the other, the development process involved differentiation from a general form. The book also included controversial facts, not least the spontaneous generation of mites through galvanic action. All this constituted an assault on the hardening boundaries between specialist and popular publication. *Vestiges* contended for the divine direction of the laws of nature, but also challenged the long-standing, uneasy compromise between science and theology.

Throughout the English-speaking world, controversy over *Vestiges* reopened discussion of the development of the individual, species and cosmos. It moved debate about transmutation based on a reproductive model into respectable drawing rooms and homes, attracting readers from Queen Victoria to the young lawyer Abraham Lincoln. The Edinburgh journalist Robert Chambers, later revealed as the author, skilfully deployed his understanding of the middle-class public to ease the reception. 'The production of a new species', the book noted, 'has never been anything more than a new stage of progress in gestation, an event as simply natural, and attended as little by any circumstances of a wonderful or startling kind, as the silent advance of an ordinary mother from one week to another of her pregnancy.'[26] This strategy was successful: when the Cambridge professor of geology accused *Vestiges* of peddling a 'filthy' doctrine, his attitude was seen as old-fashioned, even monkish.[27]

The controversy over Darwin's *On the Origin of Species* fifteen years later struck a different tone. Much of the change had to do with the growing status of science in national life. The 'development question' had become one of the dwindling range of topics that bridged polite conversation and what was increasingly seen as scientific 'shop talk'. *Origin* was accessible enough to attract the general public but too serious to be

24 [Robert Chambers], *Vestiges of the Natural History of Creation* (London, 1844), pp. 11–12, quoting John Herschel.

25 [Robert Chambers], *Explanations: A Sequel to 'Vestiges of the Natural History of Creation'* (London, 1845); M. J. S. Hodge, 'The universal gestation of nature: Chambers' *Vestiges* and *Explanations*', *Journal of the History of Biology* 5 (1972), 127–51.

26 [Chambers], *Vestiges*, p. 223; Secord, *Victorian Sensation*.

27 Secord, *Victorian Sensation*, pp. 246–7.

labelled as sensationalist.[28] Darwin possessed impeccable credentials to write on this delicate subject, as a respectable family man with monographs on geology and zoology to his credit. Even those who execrated *Origin* recognized the author's moral authority. Most readers – even such devoted proponents as the comparative anatomist Thomas Henry Huxley – rejected Darwin's mechanism of natural selection. But almost everyone acknowledged the changed tenor of debate. As the novelist George Eliot said, 'it will have a great effect in the scientific world, causing a thorough and open discussion of a question about which people have hitherto felt timid'.[29]

With relative economic prosperity and the triumph of political liberalism, the dangers of revolutionary materialism seemed distant. *Origin* could be viewed as less ambitious than previous syntheses, with the cosmological issues pushed into the final sentence and almost nothing about humans. In stressing natural selection, the work downplayed the developmental series that had been central to many previous transmutation theories, and moved towards a Malthusian understanding of populations. Death and dearth explained the origin of new forms: the unfit were less likely to be successful in the struggle for existence, and hence less likely to reproduce. Patterns of gestation became consequences of the theory, issues to explain rather than the basis of explanation. 'Embryology' was a section in the penultimate chapter, and although Darwin claimed it as his 'pet bit' (much of it was based on his researches into the bizarre sexual life of barnacles), few readers paid it much attention. Yet Darwin maintained a lifelong commitment to explaining everything (from budding in plants and polypes to the sexual crossing of orchids and human beings) through a single unifying theory of reproduction. The embryological series provided evidence for the source of variations and mechanisms of heredity, and suggested that an understanding of varieties and species could be extended to the entire living world.[30]

The tactical need to downplay sex and implications for humans in *Origin* can be seen in the lengths to which the emerging 'Darwinian' party went to avoid impropriety. Huxley had to remove references to '*emasculate* monks' and 'Uncircumcised Judaizers' from *Man's Place in Nature* before its publication in 1863.[31] Only after victory seemed secure did Darwin tackle human evolution in *The Descent of Man, and Selection in Relation to Sex* (1871), although his publisher still forced a change of title to avoid the

28 James A. Secord, 'How scientific conversation became shop talk', in Aileen Fyfe and Bernard Lightman (eds.), *Science in the Marketplace: Nineteenth-Century Sites and Experiences* (Chicago, IL, 2007), pp. 23–59.

29 Quoted in Secord, *Victorian Sensation*, p. 513.

30 Lynn K. Nyhart, 'Embryology and morphology', in Michael Ruse and Robert J. Richards (eds.), *The Cambridge Companion to the 'Origin of Species'* (Cambridge, 2009), pp. 194–215.

31 Dawson, *Darwin*, p. 11. This paragraph is based on Dawson's book and Jane Munro, '"More like a work of art than of nature": Darwin, beauty and sexual selection', in Diana Donald and Munro (eds.), *Endless Forms: Charles Darwin, Natural Science and the Visual Arts* (New Haven, CT, 2009), pp. 253–91.

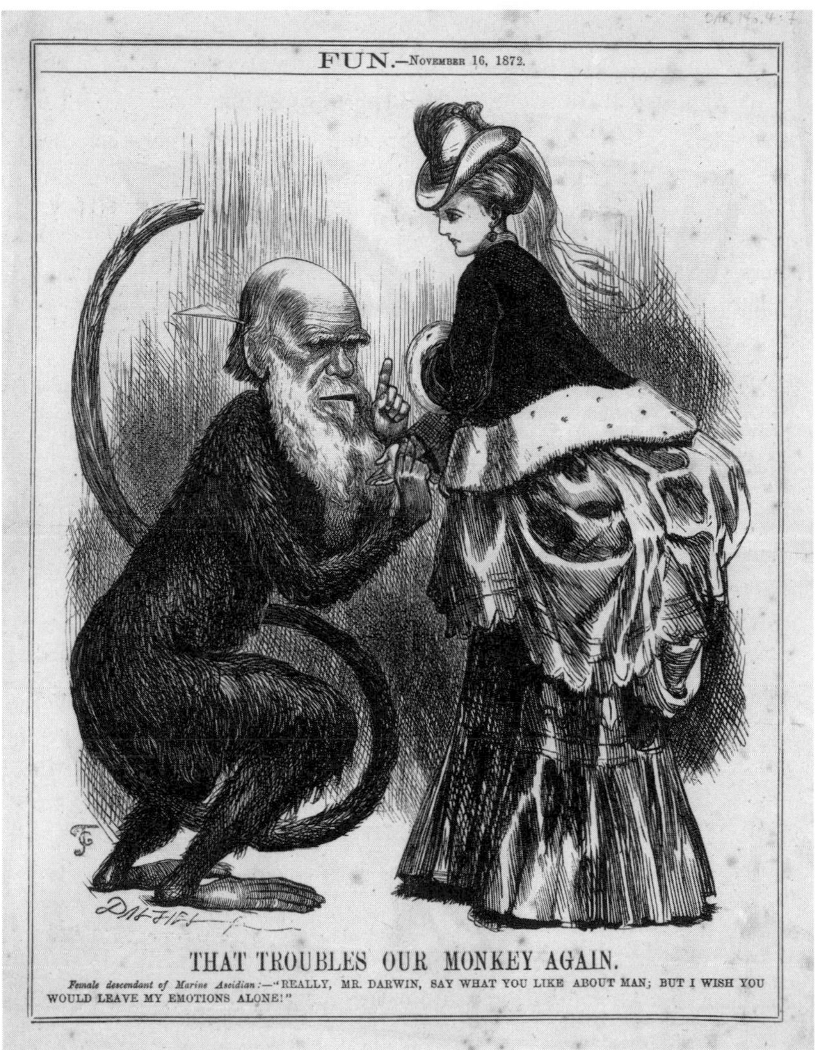
FUN.—November 16, 1872.
THAT TROUBLES OUR MONKEY AGAIN.
Female descendant of Marine Ascidian:—"REALLY, MR. DARWIN, SAY WHAT YOU LIKE ABOUT MAN; BUT I WISH YOU WOULD LEAVE MY EMOTIONS ALONE!"

Figure 26.4 'That troubles our monkey again.' Charles Darwin, with erect tail, as a perverse observer of female sexuality, in a cartoon in the comic weekly *Fun* 16, n. s. (Nov. 1872), 203. Cambridge University Library.

offending term 'sexual'.[32] The reception of *Descent* showed just how explosive combining reproduction and evolution could be (Fig. 26.4). As the *Edinburgh Review* lamented:

> ... we do him no injustice in ascribing to him the theory of Lucretius – that Venus is the creative power of the world, and that the mysterious law of reproduction, with the passions which belong to it, is the dominant force of life. He appears to

32 John Murray to Charles Darwin, 1 July 1870, in *The Correspondence of Charles Darwin*, vol. 18, ed. Frederick Burkhardt *et al.* (Cambridge, 2010), p. 194.

> see nothing beyond or above it. In a heathen poet such doctrines appear gross and degrading, if not vicious. We know not how to characterise them in an English naturalist, well known for the purity and elevation of his own life and character.[33]

Approval was tempered by distress at the moral implications of a science based on material causes: for some this verged on pornography, an analogue in science of the 'fleshly school' of avant-garde poetry and the explicit images of rape and bestiality by the Belgian artist Félicien Rops, to whom Darwin was sometimes compared. More fundamentally, close observation of exotic forms of reproduction could be seen not as a virtue, but as akin to obsessive perversion.[34]

For all these pitfalls, those in Britain eager to raise the status of science and make it a paid career welcomed the reductionist power of evolution. The new science of 'biology' – a word that came into regular use only in the late nineteenth century – encouraged the study of life from the perspective of laboratory practice, uniting form and function through a stress on development and physico-chemical explanation.[35] Biology took shape through debates about school and laboratory education as 'a publicist science *par excellence*',[36] and the term became common among those who campaigned to put science at the heart of British public life, especially in relation to eugenics. The practical and philosophical campaigns for biology, always closely related, came together in the 1880s, as evolution on a developmental model emerged as the coping stone of the new discipline and an accompanying order of population control.

Towards a New History

Circulation between genres and audiences offers potential for understanding the gradual replacement of 'generation' with 'reproduction', involving repeatable processes of heredity, procreation and development in relation to general cosmological questions. Readings of Buffon, Erasmus Darwin and other Enlightenment writers were embedded in the matrix of salon conversation and libertine free-thought. During the nineteenth century, interactions between various authors, readers and publics continued to define the meanings of reproduction; even as its study became more specialized,

33 [W. Boyd Dawkins], 'Darwin on the descent of man', *Edinburgh Review* 134 (1871), 195–235, on 234–5.

34 Nicholas Thomas, 'Licensed curiosity: Cook's Pacific voyages', in John Elsner and Roger Cardinal (eds.), *The Cultures of Collecting* (London, 1994), pp. 116–36.

35 On public discussion of laboratory science: James A. Secord, 'Spontaneous Generation and the Triumph of Experiment', Exhibit 26, this book.

36 Joseph Caron, '"Biology" in the life sciences: A historiographical contribution', *History of Science* 26 (1988), 223–68, on 253.

laboratory-based and 'biological', reproduction still provided a model for understanding origins of all kinds, from the universe to the human mind.

By 1900, narratives of evolution based on embryonic development had gained acceptance in liberal circles in urban centres across the globe as foundations for economic and imperial progress. Reproduction was central to the evolutionary models that jostled for attention. Evolution could be given a spiritual gloss, as in Henry Drummond's uplifting Protestant reading, *The Ascent of Man* (1894). It could be developed in cosmic syntheses, such as Ernst Haeckel's *The Riddle of the Universe* (1900), or in fictions about the future, including H. G. Wells's *The Time Machine* (1895). It became a 'guiding principle' in textbooks for aspiring biologists.[37]

Yet the dark undercurrent in evolutionary discussion remained, for these accounts allowed readers to contemplate science-based fantasies of eugenic cleansing, sexual miscegenation and the 'beast within'. Narratives based on reproduction continued in dialogue with controversies about sexual propriety, racial identity, the roles of women and the limits of decency. As *Thérèse philosophe* had noted long before, and as critics continued to point out, reason had its peculiar pleasures: philosophy could become pornography, observation could become obsession. The subject of origins continues to straddle boundaries of expertise, genre and morality: this is a story of passion, reason and desire, to be picked up in conversations through the present time.

37 R. J. Harvey Gibson, *A Textbook of Elementary Biology* (London, 1889), p. 353; Bernard Lightman, *Victorian Popularizers of Science: Designing Nature for New Audiences* (Chicago, IL, 2007), pp. 219–94; Daniel Pick, *Faces of Degeneration: A European Disorder,* c. *1848–1918* (Cambridge, 1989).

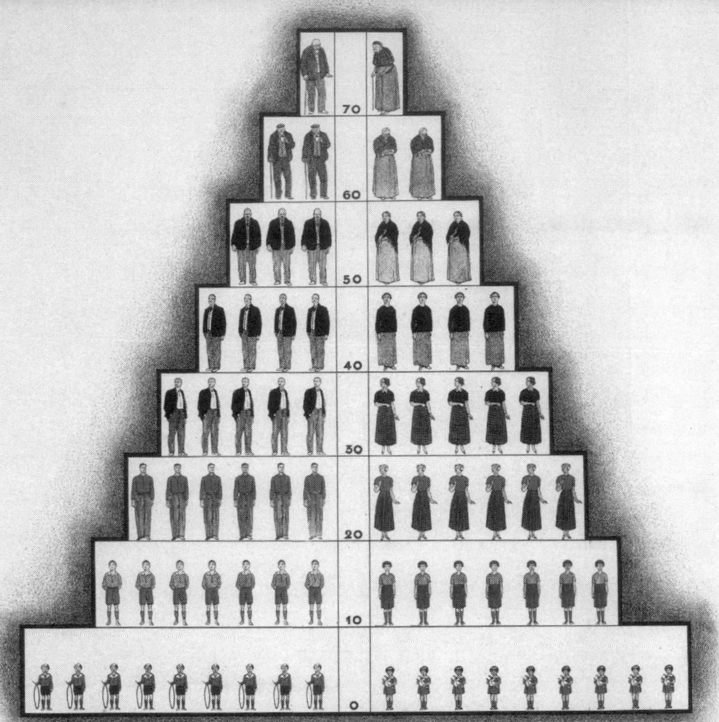

APRÈS UN SIÈCLE
DE FÉCONDITÉ NORMALE

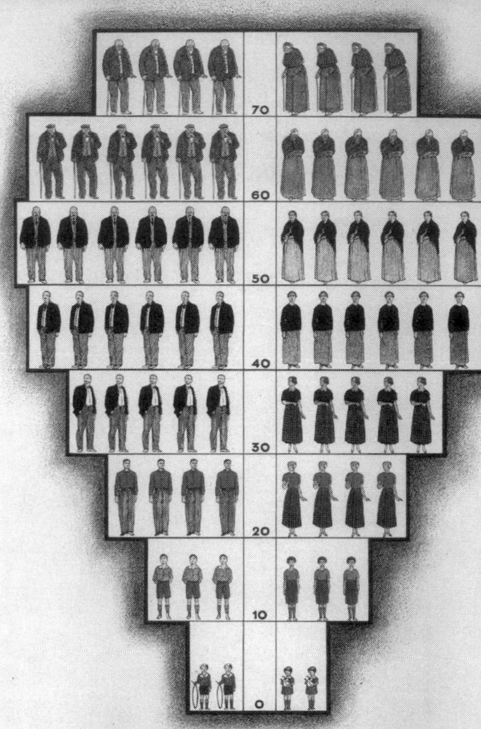

APRÈS UN SIÈCLE
DE FÉCONDITÉ INSUFFISANTE

RÉPARTITION DE LA POPULATION ENTRE LES DIFFÉRENTS GROUPES D'AGES

Il faut au moins, et en moyenne, 3 enfants par ménage
pour qu'un pays puisse vivre

ADHÉREZ A L'ALLIANCE NATIONALE
POUR L'ACCROISSEMENT DE LA POPULATION FRANÇAISE
217, Rue du Faubourg Saint Honoré_PARIS

IMP. LOUVION, PÉQUEREAU

Part IV

Modern Reproduction

'Distribution of the population between the different age groups', a poster produced in 1930 by the National Alliance for the Growth of the French Population. Channelling alarm about the declining birth-rate as a threat to national power, this pronatalist organization propagandized with images of fear and hope. On the left, the distribution 'after a century of normal fecundity'; on the right, the spectre, 'after a century of insufficient fecundity', of the country ageing and eventually dying out – a concern still present, in different contexts but related diagrams, today. 59 × 79 cm. Archives départementales de Seine-Maritime 63 Fi 148.

In the age of capital and empire between 1848 and 1939, the new framework – 'reproduction' as distinct from 'generation' – became influential against a background of huge demographic change. By 1901 many intellectuals agreed with the science-fiction writer H. G. Wells that 'the main mass of the business of human life centres about reproduction'. He was more isolated in his view that 'perhaps half the population of the world, in every generation, should be restrained from or tempted to evade reproduction', but even this was discussed. As European birth-rates fell, nation-states competed to raise the largest populations of the fittest race and worried about depopulation in their colonial possessions. Modern party politics was invented and feminist movements were founded. The Russian Revolution created a socialist alternative, temporarily including formal equality for women and legal abortion, while fascists grounded nationalism in fantasies of race. Procreation was contested across the globe, but on one thing the combatants agreed: the way a society organized reproduction was essential to making it modern. Part IV takes a fresh look at what that meant.

The major demographic facts of modern history, the large fertility declines in those industrializing nations that experienced rapid, urbanizing economic growth, were apparent to contemporaries by the late nineteenth century. (Mortality began to decline earlier, and fertility in France had been falling since the eighteenth century.) The neo-Malthusians can take some credit; those radicals sought to increase happiness and avoid Malthus's gloomy predictions by advocating what he had rejected as 'improper arts'. Termed 'contraception' from the late nineteenth century, in the early twentieth the American campaigner Margaret Sanger called it 'birth control'. Among social movements that worked to separate sex from reproduction – others defended homosexuality – the neo-Malthusians did much to spread knowledge of the possibilities, but had a less direct role in reducing fertility (Lesley A. Hall, 'Movements to Separate Sex and Reproduction', Chapter 29). Keeping their families smaller, couples now sustained a lively trade in contraceptive devices, but most did not choose the female barrier methods, the cervical caps and diaphragms, that the birth controllers preferred. The market was bigger for condoms, which also protected against the sexually transmitted infections that contributed measurably though modestly to the fertility decline, but abstinence and withdrawal were used even more, and abortion was probably widespread (Simon Szreter, 'Fertility Transitions and Sexually Transmitted Infections', Chapter 30; James M. Edmonson, 'Condoms', Exhibit 28).

Governments fought this trend. In the names of nation and empire, they passed tougher anti-abortion laws, restricted the advertising and circulation of contraceptives, and favoured larger families. Having led campaigns against abortion, physicians mostly kept their distance even from contraception until after its rebranding in the 1930s as the more respectable-sounding 'family planning' (Martin H. Johnson and Nick Hopwood, 'Modern Law and Regulation', Chapter 40). Pronatalism included measures to combat high rates of infant and especially maternal deaths – that 'deep, dark and continuous stream of mortality' lamented by William Farr of the General Register Office for England and Wales. Delivering babies had become central to general practice, but from the early twentieth century more women began to give birth in hospital, where obstetrics was consolidated at midwives' expense, especially in the United States. Initially, these institutions had worsened outcomes, but maternal mortality declined with the introduction of sulpha drugs in the 1930s. Socialists and feminists pushed governments to set up the first welfare states, and countries and colonies developed measures – by no means all effective – to enhance maternal and infant welfare, while raising the status of motherhood and rendering it more scientific (Siân Pooley, '"Pity the Poor Mother!"', Exhibit 27). Metropolitan concerns shaped imperial policies, and colonies served as testing grounds for practices then adopted at home, but movements for decolonization gathered pace after 1918 (Philippa Levine, 'Imperial Encounters', Chapter 33).

More worrying than plunging numbers were differential declines. Imperialists argued that European nations were committing 'race suicide', while population increase in Asia amounted to a 'yellow peril'. Few accepted the neo-Malthusian claim that there would soon be 'standing room only', but many saw the uneven distribution of people across the globe as putting a dangerous burden on resources, and ultimately the fertility of the soil. To relieve this pressure they variously proposed colonization or conquest, border controls or migration, labour laws or birth control (Alison Bashford, 'World Population from Eugenics to Climate Change', Chapter 34). Darwinism fed concerns about quality and provided a language for discussing the threat of degeneration that so exercised Wells. Evolutionary progress carried hopes for the future, while bad heredity, it seemed, risked dragging humanity backwards. In the early twentieth century, eugenics or racial hygiene, the science of improving the human stock, was institutionalized alongside genetics. Eugenicists wanted to breed the race – the human race and particular races – as rationally as elite farmers bred their beasts (Sarah Wilmot, 'Breeding Farm Animals and Humans', Chapter 27). Eugenics infiltrated diverse politics to varying degrees. Some national movements only inflected an existing discourse, but in the United States eugenic agitation justified race-based immigration restrictions and the sterilization of asylum patients. Under German National Socialism, physicians and geneticists collaborated not only in forced sterilization, but also in euthanasia and genocide, the most murderous biopolitical experiment (Paul Weindling, 'Pedigree of a "Schizophrenic Family"', Exhibit 29).

Laboratory sciences had developed novel approaches to reproduction, with French and German institutes taking the lead in microscopy of cells. Historians have stressed the differences between huge, static egg and tiny, motile sperm as part of an assumption, established around 1800, that the sexes differ fundamentally in kind. Yet the view that fertilization represents the fusion of one egg and one sperm depended also on recognizing similarity and equality; and on this, Florence Vienne argues, consensus was achieved only in the 1870s ('Eggs and Sperm as Germ Cells', Chapter 28). Knowledge of the cellular and biochemical changes through the menstrual cycle came in the 1920s and 1930s and was soon applied in contraception and fertility treatment (Martina Schlünder, 'Menstrual-Cycle Calendars', Exhibit 31). Laboratory experiments identified oestrogen, progesterone and testosterone as sex hormones. Collecting the raw materials (gonads and urine), measuring standard amounts and marketing drugs depended on networks linking gynaecological clinics, physiological and biochemical research laboratories and pharmaceutical industry. These produced pregnancy tests, in the form of bioassays for hormones that were available to doctors from the late 1920s, and biochemicals that they prescribed for a wide range of conditions (Jean-Paul Gaudillière, 'Sex Hormones, Pharmacy and the Reproductive Sciences', Chapter 35; Jesse Olszynko-Gryn, 'Pregnancy Testing with Frogs', Exhibit 32).

The sciences claimed a monopoly on knowledge, but themselves spoke in several voices, even as audiences expanded and diversified and the variety of interpretations grew. Proximity to sex meant that information about reproduction could still be sensitive beyond medical milieux. Rates of schooling and literacy rose, but though sex education of the young was much discussed around 1900, human reproduction entered the school curriculum to any significant extent only in the 1960s. Previously, facts about how to have and not have babies had been more at home in popular anatomy museums and the cheap, steam-printed advice books that improved postal services and door-to-door hawkers took to readerships of unprecedented size. The scale was more original than the content at first; an advice manual compiled from two sixteenth-century books in 1684 enjoyed its biggest sales in the nineteenth century (Mary E. Fissell, '*Aristotle's Masterpiece*', Exhibit 25). But the illustrated press, radio and cinema told the first mass audience about discoveries, too (James A. Secord, 'Spontaneous Generation and the Triumph of Experiment', Exhibit 26). People might occasionally talk about sex and reproduction, but there were many reasons to maintain innocence, or feign it, and many understandings competed within science and beyond. Modern knowledge gained authority from its framing as an antidote to states of ignorance that were also distinctively modern (Kate Fisher, 'Modern Ignorance', Chapter 32).

While contraception and abortion garnered more attention, a few doctors offered, more visibly from the later nineteenth century, to treat infertility. Christina Benninghaus suggests that this represents not the invention of involuntary childlessness as a medical problem, but a new sense, now that science had more to offer, of medical consumption as a solution ('Modern Infertility', Chapter 31). More than has been realized, male sterility was pathologized as well as women's, though medical interventions were generally less invasive in men. Alongside surgery and hormones, artificial insemination gradually began to be used in humans and other animals (Nick Hopwood, 'Artificial Fertilization', Chapter 39). Adoption, criticized as mired in sentiment and tainted by commerce, was remade by a set of science-based matching procedures through which social workers and psychologists administered access to children (Ellen Herman, 'Technologies of Adoption Matching', Exhibit 33).

By the 1930s, reproduction was politically prominent in polarized debates that moved between bodies politic and individual bodies, from rates in populations to difficulties in achieving families of the desired size. Aldous Huxley's novel *Brave New World* (1932), with its Central London Hatchery and 'Malthusian belts', joined Mary Shelley's *Frankenstein* (1818) as an obligatory reference for dreams-turned-nightmares of control. As numbers of Catholics grew, their church completed its formulation of a biopolitical discourse, begun in the 1870s, that defended the right of all to reproduce while blocking medical intervention. Feminists and nationalists, midwives and obstetricians contested reproduction as never before.

NICK HOPWOOD

27 Breeding Farm Animals and Humans

Sarah Wilmot

Human interference in animal breeding has a long history. Practised in antiquity, castration or gelding of horses, cattle and pigs matured into a craft skill. Though artificial insemination was rarely in evidence before 1900, experienced stud grooms had used it to breed horses for centuries. Such routines, and farmers' understandings expressed in terms such as 'heat', 'bulling', 'tupping' and 'calf-bed' for ovulation, fertile periods, insemination and the uterus, were until the mid-twentieth century largely unmediated by scientific experts or veterinarians. Change began with the advent of selective breeding and scientists' use of data from animal populations to think about human heredity and vice versa, from inbreeding maladies to eugenic possibilities. In the mid-twentieth century, a research infrastructure for a new science of reproduction was built on the farm. Livestock breeding proved a rich resource for thinking about humans, from population biology to conceptive technologies.

In this chapter, Britain is my window onto Europe-wide change and is of special interest. In the eighteenth century, Robert Bakewell introduced close inbreeding to improve livestock, inspiring an international wave of selective breeding and debates over strategies. Britain also produced the first pedigree stud- or herd-books for racehorses (1791) and cattle (1822), and among the first standard genealogical handbooks for the nobility and gentry (1769, 1826). Later, trade and empire transported British breeds, breed societies and public pedigree-keeping around the globe. In other respects Britain lagged behind, because state involvement came late, but it is representative of the widespread adoption of AI for livestock and the expansion of animal breeding science after 1945.

Artificial Selection

Theoretically, the selection choices available to livestock farmers have changed little since antiquity: random mating, negative breeding (using inferior animals not wanted for market or subsistence use) and a limited number of positive selection strategies based on desirable appearance, geographical origin or theories about inbreeding, cross-breeding and breeding value. In practice, Nicholas Russell argued, significant changes in selection strategies took place in the sixteenth century, when classical precepts, which included rules for choosing and managing the breeding pair, were imported into

England and appropriated, and in the eighteenth century, when breeders' objectives shifted from stewardship to active improvement.[1]

Classical precepts became significant in Tudor England from the reign of Henry VIII. The king and nobles created studs with imported stallions to remedy shortages in the number and quality of horses for military campaigns. Foreign, particularly Italian, horse masters and grooms accompanied the animals, bringing with them the Neapolitan riding school's ideas about preparing for a mating and how to set up a stud. Advice literature in English circulated Italian instructions on selecting shape and form. These followed the classical canon, as did much of the guidance on coat colours as markers of constitution and 'character'. In early modern cattle breeding too, most advice came from classical sources, perhaps transferred from horse breeders. In the early seventeenth century, a new generation of authors offered conflicting readings and criticism of this body of writing on breeding, but were united in the common principle that to keep the desirable features of a breed from a different region it was necessary to continue importing fresh stock.[2]

Russell identified the decline of this paradigm, in which animals (imported or native) were always in danger of decay, as the key change over the next century. Early modern breeders aimed to arrest degeneration. Practical and cosmological frameworks encouraged breeding for the status quo. Farming regimes, livestock disease and poverty often kept stock numbers too low for the breeder to select at all, and deterioration in animal condition was common. Christian teachings contributed narratives about nature running down and creating imperfection, and of animals perfect at the moment of Creation inevitably declining over time. It was a common opinion that past generations were better; few sought positive change. For the seventeenth-century breeder, astrological conditions and the imagination of the breeding pair at the time of copulation could be as important as the quality of the parent animals to the success of a mating. The paradigm shifted when breeders' objectives turned towards ideal 'types' designed by humans. This was rare before the eighteenth century, Russell argued, and changed then through 'a combination of historical understanding and a belief in positive change'.[3] By contrast, I propose that the chief innovation in animal breeding was less in ideas than in the formation of social groups. The apparatus of elite breeding, which still survives today, came into being in the eighteenth century. We might call this the formation of a 'biosocial collectivity', a heterogeneous grouping of human and nonhuman animal populations.[4]

1 Nicholas Russell, *Like Engend'ring Like: Heredity and Animal Breeding in Early Modern England* (Cambridge, 1986), pp. 11–13, 58, 70. See also Laurence M. V. Totelin, 'Animal and Plant Generation in Classical Antiquity', Chapter 4, this book.

2 Russell, *Like Engend'ring Like*, pp. 62–88, 131.

3 Ibid., pp. 12–13 (quotation), 21–2, 80–1, 99–100, 134.

4 Carol Morris and Lewis Holloway, 'Genetics and livestock breeding in the UK: Co-constructing technologies and heterogeneous biosocial collectivities', *Journal of Rural Studies* 33 (2014), 150–60.

The new biosocial world began with the foundation of 'economic' and agricultural societies. The first in Britain started in Edinburgh in 1723, and by the end of the century few counties lacked a society for agricultural improvement in which stock-breeding was discussed.[5] The aristocracy and gentry met in the more prestigious societies; smaller ones had elite patrons but drew their active membership from farmers and other rural occupations of middling status. At annual 'sheep shearings', aristocrats, such as Thomas Coke in Norfolk, hosted enormous gatherings of landlords, farmers and breeders to see improved stock, share experiences and compete for generous awards.[6] This public arena for judging livestock created the concept of and market for 'prize' cattle and sheep, and fashions in breeds.

From the 1780s, a new group of specialist painters found regular business illustrating these animals. Widely circulated as prints,[7] their portraits expressed stability, control and knowledge of breeding value; they presented a model of size, conformation, colour and fancy points for other breeders to follow. Portraits of aristocrats and gentry alongside their prize animals represented ancestry and power, identifying the qualities of elite animals and their owners, themselves often pedigreed in *Burke's Peerage* (Fig. 27.1).[8]

Racehorse breeding offers some precursors to pedigree keeping in livestock. In the eighteenth century, breeders began to keep private pedigree records for identification and age verification, important safeguards of value in horse-trading and on the racecourse, where animals competed according to age. More significantly, the importers of Arabian horses were introduced to the (ancient) Arabian breeders' practice of keeping genealogies to establish purity of lineage. By the mid-eighteenth century, the successful Thoroughbred was surrounded by a complex folklore of 'blood' lineages, with the first studbook published in 1791, pre-dating the first for cattle by thirty years.[9] Contemporaries pointed to the Thoroughbred as the model for farmers' pedigree methods, but probably livestock breeders independently combined pedigrees and inbreeding to retain the excellence of selected individuals.

5 Koen Stapelbroek and Jani Marjanen (eds.), *The Rise of Economic Societies in the Eighteenth Century: Patriotic Reform in Europe and North America* (Basingstoke, 2012).

6 Susanna Wade Martins, *A Great Estate at Work: The Holkham Estate and Its Inhabitants in the Nineteenth Century* (Cambridge, 1980), pp. 48–9.

7 Stephen J. G. Hall and Juliet Clutton-Brock, *Two Hundred Years of British Farm Livestock* (London, 1989), p. 52.

8 Harriet Ritvo, *The Animal Estate: The English and Other Creatures in the Victorian Age* (Cambridge, MA, 1987), pp. 3–6, 45–81.

9 Russell, *Like Engend'ring Like*, pp. 93–109, 220–1; John R. Walton, 'Pedigree and the national cattle herd, circa 1750–1850', *Agricultural History Review* 34 (1986), 149–70, on 152–3; Rebecca Cassidy, *The Sport of Kings: Kinship, Class and Thoroughbred Breeding in Newmarket* (Cambridge, 2002), pp. 141–2.

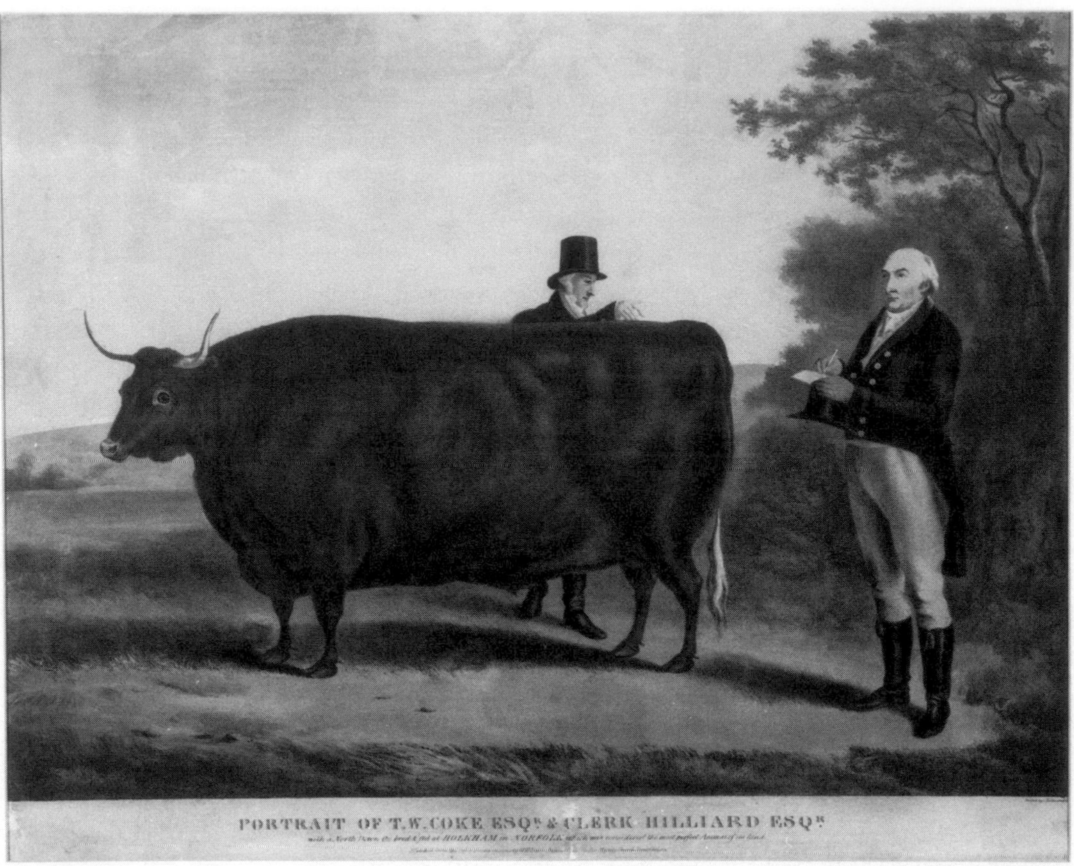

Figure 27.1 Portrait of T. W. Coke, Esq. (right), with the prize North Devon ox bred on his estate at Holkham in Norfolk, *c.* 1835. Prints such as this helped to make the owner and the breed famous. Hand-coloured lithograph drawn by William Henry Davis and printed by Charles Joseph Hullmandel. 48 × 66 cm. Museum of English Rural Life, University of Reading.

Whatever their origins, the techniques of pedigree livestock breeders involved some genealogical selection, and inbreeding in small, closed herds and flocks, to fix the traits of their ideal type. Cattle breeders founded herd-books to authenticate ancestry in public: for Shorthorn in 1822, Red Ruby Devon in 1851 and Aberdeen Angus in 1862. These dates probably mark an earlier movement; the improved Shorthorn already had roots going back eighty years (Fig. 27.2).

Beyond this growing mystique of ancestry, and the apparatus of control set up by pedigree breeders, debate continued in the nineteenth century about the stability of breeds and whether they 'degenerate' in new environments. It was common to ask whether animals (and humans) from the Old World 'degenerate' in the

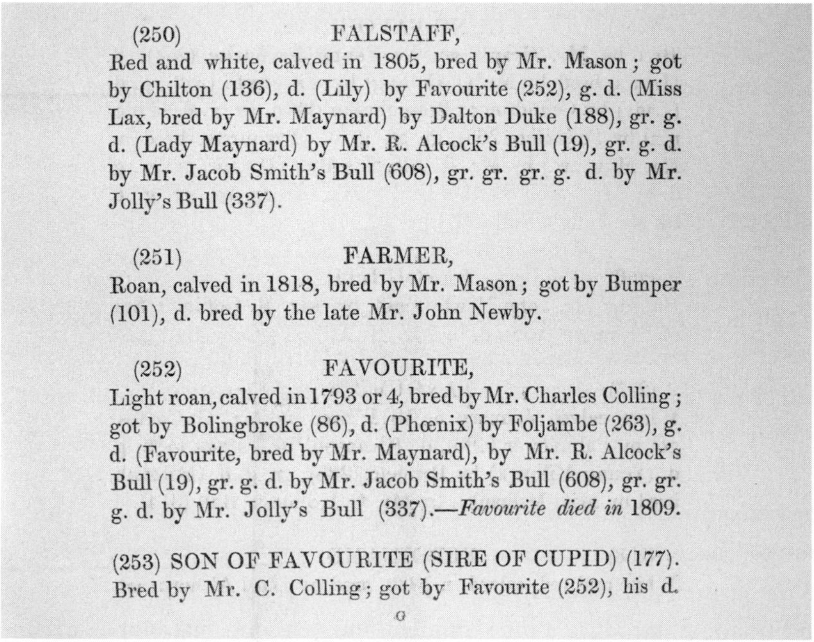

(250) FALSTAFF,
Red and white, calved in 1805, bred by Mr. Mason; got by Chilton (136), d. (Lily) by Favourite (252), g. d. (Miss Lax, bred by Mr. Maynard) by Dalton Duke (188), gr. g. d. (Lady Maynard) by Mr. R. Alcock's Bull (19), gr. g. d. by Mr. Jacob Smith's Bull (608), gr. gr. gr. g. d. by Mr. Jolly's Bull (337).

(251) FARMER,
Roan, calved in 1818, bred by Mr. Mason; got by Bumper (101), d. bred by the late Mr. John Newby.

(252) FAVOURITE,
Light roan, calved in 1793 or 4, bred by Mr. Charles Colling; got by Bolingbroke (86), d. (Phœnix) by Foljambe (263), g. d. (Favourite, bred by Mr. Maynard), by Mr. R. Alcock's Bull (19), gr. g. d. by Mr. Jacob Smith's Bull (608), gr. gr. g. d. by Mr. Jolly's Bull (337).—*Favourite died in* 1809.

(253) SON OF FAVOURITE (SIRE OF CUPID) (177).
Bred by Mr. C. Colling; got by Favourite (252), his d.

G

Figure 27.2 *Coates' Herd Book* pedigrees for Shorthorn bulls (London, 1846). Numbers gave each bull a unique identifier, which helped breeders trace ancestry. The bull Favourite became legendary for his qualities and as a representative of inbred families. Museum of English Rural Life, University of Reading.

New.[10] On English farms, 'degeneracy' was no longer expected in skilled hands, but the quality of 'improved' herds was difficult to maintain, and agricultural histories documented impermanence and decline alongside examples of progress. Theories of heredity still allowed for unpredictable outcomes, including 'maternal impression' (the effect of the mother's imagination at conception) and 'telegony' (the influence of the mother's previous mates).[11]

The stability of pedigree imagery also belied the reality of the livestock industry, of which pedigree breeders were never more than a tiny percentage.[12] 'Breed' in livestock was given physical shape by a diverse livestock economy, which collectively changed 'type' animals over time. Nevertheless, the breed societies played a formative role. Where early agricultural writers described an undifferentiated set of 'black', 'pied'

10 Philip J. Pauly, *Fruits and Plains: The Horticultural Transformation of America* (Cambridge, MA, 2007), pp. 9–32.

11 Harriet Ritvo, *The Platypus and the Mermaid, and Other Figments of the Classifying Imagination* (Cambridge, MA, 1997), pp. 107–9, 112–13.

12 Walton, 'Pedigree', 156–8; Paul Brassley, 'Livestock breeds', in E. J. T. Collins (ed.), *The Agrarian History of England and Wales*, vol. 7: *1850–1914* (Cambridge, 2000), pp. 555–69.

and 'blood-red' cattle, for modern writers regional and breed distinctions were clear.[13] By regulating size, conformation, colour and breeding policy, societies demarcated the main breed types. Pedigree breeding and breed societies changed bodies and beliefs about heredity – in humans as well as animals.

Inbreeding

Inbreeding was one of the first areas of reflexive engagement between the human sciences and farm animal reproduction. By the mid-nineteenth century, the agricultural press had already rehearsed the merits of 'in-and-in' breeding. A consensus valued inbreeding (father/daughters, brother/sisters) for 'fixing' desirable traits and transmitting them more reliably. But there were anxieties about the potential effects on animal health and fertility.

William Youatt, author of classic texts on British livestock, warned about inbreeding and animal health, and about celebrated herds and flocks that he believed had deteriorated, become bad breeders or absolutely disappeared through this cause. His advice to the farmer was 'take warning. He has been breeding too long from close affinities; and he must introduce a little different and yet congenial blood'; his animals would then 're-acquire that health and hardiness which they used to exhibit'.[14] Agricultural journalists of the mid-century informed their readers about the practical strategies of leading breeders (past and present) to avoid 'too close' inbreeding in their stock. A new generation of professionalizing veterinarians added more specific warnings about inbreeding and hereditary diseases, male and female infertility, and higher abortion rates, together with a general fear that 'high-class' breeding animals were too 'delicate'.[15]

In this later breeding literature, discourses of dysfunctional animal and human heredity interweave. An example is veterinarian Finlay Dun's 1856 article for the Royal Agricultural Society on hereditary diseases of sheep and pigs, which drew on a rich medical literature documenting the accumulation of 'morbid tendencies' in human family trees.[16] Dun incorporated tables on the inheritance of consumption and insanity in human families, with citations of Jean Lugol on scrofula, Philips on insanity and George Combe's *Constitution of Man*. As new entrants to discussions about animal breeding, the still marginal veterinarians introduced explicit human parallels partly to borrow scientific credentials from medicine.

13 Russell, *Like Engend'ring Like*, pp. 122–47; Robert Trow-Smith, *A History of British Livestock Husbandry* (London, 1959), pp. 1–4.

14 William Youatt, *Cattle: Their Breeds, Management and Diseases* (London, 1834), pp. 199–200, 525; Youatt, *Sheep: Their Breeds, Management, and Diseases* (London, 1837), p. 495 (quotation).

15 'Eastern Counties Veterinary Medical Association Minute Book', Cambridge, County Record Office, entries for 1870, 1879 and 1880.

16 Finlay Dun, 'Hereditary diseases of sheep and pigs', *Journal of the Royal Agricultural Society of England* 16 (1856), 16–45; Dun, 'On the hereditary diseases of cattle', ibid., 76–88.

Conversely, the human sciences drew on discussions of farm animal heredity. Surgeon William Lawrence's sensational *Lectures on … the Natural History of Man* (1819) may have been the first to do this in England;[17] a later generation's interest in 'close intermarriage' placed animal breeding centre stage.[18] Language indicates that this was new. Dictionaries date the first use of the word 'inbreeding' to around 1842. Bakewell's term 'in-and-in breeding' has the quality of novelty when handled by anthropologists in the mid-nineteenth century, although it had been used in agriculture for a century, and by 1800 had been translated into French and German.[19] The framing of concerns about close intermarriage also appears new. Anthropologist Eugène Dally argued that although moral and social prohibitions had been customary since antiquity, writers had remarked on the 'pretended dangers' of the practice only from around 1800. A survey of European concerns about cousin marriage also locates the key change in nineteenth-century legal and especially scientific and medical debate.[20]

The insights from 'zoologists' were nonetheless contested in anthropological debates on consanguineous marriage in the 1860s. In France, Dally's consanguinist camp refused to accept 'cross-breeding' on agricultural evidence, while using animal breeding to defend close marriages to maintain 'pure race and individual type'. The anti-consanguinist Francis Devay countered with alternative animal examples that inbreeding was dangerous; he called for regeneration of noble families through wider marriage. Similar bifurcated arguments played out in colonies, where racial mixing was either promoted as a means of improvement, bolstered with examples of mixed cattle breeds, or resisted as a danger to the parent stock.[21]

At home, medical attention expanded the original critique of royalty and aristocracy to focus on the increased incidence of mental and physical maladies in inbred families. By the 1870s, an extensive European literature on human inbreeding suggested

17 W. Lawrence, *Lectures on Physiology, Zoology, and the Natural History of Man, Delivered at the Royal College of Surgeons* (London, 1819); for Lawrence on human races: Renato G. Mazzolini, 'Colonialism and the Emergence of Racial Theories', Chapter 25, this book.

18 The first and best example is Alexander Walker, *Intermarriage* (London, 1838).

19 *OED*, s.v. *inbreeding*; Roger J. Wood, 'The sheep breeders' view of heredity before and after 1800', in Staffan Müller-Wille and Hans-Jörg Rheinberger (eds.), *Heredity Produced: At the Crossroads of Biology, Politics, and Culture, 1500–1870* (Cambridge, MA, 2007), pp. 229–50, on p. 238.

20 E. Dally, 'An inquiry into consanguineous marriages and pure races', trans. Hugh J. C. Beavan, *Anthropological Review* (1864), 65–108, on 106; A. H. Bittles, 'The bases of western attitudes to consanguineous marriage', *Developmental Medicine & Child Neurology* 45 (2003), 135–8. For earlier discussion of kin marriage: Maaike van der Lugt, 'Formed Fetuses and Healthy Children in Scholastic Theology, Medicine and Law', Chapter 12; on the law: Martin H. Johnson and Nick Hopwood, 'Modern Law and Regulation', Chapter 40, this book.

21 Francis Devay, *Du danger des mariages consanguins sous le rapport sanitaire*, 2nd edn (Paris, 1862); Damon Ieremia Salesa, *Racial Crossings: Race, Intermarriage, and the Victorian British Empire* (New York, NY, 2011); Philippa Levine, 'Imperial Encounters', Chapter 33; for earlier discussion of race mixing: Mazzolini, 'Colonialism and the Emergence of Racial Theories', this book.

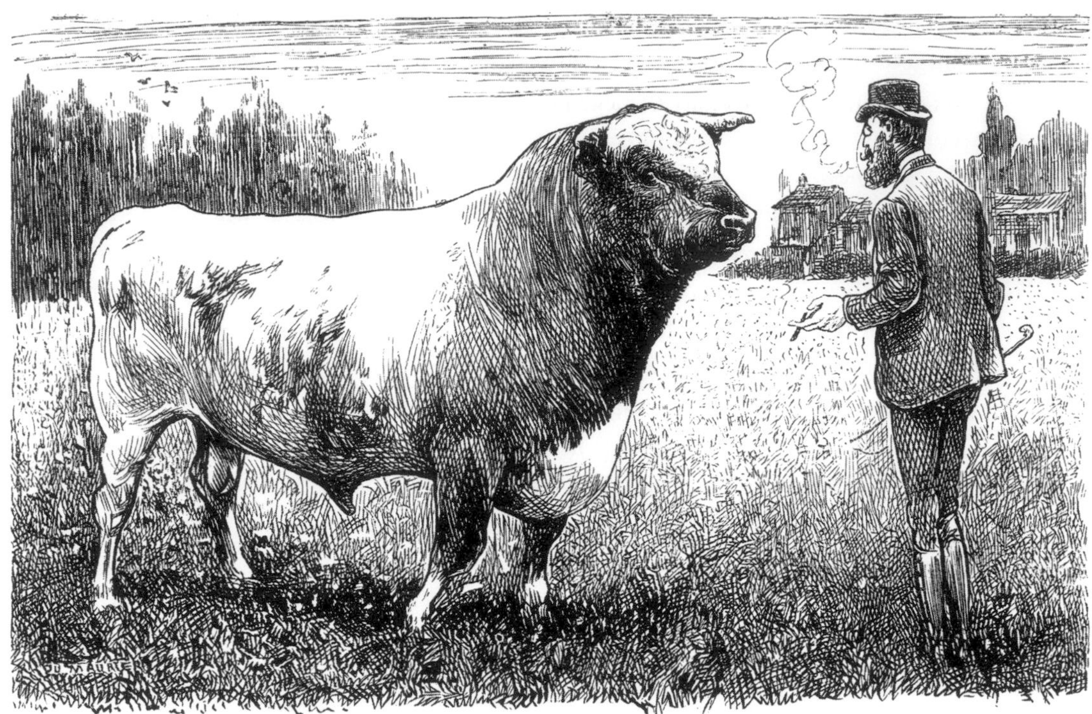

HAPPY THOUGHT! LET US ALL HAVE A VOICE IN THE MATTER.

Noble Breeder of Shorthorns. "WELL, YOU *ARE* A SPLENDID FELLOW, AND *NO* MISTAKE!"

Prize Bull. "SO WOULD *YOU* BE, MY LORD, IF YOU COULD ONLY HAVE CHOSEN YOUR PA AND MA AS CAREFULLY AND JUDICIOUSLY AS YOU CHOSE MINE!"

Figure 27.3 *Punch* cartoon comparing the breeding of nobles and of cattle. Such images were part of popular culture; Galton framed and displayed this one on his wall. *Punch* 78 (20 Mar. 1880), 126. © Punch Limited.

that insanity, imbecility, sterility, 'scrofulous and tubercular diathesis' and birth defects were more likely in children from close marriages.

From this perspective, the cousins Charles Darwin and Francis Galton, in their contributions to the literature on human breeding, merely recapitulated the worries about 'hereditary taint' and interest in 'good breeding' that were widespread in popular culture.[22] If Galton's eugenics had deep roots, his decision in the late 1860s to explore human heredity was more directly inspired by animal breeders. Galton began examining human pedigrees for 'hereditary talent and character', and germinated the idea that human qualities could be improved by institutionalized breeding (Fig. 27.3). In 1897, through the Royal Society, he tried to raise support for an experimental farm to

22 John C. Waller, 'Ideas of heredity, reproduction and eugenics in Britain, 1800–1875', *Studies in History and Philosophy of Biological and Biomedical Sciences* 32 (2001), 457–89; James Moore, *Good Breeding: Science and Society in a Darwinian Age* (Milton Keynes, 2001); Lesley A. Hall, 'Movements to Separate Sex and Reproduction', Chapter 29, this book.

investigate heredity, and Cambridge zoologist William Bateson helped him to devise a scheme of livestock breeding experiments. In 1904, Galton established the Eugenics Record Office at University College London to register 'able' families.[23]

Bateson's scheme investigated the claim that 'prepotency' (dominance) in the transmission of characters resulted from close inbreeding.[24] Bateson studied Alfred Huth's *Marriage of Near Kin* (1888), an investigation of whether or not first cousins should marry, which included pedigree data for the Shorthorn bull 'Favourite', who 'came of incestuous breeding and was bred with most of his descendants' (Fig. 27.2).[25] Huth and Bateson interwove discussion of Shorthorns, Austrian emperors and Roman families in pursuit of their different questions about the consequences of matings with close relations. Bolstered by these livestock examples, Huth challenged earlier pessimism about close intermarriage.

Between 1850 and 1900, then, human reproduction became as much a resource for thinking about animal breeding as the other way round. Comparing close matings in animals to 'incest' was not new, but drawing on data from human medicine to argue against the practice was. Advocates of 'in-and-in' breeding in animals claimed that, because the physical and health criteria that guided breeders' selections never constrained close marriage among humans, the human evidence was irrelevant, but it nevertheless shaped judgements on the farm.[26] Debates on inbreeding helped to seed an intellectual tradition of human-beast borrowings in eugenics, with a common interest in pedigree data.[27]

Public Service

In the early twentieth century, shared discourses of animal and human reproduction began to be registered on a population scale. The Europe-wide institutionalization of demography and population statistics, and the growth in Britain of the concept of a 'national herd', made it possible to speak in new ways about trends in both, and the British state finally intervened in livestock breeding.

Understanding of a nation as a 'population' was well advanced by the 1870s, when the heads of Europe's state statistical offices agreed on a standard format for decadal censuses that would allow statistical comparisons and ground nationalistic anxieties.

23 Francis Galton, *Hereditary Genius: An Inquiry into Its Laws and Consequences* (London, 1869); Pauline M. H. Mazumdar, *Eugenics, Human Genetics and Human Failings: The Eugenics Society, Its Sources and Its Critics in Britain* (London, 1992), p. 59.

24 William Bateson, 'Correspondence with Francis Galton', Norwich, John Innes Centre Archives, Bateson Letters (copies), vol. 3, nos. 240, 245, 258, 262, 266.

25 Alfred Henry Huth, *The Marriage of Near Kin* …, 2nd edn rev. (London, 1888), p. 262; Bateson, 'Correspondence', no. 240.

26 Dun, 'Cattle', 83.

27 Mazumdar, *Eugenics*, p. 89.

Birth-rates fell in most of Europe from the late 1870s, and by 1900 were a pressing concern for the rival powers of France, Germany and Britain, which debated the cumulative effects of out-migration to the colonies and the impact of urban growth on 'national efficiency'.[28]

Population surveillance of livestock was just beginning. In mid-nineteenth-century Britain, evidence was so scarce that contemporaries could not agree whether stock numbers were rising or falling.[29] Annual government statistics were introduced in 1866, beginning with simple surveys of cattle, sheep and pig numbers in every parish of England and Wales. In 1919, central government inquired specifically into breed quality, with a census of pedigree livestock.[30] Statistics fostering talk about the 'national herd' generated new anxieties about trends in livestock breeding. These related to practical problems; they also echoed worries about the human population, such as the migration of the fittest overseas.

Elite breeders were accused of tailoring their bulls to the demands of commercial breeders abroad, at the expense of the home market, which could not afford them and so relied on the residue of low-quality bulls. Increasing numbers of hill farmers abandoned the breeding of beef cattle altogether, leaving graziers dependent on imports. Struggling dairy farmers were said to resort to any old bull to get their cows into milk without worrying about offspring quality. Agricultural economists complained that while the British livestock industry exported pedigree animals all over the world, poorer animals produced the country's own meat and milk.[31]

Rather than see these problems in the livestock economy as an outcome of commercial decisions, commentators routinely invoked theories of dysfunctional reproduction. In the late nineteenth century, disquiet about the impact of 'injudicious crosses' on the quality of British horses, cattle and sheep identified sterility and abortion as a major problem.[32] By the early twentieth century, a widely held theory of inbreeding degeneration was based on the belief that each year the best British stock was exported, while import restrictions, put in place to keep diseases out, blocked the introduction of 'fresh blood'. This spurred a radical departure: the government stepped into animal breeding, beginning with the species closest to state power, the horse.

28 Michael Drake, 'Population: Patterns and processes', in Martin Pugh (ed.), *A Companion to Modern European History, 1871–1945* (Oxford, 1997), pp. 3–24, 369–71; Simon Szreter, *Fertility, Class and Gender in Britain, 1860–1940* (Cambridge, 1996).

29 E. J. T. Collins, 'The high farming period, 1850–75', in Collins, *Agrarian History*, pp. 72–137, on p. 95.

30 Ministry of Agriculture and Fisheries, *Census of Pedigree Livestock, 1919* (London, 1921).

31 K. J. J. Mackenzie, *Cattle and the Future of Beef-Production in England* (Cambridge, 1919).

32 R. J. Moore-Colyer, 'Horses and equine improvement in the economy of modern Wales', *Agricultural History Review* 39 (1991), 126–42, on 135–6; 'Veterinary Medical Association', 1870; Walter Heape, *The Breeding Industry: Its Value to the Country, and Its Needs* (Cambridge, 1906).

The royal studs of England's Tudor monarchs had not evolved into state breeding institutions, equivalent to the French and German systems of government stud-farms that offered quality stallions to private breeders, controlled and selected breeds, and supplied horses for war. Although the British army was a powerful player in the market for horses in times of crisis, it did not seek to improve breeding. Compulsory inspection of breed stock was considered an infringement of British liberty and people were convinced that, given high prices, private enterprise would deliver.[33]

Government regulation began with the Commons Act 1908, which gave horse owners on common land the right to form associations to bar non-premium stallions. The government offered incentives for the use of superior stud animals, including funding a scheme of 'public service' under which approved Thoroughbred sires were to serve mares at a low fee, under the control of a local committee. The Horse Breeding Act 1918 required all owners of stallions offered for public service to obtain a licence, at last following similar schemes in France and Germany. It also responded to a grassroots movement led by veterinarians and breed societies opposed to breeding from stallions with hereditary defects. After 1918, no stallion could move from its home base to stand for public service unless licensed free of contagious diseases and conformational faults by the Board of Agriculture and Fisheries.[34]

Cattle quality became a 'public interest' issue after World War I destabilized Britain's traditional reliance on free trade for meat supplies. The Census of Pedigree Livestock in 1919 revealed that only 2 per cent of the national herd comprised pedigree animals. In response the government made its first intervention in cattle breeding in 1920 through a Livestock Improvement Scheme, which introduced premiums for pedigree bulls.[35] Breeders were co-opted into a discourse designed to eliminate 'scrub bulls' from the nation's herds.[36] Licensing laws were imposed on breeders offering bulls for public service from 1922 (Fig. 27.4).[37]

In 1930, Francis Crew, Director of the Animal Breeding Research Department at the University of Edinburgh, commented that 'everywhere we see State intervention in the programmes of stock improvement and the genetical methods employed have been of two kinds, negative and positive'.[38] This is interesting beyond the simple point about government action. First, as we shall see, Crew belonged to a new era of state-funded

33 Margaret E. Derry, *Horses in Society: A Story of Animal Breeding and Marketing Culture, 1800–1920* (Toronto, 2006), p. 109.

34 Moore-Colyer, 'Horses', 140.

35 Ministry, *Census*; Walton, 'Pedigree', 168.

36 Shorthorn Society of the United Kingdom, 'Council and AGM Minute Book, no. 8, 1922–27', Reading, Museum of English Rural Life, 3 June 1924, 30 Mar., 4 May and 7 July 1926.

37 Bull licensing was introduced in Northern Ireland in 1922, Scotland in 1931 and England and Wales in 1934.

38 F. A. E. Crew, 'Genetical methods of livestock improvement', *Journal of the Royal Society of Arts* 78 (1930), 729–43, on 734.

MINISTRY OF AGRICULTURE, FISHERIES AND FOOD

Licensing of Bulls (England and Wales)
Regulations, 1956 and 1958

APPLICATION FOR A LICENCE TO KEEP A BULL

Name of Bull	Breed or Type	Date of Birth
		............19...... (day) (month) (year)
Is the bull pure bred? *YES/NO Is the bull registered or eligible for registration with a breed society? *YES/NO	Colour	Earmarks

Full postal address of premises at which bull is kept ....

County .... Parish ....

Nearest town or village .... and distance from farm .... miles.

If bull is to be sent to a sale within six weeks, state sale .... and date ....

FULL name of owner (in BLOCK LETTERS) ....

Figure 27.4 Extract from a bull licence application form. Owners were not allowed to keep a bull over ten months old without a licence, even if the bull was used only to serve the owner's cows. Museum of English Rural Life, University of Reading.

research departments with interests in the genetics and physiology of reproduction. Second, his 'negative' and 'positive' distinction resonated with the eugenics movement. Defined by Dr Caleb Saleeby, influential in launching the Eugenics Education Society in 1907, these terms were widely circulated and debated there.[39] The society highlighted differential birth-rates in its endeavour to promote a better-bred Britain, but was divided over the merits of encouraging the reproduction of the 'better' types versus measures to dampen the birth-rate of the so-called inferior. This raises the fascinating possibility that Crew's comment was partly intended to contribute to human eugenics debates. He was an important figure in the British section of the International Population Union, suggesting that discourses of animal and human breeding were being brought together under a variety of institutional umbrellas.[40]

39 Anthony J. Dellureficio, 'Tracing the trajectory of "positive eugenics" in Britain. Part 2', *Galton Institute Newsletter* 74 (Sept. 2010), 1–16.

40 On Crew: Alison Bashford, *Global Population: History, Geopolitics, and Life on Earth* (New York, NY, 2014), pp. 151–3.

Against this background, state direction in cattle reproduction reached its apogee in the 1940s, when the problem of improved breeding for milk production was tackled on a broad community basis, to prevent bad dairy cattle from ever being born.

Science Intervenes in the Animal Body

There was a science of animal breeding before the twentieth century, but thanks to government investment in research, new technologies now reshaped farm animal reproduction on an unprecedented scale. Adele Clarke traced the origin of this new science to the reproductive physiology inaugurated at Cambridge between 1890 and 1910, when Walter Heape and Francis Marshall united animal breeding with generative physiology and gynaecology.[41] After 1930, scientific intervention began to change interactions between farmers' and experts' knowledge of reproduction. The veterinary profession reoriented their farm practice away from the horse towards bovine reproduction, while agricultural physiologists became involved in mass livestock breeding, engineered through newly created centres for artificial insemination (AI).[42]

Heape's *The Breeding Industry* (1906) constructed animal 'infertility' as a national problem costing over £9 million annually (equivalent to perhaps £1 billion today).[43] Soon after, the government invested in special institutions for the study of animal reproduction at the University of Cambridge, where Marshall authored the first textbook, *Physiology of Farm Animals* (1920), and at Edinburgh, in the Animal Breeding Research Department (founded in 1919), where a research group on reproductive physiology was established by the late 1920s. The Agricultural Research Council developed a third centre at the National Institute for Research in Dairying at Reading. Their objective was complete knowledge of the reproductive processes of farm animals, including sperm physiology and hormones, 'to obtain practical control' of the factors regulating fertility, periodicity of breeding and lactation.[44]

Physiological research and techniques transformed breeders' barren or sterile cows, accepted as occupational hazards, into animals with 'temporary infertility'. By 1930, classic textbooks of veterinary obstetrics were rewritten with sections on contagious abortion and sterility enlarged to incorporate 'modern views', including references to

41 Adele E. Clarke, *Disciplining Reproduction: Modernity, American Life Sciences, and 'the Problems of Sex'* (Berkeley, CA, 1998).

42 Abigail Woods, 'The farm as clinic: Veterinary expertise and the transformation of dairy farming, 1930–1950', *Studies in History and Philosophy of Biological and Biomedical Sciences* 38 (2007), 462–87.

43 Heape, *Breeding Industry*, pp. 99, 105.

44 Woods, 'Farm as clinic'; T. B. Wood and F. H. A. Marshall, *Physiology of Farm Animals* (Cambridge, 1920); Sarah Wilmot, 'From "public service" to artificial insemination: Animal breeding science and reproductive research in early twentieth-century Britain', *Studies in History and Philosophy of Biological and Biomedical Sciences* 38 (2007), 411–41, on 422–3.

Marshall's and John Hammond's books on physiology of reproduction and Danish veterinarian Folmer Nielsen's research on sterility in dairy cows.[45] Veterinary panels were set up to oversee successful conception, birth and lactation on farms. Well-placed veterinary surgeons helped reproductive physiologists to gain access to traditionally closed worlds. From the 1940s, these new specialists came together in networks founded to advance the study of animal and human reproduction, notably the Society for the Study of Fertility.[46]

AI, which took off for dairy cattle in the 1940s, was the first mass reproductive intervention into farm animal bodies. Though recorded experiments date from the end of the eighteenth century, Russia's interwar programme to breed livestock on a mass scale provided the key model, and not just for livestock breeders. Galton had privately dreamed of using AI to improve human breeding in the 1890s. Experiments in the 1920s and 1930s encouraged prominent biologists such as Julian Huxley and Hermann Muller to advocate this tool of eugenic intervention under new labels including 'eutelegenesis' and 'germinal choice'.[47]

British investigations into AI in cattle began in the 1920s, but had little impact before 1940. There was no demand from breeders, pedigree societies remained wary and the government was reluctant until a wartime drive to increase milk production helped to change policy. The promise to raise productivity per cow resonated with the new efficiency and food supply agendas, and the first test AI centres opened at Cambridge and Reading in 1943.[48] In 1945, the Milk Marketing Board was charged with founding a network of centres to make the technique available to farmers nationwide. Fifteen years after it started in Cambridge, AI was breeding around 60 per cent of the dairy cattle population (Fig. 27.5).[49]

Once AI had become routine on farms, it acted as a carrier for other technologies to 'enhance fertility'. A new demand was created for 'effective veterinary-gynaecologic' services.[50] The shared networks for the study of fertility allowed techniques to transfer between species; AI research on bulls and infertility was used to fill gaps in knowledge

45 J. F. Craig, *Fleming's Veterinary Obstetrics*, 4th edn (London, 1930), p. v.

46 Wilmot, 'Public service', 430–1.

47 Helen Blackman, 'Women, savages and other animals: The comparative physiology of reproduction, 1850–1914', unpublished PhD thesis, University of Manchester (2001); Martin Richards, 'Artificial insemination and eugenics: Celibate motherhood, eutelegenesis and germinal choice', *Studies in History and Philosophy of Biological and Biomedical Sciences* 39 (2008), 211–21; Nick Hopwood, 'Artificial Fertilization', Chapter 39, this book.

48 Sheila Bowman, 'Development of artificial insemination in cattle in the United Kingdom', unpublished MPhil. thesis, University of Reading (1975).

49 Wilmot, 'Public service', 425–9.

50 Nils Lagerlöf, 'The veterinarian and the breeding and rearing of animals', in *Report of the XIVth International Veterinary Congress … 1949* (London, 1952), pp. 108–17, on p. 114.

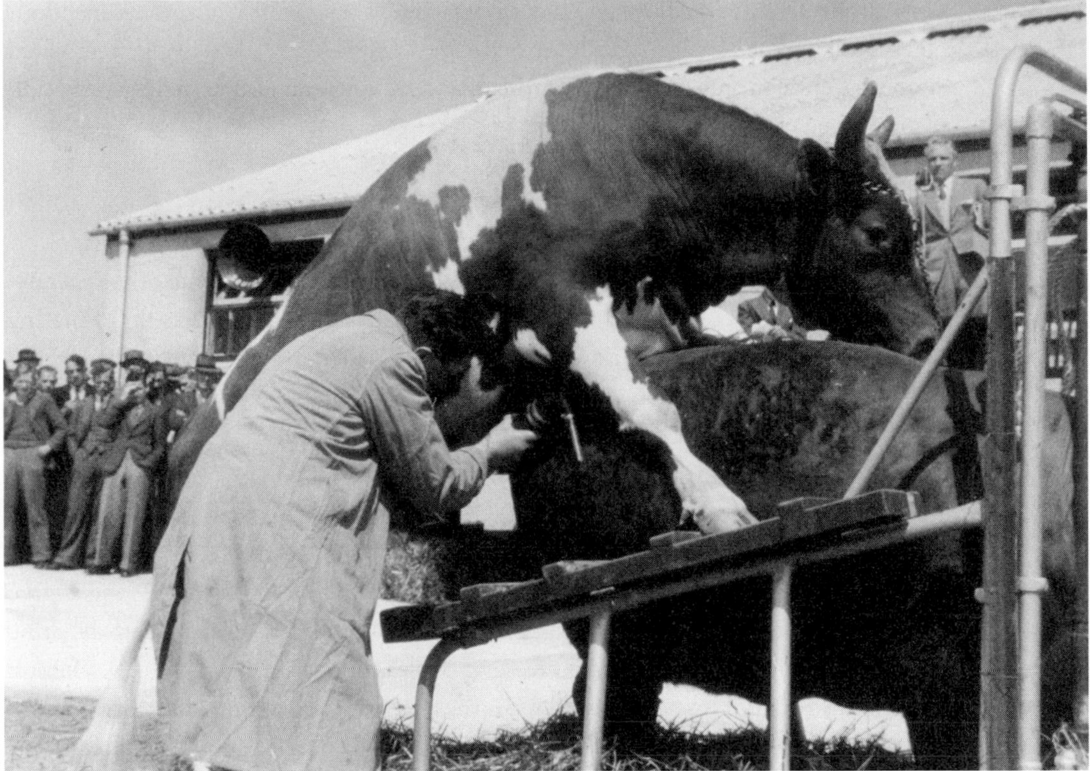

Figure 27.5 AI centre manager demonstrating semen collection in an artificial vagina while the cow is held still in a 'teaser crate' (1947). Each centre had laboratory staff to perform semen evaluation and dilution, and trained inseminators to visit local farms. Museum of English Rural Life, University of Reading.

of humans.[51] In cattle the driver was financial, since the farmer paid for only the first insemination. AI set norms for bovine reproductive efficiency and accelerated the pace of research.[52] The freezing techniques pioneered at the National Institute for Medical Research in London and the Animal Research Station in Cambridge created a global trade in semen.[53]

Research then turned to address the 'limitations' of the female by increasing the number of eggs shed and eliminating non-breeding seasons. In dairy cattle, experimentation was part of a plan to enhance the fertility of cows of high genetic worth, so that farmers could breed from only the best 10 to 20 per cent.[54] By the mid-1950s, proposed

51 Naomi Pfeffer, *The Stork and the Syringe: A Political History of Reproductive Medicine* (Cambridge, 1993), pp. 59–60, 117, 219 n. 15.

52 Wilmot, 'Public service', 430.

53 Christopher Polge, 'The work of the Animal Research Station, Cambridge', *Studies in History and Philosophy of Biological and Biomedical Sciences* 38 (2007), 511–20.

54 Wilmot, 'Public service', 432–3.

interventions in dairy cows included manipulation of the ovaries, hormone injections and embryo transfer.[55] Whereas at the start of the century dairy cows were often mated simply to get them into milk, bulls and cows were now defined by their genetic and reproductive potential.

Conclusion

Livestock breeders had long been interested in inheritance not in terms of the intricacies of ovaries, uterus or seminal fluid, but for the visible and tangible results of mating animals. Every animal was acknowledged 'for the moste parte to engender hys lyke',[56] but outcomes could also be disrupted by maternal imagination, accidental happenings and poor husbandry, and in the long run new generations were expected to decline. In the eighteenth century, breeders began to seek 'improvement' and to rely on ancestry to manage parental selection. Pedigree thinking intensified a two-way traffic with discourses on human breeding. The interplay with human concerns meant that animal breeders worried first about 'high breeding' and elite inbreeding, long before anxieties were directed at 'scrub bulls'. A late expression of this human–beast dynamic was the connection between animal breeding and eugenics in debates over AI. Though there is little evidence that doctors ever saw themselves as engaged in a similar population-scale endeavour, AI brought fertility specialists together with animal physiologists to make reproduction a cross-species field. The international research network established around AI has led to the development of superovulation, embryo transfer and cloning, ensuring that farm animal reproduction will continue as an important realm for debating and imagining human reproductive futures.[57]

55 On embryo transfer: Hopwood, 'Artificial Fertilization'.

56 Thomas Blundeville in 1565, quoted in Russell, *Like Engend'ring Like*, p. 69.

57 Gena Corea, *The Mother Machine: Reproductive Technologies from Artificial Insemination to Artificial Wombs* (New York, NY, 1985); Sarah Franklin, *Dolly Mixtures: The Remaking of Genealogy* (Durham, NC, 2007); Hopwood, 'Artificial Fertilization'; Christina Brandt, 'Cloned Frogs', Exhibit 37, this book.

28 Eggs and Sperm as Germ Cells

Florence Vienne

In 1748, the prominent naturalist Georges-Louis Leclerc, Comte de Buffon, dissected a female dog to study the fluid in its 'testicles' under the microscope. He found not the 'ovum' described by Reinier de Graaf in 1672, but the same 'moving bodies' he had himself often observed in the semen of male animals. Buffon thus contested the existence not only of ovaries and eggs, but also of the little animals, or 'animalcules', that the Dutch microscopist Antonie van Leeuwenhoek had discovered in the seventeenth century. For Buffon, Leeuwenhoek's animalcules were not living beings at all, but 'initial combinations' of organic particles. Buffon claimed that the generative organs of the two sexes were identical, and that their generative substances contained the same organic 'molecules' that animated the whole of nature.[1] By contrast, Lazzaro Spallanzani, another significant naturalist, argued that sperm were animal parasites found mainly, though not only, in the male body.[2] Where Leeuwenhoek had presented the 'spermatic animals' as preformed embryos, Spallanzani's parasite theory denied them any generative function at all. In the late eighteenth century, leading authorities still promoted diametrically opposed views of eggs and sperm and their roles in generation. When and how did the present-day understanding of the gametes as sex-specific cells that carry maternal and paternal heredity take shape?

My answer differs from Thomas Laqueur's in *Making Sex* (1990). For Laqueur, the seventeenth-century discovery of 'eggs' and 'little creatures' in the semen opened an epoch in which 'egg' and 'sperm' became 'an imaginatively convincing synecdoche for two sexes'.[3] This chapter shows, however, that physiologists did not describe eggs and sperm as products of two distinct sexes until the early nineteenth century. By considering developments in physiology, embryology and research on cells and heredity through

1 Georges-Louis Leclerc de Buffon, *Histoire naturelle, générale et particulière*, vol. 2 (Paris, 1749), pp. 203, 169. On this work of de Graaf and Buffon: Rina Knoeff, 'The Generative Parts of Women', Exhibit 16; Mary Terrall, 'A Microscopical Salon', Exhibit 20; Nick Hopwood, 'The Keywords "Generation" and "Reproduction"', Chapter 20; see further Gianna Pomata, 'Innate Heat, Radical Moisture and Generation', Chapter 14; Karin Ekholm, 'Pictures and Analogies in the Anatomy of Generation', Chapter 15; and Ekholm, 'A Placenta Painted and Engraved', Exhibit 15, this book.

2 Spallanzani, *Opuscules de physique, animale et végétale*, trans. Jean Senebier, vol. 2 (Geneva, 1777 [Italian original, 1776]), pp. 228–9.

3 Thomas Laqueur, *Making Sex: Body and Gender from the Greeks to Freud* (Cambridge, MA, 1990), pp. 171–5, on p. 171.

that century, I contend further that notions not only of incommensurable difference, but also of the similarity and equality of the sexes, shaped germ cells as we know them today. I thus propose a different chronology from Laqueur's and contest his view that a single, unified way of thinking – a 'two-sex model' – drove the modern redefinition of the body.[4] I also reassess some standard accounts in the history of biology about the emergence of our modern understanding of reproduction.

In his influential *The Logic of Life*, first published in French in 1970, François Jacob argued that cell theory 'profoundly transformed' the study of reproduction in the mid-nineteenth century. Procreation was no longer regarded as the production of a completely new being, but as formation out of an already existing organic fragment – a basic unit of life, a 'cell'. For Jacob, the formulation of cell theory immediately made it possible to think of reproduction as a process that established organic continuity between both sexes and their offspring.[5] In 1982, John Farley rebutted Jacob's argument in an exhaustive account of nineteenth-century debates over the roles of the sexes in reproduction.[6] Farley claimed that these theories largely mirrored society's views on sex. He suggested that since bearing and rearing children was seen as essentially a female occupation and sex as a bestial act, until the 1860s most biologists allowed men only a very limited role in reproduction or even denied that it needed the male sex. Yet, as we shall see, at issue in this period was not primarily the necessity of the male sex, or of copulation, but the nature of the male contribution. Prevailing notions of gender difference framed this as unlike the woman's: men did not provide anything material, but a generative or vital force. I shall argue that the decisive change that made possible our current understanding of reproduction and gametes was the conceptualization of the male contribution in material and quantitative terms. This began in the 1840s, but it took physiologists, cytologists and zoologists more than half a century to develop a model of reproduction in which both sexes played equal parts. Jacob's claim notwithstanding, they did not simply apply cell theory, but rather introduced a new concept: sex-specific germ cells each containing an equal share of hereditary material.[7]

In the nineteenth century, then, the male role in reproduction was an important object of research and debate. It is true that after the French Revolution new scientific

4 On the 'one-sex model', see esp. Helen King, *The One-Sex Body on Trial: The Classical and Early Modern Evidence* (Farnham, 2013); and, for a critique of the 'two-sex model', Heinz-Jürgen Voß, *Making Sex Revisited. Dekonstruktion des Geschlechts aus biologisch-medizinischer Perspektive* (Bielefeld, 2010).

5 François Jacob, *The Logic of Life: A History of Heredity*, trans. Betty E. Spillmann (Princeton, NJ, 1993), pp. 121–6.

6 John Farley, *Gametes & Spores: Ideas about Sexual Reproduction, 1750–1914* (Baltimore, MD, 1982).

7 Helga Satzinger, *Differenz und Vererbung. Geschlechterordnungen in der Genetik und Hormonforschung 1890–1950* (Cologne, 2009); Satzinger, 'The politics of gender concepts in genetics and hormone research in Germany, 1900–1940', *Gender & History* 24 (2012), 735–54; Bettina Bock von Wülfingen, 'Economies and the cell: Conception and heredity around 1900 and 2000', unpublished habilitation thesis, Humboldt-Universität zu Berlin (2011).

facts were produced to confine women to domesticity and motherhood. Legitimizing their exclusion from the new discourse of human and civil rights, anatomists, physiologists and physicians declared women's organs, bones, muscles and intellectual ability to be different and inferior – a view institutionalized in the founding of modern gynaecology around 1820.[8] Yet that is only part of the story. At the same time, the first investigations were undertaken to demonstrate that reproduction involved the male body in previously unknown ways.[9]

New Perspectives on Eggs and Sperm

The Frenchman Jean-Baptiste Dumas is mostly remembered as one of the founders of organic chemistry, alongside Justus Liebig. In the 1820s, however, he carried out ground-breaking studies of animal generation in collaboration with the Swiss physiologist Jean-Louis Prévost. Both researchers took seriously Buffon's microscopic investigations of the reproductive organs of women and men.[10] However, they found Buffon's view of the sperm as components of a generative material common to both sexes unacceptable: 'females do not collaborate in the act of generation by means of a fluid comparable to that provided by the males'.[11] Much of their work accordingly showed that Buffon had been wrong and de Graaf right: mammals, and not only amphibians and birds, possess ovaries containing eggs.[12] The first, and most significant, step in Prévost and Dumas's extensive studies, however, had been to examine the male reproductive organs and 'spermatic animals' of nineteen species. Whereas the majority of early nineteenth-century naturalists held sperm to be parasites, Prévost and Dumas established that the testes 'produced' sperm.[13] Illustrating their results, each of ten plates portrayed the genitals and spermatic animalcules of a different species (Fig. 28.1).

This attempt to study sperm as specific products of male bodies was new, and so was the microscopical analysis of fertilization. Early nineteenth-century physiologists

8 For example, Londa Schiebinger, *The Mind Has No Sex? Women in the Origins of Modern Science* (Cambridge, MA, 1989); Ornella Moscucci, *The Science of Woman: Gynaecology and Gender in England, 1800–1929* (Cambridge, 1990); Claudia Honegger, *Die Ordnung der Geschlechter. Die Wissenschaften vom Menschen und das Weib, 1750–1850* (Frankfurt am Main, 1991).

9 See also Christina Benninghaus, 'Modern Infertility', Chapter 31, this book.

10 Jean-Louis Prévost and Jean-Baptiste Dumas, 'Essai. Sur les animalcules spermatiques de divers animaux', *Mémoires de la Société de Physique et d'Histoire Naturelle de Genève* 1 (1821), 180–207; Prévost and Dumas, 'Nouvelle théorie de la génération', *Annales des sciences naturelles* 1 (1824), 1–29, 167–87; Prévost and Dumas, 'Deuxième mémoire sur la génération. Rapports de l'œuf avec la liqueur fécondante. Phénomènes appréciables, résultant de leur action mutuelle. Développement de l'œuf des batraciens', ibid., 2 (1824), 100–21, 129–49; Prévost and Dumas, 'Troisième mémoire. De la génération dans les mammifères, et les premiers indices de développement de l'embryon', ibid., 3 (1824), 113–38; Prévost and Dumas, 'Mémoire sur le développement du poulet dans l'œuf', ibid., 12 (1827), 415–54.

11 Prévost and Dumas, 'Troisième mémoire', 136.

12 Ibid., 114.

13 Prévost and Dumas, 'Essai', 106.

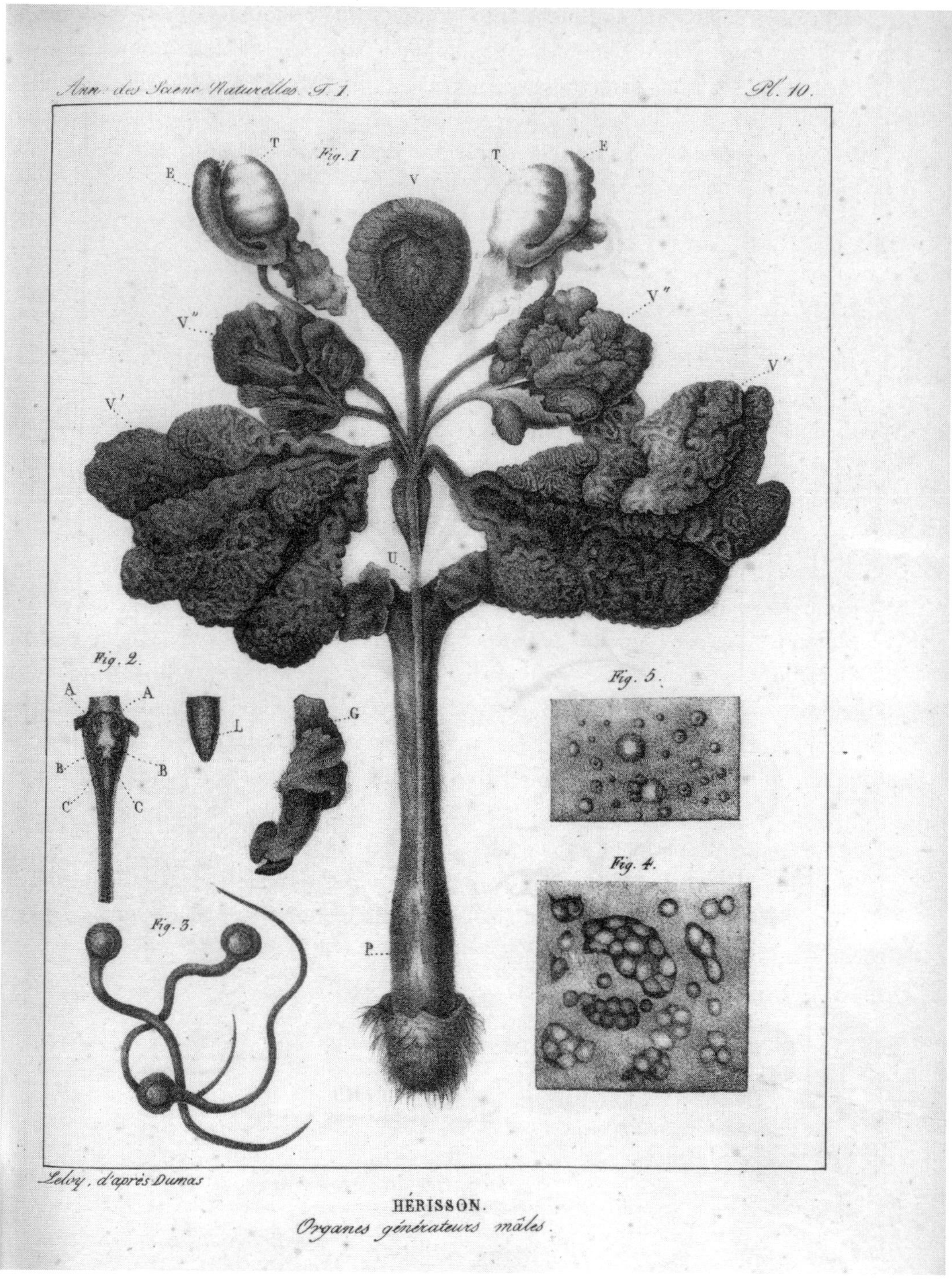

Figure 28.1 'The male sexual organs of the hedgehog' by Jean-Louis Prévost and Jean-Baptiste Dumas. This illustration was one of the first to relate the production of 'spermatic animalcules' to the anatomy of the male testicles. Lithograph from 'Nouvelle théorie de la génération', *Annales des sciences naturelles* 1 (1824), plate 10. 25 × 18 cm. Cambridge University Library.

and embryologists had equated fertilization with the act of copulation. Prévost and Dumas described fertilization as a distinct process and demonstrated its relevance to embryogenesis. Their numerous experiments on the artificial fertilization of frogs' eggs showed that only those exposed to seminal fluid underwent the transformations that culminated in the formation of an embryo. Their illustration of embryogenesis documents observations of the eggs from the first hour to five days after fertilization, dating all the changes that culminated in the appearance of the first organs back to the moment of fertilization (Fig. 28.2).[14]

In a further series of experiments, Prévost and Dumas began to describe the process of fertilization more precisely. Under the microscope, they 'saw' the spermatic animals penetrating the mucus around the ovum and coming into 'close contact' with the ovum itself.[15] Prévost and Dumas differed on what happened to the spermatic animal after fertilization: Prévost reckoned it disappeared, while Dumas argued that it went on to contribute materially to the formation of the embryo. For him, the spermatic animal was 'nothing other than the rudiment of the nervous system'.[16]

In the first half of the nineteenth century, Prévost and Dumas's work received considerable attention, but most researchers initially rejected their findings. Karl Ernst von Baer, a professor of anatomy and zoology and co-founder of modern embryology, was among their severest critics and took particular exception to Dumas's redefinition of sperm. Baer accepted that the semen was necessary 'to make the idea of the animal complete and endow it with the possibility of development', but not for any material contribution.[17] More fundamentally, Baer denied that the process of organic formation had its origin in fertilization or the generative substances. In his 1827 study, usually regarded as the definitive discovery of the human ovum, he attributed this origin to the 'fetal ovum', an entity localized in the egg, but distinct from and pre-existing the 'maternal ovum'.[18] That same year he defended the animal and parasitic character of sperm and gave them a new name, 'spermatozoa'.[19] Thus, in Baer's work the concept of organic continuity was essential, but against Dumas, he did not envisage any material continuity between male parents and their offspring.[20]

14 Prévost and Dumas, 'Deuxième mémoire', 107–21.
15 Prévost and Dumas, 'Troisième mémoire', 134.
16 Prévost and Dumas, 'Mémoire sur le développement', 452.
17 Karl Ernst von Baer, *Über Entwickelungsgeschichte der Thiere. Beobachtung und Reflexion*, part 1 (Königsberg, 1828), p. 152.
18 Karl Ernst von Baer, 'On the genesis of the ovum of mammals and of man', trans. Charles Donald O'Malley, *Isis* 47 (1956 [Latin original, 1827]), 117–53, on 147–8. De Graaf was now credited with the discovery not of the egg, but of the follicle containing it: Knoeff, 'Generative Parts of Women'.
19 Karl Ernst v. Baer, 'Beiträge zur Kenntniss der niedern Thiere', *Verhandlungen der Kaiserlichen Leopoldinisch-Carolinischen Akademie der Naturforscher* 13, no. 2 (1827), 523–762, on 640.
20 Florence Vienne, 'Seeking the constant in what is transient: Karl Ernst von Baer's vision of organic formation', *History and Philosophy of the Life Sciences* 37 (2015), 34–49.

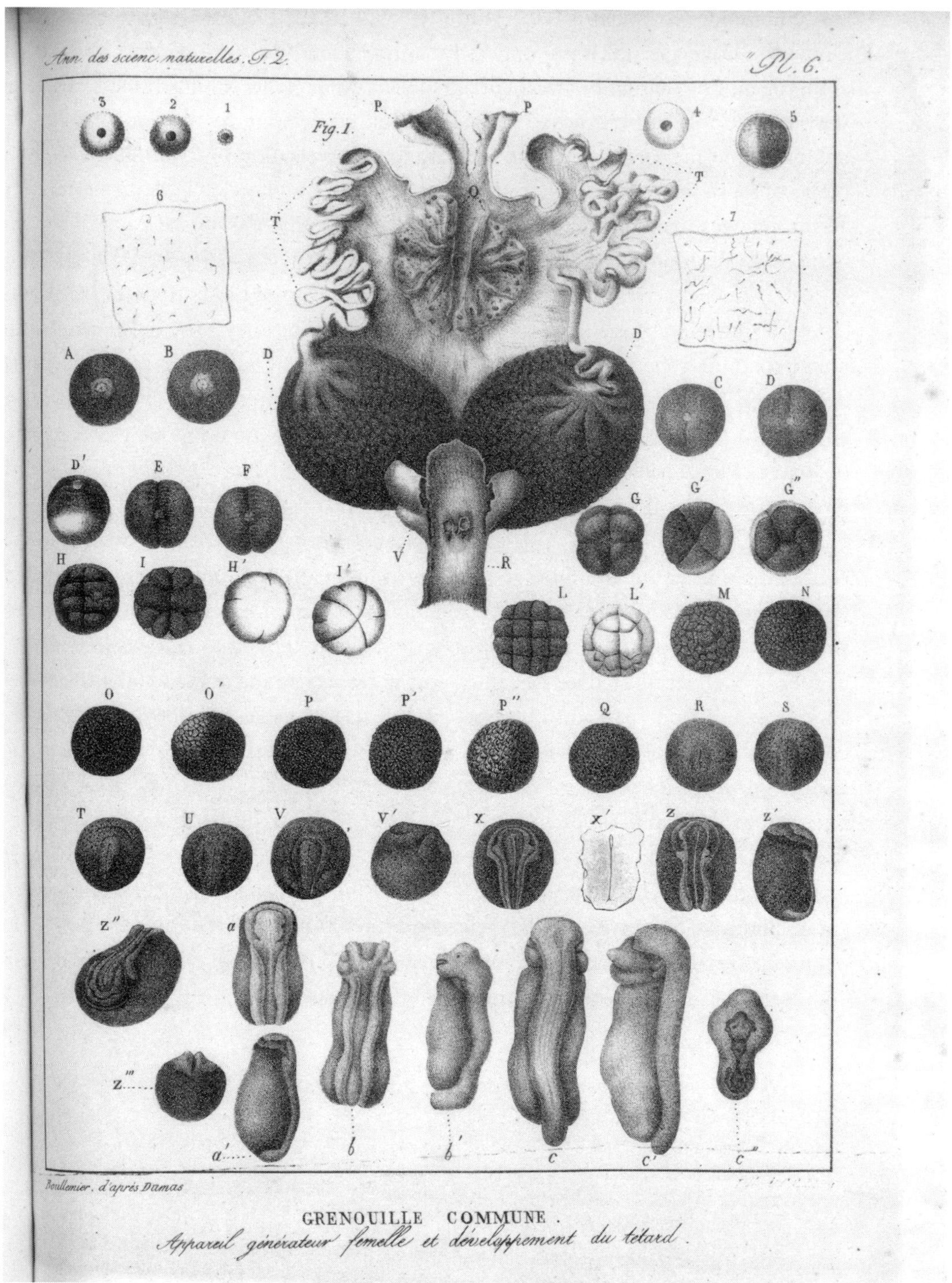

Figure 28.2 'The female sexual organs of the frog and the development of the tadpole' by Jean-Louis Prévost and Jean-Baptiste Dumas. Unlike their contemporaries, Prévost and Dumas showed embryogenesis as beginning with fertilization. Lithograph from 'Deuxième mémoire sur la génération', *Annales des sciences naturelles* 2 (1824), plate 6. 24 × 18 cm. Cambridge University Library.

The example of Baer also demonstrates that, in the early nineteenth century, research on the egg defined it not only as a distinctively female entity, but also as the seat of a basic unit of generation independent of the female body. Similarly, sperm were investigated from various perspectives: as parasites, as components of the male generative substance, and in terms of their similarities to other components of animals and plants. This last approach led the physician and naturalist Gottfried Reinhold Treviranus to play down the importance of sexual difference. He argued that the sexes differed only in their reproductive organs, not in their generative materials. Thus, unlike Prévost, Dumas and Baer, Treviranus observed in the semen not motile creatures, but organic elements no different from those in the muscles and nerves. Drawing on Buffon, he denied that the microscopic components of semen had any animal-like form or movement: the corpuscles in the semen were the same as the 'basic components' of the organism. His microscopic studies and illustrations depict these as 'extremely simple' in structure (Fig. 28.3).[21] In 1833, he even claimed that the components of the semen were 'bodies analogous to the pollen of plants'.[22]

Treviranus's search for parallels between the basic elements of all plants and animals assumed an underlying unity behind the diversity of forms. Revealing principles and laws that applied to all living nature was one of the tasks of the new science that Treviranus and others tried to instigate around 1800 under the name 'biology'.[23] In the late 1830s, the physiologist Theodor Schwann formulated a universal law of formation along these lines, one that would become the central dogma of nineteenth-century biology. Schwann's theory ascribed all physiological processes in animals and plants – including the formation of new organisms – to a unified and universal basic unit of life: the cell.[24]

Unthinkable Sperm Cells

Mid-nineteenth-century cell theory offered no basis for thinking of generation as a process that produced continuity between both parental organisms and their offspring at the cellular level. Cell theorists were concerned to explain physiological phenomena in ways that did not depend on vital forces. Instead of assuming that organic processes of

21 Gottfried Reinhold Treviranus, 'Ueber die organischen Elemente des thierischen Körpers', in Gottfried Reinhold Treviranus and Ludolf Christian Treviranus, *Vermischte Schriften anatomischen und physiologischen Inhalts*, vol. 1 (Göttingen, 1816), p. 142.

22 Gottfried Reinhold Treviranus, 'Ueber die organischen Körper des thierischen Saamens und deren Analogie mit dem Pollen der Pflanzen', *Zeitschrift für Physiologie* 5 (1833), 136–43, on 139.

23 Gottfried Reinhold Treviranus, *Biologie, oder Philosophie der lebenden Natur für Naturforscher und Aerzte*, 6 vols. (Göttingen, 1802–22); L. S. Jacyna, 'Romantic thought and the origins of cell theory', in Andrew Cunningham and Nicholas Jardine (eds.), *Romanticism and the Sciences* (Cambridge, 1990), pp. 161–8.

24 Theodor Schwann, *Mikroskopische Untersuchungen über die Übereinstimmung in der Struktur und dem Wachstume der Tiere und Pflanzen* (Leipzig, 1910 [1839]).

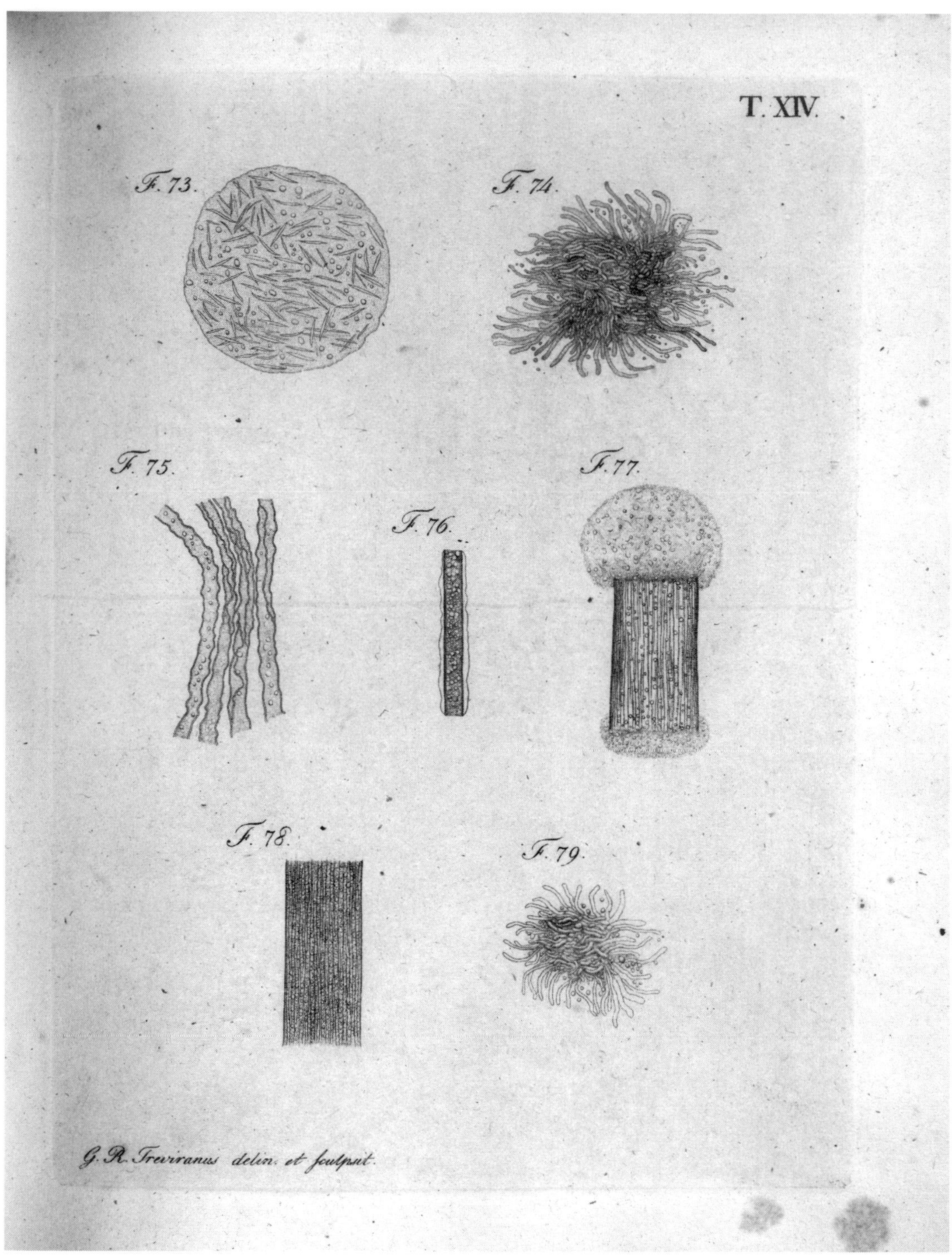

Figure 28.3 Gottfried Reinhold Treviranus's engraved drawing of frog semen (F. 73) with its 'extremely simple' elements identical to those of nerves and muscles (F. 74–9). Treviranus, 'Ueber die organischen Elemente des thierischen Körpers', in G. R. Treviranus and Ludolf Christian Treviranus, *Vermischte Schriften anatomischen und physiologischen Inhalts*, vol. 1 (Göttingen: Röwen, 1816), plate XIV. 24 × 19 cm. Cambridge University Library.

formation and development were governed by a single, immaterial principle, Schwann ascribed to each cell 'an independent life' and 'power of its own'.[25] As I have already indicated, this formative law was intended to encompass all physiological processes, including the formation of new organisms from 'egg cells' which developed independently like every other cell.[26] In Schwann's view, no male contribution was needed, but other researchers continued to insist that the agency of the sperm was necessary to trigger the development of the egg.

In an 1848 lecture on 'woman and the cell' to the Berlin Society for Midwifery, Rudolf Virchow, later known as the founder of cellular pathology, stated that the sperm was required in order to bestow 'real, independent life' on the cell, which was otherwise only '*capable*' of life.[27] In other words, the egg cell differed from other cells in not being an autonomous individual, but in attaining the power to develop into an embryo through the man, or more precisely through the male generative substance. It has often been shown that Virchow's interpretation of the organism as an entity composed of equal and autonomous cells – 'individuals', or 'citizens' – was shaped by his politics. All his life, Virchow campaigned for the abolition of the authoritarian absolutist state and the founding of a democratic, liberal social order.[28] When it came to gender, however, he was evidently satisfied with the existing states of affairs, in physiology as in society. Since 1800, physicians, especially gynaecologists, had argued that the essence of femininity was merely dependent on the ovary, and Virchow's lecture just repeated that position. The whole existence of woman, he explained, was directed towards motherhood. As a 'virgin' she wished for nothing more than to engender 'living clusters of cells: children'.[29] Virchow was translating prevailing notions of gender into the language of cells, not founding a new cellular order of the sexes.

Like most mid-nineteenth-century physiologists, Virchow regarded the egg as a cell, but not the sperm. In this he followed his teacher, the physiologist Johannes Müller, who in 1840 had declared egg and sperm incommensurable and complementary generative materials, and repudiated the possibility that the sperm too contained 'primal cells'.[30] None of the leading physiologists of this period adopted the approach of Buffon or Treviranus and put sperm on a par with the other elementary parts of organisms. Drawing instead on Prévost and Dumas, they described sperm as a component and

25 Ibid., p. 189. 26 Ibid., p. 214, also pp. 189–90.

27 Rudolf Virchow, 'Der puerperale Zustand. Das Weib und die Zelle', in *Rudolf Virchow. Sämtliche Werke*, ed. Christian Andree, vol. 16: *Gesammelte Abhandlungen zur wissenschaftlichen Medicin*, part 2 (Hildesheim, 2007), pp. 735–79, on p. 753.

28 For example, Eva Johach, *Krebszellen und Zellenstaat. Zur medizinischen und politischen Metaphorik in Rudolf Virchows Zellularpathologie* (Freiburg, 2008).

29 Virchow, 'Der puerperale Zustand', p. 752; Constantin Goschler, *Rudolf Virchow. Mediziner – Anthropologe – Politiker* (Cologne, 2002), pp. 111–25.

30 Johannes Müller, *Handbuch der Physiologie des Menschen*, vol. 2 (Koblenz, 1840), p. 655.

fertilizing factor of the semen, and even as the product of a process of cellular formation. But the form of the sperm and the peculiar, rapid movements they observed with fascination through the microscope in their view only emphasized its difference from other cells, and especially from the egg.[31]

However, if the majority of mid-nineteenth-century physiologists found it difficult or even impossible to see sperm as cells, they neither ruled out continuity between the paternal organism and the next generation, nor ignored the more general question of heredity.[32] Virchow and Müller, for example, had no doubt that the father transmitted traits such as skin colour, deformities and illnesses to his offspring 'through the semen'.[33] As Müller put it, 'the form of the father' had to be 'already contained in the semen, just as the form of the mother is contained in the mother's germ'.[34] They did not find this assumption incompatible with the view that the egg alone functioned as a germ cell, the semen as an agent. Only those who posed the question of the male contribution to reproduction in quantitative terms experienced a contradiction.

Cellular Equality and Difference

'If the sperm is nothing more than an agent of impulsion, how can the immense influence of the male on the product of conception be explained?' asked the French professor of clinical surgery Claude François Lallemand in 1841.[35] Lallemand was a recognized authority on spermatorrhœa. Defined as excessive seminal losses caused by too much sexual activity, especially masturbation, the disease was understood to cause all sorts of psychic and physical disorders.[36] By undertaking microscopic observations of the semen of his patients, Lallemand demonstrated that these disorders affected the number, shape and motility of the 'zoosperms' and ultimately the men's fertility. He extended these findings by conducting exhaustive microscopic studies of the semen of various animal species in collaboration with the leading French zoologist Henri Milne-Edwards. Milne-Edwards is known for having introduced the economic concept of the 'division of labour' into physiology and reproduction research.[37] In

31 Albert Kölliker, *Beiträge zur Kenntniss der Geschlechtsverhältnisse und der Samenflüssigkeit wirbelloser Thiere, nebst einem Versuch über das Wesen und die Bedeutung der sogenannten Samenthiere* (Berlin, 1841).

32 For the argument that the physiology of generation paid scant attention to heredity: Frederick B. Churchill, 'From heredity theory to *Vererbung*: The transmission problem, 1850–1915', *Isis* 78 (1987), 337–64.

33 Virchow, 'Der puerperale Zustand', p. 742.

34 Müller, *Handbuch der Physiologie*, p. 654.

35 Claude François Lallemand, 'Observations sur le rôle des zoospermes dans la génération', *Annales des sciences naturelles* 15 (1841), 262–307, on 277.

36 Claude Robert Darby, 'Pathologizing male sexuality: Lallemand, spermatorrhea, and the rise of circumcision', *Journal of the History of Medicine and Allied Sciences* 60 (2003), 283–319.

37 Camille Limoges, 'Milne-Edwards, Darwin, Durkheim and the division of labour: A case study in reciprocal conceptual exchanges between the social and the natural sciences', in I. Bernhard Cohen (ed.),

line with Milne-Edwards, Lallemand claimed that if in higher organisms reproduction involved two distinct individuals with specific sexual organs, the 'division of labour' implied that both sexes provided 'the material' necessary for the production of offspring. Lallemand wrote about not the engendering, but the 'production of a new being' on which both sexes exerted an '*equal* influence'. Articulating the issue of sexual reproduction in economic terms led him to propose a new research agenda. Unlike the physiologists who, as we have seen, comprehended eggs and sperm as incommensurable generative substances, Lallemand investigated them as organic entities with analogous functions and properties. Sperm, and not only the egg, had to be regarded as supplying 'organized material'. In turn, 'the egg, like the spermatic animal, would be alive' and possess 'an independent life'.[38]

This new view of reproduction, with its fresh perspective on egg and sperm, initially faced considerable resistance. This is shown by the interest in and the extension of Prévost and Dumas's microscopical observations and experiments. During the 1840s and 1850s, several British and German researchers observed sperm in the egg, and the theory gained ground that in fertilization the 'spermatozoa' penetrated the ovum.[39] Some assumed that the sperm then dissolved immediately, and ruled out a material contribution to the embryo, but others used these findings to claim that the 'spermatozoa' were more than just bearers of a male 'force' or 'vitality'.[40] They were also 'bearers of the father's characteristics', just as the egg was the 'bearer of the female's characteristics'.[41] During this debate, the physician Ferdinand Keber not only expressed his conviction that both sexes must contribute 'in equal measure' to the future child. He also, for the first time, defined the sperm as a cell: 'a simple cell, reminiscent of the protozoa … that detaches itself from the paternal organism'.[42] Introducing the notion of a male cell marked a far-reaching change from Schwann's cell theory: new life did not originate from a gender-neutral autonomous basic unit of life, but from two sex-specific germ cells.

The Natural Sciences and the Social Sciences: Some Critical and Historical Perspectives (Dordrecht, 1994), pp. 317–43; Frederick B. Churchill, 'Sex and the single organism: Biological theories of sexuality in mid-nineteenth century', *Studies in History of Biology* 3 (1979), 139–77.

38 Lallemand, 'Observations sur le rôle', 296, 299, 279, 281; Lallemand, 'Observations sur l'origine et le mode de développement des zoospermes', *Annales des sciences naturelles* 15 (1841), 30–101, on 97.

39 For example, Martin Barry, 'Spermatozoa observed within the mammiferous ovum', *Philosophical Transactions of the Royal Society* 133 (1843), 33; Henry Nelson, 'The reproduction of the *Ascaris mystax*', ibid., 142 (1852), 563–94; George Newport, 'On the impregnation of the ovum of the amphibia. (Second series, revised.) And on the direct agency of the spermatozoon', ibid., 143 (1853), 233–89; Ferdinand Keber, *Ueber den Eintritt der Samenzellen in das Ei. Ein Beitrag zur Physiologie der Zeugung* (Königsberg, 1853); Georg Meissner, 'Beobachtungen über das Eindringen der Samenelemente in den Dotter', *Zeitschrift für wissenschaftliche Zoologie* 6 (1855), 208–64.

40 Newport, 'On the impregnation of the ovum', 234.

41 Meissner, 'Beobachtungen über das Eindringen der Samenelemente', 261.

42 Keber, *Ueber den Eintritt der Samenzellen*, pp. 54, 49.

Paradoxically, this version of cell theory soon proved obstructive to the claim that both sexes contributed equally to reproduction. In the 1870s, it was observed that only one sperm, not several, penetrated the egg; two cells, thus two generative substances, of greatly different dimensions now faced each other.[43] How could the seminal filaments, 'so tiny' compared with the egg cell, 'transmit the characteristics of the male organism'? Given this size difference, and the assumption that a single sperm 'contains everything that enables inheritance from the paternal organism',[44] in the final third of the nineteenth century the view gained currency that heredity was tied to the cell nucleus alone – an entity within the cell that, unlike the germ plasm, was of equal size in egg and sperm.[45]

Staffan Müller-Wille and Hans-Jörg Rheinberger have argued that 'the shifting of the hereditary processes into the nucleus of the cell and, with the beginning of the twentieth century, onto processes of exchange among chromosomes can be read as a desperate effort to single out a level at which the female and the male enjoyed equality despite the overwhelming evidence to the contrary'. They interpret this as 'a massive break' in the history of heredity which at last cast doubt on the notion, current since antiquity, that the two parents made asymmetrical contributions to the products of generation.[46] In fact, in the eighteenth century Buffon had explained the child's resemblance to both its mother and its father by interpreting the generative organs and substances of women and men as similar in kind and equal in value. To this end, he sought evidence that 'moving bodies' were present in both the female and the male semen. The two seminal fluids – and this was Buffon's principal finding – were two 'equally active' materials.[47] With this claim, Buffon rejected the many theories of generation that since classical times had envisaged an asymmetrical contribution from the two sexes, including the Aristotelian dichotomy between female matter and a male animating principle. As we have seen, early nineteenth-century embryologists and physiologists did not follow Buffon, but went back to this dichotomy. Even when, in the second half of the century, biologists began to regard the contribution of both sexes to reproduction as equivalent, they did not make a radical break with all notions of sexual difference.

Indeed, research on reproduction undertaken between 1850 and 1900 established that the formation of a new living being originated from two generative substances equal in value but different in kind. To define egg and sperm as cells of the same kind would have meant extinguishing all sexual difference on the cellular level, something

43 Hermann Fol, 'Sur le commencement de l'hénogénie chez divers animaux', *Archives des sciences physiques et naturelles* 58 (1877), 439–72.

44 Albert Kölliker, 'Die Bedeutung der Zellenkerne für die Vorgänge der Vererbung', *Zeitschrift für wissenschaftliche Zoologie* 42 (1885), 1–46, on 12, 2.

45 Wülfingen, 'Economies and the cell'; Staffan Müller-Wille and Hans-Jörg Rheinberger, *A Cultural History of Heredity* (Chicago, IL, 2012).

46 Müller-Wille and Rheinberger, *Cultural History*, p. 93; also Satzinger, *Differenz und Vererbung*, pp. 40–152.

47 Buffon, *Histoire naturelle*, pp. 203, 329, also pp. 67–91.

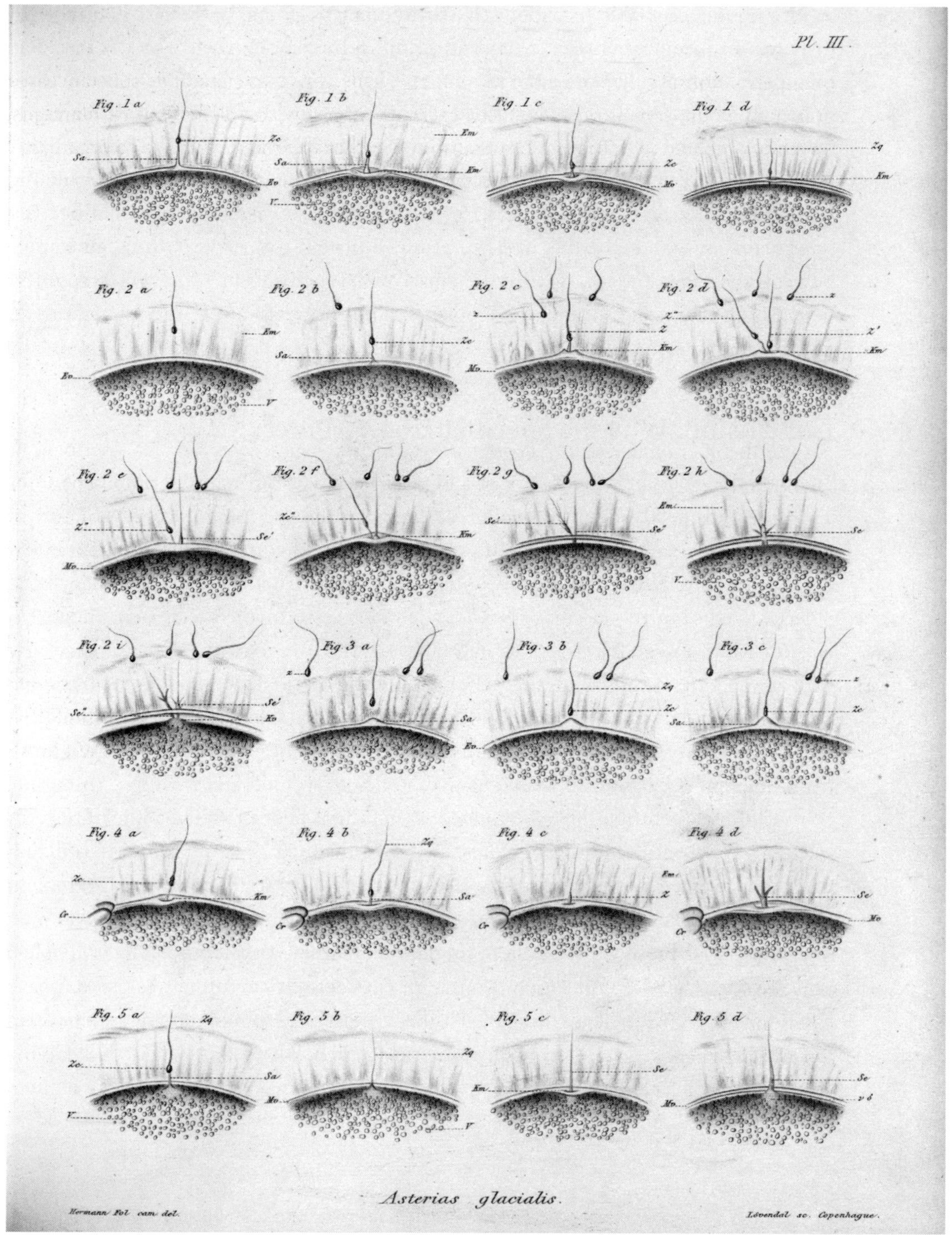

Figure 28.4 A small but agile tail-bearing 'spermatozoon' penetrating the egg of the spiny starfish, many times larger than itself. Engraving after drawing by Hermann Fol from 'Recherches sur la fécondation et le commencement de l'hénogénie chez divers animaux', *Mémoires de la Société de Physique et d'Histoire Naturelle de Genève* 26 (1879), plate 3. 26 × 20 cm. Cambridge University Library.

apparently unacceptable to biologists. Treviranus was probably the last naturalist to dispute the analogies between sperm and animals. The physiologists who studied spermatozoa after him interpreted the movement of the sperm as signalling a special force of life and generation that distinguished it from other organic elements and especially from the egg. Since the 1850s, the animal-like shape and motility of sperm has constantly been cited to emphasize the distinctiveness of the male germ cell and its fertilizing role. An illustration by the zoologist Hermann Fol shows small but agile, tail-bearing 'spermatozoa' – the name that came to prevail in the 1870s – approaching an immobile egg cell many times larger than themselves (Fig. 28.4). Only one will succeed in penetrating the surface of the egg. Similar images can be found in representations of fertilization today.[48]

Conclusion: Why the Spermatozoon Matters

The present understanding of the egg and the sperm as germ cells did not arise out of a single, undisputed way of thinking. The figure of the spermatozoon, as we know it, reveals with particular clarity how various, and sometimes contradictory, ideas about the distinctions, similarities and equality of the sexes can be articulated in one and the same object. Like the egg, the sperm is a cell. This definition rests on the notion of a fundamental similarity between the generative substances of the two sexes and their commonality with all other basic units of life. At the same time, the spermatozoon differs from the egg cell and other cells in being produced exclusively in the male body and containing the father's hereditary material. It thus stands for efforts since the eighteenth century to move from differences between the reproductive bodies of women and men to a materially equivalent male contribution to reproduction. In today's understanding of the male germ cell, however, we still find sperm represented as something like animals, an idea dating from the seventeenth and eighteenth centuries. The animal-like form and movement of the sperm cells is interpreted as indicating a specifically male generative power – an interpretation that echoes the Aristotelian notion of an active male animating principle – against which understandings, for example, of eggs actively capturing weak sperm have had to struggle.[49] Ultimately, the figure of the spermatozoon should prompt us to reassess the assumption of a 'watershed' or an 'epistemological break' in the sciences of the living around 1800. This view obscures the way that, over the course of the nineteenth century, 'premodern' ideas persisted and were integrated into a new conceptual framework.

48 On interventions in fertilization: Benninghaus, 'Modern Infertility'; Nick Hopwood, 'Artificial Fertilization', Chapter 39, this book.

49 Emily Martin, 'The egg and the sperm: How science has constructed a romance based on stereotypical male–female roles', *Signs* 16 (1991), 485–501.

29 Movements to Separate Sex and Reproduction

Lesley A. Hall

The separation between sex and reproduction, through widespread availability of effective contraceptives and legal abortion, the rise of assisted reproduction and the increased acceptability of homosexuality, has become a major, if far from universal, feature of the modern world. Campaigning movements played a significant role in advancing the case, agitating to change laws and pioneering services. Until the 1930s, arguments by neo-Malthusians, eugenicists and radical sex reformers met with resistance from governments and hostility from medical professionals concerned to preserve their respectability. Birth control campaigners differed among themselves and had complex relations with other progressive social movements, while opposition has ranged from religious objectors and nationalist pronatalism around 1900 to attacks on abortion providers and homophobic legislation in the twenty-first century. Though the impact of campaigns for birth control upon its practice continues to be debated, they did much to disseminate the possibility and prefigure provision.

The Rise of Neo-Malthusianism

The Enlightenment philosopher the Marquis de Condorcet justified deploying artificial means to restrain population growth and avoid misery in 1794. Yet it was Thomas Robert Malthus's *Essay on the Principle of Population*, gloomily delineating a tense relationship between fecundity and available resources four years later, and contending that the proliferation of the poor could be remedied only by 'moral restraint', which rendered population decision-making a topic for respectable conversation.[1]

The generally accepted narrative of the origins of a 'neo-Malthusian' movement positions this as a predominantly economic response among early nineteenth-century British radicals and free-thinkers resistant to the strong class bias of Malthus's recommendations. It emerged in a context of proliferating ideas about reproduction, sexual pleasure and the role of science. The Romantics responded to recent developments in the science of reproduction, and positioned non-reproductive and mutual sexual pleasure as the highest form of rapture.[2] Mary Shelley's 1818 novel *Frankenstein* became

1 Angus McLaren, *A History of Contraception from Antiquity to the Present Day* (Oxford, 1990), pp. 181–2; Andrea Rusnock, 'Biopolitics and the Invention of Population', Chapter 23, this book.

2 Richard C. Sha, *Perverse Romanticism: Aesthetics and Sexuality in Britain, 1750–1832* (Baltimore, MD, 2009).

an archetypal vision of the horrors of reproduction without sex. Like the Romantics, Jeremy Bentham, whose utilitarian philosophy was influential in radical circles, saw sexual pleasure as a good in itself, distinct from its reproductive purpose. His thoughts on the decriminalization of homosexual acts (at that time a capital crime) were not published in his lifetime, but he discussed them with members of his circle and they may have spread in manuscript.[3] The first published defences of homosexuality were by Karl Heinrich Ulrichs and Karl-Maria Kertbeny during the 1860s, when the case for contraception was beginning to be debated more widely.

Neo-Malthusian activists such as Francis Place and Richard Carlile advanced the notion – utopian, perhaps even science-fictional, given the unreliable methods available then – that contraception offered a way out of Malthus's bind and would maximize the felicities of sexual intercourse (Fig. 29.1). The first activists were few, and their ideas contentious even among free-thinkers and radicals. The association with resistance to authority, in both politics and matters of health and personal relations, hardly curried favour with the powers that be. Radical publications with limited circulation led the way, although Place's 'diabolical handbills', not merely advocating contraception but providing practical advice, were intended for wide dissemination.[4] As with pronatalist movements, the effect on praxis remains moot, but discussing choice in reproduction did render the notion visible.[5]

The ideas were taken up within the utopian socialism of Robert Owen, whose son, Robert Dale Owen, moved to the United States and in 1830 published *Moral Philosophy* in New York. Championing a self-help approach to family limitation in tune with Owenite philosophy, the book circulated widely over the next decades. Dale Owen suggested that single as well as married women were entitled to this knowledge, following the feminist and free-love ideology of Owenism.[6] He influenced the Massachusetts physician Charles Knowlton, who brought out his own tract, *Fruits of Philosophy*, in Rhode Island in 1832. Establishing a tradition of idealistic non-profit and legally risky self-publication, Knowlton was prosecuted, fined and imprisoned for publishing an obscene work.[7]

Abortion, once a concealed folk practice, was increasingly criminalized: in England, Lord Ellenborough's Act 1803 made the administration with a view to

3 Philip Schofield, Catherine Pease-Watkin and Michael Quinn (eds.), *The Collected Works of Jeremy Bentham: Of Sexual Irregularities, and Other Writings on Sexual Morality* (Oxford, 2014).

4 Peter Fryer, *The Birth Controllers* (London, 1965), pp. 43–86.

5 Simon Szreter, 'Fertility Transitions and Sexually Transmitted Infections', Chapter 30, this book.

6 Barbara Taylor, *Eve and the New Jerusalem: Socialism and Feminism in the Nineteenth Century* (London, 1983).

7 Robert Jütte, *Contraception: A History*, trans. Vicky Russell (Cambridge, 2008), pp. 106–7; Janet Farrell Brodie, *Contraception and Abortion in Nineteenth-Century America* (Ithaca, NY, 1994), pp. 89–106.

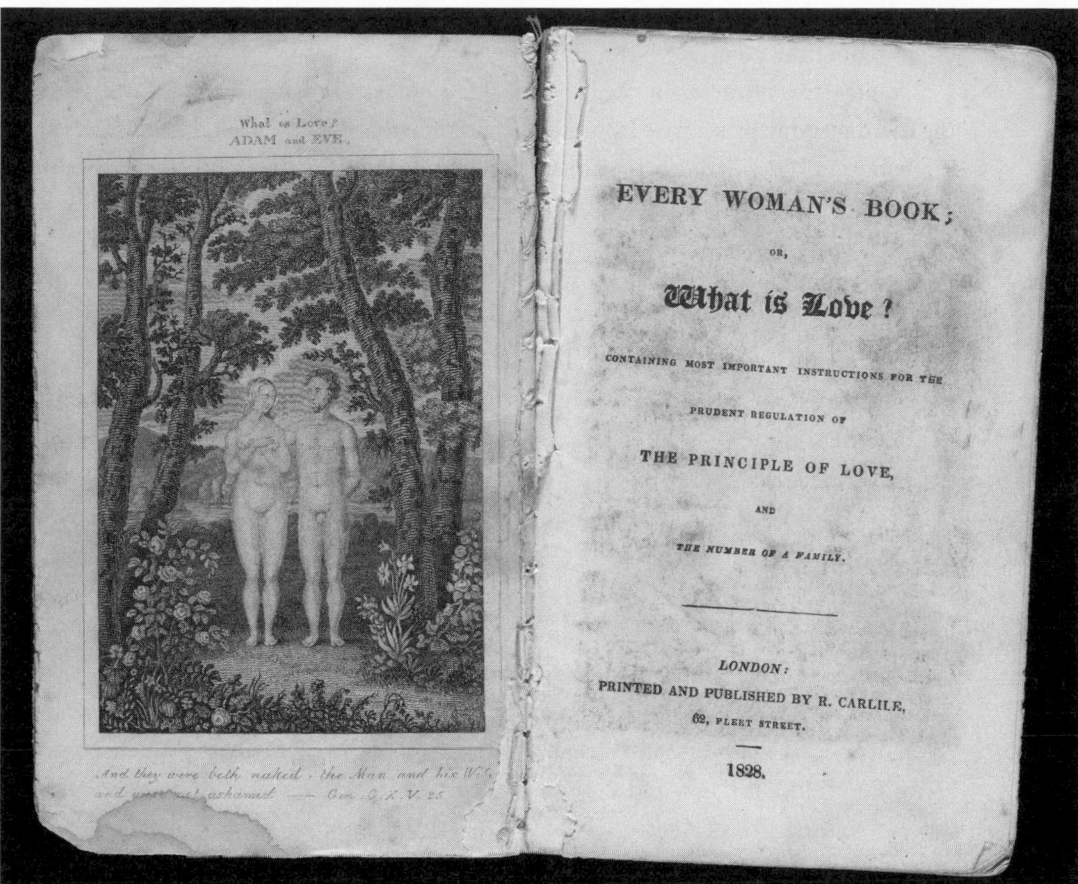
What is Love?
ADAM and EVE.

EVERY WOMAN'S BOOK;

OR,

What is Love?

CONTAINING MOST IMPORTANT INSTRUCTIONS FOR THE PRUDENT REGULATION OF

THE PRINCIPLE OF LOVE,

AND

THE NUMBER OF A FAMILY.

LONDON:
PRINTED AND PUBLISHED BY R. CARLILE,
62, FLEET STREET.

1828.

Figure 29.1 The frontispiece and title-page of Richard Carlile's *What Is Love?* For Carlile, birth control provided practical underpinning for his ideology of free love. Carlile, *Every Woman's Book; or, What Is Love?* (London: Carlile, 1828). 17 × 20 cm. Wellcome Library, London.

inducing a miscarriage of 'deadly poison, or other noxious and destructive substance or thing' to a woman quick with child a capital crime; it also introduced penalties for abortion prior to quickening, previously no crime at all. It is unclear that this had any pronatalist intention. Particularly in North America, the medical profession, anxious to assert its respectable status, campaigned against a practice rhetorically associated with lower-class or immigrant midwives. Contraception, however, was not illegal in most jurisdictions during the nineteenth century, perhaps because it was hard to police, but public advocacy always risked prosecution under laws against obscenity and indecency. Lawmakers extended their reach, but did not prevent the proliferation of commercial enterprises, for which the occasional fine was the cost of doing business. The obscenity laws weighed more heavily upon the activities of those idealistically committed to enlightening the public.[8]

State responses to the alleged problem of over-breeding among the poor took the form of punitive welfare legislation: the English New Poor Law of 1834 insisted on segregation of the sexes in workhouses. Most branches of Christianity deemed deliberate interference with conception an attempt to thwart God's will. Catholic priests were advised to use the confessional to ascertain whether parishioners were practising contraception, without putting ideas into their heads.[9] Medics were largely antagonistic, or at best silent, on the subject. Neo-Malthusianism was associated with lay groups suspicious of medical claims to authority, and most doctors positioned themselves as guarding morals as well as health.[10]

Britain continued to play a central role in the development of an organized neo-Malthusian campaign and the production of literature about it. In 1854, the doctor George Drysdale published *Physical, Sexual and Natural Religion* (reissued in 1861 as *Elements of Social Science*), a treatise advocating contraception for individual and social benefit, and describing methods.[11] He and his brother, Charles Robert, and the latter's wife, Alice Vickery, one of the first modern women doctors, became strong proponents of a neo-Malthusianism which, though still embedded in secularism, was detached from the radicalism of earlier propagandists and increasingly presented 'prudential restraint' as a valuable remedy against socialism.[12] The neo-Malthusian case gained more attention, although with significant push-back from the establishment and hostility even among free-thinkers.

George Drysdale's work enjoyed international circulation, with translations into French (1869), German (1871) and other European languages, including Russian.[13] It was never prosecuted, but in 1877 his secularist colleagues, Charles Bradlaugh and Annie Besant, republished Knowlton's *Fruits of Philosophy* with Drysdale's additional notes, provoking a test of the law. The result was a somewhat equivocal win: the book was deemed to be obscene but Bradlaugh and Besant's motives good.[14] The case did not guarantee impunity for works on birth control: a number of subsequent cases had more

8 Barbara Brookes, *Abortion in England, 1900–1967* (London, 1988), p. 24; Leslie J. Reagan, *When Abortion Was a Crime: Women, Medicine, and Law in the United States, 1867–1973* (Berkeley, CA, 1997), pp. 80–131; Jesse Olszynko-Gryn, 'Technologies of Contraception and Abortion', Chapter 36; Martin H. Johnson and Nick Hopwood, 'Modern Law and Regulation', Chapter 40; James M. Edmonson, 'Condoms', Exhibit 28, this book.

9 Jütte, *Contraception*, pp. 140–4.

10 R. A. Soloway, *Birth Control and the Population Question in England, 1877–1930* (Chapel Hill, NC, 1982), pp. 112–32.

11 J. Miriam Benn, *The Predicaments of Love* (London, 1992), pp. 3–77.

12 Ibid., pp. 81–4, 106–15, 164–81. 13 Ibid., pp. 286–7.

14 Rosanna Ledbetter, *A History of the Malthusian League, 1877–1927* (Columbus, OH, 1976), pp. 25–55.

adverse outcomes. It did stimulate the formation the following year of the Malthusian League, which promoted public awareness. The league eschewed direct practical advice, though several Malthusians went into business supplying contraceptives.[15] The Drysdales' economic stance hindered the league's gaining favour in the growing labour movement, although given the lack of alternatives individual socialists did join.[16]

In the United States, arguments for voluntary parenthood were predominantly part of a broader agenda of sexual emancipation, and a flourishing commercial sector disseminated information and products of dubious value. By the late nineteenth century, as a result of complex economic, social and racial anxieties and the rise of active social purity movements leading to the Comstock Laws of 1873, the selling and advertising of contraceptives and abortifacients was criminalized, driving the trade underground and exposing campaigners to legal penalties. While state authorities tried to suppress voluntary contraceptive practice, some American doctors sterilized the 'unfit'. During the first decades of the twentieth century, many states passed laws mandating sterilization for categories of people they believed should not reproduce. They also restricted marriage.[17]

In 1879 Drysdale convened a neo-Malthusian conference during the International Medical Congress in Amsterdam. This stimulated interest among French and German doctors, and led to the formation of the Dutch Nieuw-Malthusiaansche Bond (Neo-Malthusian League) in 1881. In 1882, pioneer Dutch woman doctor Aletta Jacobs began fitting women with the pessary recently invented by German physician Wilhelm Mensinga.[18] Left-wing libertarian Paul Robin imported the neo-Malthusianism he had discovered during exile in London to France. He published extensively, opened a dispensary to supply women with contraceptives, and founded the Ligue de la régénération humaine (League for Human Regeneration) in 1896. Given long-standing French anxieties about depopulation across the political spectrum, this occupied a marginal position: organizations founded to improve social morality had pronatalist aims, and from 1896 the Alliance nationale pour l'accroissance de la population française (National Alliance for the Growth of the French Population) preached a specifically anti-Malthusian agenda.[19]

In 1900, Robin initiated a series of international Malthusian conferences, and an International Federation of Neo-Malthusian Leagues was formed. By 1910, 'contributing

15 Fryer, *Birth Controllers*, pp. 167–72, 235–6.

16 Soloway, *Birth Control*, pp. 70–90.

17 Daniel J. Kevles, *In the Name of Eugenics: Genetics and the Uses of Human Heredity* (Cambridge, MA, 1995), pp. 99–112.

18 Ledbetter, *Malthusian League*, pp. 172–80.

19 Angus McLaren, *Sexuality and Social Order: The Debate over the Fertility of Women and Workers in France, 1770–1920* (New York, NY, 1983), pp. 93–109 and 176–7. The illustration on p. 390, this book, depicts a poster produced by the Alliance nationale.

leagues' came from Belgium, Switzerland, Spain, Portugal, Sweden and Hungary. In 1913, the American Society of Medical Sociology joined, and by 1914 there were affiliated organizations in Brazil, Cuba, Italy and Algeria.[20]

Relations with Other Social Movements

Alongside organized and articulate movements advocating legal and effective contraception, others developed measures to restrict if not ban the dissemination of information. Most industrialized nations had experienced perceptible population decline by 1900. Allied to the wider political and social anxieties of the *fin de siècle*, this caused authorities to view neo-Malthusianism with profound suspicion, especially when associated with other radical causes.

The equivocal relationship of contraception to political radicalism continued well into the twentieth century. Preaching a gospel of prudential restraint echoed rather too closely conservative disparagement of the fecklessly breeding poor. Proponents countered that workers should be empowered with knowledge that was being withheld from them, and this fitted into a wider plebeian culture of alternative health practice and resistance to medical authority. Refusing to maintain the supply of cheap labour and cannon-fodder for capitalism counted as a revolutionary act.[21]

The relationship between the rising women's movement and Malthusianism was complex. Limiting and spacing pregnancies for women's well-being had long been a neo-Malthusian motif. By the later nineteenth century, women were advancing a strong case for wives to control the number of children they bore. However, in the context of controversy over the dangers of male lust and associated venereal diseases, the active social purity movements in North America and much of Europe argued that artificial devices would merely enable men to indulge themselves without fear of consequences. Individual women might advocate contraception – Vickery founded a Women's Branch of the International Malthusian League in 1905 on feminist grounds – but others wished to promote marital restraint and keep sex for conception.[22]

A new twist to population debates was given by the rise of discourses of degeneration and the eugenic theories adumbrated by Charles Darwin's cousin, Francis Galton – another 'science fiction' with its uncomplicated pre-Mendelian notions of hereditary transmission and simplistic solutions. Classic Malthusianism had always had the subtext that the wrong elements within the population were over-breeding. Eugenics asserted that the 'unfit' proliferated while the 'fit' limited their families, in part

20 Ledbetter, *Malthusian League*, pp. 169–201; further: Alison Bashford, 'World Population from Eugenics to Climate Change', Chapter 34, this book.

21 Ledbetter, *Malthusian League*, pp. 87–119.

22 Soloway, *Birth Control*, pp. 133–55; Benn, *Predicaments*, pp. 182–96.

because 'selfish' middle- and upper-class women were failing in their reproductive duty. This did not, however, predicate enthusiasm for birth control. The worry was that the fit were already too effectively practising contraception, whereas the teeming masses were incapable of prudence and self-discipline. Imbricated in these debates was the continuing threat to public health and national well-being posed by diseases which, if not hereditary, were nonetheless perceived as congenital and familial, such as tuberculosis and especially syphilis. A feminist eugenics proposed that the problem was largely due to pressures affecting women's choices in marriage and that if unconstrained by financial need or conventional values, they would choose fit mates for healthy offspring.[23] Few, however, went as far as Helene Stöcker and her Bund für Mutterschutz (League for the Protection of Mothers) in advocating women's right to motherhood outside wedlock.[24]

Stöcker's league was one of a number of organizations and groups that prior to the Great War already promoted a new, modern, scientific and rational approach to sexual problems in society. The Drysdales were involved with movements for broader reform, in particular the Legitimation League of the 1890s, which agitated for better rights for the illegitimate and sexual emancipation.[25] Such groups, among which there was significant international exchange, discussed contraception dispassionately alongside the double moral standard, problems of marriage and divorce, sexual enlightenment of the young and even the decriminalization of homosexuality. They re-emerged after the war, when a World League for Sexual Reform held several international conferences and maintained national branches of varying vitality.[26]

During the war, two women had developed a new dimension to the question of birth control. These charismatic publicists reframed the subject around women's health, a fresh approach to motherhood and eroticized marriage between equal companions as a foundation of social stability in a troubled world. Margaret Sanger, an American nurse, inspired by her own experiences and anarchist Emma Goldman's radical oratory to open a birth control clinic in New York, fled to Europe in 1914 to escape arrest under

23 Kevles, *In the Name of Eugenics*, pp. 87–9; Susanne Klausen and Alison Bashford, 'Fertility control: Eugenics, neo-Malthusianism and feminism', in Bashford and Philippa Levine (eds.), *The Oxford Handbook of the History of Eugenics* (Oxford, 2010), pp. 98–115; Sarah Wilmot, 'Breeding Farm Animals and Humans', Chapter 27; Szreter, 'Fertility Transitions', this book.

24 Amy Hackett, 'Helene Stöcker: Left-wing intellectual and sex reformer', in Renate Bridenthal, Atina Grossmann and Marion Kaplan (eds.), *When Biology Became Destiny: Women in Weimar and Nazi Germany* (New York, NY, 1984), pp. 109–30.

25 Benn, *Predicaments*, pp. 154–9.

26 Lesley A. Hall, '"Disinterested enthusiasm for sexual misconduct": The British Society for the Study of Sex Psychology, 1913–1947', *Journal of Contemporary History* 30 (1995), 665–86; Ralf Dose, 'The World League for Sexual Reform: Some possible approaches', in Franz X. Eder, Lesley A. Hall and Gert Hekma (eds.), *Sexual Cultures in Europe: National Histories* (Manchester, 1999), pp. 242–59.

the Comstock Laws. She made significant contacts with the British Malthusian League, and learnt about the Mensinga pessary from Aletta Jacobs. She also met British scientist Marie Stopes, who, as her marriage imploded, was working on the manuscript of the epoch-making manual *Married Love* (1918).[27]

The iconic images of Sanger and Stopes as martyred pioneers giving women control over their reproductive capacities, and their role as the public face of 'The Cause', occluded lower-profile campaigners spreading the message, agitating for legislative change and establishing clinic systems. But by repositioning the matter away from the gloomy Malthusian economic model and threatening associations with radicalism, they did make it very difficult to ignore.[28] Both established organizations in 1921, invoking Sanger's new term 'birth control'. Sanger set up the American Birth Control League, and Stopes inaugurated her Society for Constructive Birth Control at a large public meeting in London. They had already founded clinics (Fig. 29.2).

With other individuals and organizations, they lobbied for legislative change, spread the gospel of contraception by a range of means, established more clinics, and began to promote research into methods and their reliability. The birth control movement considered female occlusive devices the best and most reliable, as well as desirable for feminist reasons. While also perceived as preferable to male methods on erotic grounds, the need for professional fitting and pre-coital preparation militated against widespread acceptance.[29]

Advances and Backlashes

Activists differed over relations with the medical profession. With some exceptions, doctors were still hostile towards, and ignorant about, contraception, even if they achieved notably small families themselves. However, developing models of public health, and concerns over maternal well-being, provided a means to engage medical sympathies. Sanger created alliances with the profession, whereas Stopes advocated nurses trained in birth control, who she believed would be more acceptable to her target constituency, a model which never gained much traction.

In Weimar Germany, lay activists had early set up sexual information centres and distribution networks. As contraception became more acceptable, medical professionals lent it increasing support, leading to the imposition of medical authority and greater regulation, along with significant elements of racial hygiene and eugenics, including

27 Peter C. Engelman, *A History of the Birth Control Movement in America* (Santa Barbara, CA, 2011), pp. 23–59.

28 Soloway, *Birth Control*, pp. 208–32.

29 Olszynko-Gryn, 'Technologies of Contraception and Abortion'.

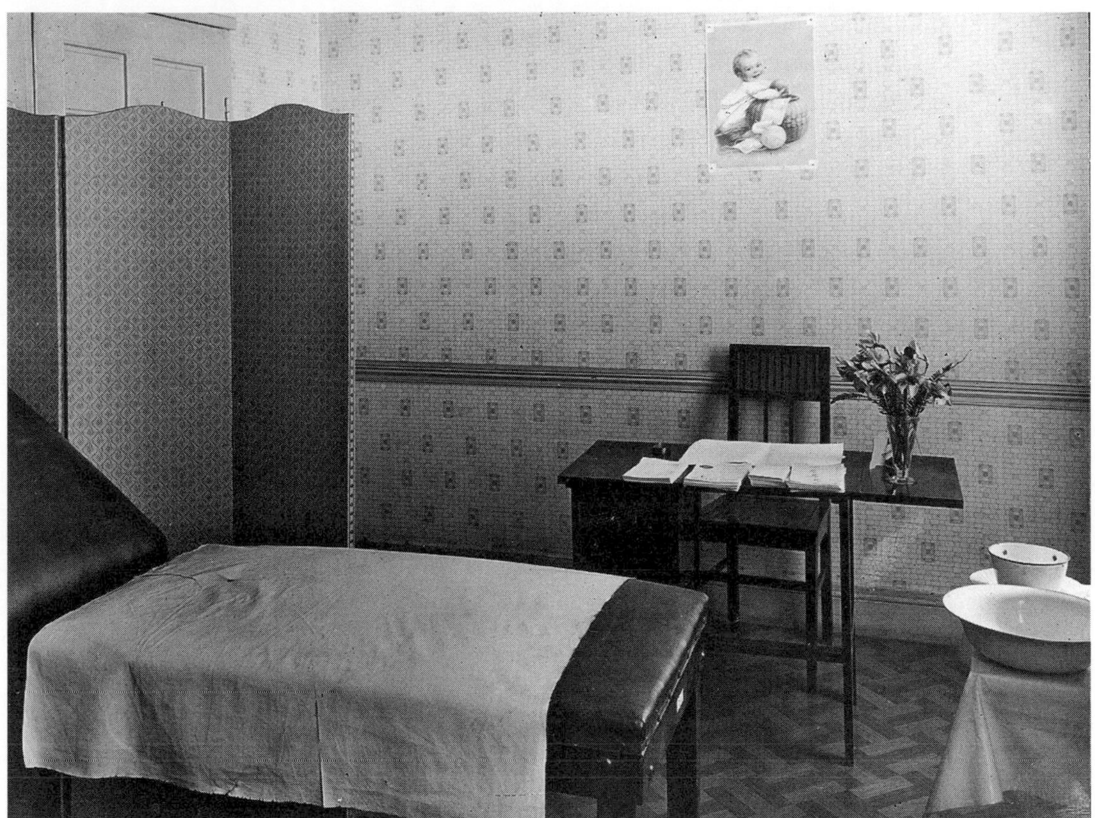

Figure 29.2 Interior of Marie Stopes's Mothers' Clinic, late 1920s. Stopes's vision associated contraception with maternal fulfilment, conjugal bliss – and happy babies. 15 × 20.5 cm. Wellcome Library, London: Stopes Papers, PP/MCS/C.45.

arguments for sterilization of 'inferior' members of society, even before the rise of the Nazis to power in 1933.[30]

A key element in birth control advocacy was dissociating it from abortion, on the basis that the former would do away with the latter and its deleterious effects on women's health and fertility. The legal status of abortion varied in different national and even regional jurisdictions, being permitted in specific circumstances in some and completely illegal in others. Developments in surgery and antisepsis had made it relatively safe, but this did not change medical attitudes. The topic was associated with immorality, even though most women who sought it were married, and with sleazy

30 Franz X. Eder, 'Sexual cultures in Germany and Austria, 1700–2000', in Eder, Hall and Hekma, *Sexual Cultures*, pp. 138–72; Jütte, *Contraception*, pp. 171–3; Atina Grossmann, *Reforming Sex: The German Movement for Birth Control and Abortion Reform, 1920–1950* (Oxford, 1995); Paul Weindling, 'Pedigree of a "Schizophrenic Family"', Exhibit 29, this book. A German march for abortion-law reform in 1929 is depicted as one of the frontispieces to this book.

commercial exploitation. Most countries had a thriving subterranean trade in 'women's pills' of little or no efficacy. Illicit abortion was widespread, both by women operating upon themselves and 'backstreet' abortionists. Some doctors also engaged in this profitable if stigmatized practice. Few birth control activists during the 1920s included decriminalization among their aims. The Bolsheviks' legalization of abortion in Russia in 1920 was not a favourable association for campaigners seeking to make control over reproduction about conventional family life.[31]

Traditional attitudes rooted in Roman Catholicism, and population anxieties, led some European nations to resist contraception, and many experienced an organized pronatalist backlash after the Great War. Even in the United Kingdom, a League of National Life was founded in 1926 to combat contraception. In France in 1920, the National Assembly made contraception illegal, although this did not raise the persistently low French birth-rate. French neo-Malthusians were marginalized and persecuted, though the (Lamarckian) eugenics movement remained fairly active.[32] Italian Fascism clamped down upon liberalization. In 1927, Benito Mussolini inaugurated a wide-ranging pronatalist programme including incentives for large families and higher taxation for the unmarried, and in 1930 he criminalized birth control propaganda.[33] In Spain, the church continued to wield significant influence until the advent of the Republic, although some groups in Catalonia were already promoting contraception along with other sexually and politically radical ideas. Spanish anarchists positioned eugenics as a form of resistance to the power of the priesthood and as a means to ensure the rights of the individual to knowledge and healthy offspring.[34]

Although Malthusianism had been seen as anti-worker, a major element in arguments during the 1920s was the plight of the working-class woman overburdened with too frequent pregnancies, who resorted to the dangerous methods of termination mentioned in letters to Sanger and Stopes and reported by other activists. By contrast, middle-class women could, allegedly, obtain the necessary advice from their physicians. Although the reluctance of the vast majority of the medical profession to engage with birth control would have made this rare, it provided a useful rhetorical strategy given prevalent concerns over middle-class women failing to perform their eugenic

31 Reagan, *When Abortion Was a Crime*, pp. 132–92; Brookes, *Abortion in England*, pp. 2–7; Angus McLaren, *Birth Control in Nineteenth-Century England* (London, 1978), pp. 231–53; Cornelie Usborne, *Cultures of Abortion in Weimar Germany* (New York, NY, 2007); Johnson and Hopwood, 'Modern Law and Regulation'; Olszynko-Gryn, 'Technologies of Contraception and Abortion'.

32 McLaren, *Sexuality and Social Order*, pp. 180–3; William H. Schneider, *Quality and Quantity: The Quest for Biological Regeneration in Twentieth-Century France* (Cambridge, 1990).

33 Bruno P. F. Wanrooij, 'Italy: Sexuality, morality and public authority', in Eder, Hall and Hekma, *Sexual Cultures*, pp. 114–37.

34 Richard Cleminson, *Anarchism, Science and Sex: Eugenics in Eastern Spain, 1900–1937* (Oxford, 2000).

duty. Continuing resistance on the left was tackled by positioning the dangers of motherhood as an occupational health problem that birth control would alleviate.[35]

Birth control movements had complex relationships to the state. In the United States and Canada, the issue was the lifting of existing restrictions on promotion and provision. In Sweden, campaigners mostly involved in left-wing politics preferred a syndicalist system of clinics outside the state medical system on ideological grounds: Sweden, like other Nordic social democracies, was an early adopter of eugenic sterilization legislation.[36] In the UK, pioneers such as Stopes saw themselves as creating a clinic model for eventual adoption by a state medical service, but although birth control advice in local authority maternal welfare services was authorized in 1930, until the 1970s most provision remained through the clinics of the National Birth Control Association, renamed the Family Planning Association in 1939.[37] The increasing absorption of birth control into state medical provision in Germany made it easy for the Nazi regime to redirect this into policies favouring the racial agenda of the Reich.[38]

Becoming Respectable, Shifting Emphases

By 1930, birth control had ceased to be radical and become almost conventional in large parts of northern Europe and North America. Even religious bodies were conceding limited support. The Lambeth Conference of the Anglican church in 1930 allowed contraception a place in marriage, although in the same year Pope Pius XI responded with the encyclical *Casti connubii* explicitly prohibiting Catholics from employing contraception and re-emphasizing the ban on abortion.[39]

Some campaigning groups and individuals settled down to founding and running clinics or lobbying public health officials to do so. Since contraceptive provision no longer demanded extreme discretion, research into best practice and efficacy could be undertaken. The UK National Birth Control Association probably had more impact through its list of approved products that met rigorous standards and were commercially available via retail chemists than through their clinics which only ever reached a small segment of the potential constituency.

35 Soloway, *Birth Control*, pp. 280–303.

36 Doris H. Linder, *Crusader for Sex Education: Elise Ottesen-Jensen (1886–1973) in Scandinavia and on the International Scene* (Lanham, MD, 1996), pp. 105–11; Mattias Tydén, 'The Scandinavian states: Reformed eugenics applied', in Bashford and Levine, *Oxford Handbook*, pp. 363–76.

37 Audrey Leathard, *The Fight for Family Planning: The Development of Family Planning Services in Britain, 1921–1974* (London, 1980).

38 James Woycke, *Birth Control in Germany, 1871–1933* (London, 1988), pp. 151–5.

39 On the Anglicans: Soloway, *Birth Control*, pp. 233–55; on Catholic opposition: Bashford, 'World Population'.

The growing scholarship on individual clinics suggests that, whatever the public rhetoric justifying birth control, they considered themselves service providers whose clients' needs came first. These came to include assistance in cases of infertility or subfertility as well as over-fertility, and marital counselling.[40] By the late 1940s a few doctors were providing donor insemination for infertile couples (not for the eugenic purposes some had posited between the wars), a further dissociation between sexual activity and reproduction prefiguring later developments in assisted fertility. Though never widespread, exaggerated press claims notwithstanding, people now knew that artificial insemination was an option.[41]

Other activists, including Sanger and Stopes, took their campaign onto a global stage. International conferences were held (Fig. 29.3), and from 1929 a London-based Birth Control International Information Centre acted as a clearing-house. Nascent birth control movements in several Asian countries negotiated tensions between a commitment to modernity and science and nationalist movements suspicious of contraception as a colonialist import.[42]

By the 1930s, hitherto opposed forces converged on common aims. Both birth controllers and eugenicists were interested in the development of a simple and reliable form of contraception. The eugenics movement tended to have money and establishment credentials, but birth control had widespread popular support. The concept of 'planning' – the main UK and US organizations were renamed Family Planning and Planned Parenthood respectively – embodied a mindset in which lives and families would no longer be haphazard. However, tensions remained between groups with coercive agendas of stopping the wrong sort from breeding, and those focused on the democratization of individual choice. This theme continued after World War II with the rise of fears over global overpopulation and the interventions of non-governmental organizations.[43]

40 Cathy Moran Hajo, *Birth Control on Main Street: Organizing Clinics in the United States, 1916–1939* (Urbana, IL, 2010); Deborah A. Cohen, 'Private lives in public spaces: Marie Stopes, the Mothers' Clinics and the practice of contraception', *History Workshop Journal* 35 (1993), 95–116; Tania Macintosh, 'An abortionist city: Maternal mortality, abortion and birth control in Sheffield, 1920–1940', *Medical History* 44 (2000), 75–97.

41 Nick Hopwood, 'Artificial Fertilization', Chapter 39, this book.

42 Sarah Hodges (ed.), *Reproductive Health in India: History, Politics, Controversies* (New Delhi, 2006); Sanjam Ahluwalia, *Reproductive Restraints: Birth Control in India, 1877–1947* (Urbana, IL, 2008); Karl Ittmann, *A Problem of Great Importance: Population, Race, and Power in the British Empire, 1918–1973* (Berkeley, CA, 2013); Sabine Frühstück, *Colonizing Sex: Sexology and Social Control in Modern Japan* (Berkeley, CA, 2003), pp. 116–84.

43 Linder, *Crusader for Sex Education*, pp. 171–95, 217–42; Matthew Connelly, *Fatal Misconception: The Struggle to Control World Population* (Cambridge, 2008); Ittmann, *Problem of Great Importance*; Bashford, 'World Population'; Olszynko-Gryn, 'Technologies of Contraception and Abortion'; Nick Hopwood, 'Globalization', Chapter 43, this book.

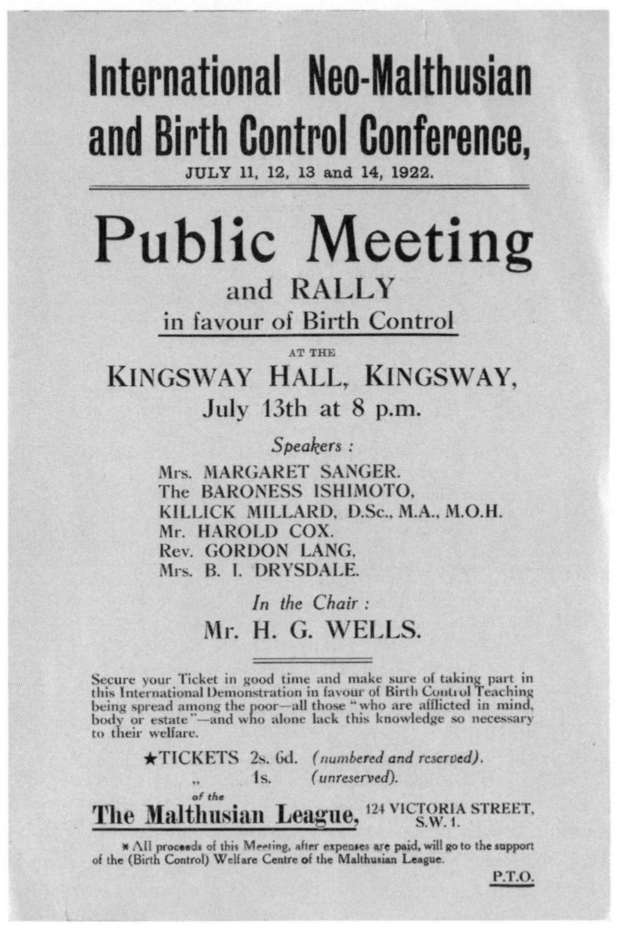

Figure 29.3 Poster for the International Neo-Malthusian Conference 1922. At this meeting, the socialist feminist Stella Browne made her controversial plea for the legalization of abortion as an intrinsic element of the birth control cause. 19 × 12.5 cm. Wellcome Library, London: Eileen Palmer Papers, PP/EPR/B.1.

Access to abortion still varied. Availability in the Soviet Union was restricted under Stalin. An Abortion Law Reform Association was formed in Britain in 1936, but *Rex v. Bourne* (1938), by supporting clinical judgements as to the deleterious effect of continuing pregnancy on a woman's physical or mental health, provided doctors as much legality as they wanted. A number of Nordic countries legalized abortion under certain conditions, such as a board adjudicating individual cases. It was not until the 1960s, in part as a result of the thalidomide scandal and the resurgence of an active women's movement in North America and Europe, that vigorous demands for the reform of the laws emerged (Fig. 29.4). These were countered by the rise of 'pro-life' groups that vehemently opposed change. They later campaigned to repeal or limit legal provisions by positioning themselves as advocates of the fetus: a new development,

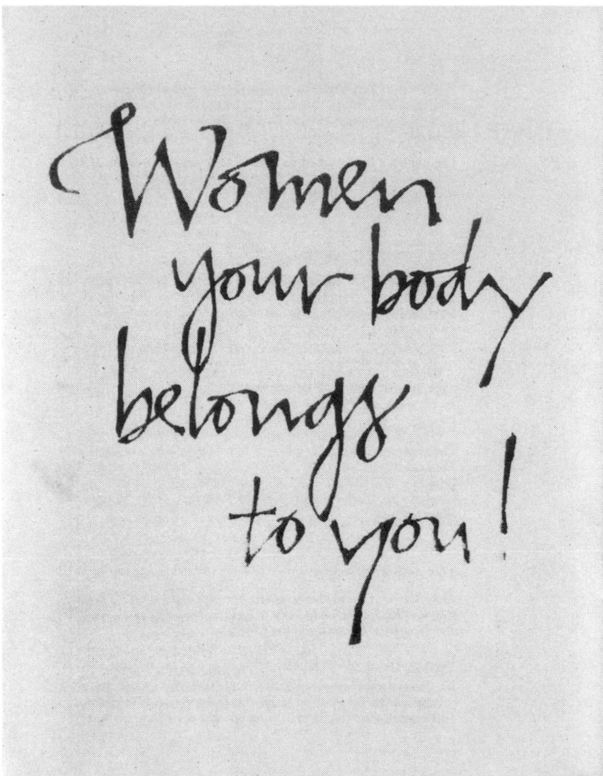

Figure 29.4 Cover of an Abortion Law Reform Association campaign leaflet, probably from the 1970s. Even once abortion had been legalized it remained necessary to campaign for adequate provision and awareness. 21 × 16 cm. Wellcome Library, London: Abortion Law Reform Association Archives, SA/ALR/H.70.

since there had been no reason for anti-abortion militancy when abortion was illegal and stigmatized.[44]

By the 1960s, marital family planning was widely accepted in the developed world. The next frontier was contraception for the unmarried. With the advent of the pill, birth control became increasingly medicalized, but the women's liberation movement and larger agitation for patient empowerment brought a critical reaction. This focused on the safety of specific methods, and on coercive practices of sterilization and long-term hormonal contraception affecting women from ethnic minorities, and fostered the development of grassroots women's health activism. Post-coital contraception and

44 Leathard, *Fight for Family Planning*, pp. 130–2; Keith Hindell and Madeleine Simms, *Abortion Law Reformed* (London, 1971), pp. 95–107; Rickie Solinger (ed.), *Abortion Wars: A Half Century of Struggle, 1950–2000* (Berkeley, CA, 1998); Sarah Franklin, 'Feminism and Reproduction', Chapter 42, this book.

steroidal medical abortion have evoked controversy more recently.[45] Now that a large commercial sector profits from the desire for assisted fertility, same-sex couples are able to engender children through a variety of means not involving intercourse with the other parent.[46] There have even been suggestions that in future the distinction between gay and straight may be superseded by a division into parent and non-parent.

The situation today is thus very different from the world of the early neo-Malthusians. Their science fictions have become everyday fact. Many of the campaigners discussed in this chapter aimed to render themselves redundant, and to a significant extent, their roles have mutated. Nonetheless, in spite of this general shift from activism to providing services or educational resources, it remains necessary, in the second decade of the twenty-first century, to campaign for the preservation or creation of access to safe abortion and to ensure that the availability of contraception is not impeded by the religious beliefs of pharmacists or health insurance providers.

45 Wendy Kline, *Bodies of Knowledge: Sexuality, Reproduction, and Women's Health in the Second Wave* (Chicago, IL, 2010); Kathy Davis, *The Making of* Our Bodies, Ourselves*: How Feminism Travels across Borders* (Durham, NC, 2007); Olszynko-Gryn, 'Technologies of Contraception and Abortion'; Wendy Kline, '*Our Bodies, Ourselves*', Exhibit 35, this book.

46 Hopwood, 'Artificial Fertilization'.

30 Fertility Transitions and Sexually Transmitted Infections

Simon Szreter

Early twentieth-century worries about the demographic effects of what were then called 'venereal diseases' contrast intriguingly with their neglect ever since. After the spike in incidence during World War I, sexually transmitted infections (STIs) seem to have been reconfigured in western Europe, North America and Australasia primarily as a manageable public health problem focused on the control of syphilis with less attention to the non-fatal gonorrhoea.[1] (Chlamydia was not identified as an STI until the 1960s.) The long-term fertility declines that occurred in developed nations came to be viewed as caused by the diffusion of new contraceptive technology. Only for some populations in less developed countries did STIs continue to be considered a potentially serious threat to fertility.

Public health concern with venereal disease increased temporarily in the United States in the late 1930s and in all belligerent countries during World War II. It then subsided, because – with the same over-confidence as in salvarsan and neosalvarsan to treat syphilis in the 1910s and 1920s – antibiotics were initially perceived as 'magic bullets' for syphilis and gonorrhoea.[2] Also in the 1940s there emerged a consensus, soon dominant, on demographic change in modern history, the demographic transition theory. This purported to offer an integrated general model of linked change in both mortality and fertility, driven by economic, technological and cultural 'modernization', a view apparently confirmed in the 1970s by the theory of epidemiological transition.[3] These theories envisaged the decline of venereal diseases, and communicable diseases more generally, as following from rising per capita incomes and advances in medical science. However, no research has ever tested this assumption for the historic fertility declines of the developed nations. Nor has any estimate of the population prevalence of sexually transmitted diseases in the period before 1914 ever

1 Allan M. Brandt, *No Magic Bullet: A Social History of Venereal Disease in the United States since 1880*, expanded edn (New York, NY, 1987); Milton Lewis, *Thorns on the Rose: The History of Sexually Transmitted Diseases in Australia in International Perspective* (Canberra, 1998); Roger Davidson, *Dangerous Liaisons: A Social History of Venereal Disease in Twentieth-Century Scotland* (Amsterdam, 2000).

2 Brandt, *No Magic Bullet*, pp. 161–82.

3 Frank W. Notestein, 'Population: The long view', in Theodore W. Schultz (ed.), *Food for the World* (Chicago, IL, 1945), pp. 36–57; George Weisz and Jesse Olszynko-Gryn, 'The theory of epidemiologic transition: The origins of a citation classic', *Journal of the History of Medicine and Allied Sciences* 65 (2010), 287–326.

been published, probably because of the extreme difficulty of identifying plausible data. After first reviewing the history of ideas about the possible relationship between the venereal diseases and fertility declines, this chapter presents some new research on venereal disease prevalence in England and Wales before 1914 and reflects on the possible implications for fertility.

Early Twentieth-Century Concerns about Venereal Disease

In the history of reproduction, the major demographic event of the modern period has been a precipitous and apparently permanent general reduction of fertility in every national population that has experienced rapid and sustained urbanizing economic growth; and conversely the absence of a similar fall in fertility in most populations with a predominantly agrarian, rural-dwelling or extractive economy. Having stated this generalization, it is necessary immediately to acknowledge the exceptional history of France, where fertility declined permanently from the second half of the eighteenth century, before the French Revolution and before urbanizing economic growth.[4] This produced fearful public discussions of depopulation and proposals for remedial government policies to promote marriage and increase family size. In early nineteenth-century England, by contrast, Malthusians successfully argued for the opposite policies: cutting back the long-standing welfare legislation, the Poor Laws, to discourage large families among the poor.[5]

In most northern European countries, fertility began to exhibit a pattern of secular decline from the last quarter of the nineteenth century; the trend set in somewhat earlier in the United States. In Britain, early analysts included the economist Edwin Cannan, who published a projection of the impending fall in the population growth rate, and the social Darwinist statistician Karl Pearson.[6] Given the series of major advances since 1860 in germ theory, alongside growing acceptance of evolutionary theory, decline in the nation's fertility was interpreted initially in biological terms. Pearson's claims that the nation's demographic patterns reflected the degeneration of the reproductive stock of the social elite were taken seriously enough to form the initial terms of reference of the influential Interdepartmental Committee on Physical Deterioration of 1903–4. However, the committee's chief conclusions and policy recommendations, such

4 David R. Weir, 'New estimates of nuptuality and marital fertility in France, 1740–1911', *Population Studies* 48 (1994), 307–31.

5 Joseph J. Spengler, *France Faces Depopulation* (Durham, NC, 1938); on the Malthusians: Lesley A. Hall, 'Movements to Separate Sex and Reproduction', Chapter 29, this book.

6 Edwin Cannan, 'The probability of the cessation of the growth of the population in England and Wales during the next century', *Economic Journal* 5 (1895), 505–15; Karl Pearson, 'Reproductive selection', in his *The Chances of Death and Other Studies in Evolution*, vol. 1 (London, 1897), pp. 63–102.

as free school meals for the poor, diametrically opposed Pearson's elitist hereditarian eugenics.[7]

Several other biological theories competed in the 1900s and 1910s to account for the downward trend in national fertility.[8] The only one to generate sufficient public interest to induce the national government to commission another official inquiry pointed to venereal disease. The most vociferous champions of the importance of venereal disease were feminists. Victorian feminism had cut its teeth on this issue in fighting a long and ultimately successful campaign against the Contagious Diseases Acts of 1864–86, which had temporarily created a continental-style system for policing prostitution involving compulsory medical inspection of suspected prostitutes and detention for treatment in 'lock' hospitals.[9] By the Edwardian decade, suffragettes were linking their argument for the female vote with denunciation of male sexual irresponsibility and the consequent 'race suicide' of birth-rate decline.[10]

The link with venereal diseases was most forcefully articulated in Christabel Pankhurst's excoriating polemic of 1913, *The Great Scourge*, which also gave prominent publicity to gonorrhoea, rather than syphilis, as a particular danger to female fertility. Claiming that medical authorities widely accepted that gonorrhoea was acquired before or during marriage by 75–80 per cent of men, Pankhurst cited the view of the American venerologist, Dr Prince Morrow, 'that men are ultimately responsible for from 50 to 75 per cent. of sterile marriages … Such being the connection between the problem of what is called "race suicide" and the infection of women in marriage'.[11] Four years later, in his Lettsonian Oration, the senior figure in academic medicine in the British Empire, Sir William Osler, Regius Professor at Oxford, publicly endorsed the statistics cited by Pankhurst: 'The gonococcus was … the greatest known preventer of life; one of its cruel properties was to sterilize a very considerable proportion of its hosts … Conservative estimate placed the percentage of sterility in women due to gonorrhoea at 50 [per cent].'[12]

The Royal Commission on Venereal Diseases of 1913–16 had been lobbied vigorously by such leading medical men as Osler, Sir William Morris and Sir Arthur Newsholme, the government's Chief Medical Officer.[13] This reflected their new

7 Simon Szreter, *Fertility, Class and Gender in Britain, 1860–1940* (Cambridge, 1996), pp. 182–237.

8 Ibid., pp. 263, 269.

9 Judith R. Walkowitz, *Prostitution and Victorian Society: Women, Class and the State* (Cambridge, 1980); Alain Corbin, *Women for Hire: Prostitution and Sexuality in France after 1850* (Cambridge, MA, 1990); Peter Baldwin, *Contagion and the State in Europe, 1830–1930* (Cambridge, 1999), pp. 355–523.

10 Lucy Bland, *Banishing the Beast: English Feminism and Sexual Morality, 1870–1914* (Harmondsworth, 1995); Susan Kingsley Kent, *Sex and Suffrage in Britain, 1860–1914* (London, 1990).

11 Christabel Pankhurst, *The Great Scourge and How to End It* (London, 1913), pp. 10, 17, 101–2 (quotation).

12 Sir William Osler, 'The campaign against venereal disease' (Report of the Annual Lettsonian Oration), *British Medical Journal* 1 (26 May 1917), 694–6.

13 Richard Davenport-Hines, *Sex, Death and Punishment: Attitudes to Sex and Sexuality in Britain since the Renaissance* (London, 1990), pp. 210–44; David Evans, 'Tackling the "hideous scourge": The creation of the

confidence in the capacity of medicine to control the diseases following the identification of the syphilis spirochaete in 1905. By 1913, both August Wassermann's laboratory test and an effective treatment, Paul Ehrlich's salvarsan and neosalvarsan, were available, though there was still nothing comparable for the gonococcus.[14] In 1917, with almost unprecedented alacrity, the wartime government implemented the Royal Commission's costly principal proposal, an innovative and well-publicized national system of largely Exchequer-funded free and confidential treatment (Fig. 30.1).[15]

Demographic Transition Theory

With the establishment of a public health management regime for syphilis based on effective treatment, the interwar period saw the evaporation of scientific concerns that the nation's secular fertility decline might have a basis in venereal disease.[16] At the 1911 census, the British government, perplexed by the headlong decline in the nation's birthrate, had sanctioned an official survey of the fertility of marriage. The analysis and interpretation of this vast body of data by the official statistician, T. H. C. Stevenson, took the interpretation of fertility decline on a new, non-biological track that was endorsed by the independent research of Britain's most influential social scientist, William Beveridge, director of the London School of Economics (Fig. 30.2). Their explanation was the diffusion through Britain's socially graded, hierarchical society of new ideas regarding the acceptability of family planning and the accessibility of novel contraceptive technologies. In France and the United States, with their more explicitly egalitarian ideological inheritances, an even more thoroughgoing sociological thesis of voluntary fertility restriction driven by self-improving, individualist behaviour and the 'democratization' of birth control also became the orthodox interpretation of fertility decline in the interwar decades: aspirations to affluence and barrier methods, or cars and condoms.[17]

venereal disease treatment centres in early twentieth-century Britain', *Social History of Medicine* 5 (1992), 413–33, on 414–16.

14 J. D. Oriel, *The Scars of Venus: A History of Venereology* (London, 1994), pp. 71–101. On the patchy scientific knowledge of general practitioners before 1916: Anne Rebecca Hanley, 'Development and dissemination of venereological knowledge among English medical professionals, 1886–1913', unpublished PhD thesis, University of Cambridge (2014).

15 John M. Eyler, *Sir Arthur Newsholme and State Medicine, 1885–1935* (Cambridge, 1997), pp. 277–94. The best study of venereal disease medicine and policy in Britain after 1918 is Davidson, *Dangerous Liaisons.* See also James M. Edmonson, 'Condoms', Exhibit 28, this book.

16 An official review of the 'causes of infertility' during the fertility decline offered no substantive conclusions on this: *Papers of the Royal Commission on Population*, vol. 1 (London, 1949), pp. 90–2.

17 Norman E. Himes, *Medical History of Contraception* (London, 1936); Szreter, *Fertility, Class and Gender*, pp. 9–21, 262–71; Simon Szreter, 'The official representation of social classes in Britain, the United States, and France: The professional model and "les cadres"', *Comparative Studies in Society and History* 35 (1993), 285–317.

THE HIDDEN PLAGUE

By order of the Government the Town Council is starting a campaign against Venereal Diseases.

This is in the interests of

PERSONAL HEALTH
and
NATIONAL EFFICIENCY

It is up to you to **HELP** where and when you can.
A Royal Commission has declared that Venereal Diseases are sapping the vitality of the Nation.
They say that not less than one-tenth of the population in large cities are infected with Syphilis, acquired or congenital, while those infected with Gonorrhoea greatly exceeds this.

THINK OF IT

These two diseases are the chief causes of-

BLINDNESS
DEAFNESS
MENTAL
ENFEEBLEMENT

Figure 30.1 Transcript of a cinema announcement authorized by Dundee Corporation in 1917. When the Royal Commission on Venereal Diseases revealed widespread infection, the government initiated a novel centrally funded public-health response that included publicizing the findings. Ten Dundee cinemas were approached, but four apparently refused to show the announcement. Dundee City Archives.

Birth-rates continued downwards in many countries through the economically troubled interwar decades, and the total fertility rate, the average number of live births per woman during her lifetime, reached a nadir of just 2.0 in late 1930s Britain. International discussion of the causes of this historic and continuing fertility decline tended to focus on class differentials, now understood as representing the diffusion of volitional birth control and consumerist values and knowledge of modern contraceptives.[18] This was the context from which emerged the influential postwar orthodoxy, the so-called theory of demographic transition. Following earlier French and American work from the first decade of the twentieth century, demographers in the Princeton Office of Population Research, under its founding director Frank Notestein, produced the classic formulation

18 Margaret Sanger (ed.), *Proceedings of the World Population Conference …* (London, 1927), pp. 130–207.

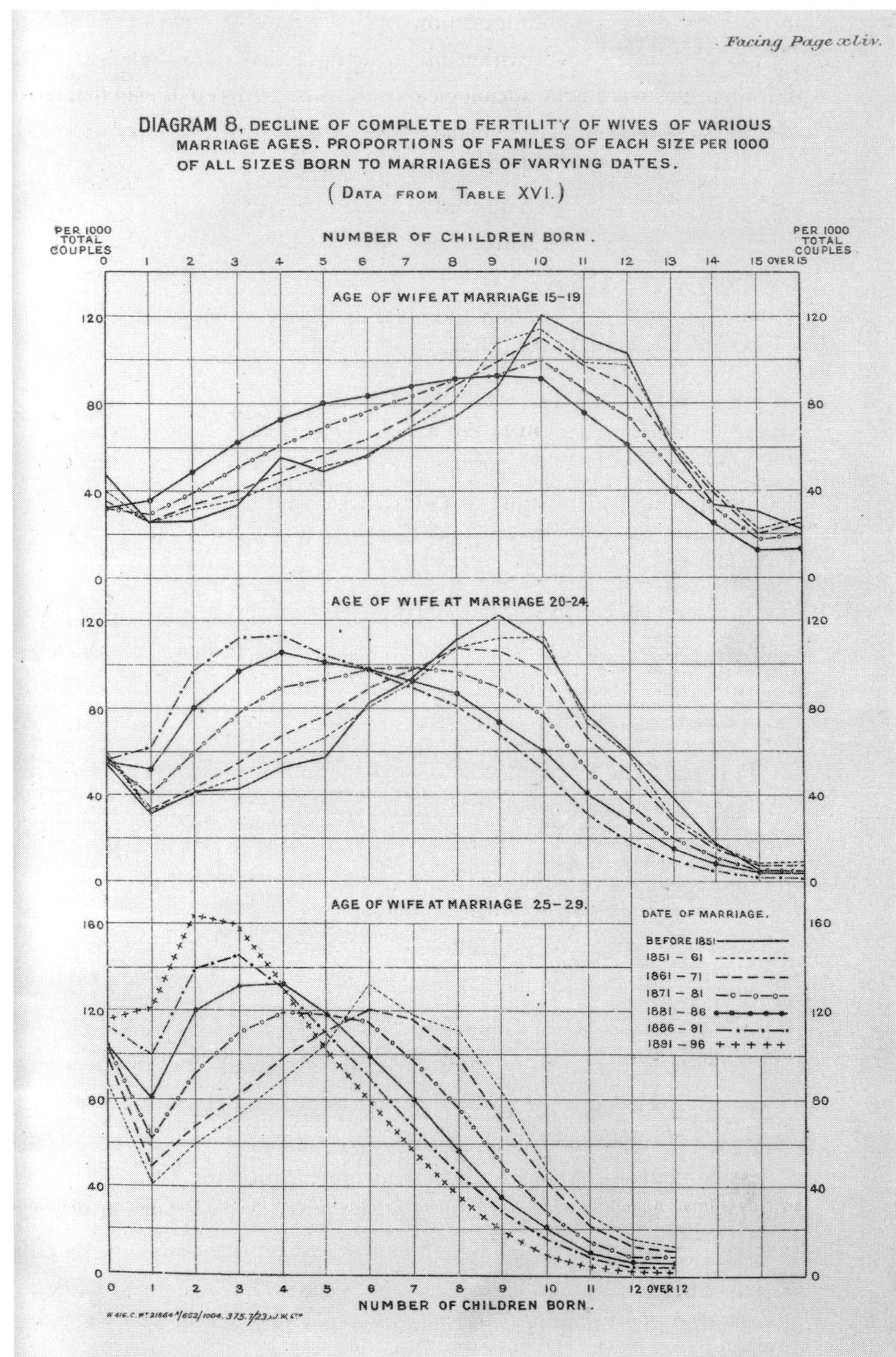

Figure 30.2 T. H. C. Stevenson's diagram shows women's reports of the distribution of numbers of live births at three different ages at marriage and at different durations of marriage. Women marrying after the 1870s reported fewer and fewer births. From Census of England and Wales 1911, *Fertility of Marriage Report Part II*, diagram 8, facing p. xliv. 29 × 20 cm. Cambridge University Library.

in 1944–5.[19] Demographic transition theory sought to make sense of historic falls in fertility by locating them within the general framework of modernization theory, the dominant postwar liberal sociological consensus.[20] This envisaged that fertility declined as a direct response to the beneficial results of 'modernizing' and urbanizing economic growth: higher per capita incomes, increasing educational enrolments, more social mobility and aspirations, improved medical science, greater survivorship of infants and the rise of secular individualism leading to increased access to and acceptability of contraception.

Demographic transition theory was rapidly adopted as a predictive tool with which to devise population policies to induce market-oriented economic development in the world's many less developed countries, at a time when these were being encouraged to negotiate decolonization and become independent liberal democracies.[21] In relation to fertility, policy focused on how to achieve change from a 'traditional' state of uncontrolled 'natural' fertility to a society of 'modern' family planners, as was believed to have happened in recent European history. Within this policy-oriented framework the Princeton office developed the Coale–Hoover model by integrating demographic transition theory with post-Keynesian economic development theory.[22] Using the example of India's future, this demonstrated that a proactive family planning policy was a priority to achieve national economic growth (Fig. 30.3).

Ansley Coale succeeded Notestein as director of the Office of Population Research in 1959 and initiated the European Fertility Project, an ambitious statistical survey of the historic fertility declines in 700 'provinces' (equivalent to British counties) in twenty-five European nations, including Russia.[23] This project deployed a new suite of 'Princeton' fertility indices developed by Coale and James Trussell, designed to track and date across each province the transition from uncontrolled 'natural' fertility to modern, controlled fertility. Following the lead of the French historical demographer Louis Henry, this was defined as parity-specific regulation of fertility: the curtailment of further births (parities) once a target number had been achieved. It was intended that a range of socio-economic and cultural variables could then be correlated with

19 Dennis Hodgson, 'Demography as social science and policy science', *Population and Development Review* 9 (1983), 1–34; Jean-Claude Chesnais, *La transition démographique: Étapes, formes, implications économiques. Étude de séries temporelles (1720–1984) relatives à 67 pays* (Paris, 1986).

20 Nils Gilman, *Mandarins of the Future: Modernization Theory in Cold War America* (Baltimore, MD, 2003).

21 Simon Szreter, 'The idea of demographic transition and the study of fertility change: A critical intellectual history', *Population and Development Review* 19 (1993), 659–701.

22 Ansley J. Coale and Edgar M. Hoover, *Population Growth and Economic Development in Low-Income Countries: A Case Study of India's Prospects* (Princeton, NJ, 1958); Richard M. Smith, 'Marriage and Fertility in Different Household Systems', Chapter 24, this book.

23 There were many publications on individual countries and a summary volume: Ansley J. Coale and Susan C. Watkins (eds.), *The Decline of Fertility in Europe. The Revised Proceedings of a Conference on the Princeton European Fertility Project* (Princeton, NJ, 1986).

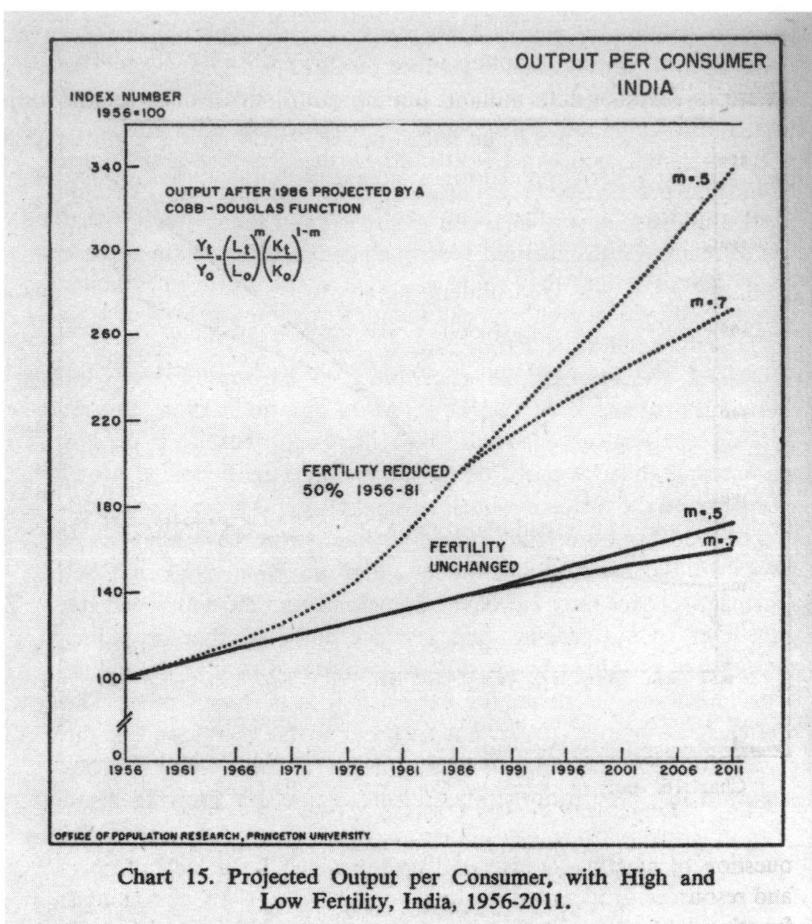

Figure 30.3 Ansley J. Coale and Edgar M. Hoover's graph, which predicted that unrestrained Indian fertility would limit output per consumer (per capita economic growth) owing to rising consumption needs; whereas family planning would allow greater savings and investment and thus faster economic growth. From Coale and Hoover, *Population Growth and Economic Development in Low-Income Countries …* (Princeton, NJ: Princeton University Press, 1958), p. 328. 14 × 12 cm.

these measures of behavioural change to assess the factors most associated with the shift from natural to controlled fertility.

With the widely appreciated policy importance of devising ways to encourage family planning among the world's poor, and the extension into most historical work of the methods of Henry and of Coale and Trussell, the demographic study of both historical and contemporary reproductive change was dominated from the 1950s to the 1980s by attempts to discern the signs of parity-specific family limitation. However, it was also known that levels of 'natural' fertility varied even in the absence of parity-specific control due to such factors as differences in the norms of duration for breast-feeding.

To study this, a separate framework of analysis focused on 'the proximate determinants of fertility'.[24] Most demographers would identify sexually transmitted infections (STIs) as such a 'proximate determinant': one of a number of diseases known potentially to affect the 'natural' fertility level. Yet, while the proximate determinants framework can in theory model the likely demographic effects of a disease such as gonorrhoea, very few have tried to study empirically its impact on reproduction during the modern fertility declines.[25] Since the mid-1980s, the attention of demographers and epidemiologists has been monopolized, understandably, by the more urgent need to respond to the emerging public health catastrophe of the most recently identified STI, HIV/AIDS.[26]

STIs and Infertility in the Colonies: Different Demographic Transitions

If analysts of the developed countries were less concerned to explore the possible relationship between reproductive patterns and STIs after 1920, this paradoxically gained interest among various colonial medical authorities and then anthropologists and historical demographers. Contemporaneous with metropolitan anxieties over 'physical deterioration' of the imperial nation, in 1908 a high-profile revelation of 'epidemic' syphilis in the Ugandan kingdom of Buganda had initiated a decades-long debate over its social and moral causes, raising analogous issues relating to the breakdown of patriarchal authority, here in the colonial context of British indirect rule.[27] During the 1930s, worries about syphilis and increasingly gonorrhoea became prevalent across East and central Africa, amounting by the 1950s to 'a mini-industry of colonial research' on infertility among the Mongo in the Belgian Congo.[28]

From the 1950s, studies of populations in Africa and Oceania began to challenge some policy applications of the orthodox demographic transition model, including its slighting of non-volitional effects on fecundity. Colonial medical officers and African chiefs were correct in believing that venereal diseases had become so prevalent in some populations between 1900 and 1950 that they reduced fertility significantly. When effective antibiotic treatment was finally disseminated under late colonialism in the 1950s,

24 Kingsley Davis and Judith Blake, 'Social structure and fertility: An analytic framework', *Economic Development and Cultural Change* 4 (1956), 211–35; John Bongaarts and Robert G. Potter, *Fertility, Biology, and Behavior: An Analysis of the Proximate Determinants* (New York, NY, 1983).

25 The most comprehensive demographic treatment of this subject: Joseph A. McFalls, Jr and Marguerite Harvey McFalls, *Disease and Fertility* (Orlando, FL, 1984), esp. pp. 467–500.

26 John Iliffe, *The African AIDS Epidemic: A History* (Athens, OH, 2006).

27 Megan Vaughan, *Curing Their Ills: Colonial Power and African Illness* (Stanford, CA, 1991), pp. 132–40; on venereal disease in the colonies, see further Philippa Levine, 'Imperial Encounters', Chapter 33, this book.

28 Vaughan, *Curing Their Ills*, pp. 140–9; Nancy Rose Hunt, 'Rewriting the soul in a Flemish Congo', *Past & Present* 198 (2008), 185–215, on 188.

fertility rates rose significantly.[29] It is also claimed that a subfertility band across equatorial central Africa is due primarily to the prevalence of sexually transmitted diseases.[30] However, the geographical extent of such a band remains open to question, while the thesis of the primacy of the decline of STIs in accounting for subsequent rises in fertility has received only partial support in the most recent and rigorous historical demographic research on regions of Uganda and northern Tanzania for the period 1900–80.[31] Meanwhile, in Oceania in the 1950s, Roy Scragg proved that high levels of subfertility and sterility in some island populations were due to high levels of gonorrhoea; by the 1970s, fertility rates were shown to be rising after the mass introduction of penicillin.[32] These studies indicate that fertility has varied significantly with the prevalence of STIs. So in less developed countries the impact of contact with the economic and cultural forces of 'modernization' could be nothing like the straightforward pattern predicted by demographic transition theory. It could result in an initial rise in mortality and in diseases, including fertility-reducing STIs, and then a decrease, thereby causing fertility to fall and then rise.

New Estimates of STIs and Infertility During the Demographic Transition in England and Wales

These findings may be significant for the demographic transitions of populations experiencing rapidly urbanizing economic growth in Europe and North America from the late eighteenth to the early twentieth centuries. There were no antibiotics in the overcrowded factory towns and mining districts. In most countries, centres of industry grew by unplanned, chaotic in-migration of waves of young adults from rural districts; and especially women's incomes were often insecure because of periodic unemployment crises. These are the same economic 'preconditions' for the spread of STIs as have been identified in many surveys of Asian and Pacific populations experiencing

29 John Iliffe, *Africans: The History of a Continent* (Cambridge, 1995), p. 240; Anne Retel-Laurentin, 'Sub-fertility in black Africa: The case of the Nzakara in Central African Republic', in B. Kwaku Adadevoh (ed.), *Sub-Fertility and Infertility in Africa* (Ibadan, 1974), pp. 69–75; Anatole Romaniuk, 'Increase in natural fertility during the early stages of modernization: Evidence from an African case study, Zaire', *Population Studies* 34 (1980), 293–310.

30 Odile Frank, 'Infertility in sub-Saharan Africa: Estimates and implications', *Population and Development Review* 9 (1983), 137–44; John C. Caldwell and Pat Caldwell, 'The demographic evidence for the incidence and cause of abnormally low fertility in tropical Africa', *World Health Statistics Quarterly* 36 (1983), 2–34; Ulla Larsen, 'Sterility in sub-Saharan Africa', *Population Studies* 48 (1994), 459–74.

31 Shane Doyle, *Before HIV: Sexuality, Fertility and Mortality in East Africa, 1900–1980* (Oxford, 2013), pp. 105–38. Doyle points out that the decline in birth spacing pre-dated antibiotics and was due to better maternal health and nutrition and shortening of breast-feeding associated with improved female education and employment prospects.

32 Ronald H. Gray, 'Biological factors other than nutrition and lactation which may influence natural fertility: A review', in Henri Leridon and Jane Menken (eds.), *Natural Fertility …* (Liège, 1977), pp. 217–51, on p. 240; Roy F. R. Scragg, 'Depopulation in New Ireland: A study of demography and fertility', MD thesis, University of Adelaide (reprinted, Port Moresby, 1954).

trade-based urbanization.[33] No reliable statistics of STI prevalence in early nineteenth-century British towns have yet been produced. However, T. J. Wyke's research has confirmed that provincial medical leaders considered venereal disease such a threat that during the first half of the nineteenth century, several of the largest of these growing cities, including Glasgow, Newcastle, Manchester, Liverpool and Leeds, built philanthropically funded lock hospitals specifically to treat venereal disease. These emulated the London Lock, which had opened in 1747.[34]

Since Wyke's pioneering publications on hospital treatment, a wide range of excellent and innovative research on venereal disease in late Victorian Britain has tackled the politics of gender, bacteriological science and psychiatry, prostitution and poverty, and public health and social policy.[35] The literature on the demographic transition and the associated steep fertility declines in Britain remains disconnected from these histories of venereal diseases, mainly because demographers have lacked robust epidemiological evidence. Yet a recent effort to produce an empirically derived estimate of the prevalence of syphilis has indicated an overall cumulative population prevalence of between 7.1 and 8.6 per cent among adult men in their mid-thirties in England and Wales in the years 1911–12.[36] On this basis we can make an informed assessment of the quantitative impact of venereal diseases on the fertility of the population at that time.

Of course, it was gonorrhoea, not syphilis, that exerted the principal direct effect on infertility by causing pelvic inflammatory disease. It is possible, however, to use the estimated syphilis rate to derive an estimate of the likely prevalence of gonorrhoea in England and Wales between 1910 and 1914, since there is helpful contemporary evidence for the comparable population of Sweden, where both diseases were compulsorily notified. The Swedish data for the two most comparable years, 1918 and 1919, indicates that the prevalence of gonorrhoea among men was almost four times greater than that of syphilis, suggesting a rate of 27–34 per cent for men aged 30–35 in England and Wales.[37] However, the same Swedish data and a single, relevant study from

33 Milton Lewis, Scott Bamber and Michael Waugh (eds.), *Sex, Disease and Society: A Comparative History of Sexually Transmitted Diseases and HIV/AIDS in Asia and the Pacific* (London, 1997), pp. 14–15.

34 Kevin P. Siena, *Venereal Disease, Hospitals and the Urban Poor: London's 'Foul Wards', 1600–1800* (Rochester, NY, 2004), p. 181; T. J. Wyke, 'The Manchester and Salford Lock Hospital, 1818–1917', *Medical History* 19 (1975), 73–86.

35 Walkowitz, *Prostitution*; Frank Mort, *Dangerous Sexualities: Medico-Moral Politics in England since 1850* (London, 1987); Bland, *Banishing the Beast*; Kent, *Sex and Suffrage*; Baldwin, *Contagion*, pp. 355–523; Gayle Davis, *'The Cruel Madness of Love': Sex, Syphilis and Psychiatry in Scotland, 1880–1930* (Amsterdam, 2008); Philip Howell, *Geographies of Regulation: Policing Prostitution in Nineteenth-Century Britain and the Empire* (Cambridge, 2009); Eyler, *Sir Arthur Newsholme*; Davidson, *Dangerous Liaisons*.

36 Simon Szreter, 'The prevalence of syphilis in England and Wales on the eve of the Great War: Re-visiting the estimates of the Royal Commission on Venereal Diseases 1913–1916', *Social History of Medicine* 27 (2014), 508–29.

37 For the Swedish data for 1918–19: Gunnar Dahlberg, 'Venereal diseases in Sweden 1913 to 1937', *American Journal of Hygiene* 33 (1941), 51–63, table 1; on the long Swedish history of venereal disease controls: Anna Lundberg, *Care and Coercion: Medical Knowledge, Social Policy and Patients with Venereal Disease in Sweden, 1785–1903* (Umeå, 1999).

Britain on one section of the population in early 1914 suggest that female rates of infection with venereal diseases in general may have been approximately one-half of male rates, which would give an estimate of 13.5–17 per cent for women of comparable ages.[38]

Modern research has found that in a population of women experiencing repeated childbearing (more than one live birth), about 30 per cent of those with gonorrhoea usually progress to pelvic inflammatory disease.[39] Furthermore, among those women contracting pelvic inflammatory disease, if this is untreated for three days (as it would have been for virtually all women in Britain before 1914), there is a further 30 per cent chance that tubal blockage sterility will result.[40] This implies that 1 in 11 of all women who became infected with gonorrhoea are likely to have become sterile owing to pelvic inflammatory disease. If our best estimate is that by age 35, 15.25 per cent had been infected, gonorrhoea would have rendered about 1.4 per cent (0.909 × 15.25 per cent) of all women infertile.

A final non-trivial factor to add to these estimates is the less well-known capacity of gonorrhoea to cause male infertility, primarily through the complication of epididymitis, and less frequently prostatitis and secretory gland involvement. About a fifth of untreated cases of gonorrhoea in men lead to epididymitis, and about one-third to one-half of such cases result in sterility.[41] An estimated male rate of gonorrhoea infection of 30.5 per cent implies sterility in as many as 2.5 per cent of men between about 1910 and 1914.

Fertility and Fear of Venereal Diseases

Contemporaries such as Christabel Pankhurst and Sir William Osler were thus not mistaken in their concerns about gonorrhoea. STIs were probably prevalent enough to have caused sterility among about 1.5–2.5 per cent of women and men of prime childbearing age in England and Wales on the eve of the Great War. However, interwar and postwar demographers have also been broadly correct that the biological impact was not on a scale to account for more than a modest part of the overall sharp reduction in the national birth-rate that had seen the total fertility rate halved from over 5.0 live births per woman to little more than 2.5 by 1911.

We may conclude, therefore, that while the impact of STIs on reproduction has been significant in Britain, continental Europe and many other regions of the world, overall their greatest demographic impact may have been less through direct biological effects and more through the fears they generated, especially when medically and

38 Szreter, 'Prevalence of syphilis', pp. 526–7.

39 Richard L. Sweet and Harold C. Wiesenfeld (eds.), *Pelvic Inflammatory Disease* (London, 2006), p. 21.

40 The Lund 24-year prospective cohort study, 1964–88: ibid., pp. 70–2.

41 McFalls and McFalls, *Disease and Fertility*, pp. 298–301, 308.

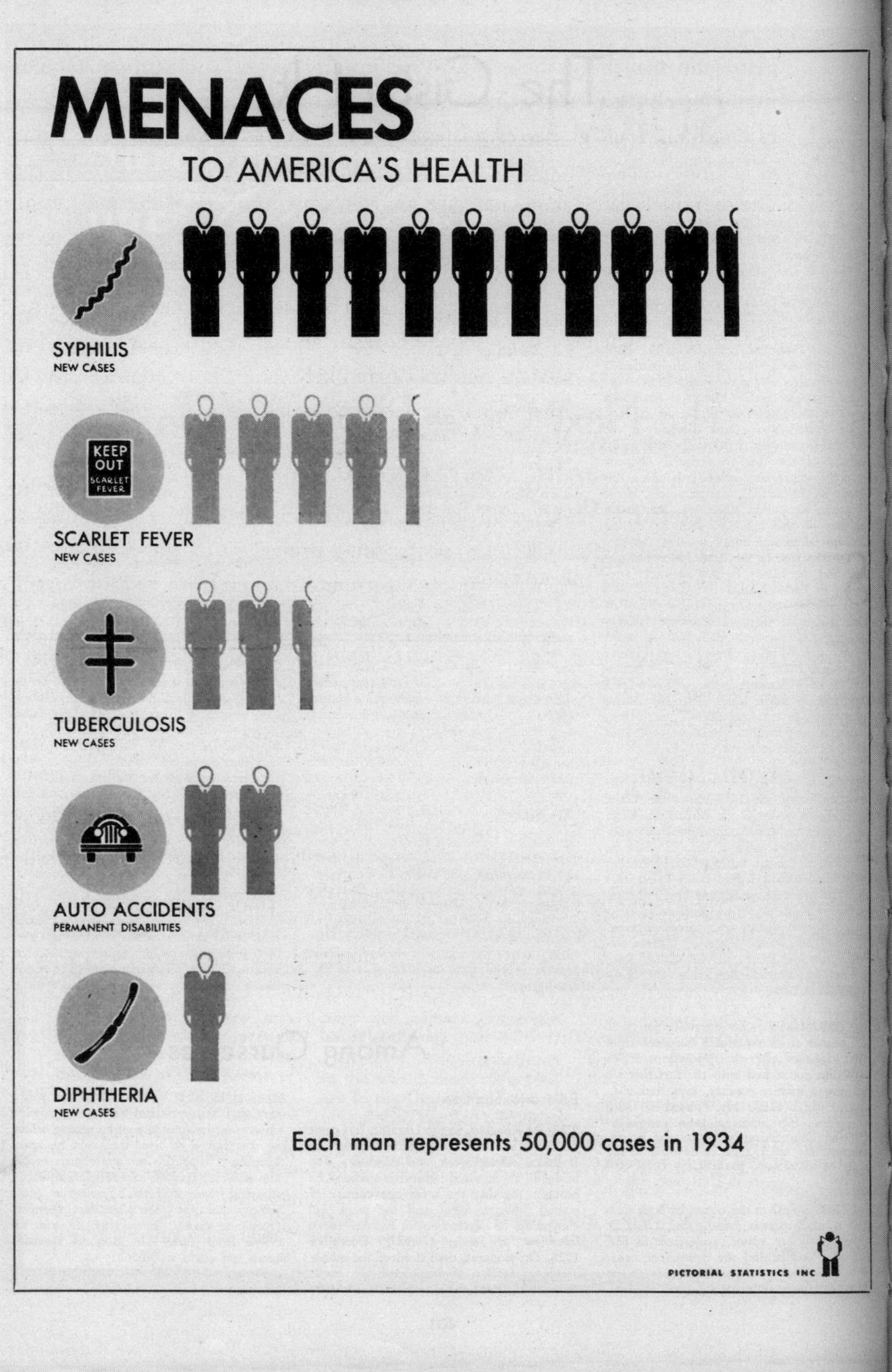

Figure 30.4 Launching Thomas Parran's crusade against syphilis, this graphic depicted its greater case incidence, among the sexes combined, than other serious and potentially fatal conditions. Appearing in a progressive public welfare journal, it is by Rudolf Modley, the leading American representative of the Isotype movement to make social facts visually engaging. From Parran, 'The next great plague to go', *Survey Graphic* 25 (1936), 404–11, 442–3, on 404. Social Welfare History Archives, University of Minnesota Libraries.

politically mediated as these were in early and mid-twentieth-century colonial Africa.[42] In modern British history, this influence on demographic behaviour was perhaps most explicitly exerted by the feminist movement, who warned their sisters that 'Healthy girls enter into marriage without the smallest idea of the risk they are incurring'.[43] The extremely late age of marriage among large numbers of the most educated and privileged men and women by the early twentieth century may also have reflected an awareness of the risks to spouses and offspring, gained from the specialist private medical advice that they alone could afford. This knowledge was often gendered, with male doctors and patients controversially concealing venereal disease from their wives.[44] Subsequently, all combatant nations during the Great War recognized the validity of the feminist strategy of publicizing the dangers of these previously secret, shameful diseases as vital to protecting the fighting fitness of their troops.[45]

With the availability of effective treatments this also led to the deliberate fostering of public anxiety over venereal disease in peacetime, for instance in the interwar United States through the public health propaganda campaigns of Thomas Parran, President Franklin D. Roosevelt's newly appointed Surgeon-General (Fig. 30.4). Several American state legislatures mandated chastity, or at least a clean Wassermann test, for young people, as a condition of obtaining a marriage licence, requirements that were not finally abandoned until the 1970s.[46]

Conclusion

Perceptions of the importance of venereal diseases have been diverse and the degree of scientific and public health response very varied throughout the modern era of population change addressed by the theory of demographic transition. The secrecy surrounding their sexual transmission, and the relatively late unravelling of their aetiological complexity by medical science, have produced a chronic deficit of reliable historical epidemiological data. The role of STIs in the secular fertility declines consequently remains under-explored because of the great difficulty in evaluating their impact on changes in reproduction. Yet although the plunge in birth-rates between the 1870s and 1930s was due to many factors, it seems likely that venereal diseases, and contemporaries' enhanced fears of these diseases, played a significant part.

42 Vaughan, *Curing Their Ills*, pp. 129–54.

43 Pankhurst, *Great Scourge*, p. 10.

44 Jill Harsin, 'Syphilis, wives, and physicians: Medical ethics and the family in late nineteenth-century France', *French Historical Studies* 16 (1989), 72–95. Pankhurst's *Great Scourge* also complained bitterly on this score.

45 Brandt, *No Magic Bullet*, pp. 52–121.

46 McFalls and McFalls, *Disease and Fertility*, pp. 333, 341; Brandt, *No Magic Bullet*, pp. 122–60.

31 Modern Infertility

Christina Benninghaus

What was infertility in the early twentieth century, when science held unprecedented promise and religious belief faded; when welfare states expanded, and spending power and consumption increased; when urban centres grew, birth control spread and sexual experimentation became more acceptable; when experts offered advice on all aspects of life and degeneration was a widely shared concern? What did it mean to be infertile in this rapidly changing world? Was there something specifically modern in the experience of reproductive failure? Or is infertility better understood as an age-old phenomenon that changed little until in vitro fertilization and related technologies revolutionized reproduction in the 1980s?

In this chapter, I propose that the decades around 1900 transformed experiences of infertility. To show how infertility became 'modern', I will look at long-term changes in perception and treatment, and place experiences increasingly shaped by medicine within a broader reproductive culture. I begin, however, with two cases from the mid-1920s. They come from Germany, a society that around 1900 was modernizing at breakneck speed. Industrialization and urbanization uprooted traditional forms of social and family life, leading to class conflict and making space for science, expert advice and commercial culture to shape and respond to revolutions in sexuality and reproduction.

Fighting Childlessness, *c.* 1925

Karoline Homberger, the 31-year-old wife of Friedrich, a day-labourer, was angry. Early in 1925, she had spent five weeks at the Tübingen university hospital because she wanted a baby. She had been treated with baths, enemas and diathermy, in which electrically produced heat was directed towards her abdomen. An earlier test had shown no traces of gonorrhoea, and insufflation of the fallopian tubes – a recently invented procedure in which air was pumped into the uterus – detected no blockage. Her husband's sperm contained living spermatozoa. A second uterine abrasion had been performed to encourage blood circulation towards the womb. According to her doctors, nothing more could be done. But as the discharge notes state, Karoline was 'very indignant' about being sent home, since one of the professors had mentioned the possibility of an operation to cure her childlessness.[1] At the time, surgery was used to reposition a displaced uterus and to widen a tight cervix. Very occasionally, tubal microsurgery or ovarian transplantations were performed. Such extreme measures were not indicated in Karoline's case, especially as an earlier miscarriage suggested that she could become pregnant, but she and her husband did not wish to wait. They wanted a definite diagnosis. In a letter, Friedrich begged the experts 'finally to determine the real causes of her illness especially with regard to her abdominal complaints (*Unterleibsleiden*)'. During five years of marriage, the couple had consulted several doctors, and Karoline had attended the outpatient clinic in Tübingen and stayed in hospital three times. Medical insurance had covered the treatment costs.

In another case, in May 1927 a chemist from Köslin in Western Pomerania (now in Poland) approached the adoption agency of the Child Rescue Association (Kinderrettungsverein) in Berlin.[2] Mr Meier was sterile because of a war injury. To end their childlessness and cover up his sterility, and possibly also impotence, he and his wife had decided to adopt a child of a 'most tender age' and to present him or her to their family and friends as their own. This was unusual. Most adoptive parents preferred toddlers who were already past the most dangerous and demanding early months and showed signs of healthy development (Fig. 31.1).

After the Meiers had rejected several children as unsuitable, the agency found a solution. A 27-year-old office worker, Ilse Gerber, was expecting her second illegitimate child, by a policeman, that autumn. She approached the association's social worker when her marriage plans fell through and her father would not allow her to keep her baby. Since the association had already organized the adoption of her first child, Ilse was familiar with the standard procedure. But this time, an especially elaborate scheme was put in place. The Meiers paid for Ilse's hospital stay, provided baby clothes and chose the child's name. After the birth, the social worker, Miss Renner, assumed the role of the child's guardian and gave her consent to an adoption contract between Ilse and the Meiers, which the local district court approved. Within ten days, the Meiers returned to Köslin with little Wilhelm, whose papers gave no hint of his adoptive status.

Their social backgrounds and reproductive goals differed, but the Hombergers, the Meiers and Ilse Gerber all regarded reproduction as a matter less of chance or providence than of choice. They could rely on an expanding welfare state and experts willing to help. They were not necessarily successful in getting pregnant, avoiding unwanted pregnancies or fathering a child, but they were resourceful and determined and lived in a culture that would support their quest.

1 Universitätsarchiv Tübingen, 317/217, no. 166.

2 Landesarchiv Berlin, Pr. Br. Rep 106, case 369 (all names altered).

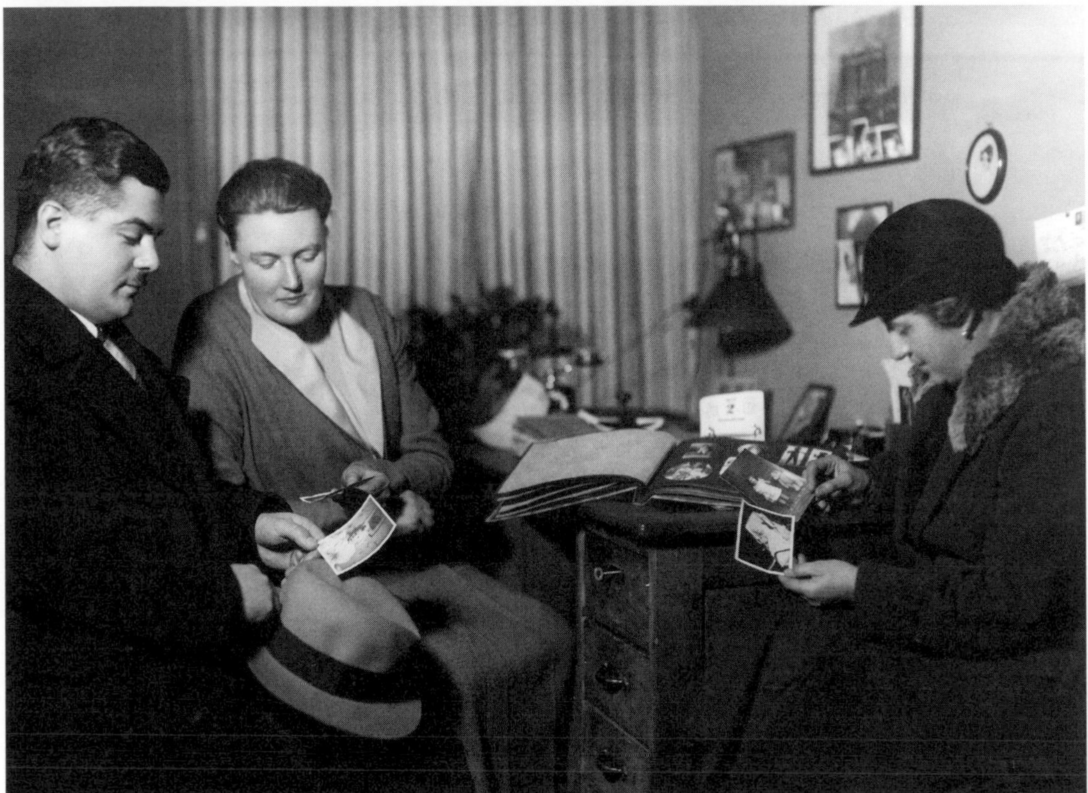

Figure 31.1 Photograph in a fashion magazine of a childless couple looking at pictures of adoptable children in a Berlin agency run by the Landeswohlfahrts- und Jugendamt (State social security and youth office). The accompanying article underlines that plenty of children, all regularly checked by a physician, were available for adoption without a fee. From *Das Neueste von der Mode* (Dec. 1932), 10. Copyright Ullstein Bild / Jenny Schneider.

Histories of Infertility

Infertility may have taken on a modern meaning in the decades around 1900, but reproductive difficulties had been experienced throughout history. Many people waited for years for a desired pregnancy or had to cope with repeated miscarriages and, for some, such problems led to permanent childlessness. Rates depended on patterns of family formation. Statistical information is scarce, but even in societies in which couples married very young, average levels of infertility rarely fell below 5 per cent.[3]

Although unintended childlessness has existed everywhere, it has not received much historical attention until recently. It does not feature prominently in studies of the history of the family, and compared with abortion, infanticide, contraception

3 Donald T. Rowland, 'Historical trends in childlessness', *Journal of Family Issues* 28 (2007), 1311–37.

or man-midwifery, has been little studied by historians of medicine or gender.[4] This can partly be attributed to the political agenda that informed feminist research on medicine, reproduction and motherhood in the 1980s and 1990s, but it also reflects the limitations of the sources. At least in the emerging bourgeois societies of western Europe, those struggling to have children do not seem to have left much of a record about their feelings and thoughts or the often intertwined social, medical and religious strategies through which they tried to overcome or cope with their sterility. Their diaries and letters tended to avoid the topic of unintended childlessness, and the papers of those who died childless were seldom preserved. The subject rarely inspired novelists, nor did it capture the attention of early social scientists. Infertility was hardly ever perceived as political.[5]

Looking back from the early twenty-first century, this silence might appear odd. For decades the ethical, political and economic challenges posed by new reproductive technologies have fed a growing stream of publications on infertility. A century ago, by contrast, people regarded infertility as better kept private to avoid embarrassment and distress.

While personal accounts are rare, historians have tapped into medical sources. They have challenged the assumption of only recent medicalization by showing that medical discussions of, and intervention in, reproductive failure go back to ancient Greece.[6] They have also discovered that sterility was by no means always blamed on women, even if most treatments seem to have targeted female bodies.[7] Ancient, medieval and early modern medicine offered various remedies to counter reproductive difficulties and tests to determine whether to hold husband or wife responsible for childlessness. Conception could be facilitated by internal medicine, baths and pessaries. If infertility was due to an imbalance of humours, to obesity or to a lack of sexual pleasure, it might be overcome by changing diet, moving to a different area or some sexual experimentation. Many medical authorities claimed that simultaneous orgasm was a prerequisite for conception.[8]

4 But see Naomi Pfeffer, *The Stork and the Syringe: A Political History of Reproductive Medicine* (Cambridge, 1993); Elaine Tyler May, *Barren in the Promised Land: Childless Americans and the Pursuit of Happiness* (Cambridge, MA, 1995); Margaret Marsh and Wanda Ronner, *The Empty Cradle: Infertility in America from Colonial Times to the Present* (Baltimore, MD, 1996); Gayle Davis and Tracey Loughran (eds.), *The Palgrave Handbook of Infertility in History: Approaches, Contexts and Perspectives* (London, 2017).

5 For Britain: Pfeffer, *Stork and Syringe*.

6 Rebecca Flemming, 'The invention of infertility in the classical Greek world: Medicine, divinity, and gender', *Bulletin of the History of Medicine* 87 (2013), 565–90, on 567.

7 Jennifer Evans, '"They are called imperfect men": Male infertility and sexual health in early modern England', *Social History of Medicine* 29 (2016), 311–32.

8 Helen King, 'Women and Doctors in Ancient Greece', Chapter 3; Katharine Park, 'Managing Childbirth and Fertility in Medieval Europe', Chapter 11; Peter Murray Jones, 'Generation between Script and Print', Chapter 13; Lauren Kassell, 'Fruitful Bodies and Astrological Medicine', Chapter 16, this book; on obesity: Sarah

To regard infertility as a medical problem did not preclude magical and religious thinking; spiritual and medical approaches had long been intertwined.[9] Zedler's mid-eighteenth-century encyclopaedia devoted eighteen columns to '*Unfruchtbarkeit*' (infertility, barrenness). These offered detailed descriptions of diagnosis and treatment but warned readers that children were not 'a mere work of nature' to be influenced by men but 'a gift, present and blessing of the lord'.[10] Around the same time, the physician Johann Peter Storch, on whose case histories Barbara Duden based *The Woman beneath the Skin*, included prayers for the infertile in his midwifery book.[11]

Biblical stories and sermons, prayers and meditations provided those experiencing reproductive difficulties with narratives about childless couples that offered scripts for dealing with infertility. Even in these normative texts, peace of mind was hard to attain; they regularly portrayed accepting the barrenness of a union as drawn out and emotionally draining. The faithful struggled to derive comfort from religion. Time and again, Wilhelmine Heyne-Heeren, the young Protestant wife of a Göttingen historian, told herself that only God could know what was best. 'And when this has helped a little, and I seem to have overcome this desire, and I visit one of my acquaintances, all of whom have children, and see how the mothers fuss over them, well, then everything is lost again and I must start from the beginning.'[12] Not only today, but also in the eighteenth and nineteenth centuries, accepting one's childlessness was easier said than done.[13]

Infertility and the Rise of Scientific Medicine

During the nineteenth century, religious interpretations of infertility did not disappear, but their authority declined. In medicine, localized disease concepts replaced humoral pathology. For the treatment of unintended childlessness – once known as 'barrenness' but now increasingly called 'sterility' – this meant an expectation of disease, malformation or malfunctioning of male and female genitalia. By mid-century, gynaecologists in France, Britain, Germany and the United States advocated bimanual examination of the pelvis and use of the speculum. At first, this did not necessarily imply a special interest

Toulalan, '"To[o] much eating stifles the child": Fat bodies and reproduction in early modern England', *Historical Research* 87 (2014), 65–93.

9 Flemming, 'Invention of infertility'.

10 'Unfruchtbarkeit', in Johann Heinrich Zedler (ed.), *Grosses Vollständiges Universal-Lexikon*, vol. 49 (Leipzig and Halle, 1746), cols. 1294–314.

11 Johann Storch, *Unterricht vor Heb-Ammen …* (Gotha, 1746); Barbara Duden, *The Woman beneath the Skin: A Doctor's Patients in Eighteenth-Century Germany*, trans. Thomas Dunlap (Cambridge, MA, 1991).

12 M. Eckardt (ed.), *Briefe aus alter Zeit. Wilhelmine Heyne-Heeren an Marianne Friederike Bürger 1794–1803* (Hannover, 1913), p. 71.

13 Barbara Beck, *Mathilde Großherzogin von Hessen und bei Rhein, geb. Prinzessin von Bayern (1813–1862). Mittlerin zwischen München und Darmstadt* (Darmstadt, 1993), p. 140.

in surgery. Inflammation of the ovaries or uterus could also be treated with traditional therapies including baths and the application of leeches.[14] But with the introduction of anaesthetics and antisepsis, gynaecological treatment became more invasive. Surgery was now directed at the cervix as well as the vagina and hymen. The idea that a tight cervix needed to be widened to allow sperm to pass more easily into the uterus, an intervention most vociferously advocated by the American surgeon James Marion Sims, rapidly gained acceptance. During the 1860s and 1870s, it was practised all over Europe. Later, doctors discussed the malposition of the uterus as a major cause of sterility, and women found their wombs manipulated by pessaries, probes and massages, and from 1882 also by surgery.[15]

While female bodies were at the centre of attention, this excluded men and their genitals from neither scrutiny nor treatment. More research is needed to determine to what extent microsurgery on spermatic ducts, electrotherapy on testes and sperm testing were performed, and there is some indication of national differences. The hypothesis of the American gynaecologist Emil Noeggerath that ascribed marital infertility to gonorrhoea was perhaps more readily accepted in Germany, his country of origin and home of bacteriology, than in the anglophone world.[16] Sperm testing seems to have been rare in Britain, but in Germany it started in the 1880s to be regarded as an indispensable part of any rational approach to infertility. By this time, the case histories and statistics published in 1879 by Ferdinand Kehrer, professor of gynaecology at the University of Giessen, were generally accepted as indicating that one-third of all cases of marital infertility could be attributed to the husband's sterility.[17] Female sterility was now also often understood as resulting from gonorrhoea transmitted to an 'innocent' woman by a promiscuous husband. In the following decades, medical textbooks and articles and popular health manuals drove home the message that male sterility was far more common than hitherto imagined and could be easily diagnosed.[18]

From the mid-1860s onwards, the medical literature frequently discussed the possibilities of artificial insemination. To use a syringe or probe to introduce sperm into the vagina or the uterus seemed a particularly promising approach when the husband's

14 Carl Mayer, 'Einige Worte über Sterilität ...', *Archiv für pathologische Anatomie und Physiologie* 10 (1856), 115–43.

15 On developments in infertility treatment: Marsh and Ronner, *Empty Cradle*; on gynaecology more generally: Ornella Moscucci, *The Science of Woman: Gynaecology and Gender in England, 1800–1929* (Cambridge, 1990).

16 Elliott Bowen, 'Limits of the lab: Diagnosing "latent gonorrhea", 1872–1910', *Bulletin of the History of Medicine* 87 (2013), 63–85.

17 Pfeffer, *Stork and Syringe*, p. 40; Christina Benninghaus, 'Beyond constructivism? Gender, medicine and the early history of sperm analysis, Germany 1870–1900', *Gender & History* 24 (2012), 647–76, on 659–60; further: Florence Vienne, 'Eggs and Sperm as Germ Cells', Chapter 28; Simon Szreter, 'Fertility Transitions and Sexually Transmitted Infections', Chapter 30, this book.

18 For example, Hope Bridget Adams, *Das Frauenbuch. Ein ärztlicher Ratgeber für die Frau in der Familie und bei Frauenkrankheiten* (Berlin, 1896).

penis was malformed. However, even the usual recommendation, insemination with the husband's sperm, met with considerable ethical criticism. In the 1880s, French doctors reported hundreds of successful treatments, an intervention into the natural act of procreation which struck Catholics especially as problematic. After several inquiries, in 1897 the Vatican declared artificial insemination incompatible with Catholic beliefs, a ban repeated in an encyclical of 1930.[19]

While artificial insemination inspired debate and triggered expectations, the extent of practice is unclear; practitioners were particularly reluctant to publish unsuccessful experiments. Until the mid-1920s, they often tried shortly before or after menstruation, times wrongly believed to be especially fertile. Only after World War II, when the female cycle had been understood and donor insemination had become acceptable, did artificial insemination develop into a standard infertility treatment.[20]

In the early twentieth century, hormones began to be credited with roles in reproduction. By the 1920s, doctors routinely offered infertility patients glandular extracts to increase their potency and fertility, but these were not strong enough to induce ovulation, and only from the 1930s did more powerful, synthetic hormones come in.[21] The 1920s saw the rapid introduction of transuterine tubal insufflation to determine whether the fallopian tubes were open or obstructed. Together with new means of visualizing tubal blockages by X-rays, more sophisticated sperm testing and bacteriological tests for venereal disease, tubal insufflation shifted power relations towards doctors. The latter could now confront patients with information about their fertility that did not resonate, or was even at odds, with their bodily experiences.

Expectations, Access and Hope

For many female patients, going through infertility treatment must have been an ordeal. Having to speak to a male doctor about their periods and – even worse – their sex life challenged notions of decency. Many women dreaded the gynaecological examinations by touch and sight. Even comparatively safe diagnostic procedures could be painful. Treatments could be dangerous. Yet studies of hospitals and private practices carried out in the early twentieth century, as well as recent archival research, suggest that the demand for infertility treatment was on the rise. In the Tübingen university hospital, for example,

19 Emmanuel Betta, *L'altra genesi: Storia della fecondazione artificiale* (Rome, 2012); further: Nick Hopwood, 'Artificial Fertilization', Chapter 39, this book.

20 Martin Richards, 'Artificial insemination and eugenics: Celibate motherhood, eutelegenesis and germinal choice', *Studies in History and Philosophy of Biological and Biomedical Sciences* 39 (2008), 211–21; on the cycle: Martina Schlünder, 'Menstrual-Cycle Calendars', Exhibit 31, this book.

21 Christer Nordlund, *Hormones of Life: Endocrinology, the Pharmaceutical Industry, and the Dream of a Remedy for Sterility, 1930–1970* (Sagamore Beach, MA, 2011); Jean-Paul Gaudillière, 'Sex Hormones, Pharmacy and the Reproductive Sciences', Chapter 35, this book.

as many as 150 cases of sterility were diagnosed and treated in 1925, compared with only thirty or forty in 1913. The university hospital at Giessen treated fewer patients for sterility, but the number doubled from fifteen per year before World War I to more than thirty after the war.[22] Other studies showed similar increases. These partly reflect the greater accessibility of health care, but not only did the absolute numbers of infertility patients rise, so did their proportion among gynaecology patients in general.[23] In Tübingen, unusually popular with women experiencing reproductive difficulties, infertility accounted for 2.5 per cent of all gynaecological patients in 1910, but over 8 per cent in 1925.

Why did people submit to painful and dangerous treatments? It might be tempting to attribute the rising demand for infertility treatment to social pressures and an increasing political interest in reproduction. Eugenic thinking was becoming more widespread, and dwindling birth-rates caused concern. Infertility experts cashed in on these new fears in the 1920s, claiming that their research and practice could contribute to solving the population crisis. But the 1920s not only witnessed the spread of 'scientific motherhood' and the invention of Mother's Day; this was also the era of the Modern Girl, consumerism and mass culture. For the first time, some people decided to embrace voluntary childlessness as a real option in its own right (Fig. 31.2).[24] Rather than assuming that infertility patients simply gave in to a motherhood mandate, to family pressures and ruthless gynaecologists eager to reshape female bodies, their expectations and motives warrant closer examination.

In the early twentieth century, medical knowledge about reproductive processes – the relationship between menstruation and ovulation, the timing and place of conception, the functioning of the endocrine system – was still limited. Some sterility treatments were based on false theories and some were likely to cause harm, but physicians tried to standardize diagnosis and treatment and valued scientific research. Statistical evidence of the frequency of infertility and its connection to age had been collected since the 1860s and 1870s.[25] To refine understanding of the normal structure of the reproductive system and to study human sperm, pathologists conducted hundreds of postmortems on women and men.[26] Medical handbooks from the 1890s and especially the 1920s cited impressive numbers of relevant publications.

22 Friedrich Weinfeld, *Beitrag zur Pathologie und Behandlung der weiblichen Sterilität an Hand der Erfahrungen der Universitätsklinik Gießen in den Jahren 1918–1926*, medical dissertation, University of Giessen (1927), p. 4.

23 In Tübingen, this proportion rose from under 2 to more than 6 per cent for third-class patients and from 6 to 16 per cent for private patients: Universitätsarchiv Tübingen, 317/632, 634, 638, 640, 642 and 644–5 (Hauptbücher III. Klasse), and 317/662–8 (Hauptbücher P.P.).

24 Christina Benninghaus, '"No, thank you, Mr Stork!" Voluntary childlessness in Weimar and contemporary Germany', *Studies in the Maternal* 6 (1) (2014), http://doi.org/10.16995/sim.8; on scientific motherhood: Siân Pooley, '"Pity the Poor Mother!"', Exhibit 27, this book.

25 J. Matthews Duncan, *Fecundity, Fertility, Sterility and Allied Topics*, 2nd edn (Edinburgh, 1871).

26 At the pathological institute in Vienna, Hermann Beigel dissected 600 cadavers of women of childbearing age: Beigel, *Pathologische Anatomie der weiblichen Unfruchtbarkeit (Sterilität), deren Mechanik und Behandlung* (Braunschweig, 1878).

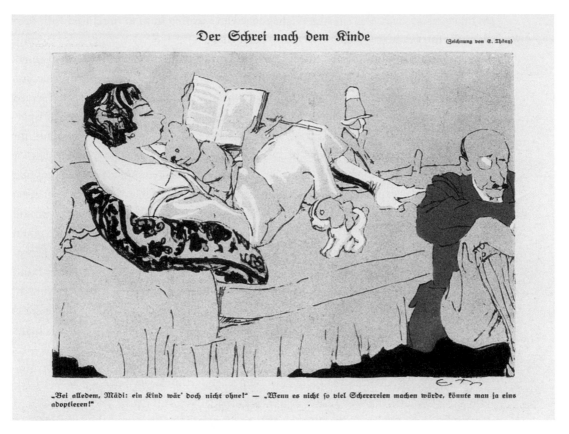

Figure 31.2 Caricature from a satirical magazine. By the mid-1920s, 'new women' could be shown as happy to hold teddies or pets, but unwilling to fulfil a partner's 'cry for a child'. Even adoption would 'take too much trouble'. From *Simplicissimus* 32 (13 Feb. 1928), 619, courtesy of Herzogin Anna Amalia Bibliothek Weimar and by kind permission of Dr Dagmar von Kessel, Munich.

It is not clear to what extent infertility patients were aware of these developments, but they certainly knew that scientific medicine was making progress. The rise in diagnostic possibilities, thanks to bacteriology and the invention of X-rays and other instruments, enhanced the authority of doctors and boosted patients' expectations, even if treatment lagged behind diagnosis. A negative prognosis could at least provide a starting point for considering alternative routes to parenthood. In German law, couples who wanted to adopt had to be childless and over 50, but during the Weimar Republic those who had not reached that age could adopt if a doctor certified that they were believed to be sterile. Other possible solutions included divorce and remarriage or an extra-marital affair. Such emotionally fraught and socially daring strategies were not new, but they could now be guided by expert advice. As hospital case records from the early 1930s reveal, some married women asked for an assessment of their fertility because they wanted to make sure that they could get pregnant with a different partner.

In other cases, advice was already sought before the wedding so as to minimize the risk of reproductive failure.[27]

Sims did not investigate whether or not his 'uterine surgery' had worked, as Elaine Tyler May, Margaret Marsh and Wanda Ronner have pointed out, but many gynaecologists involved in infertility diagnosis did attempt follow-up studies analogous to those performed for cancer treatment. Kehrer contacted former patients to find out whether his cervical operations had helped to relieve painful menstruations and promote fertility. In the early twentieth century, larger follow-up studies became common, with rather encouraging results. For instance, of 173 patients treated for infertility at Giessen university hospital between 1905 and 1918, 109 were later tracked down to participate in a study, and of these, 42 (or 38.5 per cent) had become pregnant after their treatment.[28] Most reports were less positive, but could still claim success rates of 25 per cent.[29] Physicians knew that not all of these pregnancies could be attributed to the treatment, but with the increase in numbers of patients and of procedures, ever more women became pregnant after receiving infertility treatments of one kind or another. For them, these were technologies of hope.[30]

Modern Bodies, Expert Advice and Reproductive Choices

Karoline and Friedrich Homberger trusted in medicine, and those couples who decided to embark on medical treatment often appear determined, in Germany as at a London hospital.[31] These patients' knowledge and trust had been fostered by a plethora of publications, exhibitions and talks which for decades had trumpeted the usefulness of science, including physiology and anatomy.[32] The international exhibitions organized by the German Hygiene Museum in 1911 and 1930 drew millions of visitors. Alongside touring exhibitions, brochures, books, slide shows and soon also films, they popularized biological knowledge. They also introduced the public to the complexities of diagnostic techniques including the chemical analysis of urine and staining methods used in bacteriology. Images relating to female disorders suggested that gynaecologists could diagnose a whole array of different ailments simply by knowing how to look, for example, at the cervix through a speculum (Fig. 31.3). Unlike wax models showing the signs and effects of venereal disease, such images did not teach ordinary people to spot disease in a potential

27 Universitätsarchiv Tübingen, 317/853, nos. 126 and 209.

28 Alexander Kapp, *Beiträge zur Frage der weiblichen Sterilität und deren Behandlung* (Giessen, 1921).

29 For example, Gertrud Förstner, *Über Ursachen und Behandlung primärer Sterilität*, medical dissertation, University of Tübingen (1930).

30 For a comparable argument for cancer: Ilana Löwy, '"Because of their praiseworthy modesty, they consult too late": Regime of hope and cancer of the womb, 1800–1910', *Bulletin of the History of Medicine* 85 (2011), 356–83.

31 Pfeffer, *Stork and Syringe*, p. 45.

32 Most recently: Sybilla Nikolow (ed.), *Erkenne Dich Selbst! Strategien der Sichtbarmachung des Körpers im 20. Jahrhundert* (Cologne, 2015).

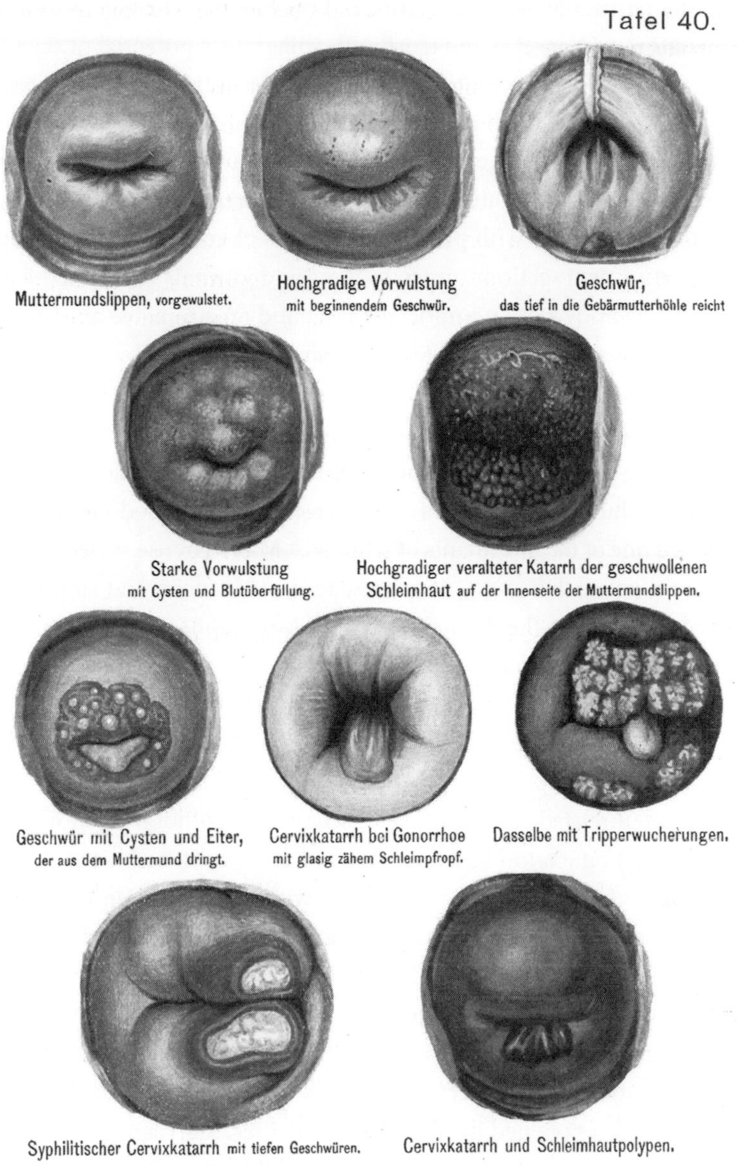

Figure 31.3 'The cervix showing various forms of catarrh' in a plate from Jenny Springer's popular health manual *Die Ärztin im Hause* (The woman doctor in the home). First published in 1910, it had sold some half-million copies by 1930. This illustration, plate 40 in an edition issued by Groh of Dresden in 1911, offered readers an unfamiliar view usually reserved to doctors: the cervix 'seen through the speculum'.

sexual partner or themselves, nor did they work as deterrents. Rather, they served as an invitation to marvel at and trust in the diagnostic potential of scientific medicine.

Bodies as represented within the health advice literature around 1900 were legible and malleable. Drawings explained how contraceptives needed to be inserted or how a pessary could change the position of the womb; they showed hands and instruments in the act of manipulating the body (Fig. 31.4). During the Weimar Republic such illustrations resonated with prominent images of enhancement through diets and sports.[33] Advertisement sections of newspapers and journals reflected the growing belief that an attractive body was an important asset and an attainable aim.

Experiences of infertility were shaped not only by medicine and concepts of the body, but also by changing attitudes to reproduction. In the early twentieth century, average family size fell while childlessness rose. Some of this increase might have been due to mounting infertility, but a growing number of couples did not want children at all or at least not during the first years of marriage. 'We have a modern marriage, we don't need kids', replied one of the informants of sexologist Max Marcuse.[34] Demographic studies show that some nineteenth-century couples spaced pregnancies and stopped having children once they had reached the desired number.[35] Around 1900, and within one generation, average numbers of children halved as even the working classes embraced the two-child ideal.

With many couples practising birth control or resorting to abortion, those experiencing reproductive difficulties also tried to create the families they wanted. Countries throughout Europe passed modern adoption laws, as more and more couples decided to raise an unrelated child. *Wahlelternschaft* – parenthood by choice – created nuclear families based on emotional ties, and is not to be confused with existing forms of fostering, in which children in need were placed with family or friends or with foster mothers who sought an extra income but usually had biological children themselves. As agency records indicate, some couples considering adoption approached their project as frankly as their peers who decided to keep their families small. Often impatient, adoptive parents expected to be given a choice, and adoption agencies promised to offer only quality children.[36]

By the 1920s, expert advice was becoming common in everyday life. Marriage advice centres opened in many German cities. Marriage guides promised better sex and

33 Michael Hau, *The Cult of Health and Beauty in Germany: A Social History, 1890–1930* (Chicago, IL, 2003).

34 Max Marcuse, *Der Eheliche Präventivverkehr, seine Verbreitung, Verursachung und Methodik. Dargestellt und beleuchtet an 300 Ehen* (Stuttgart, 1917), p. 23.

35 Philip Kreager, 'Where are the children?', in Kreager and Elisabeth Schröder-Butterfill (eds.), *Ageing Without Children: European and Asian Perspectives* (New York, NY, 2004), pp. 1–47; Szreter, 'Fertility Transitions and Sexually Transmitted Infections'.

36 On Britain and the United States: Jenny Keating, *A Child for Keeps: The History of Adoption in England, 1918–45* (Basingstoke, 2009); Deborah Cohen, *Family Secrets: Living with Shame from the Victorians to the Present Day* (London, 2013); Ellen Herman, *Kinship by Design: A History of Adoption in the Modern United States* (Chicago, IL, 2008). Compare adult adoption in antiquity: Tim Parkin, 'The Ancient Family and the Law', Chapter 6, this book.

674 *WOMB, MASSAGE OF*

developed and continued and violent pains of menstruation are removed, or at least mitigated. This massage of the uterus is extended over a period of five to ten minutes, the patient lying on her back with the legs and thighs flexed. The operator is sitting by her side. The sittings should be repeated three to six times per week for a period of one, two or even three months. If it is only a matter of improvement and invigoration of tissue change, a treatment of a few weeks will usually suffice. In the presence of adhesions, however, and distinct displacement, a longer period of treatment is necessary. This massage is very difficult and requires extensive physiological and anatomical knowledge, and ought, therefore, only to be performed by experienced physicians and with the greatest care. Since this form of treatment, when performed by male physicians, is very offensive to womanly delicacy, it is naturally creating a want for more female physicians; it ought to be one of the principal duties of female physicians to master just these methods of healing. Fig. 328 shows the position of the patient during massage and Figs. 329 and 330 the position of the hands of the physician, and the method of influencing the uterus through the same.

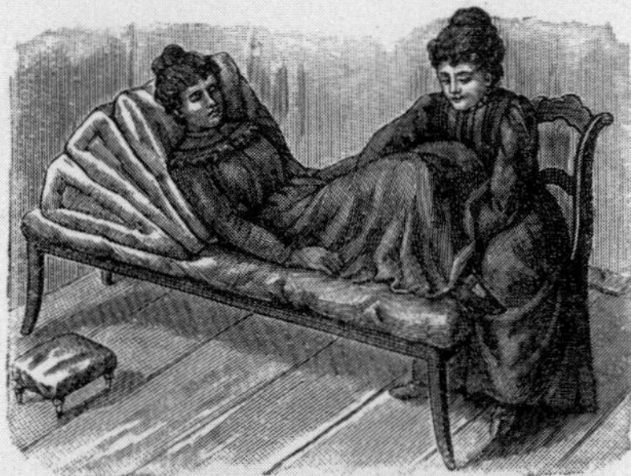

Fig. 328. Position for examination and massage. (Thure-Brandt.)

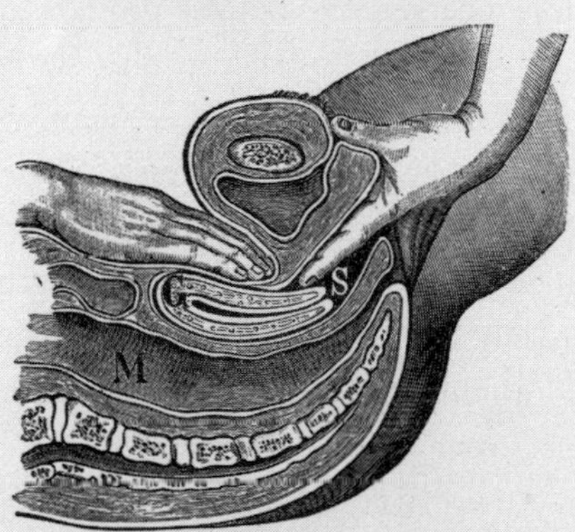

Fig. 329. Massage of the womb. M—Rectum. G—Womb. S—Vagina. Massage of the anterior wall of the womb, before reposition.

Figure 31.4 'A course of massage treatments', one of the most popular health advice books suggested, could increase 'the capacity to conceive on the part of a previously indolent uterus'. First published in 1901 and translated from German into several languages, this manual sold millions. From Anna Fischer-Dueckelmann, *The Wife as the Family Physician …* (Milwaukee, WI: International Medical Book Co., 1908), p. 674. 24 × 17 cm. Cambridge University Library.

marital bliss. Just as tests told school leavers which profession would suit them, so couples considering adoption hoped to be 'matched' with children who would fit into their families.[37] Those suffering reproductive difficulties had reason to expect expert help.

In Vitro Fertilization: A Revolution?

Historical change – however revolutionary – always relies on long-term continuities and recurrent phenomena. Even cutting-edge research in science and medicine builds on established knowledge, and on routines, instruments and institutions. While new technologies can produce or accelerate social change, they may also match, mirror or embody longer-term developments that are as hard to pinpoint as changes in mentalities.

For infertility, in vitro fertilization (IVF) has, despite its uncertain outcomes, often been presented as a watershed, ushering in a 'new era of reproductive intervention and management'. 'Rather than being a hopeless condition, infertility has become subject to a new order, in which conception is something that can be *achieved*.'[38] Yet decades before the advent of IVF, couples hoping to overcome their reproductive difficulties looked to medicine and insisted on the best available treatment. Those visible in hospital records and medical case histories embarked on veritable projects to overcome their infertility. The Hombergers and their peers, who often consulted several doctors and repeatedly returned to access new forms of diagnosis and treatment, apparently already saw their quest for a child as something like an obstacle course. Their expectations matched the promises of popular medicine and the more general reconceptualization of reproduction as a matter of choice and design that was at the root of eugenics and informed contemporary thinking more broadly.[39] The rise of the welfare state brought fertility diagnosis and infertility treatment, including sperm testing and tubal insufflation, surgery, hormonal treatment and artificial insemination, as well as expert-led adoptions, increasingly within reach. The widespread use of contraception, public engagement with eugenic ideas and newly institutionalized forms of adoption all worked with an understanding of reproduction as a matter of design and expert advice. The swift normalization of IVF has puzzled sociologists, but in historical perspective, IVF was made possible by a long-term association of reproduction, medicine and a culture of choice and design that had been fundamental to modernity since the early twentieth century.

37 Ellen Herman, 'Technologies of Adoption Matching', Exhibit 33, this book.

38 Sarah Franklin, *The Reproductive Revolution: How Far Have We Come?* (London, 2008), p. 9. Further on IVF: Hopwood, 'Artificial Fertilization'; Nick Hopwood, '"It's a Girl"', Exhibit 38, this book.

39 Angus McLaren, *Reproduction by Design: Sex, Robots, Trees, and Test-Tube Babies in Interwar Britain* (Chicago, IL, 2012). On the appropriation of biopolitical thinking: Edward Ross Dickinson, 'Biopolitics, fascism, democracy: Some reflections on our discourse about "modernity"', *Central European History* 37 (2004), 1–48.

32 Modern Ignorance

Kate Fisher

Sexual Ignorance, a Modern Invention

The past three centuries have seen significant changes in what people know about sex, reproduction and birth control and how they know it. Medical understandings and approaches have been transformed. Innovations in literary, print and media cultures, and a proliferation of material, including cheap pornography, newspapers and books, have provided a wide variety of ways of learning about sex and reproduction. In the last century, when film, television and digital media added yet more means of consuming knowledge, the perception became common of a sudden and profound shift. Histories frequently characterize the western world prior to the revolution of the 1960s as mired in sexual and reproductive ignorance.[1] Despite widespread acceptance of Michel Foucault's re-evaluation of the 'repression' of sexuality in the nineteenth century as a process through which sex was inserted into social and cultural life, historians have pointed out how regulations and restrictions left many unaware or confused.[2] Powerful stories demonstrate the effect of deep ignorance on sexual and reproductive lives. Disastrous wedding nights, for example, figure regularly in history and fiction. Think of John Ruskin and Effie Gray in 1848, or Edward Mayhew and Florence Ponting in Ian McEwan's *On Chesil Beach*, set in 1962.[3]

To conceptualize knowledge of sex and reproduction as requiring a journey out of ignorance derives from a distinctively modern understanding. It makes sense only

1 For example, Hera Cook, *The Long Sexual Revolution: English Women, Sex, and Contraception, 1800–1975* (Oxford, 2004); Lutz D. H. Sauerteig and Roger Davidson (eds.), *Shaping Sexual Knowledge: A Cultural History of Sex Education in Twentieth-Century Europe* (London, 2009). This chapter will focus on the anglophone west, but include some continental European examples; notes will indicate comparisons with other regions.

2 Michel Foucault, *The History of Sexuality*, vol. 1: *The Will to Knowledge*, trans. Robert Hurley (London, 1979); Simon Szreter, 'Victorian Britain, 1831–1963: Towards a social history of sexuality', *Journal of Victorian Culture* 1 (1996), 136–49; Catherine Cocks, 'Rethinking sexuality in the progressive era', *Journal of the Gilded Age and Progressive Era* 5 (2006), 93–118.

3 Marie-Luise Kohlke, 'Sexsation and the neo-Victorian novel: Orientalising the nineteenth century in contemporary fiction', in Kohlke and Luisa Orza (eds.), *Negotiating Sexual Idioms: Image, Text, Performance* (Amsterdam, 2008), pp. 53–78; Ian McEwan, *On Chesil Beach* (New York, NY, 2007), pp. 96–7; Peter Mathews, 'After the Victorians: The historical turning point in McEwan's *On Chesil Beach*', *Critique: Studies in Contemporary Fiction* 53 (2011), 82–91.

once an emphasis on core facts has replaced a premodern view of knowledge as a pluralistic mix of natural wisdom, bodily awareness, scholarly learning, lore and experience.[4] This transition saw the gradual and fragmented separation of authoritative science – the facts of life – from lay beliefs and superstitions.[5] References to the 'secrets of women' within a framework of 'generation' became increasingly rare, while texts claiming scientific expertise about what was now called 'reproduction' became increasingly common.[6] This transformation fundamentally altered not just how people learned, but also what there was to know, and in a way that altered embodied experience. Newly constructed facts recast understandings of the differences between male and female bodies, their reproductive roles and sexual desires.[7] The focus on learning about sex and reproduction as an empirical exploration was accompanied by a politicized debate over who should be allowed to know.[8]

In writing a history of communicating sexual knowledge, it is tempting to narrate the massive changes in types of material available, the proliferation of a widespread and diverse culture of medical advice about sex, reproduction and bodily management, the contestations over sex education and the burgeoning of a highly sexualized popular culture. Yet that would miss the bigger transformation. This chapter instead places knowledge about sex and reproduction in debates about what should be known, by whom and in what format. It explores the politics of such knowledge in contests between different authorities. Rather than asking how much people knew about sex and reproduction and how the amount changed, it examines what was involved in acquiring the knowledge; how, that is, within competing frameworks, individuals translated, assimilated and consumed reproductive information as they built their own understandings and identities.[9]

4 Mary Fissell and Roger Cooter, 'Exploring natural knowledge: Science and the popular', in Roy Porter (ed.), *The Cambridge History of Science*, vol. 4: *Eighteenth-Century Science* (Cambridge, 2003), pp. 129–58.

5 Ralph O'Connor, 'Reflections on popular science in Britain: Genres, categories, and historians', *Isis* 100 (2009), 333–45.

6 Katherine Crawford, *European Sexualities, 1400–1800* (Cambridge, 2007); on the 'secrets' literature: Peter Murray Jones, 'Generation between Script and Print', Chapter 13, this book.

7 Ivan Crozier, 'Introduction: Bodies in history – the task of the historian', in Crozier (ed.), *A Cultural History of the Human Body in the Modern Age* (Oxford, 2010), pp. 3–22. On the construction of ignorance: Robert N. Proctor and Londa Schiebinger (eds.), *Agnotology: The Making and Unmaking of Ignorance* (Stanford, CA, 2008); Schiebinger, 'Agnotology and exotic abortifacients: The cultural production of ignorance in the eighteenth-century Atlantic world', *Proceedings of the American Philosophical Society* 149 (2005), 316–43.

8 Patricia Crawford, 'Sexual knowledge in England, 1500–1750', in Crawford (ed.), *Blood, Bodies and Families in Early Modern England* (Harlow, 2004), pp. 54–79; Roy Porter, 'Forbidden pleasures: Enlightenment literature of sexual advice', in Paula Bennett and Vernon A. Rosario II (eds.), *Solitary Pleasures: The Historical, Literary, and Artistic Discourses of Autoeroticism* (New York, NY, 1995), pp. 75–98.

9 James A. Secord, 'Knowledge in transit', *Isis* 95 (2004), 654–72; further: Nick Hopwood *et al.*, 'Introduction: Communicating reproduction', *Bulletin of the History of Medicine* 89 (2015), 379–405; James A. Secord, 'Talking Origins', Chapter 26, this book.

Communicating about Sex and Reproduction

From the eighteenth century, ignorance has provided the dominant frame for understanding the communication and acquisition of knowledge about sex and reproduction.[10] The new framework is apparent in the reconceptualization of readers of books on these matters as ill-informed. Many early modern texts assumed that women already knew about generation.[11] Editions of the long-lived advice manual *Aristotle's Masterpiece* initially represented sexual knowledge as a woman, and addressed the queries of those (men) who did not have direct or experiential knowledge of women's bodies.[12] Around 1750, by contrast, the *Masterpiece* increasingly cast readers as young women naturally ignorant and in need of expert enlightenment. The figure of the shy and ill-informed mother came to justify the publication of popular medical texts. Thomas Bull's *Hints to Mothers* aimed to answer questions that young married women were too 'delicate' to ask their 'medical advisors' directly. H. Arthur Allbutt's accessible, affordable and widely advertised *Wife's Handbook*, famous for providing advice on contraception as well as health, marriage and pregnancy, framed its 'newly-wed' female reader as 'ignorant' of reproduction, a theme that continued in advice literature into the twentieth century.[13] Current pregnancy manuals and sex education materials still imagine (especially female) readers as in need of science to interpret bodily experiences and disentangle truth from rumour and gossip.[14]

Sexual knowledge was politicized. From the later eighteenth century, and increasing in intensity through the nineteenth, we find discussion of the meanings and effects of sexually themed material.[15] What different groups knew and should know about sex

10 Eve Kosofsky Sedgwick, *Epistemology of the Closet* (Berkeley, CA, 1990), p. 68. On the need to put the 'epistemology of sex', that is, the structural dynamic between knowledge and ignorance, at the heart of the history of sexuality: Valerie Traub, *Thinking Sex with the Early Moderns* (Philadelphia, PA, 2015).

11 Mary E. Fissell, 'Making a masterpiece: The Aristotle texts in vernacular medical culture', in Charles E. Rosenberg (ed.), *Right Living: An Anglo-American Tradition of Self-Help Medicine and Hygiene* (Baltimore, MD, 2003), pp. 59–87.

12 Mary E. Fissell, '"Hairy women and naked truths": Gender and the politics of knowledge in *Aristotle's Masterpiece*', *William and Mary Quarterly*, 3rd ser., 60 (2003), 43–74; Fissell, '*Aristotle's Masterpiece*', Exhibit 25, this book.

13 Thomas Bull, *Hints to Mothers on the Management of Health During the Period of Pregnancy, and in the Lying-In-Room* (London, 1837), pp. iii–iv; H. Arthur Allbutt, *The Wife's Handbook …*, 2nd edn (London, 1886), p. 30; John Peel, 'Contraception and the medical profession', *Population Studies* 18 (1964), 133–45.

14 The expansion of medical and other material on the proper conduct of pregnancy and birth also reflects the investments of nation-states in population regulation and the national health: Dorothy Porter, *Health, Civilization and the State: A History of Public Health from Ancient to Modern Times* (London, 1999).

15 French erotica stopped presenting girls' sexual curiosity positively: Dorelies Kraakman, 'Reading pornography anew: A critical history of sexual knowledge for girls in French erotic fiction, 1750–1840', *Journal of the History of Sexuality* 4 (1994), 517–48.

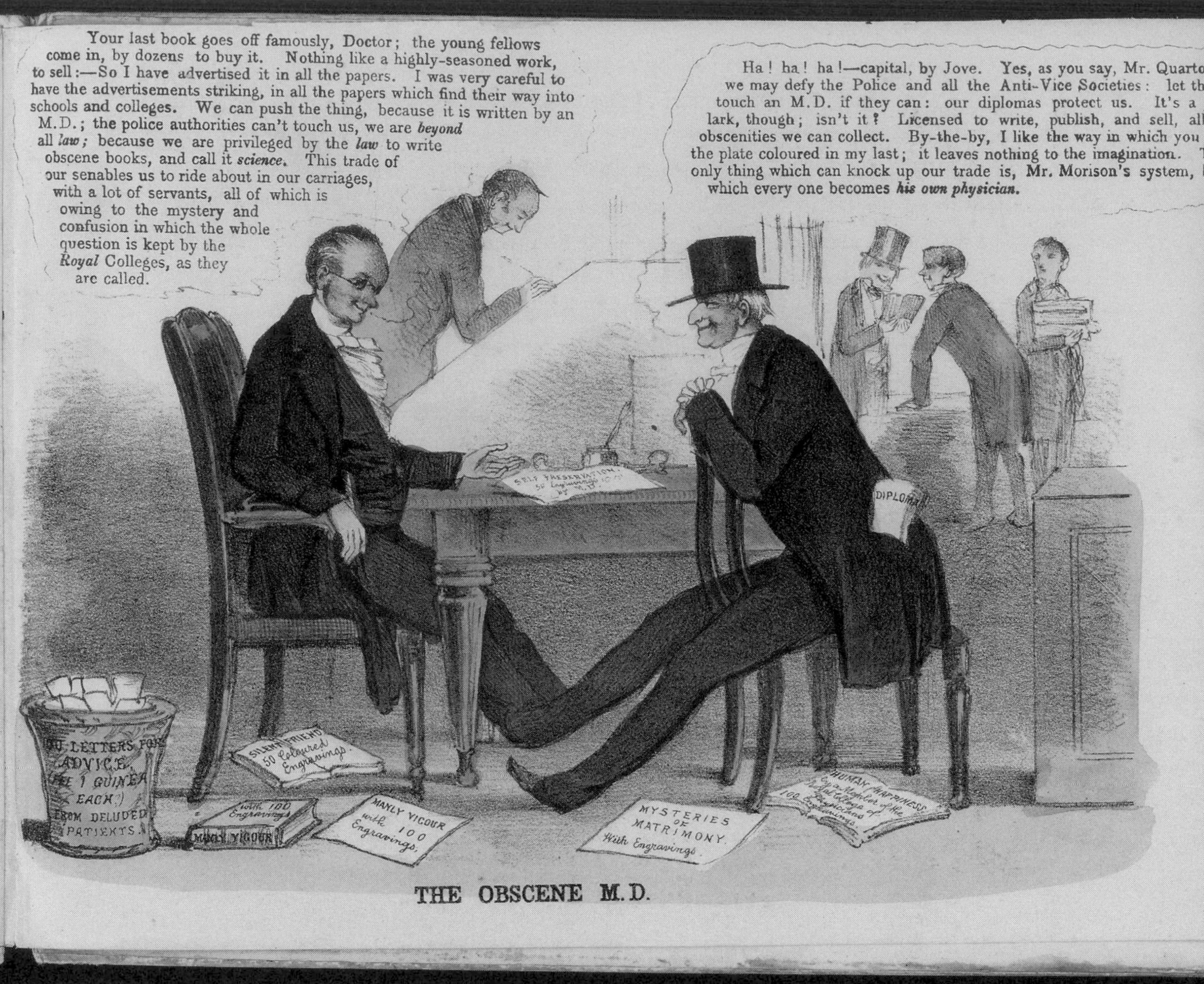

Figure 32.1 A doctor and his publisher celebrate the success of their 'highly-seasoned work'. Advertising James Morison's vegetable pills, this coloured lithograph satirizes the publication of obscenity under the cloak of medical authority. Strewn across the floor are works entitled 'mysteries of matrimony', 'manly vigour' and 'human happiness'. Produced by the British College of Health, 1852. Wellcome Library, London.

and reproduction became a potent social question.[16] Where to talk about these matters, in what circumstances and to whom was frequently regulated.[17] Debate about the

16 Lisa Forman Cody, *Birthing the Nation: Sex, Science, and the Conception of Eighteenth-Century Britons* (Oxford, 2005).

17 The recent history of sexuality has been much concerned with the gradual, fragmented yet profound shift to this distinctively modern way of thinking about sexual knowledge: Michael McKeon (ed.), 'Sex: A thematic issue', *Signs* 37, no. 4 (2012).

politics of publishing was invigorated: the potential impact on vulnerable readers and viewers became a particular anxiety, and the category of pornography was invented for texts that required special treatment, for example, through new censorship laws.[18] Museums amassed secret cabinets to house the material they would not show. Those texts discussing sex and reproduction, even when seeking to disseminate respectable medical knowledge, might nonetheless be attacked for failing to preserve enough ignorance. Allbutt was struck off the medical register because his book sold 'at so low a price as to bring the work within the reach of the youth of both sexes, to the detriment of public morals' (Fig. 32.1).[19]

Thus debates about what to publish and for whom were increasingly structured by the expectation of an ignorant populace. Many lauded naivety as essential to a morally respectable nation; but during the nineteenth century, others launched a concerted attack on ignorance as producing prostitution, masturbation and promiscuity, the very social evils that silence about sex and reproduction was supposed to prevent.[20] As early as 1826, the radical republican Richard Carlile's prison-penned *Every Woman's Book* challenged the value of sexual ignorance and offered information about pleasure and contraception.[21] From around 1900, birth control campaigners, Christian reformers, feminists, advocates of free love and of sexual purity, social hygienists, sexual scientists, psychiatrists, eugenicists, educationalists and socialists began to claim that some degree of sex education was necessary to counter 'unwholesome' sources which encouraged 'immoral behaviour'.[22] Knowledge could be prurient, but ignorance

18 Walter M. Kendrick, *The Secret Museum: Pornography in Modern Culture* (New York, NY, 1987); for an earlier dating: Joan E. DeJean, *The Reinvention of Obscenity: Sex, Lies, and Tabloids in Early Modern France* (Chicago, IL, 2002). On attempts to shelter young people from sexual knowledge: Nicola Kay Beisel, *Imperiled Innocents: Anthony Comstock and Family Reproduction in Victorian America* (Princeton, NJ, 1997); Colin Heywood, 'Innocence and experience: Sexuality among young people in modern France, *c.* 1750–1950', *French History* 21 (2007), 44–64.

19 'Allbutt v. General Council of Medical Education and Registration of the United Kingdom, and another', *British Medical Journal* 1 (2 Feb. 1889), 270; see further Peel, 'Contraception and the medical profession'.

20 Frank Mort, *Dangerous Sexualities: Medico-Moral Politics in England since 1830*, 2nd edn (London, 2000); Lisa Z. Sigel, *Making Modern Love: Sexual Narratives and Identities in Interwar Britain* (Philadelphia, PA, 2012), p. 48.

21 M. L. Bush, *What Is Love? Richard Carlile's Philosophy of Sex* (London, 1998); Lesley A. Hall, 'Movements to Separate Sex and Reproduction', Chapter 29, this book.

22 Leigh Ann Wheeler, 'Rescuing sex from prudery and prurience: American women's use of sex education as an antidote to obscenity, 1925–1932', *Journal of Women's History* 12, no. 3 (2000), 173–95. On middle-class concerns about working-class sexual awareness, see Peter Gurney, '"Intersex" and "dirty girls": Mass-Observation and working-class sexuality in England in the 1930s', *Journal of the History of Sexuality* 8 (1997), 256–90; and on Japanese reinterpretations of these debates, Sepp Linhart and Sabine Frühstück (eds.), *The Culture of Japan as Seen Through Its Leisure* (Albany, NY, 1998); Frühstück, *Colonizing Sex: Sexology and Social Control in Modern Japan* (Berkeley, CA, 2003).

was dangerous.[23] In the twentieth century, a wide variety of educational materials provided descriptions of men's and women's anatomies, fertilization, stages of pregnancy and bodily changes associated with sex, as well as information about orgasms and pleasure, in order to give the ignorant basic instruction in the facts of life (Fig. 32.2).[24]

Authorizing Knowledge

Essential to the authorization of scientific knowledge of sex and reproduction was the delegitimization of experience, so that 'sexual' was no longer synonymous with 'carnal' knowledge. Late eighteenth-century obstetrics devalued knowledge about the birthing body derived from being a mother and attacked midwives for failing to achieve the required detachment because they drew upon their own experiences when helping other women.[25] Yet the view has endured that the physicality of sex and reproduction cannot be explained, but only experienced, and medical authorities were and are less likely to have their advice heeded when it contradicts embodied knowledge.[26]

The range of competing authorities and the ways individuals evaluated them were central to the communication of sexual and reproductive knowledge. Of particular significance was the growing, yet precarious influence of medicine. Many historians have characterized the past three hundred years, particularly the last century, as a period of medicalization, when doctors gained a monopoly on reliable knowledge and denigrated other material as irrational, quack or disreputable. Bull's much republished *Hints to Mothers* offered a plain summary of medical opinion to counteract the erroneous information purveyed by 'ignorant persons'.[27] Colonial medicine frequently condemned native knowledge as dangerously primitive, irrational and ignorant.[28]

23 Sauerteig and Davidson, *Shaping Sexual Knowledge*; Helen Lefkowitz Horowitz, *Rereading Sex: Battles over Sexual Knowledge and Suppression in Nineteenth-Century America* (New York, NY, 2002); Robin E. Jensen, *Dirty Words: The Rhetoric of Public Sex Education, 1870–1924* (Urbana, IL, 2010).

24 This knowledge also constructed ignorance: Nancy Tuana, 'Coming to understand: Orgasm and the epistemology of ignorance', *Hypatia* 19 (2004), 194–232.

25 Lisa Forman Cody, 'The body in birth and death', in Carole Reeves (ed.), *A Cultural History of the Human Body in the Enlightenment* (London, 2012), pp. 13–32, on pp. 22–3; also Crawford, *European Sexualities*, p. 129; further: Mary E. Fissell, 'Man-Midwifery Revisited', Chapter 22; Philippa Levine, 'Imperial Encounters', Chapter 33; Salim Al-Gailani, 'Hospital Birth', Chapter 37; Ludmilla Jordanova, 'Man-Midwifery Dissected', Exhibit 22, this book.

26 C. H. Browner and Nancy Press, 'The production of authoritative knowledge in American prenatal care', *Medical Anthropology Quarterly* 10 (1996), 141–56.

27 Bull, *Hints to Mothers*, p. iii; Hilary Marland and Anne Marie Rafferty (eds.), *Midwives, Society and Childbirth: Debates and Controversies in the Modern Period* (London, 1997); K. K. Barker, 'A ship upon a stormy sea: The medicalization of pregnancy', *Social Science & Medicine* 47 (1998), 1067–76; Janet Greenlees and Lynda Bryder (eds.), *Western Maternity and Medicine, 1880–1990* (London, 2013).

28 Felicity Nussbaum, *Torrid Zones: Maternity, Sexuality, and Empire in Eighteenth-Century English Narratives* (Baltimore, MD, 1995); Andrew P. Lyons and Harriet Lyons, *Irregular Connections: A History*

the KINSEY REPORT and YOUR WIFE

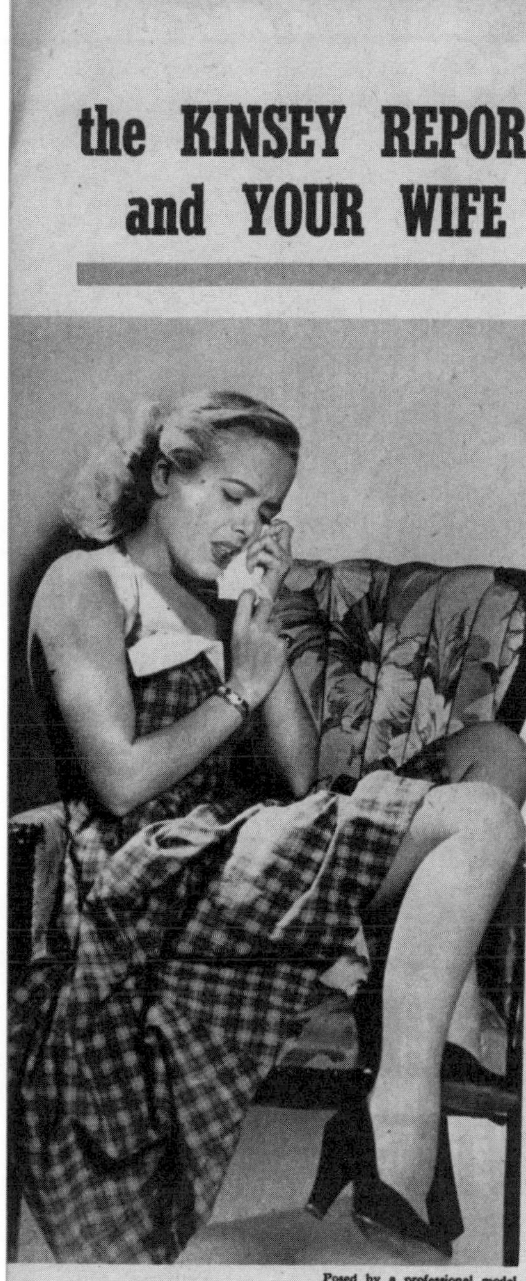

Posed by a professional model

In the past, ignorance and uncertainty have made many young wives unhappy, have caused divorces.

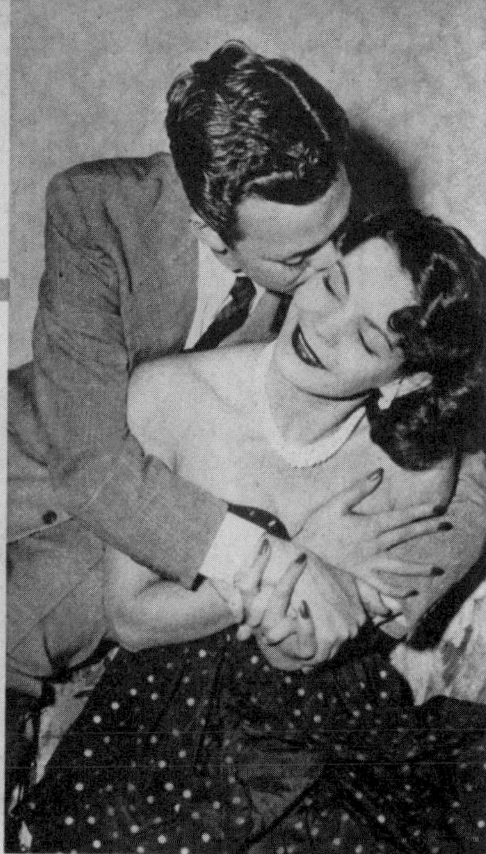

Posed by Professional Models

Doctor Kinsey hopes that the knowledge contained in his book will make marriages more successful.

THE BOOK THAT, is considered by many scientific authorities to be the most important single volume of the century is due on the stands within a few weeks. That book is the Kinsey report on sexual behavior in the human female.

The value of this study in feminine behavior, of course, lies basically in the effect it will have on marital and pre-marital relationships. In short, while the work will include case histories of females of all types and all ages, its fundamental worth lies in what it will mean to your wife and to your marriage. Women will be able to better understand, from a purely factual viewpoint, what the habits and actions of other women are. And marriages will have a chance to become more mature and happier through this knowledge.

It's a paradox that this genuinely world shaking volume is being put into its final form at this moment by a soft spoken, scholarly gentleman whose chief interests in life are music and gardening, a quiet, infinitely patient man whose passion for facts and truth once led

12

Figure 32.2 An article in the short-lived American men's magazine *Action* champions Alfred Kinsey's *Sexual Behavior in the Human Female* as an antidote to the ignorance that, it claimed, blighted marriages and caused divorce. The report was very widely discussed (Chapter 41, this book). R. B. Armstrong, 'The Kinsey Report and your wife', *Action* 1, no. 5 (Oct. 1953), 11–15 and 49, on 12. 26 × 20 cm.

Since the nineteenth century, scientific and medical research into fertility, conception and contraception, fetal development and the management of pregnancy and labour has not just transformed knowledge of sex and reproduction. Such innovations in ways of seeing and monitoring the reproductive body as microscopy, hormonal tests and ultrasound also changed perceptions of bodies in ways that directly challenged women's experiential understanding.[29] These techniques produced powerful visualizations of the interior truths of reproduction that bypassed the testimony of the pregnant woman herself (Fig. 32.3).[30] Home pregnancy tests, which were developed and commercialized in response to consumer demand in the 1970s, served nonetheless to bring medical ways of knowing into the earliest stages of pregnancy.[31] The pill, which needs to be prescribed by health practitioners and requires medical monitoring, while working in imperceptible ways on ovulation, has similarly reshaped contraceptive knowledge.[32]

Yet medical voices were a cacophony themselves; men and women found themselves confronted by various medical authorities, including local doctors, hospital specialists, pharmacists, herbalists, midwives, obstetricians, advice books, pharmaceutical advertisements and newspaper reports. Moreover, these formal and informal medical sources were in dynamic dialogue with parents, friends, neighbours and work colleagues.[33] Pregnant and labouring women came into contact with different medical standpoints in the doctor's surgery, obstetric clinic, antenatal class and midwife's visit. They found different translations of medical opinion in, for example, pharmaceutical-sponsored pamphlets, women's magazines, pregnancy guides, newspapers, television and the internet. They confronted perspectives from mothers, husbands, friends

of Anthropology and Sexuality (Lincoln, NE, 2004); Megan Vaughan, *Curing Their Ills: Colonial Power and African Illness* (Stanford, CA, 1991); Liat Kozma, '"We, the sexologists …": Arabic medical writing on sexuality, 1879–1943', *Journal of the History of Sexuality* 22 (2013), 426–45; Levine, 'Imperial Encounters'.

29 Barbara Duden, *Disembodying Women: Perspectives on Pregnancy and the Unborn*, trans. Lee Hoinacki (Cambridge, MA, 1993); Nick Hopwood, 'Embryology', in Peter J. Bowler and John V. Pickstone (eds.), *The Cambridge History of Science*, vol. 6: *The Modern Biological and Earth Sciences* (Cambridge, 2009), pp. 285–315. For the impact of medical changes on the very concept of reproduction: Angus McLaren, *Reproduction by Design: Sex, Robots, Trees, and Test-Tube Babies in Interwar Britain* (Chicago, IL, 2012).

30 Jennifer Shaw, 'The birth of the clinic and the advent of reproduction: Pregnancy, pathology and the medical gaze in modernity', *Body & Society* 18 (2012), 110–38.

31 Sarah A. Leavitt, '"A private little revolution": The home pregnancy test in American culture', *Bulletin of the History of Medicine* 80 (2006), 317–45; further: Jesse Olszynko-Gryn, 'Pregnancy Testing with Frogs', Exhibit 32, this book.

32 Andrea Tone, 'Medicalizing reproduction: The pill and home pregnancy tests', *Journal of Sex Research* 49 (2012), 319–27.

33 Lucinda McCray Beier, *Health Culture in the Heartland, 1880–1980: An Oral History* (Urbana, IL, 2009); Angela Davis, *Modern Motherhood: Women and Family in England,* c. *1945–2000* (Manchester, 2012).

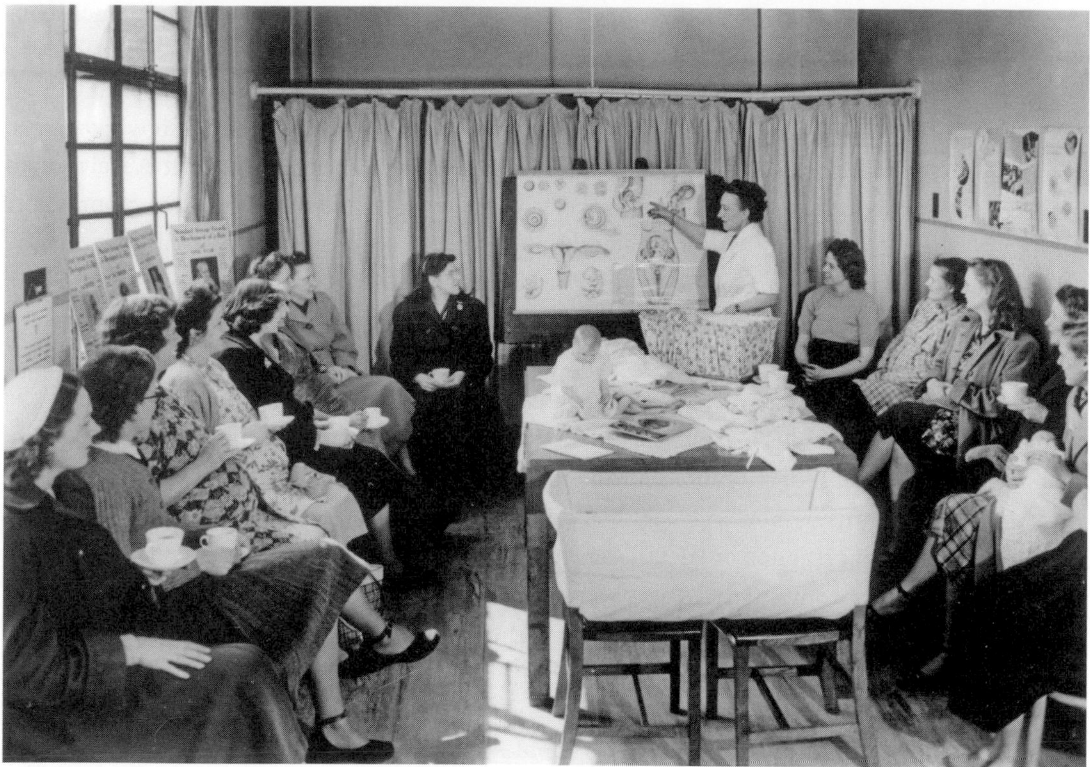

Figure 32.3 A nurse explains the embryology of pregnancy to women at a maternity welfare centre in Paddington, London, around 1950. Across Europe from the early twentieth century, maternity and child welfare centres had offered mothers and mothers-to-be advice about pregnancy, birth and domestic hygiene. London Metropolitan Archives, City of London.

and latterly social media.[34] And they obtained significant knowledge through their own bodily experiences of pregnancy and childbirth.[35] Twentieth-century medical frameworks intensified the sense that pregnancy and birth were complex matters about which there is much to know or feel ignorant. They did not diminish the complexity of the various interacting and competing claims.[36]

Abortion provides a powerful example. In twentieth-century women's experiences, a medico-scientific understanding of the development of the embryo and fetus and the process of terminating a pregnancy coexisted with different ways of knowing about

34 Robbie E. Davis-Floyd and Carolyn F. Sargent (eds.), *Childbirth and Authoritative Knowledge: Cross-Cultural Perspectives* (Berkeley, CA, 1997); Sarah Pedersen and Janet Smithson, 'Mothers with attitude – How the Mumsnet parenting forum offers space for new forms of femininity to emerge online', *Women's Studies International Forum* 38 (2013), 97–106.

35 Browner and Press, 'Production of authoritative knowledge'.

36 Leona VandeVusse, 'Decision making in analyses of women's birth stories', *Birth* 26 (1999), 43–50; Della Pollock, *Telling Bodies, Performing Birth: Everyday Narratives of Childbirth* (New York, NY, 1999).

fertility, infertility and pregnancy. For example, what from the perspective of menstrual cycles might look like an induced miscarriage could be understood as the restoration of regularity and bodily balance.[37]

Medical understandings of sex and reproduction always competed with alternative authorities, such as trusted interpersonal contacts. The attraction of medical modernity might be undermined by a rhetoric that constructed other voices as grounded in tradition, ancient wisdom, natural knowledge or old-fashioned, passed-down truths. The appeal became explicit through, for example, the trust placed in illegal abortionists, the rise of the natural childbirth and home birth movements in postwar Britain and America, the success there of Chinese herbal medicine, and the survival of independent midwifery, unsupported by hospital obstetrics.[38] From the mid-nineteenth century, an enduring counter-narrative exoticized eastern cultures as holding secret knowledge of sex and reproduction, absent from the west and capable of challenging western morality, and this became a strong theme in the 1960s and 1970s.[39] Thus, while medics denigrated unorthodox or lay knowledge as ignorant, its construction as alternative gave it a counter-conventional status and appeal.

Deciphering Knowledge and Experiencing Ignorance

These politics reshaped learning about sex: they constructed knowledge as a secret about which few could speak with authority. Those who sought to find out about sex and reproduction had to explore and decode such information as was available in what Anna Clark calls 'twilight moments'. By this she means the oblique circulation of knowledge through 'half-understood' 'gestures' in the gentleman's pornographic library and the red-light district, on the seaside pier and the factory floor.[40] Post-Enlightenment Europe was distinctive not in the repression of sexuality, but in the endless production of materials about sex and reproduction in a way so mediated or regulated that these

37 Cornelie Usborne, *Cultures of Abortion in Weimar Germany* (New York, NY, 2007), pp. 152–8; Jesse Olszynko-Gryn, 'Technologies of Contraception and Abortion', Chapter 36, this book.

38 Haiming Liu, 'Chinese herbalists in the United States', in Sucheng Chan (ed.), *Chinese American Transnationalism: The Flow of People, Resources, and Ideas between China and America During the Exclusion Era* (Philadelphia, PA, 2005), pp. 136–55; Wendy Kline, *Bodies of Knowledge: Sexuality, Reproduction, and Women's Health in the Second Wave* (Chicago, IL, 2010); Jon Adams and Philip Tovey, *Complementary and Alternative Medicine in Nursing and Midwifery: Towards a Critical Social Science* (London, 2014); Wendy Kline, 'Communicating a new consciousness: Countercultural print and the home birth movement in the 1970s', *Bulletin of the History of Medicine* 89 (2015), 527–56; Al-Gailani, 'Hospital Birth'.

39 Ben Grant, 'Translating/"the" *Kama Sutra*', *Third World Quarterly* 26 (2005), 509–16; Leon Antonio Rocha, 'Scientia sexualis versus ars erotica: Foucault, van Gulik, Needham', *Studies in History and Philosophy of Biological and Biomedical Sciences* 42 (2011), 328–43.

40 Anna Clark, 'Twilight moments', *Journal of the History of Sexuality* 14 (2005), 139–60.

matters were made secret at the same time.[41] This challenged people to uncover or decipher this knowledge.

Readers of nineteenth and early twentieth-century medical books and marriage manuals struggled to interpret texts that were euphemistic, or used Latin or French to discuss sex and desire.[42] Some books provided clues to inventive reading or hints for reading in reverse.[43] Readers might be guided by introductions reassuring them that the material inside was not pornographic or warning that it was appropriate only for certain types of reader. Admonitions to avoid certain sexual practices could inspire new methods of avoiding pregnancy. Information about abortifacient drugs might be obtained by scrutinizing warnings of the dangers of taking while pregnant; and from the mid-nineteenth to the mid-twentieth centuries, pills to prevent menstrual obstruction were widely advertised.[44]

Uncovering secrets also meant creative exploration, for example, by reading cheap novels, seeking out pornography or absorbing newspaper reports of sexual crimes.[45] Authors and readers actively blurred the distinction between medicine and pornography; erotic writers, for example, borrowed the language of science to imply an overlap in their roles as producers of authoritative knowledge.[46] Coded messages and euphemistic labels challenged people to decipher the knowledge that lay beneath. The popular anatomical museums of the late eighteenth to the early twentieth century were places of medical education and for the enjoyment of lurid, exotic and sexualized displays, including partly dissected Venuses, embryological models, diseased genitals, waxworks of obstetric operations and plaster casts of the exoticized faces and bodies of non-European people.[47] By the 1930s, the public visibility of contraception extended to condom vending machines outside barbers' and chemists' and in men's toilets (Fig. 32.4).

The acquisition of information affected social and gender identities. Those twilight places where people could learn about sex also disciplined hearing and reading,

41 Foucault, *History of Sexuality*.

42 Roy Porter and Lesley Hall, *The Facts of Life: The Creation of Sexual Knowledge in Britain, 1650–1950* (New Haven, CT, 1995), pp. 83–90, 128–31; Sally Alexander, 'The mysteries and secrets of women's bodies', in Mica Nava and Alan O'Shea (eds.), *Modern Times: Reflections on a Century of English Modernity* (London, 1996), pp. 161–75; Jensen, *Dirty Words*, pp. 1–35.

43 Porter and Hall, *Facts of Life*, p. 104.

44 Olszynko-Gryn, 'Technologies of Contraception and Abortion'.

45 William A. Cohen, *Sex Scandal: The Private Parts of Victorian Fiction* (Durham, NC, 1996).

46 Karen Harvey, *Reading Sex in the Eighteenth Century: Bodies and Gender in English Erotic Culture* (Cambridge, 2004). See also Roberta McGrath, *Seeing Her Sex: Medical Archives and the Female Body* (Manchester, 2002).

47 Richard D. Altick, *The Shows of London* (Cambridge, MA, 1978); Elizabeth Stephens, 'Pathologizing leaky male bodies: Spermatorrhea in nineteenth-century British medicine and popular anatomical museums', *Journal of the History of Sexuality* 17 (2008), 421–38; Alan W. Bates, '"Indecent and demoralising representations": Public anatomy museums in mid-Victorian England', *Medical History* 52 (2008), 1–22.

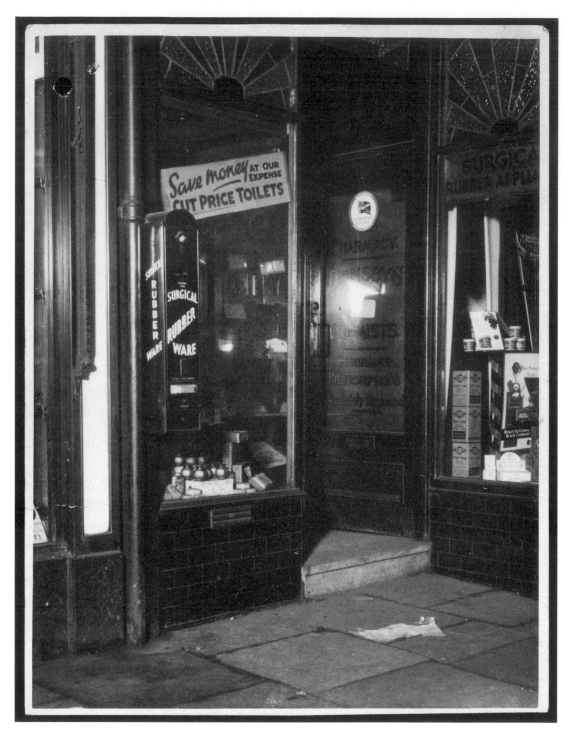

Figure 32.4 Photograph showing a slot machine for 'surgical rubber ware' outside Dunsby's Chemists in central London in 1932–4. Wellcome Library, London.

sustaining social hierarchies and reinforcing gendered codes of respectability.[48] Knowledge of the secrets of sex and reproduction might imply improper reading or illicit experience. Households that owned medical advice books, marriage manuals or pornography often kept them in locked cupboards or hidden in drawers, and those who came across them remembered reading in snatched glances in the dark.[49] Part of obtaining information was learning about its appropriate use. Warnings of the dangers and perils of sexual knowledge inflect the writings of physicians, clergymen, pharmaceutical suppliers and teachers. Producing, circulating and gossiping about sex and reproduction was often a form of resistance or rebellion, entered into with trepidation or transgressive zeal.

Men and women did tell neighbours where to find secret abortionists over a back wall, and gossiped about affairs, babies, pregnancies and contraception in the pub, shops, park and workplace. Yet two women who talked openly about sex in a factory in England in the 1930s shocked their peers, who subsequently doubted their respectability and moral values.[50] A headmistress giving evidence to the London County Council inquiry on sex hygiene teaching in 1914 argued that 'bold' girls who had obtained information from unsuitable sources had to be controlled to preserve the moral health of the boys with whom they consorted.[51] Fear of being labelled 'loose' may have led other (less bold) girls to act innocent instead. Peter Gay characterized the Victorian age as one of 'learned ignorance', an identity which women 'desired … and assiduously fostered'.[52] Men who found out about contraception in the army sometimes kept such knowledge for the brothel and away from their own marriages. In these and other ways, ignorance was culturally produced and socially maintained.

Conclusion

The past three centuries have seen major changes in the production and consumption of medical knowledge, the rise of an industry devoted to telling women and men what to expect from sex, pregnancy and birth, and the introduction of formal sex education. Charting this increased volume of information about sex and reproduction is central to recent historical inquiry. Yet, the period is distinctive not only for this expansion in information, but also for the construction of sexual knowledge as a set of truths that had to be learned in order to make good a deficit of facts. This framework is fundamental to understanding experiences, choices, beliefs and identities.

48 Clark, 'Twilight moments'.

49 Kate Fisher, *Birth Control, Sex and Marriage in Britain, 1918–1960* (Oxford, 2006), pp. 42–3.

50 Simon Szreter and Kate Fisher, *Sex before the Sexual Revolution: Intimate Life in England, 1918–1963* (Cambridge, 2010), pp. 87, 97–8.

51 Mort, *Dangerous Sexualities*, p. 149.

52 Peter Gay, *The Bourgeois Experience: Victoria to Freud*, vol. 1 (New York, NY, 1984), p. 281.

Just as the 'epistemology of the closet' has been recognized as structuring twentieth-century homosexual identities, so an 'epistemology of sexual ignorance' underpinned how people made sense of sex and reproduction as they developed their own identities in relation to contestations around authority and gendered notions of respectability.[53] The conceptualization of knowledge as requiring a journey out of ignorance politicized the processes of producing and circulating information and was accompanied by intense debates about the purpose and effects of learning about sex and reproduction. By understanding these politics, historians can effectively integrate knowledge and lived experience. For obtaining sexual and reproductive knowledge involved (and still involves) engaging with these politics: choosing how to react to the various cultures of dissemination, determining where to look and what to look for, deciding what to believe and what to reject, what to broadcast to others and what to avoid knowing or appearing to know. This engagement is at the heart of sexual, personal and reproductive identities.

53 Sedgwick, *Epistemology of the Closet.*

33 Imperial Encounters

Philippa Levine

'What is the use of an Empire if it does not breed and maintain in the truest and fullest sense of the word an Imperial race?'[1] So remarked the British liberal politician Herbert Asquith in 1901. Reproduction was central to sustaining empire, whether in ensuring new supplies of soldiers and labourers or a healthy ruling class. In this era of high imperialism, the politics of nationalism intersected with the idea of separate spheres for men and women to frame reproduction as women's work. Medicalized childbirth and maternal and infant welfare were trumpeted as modern innovations that would improve the health of nations and empires as well as of individuals.

A similar rhetoric was at work in the colonies. In India, the 'citizen-mother' embodied the spirit of the nation.[2] In Egypt, an ideology of republican motherhood emphasized the importance of maternity and domesticity for that modernizing nation, even as colonial influence persisted.[3] By the start of the twentieth century, reproduction had become a significant site of state intervention. States increasingly involved themselves in childbirth practices and the care of mothers and infants, the prevention and termination of pregnancies and the rearing of children, as well as who could and should reproduce. They were invariably more lavish with ideals than with funding, but, by the early twentieth century, reproduction was firmly on the political agenda of the imperial powers, and its importance would continue to grow.

Colonial interest in reproduction had deep roots. Registration of births, deaths and marriages, along with census data, had been expanding enterprises from at least the eighteenth century, while plantation slavery saw some of the earliest colonial attempts to control women's reproductive capacities. The heritability of slave status encouraged planters to enlarge their slave holdings by 'breeding' their female slaves.[4] After Britain

1 'Liberals, forward! March!!', *Westminster Review* 156 (1901), 370–84, on 376, quoting Asquith's speech at the Hotel Cecil in London.

2 Maneesha Lal, '"The ignorance of women is the house of illness": Gender, nationalism, and health reform in colonial north India', in Mary P. Sutphen and Bridie Andrews (eds.), *Medicine and Colonial Identity* (London, 2003), pp. 15–40, on p. 16.

3 Hibba Abugideiri, *Gender and the Making of Modern Medicine in Colonial Egypt* (Farnham, 2010), pp. 10–11; Omnia El Shakry, *The Great Social Laboratory: Subjects of Knowledge in Colonial and Postcolonial Egypt* (Stanford, CA, 2007), p. 174.

4 Jennifer L. Morgan, *Laboring Women: Reproduction and Gender in New World Slavery* (Philadelphia, PA, 2004), p. 56.

abolished the slave trade in 1807, a registry system was introduced in the sugar colonies to track falling slave numbers, which led ultimately to the legalization of slave marriages that reformers hoped would foster Christian family growth and planters anticipated would maintain numbers in the absence of new purchases.[5] Individual slave owners adopted such techniques, but imperial expansion affected reproduction most through the increasing reach and power of the state. In many arenas, the colonial state played an active role in regulating a broad range of sexual and reproductive activity. Interventions were often more prominent in reproduction than in other medicalized situations. As empires grew in the nineteenth century, colonial officials, entrepreneurs and missionaries took a greater interest in reproduction, whether to develop settler populations or to ensure labour supplies in extractive colonies. Both state and private sectors appreciated the vital importance of reproduction in maintaining colonial pre-eminence, and greater intervention paralleled a rising confidence in technological solutions, though with very uneven results.

Depopulation and Overpopulation

Responses to thinning slave numbers in the early nineteenth-century Caribbean represent fears of depopulation that lasted throughout the imperial era. In many European colonies, low birth-rates and high infant mortality rates threatened the stability and profitability of imperial assets and the claims of imperial states. As birth-rates plummeted in much of equatorial and East Africa, the Pacific and parts of Asia, diminishing populations threatened labour needs. Commentators blamed poor hygiene, minimal technology, and 'primitive' ignorance and superstition (Fig. 33.1), as well as what they saw as the prevalence of venereal diseases among indigenous peoples. Horror stories of insanitary deliveries and postnatal care abounded, remarkably similar in tone and substance from colony to colony, and routinely ignoring the ways in which colonial rule itself shaped population decline by disrupting kin networks, relocating peoples, introducing new pathogens and inducing ecological change.

Imperial expansion transformed reproductive practices as well as fertility. Notable changes in family structure and marriage patterns followed the massive increase in migration consequent upon imperial rule. Long after the Atlantic slave trade ended, the indenture, first of male labourers and then of women, disrupted marriage cycles. By the mid-nineteenth century, ships supplying indentured labour from India were required

5 Katherine Paugh, 'The politics of childbearing in the British Caribbean and the Atlantic world during the age of abolition, 1776–1838', *Past & Present* 221 (2013), 119–60, on 153. See also Sasha Turner, 'Home-grown slaves: Women, reproduction, and the abolition of the slave trade, Jamaica 1788–1807', *Journal of Women's History* 23, no. 3 (2011), 39–62; and Barbara Bush-Slimani, 'Hard labour: Women, childbirth and resistance in British Caribbean slave societies', *History Workshop Journal* 36 (1993), 83–99.

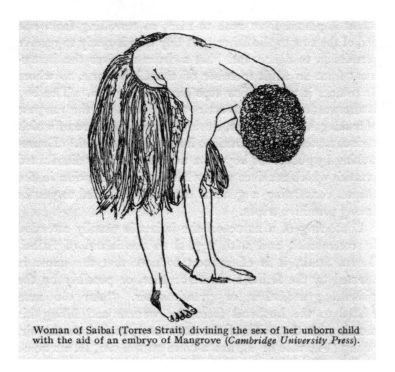

Figure 33.1 A Saibai Island woman 'divining the sex of her unborn child with the aid of an embryo of Mangrove'. The anthropologist Wilfrid Hambly used this drawing, made by Mrs A. Solomon for the *Reports of the Cambridge Anthropological Expedition to Torres Straits* (1905), to illustrate birth customs in his *Origins of Education among Primitive Peoples* (London: Macmillan, 1926), p. 64. 9.5 × 10 cm.

to fulfil a quota of women to ensure the stability of plantation life. Increased global contact introduced new diseases which often compromised fertility, while migration tended to raise the incidence of venereal diseases. Poverty and malnutrition exacerbated the effects of these changes on fertility patterns; so could the encouragement by missionaries especially, and by colonizing cultures more generally, of nuclear family models which emphasized quality over quantity.

Colonial rule eroded the birth spacing traditionally achieved in many regions of Africa through a mix of prolonged breast-feeding, polygyny and a postpartum taboo on sex.[6] Migration forced men in particular to seek work away from home, frequently in environments where women were forbidden. They could return home rarely, and often only with their employers' permission, leaving women to raise children without

6 Ron J. Lesthaeghe, 'Production and reproduction in sub-Saharan Africa: An overview and organizing principles', in Lesthaeghe (ed.), *Reproduction and Social Organization in Sub-Saharan Africa* (Berkeley, CA, 1989), pp. 13–59, on p. 17; Helen Bradford, 'Herbs, knives and plastic: 150 years of abortion in South Africa', in Mark Walker and Teresa A. Meade (eds.), *Science, Medicine, and Cultural Imperialism* (New York, NY, 1991), pp. 120–47, on p. 131.

them. Colonial encouragement of monogamous marriages destabilized older family formations, while in many areas the rise of cash-crop agriculture and of taxation encouraged late marriage, further reducing fertility. In these circumstances, young men were disinclined to shoulder the financial burdens of marriage, while fathers valued the labour of their unmarried daughters. Changes in bride-wealth practices in Africa also altered marriage patterns. Where bride-wealth faltered, men had little incentive to marry, and where it rose rapidly, marriage was delayed for those unable to offer enough to prospective grooms.[7]

The spectre of depopulation haunted Europe's colonies of extraction, where indigenous labour was needed to keep the raw materials of industrial wealth flowing. Settler colonies, by contrast, strove to increase European numbers and limit indigenous population growth. In early settler communities, men vastly outnumbered women. Small-scale efforts in the mid-nineteenth century to balance sex ratios by encouraging the migration of single white women yielded slow results, and even in the early twentieth century there were still many more men than women in most settler lands.[8] As sex ratios gradually began to equalize, reproduction was cast as a national duty, firmly inserting the state's interest and involvement in reproduction into a new imperial-national rhetoric. The scattered provision of maternity hospitals by philanthropic organizations typical of the nineteenth century gave way, slowly, to state funding and state interest in reproduction. By the early twentieth century, clinics and training schemes were emerging, though funding was rarely generous, notwithstanding the recommendation of the *British Medical Journal* in 1901, shortly before Asquith's speech, that 'a steadily declining birth rate … requires the consideration of all who have the well-being of the country and the empire at heart'.[9]

The perceived need to ensure that white settlers were of good 'stock', fit to create and maintain imperial possessions, made babies 'valuable assets in the emerging struggle for supremacy'.[10] Addressing the New Zealand branch of the British Medical Association as its President in 1906, the Christchurch surgeon Charles Morton Anderson warned that in Germany and Japan 'the natural increase is in a much greater ratio than our own'. He concluded that 'if the empire is to be maintained, we must rely, not simply on our navy and army, or on both, nor yet upon physique, but on numbers also'.[11]

7 Richard M. Smith, 'Marriage and Fertility in Different Household Systems', Chapter 24, this book.

8 Adele Perry, *On the Edge of Empire: Gender, Race, and the Making of British Columbia, 1849–1871* (Toronto, 2001); Rita S. Kranidis, *The Victorian Spinster and Colonial Emigration: Contested Subjects* (New York, NY, 1999).

9 'The preliminary census returns', *British Medical Journal* 1 (11 May 1901), 1159.

10 Milton Lewis, 'The "health of the race" and infant health in New South Wales: Perspectives on medicine and empire', in Roy M. MacLeod and Milton Lewis (eds.), *Disease, Medicine, and Empire: Perspectives on Western Medicine and the Experience of European Expansion* (London, 1988), pp. 301–15, on p. 301.

11 Morton Anderson, 'Declining birth rate in "the Britain of the South"', *New Zealand Medical Journal* 119 (Feb. 2006), 66–7, on 67, reprinted from ibid., 5 (1906).

Anderson's comments raised a panic about the 'crisis' of depopulation that paralleled concern about its opposite, overpopulation. Reproductive success in East Asia, especially in areas mostly resistant to colonization such as China and Japan, stirred fears of racial swamping. A literary genre foretelling the fate of a globe overrun by Asians found a receptive audience in the west.[12] These 'yellow peril' writings peddled an anxious image of a powerful Europe blocked in its path, on the one hand, by a shrinking supply of cheap colonial labour, and on the other, by the menace of an overly fecund but alien rival. In Australasia, federal and state governments initiated limits on immigration and offered white families welfare.[13]

'Dying race' theory, first articulated in the eighteenth century, thus found fertile soil.[14] The belief that 'primitive' peoples would be unable to withstand the onset of modernity had found special favour in white settler colonies where the disappearance of the indigenous peoples who were increasingly unnecessary for profitability was seen to enhance white opportunities. In the 1830s and 1840s, British activists raised concerns about the damage done to vulnerable populations by colonial rule and by individual colonists, urging the Colonial Office to take precautions to ensure the survival of aboriginal peoples. For many settlers, however, the disappearance of local populations was a sign of civilization and success. Attitudes to reproduction thus varied: where colonists needed an abundant supply of local labour, as they did in the extractive colonies, low fertility was a problem, while in settler colonies, locals often constituted a nuisance best eliminated, reduced or relocated to the margins.

Low fertility was frequently read as an effect of venereal disease, long a source of anxiety among both civil and military colonial administrations. Imperial powers routinely sought to regulate prostitution as a means of controlling venereal disease, but limited understanding of the origin, diagnosis and control of such illnesses prior to the twentieth century, coupled with a pervasive view of colonial populations as hypersexual, resulted in persistent overdiagnosis especially of syphilis, which was easily confused with other treponemas such as yaws and pinta.[15] Moreover, the use on pregnant women of mercury, the most common treatment for syphilis prior to World War I,

12 For example, Lothrop Stoddard, *The Rising Tide of Color Against White World-Supremacy* (New York, NY, 1920); Étienne Dennery, *Foules d'Asie: Surpopulation japonaise, expansion chinoise, émigration indienne* (Paris, 1930); Charles H. Pearson, *National Life and Character: A Forecast* (London, 1893); further: Alison Bashford, 'World Population from Eugenics to Climate Change', Chapter 34, this book.

13 Alison Bashford, *Imperial Hygiene: A Critical History of Colonialism, Nationalism and Public Health* (Basingstoke, 2004), p. 172; Lewis, '"Health of the race"'.

14 On early race theories more generally: Renato G. Mazzolini, 'Colonialism and the Emergence of Racial Theories', Chapter 25, this book.

15 Michael Tuck, 'Syphilis, sexuality, and social control: A history of venereal disease in colonial Uganda', unpublished PhD thesis, Northwestern University (1997); Philippa Levine, *Prostitution, Race and Politics: Policing Venereal Disease in the British Empire* (New York, NY, 2003); Simon Szreter, 'Fertility Transitions and Sexually Transmitted Infections', Chapter 30, this book.

compromised the health of the fetus; active public health campaigns thus sometimes exacerbated the problem.

The suspicion that African women routinely practised abortion lessened the contradiction between falling colonial birth-rates and stereotypes of black hypersexuality; women were getting pregnant, but not having babies.[16] A ban on abortion became a hallmark of modern civilization; in the 1830s it was one way in which the increasingly chaotic Ottoman Empire signalled its modernization.[17] Ironically, it was just as medical advances made clinical termination safer in the early twentieth century that laws banning abortion other than to save the life of the mother became widespread.[18]

By the early twentieth century, after Darwinism had ushered in new ways to consider heredity, these anxieties over depopulation and overpopulation became associated with a eugenics movement concerned that the 'wrong' people were reproducing most and that the quality of ruling elites might be degenerating. Colonial eugenics often focused on mixed-race coupling; some colonies forbade interracial sex in part to limit 'hybrid' populations.[19]

Eugenics was also closely associated with family limitation. Birth control slowly became more widespread, although the idea of contraception as a preventive tool was never universal. In many parts of Africa, birth control was and remains a means to improve maternal health and thus future reproductive potential, a more technological version of earlier methods of birth spacing.[20] In former slave colonies in the Caribbean, early advocates faced opposition on multiple fronts: from religious opponents and from those who read into birth control a eugenic intent to curb black populations.[21] The practice has also had two histories in the United States: a white narrative of increased female decision-making and a black story of increased state control.[22]

16 Nancy Rose Hunt, '"Le bébé en brousse": European women, African birth spacing and colonial intervention in breast feeding in the Belgian Congo', *International Journal of African Historical Studies* 21 (1988), 401–32, on 406.

17 Ruth A. Miller, 'Rights, reproduction, sexuality, and citizenship in the Ottoman Empire and Turkey', *Signs* 32 (2007), 347–73, on 373; Tuba Demirci and Selçuk Akşin Somel, 'Women's bodies, demography, and public health: Abortion policy and perspectives in the Ottoman Empire of the nineteenth century', *Journal of the History of Sexuality* 17 (2008), 377–420; also Miri Shefer-Mossensohn and Rebecca Flemming, 'Generation in the Ottoman World', Chapter 19, this book.

18 Martin H. Johnson and Nick Hopwood, 'Modern Law and Regulation', Chapter 40, this book.

19 Jock McCulloch, *Black Peril, White Virtue: Sexual Crime in Southern Rhodesia, 1902–1935* (Bloomington, IN, 2000); Amirah Inglis, *The White Women's Protection Ordinance: Sexual Anxiety and Politics in Papua* (New York, NY, 1975). On eugenics in relation to animal breeding: Sarah Wilmot, 'Breeding Farm Animals and Humans', Chapter 27, this book.

20 Caroline H. Bledsoe, *Contingent Lives: Fertility, Time, and Aging in West Africa* (Chicago, IL, 2002).

21 Nicole C. Bourbonnais, *Birth Control in the Decolonizing Caribbean: Reproductive Politics and Practice on Four Islands, 1930–1970* (New York, NY, 2016).

22 Dorothy Roberts, *Killing the Black Body: Race, Reproduction, and the Meaning of Liberty* (New York, NY, 1997), p. 4.

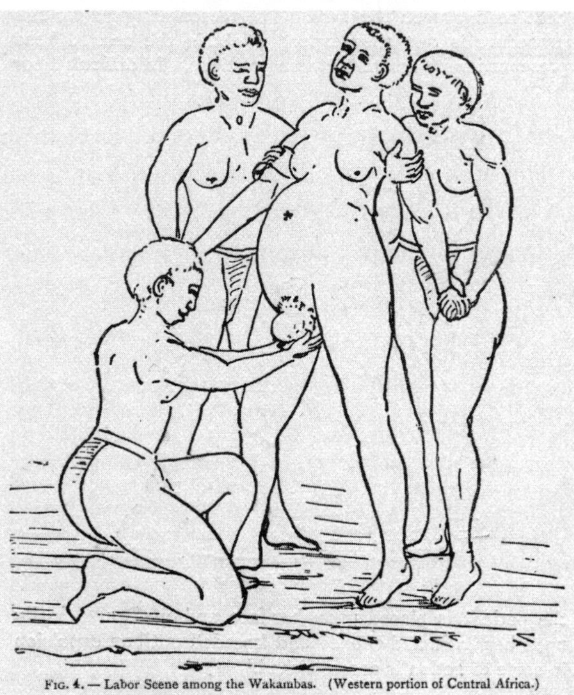

Fig. 4. — Labor Scene among the Wakambas. (Western portion of Central Africa.)

Figure 33.2 An African delivery scene from *Labor Among Primitive Peoples* by the noted American gynaecologist George Julius Engelmann. He offered many drawings of what he regarded as primitive birth practices, mostly in European colonies, which fed existing assumptions about childbirth beyond the west. From Engelmann, *Labor Among Primitive Peoples* (St Louis, MO: Chambers, 1883), p. 63.

Childbirth and Motherhood

The effects of colonial rule in the late nineteenth and early twentieth centuries were most visible on childbirth. The vast majority of women throughout the world continued to give birth at home until at least the mid-twentieth century, but the medicalization of obstetrics steadily grew.[23] The medical profession was centrally concerned with what doctors regarded as widespread and dangerously unprofessional modes of delivery (Fig. 33.2). Formal medical training was a closely guarded male preserve almost everywhere, and women's entry into the profession was slow and difficult. Yet despite the paucity of the obstetrical education that male doctors themselves received, they actively lobbied for the training and regulation of female midwives at home and in the colonies.

Women skilled in delivering babies in non-medicalized societies generally knew herbal and other remedies but had none of the formal training increasingly regarded

23 Salim Al-Gailani, 'Hospital Birth', Chapter 37; Nick Hopwood, 'Globalization', Chapter 43, this book.

as necessary in the west.[24] Critiques of the female birth attendant were loud, constant, vitriolic and near-universal, even among women doctors.[25] She was castigated as backward, superstitious, filthy, ignorant and dangerous, and blamed for mishandling deliveries, spreading disease through unhygienic practices and procuring abortions. She was the 'ubiquitous negative symbol' of all that modern western medicine rejected.[26] Writing in 1883, the German-American doctor George Engelmann described midwives as unchanged over time, distanced from modern obstetrical practice and unaware of new technologies.

> [T]hese good women were as unskilful thirty-five centuries ago as they can still be found at the present day. From all that we have seen it appears that the *Yi* of India, the *Dye* of Syria, the herb-knowing hag of Mexico, and the midwife of the Bible are very much the same in their habits, their qualifications, and their knowledge. It is the same habitual old woman who figures in all countries and at all times.[27]

A strong and tenacious link between poverty and uncleanliness fed the constant demonization of the birth attendant. Doctors bemoaned their difficulties in training unschooled, illiterate women in modern medical methods. Yet western midwife education in the colonies was rarely more than nugatory. Early training schemes were highly localized, some introduced by medical missionaries, others by local authorities. Not surprisingly, given the positive attitude to midwifery in the Netherlands and France, some of the earliest colonial training began at the Cape and in the Dutch East Indies,

24 In many cases they probably could and did advise on or assist with terminations as well as deliveries, although abortion was in some places in male hands: Lynn M. Thomas, *Politics of the Womb: Women, Reproduction, and the State in Kenya* (Berkeley, CA, 2003), p. 34.

25 Among many, see Lenore Manderson, 'Blame, responsibility and remedial action: Death, disease and the infant in early twentieth-century Malaya', in Norman G. Owen (ed.), *Death and Disease in Southeast Asia: Explorations in Social, Medical and Demographic History* (Singapore, 1987), pp. 257–82; Dagmar Engels, 'The politics of childbirth: British and Bengali women in contest, 1890–1930', in Peter Robb (ed.), *Society and Ideology: Essays in South Asian History Presented to Professor K. A. Ballhatchet* (Delhi and New York, NY, 1993), pp. 222–46, on pp. 226–7; Geraldine Forbes, 'Managing midwifery in India', in Dagmar Engels and Shula Marks (eds.), *Contesting Colonial Hegemony: State and Society in Africa and India* (London, 1994), pp. 152–72, on p. 154; Sandhya Shetty, '(Dis)locating gender space and medical discourse in colonial India', *Genders* 20 (1994), 188–230, on 196; Harriet Deacon, 'Midwives and medical men in the Cape Colony before 1860', *Journal of African History* 39 (1998), 271–92, on 275; Anshu Malhotra, 'Of dais and midwives: "Middle-class" interventions in the management of women's reproductive health. A study from colonial Punjab', *Indian Journal of Gender Studies* 10 (2003), 229–59; Seán Lang, 'Drop the demon dai: Maternal mortality and the state in colonial Madras, 1840–1875', *Social History of Medicine* 18 (2005), 357–78; and Juanita De Barros, *Reproducing the British Caribbean: Sex, Gender, and Population Politics after Slavery* (Chapel Hill, NC, 2014), pp. 68–71.

26 Maneesha Lal, 'The politics of gender and medicine in colonial India: The Countess of Dufferin's Fund, 1885–1888', *Bulletin of the History of Medicine* 68 (1994), 29–66, on 48; Margaret I. Balfour and Ruth Young, *The Work of Medical Women in India* (London, 1929).

27 George J. Engelmann, *Labor Among Primitive Peoples* (St Louis, MO, 1883), p. 17.

although state-funded midwifery classes also started in the Ottoman Empire in 1842 and in Egypt (under French supervision) in the 1830s. The earliest Dutch initiative was probably that undertaken by missionaries in Batavia in 1817, with a larger school of midwifery following in 1850.[28] Late in the century, training programmes emerged in Queensland, Jamaica, British Guiana and Uganda. More followed in the early twentieth century: in Senegal, Ceylon, the Sudan, Tanganyika and Barbados. Midwife registration began in the 1890s in Britain, Egypt, South Africa, Malaya and Australia among other countries, while in the Canadian province of Quebec doctors led an effort in the 1870s to eliminate midwifery entirely.[29]

It was not only midwives whose unhygienic and unmodern practices were blamed for high infant and maternal mortality rates. Colonial as well as poor mothers in the metropole were also typically rebuked as ignorant, unclean and unhealthy.[30] Feeding practices came in for particular criticism. Hygiene concerns spurred the promotion of breast-feeding. Fears over contaminated milk had some basis, given that refrigeration was everywhere limited well into the twentieth century. The French *goutte de lait*, or milk depot, became the model for schemes in the Belgian Congo, British India, Australia and Canada. In an early twentieth-century postcard, African mothers are bathing their babies; they also learned other forms of hygiene and received sterilized milk (Fig. 33.3).

Tinned milk from Europe and America was heavily advertised and widely available in the colonies, though aimed largely at Europeans and local elites for whom breast-feeding was uncongenial. Poor women generally breast-fed, but an inadequate diet could reduce the nutritional value of their milk. In the colonies, where the niceties of separate-sphere ideology seldom applied, many women with children also worked outside the home, disrupting feeding routines. They were often forced to rely on alternatives, despite the expense and doctors' warnings that tinned milk or solid foods given too early were detrimental to young babies.[31]

The same officials generally looked askance at traditional postnatal practices, including the cutting and disposal of the umbilical cord, and the early feeding and swaddling of newborns, lending credence to claims that inadequate mothering, fuelled by custom and ignorance, was to blame for the stubbornly high infant mortality rates

28 Susan Abeyasekere, 'Death and disease in nineteenth century Batavia', in Owen, *Death and Disease*, pp. 189–209, on p. 198.

29 Helene Laforce, 'The different stages of the elimination of midwives in Quebec', in Katherine Arnup, Andrée Lévesque and Ruth Roach Pierson (eds.), *Delivering Motherhood: Maternal Ideologies and Practices in the 19th and 20th Centuries* (London, 1990), pp. 36–50, on p. 41.

30 De Barros, *Reproducing the British Caribbean*, pp. 80, 84–5.

31 Judith Richell, 'Ephemeral lives: The unremitting infant mortality of colonial Burma, 1891–1941', in Valerie Fildes, Lara Marks and Hilary Marland (eds.), *Women and Children First: International Maternal and Infant Welfare, 1870–1945* (London, 1992), pp. 133–53, on p. 136.

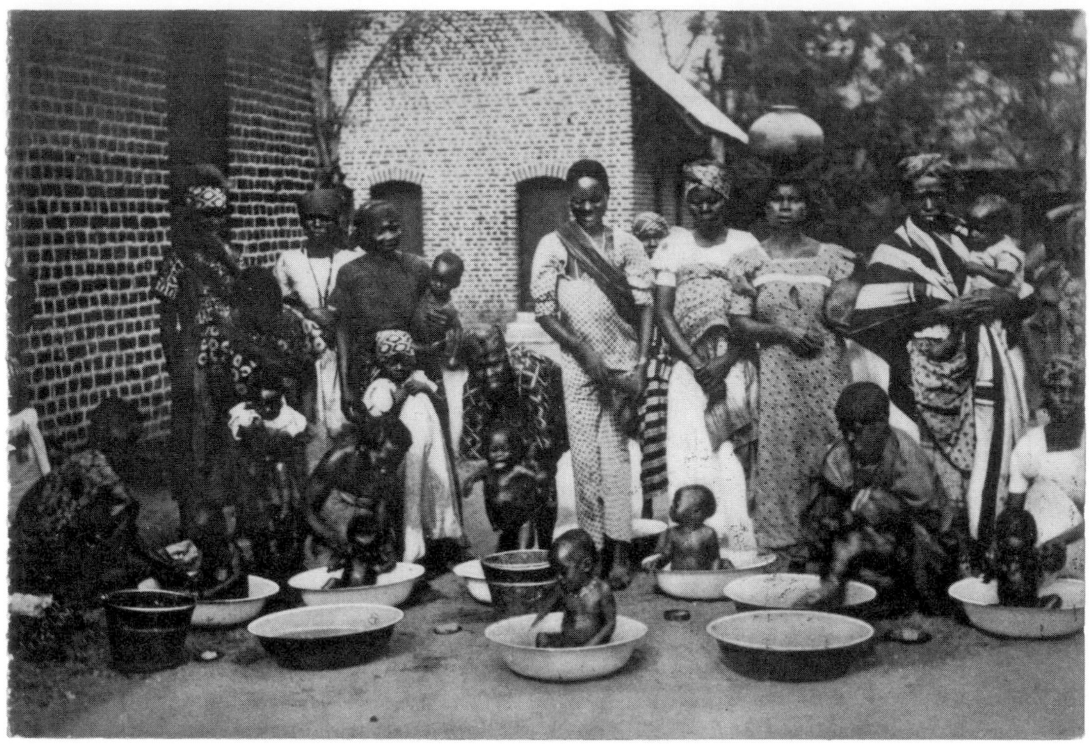

Figure 33.3 Postcard of a *goutte de lait* in the Belgian Congo. Missions such as that run by the Jesuits at Kwango, and pictured here, promoted these milk depots as a way to mitigate high infant mortality rates. The first was established in 1912 in Kisantu. 9 × 13 cm.

of the early twentieth century. In South Africa, black infants always died at a higher rate than whites – in the 1920s a staggering ten times higher at a time when rates were finally declining in many areas. The refusal of colonial as well as domestic officials to move beyond the trope of poor mothering was common; instead of addressing economic and environmental inequities, they often encouraged an ideology of mothercraft (Fig. 33.4).

Mothercraft guided a multiplicity of early twentieth-century schemes, including training classes in the new infant welfare clinics, health visiting schemes reminiscent of Victorian charity visiting and mothercraft curricula for schoolgirls. Hygiene training became commonplace in Indian schools, though few girls from poor families would have benefited since they were rarely schooled.[32] Mary Blacklock, the sole female

32 Mark Harrison, *Public Health in British India: Anglo-Indian Preventive Medicine, 1859–1914* (Cambridge, 1994), p. 96.

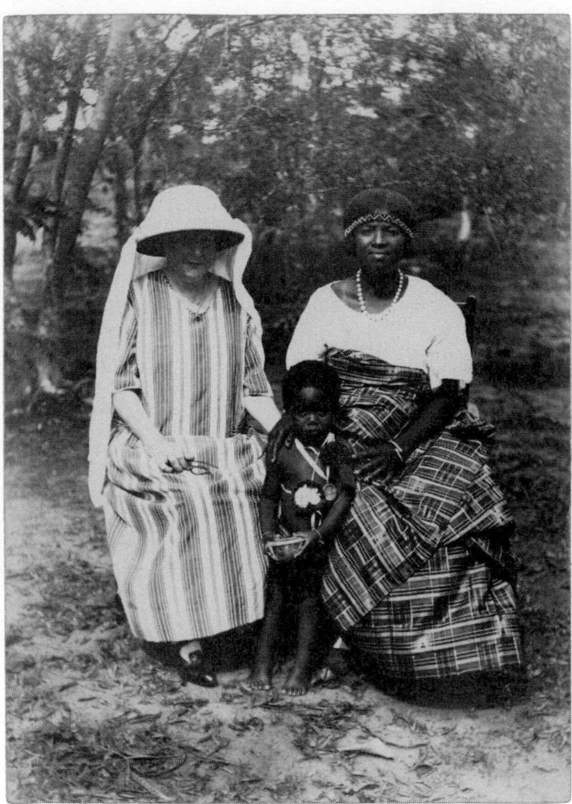

Figure 33.4 A baby show in Accra (then Gold Coast) in the 1920s. Such shows, part of mothercraft training, were by then widespread in African colonies. Queen Mary sent the silver bowl via Mrs Armstrong, the 'English lady' seen here. Photograph by Justus A. C. Holm, Smyly Collection, Royal Commonwealth Society, Y30448L/42, Cambridge University Library.

member of Britain's Colonial Advisory Medical Committee, promoted domestic training of African girls as the best means to reduce infant mortality rates and improve overall health.[33] Medical personnel, teachers and missionaries across Africa touted the benefits of mothercraft and hygiene training.[34]

The aim was the making of modern mothers attuned to the needs not only of their babies and families but also of the state.[35] This ideology of what Debby Gaitskell has called 'sanitized modernity' was widespread, and as actively pursued in Egypt and

33 Mary G. Blacklock, 'Co-operation in health education', *Africa* 4 (1931), 202–8, on 206.

34 Jean Allman, 'Making mothers: Missionaries, medical officers and women's work in colonial Asante, 1924–1945', *History Workshop Journal* 38 (1994), 23–47.

35 Anna Davin, 'Imperialism and motherhood', *History Workshop* 6 (1978), 9–65; see also Siân Pooley, '"Pity the Poor Mother!"', Exhibit 27, this book.

the Sudan as in Europe.[36] But the vision of the healthy productive family rang hollow in the colonies of all the major European powers, where the economic realities of imperialism disrupted family lives. The labour value of colonial peoples counted for more than the 'family values' claims that cloaked the new emphasis on reproduction.

Perhaps surprisingly, missionaries played only a minor role in childbirth and antenatal care in nineteenth-century colonies, though their medical enterprises were otherwise often important. Missionary doctors were rarely called to attend deliveries, demonstrating a clear preference among colonized women for local childbirth traditions and helpers.[37] While this must have been a source of frustration for missions, given the centrality of motherhood and family in Christian discourse, surprisingly few wrote about the issue.[38] Patients often moved between western and indigenous medicine, but childbirth remained mostly in local hands, suggesting that despite western intervention, women's choices still counted.

Conclusion

In an age when imperial power was the pinnacle of global achievement, reproduction became a core concern. As the hold of the European empires deepened and rivalry between them magnified in the later nineteenth and early twentieth centuries, women were increasingly cast as the reproductive foot soldiers in a largely European race to conquer the globe. Building on existing and sometimes long-standing attention to reproduction, articulated through expanding registration procedures, census statistics and medical regulation, national rivalries in the era of high imperialism precipitated what Hilary Marland has called the 'resolute intrusion of the state in female health matters'.[39]

Women's civic responsibilities were tied to motherhood and, in the metropolis as in the colonies, women became a prominent focus of state attention, because they were having either too few babies or too many for national or imperial interests – or because they might. The prejudiced stereotypes of indigenous hypersexuality and careless

36 Debby Gaitskell, '"Getting close to the hearts of mothers": Medical missionaries among African women and children in Johannesburg between the wars', in Fildes, Marks and Marland, *Women and Children First*, pp. 178–99, on p. 180; Abugideiri, *Gender and the Making of Modern Medicine*; Janice Boddy, 'Barbaric custom and colonial science: Teaching the female body in the Anglo-Egyptian Sudan', *Social Analysis* 47 (2003), 60–81, on 63.

37 Markku Hokkanen, *Medicine and Scottish Missionaries in the Northern Malawi Region, 1875–1930: Quests for Health in a Colonial Society* (Lewiston, NY, 2007), pp. 286–91.

38 David Hardiman, *Missionaries and Their Medicine: A Christian Modernity in Tribal India* (Manchester, 2008), esp. p. 144.

39 Hilary Marland, 'Women, health, and medicine', in Mark Jackson (ed.), *The Oxford Handbook of the History of Medicine* (Oxford, 2013), pp. 484–502, on p. 484.

parenting clashed with the real and often devastating effects of poverty and colonialism at a moment when both technological change and a surge in welfare politics might have permitted a profound change in the management of reproduction and the lives of women. On the ground, the penny-pinching of quotidian politics frequently rendered the vision of improved maternity and motherhood irrelevant, but, at home as well as in the colonies, colonial states maintained their new-found interest in controlling reproduction efficiently. This was bolstered by the discourse of eugenics and an ever-strengthening public health establishment for whom infant mortality represented an urgent challenge. The emergence, in the wake of Darwinian theory, of fears around degeneration – expressed in alarm over both depopulation and overpopulation – and the hope that eugenic practices could halt 'bad' and encourage 'good' reproduction signals a fundamental shift, especially to the conviction that reproduction could be improved by state and medical intervention. Such approaches exacted a heavy physical, political and economic toll on women.

Reproduction was rhetorically important to the empire, notably in the wake of the South African War with which the twentieth century began, but there was far more talk than action. The minimal obstetrical and gynaecological training of medical students and the shaky hold of midwifery training schemes, the overdiagnosis of syphilis as the cause of infertility and the failure to understand reproduction in cultural context (from conception through delivery to after-care) all inhibited material progress even as the available technologies of childbirth improved. These ideas and practices, ushered in through a strange brew of imperial anxiety and genuine humanitarian concern, rarely helped those who bore the next generation: the slave woman forced to breed slaves, the African woman whose husband worked in a distant mining compound or the Indian woman picking tea immediately after giving birth. Their future under colonial governance was far less certain and by no means always helped by the new approaches to reproduction.

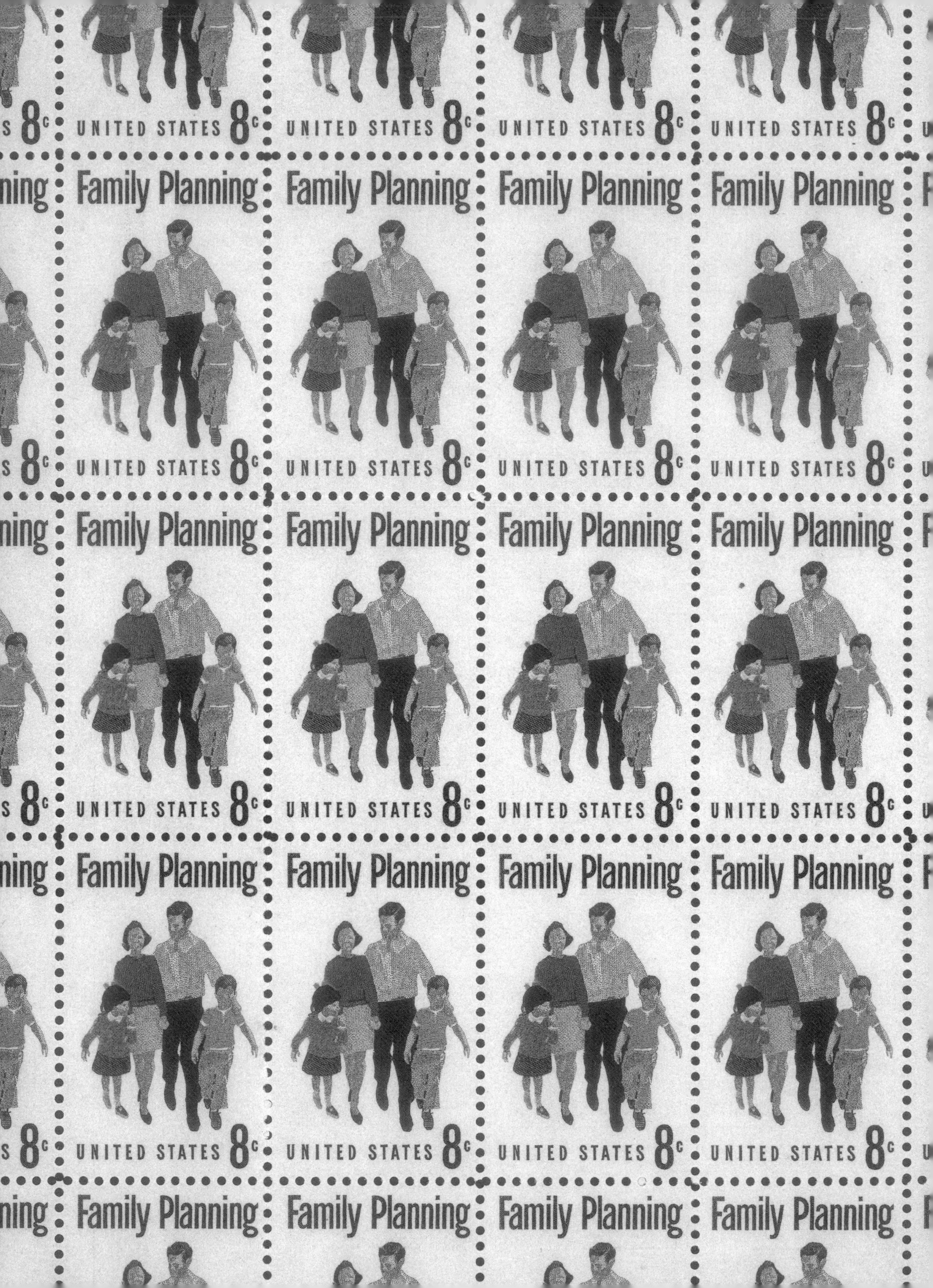
Family Planning
UNITED STATES 8c

Part V

Reproduction Centre Stage

Family planning stamps. In 1972 the United States Postal Service, following several in Asia (see Fig. 43.3), recognized the acceptability of planned parenthood. Population controllers having put most effort into reducing reproduction in 'less developed countries' and among African Americans, the stamp promoted a white nuclear family as the norm. The Postmaster General reminded 'all members of society of the current world environmental situation and the need for planning to have a better America and a better world'. Designer: Charles Reid; engravers: Joseph S. Creamer, Jr (vignette) and Kenneth C. Wiram (lettering). From a mint fifty-stamp sheet, each one 3.7 × 2.1 cm.

Already a coherent topic of importance in national and international politics by the outbreak of World War II in 1939, reproduction moved centre stage as science and medicine claimed ever larger roles in and after the conflict. We can identify two contrasting phases of change. During the postwar (baby) boom in the west, childbirth and contraception were further medicalized, and the United States, locked in Cold War with the Soviet Union, began to lead industrialized countries in exporting population control to the now increasingly decolonized 'Third World'. From the late 1960s, social movements, especially feminism, challenged medical authority and produced a new politics of reproduction, which was then reconfigured during economic restructuring and the rise of neoliberalism. Part V analyses these changes, revisiting those innovations that historians have studied most, including hospital birth and the oral contraceptive pill, and exploring other major novelties, such as contraceptives that were more widely used and technologies of assisted conception.

Postwar governments established more comprehensive welfare and health-care systems and funded large-scale research. Especially in Europe, communitarianism and state action defined the era; medical authority rose to a peak. The term 'biomedicine' describes the regime, based on wartime models, which combined biological research, medical care, industry and state regulation in a variety of feedback loops. In obstetrics, where the aim had been to provide a safety-net to catch the few cases that needed intervention, antenatal monitoring and surveillance of every pregnancy became the ideal. Childbirth, in the 1930s still mostly at home in Europe and even the United States, entered the hospital to varying degrees around the world, but globalization relied on adaptation to local conditions (Salim Al-Gailani, 'Hospital Birth', Chapter 37). Maternal mortality finally declined in industrialized countries, but as women invested more in fewer pregnancies, they were taught new fears, including of age as a risk factor for Down syndrome (Ilana Löwy, 'Prenatal Diagnosis, Surveillance and Risk', Chapter 38).

While the war and the postwar decade reinforced pronatalism and marriage, which enjoyed unmatched popularity in Europe and North America, contraception was generally accepted as a means of ensuring that children were wanted, healthy and legitimate. Physicians overcame their reluctance to prescribe birth control, now reframed as a moral duty, and installed themselves as gatekeepers to medical technologies. The pill, the most famous product of the reproductive sciences, went on sale in the United States in 1957. Part of the more general separation of sexual activity from procreation, the pill was associated with a 'sexual revolution' that for many groups happened only later; but in Britain, for example, it did represent a significant shift from male to female responsibility for contraception – by extending women's existing practice of menstrual regulation. It was soon joined by other medical products and procedures, especially new intrauterine devices and quicker sterilizations, today the most used methods worldwide (Jesse Olszynko-Gryn, 'Technologies of Contraception and Abortion', Chapter 36).

The crimes of National Socialism cast a long shadow, but eugenics survived in other forms. Geneticists, who had begun in the 1930s to approach race in terms of gene frequencies within populations, took over eugenics institutes and journals (Jenny Bangham, 'Populations, Genetics and Race', Exhibit 30); the profession of genetic counselling was established. Neo-Malthusianism morphed into population control as American-led agencies warned that exploding numbers would push developing countries into Soviet arms. International bodies, including the United Nations and the World Health Organization, developed population policies, often in cooperation with American philanthropies such as the Rockefeller and Ford Foundations. Catholic and communist distrust limited the effects, but in the 1960s a fragile consensus, also among the nationalist leaders of newly independent countries, allowed contraception into United Nations development projects and to be funded by the US Agency for International Development (USAID), especially in India. With personal freedom, family planning and limits to growth all pressing issues, mass-market paperbacks, notably Paul R. Ehrlich's *The Population Bomb* (1968), and films such as *Z.P.G.* (1972) and *Soylent Green* (1973), mediated a 'Malthusian moment', its slogan 'Make love, not babies' (Alison Bashford, 'World Population from Eugenics to Climate Change', Chapter 34; Patrick Ellis, '*Z.P.G.*', Exhibit 36).

Inaugurating the second phase in the rise of reproductive politics, a sea-change in attitudes began in the 1960s, when the huge baby-boom generation became teenagers and insisted on dispensing with such formalities as marriage, and gained momentum in the 1970s. Feminist campaigners radicalized reform initiatives within the professions – these were the main impetus behind the 1967 Abortion Act in Britain – and generalized them beyond family planning circles. Struggles for contraception and abortion-law reform scored signal successes, above all the 1973 US Supreme Court judgement in the case of *Roe v. Wade* that ruled state-level anti-abortion laws unconstitutional because they violated a woman's right to privacy (Martin H. Johnson and Nick Hopwood, 'Modern Law and Regulation', Chapter 40). This and a companion ruling also extended medical autonomy, and critics lambasted 'medicalization'; hospital birth and contraceptive safety were debated as part of a more general claiming of patients' rights. Women's health movements organized alternatives to 'malestream' medicine and worked to make services more sensitive to their needs, especially through a bestselling manual (Wendy Kline, '*Our Bodies, Ourselves*', Exhibit 35). Theoretically as well as practically, feminism put reproduction on the agenda as integral to modern economies and societies, and sought to liberate women from the assumption that reproduction was naturally their domain (Sarah Franklin, 'Feminism and Reproduction', Chapter 42).

By the mid-1970s, when western consumers were boycotting multinationals that sold formula milk in the Third World, the short-lived consensus on population and birth control had shattered. Feminist activists fought for 'reproductive rights', while some population controllers pursued yet more coercive programmes, most notoriously during the Indian Emergency and then through China's one-child policy. By contrast, the last International Conference on Population Control and Development, held in Cairo in 1994, promoted a paradigm of reproductive health that stressed women's freedom to decide about their fertility. But anti-abortionists were already pushing for recognition of the personhood of fetuses that were now more publicly visible: antenatal monitoring had constructed a 'fetal patient', photojournalism put aborted fetuses on magazine covers, and frank sex education had entered schools (Solveig Jülich, '"Drama of Life before Birth"', Exhibit 34). In the United States, the New Right made opposition to abortion a pillar of its coalition and, by banning federal funding of organizations that provide abortion counselling or referrals, Republican presidents have since 1984 restricted international action too. Climate change has recently renewed the urgency of concern over global population growth, even as the rate slowed. Since 1980, ever more countries have reproduced themselves only thanks to immigration.

Meanwhile, the oil crisis of 1973 had marked the end of the long postwar economic boom and the beginning of a period of capitalist restructuring, the other underlying shift of these decades. Although private funding had long played key roles alongside state interventions in reproduction, most debates assumed, on both sides, that the issue was whether or not governments should exercise more control. The rationalization of animal breeding served as model and warning, especially from the 1930s, when laboratory science began to transform livestock production through artificial insemination. Funding from agricultural and population control interests let fertility researchers found centres, societies and journals at the intersection of academic biology, clinical and veterinary medicine, industrialized agriculture and pharmaceutical industry (Sarah Wilmot, 'Breeding Farm Animals and Humans', Chapter 27; Nick Hopwood, 'Artificial Fertilization', Chapter 39). Biology produced such controversial novelties as cloning, recombinant DNA and in vitro fertilization (IVF) (Christina Brandt, 'Cloned Frogs', Exhibit 37; Nick Hopwood, '"It's a Girl"', Exhibit 38). But by the time that medical scientists could reliably fertilize human eggs outside the body, state planning was going out of fashion. The end of the Cold War in 1989 consolidated neoliberalism; governments did less, while global corporations, non-governmental organizations and supranational institutions gained power. Over the next quarter-century, maternal and neonatal mortality almost halved worldwide, but remained high in some regions as inequality increased.

Biomedicine expanded through this era of globalization. From 1980, IVF clinics were founded as hubs of a 'reproductive medicine' dependent on transnational transfers of people, practices and products, with differences in regulations between countries driving much travel (Nick Hopwood, 'Globalization', Chapter 43). This industry is one of several linked innovations of the period since 1960. John Forrester asks to what extent Michel Foucault's analysis of the field of the sexual – the dominant paradigm for the past forty years – might usefully be renovated to encompass these connections and dislocations ('Sex, Gender and Babies', Chapter 41). Or have the successes of the contraceptive revolution, the gay and feminist movements, the market in assisted reproductive technologies, the concept of 'gender' and practices of gender reassignment altered the world too much?

Biomedicine did not just expand; it also intensified and adjusted to incorporate enhancements of reproductive health and a culture of managing risks in increasingly privatized systems, with more sources of authority and arm's-length regulation by states. As surveillance deepened, prenatal diagnosis made pregnancy more tentative; in some communities, it fostered abortion for sex selection. More recently, environmental effects on inheritance have become a hot field of research into risks, especially of obesity (Tatjana Buklijas, 'Developmental Origins of Health and Disease', Exhibit 39). In a medical world no longer dominated by physicians, consumers' voices are now formally recognized, including in regulatory institutions (Jean-Paul Gaudillière, 'Sex Hormones, Pharmacy and the Reproductive Sciences', Chapter 35). Science routinely assists nature, but has supplemented not supplanted religious and other rites (Jessica Hughes and Rebecca Flemming, 'The Room of the Ribbons', Exhibit 40). Media debate has become an essential part of gaining consent to any innovation; today, reproduction happens on screens as well as in bedrooms, clinics and barns.

NICK HOPWOOD

34 World Population from Eugenics to Climate Change

Alison Bashford

It is well known that population growth accelerated at an unprecedented rate over the twentieth century. That the planet now sustains approaching eight billion people is often bemoaned. But when pressed, it is difficult for policymakers, politicians, the public and sometimes scholars to pin down just what makes population growth problematic, and even harder for them to find solutions. As political and intellectual history, the world population problem is a complicated object of inquiry too. It is a tight knot of tangled motivations, humanitarian aims and hidden agendas, some obvious and odious to us now, others less so. Unlikely alliances formed as multiple interest groups joined funding, research and lobbying forces, attempting to understand and to modify fertility and mortality rates on regional and world levels. At the same time, unexpected transnational allies blocked advocacy of voluntary fertility control, and rejected the very idea that world population growth constituted a problem for intervention.

This chapter traces the ways in which population came to be seen as an international and global problem over the twentieth century and into the present.[1] It focuses on the organizations and institutions through which world population was examined as well as politicized, including the chequered uptake of reproduction and population matters within the League of Nations, the United Nations (UN) and their multiple agencies. Philanthropic foundations and then non-governmental organizations (NGOs) weighed in earlier and more strongly, with discussion, research and activity that involved a range of population experts from geographers to birth control researchers, economists to ecologists. Throughout, sexual and gender politics were linked to a changing global political economy, intimate relations to international relations, and population growth to political unrest. Population growth and aspirations to control it at a world level thus became the business of major movements, from eugenics to feminism to environmentalism.

1 For the earlier history: Rebecca Flemming, 'States and Populations in the Classical World', Chapter 5; Peter Biller, 'The Multitude in Later Medieval Thought', Chapter 10; Philip Kreager, 'The Emergence of Population', Chapter 18; Andrea Rusnock, 'Biopolitics and the Invention of Population', Chapter 23, this book.

Global Malthusians and World Eugenics

Around 1800, Malthus's *Essay on the Principle of Population* linked the regulation of human population growth and world history. In this early limits-to-growth argument, Malthus wrote about the world as an island, in which spatial limits on cultivable land, and hence food, necessarily affected population.[2] That forced the constant regulation of fertility and mortality. Early twentieth-century 'neo-Malthusians' took this idea and sought to shift the means of that regulation from uncontrolled to planned measures, and from death (infanticide, abortion, starvation, disease, infant mortality) to the prevention of life (new forms of contraception). They included economists such as Radhakamal Mukerjee in India, demographers such as Warren Thompson in the United States, medical practitioners such as the Drysdale family in Britain, geneticists such as Edward East and feminists such as Margaret Sanger.[3] Rightly or wrongly, they perceived this shift as good political economy, the best intervention into the problem of poverty. The neo-Malthusians of the early twentieth century thus understood their work not only as humanitarian, but also as improving and civilizing. By the end of the century, however, it was the reproductive rights tradition of argument for birth control, as distinct from the food security or geopolitical security cases, that had achieved phenomenal success.

Neo-Malthusians harboured international ambitions, pursued organizationally through the establishment of an International Neo-Malthusian Bureau at the Hague in 1910, and intellectually through connections to early twentieth-century internationalism. For British, Dutch, Indian and French Malthusians, controlling fertility on a large scale and in many different parts of the globe would contribute to world peace. Along with many economists, they reasoned that population growth driving overpopulation in relation to the productivity of land in one region, vis-à-vis optimal population in relation to land in another region, was a key driver of international tension and war. Their utopian vision in which fertility was reduced, freeing up enough food for all, was part of an aspirational world federation. Cosmopolitan politics – the powerful idea of 'one world' – and population politics have long been linked. Thus the neo-Malthusians dreamed of a League of Low Birth-Rate Nations, a nominally inclusive, expanding group in which the fertility decline already evident in France, the United Kingdom, the Australasian colonies and North America would become a much wider trend. Led by Europeans, soon influentially to involve Americans, and early including Indian economists, neo-Malthusians envisaged fertility decline as a world-scale programme through

2 T. R. Malthus, *An Essay on the Principle of Population* ..., 2nd edn (London, 1803); Alison Bashford, *Global Population: History, Geopolitics, and Life on Earth* (New York, NY, 2014).

3 Lesley A. Hall, 'Movements to Separate Sex and Reproduction', Chapter 29, this book.

mass education of the poor; contraceptive advice and new technologies were, they argued, already available to monied men and women.

This neo-Malthusian zeal for a new internationalism, a 'brotherhood of man', dovetailed with a politicizing of birth control for women. Picking up French republican feminism, on the one hand, and the political economy of John Stuart Mill, on the other, neo-Malthusians proposed that, as a matter of individual human 'liberty' and even 'right', women should have the means and freedom to control their reproductive lives. This, too, was early a world-level enterprise, and birth control lobbyists linked arguments about women's reproductive autonomy to political outcomes in the international sphere as a matter of course. Margaret Sanger's 1922 manifesto for the American Birth Control League, for example, had an international agenda: 'to study Birth Control in its relations to the world population problem, food supplies, national and racial conflicts, and to urge upon all international bodies organized to promote world peace, the consideration of these aspects of international amity'.[4]

Although often assessed as conflicting ideologies, the feminism and eugenics that Sanger espoused were easily and widely reconciled as programmes for progressive human transformation, at individual and population levels. Many left-wing economists and biologists pushed fertility regulation as key to human welfare and improvement. It was a commonplace in the early twentieth century to suggest that a (quantitative) transition to low birth-rates and low infant mortality rates was the necessary precursor to a qualitative transition to a fitter population. As eugenicists and Malthusians both had it, frequent childbirth manifested as unhealthy newborns, likely to die in infancy. Precisely this formulation of bioeconomic 'waste' and 'inefficiency' was to be repeated in American sociologist Kingsley Davis's ecologically informed rendition of demographic transition theory in 1945.[5] In these earlier decades, preventing the reproduction of the world's 'degenerates or defectives, its derelicts and its poor', was called, by some, not eugenics but 'New Malthusianism', ready to be rolled out on a global stage.[6]

The history of eugenics is well documented and understood, but its links to internationalism, its world-scale ambitions and global vision are less often noted. Nor are eugenics and environmentalism often understood to be linked, yet the political and epistemological connections were strong, not least through ecological methods that counted the life and death of organisms in relation to each other, and to their spatially

4 Margaret Sanger, *The Pivot of Civilization* (New York, NY, 1922), appendix: 'Principles and aims of the American Birth Control League'.

5 Kingsley Davis, 'The world demographic transition', *Annals of the American Academy of Political and Social Science* 237 (1945), 1–11; Simon Szreter, 'Fertility Transitions and Sexually Transmitted Infections', Chapter 30, this book.

6 Sir George Handley Knibbs, *The Shadow of the World's Future* ... (London, 1928), p. 114; see also Philippa Levine, 'Imperial Encounters', Chapter 33, this book.

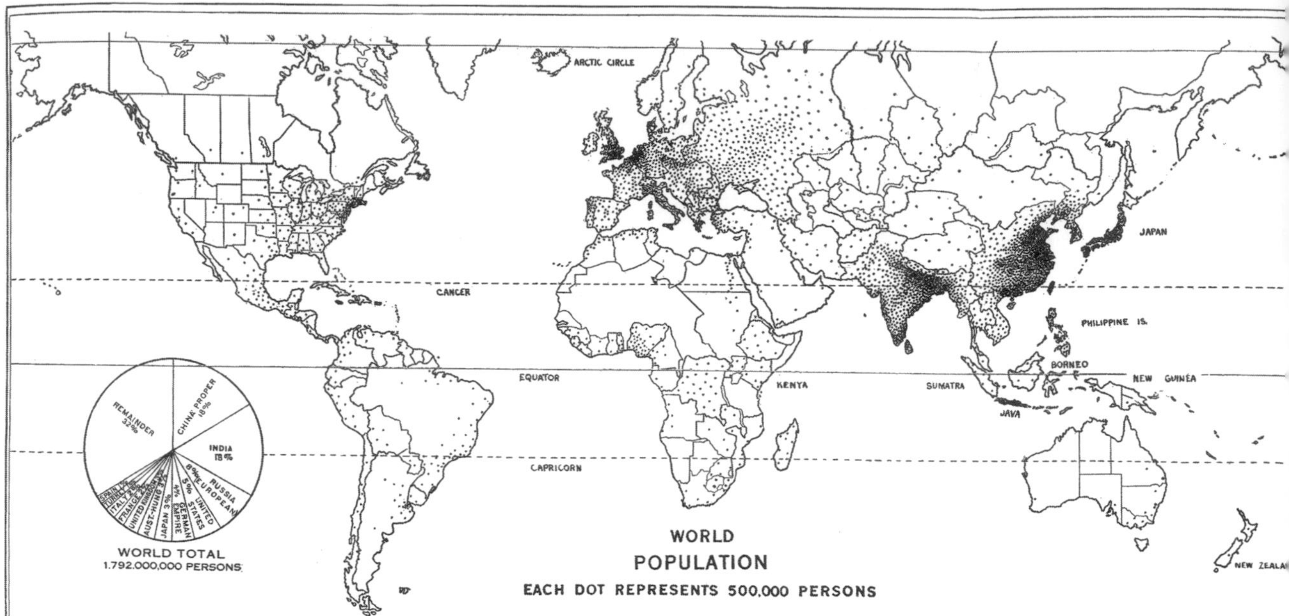

Reproduced, by permission, from *Geography of World Agriculture*, by V. C. Finch and O. E. Baker.

Figure 34.1 Warren Thompson's map of world population density. As was common in the interwar period, it reveals three major 'danger spots' in Thompson's terminology: East Asia, South Asia and Europe. From Thompson, *Danger Spots in World Population* (New York, NY: Knopf, 1929), facing p. 4.

limited environment.[7] Such ideas spilled into the political domain. In 1919, the *Journal of Heredity* published 'Immigration restriction and world eugenics', an article that captured the powerful crossover of political economy, natural history and nationalist geography.[8] The author, lawyer Prescott Hall, predictably advocated immigration restriction to the United States. But his political aspirations rested on a Malthusian and ultimately ecological argument, in which land and space correlated with increased fertility and population growth. Malthus himself had made this general point with respect to North America. Hall's early twentieth-century plan was to reserve that space for American 'natives', meaning Anglo-derived families.

This was just one of several ways in which eugenics and immigration restriction functioned on an intercontinental stage. Another constituted perhaps the most sustained manifestation of eugenics over many decades and into the present: the clauses in

7 Thomas Robertson, *The Malthusian Moment: Global Population Growth and the Birth of American Environmentalism* (New Brunswick, NJ, 2012), pp. 13–35.

8 Prescott F. Hall, 'Immigration restriction and world eugenics', *Journal of Heredity* 10 (1919), 125–7.

immigration acts that excluded or deported people with mental illnesses.[9] And yet commentators on world population were just as likely to oppose race-based immigration restriction. In these years, population was assessed as much spatially (in terms of density) as temporally (growth over time), and many demographers saw differential densities between regions as problematic. Early to mid-twentieth-century solutions thus encompassed not only interventions into fertility, but also mass migration to even out the 'danger spots' where overcrowded regions abutted underutilized, undercultivated lands (Fig. 34.1). Many argued that immigration restriction acts compounded the problem, blocking migration into undercultivated and underpopulated regions. Such early demographers as Sripati Chandrasekhar and Warren Thompson decried immigration acts as short-sighted nationalist measures that stopped the peace-securing free movement of humans across the globe.[10]

Population and the League of Nations

Hall had called for 'world eugenics' in response to the formation of the League of Nations, attempting like many others to have eugenic ideas and ideals incorporated into the work of the league's assembly and its various agencies. They would all fail. Eugenics was too closely linked to birth control and sterilization for Catholic member states to do anything but decry it. *Casti Connubii* (Of chaste wedlock), the 1930 encyclical of Pope Pius XI, pronounced directly and damningly on birth control, placing the Vatican at the forefront of transnational opposition. But it is perhaps more intriguing to note that the church also led resistance to coerced eugenic sterilization. While it undermined women's right to control conception, it defended in this period all people's right (or duty) to reproduce (though not all medical interventions to this end).[11]

During the 1920s and 1930s, the secretariat of the League of Nations approached and retreated from the issue of world population growth, time and again. Population matters were most easily incorporated as an economic phenomenon – optimum population was defined according to standards of living and levels of employment, although occasionally health-based criteria, especially longevity and infant mortality rates, signalled under- or overpopulation. In these decades, population and the movement of

9 Alison Bashford, 'Insanity and immigration restriction', in Catherine Cox and Hilary Marland (eds.), *Migration, Health and Ethnicity in the Modern World* (New York, NY, 2013), pp. 14–35.

10 S. Chandrasekhar, *Hungry People and Empty Lands: An Essay on Population Problems and International Tensions* (Baroda, 1952).

11 *Casti Connubii, Encyclical of Pope Pius XI on Christian Marriage* (1930); on sterilization, further: Jesse Olszynko-Gryn, 'Technologies of Contraception and Abortion', Chapter 36; and Paul Weindling, 'Pedigree of a "Schizophrenic Family"', Exhibit 29; and for Catholic opposition to artificial insemination: Nick Hopwood, 'Artificial Fertilization', Chapter 39, this book.

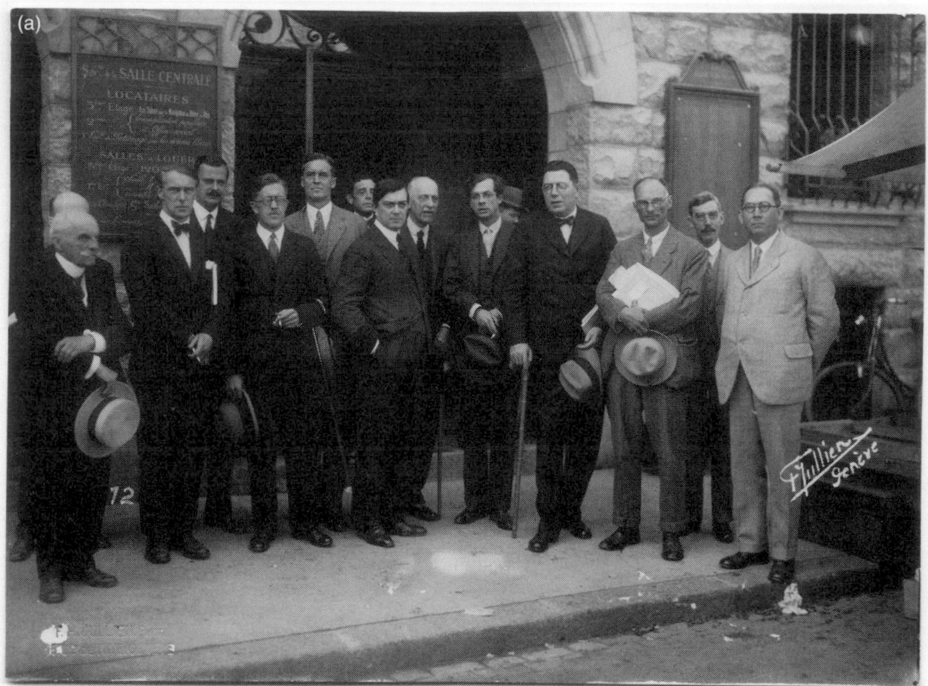

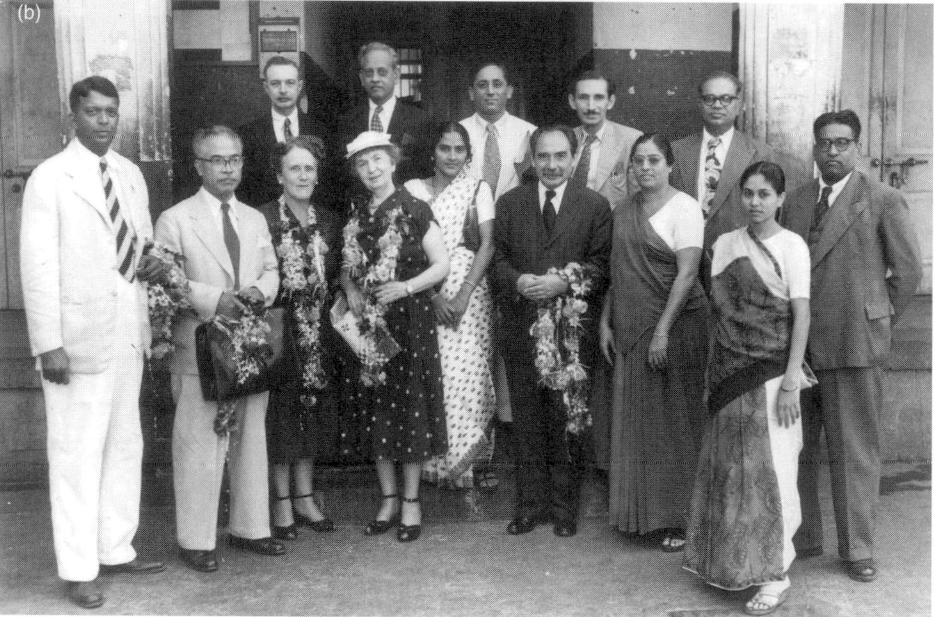

Figure 34.2 Between the 1920s and the 1950s, the participants in world population meetings diversified considerably. (a) The World Population Conference organized by Margaret Sanger in Geneva in 1927; (b) the founding meeting of the International Planned Parenthood Federation in Bombay, 1952. Photographs by F. H. Jullien, Geneva, and Asian Photos, Bombay, courtesy of the Margaret Sanger Papers, Sophia Smith Collection, Smith College, Northampton, MA.

labour across the world were regularly connected. For this reason, of all the league's associated bodies, the International Labour Office was perhaps closest to intervening in the question of world population.

The league's Health Committee also, on occasion, addressed the control of reproduction, attempting to render it an international issue. In 1930, the same year as *Casti Connubii*, a senior medical officer in the UK Ministry of Health, Dame Janet Campbell, was commissioned to study maternal and infant mortality for the League of Nations Health Committee. By endorsing contraception, at the very least where a woman's physical health indicated the need, her 1932 report sparked a major controversy, fuelled by the Catholic press, Catholic doctors' organizations and Catholic welfare groups, and fought between Irish and Italian delegations, on the one hand, and the putatively independent Health Committee, on the other.[12] Opponents argued successfully that interruption or prevention of conception was illegal in many, if not most, constituent nations and in any case was against the moral codes of millions, so could not be represented or recommended by an international body such as the Health Committee.

This explains the real caution with which league officers had approached the World Population Conference, provocatively held in Geneva, home of the league, in 1927 (Fig. 34.2a). The meeting had a global scope, announcing the core problem for discussion: 'The earth, and every geographical division of it, is strictly limited in size and in ability to support human populations.'[13] Yet birth control propaganda had been refused at that key meeting of international experts, notwithstanding either Sanger's central role or its provenance in a series of International Neo-Malthusian meetings. That conference still spawned two important international organizations that grappled with population growth in very different ways. One was the Birth Control International Information Centre, a London-based internationalization of women's advocacy groups that functioned through the 1930s. The other, quite different, was the International Union for the Scientific Investigation of Population Problems, an organization run by biologists, economists and physicians that attempted to set politics to one side. This proved impossible, especially in the 1930s when fascist statesmen in particular were politicizing reproduction in starkly pronatalist terms.

Disparities in population density had long been comprehended as contributing to international tensions, and indeed to war. The escalation of *Lebensraum* (living space) arguments in Nazi Germany, following Mussolini's policies of demographically based colonial expansion and land reform, had rendered the relation between reproduction,

12 League of Nations Archives, Geneva, Box R6003 (Health Section): Draft Report, Committee on Maternal Welfare and the Hygiene of Infants and Children (1931), p. 25.

13 Margaret Sanger (ed.), *Proceedings of the World Population Conference …* (London, 1927), p. 5.

states and territorial claims firmly an international relations issue, and one that the league, ultimately, could not ignore.[14] In the late 1930s, the assembly finally established a Demographic Committee to assess population, war and world distributions of natural resources. The committee was chaired by Alexander Carr-Saunders of the London School of Economics, himself deeply interested and schooled in the control of human reproduction, but all league-endorsed work had to tread carefully when it came to population.[15]

The United Nations, from Resistance to Promotion of Population Control

In the event, the Demographic Committee, created on the cusp of war in 1939, was relocated to the Office of Population Research at Princeton University. There, international conversation on world population growth and reproduction grafted readily onto prior US demographic research. The result was a dovetailing of League of Nations endeavours and the ideas that Frank Notestein and Kingsley Davis were just then refining on demographic transition, development and modernization.[16] Notestein had established the Office of Population Research in 1936. A decade later, he headed the new UN Population Division, part of its Economic and Social Council. This was already a greater acknowledgement of population growth as a world problem than the league had ever allowed, although the Population Division's function was to be purely statistical for some years yet. Catholic nations, as well as the USSR, about which Notestein had just published, still watched warily.

As well might they, since in other sections and agencies of the UN, public figures long involved in politicizing and promoting a world population problem within the international public sphere were now in leading roles. John Boyd Orr, physician and nutritionist, directed the Food and Agriculture Organization (FAO), where he linked the questions of postwar population growth and world food production, consumption and distribution. Biologist Julian Huxley, appointed Director-General of the UN Educational, Scientific and Cultural Organization (UNESCO), co-operated with Boyd Orr to put population control on the UN agenda. Both felt licensed by the uptake of ideas

14 Maria Sophia Quine, 'Racial "sterility" and "hyperfecundity" in fascist Italy: Biological politics of sex and reproduction', *Fascism* 1 (2012), 92–144.

15 A. M. Carr-Saunders, *World Population: Past Growth and Present Trends* (Oxford, 1936); Richard Symonds and Michael Carder, *The United Nations and the Population Question, 1945–1970* (London, 1973).

16 Frank W. Notestein *et al.*, *The Future Population of Europe and the Soviet Union: Population Projections, 1940–1970* (Geneva, 1944); Simon Szreter, 'The idea of demographic transition and the study of fertility change: A critical intellectual history', *Population and Development Review* 19 (1993), 659–701; Szreter, 'Fertility Transitions'.

about world federalism and world peace in the earliest years of the UN. For example, Boyd Orr's *Food: The Foundation of World Unity* (1946) linked population, food security and systems of world governance.[17]

Both were too optimistic, however, and paid with their jobs. The control of reproduction through any technical method was still highly controversial. Soviet delegations successfully opposed the Malthusian principles on which Huxley based his case for population control: poverty, the Soviets argued, was about the maldistribution of wealth and ownership of the means of production, not fertility and mortality rates. Thus, when the World Health Organization (WHO) embarked on a small trial in India in the early 1950s, member states objected. Even though this trial was limited to the rhythm method, and came at the invitation of the Indian government, it was too controversial to repeat.[18]

The WHO, like UNESCO and the FAO, was defeated in its early bids for reproductive control to be part of any technical assistance programme. By 1954, however, there was enough worldwide discussion of population growth for the UN to endorse a major conference, held in Rome. By 1969 the UN Fund for Population Activities had been established, under the UN Development Fund.

Philanthropy, Foundations and NGOs

Conversation in the international public sphere was in part turned around by the influential efforts of US philanthropy, including the Ford Foundation and the Scripps Foundation. John D. Rockefeller III influentially pressed US involvement in population control. Various arms of the Rockefeller Foundation had been involved in international health since the beginning of the twentieth century, but John D. Rockefeller III had developed particular interests in East Asia. In 1952, at his behest and under the auspices of the National Academy of Sciences, leading American demographers, economists, physicians and agriculturalists gathered in Williamsburg, Virginia, to think through world population growth and strategies for its control. The question of demographic transition and its relation to economic development was at the very core of discussion. Debate turned also to new technologies of contraception and new strategies for increasing food production. Various Rockefeller enterprises had been key to research and

17 Bashford, *Global Population*, pp. 181–304; on UNESCO and population genetics: Jenny Bangham, 'Populations, Genetics and Race', Exhibit 30, this book.

18 John Farley, *Brock Chisholm, the World Health Organization, and the Cold War* (Vancouver, 2008); Matthew Connelly, *Fatal Misconception: The Struggle to Control World Population* (Cambridge, MA, 2008); Nick Hopwood, 'Globalization', Chapter 43; on the rhythm method: Martina Schlünder, 'Menstrual-Cycle Calendars', Exhibit 31, this book.

development in the so-called green revolution, as well.[19] The Population Council was the main outcome of this initiative.

US foundations were typically driven by anti-communism in these years. Although historians tend to approach this as a hidden agenda that their scholarship uncovers, in fact high-level actors in the field were explicit about the link between population control and Cold War politics as they successfully lobbied the American government to fund family planning as part of international development. The Cold War context was key to influential US backing of international family planning programmes, but the connection between world population growth, war and peace had been argued at least from World War I. In other words, internationalism routinely turned into anti-communism for those thinking about world population. For example, the Dixie-Cup millionaire Hugh Moore, who drove strong population control (in particular, voluntary sterilization) programmes in the 1950s and 1960s on an anti-communist line, had been an interwar advocate of internationalism. From that interwar linking of Malthusianism, pacifism and internationalism, as much as from the Cold War itself, Moore launched his millions, via the Hugh Moore Fund, into the population field. The connection between population growth, famine and political unrest was eventually persuasive in Washington, DC, and family planning became a formal part of US foreign policy, implemented through the Food for Peace programme.[20]

The politics of postwar world population programmes are often assessed as starkly divided. On the one hand, feminist-oriented initiatives promoted individual women's health and well-being through 'family planning', with the significant establishment of the International Planned Parenthood Federation in 1952 (Fig. 34.2b). On the other, organizations interested in 'population control' such as the Population Council are presented as having fairly crude political security agendas. In truth, personnel and agendas crossed between these domains. Both are typically interpreted as being driven by elite groups, their ambitions secured on and through the bodies and lives of the subaltern poor, and often enabled by racialized presumptions. There is much evidence of just that, and the link between early twentieth-century eugenics and later twentieth-century population control is clear.[21] And yet there is a reverse chronology too: global Malthusianism itself pre-dated and created early eugenics. We should perhaps be unsurprised that postwar liberal figures like biologist and writer Julian Huxley continued to claim eugenics as a progressive, improving, even humanitarian programme in the postwar years, that is, even after the Holocaust and the trial of Nazi doctors. It was the

19 John H. Perkins, *Geopolitics and the Green Revolution: Wheat, Genes, and the Cold War* (Oxford, 1997).

20 John Sharpless, 'World population growth, family planning, and American foreign policy', *Journal of Policy History* 7 (1995), 72–102.

21 For example, Ian Dowbiggin, *The Sterilization Movement and Global Fertility in the Twentieth Century* (Oxford, 2008).

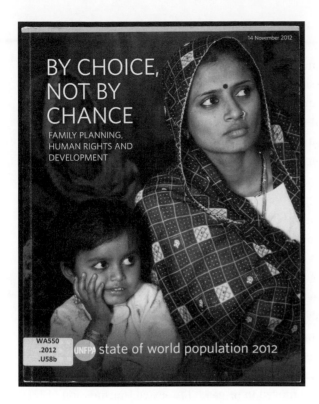

Figure 34.3 Mother and child, Pakistan, an image of assertive choice, representing the post-Cairo agenda, on the cover of the United Nations Population Fund report, *By Choice, Not by Chance*, 14 Nov. 2012, courtesy of UNFPA and Peter Barker (Panos Pictures). Wellcome Library, London.

internationalist and pacifist argument that was mobilized yet again. Popular and expert studies on world population, world war and world peace proliferated after World War II, just as they had after World War I.

As a general trend, postwar geopolitical rationales for population control as a means to international security have diminished, alongside the economic rationales centred on development and national planning and even food-and-agriculture arguments for family planning. They have all been trumped by the success of the feminist tradition of presenting reproductive rights as human rights. This has proven strategically useful, even though the history of the inclusion of reproduction within human rights definitions has been chequered at best. In 1948, the Universal Declaration of Human Rights itself codified the right *to reproduce* and left aside any right to knowledge or technology that enabled the *prevention* of conception. Article 16 reads: 'Men and women of full age, without any limitation due to race, nationality or religion, have the right to marry and to found a family.' This made sense in the immediate postwar period in response to involuntary sterilizations, child removals and laws against marriage. By the late 1960s it seemed inadequate, and from the 1970s onwards, the UN increasingly endorsed a right to contraceptive knowledge, notably at the landmark International Conference on Population and Development held in Cairo in 1994 (Fig. 34.3). But this was never unopposed;

the Holy See and delegates from some Islamic nations strongly objected to the liberalization of contraception and abortion policy and practice in many polities.[22]

The work of numerous foundations has been continuous over the twentieth century, despite changing titles, mission statements and to some extent geographies. For example, the activity in family planning of the Procter and Gamble heir, Clarence Gamble, evolved from 1930s Puerto Rico to 1940s Japan to 1950s India, and into the present-day NGO, Pathfinder International.[23] The 1930s Sterilization League morphed into EngenderHealth, an NGO that currently works in family planning, maternal health and HIV, mainly but not only in Africa.[24] Other organizations remain intact – the Population Council, for example. It is typical of population NGOs, as of the UN Population Fund, to have shifted from a squarely birth control agenda (medical and technological research, social science research on 'motivation' and fertility effects) to a more expansive remit of women's health and reproductive health delivery, and finally to research and primary care in what came to be termed 'reproductive health' and 'sexual health'. The latter emerged in the 1980s when HIV/AIDS prevention and treatment were taken up by organizations previously concerned with birth control and family planning. The Population Council's trajectory is typical. It began with training in demography, and continued with biomedical research into human reproduction and sociological research into 'motivations' and 'attitudes' to family planning. From development of intrauterine devices in the early 1960s, it moved to research the sexual transmission of HIV in the mid-1980s, announced the Norplant contraceptive implant in 1990, and worked on a programme for health needs of men who have sex with men in Kenya in 2006, treatments for pre-eclampsia in Nigeria in 2008 and child marriage in 2009.[25]

The tradition of US foundations' involvement has been extended more recently through the Bill & Melinda Gates Foundation.[26] In this case, in a reverse trajectory of programme development, a foundation concerned to improve health, with a focus on HIV, malaria and tuberculosis, has lately incorporated family planning within its remit. Associated with or at least parading Melinda Gates in particular, this influential foundation inherits the women's health and individual rights rationale for family planning that originated with the feminist Malthusians and re-emerged strongly after the Cairo conference in 1994. There the discourse of population control was displaced

22 John F. May, *World Population Policies: Their Origin, Evolution, and Impact* (Dordrecht, 2012).

23 Laura Briggs, *Reproducing Empire: Race, Sex, Science, and U.S. Imperialism in Puerto Rico* (Berkeley, CA, 2002); Ilana Löwy, 'Defusing the population bomb in the 1950s: Foam tablets in India', *Studies in History and Philosophy of Biological and Biomedical Sciences* 43 (2012), 583–93.

24 Dowbiggin, *Sterilization Movement*.

25 Timeline, Population Council, www.popcouncil.org/about/timeline, accessed 29 July 2015; on Norplant: Olszynko-Gryn, 'Technologies of Contraception and Abortion'.

26 'What we do: Family planning strategy overview', Bill & Melinda Gates Foundation, www.gatesfoundation.org/What-We-Do/Global-Development/Family-Planning, accessed 21 Nov. 2013.

by one of individualized family planning, although efforts to dispose of 'population control' cleaved these movements rather more sharply in retrospect than they ever really were.

The eugenic past of population organizations is simple to identify, a matter of fact more than interpretation. The difficulty lies in adjudicating what this means for the present. Claims abound that population NGOs represent a straightforward substitution of eugenic prejudices for racial prejudices about the global south – coerced sterilizations of the poor and disenfranchised in the interwar west became sterilizations in the postwar Third World. And yet it is these organizations that promote gender equity more than any other kind of international entity, and that recognize the problems of, and the problems that flow from, women's disempowerment. It is hardly problematic, in and of itself, that the Population Council produced a sex-education package in 2010 announced as 'an innovative resource that places gender issues and human rights at the heart of sex and HIV education'.[27] The difficulty lies with the tenacious world geography in which poverty maps onto non-whiteness, making the developing world the main target for all NGOs. Historians and policymakers alike often forget, however, that in the first half of the twentieth century it was European density and European population growth that constituted a heavily problematized 'danger spot'.[28] Thus the rubric of 'world population' itself has shifted markedly over the twentieth century to signify population in developing countries specifically.

Population and Earth Politics

Between 1948 and 1968, an explosion of books and agendas linked population and political ecology. They extended earlier concerns about soil erosion and conservation, linked to the agricultural pressures of ever more mouths to feed. Studies emerging from the dust bowl experience such as *The Rape of the Earth: A World Survey of Soil Erosion* (1939) set the terms for postwar and post-atomic writing. Fairfield Osborn's *Our Plundered Planet* (1948), for example, escalated the whole question of population to global catastrophe, anticipating Stanford biologist Paul Ehrlich's *Population Bomb* (1968). Ehrlich borrowed title and image, with acknowledgement, from Hugh Moore, whose pamphlet Ehrlich noted had been distributed in two million copies; Ehrlich's own book sold as many (Fig. 34.4).[29] In general, plant and animal ecologists, not demographers or economists, were raising the stakes at this point, followed by no-growth economics and

27 Timeline, Population Council.

28 For example, Warren S. Thompson, *Danger Spots in World Population* (New York, NY, 1929).

29 G. V. Jacks and R. O. Whyte, *The Rape of the Earth: A World Survey of Soil Erosion* (London, 1939); Fairfield Osborn, *Our Plundered Planet* (New York, NY, 1948); Paul R. Ehrlich, *The Population Bomb* (New York, NY, 1968).

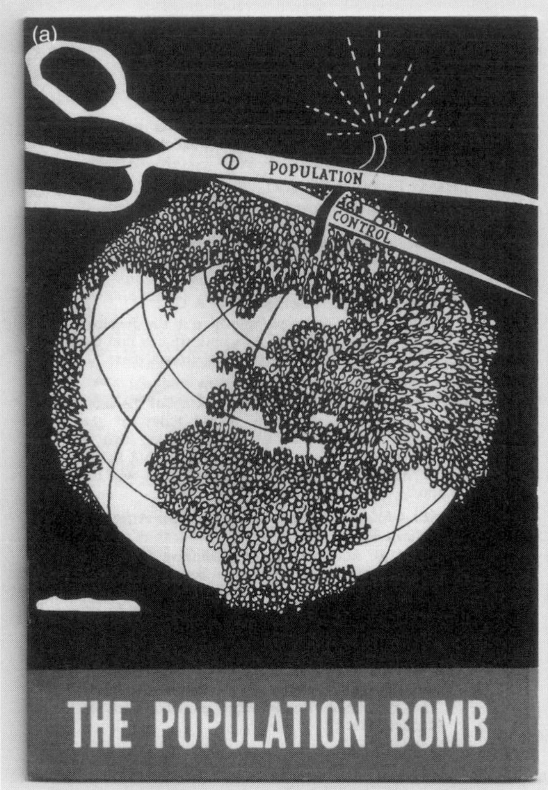

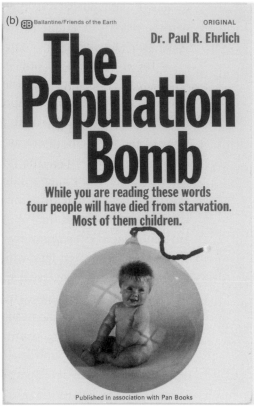

Figure 34.4 Population bombs on covers. (a) The Moore Fund's 1954 pamphlet, 'prepared by an informal group of business, labor and professional men concerned with preserving world peace, arresting Communism and improving the lot of people in overpopulated countries'. (b) Ehrlich's book in a UK paperback edition (London: Ballantine / Friends of the Earth in association with Pan Books, 1971).

zero-population-growth demography (originally from Kingsley Davis).[30] The serious matter of soil erosion explains the increasingly common crossover of personnel between conservation and birth control groups. William Vogt, for example, directed both the Conservation Foundation and the Planned Parenthood Federation of America.[31]

Connecting population growth and environmental politics became increasingly fraught over the 1970s and 1980s. Feminist opposition to the whole field of population control aligned with new historical work on sterilization and eugenics in the United States, Nazi Germany and Canada. This history is often linked to the Indian government's active sterilization campaigns especially in the Emergency Period (1975–7),

30 Derek S. Hoff, *The State and the Stork: The Population Debate and Policy Making in US History* (Chicago, IL, 2012), pp. 164–94; Patrick Ellis, '*Z.P.G.*', Exhibit 36, this book.

31 Robertson, *Malthusian Moment*.

and later China's much publicized one-child policy.[32] This difficult twentieth-century history of state power and citizens' reproductive bodies became a political quagmire that considerably reduced the impact of books about population bombs.

Climate change has since turned this around, countering the discomfort that accompanied population talk in the last decades of the twentieth century. Environmental limits are back in discussion in the international public sphere, connected to population growth, population structure and global consumption. Postwar global political ecology should be understood as a rehearsal for all of this: apocalyptic visions of population growth, soil erosion and planetary destruction directly anticipated current invocations of an Anthropocene. In 1949, the London edition of Vogt's *Road to Survival* ran with the subtitle: 'On the problem of man's destruction of the earth's surface and its products'.

The planetary consciousness that governs twenty-first-century population politics – Population Action International's 'Healthy People, Healthy Planet' is just one rendition – would seem to stem from a history of environmentalism.[33] A truer historical lineage traces a geopolitical world population problem, including eugenics, which itself gave rise to late twentieth-century environmentalism. Experts on population had long envisaged limited space on earth.

32 Mohan Rao, *From Population Control to Reproductive Health: Malthusian Arithmetic* (New Delhi, 2004); Betsy Hartmann, *Reproductive Rights and Wrongs: The Global Politics of Population Control and Contraceptive Choice* (New York, NY, 1987); Hopwood, 'Globalization'; Weindling, 'Pedigree'.

33 'What we do', Population Action International, http://populationaction.org/what-we-do/, accessed 16 Nov. 2013.

35 Sex Hormones, Pharmacy and the Reproductive Sciences

Jean-Paul Gaudillière

Authored by the American sociologist Adele Clarke in 1998, *Disciplining Reproduction* transformed historical writing on the reproductive sciences. Clarke revealed how practical work and concerns about reproductive bodies fed mid-twentieth-century biology, and advanced the idea that the new domain of the reproductive sciences owed much of its influence to the circulation of biological materials, tools, techniques, people and concepts between the three social worlds of biology, medicine and agriculture. This had given a problematic field legitimacy.

The notion that the reproductive sciences emerged as a boundary domain captures the fragility of a body of knowledge which has intervened in fertility, sex and gender and promised innovative means of improving human and animal populations. As Clarke argued for the United States, the problems of reproduction – beyond the medical management of women's diseases and childbirth – became a target for a flurry of research initiatives after World War I. Yet outside a few textbooks and institutions, the phrase 'reproductive sciences' was not much used before the 1980s, though 'reproductive biology' had gained currency since the 1960s.[1] Until the end of the twentieth century these were less than a discipline with its body of knowledge, learned society, research institutes and journals. But they were more than a loose conglomeration of scientists with their own agendas, interests and affiliations. So what linked such disparate social worlds as biology, medicine and agriculture?

Clarke drew attention to the way that, between the early 1920s and the late 1940s, the physiological specialty of endocrinology became a shared reference point:

> As the centerpiece of the reproductive sciences, endocrinology provided … several structural and strategic advantages. These included … a core, widely recognizable research activity … that appeared distant from the social issues of human sexuality and reproduction …; a biochemical instead of a 'merely' physiological thrust and strong working alliances with sophisticated biochemists …; a common denominator and a common language across biology, medicine and agriculture; and the promise of a host of valuable technoscientific interventions into reproductive phenomena.[2]

1 See further Nick Hopwood, 'The Keywords "Generation" and "Reproduction"', Chapter 20, this book.

2 Adele E. Clarke, *Disciplining Reproduction: Modernity, American Life Sciences, and 'the Problems of Sex'* (Berkeley, CA, 1998), p. 129. The book originated in Clarke's 1985 PhD dissertation.

Most, if not all, subsequent studies of mid-twentieth-century reproductive sciences may be read as confirming this general insight. But this large literature has also pushed the argument further, especially in relation to the most studied objects in endocrinology and research on reproduction, the sex hormones.

By the early 1920s, knowledge of reproduction, though present in many disciplines, was concentrated in two areas of the life sciences: physiology and the study of heredity. The first was deeply entrenched in medicine, epistemically as well as institutionally, while the second was more directly associated with agriculture and the management of plants and animals, though eugenics claimed to extend genetics to human populations. Both offered a general perspective on reproductive issues, linking experimental knowledge with interventions respectively dominated by surgery and breeding. By the late 1940s, however, physiology, in the form of endocrinology, had won. Observers inclined to a political and cultural reading may imagine this victory as a direct consequence of the increasingly controversial status of eugenics, and thus of the mounting difficulty of mobilizing genetics to control human bodies, at least at the population level. The recent literature tells us that the change was more material. With the sex hormones, endocrinology gave biologists, physicians and animal breeders widely circulating tools that shared loose general meanings but had specific local applications in the social worlds involved in making the reproductive sciences.

This chapter therefore seeks to revisit Clarke's argument about the role of endocrinology by focusing on the trajectories, multiple uses and diverse roles played by sex hormones in the twentieth-century history of the reproductive sciences. It enlarges the horizon in three ways. First, it brings in the European scene. Second, benefiting from new historical writing on drugs and therapeutic agents, it argues for the critical impact of industrial pharmacy, a social world missing from Clarke's scheme. Third, it shows how taking into account the centrality of biochemically defined sex hormones helps us understand the most recent transformation of the reproductive sciences, their increasing marketization, encompassing of risk prevention and incorporation of activism – in a word, their 'biomedicalization'.

The studies reviewed here thus differentiate between various ways in which sex-related substances have shaped our life and health. They distinguish three eras: of professionals and physiological practices, of industrialists and biochemists, and of consumers, public regulation and experts in risk (Fig. 35.1).

Sex Hormones in the Laboratory: Molecules and Gender

In an insightful article also published in 1998, Nelly Oudshoorn updated her celebrated archaeology of the sex hormones by arguing that these were pivotal in the ability of science to redefine reproduction as a problem of molecules. That is because, as biological

	1880–1920	1920–70	1970–
Main actors and arenas	Physicians and pharmacists	Pharmaceutical industry	Consumers and regulatory bodies
Dominant form of knowledge	Physiology	Biochemistry and organic chemistry	Epidemiology and clinical research
Biotech goals	Isolation	Standardization, synthesis	Enhancement and risk management
Pharmaceuticals	Rare biological extracts	Mass-produced steroids	Contraceptives and replacement therapies

Figure 35.1 Sex-related substances in the twentieth century.

raw materials manipulated through isolation technologies, they could serve the identification of the natural as well as the production of the artificial.[3] I therefore begin after World War I, when physiologically active preparations of ovaries and testes were first turned into purified substances.

The sex hormones typify those molecules of biological origin that gained prominence between the 1910s and the 1940s. Heiko Stoff and others have suggested that this was the age of the 'biologicals', with the sex steroids one of a series of potent biological agents including other hormones, such as insulin, as well as vaccines, antisera, enzymes and vitamins.[4] Beyond their novelty, the biologicals were distinguished by their origins in living organisms and connections to physiological processes. They were wonder molecules in two different ways. First, as biological entities, they acted in small quantities to control or modify astonishingly complex phenomena in living beings, thus participating in the regulation of major bodily functions from nutrition to immune resistance. Second, as technological entities that could be isolated and administered in one form or another, they promised successful and multipurpose interventions to alleviate diseases, control growth or improve reproduction. Within this landscape, the sex hormones occupied a peculiar niche since – thanks to the biochemists – they soon became molecules, that is, substances which could be crystallized and assigned a chemical structure as steroids.

Nothing better testifies to the technological work performed to define the sex hormones than the commitment of endocrinologists and biochemists to the development of assays and standards. Although hormones were tested on animals before

3 Nelly Oudshoorn, 'Hormones, technique et corps: L'archéologie des hormones sexuelles (1923–1940)', *Annales HSS* 53 (1998), 775–93; Oudshoorn, *Beyond the Natural Body: An Archeology of Sex Hormones* (New York, NY, 1994). See also Fig. 1.3, this book.

4 Alexander von Schwerin, Heiko Stoff and Bettina Wahrig (eds.), *Biologics: A History of Agents Made from Living Organisms in the Twentieth Century* (London, 2013); Stoff, *Wirkstoffe. Eine Wissenschaftsgeschichte der Hormone, Vitamine und Enzyme, 1920–1970* (Stuttgart, 2012).

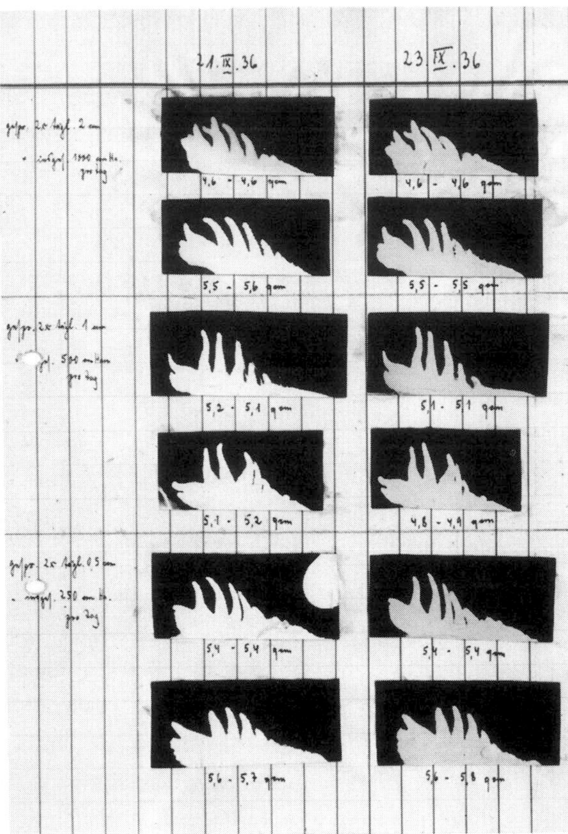

Figure 35.2 Record of the chicken crest assay for 'male' potency. The test compared the surface area of the crest of a castrated chicken before and after inoculation with the material to be assayed. For each dosage, two birds were injected. This page of a laboratory notebook from 1936 shows measurements taken at two-day intervals by illuminating the crests placed on photographic paper. Schering Archives, Bayer AG, Berlin.

the 1920s, only between the world wars did laboratory scientists turn the isolation of extracts from glands into a problem of standard protocols, quantified outputs and molecular fractions. As Oudshoorn argued, biological assays of hormonal activity, such as the Allen–Doisy mouse test for the follicular hormone and the chicken crest assay, became standard then (Fig. 35.2).[5]

Beyond standardization, biochemists gained the significant ability to differentiate and multiply the sex steroids. The purification paradigm not only implied collecting biological materials of various origins to prepare stable and homogeneous compounds; biochemists also dreamed of deciphering the processes by which the sex steroids were elaborated in nature. Two strategies were essential: first, to diversify the extraction protocols in order to isolate minute amounts of substances bearing chemical analogies to the three major sex steroids – oestrogens, progesterone and testosterone – and to find putative precursors; second, to develop reaction pathways modifying the 'natural'

5 Oudshoorn, *Beyond the Natural Body*; Jean-Paul Gaudillière, 'The visible industrialist: Standards and the manufacture of sex hormones', in Christoph Gradmann and Jonathan Simon (eds.), *Evaluating and Standardizing Therapeutic Agents, 1890–1950* (London, 2010), pp. 174–201.

hormones by changing the functional groups attached to the main core as well as exploring pathways that might play a role in the natural synthesis of the hormones in the producing cells. Artificial chemical variation and studies of natural metabolism were thus intimately connected, as we see in the decade-long work on dehydroandrosterone and its derivatives that the German biochemist and Nobel laureate Adolf Butenandt performed in his Berlin institute in the late 1930s.[6]

In her initial study, Oudshoorn also insisted that the science of hormones was gendered: within a long-term tendency to organize and interpret all physiological investigations of reproduction according to a bipolar and biological understanding of gender, the existence of gynaecology as a medical specialty focusing on women's reproductive lives directed special attention and investment towards the female hormones.[7] The standard biological assays for 'male' or 'female' potency guaranteed scientists and clinicians that they could label a given preparation 'male' or 'female'.

The interwar development of metabolic studies as well as the proliferation of new steroids originating in either purification or artificial synthesis endangered this form of gendering. The discovery of many more steroids added a series of molecules not primarily associated with reproduction, such as the hormones originating in the adrenals; it also blurred the biochemical – if not the medical – distinction between the sexes. By the mid-1930s, it was accepted that male hormones could be found in female bodies and vice versa, and that some of the new analogues were active in both male and female assays. Since these ambivalent or 'hermaphrodite' hormones were not only artificial products elaborated by chemists, but could sometimes be isolated from normal human bodies, their mere existence destabilized the bipolar organization of testing.

Biochemists like Butenandt worked out a solution that distinguished two dimensions in the molecular determination of the sexes.[8] On the one hand, they readily admitted that there was a continuum between male and female. On the other, a differentiation-oriented understanding of metabolism limited the consequences of this molecular continuum for the bipolar understanding of physiology and reproduction. In a strict parallel to the notion that the development of sex organs starts with undifferentiated embryonic structures with both male and female potentialities, the biochemists admitted that the cellular synthesis of sex steroids starts with undifferentiated molecules (most importantly, cholesterol), which are gradually modified to acquire new side

6 Jean-Paul Gaudillière, 'Better prepared than synthesized: Adolf Butenandt, Schering AG and the transformation of sex steroids into drugs (1930–1946)', *Studies in History and Philosophy of Biological and Biomedical Sciences* 36 (2005), 612–44.

7 Anne Fausto-Sterling, *Myths of Gender: Biological Theories about Women and Men*, 2nd edn (New York, NY, 1992); Fausto-Sterling, *Sexing the Body: Gender Politics and the Construction of Sexuality* (New York, NY, 2000); on the history of the concept of 'gender': John Forrester, 'Sex, Gender and Babies', Chapter 41, this book.

8 Gaudillière, 'Better prepared than synthesized'.

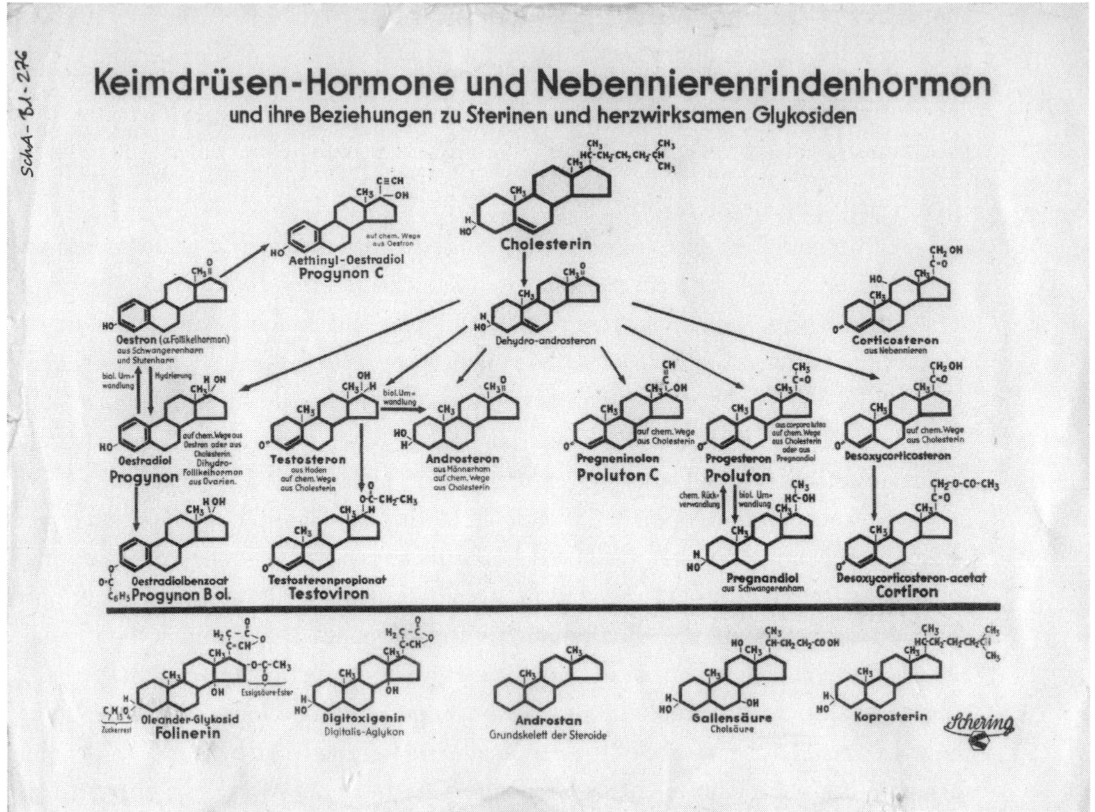

Figure 35.3 Bio-industrial pathways. The long-term collaborations between biochemists and pharmaceutical companies resulted in a two-way traffic of molecules, protocols, experimental results, technicians and money. This infrastructure strengthened the idea of natural biochemical pathways as mimicking industrial processes. Butenandt's late 1930s scheme for the derivation of all sex steroids from cholesterol matched Schering's production lines. Schering Archives, Bayer AG, Berlin.

chains that confer increasingly differentiated sexual potency. This progressive 'sexing' of the reproductive steroids was imagined to take place in every reproductive cell but very differently in male and female bodies, thus explaining the presence of all intermediates in every single body and the clear hierarchies in their concentrations.

The sophisticated combination of organ collection, biochemical separation, chemical synthesis and standardized bioassays that characterized the expansion of the laboratory-defined sexes eventually led to a major reconfiguration of reproductive physiology. As Clarke pointed out, the 1930s and 1940s were the years not only of the sex steroids but also of the pituitary as the master gland controlling the entire biochemical and cellular apparatus responsible for mammalian reproductive life. This development depended on the new material and, one should add, industrial culture of endocrinology.

Sex Hormones in the Factory

The sex steroids were industrialized in the interwar period, when a whole palette of new products came onto the market. These were no longer organ extracts, but pure hormones isolated or partly chemically synthesized, usually from cholesterol. Industrially produced and molecularly defined, the substances were credited with potent effects on the reproductive systems of humans and other mammals. The speed of industrial innovation is impressive. The follicular hormone was prepared from women's urine from the late 1920s onwards, and from mares' urine in the early 1930s. The most active ingredient and main vertebrate oestrogen, oestradiol, was marketed a couple of years later, oestradiol derivatives in the late 1930s, progesterone around 1938 and testosterone and androsterone in the mid-1930s. Finally, entirely synthetic products showing oestrogen-like effects became available in the late 1930s (Fig. 35.3). There are also the corticosteroids, prepared through the same family of processes and by the same scientists; their diversification led to the production of cortisone soon after World War II. Uses were not limited to treating diseases but included numerous examples of bodily enhancement. Against expectations, given the initial domination of gynaecology, the male hormones, led by testosterone, claimed a significant market share.[9]

In contrast to organ extracts, which were often marketed by relatively small firms, sometimes started by single pharmacists, the pure sex hormones were manufactured by large companies whose commercial fates were linked to their expertise in the invention, production and sale of these biologicals: Organon in the Netherlands, Ciba in Switzerland, Schering and Boehringer in Germany, Roussel-Uclaf in France and Merck in the United States. Rather than depending on external collaboration with biologists or chemists, these concerns developed large infrastructures for in-house research. Recent histories have therefore explored the trajectory of the sex hormones as exemplifying industrial pharmacy based on biology.

The issue has been addressed in two ways. A first approach, focused on laboratories, has located the companies within the nexus of biological, medical and eventually also agricultural research that brought sex hormone molecules to the world. This was Oudshoorn's strategy in her 1994 book on how the establishment of Organon was enabled by the pharmacologist Ernst Laqueur's dense network of collaborations with hospitals and slaughterhouses that made it possible to supply raw materials and find medical uses for the products. A second, more recent approach has been to focus not on the research network, but on the companies themselves, and to take into account their scientific, technological and commercial work, in order to understand how the trajectory of the sex hormones was determined by this industrial context and also changed it. The history of the reproductive sciences has thus become part of the history of pharmacy.

9 John Hoberman, *Testosterone Dreams: Rejuvenation, Aphrodisia, Doping* (Berkeley, CA, 2005).

Company archives are indispensable but often unavailable; recent investigations have favoured Swiss and German producers, beginning with Ciba and Schering.[10] Since the former was a large chemical firm, which gradually shifted into therapeutic products from its base in organic chemistry, Schering provides the clearer example of the biological mode of drug innovation.

Created by a family of pharmacists, Schering produced ready-made drugs as well as the bulk chemicals from which pharmacists prepared the compounds in the German pharmacopoeia.[11] Biological derivatives, especially plant extracts, loomed large in Schering's catalogue before World War I; knowledge of biological molecules was critical to the firm. The in-house laboratories thus included not only chemists but soon also a large biological section. In the early 1920s, in connection with its marketing of Progynon, a female hormone first made from sow ovaries and later isolated from urine, Schering added to the central laboratory a section for 'animal research', that is, breeding rats, rabbits and chickens and using them to check the potency and quality of production batches. Typically of sciences within research-intensive industries, the testing section soon evolved to include physiological experiments. For example, Karl Junkmann and Walter Holweg contributed to the discovery of feedback regulation by linking the pituitary and the ovaries to generate a vision of the female cycle as a series of changes in the secretion and circulation of physiologically active chemicals.[12]

Another important dimension in the industrial life of the sex hormones is their status as property. Though sold on the market, drugs were excluded from intellectual property legislation in most European countries until World War II.[13] The exclusion was grounded in two different motives and social worlds. On the one hand, many physicians and health authorities perceived patents on drugs as detrimental to public health, since monopoly would result in high prices and reduced access. On the other, pharmacists and their professional organizations opposed any regulation that would limit their opportunities to prepare the drugs in their own pharmacies and the role of the pharmacopoeia as a shared compendium of recipes.

10 Christina Ratmoko, *Damit die Chemie stimmt. Die Anfange der industriellen Herstellung von weiblichen und männlichen Sexualhormonen 1914–1938* (Zurich, 2010); Lea Haller, *Cortison. Geschichte eines Hormones, 1900–1955* (Zurich, 2012); Jean-Paul Gaudillière, 'Biochemie und Industrie. Der "Arbeitskreis Butenandt-Schering" im Nationalsozialismus', in Wolfgang Schieder and Achim Trunk (eds.), *Adolf Butenandt und die Kaiser-Wilhelm-Gesellschaft. Wissenschaft, Industrie und Politik im 'Dritten Reich'* (Göttingen, 2004), pp. 198–246; Jean-Paul Gaudillière, 'Une marchandise scientifique? Savoirs, industrie et régulation du médicament dans l'Allemagne des années trente', *Annales HSS* 65 (2010), 89–120.

11 Wolfgang Wimmer, *'Wir haben fast immer was Neues.' Gesundheitwesen und Innovationen der Pharma-Industrie in Deutschland, 1880–1935* (Berlin, 1994).

12 Gaudillière, 'Better prepared than synthesized'; Martina Schlünder, 'Menstrual-Cycle Calendars', Exhibit 31, this book.

13 Jean-Paul Gaudillière, 'How pharmaceuticals became patentable: The production and appropriation of drugs in the twentieth century', *History and Technology* 24 (2008), 99–106.

As new biologicals, however, hormones were not included in the pharmacopoeia or prepared in pharmacies; they were made in large factories. Like the earlier vaccines, their production was regulated ad hoc by inspections and the surveillance of facilities. This conjunction of biological research and industrial processing in turn favoured the increasing use of process patents to control the hormone market. Firms including Schering, Ciba, Roussel and Organon applied for patents on their protocols for purification and isolation. This practice was generalized when (partial) chemical synthesis and metabolic studies diversified the molecules. A strong looping effect thus came to link biochemical research and the creation of exclusive rights in its products. Once patents on the making of hormones were accepted, in spite of the argument that controlling processes could imply a monopoly, studying the sex steroids to diversify their range became all the more interesting, and this in turn helped multiply the patents. In the late 1930s, Schering owned four dozen items of intellectual property related to the synthesis of sex steroids. The appropriation of these molecules – along with sera and vitamins – thus provided the experience that patent specialists from industry, lawyers and engineers needed in order to argue for a change in the law, which after World War II was achieved in most of continental Europe.[14]

Sex Hormones in Public: Risk Management and Risky Technologies

Historical writing on the reproductive sciences documents much traffic to and from medical practice, with clinical data repeatedly turned into objects of fundamental research and laboratory tools or targets transformed into means of intervention. The golden decades of sex hormone molecules increased the density of these circulations, as histories of the contraceptive pill have shown.[15] This nexus in turn raised new problems and controversies that are well illustrated by the development and critique of hormone replacement therapy (HRT) for managing the female menopause and other conditions newly deemed 'risky'.[16]

As powerfully recounted by Elizabeth Watkins for the United States, HRT was predicated upon the isolation, synthesis and mass circulation of oestrogens and progesterone

14 Jean-Paul Gaudillière, 'Professional or industrial order? Patents, biological drugs, and pharmaceutical capitalism in early twentieth-century Germany', *History and Technology* 24 (2008), 107–33.

15 Andrea Tone, *Devices and Desires: A History of Contraceptives in America* (New York, NY, 2001); Lara V. Marks, *Sexual Chemistry: A History of the Contraceptive Pill* (New Haven, CT, 2001); Elizabeth Siegel Watkins, *On the Pill: A Social History of Oral Contraceptives, 1950–1970* (Baltimore, MD, 1998). Especially for histories of contraception beyond the pill: Jesse Olszynko-Gryn, 'Technologies of Contraception and Abortion', Chapter 36, this book.

16 For risk in relation to prenatal testing: Ilana Löwy, 'Prenatal Diagnosis, Surveillance and Risk', Chapter 38, this book.

in the 1930s and 1940s. But if the idea of using pure steroids to ease the menopausal transition was familiar to pharmaceutical industrialists in the 1930s, HRT is typical of the affluent, urbanized, longer-living societies of the postwar west.[17] Only then was the interwar model of menopause as a normal life stage, with the focus on short-term treatment and extreme cases, marginalized in favour of the long-term and large-scale prescription of oestrogens to middle-aged women. In the United States, the successful advocates of this practice were prominent gynaecologists, among whom Robert Wilson stands out. A New York physician, he established the Wilson Research Foundation in 1963 with industry support, having authored a famous book, *Feminine Forever*, in 1962. This 'plea for the maintenance of adequate estrogen from puberty to grave' was widely echoed in women's magazines through sad cases of suffering and miraculous tales of therapy assessed by Wilson's 'feminine index', which was based on the microscopic examination of vaginal cells.

Oestrogen or hormone replacement therapy is not only a success story, however. In the late 1970s, the practice was strongly criticized following the publication of clinical and epidemiological results that correlated oestrogen prescription and increased risk of endometrial cancer. These articles appeared at a specific moment in the history of American medicine, with the development of women's health organizations, the battle for the legalization of contraception and abortion, and critiques of the side-effects of the pill. They stirred public controversy and mobilized women.

Feminists such as journalist Barbara Seaman indicted the wholesale use of sex hormones as the 'greatest experiment ever performed on women' for the benefit of industry and a segment of the medical profession.[18] Feminist magazines insisted that HRT was unnecessary and valorized more 'natural' ways of living through the transition years. The disclosure of the oestrogen–endometrial cancer link and this public mobilization put the Food and Drug Administration under fire, and in spring 1976 the agency started to move in the direction of mandating patient package inserts for all oestrogen products and not just oral contraceptives. On the medical side, the controversy resulted in a steep drop in prescription numbers, from 28 million to 14 million in five years.

The great paradox of HRT is that it survived this criticism, thus revealing the complex links between activism and consumption, and the interwoven identities of the sex hormones as both potentially dangerous and promising control. By 1980, the prescription of oestrogens was back at its early 1970s level, thanks to a renewed medical discourse. This built on the invention of combined preparations (oestrogens plus progesterone) to reduce the risk of endometrial cancer, and the availability of imaging

17 Elizabeth Siegel Watkins, *The Estrogen Elixir: A History of Hormone Replacement Therapy in America* (Baltimore, MD, 2007).

18 Barbara Seaman, *The Greatest Experiment Ever Performed on Women: Exploding the Estrogen Myth* (New York, NY, 2003).

techniques for measuring the bone loss and objectifying the osteoporosis associated with menopause. The medical target shifted from the treatment of deficiency to the mass prevention of risk.

The rise of HRT might seem to be a clear-cut case of 'medicalization'. Menopause, previously a normal life stage addressed through self- and social help, was turned into an abnormal loss of 'femininity', a deficiency disease to be handled through regular medical check-ups and drug prescriptions. Yet, in a medical world no longer dominated by the professions, HRT was rather a product of the postwar chemotherapeutic revolution with its huge investment in research, new classes of drug and growing markets, and of the transformation of pharmacy into one of the most profitable and visible industrial sectors.

The large number of advertisements or sponsored articles that oestrogen producers placed in women's magazines testifies to the power of the drug industry, but the firms did more than mere 'propaganda'. The postwar years also saw another major transformation of pharmaceutical research and development with the generalization of molecular screening and the advent of 'scientific marketing'.[19] This mobilized 'science' in two ways. First, science provided a set of resources to 'rationalize' marketing and convert it into a system of action, a planning practice based on economic research into prices, sales and prescriptions as well as sociological and psychological studies of patients' and doctors' behaviours. Second, the science mobilized for marketing increasingly originated in the massive research and development apparatus developed by drug companies, both in-house in the form of chemical, biological and pharmacological laboratories, and externally with the series of phase I, II, III and even IV clinical trials required by governmental regulators. This close integration of clinical research and marketing changed how the value of drugs was defined. It created a situation in which industrial entrepreneurs provided most, if not all, of the clinical data on which administrative control was – and still is – supposed to operate.

The specificity of the situation has been captured in a recent scheme that Adele Clarke and her colleagues have offered for the analysis of contemporary changes in medicine.[20] As an alternative to medicalization, they refer to 'biomedicalization'. This is not just a linkage between biology and medicine. In addition to the new role of markets, they insist on: the mounting visibility of health risks, both as epidemiological factors involved in disease causation and as targets of preventive interventions that include chemotherapeutics; the rise of patient activism, in particular the women's health

19 Jean-Paul Gaudillière and Ulrike Thoms, 'Pharmaceutical firms and the construction of drug markets: From branding to scientific marketing', *History and Technology* 29 (2013), 105–15.

20 Adele Clarke *et al.*, 'Biomedicalization: Technoscientific transformations of health, illness, and U.S. biomedicine', *American Sociological Review* 68 (2003), 161–94; see also Martin H. Johnson and Nick Hopwood, 'Modern Law and Regulation', Chapter 40; and Forrester, 'Sex, Gender and Babies', this book.

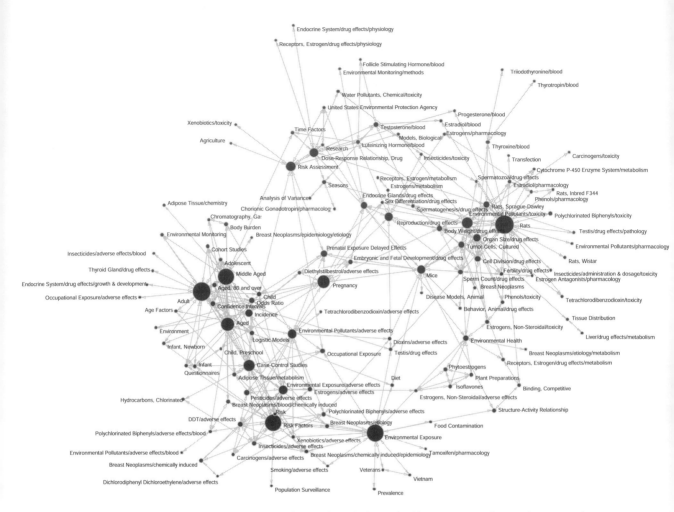

Figure 35.4 Links (co-occurrences) between keywords in the biomedical literature on endocrine disruption. These reveal the centrality of DES, reinvented as an endocrine disruptor in the 1990s, and the role that this sex hormone analogue played in mediating between the various research domains participating in the construction of the new toxicological paradigm. © Jean-Paul Gaudillière.

movement, which seeks better care and also provides critical expertise in the public sphere; and the extension of the domain of biomedicine beyond the management of diseases to the prevention of risk and the enhancement of bodily capabilities.

This juncture is exemplified by the ups and downs of a molecule that has attracted much historical attention, although it is not a sex steroid but an analogue of different structure: diethylstilbestrol (DES). Charles Dodds and his colleagues in London and Oxford first synthesized DES in 1938. Cheap and easy to produce, it rapidly became a substitute – and competitor – for industrial oestrogens. As early as the late 1940s, gynaecologists used DES for a variety of indications.[21] In the 1950s, following pioneering work by animal nutritionists, DES use was extended to agriculture as a way to accelerate growth. The most important reproductive indication – in terms of prescription numbers – was for managing the risk of spontaneous abortion during pregnancy, that is, as a 'replacement' therapy for a condition which, like menopause, was attributed to oestrogen deficiency.

Large-scale use of DES was never considered trivial, but only a small minority of physicians expressed concern that, as early as the 1930s, laboratory experiments with mice had shown that oestrogens in general, and DES in particular, could induce tumours in animals. This became a scandal in 1971, when it was discovered that DES caused vaginal cancer in young women whose mothers had taken the drug during pregnancy. The history of DES in the United States is paradigmatic of the intervention of feminist and consumer movements. It also illustrates the biomedical regime of risk management that emerged during the 1960s and 1970s, and strongly reinforced the role of public expertise.[22] Court cases as well as such political arenas as congressional hearings were decisive for the production of legitimate evidence regarding the magnitude of the risks and the measures needed to control them. The DES trials thus legitimized a 'precautionary' approach to cancer risks, which not only directed attention to the effects of low doses, but also constructed a model for expertise in reproductive disorders of chemical origin. The main legacy is the very recent incorporation of DES into the new and controversial category of endocrine disruptors, those artificial analogues of sex hormones which have been massively released into the environment for decades and now prove to have profoundly 'disrupting' effects on the reproductive physiology of animals and humans (Fig. 35.4).[23]

Conclusion

The interwar period turned the early twentieth-century organ extracts into pure, partly synthesized molecular entities. This transformation was practical, social and, crucially, industrial as well as biochemical. Recent historical writing on sex hormones has thus added a fourth major social world to those that Clarke associated with the twentieth-century reproductive sciences: the pharmaceutical industry. Drug producers in the 1920s started a long-term process of scaling-up, investing in large in-house research

21 Susan E. Bell, 'The synthetic compound diethylstilbestrol (DES), 1938–1941: The social construction of a medical treatment', unpublished PhD thesis, Brandeis University (1980).

22 Jean-Paul Gaudillière, 'DES, cancer and endocrine perturbation: Ways of regulating, chemical risks and public expertise in the United States', in Soraya Boudia and Nathalie Jas (eds.), *Powerless Science? Science and Politics in a Toxic World* (New York, NY, 2014), pp. 65–94.

23 Nancy Langston, *Toxic Bodies: Hormone Disruptors and the Legacy of DES* (New Haven, CT, 2010).

facilities, mass marketing and committing to the synthesis of an ever-greater number of sex-related molecules. These sex steroids became prototypes in a new infrastructure aimed at making knowledge that would put products on markets while fostering uses ranging from treating newly defined pathologies to doping in sport and promoting animal growth.

As it expanded, this infrastructure established a regime of laboratory investigations characterized by intense circulation between academic and industrial settings, and practical and metaphorical linkages between reproductive organs and factories. Two decades later, in the postwar era, the 'therapeutic revolution' built on that basis vastly expanded the uses of female sex hormones for 'medical' purposes, contraception included. The generalization of scientific marketing then provided the pharmaceutical industry with new means of framing medical practice, while reinforcing its pivotal position between reproductive biology and medicine as provider of molecules and organizer of clinical research. The unintended outcome of this strengthened nexus was the mounting visibility of side-effects and the public critique of the 'pharmaceuticalization' of what could be viewed as normal events in women's lives. According to recent historians, the increased consumption of sex steroids, as well as critiques thereof, may be viewed as integral elements in a late twentieth-century governance of health that focuses on risks, and as representative of a more general process of biomedicalization. Sex hormones have become simultaneously technologies of risk management and risky technologies. Highlighting the *longue durée* of biotechnological practices with their range of projects at the boundaries between research and production, academic institutions and markets, biology and pharmaceutical or agricultural capitalism, recent studies of the twentieth-century reproductive sciences have contributed to a much-needed historical and critical evaluation of a world of biological promises that is still pervasive today.

36 Technologies of Contraception and Abortion

Jesse Olszynko-Gryn

Soon to turn 60, the oral contraceptive pill still dominates histories of technology in the 'sexual revolution' and after.[1] 'The pill' was revolutionary for many, though by no means all, women in the west, but there have always been alternatives, and looking globally yields a different picture.[2] The condom, intrauterine device (IUD), surgical sterilization (male and female) and abortion were all transformed in the twentieth century, some more than once. Today, female sterilization (tubal ligation) and IUDs are the world's most commonly used technologies of contraception. The pill is in third place, followed closely by the condom. Long-acting hormonal injections are most frequently used in parts of Africa, male sterilization by vasectomy is unusually prevalent in Britain, and about one in five pregnancies worldwide ends in induced abortion. Though contraceptive use has generally increased in recent decades, the disparity between rich and poor countries is striking: the former tend to use condoms and pills, the latter sterilization and IUDs.[3]

Contraception, a term dating from the late nineteenth century and since then often conflated with abortion, has existed in many forms, and techniques have changed and proliferated over time. Diverse local cultures have embraced new technologies while maintaining older practices. Focusing on Britain and the United States, with excursions to India, China and France, this chapter shows how the patterns observed today were established and stabilized, often despite persistent criticism and reform efforts. By examining past innovation, and the distribution and use of a variety of tools and techniques, it reconsiders some widely held assumptions about what counts as revolutionary and for whom. Analytically, it takes up and reflects on one of the main issues raised by feminists and social historians: the agency of users as patients and consumers faced with choice and coercion.[4] By examining practices of contraception alongside those of abortion, it revisits the knotty question of technology in

1 Heather Prescott, 'The pill at fifty: Scientific commemoration and the politics of American memory', *Technology and Culture* 54 (2013), 735–45.

2 David Edgerton, *The Shock of the Old: Technology and Global History since 1900* (London, 2006).

3 Jacqueline E. Darroch, 'Trends in contraceptive use', *Contraception* 87 (2013), 259–63.

4 For example, Linda Gordon, *Woman's Body, Woman's Right: A Social History of Birth Control in America* (New York, NY, 1976); Johanna Schoen, *Choice and Coercion: Birth Control, Sterilization, and Abortion in Public Health and Welfare* (Chapel Hill, NC, 2005).

the sexual revolution and the related themes of medical, legal, religious and political forms of control.[5]

Supply and Demand

Respectable women in Victorian Britain projected a culture of modesty and sexual innocence,[6] but techniques of self-discipline depended on reproductive knowledge and constituted technologies in their own right. Some called for domestic tools such as a calendar or thermometer, others for a visit to the herbalist or chemist.[7] In the absence of pregnancy testing, the first trimester was an uncertain time for many women and their physicians.[8] Though in past centuries women took emmenagogues more to promote conception than to remove an unwanted pregnancy, by the late nineteenth century many thousands of women every year were using widely advertised 'female pills' as abortifacients (Fig. 36.1).[9] Other common methods of inducing miscarriage included falling down the stairs, drinking gin or pennyroyal tea, dilating the cervix with slippery elm bark, and ingesting lead, ergot or quinine; few had access to surgical abortions.[10] Statistics do not exist for earlier decades, but estimates based on official inquiries from the 1930s range from 60,000 to 125,000 abortions a year for England and Wales even though the practice had been outlawed in the nineteenth century.[11]

As birth control campaigners complained, many working-class women regulated fertility around menstruation more than intercourse and did not distinguish (illegal) abortion from (increasingly tolerated) contraception. Although in the interwar years networks of clinics on both sides of the Atlantic promoted prescription-only female

5 On movements: Lesley A. Hall, 'Movements to Separate Sex and Reproduction', Chapter 29; and on the law: Martin H. Johnson and Nick Hopwood, 'Modern Law and Regulation', Chapter 40, this book. On contraception and abortion in earlier times: Helen King, 'Women and Doctors in Ancient Greece', Chapter 3; Marie-Hélène Congourdeau, 'Debating the Soul in Late Antiquity', Chapter 8; Katharine Park, 'Managing Childbirth and Fertility in Medieval Europe', Chapter 11, this book.

6 Kate Fisher, 'Modern Ignorance', Chapter 32, this book.

7 On calendars: Lauren Kassell, 'Jane Dee's Courses in John Dee's Diary', Exhibit 14; Martina Schlünder, 'Menstrual-Cycle Calendars', Exhibit 31, this book.

8 Jesse Olszynko-Gryn, 'Pregnancy Testing with Frogs', Exhibit 32, this book.

9 Jennifer Evans, '"Gentle purges corrected with hot spices, whether they work or not, do vehemently provoke venery": Menstrual provocation and procreation in early modern England', *Social History of Medicine* 25 (2012), 2–19; Jeffrey Weeks, *Sex, Politics and Society: The Regulation of Sexuality since 1800*, 3rd edn (Harlow, 2012), pp. 87–8.

10 Barbara Brookes, *Abortion in England, 1900–1967* (London, 1988); Leslie J. Reagan, *When Abortion Was a Crime: Women, Medicine, and Law in the United States, 1867–1973* (Berkeley, CA, 1997); Cornelie Usborne, *Cultures of Abortion in Weimar Germany* (New York, NY, 2007).

11 Simon Szreter, *Fertility, Class and Gender in Britain, 1860–1940* (Cambridge, 1996), p. 428.

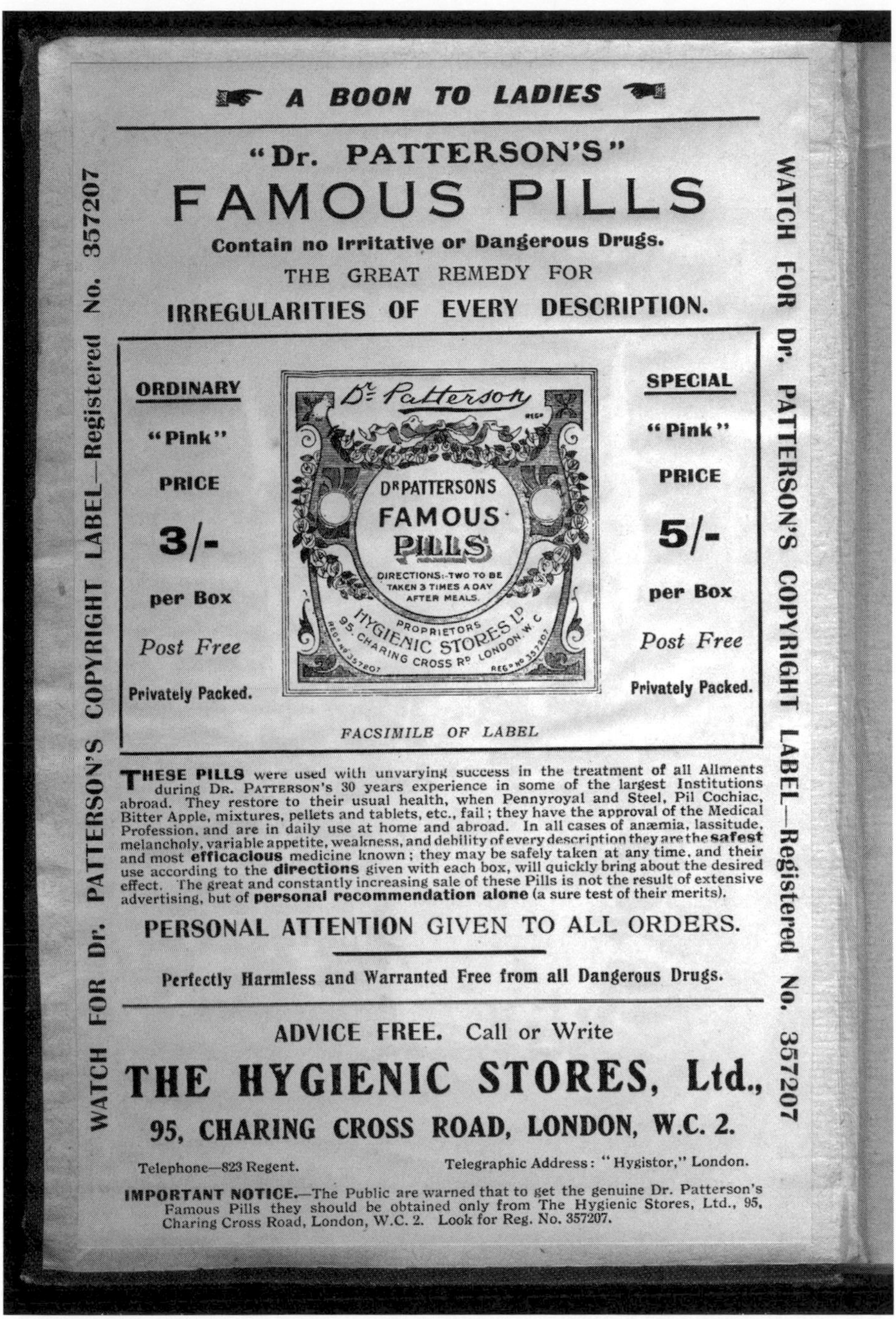

Figure 36.1 Advertisement for Dr Patterson's 'famous' pills, one of the more popular remedies for female 'irregularities'. Mention of such well-known abortifacients as pennyroyal indicated the function. This advertisement was stuck after publication inside a copy of *Married Love* (first published in 1918), the bestselling manual by Marie Stopes, who publicly opposed abortion although she sometimes helped individual women. 19 × 13 cm. Nick Hopwood's collection.

barrier methods (cervical caps, diaphragms and pessaries), women continued to view menstrual regulation as 'natural', but birth control as 'artificial' and sinful.[12] Many couples in Britain rejected 'modern' appliances as expensive and impractical, embracing instead the unreliability of 'being careful' as a means of reducing the odds of pregnancy without cheating fate or God. Viewed by some as a pleasure-enhancing sexual skill, withdrawal (coitus interruptus) was familiar, socially acceptable, easy-to-understand and conformed to the gender norm of male responsibility. Along with abstinence and the rhythm method ('Vatican roulette'), withdrawal could also be aligned with Catholicism's vague injunction to self-control.[13]

It was not the medically approved devices pushed by campaigners but those pedalled by entrepreneurial vendors that found the largest share of the market. Men of all classes used 'skins' made from animal guts and, from the 1840s, sheaths of vulcanized rubber. The industrial mass production of thinner, more comfortable and disposable latex condoms was a major innovation of the 1920s; by the 1930s, large rubber companies around Britain produced millions every year. Previously mainly imported from Germany, these sold openly from pubs, barbers, cinemas, dance halls, arcades, tobacconists and vending machines. Wartime campaigns against venereal disease and military contracts helped position the London Rubber Company as Britain's dominant manufacturer. The company supplied Durex to thousands of chemists in the 1940s and made 95 per cent of the hundred million condoms sold in that country alone in 1968.[14]

The United States was also a 'nation of condoms'. Despite the federal Comstock Act passed in 1873 to prohibit the mailing or transport of contraceptive products and information, Americans had access to a lively underground trade. Avoiding the expense and inconvenience of a doctor's visit, consumers purchased vaginal jellies, foam tablets, suppositories, douches (most notoriously, the household cleaning product Lysol) and especially condoms directly from drug stores, mail-order catalogues and travelling pedlars.[15] Following Margaret Sanger's arrest for opening the nation's first birth control

12 Hall, 'Movements to Separate Sex and Reproduction'; Atina Grossmann, *Reforming Sex: The German Movement for Birth Control and Abortion Reform, 1920–1950* (Oxford, 1995); Peter Neushul, 'Marie C. Stopes and the popularization of birth control technology', *Technology and Culture* 39 (1998), 245–72; Cathy Hajo, *Birth Control on Main Street: Organizing Clinics in the United States, 1916–1939* (Urbana, IL, 2010).

13 Kate Fisher, *Birth Control, Sex and Marriage in Britain, 1918–1960* (Oxford, 2006); Simon Szreter and Fisher, *Sex before the Sexual Revolution: Intimate Life in England, 1918–1963* (Cambridge, 2010); Schlünder, 'Menstrual-Cycle Calendars'.

14 Claire L. Jones, 'Under the covers? Commerce, contraceptives and consumers in England and Wales, 1880–1960', *Social History of Medicine* 29 (2016), 734–56; James M. Edmonson, 'Condoms', Exhibit 28, this book; Fig. 32.4 depicts a vending machine.

15 Andrea Tone, 'Making room for rubbers: Gender, technology, and birth control before the pill', *History and Technology* 18 (2002), 51–76, on 60.

clinic in Brooklyn in 1916, a New York judge ruled in favour of contraceptive use to prevent venereal disease (prophylaxis) only. The condom business boomed in the 1920s. Standards imposed by the Food and Drug Administration (FDA) pushed small-timers out of business, effectively centralizing production in the late 1930s. In 1950, two companies controlled half the $100 million market. By 1958, sales had risen to $150 million, compared with $20 million for female contraceptives.[16] This situation changed abruptly with the advent of the prescription-only pill in 1960.

Medicalization and Population Control

Sanger's medical solution to overpopulation was developed in the mid-1950s with the support of wealthy philanthropist Katharine Dexter McCormick. The first commercial oral contraceptive, the pharmaceutical company Searle's Enovid, combined mestranol, an oestrogen, and norethynodrel, a progestin, to inhibit female fertility. It was tested in Massachusetts and then on a much larger scale in the US territory of Puerto Rico.[17] Though abandoned by population controllers as too expensive and excessively reliant on patient compliance, 'the pill' proved unexpectedly popular with affluent consumers, who were used to going to the doctor (Fig. 36.2). In 1955, about half of the American women who used contraception reported relying on either condoms (27 per cent) or a diaphragm (25 per cent). Ten years later, 27 per cent used the pill, 18 per cent condoms and just 10 per cent a diaphragm.[18]

The first decade of medicalized contraception coincided with the liberalization of laws and policies. Though the Comstock Act was overturned in 1936, thirty states still had statutes prohibiting or limiting the advertisement and sale of contraceptives in 1960. Five years later, the Supreme Court ruled in *Griswold v. Connecticut* that married couples had a right to privacy and, by extension, the right to purchase and use birth control. This judgement superseded most proscriptive state laws, but Massachusetts continued to ban the distribution of contraceptives to unmarried individuals. In 1972, the Supreme Court extended the right of privacy in matters of birth control to the unmarried in the *Eisenstadt v. Baird* decision and reversed the last of the state laws against contraception.[19]

16 Ibid., 72.

17 Lara V. Marks, *Sexual Chemistry: A History of the Contraceptive Pill* (New Haven, CT, 2001).

18 These surveys did not include men: Elizabeth Siegel Watkins, *On the Pill: A Social History of Oral Contraceptives, 1950–1970* (Baltimore, MD, 1998), pp. 61–2.

19 John W. Johnson, Griswold v. Connecticut: *Birth Control and the Constitutional Right to Privacy* (Lawrence, KA, 2005); David J. Garrow, *Liberty and Sexuality: The Right to Privacy and the Making of* Roe v. Wade (Berkeley, CA, 1994); Johnson and Hopwood, 'Modern Law and Regulation'.

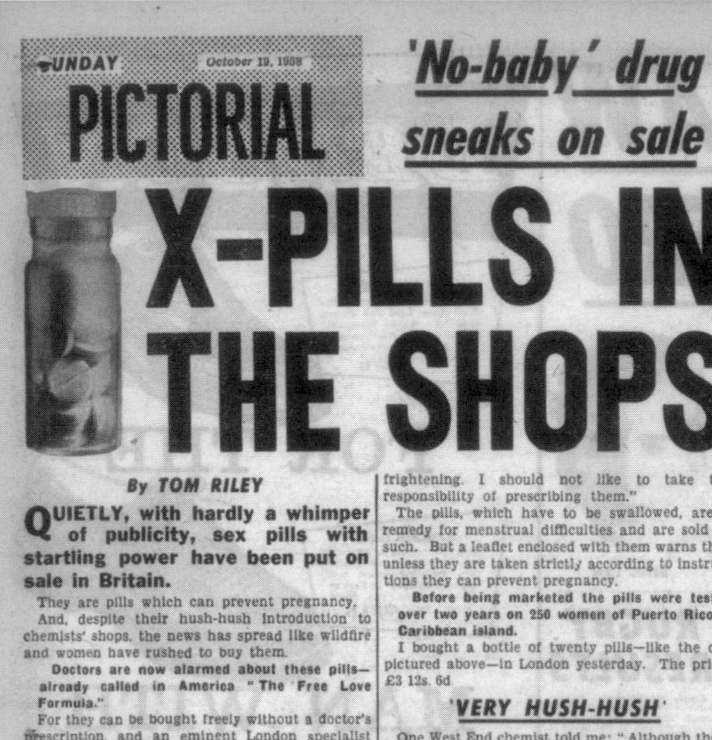

SUNDAY October 19, 1958

PICTORIAL

'No-baby' drug sneaks on sale

X-PILLS IN THE SHOPS

By TOM RILEY

QUIETLY, with hardly a whimper of publicity, sex pills with startling power have been put on sale in Britain.

They are pills which can prevent pregnancy.

And, despite their hush-hush introduction to chemists' shops, the news has spread like wildfire and women have rushed to buy them.

Doctors are now alarmed about these pills—already called in America "The Free Love Formula."

For they can be bought freely without a doctor's prescription, and an eminent London specialist warned last night:—

"There are terrible hidden dangers if these pills are wrongly used. No one yet knows what their long-term effect may be.

"They are unusually potent. They are very frightening. I should not like to take the responsibility of prescribing them."

The pills, which have to be swallowed, are a remedy for menstrual difficulties and are sold as such. But a leaflet enclosed with them warns that unless they are taken strictly according to instructions they can prevent pregnancy.

Before being marketed the pills were tested over two years on 250 women of Puerto Rico, a Caribbean island.

I bought a bottle of twenty pills—like the one pictured above—in London yesterday. The price: £3 12s. 6d.

'VERY HUSH-HUSH'

One West End chemist told me: "Although these pills are supposed to be very hush-hush and have been advertised only in the medical Press, women have somehow got to know about them."

Sir Hugh Linstead, M.P., secretary of the Pharmaceutical Society, said: "If there is a rush for these pills we shall certainly consider steps to prevent them from falling into wrong hands."

THE PICTORIAL SAYS: We do not name the pill, for obvious reasons.

But it is appalling that such an important scientific achievement—with its possible dangers through inexpert use—should be allowed to sneak into the country. The pills ought to be on the by-prescription-only list—**NOW.**

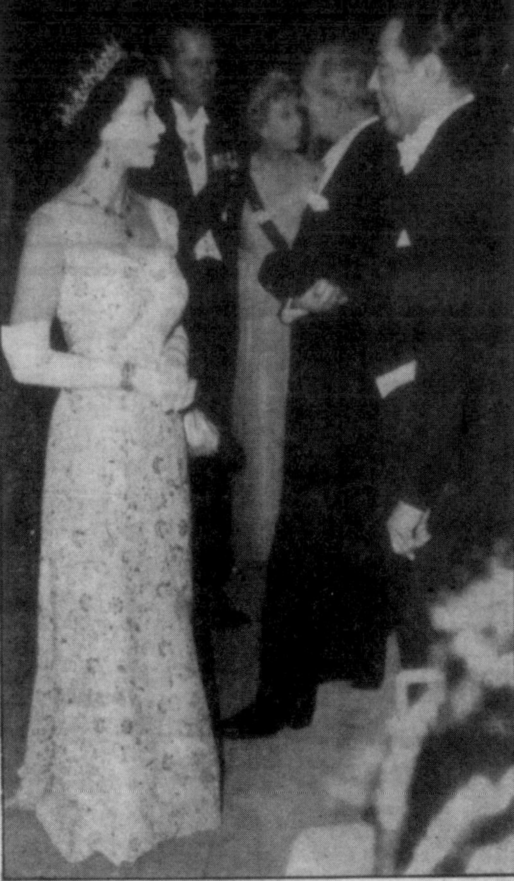

QUEEN MEETS DUKE

THE Queen, a glittering figure in a magnificent evening gown, chats with the great American jazzman Duke Ellington last night in Leeds Civic Hall.

"The Duke" rushed to the hall after a concert he and his band had given as part of the city's Music Festival.

After "The Duke" had been presented to the Queen, Prince Philip told him: "I was sorry I missed 'Take the A Train.' It is one of my favourites."

Russia's ace jet crashes

MOSCOW admitted last night that a TU 104 jet airliner—Russia's rival to Britain's Comet—had crashed, killing everyone

Figure 36.2 Article in the Sunday edition of a popular British tabloid (the predecessor of the *Sunday Mirror*) warning that 'frightening' 'X-pills' had been 'allowed to sneak into the country'. Three years before Enovid was marketed as a contraceptive, the FDA had approved it for the treatment of menstrual disorders. Tom Riley, 'X-pills in the shops', *Sunday Pictorial*, 19 Oct. 1958, back page. Mirrorpix.

The optimism that greeted the pill faded as medical concerns mounted over potentially fatal side-effects, including thrombosis and cancer. Books such as Barbara Seaman's *The Doctors' Case Against the Pill* (1969) and Wisconsin Senator Gaylord Nelson's congressional hearings on its safety (1970) galvanized public debate in the United States, while the UK government restricted higher dosages.[20] And yet, even as its safety came into question, the pill encouraged women to become more active patients and empowered them to challenge medical authority. Frequent claims notwithstanding,[21] no single technology launched a 'sexual revolution', but oral contraception, in concert with a host of social, cultural and political changes, did help to make women's lives in the 1980s very different from those of their mothers in the 1950s.

Far from sweeping alternatives away, the pill emboldened researchers to develop new technologies, including the modern IUD.[22] Though devices such as Gräfenberg's ring, made from silkworm gut and silver wire, were available from the early twentieth century, few doctors were willing to fit them.[23] After Israeli and Japanese clinicians reported positive results with new materials in 1959, the Population Council, an NGO created in the United States in 1952 to focus on world population growth, funded numerous projects to bring these devices to market. As with the pill, IUDs were intended as cheap, effective contraception for poor, uneducated women in 'developing' countries, where coercive family planners inserted them routinely after childbirth and abortion. In 'the west', in contrast, middle-class, educated white women, including many of those coming off the pill, increasingly opted for the copper and plastic devices as a non-hormonal alternative (Fig. 36.3).[24]

In the early 1970s, however, the 'Dalkon Shield scandal' severely damaged the reputation of IUDs in the United States. First marketed there and in Puerto Rico in 1971, the Dalkon Shield featured prongs, which prevented expulsion from the uterus but increased the chance of perforating the uterine wall, and a multifilament tail string, which extended into the vagina to aid removal but purportedly allowed bacteria to travel, or 'wick', into the uterus. It was withdrawn from the US market in 1974 amidst allegations of pelvic infections and other potentially fatal complications as well as hundreds

20 Watkins, *On the Pill*; Marks, *Sexual Chemistry.*

21 For example, Jonathan Eig, *The Birth of the Pill: How Four Crusaders Reinvented Sex and Launched a Revolution* (New York, NY, 2014).

22 Edgerton, *Shock of the Old*, p. 24.

23 Caroline Rusterholz, 'Testing the Gräfenberg ring in interwar Britain: Norman Haire, Helena Wright, and the debate over statistical evidence, side effects, and intra-uterine contraception', *Journal of the History of Medicine and Allied Sciences* 72 (2017), 448–67.

24 Chikako Takeshita, *The Global Biopolitics of the IUD: How Science Constructs Contraceptive Users and Women's Bodies* (Cambridge, MA, 2012); on the Population Council: Alison Bashford, 'World Population from Eugenics to Climate Change', Chapter 34, this book.

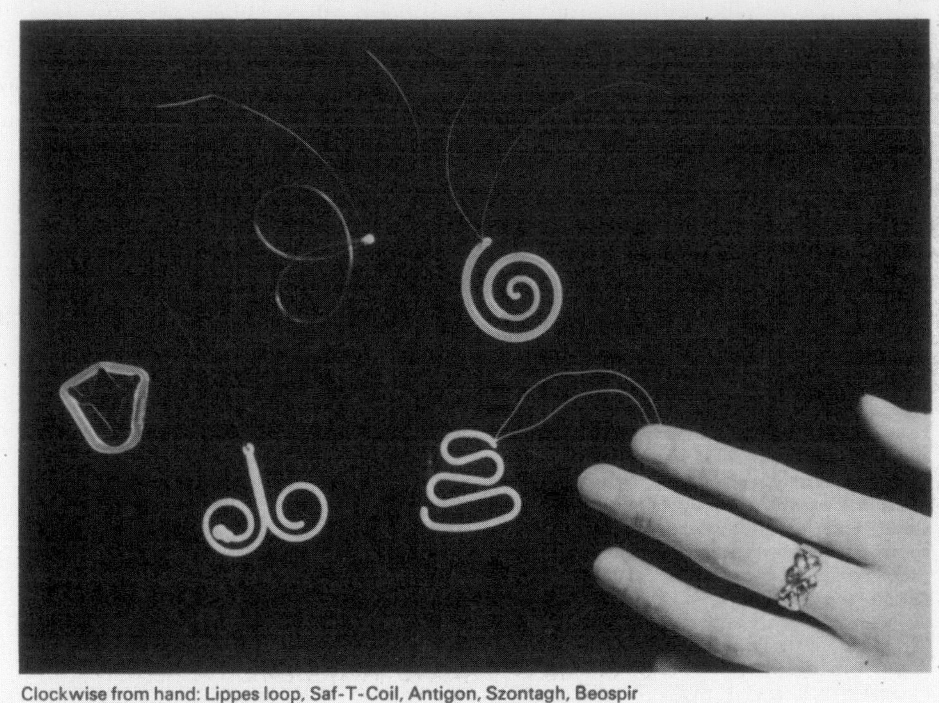

Clockwise from hand: Lippes loop, Saf-T-Coil, Antigon, Szontagh, Beospir

Figure 36.3 A conspicuously married woman's hand displaying IUDs in a consumer survey. From *Contraceptives: A Which? Supplement*, 3rd edn (London, 1970), p. 29. The copyright in this material is owned and/or licensed by Which? Limited and has been reproduced here with their permission. The material and logo must not be reproduced in whole or in part without the written permission of Which? Limited.

of thousands of lawsuits against the manufacturer, A. H. Robins.[25] Not until the early 2000s did Mirena, a Finnish innovation and the first widely available hormone-releasing IUD, reinvigorate the US market.[26] Though the proportion of female contraceptors choosing long-acting reversible methods (mainly Mirena and subsequent variants) more than tripled in the United States between 2002 (2.4 per cent) and 2009 (8.5 per cent), it remained lower than in Britain (11 per cent), France (23 per cent), Norway (27 per cent) and China (41 per cent), where copper devices continued to dominate.[27]

Reproductive technologists had high hopes not only for IUDs, but also for long-acting hormonal injections (Depo-Provera), implants (Norplant), vaginal rings

25 Andrea Tone, *Devices and Desires: A History of Contraceptives in America* (New York, NY, 2001), pp. 261–83.
26 Takeshita, *Global Biopolitics of the IUD*, pp. 138–9, 141.
27 Lawrence B. Finer, Jenna Jerman and Megan L. Kavanaugh, 'Changes in use of long-acting contraceptive methods in the United States, 2007–2009', *Fertility and Sterility* 98 (2012), 893–7.

and patches. Clinical trials began in 1969 in Chile; Finland was the first country to approve and market Norplant for general use in 1983. Like Mirena later, it came out of a collaboration between the Population Council and the Finnish pharmaceutical company Leiras Oy. The United States became the seventeenth nation to sanction sale and use in 1990, and almost immediately the implants became embroiled in controversy over the potential coercion of poor, black women. Although no more than 2 per cent of American women of reproductive age (about a million) ever used it as their method of choice, by 1996 some 50,000 individuals had joined class-action lawsuits against the manufacturer claiming restitution for pain and suffering.[28] Norplant sales were discontinued in the United States in 2002, but Bayer and the Bill & Melinda Gates Foundation have made its WHO-approved successor product, Jadelle, available to millions of women worldwide through the recently launched Implant Access Program. In Brazil, personalized implants tailor-made in specialized pharmacies are today an increasingly popular upper-class contraceptive choice.[29]

Surgical Solutions

Though even more controversial than implants and injections, sterilization and abortion are amongst the most common methods of avoiding pregnancy and childbirth in the world today. How did such divisive operations become so widespread? Used coercively in the first half of the twentieth century in the service of eugenics, to prevent the 'unfit' from reproducing, sterilization retained legitimacy to become the most popular form of contraception for married couples in the United States by 1975.[30] Not only women but men too chose sterilization as concerns about oral contraception reframed vasectomy as a manly operation (Fig. 36.4). Developed in China in 1974 and introduced to the United States in 1986, 'no-scalpel' vasectomy was praised by *Men's Health* magazine in 1996 as a painless procedure that spilled 'not even a single drop of blood'.[31]

Laparoscopy – a form of minimally invasive ('keyhole') surgery performed through a small incision in the female abdomen – made tubal ligation less expensive

28 Elizabeth Siegel Watkins, 'From breakthrough to bust: The brief life of Norplant, the contraceptive implant', *Journal of Women's History* 22 (2010), 88–111; Wendy Kline, 'Bodies of evidence: Activists, patients, and the FDA regulation of Depo-Provera', *Journal of Women's History* 22 (2010), 64–87; William Green, *Contraceptive Risk: The FDA, Depo-Provera, and the Politics of Experimental Medicine* (New York, NY, 2017).

29 Emilia Sanabria, *Plastic Bodies: Sex Hormones and Menstrual Suppression in Brazil* (Durham, NC, 2016).

30 Rebecca M. Kluchin, *Fit to Be Tied: Sterilization and Reproductive Rights in America, 1950–1980* (New Brunswick, NJ, 2009), p. 1; Paul Weindling, 'Pedigree of a "Schizophrenic Family"', Exhibit 29, this book.

31 Sarah Shropshire, 'What's a guy to do? Contraceptive responsibility, confronting masculinity, and the history of vasectomy in Canada', *Canadian Bulletin of Medical History* 31 (2014), 161–82, on 176.

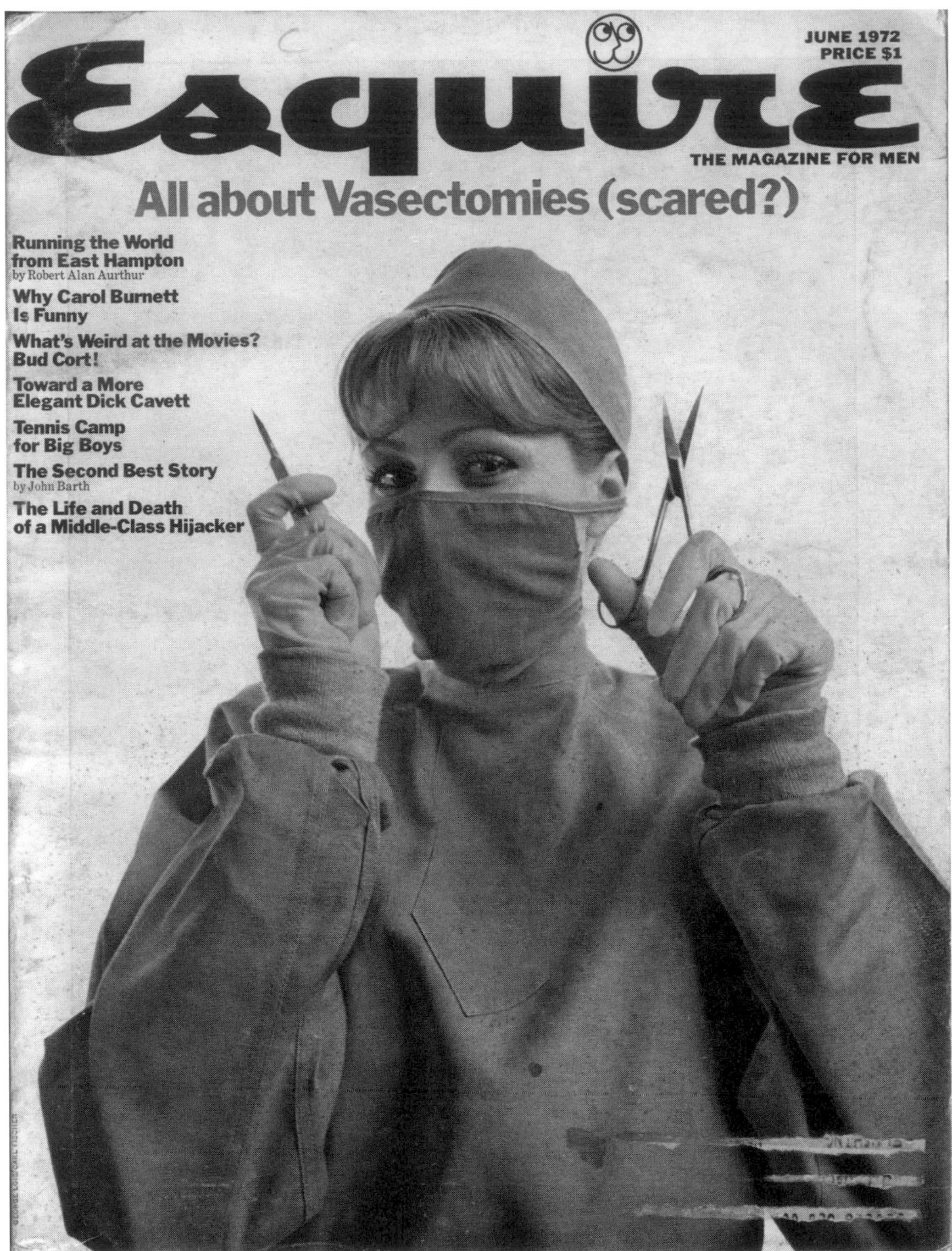

Figure 36.4 Cover of *Esquire* (June 1972), the then iconic American men's magazine, promoting a piece about vasectomies by showing a woman in surgical gear as she brandishes a scalpel and scissors. During the shoot with photographer Carl Fischer and designer George Lois, the model exclaimed: 'I'd like to do this to my ex-boyfriend!' (Lois to author, 20 Oct. 2015). Reprinted with permission from Hearst Corporation and George Lois.

United States Patent [19] — [11] **4,112,951**

Hulka et al. — [45] **Sep. 12, 1978**

[54] **SURGICAL CLIP**

[75] Inventors: **Jaroslav Fabian Hulka,** Chapel Hill, N.C.; **George Selden Clemens,** Northfield, Ill.

[73] Assignee: **Research Corporation,** New York, N.Y.

[21] Appl. No.: **652,616**

[22] Filed: **Jan. 26, 1976**

[51] **Int. Cl.**[2] **A61B 17/12**

[52] **U.S. Cl.** **128/346;** 24/251; 128/325

[58] **Field of Search** .... 24/251; 128/321, 325, 128/346; 339/255 P, 261; 251/9

[56] **References Cited**

U.S. PATENT DOCUMENTS

475,257	5/1892	Thuge	24/251 UX
1,832,879	11/1931	Ruskin	128/321
2,036,461	4/1936	Darby	339/255 P X
3,090,029	5/1963	Stroebel	339/255 P
3,398,746	8/1968	Abramson	128/321 X
3,687,131	8/1972	Rayport et al.	128/346 X
3,882,854	5/1975	Hulka et al.	128/6
3,950,829	4/1976	Cohen	24/251 X
4,064,881	12/1977	Meredith	128/325

FOREIGN PATENT DOCUMENTS

D971,659	6/1975	United Kingdom	128/346

Primary Examiner—Robert W. Michell
Assistant Examiner—Michael H. Thaler
Attorney, Agent, or Firm—Harold L. Stowell

[57] **ABSTRACT**

A surgical clip, particularly adapted to produce necrosis in Fallopian tube tissue, consists of jaws hinged adjacent one end and a U-shaped spring which holds the jaws open in one position and exerts a closing pressure on the jaws in another position. When the spring is in the jaws closing position, the bridge portion thereof in conjunction with side flanges carried by one of the jaws provides a smoothly contoured hinge end thereby reducing to a minimum zones for the entrapment of tissue which might be the cause of adhesions.

5 Claims, 4 Drawing Figures

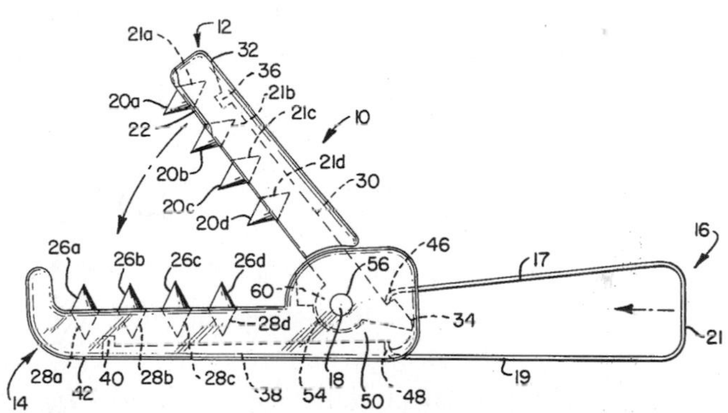

Figure 36.5 United States patent 4,112,951 (12 Sept. 1978) for a plastic, spring-loaded clip designed by gynaecologist Jaroslav Hulka 'to produce necrosis in Fallopian tube tissue'. Mass-produced by Richard Wolf, a leading surgical instruments company, the 'Hulka clip' became the most important source of patent royalties to the University of North Carolina, where Hulka was based, in the 1980s.

and less risky, but still more invasive and traumatic than vasectomy, by avoiding general anaesthesia and hospitalization. In the early 1970s, the US Agency for International Development (USAID) funded the development of portable outpatient technologies of female sterilization for use in makeshift 'camps'. Specialized equipment that fitted in a suitcase was deployed on a massive scale in rural India, where one enthusiastic surgeon claimed to have sterilized over 250,000 women between 1979 and 1989 (Fig. 36.5). Despite continual disclosures of coercion and even deaths, population control programmes have stabilized female sterilization as the world's commonest method of preventing pregnancy. In India and Puerto Rico, for example, tubal ligation is known simply as 'the operation'.[32]

Today, surgeons not only control fertility by operating on male and female bodies, but also routinely remove the contents of women's wombs. Of an estimated 205 million pregnancies worldwide in 2003, 20 per cent ended in induced abortion. The ratio of terminations to live births stands at 31 to 100 globally, but varies regionally; it is 1 to 5 in North America and 105 to 100 in eastern Europe, a legacy of Soviet-era policies that limited access to contraception but made abortion widely available.[33] From the mid-nineteenth century, licensed physicians increasingly used cervical dilators, curettes (hooked scraping tools) and other surgical instruments to perform abortions. By the early twentieth century, dilation and curettage (D&C), which involves opening the cervix and scraping out the uterine contents, combined with asepsis, anaesthesia, analgesia and later antibiotics, had become the standard medical practice for first-trimester terminations. D&C remained dominant in the west until the early 1970s, when it was supplanted by vacuum aspiration, another Chinese innovation.

China was one of few countries in the 1950s with an active, state-sponsored 'planned birth' programme (*jihua shengyu*) for researching new techniques of fertility control.[34] Designed in 1958 for use in rural China, the 'negative pressure' technique involved heating a glass bottle with a match to create a vacuum in the absence of electric power. Physicians in Japan, the Soviet Union and eastern Europe were early adopters as abortion technology travelled east to west.[35] A Los Angeles gynaecologist recalled his enthusiasm on hearing about vacuum aspiration in the mid-1960s, when the profession was still dominated by men. At a national conference in Chicago, a colleague told of completing a miscarriage for a Soviet diplomat's wife in Washington, DC. As he 'began inserting the instruments to remove the last of the pregnancy, a Soviet doctor, who had accompanied the patient to the operating theatre for reasons of protocol, asked: "How come you don't vacuum her?" None of us had ever heard of this vacuum machine before. I couldn't wait to get my hands on one.'[36]

32 Jesse Olszynko-Gryn, 'Laparoscopy as a technology of population control: A use-centred history of surgical sterilization', in Heinrich Hartmann and Corinna R. Unger (eds.), *A World of Populations: Transnational Perspectives on Demography in the Twentieth Century* (New York, NY, 2014), pp. 147–77.

33 Gilda Sedgh *et al.*, 'Legal abortion worldwide: Incidence and recent trends', *International Family Planning Perspectives* 33 (2007), 106–16.

34 Michelle Murphy, *Seizing the Means of Reproduction: Entanglements of Feminism, Health, and Technoscience* (Durham, NC, 2012), p. 155.

35 Tanfer Emin Tunc, 'Designs of devices: The vacuum aspirator and American abortion technology', *Dynamis* 28 (2008), 353–76.

36 Quoted in Cynthia Gorney, *Articles of Faith: A Frontline History of the Abortion Wars* (New York, NY, 1998), p. 197.

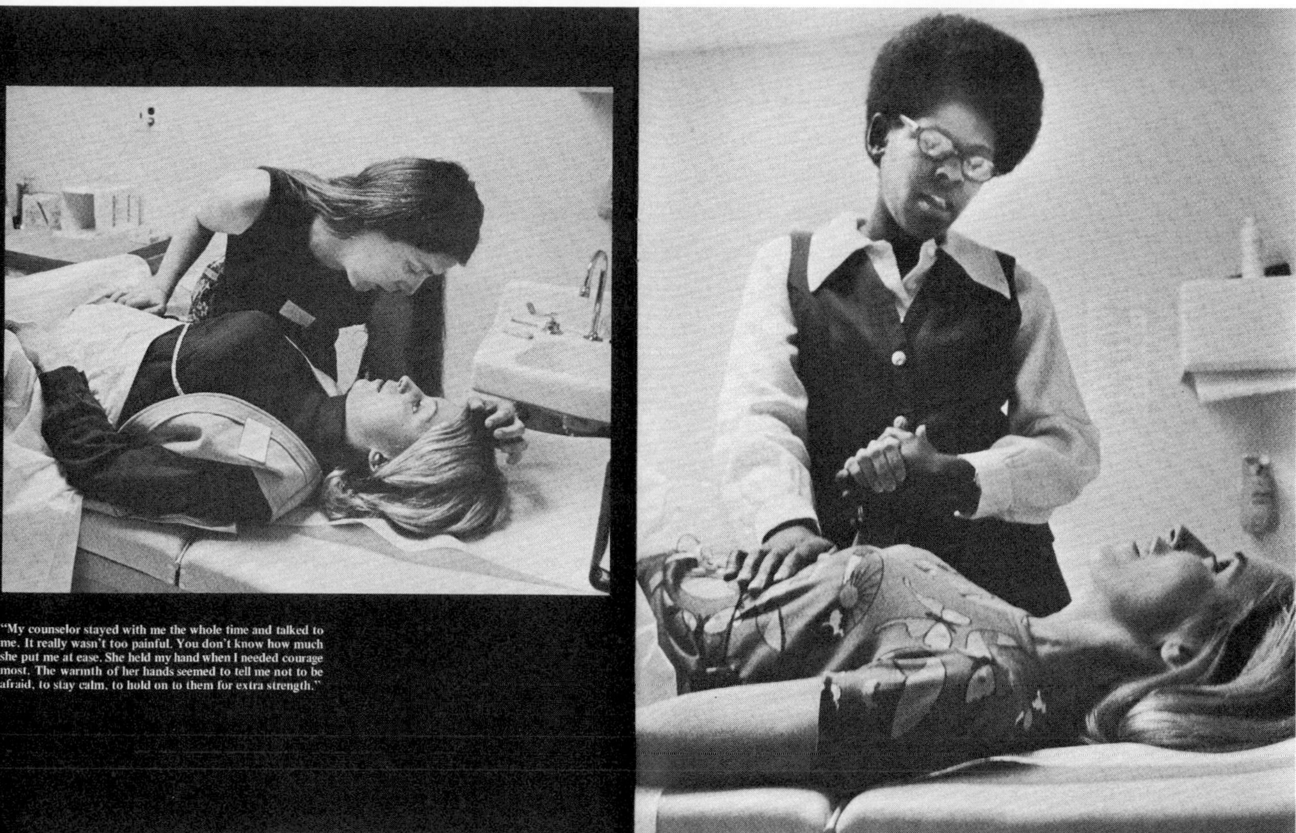

"My counselor stayed with me the whole time and talked to me. It really wasn't too painful. You don't know how much she put me at ease. She held my hand when I needed courage most. The warmth of her hands seemed to tell me not to be afraid, to stay calm, to hold on to them for extra strength."

Figure 36.6 Spread from a pamphlet produced *c.* 1972 by Preterm, a nonprofit clinic that opened in Washington, DC, shortly after the District of Columbia decriminalized abortion. Emphasizing compassion and counselling, the photographs portray women helping women and racial harmony. Reprinted with permission from Preterm and the Jaroslav Hulka Papers, David M. Rubenstein Rare Book & Manuscript Library, Duke University.

Before long, Americans constructed their own devices for domestic and overseas use. Harvey Karman, a controversial lay abortionist in Santa Monica, patented a narrow, flexible, plastic tube that removed the need for cervical dilation and electricity. In nearby Los Angeles, feminist Lorraine Rothman assembled parts purchased at grocery, hardware and pet stores into the patented *Del-em* for do-it-yourself 'menstrual extraction'. Cheap plastic technologies made abortion affordable for the network of outpatient clinics that activists established around the country (Fig. 36.6). Meanwhile, various states had relaxed their abortion laws, and USAID contracted the mass production of thousands of disposable kits, based on Karman's patent, for export.[37] In 1973, the landmark ruling, *Roe v. Wade*, decriminalized abortion nationwide, but the 1973 Helms amendment prohibited federal

37 Murphy, *Seizing the Means*, pp. 150–76.

foreign aid from subsidizing abortion.[38] NGOs continued to distribute the kits, including in the new country of Bangladesh, where the government had temporarily legalized abortion for women who had been raped during the Liberation War.[39]

Under the Reagan presidency, religious conservatives in the Republican Party successfully restricted abortion access at the state and federal levels while 'pro-life' activists picketed clinics and 'rescued' unborn 'babies'. Militants turned violent in the 1990s, bombing clinics and assassinating physicians. For 'pro-choice' activists, this state of siege made access to pharmaceutical alternatives more pressing than ever.[40] But research had slowed down, especially in the United States, where the threat of class-action lawsuits, increasing government regulation, a seemingly saturated market and greater public scrutiny dampened enthusiasm.

As the number of US companies actively researching contraception fell from nine in 1980 to just one, Ortho Pharmaceutical, in 1990,[41] the World Health Organization (WHO) took the lead. Beginning in the 1970s, the WHO had built an international network of laboratories to develop new forms of contraception and abortion, including controversial anti-fertility 'vaccines' and male methods involving synthetic hormones.[42] Clinical trials on men were stymied, however, by the absence of an existing infrastructure for testing male contraceptives, low acceptance of any risk by either clinicians or study participants, and the ethical dilemma that failures would impregnate women, not the men enrolled in the trials.[43] No male pill materialized, but a new generation of female pills expanded women's choices and rekindled old debates about the boundary between contraception and abortion.

'Emergency' Contraception and Pharmaceutical Abortion

Heralded in the *New York Times* back in 1966 as a 'second revolution in birth control', the 'morning-after' pill was promoted by 'fathers' of 'the pill' Gregory Pincus and Min Chueh Chang as a convenient back-up, but condemned by their former collaborator,

38 Sneha Barot, 'Abortion restrictions in US foreign aid: The history and harms of the Helms Amendment', *Guttmacher Policy Review* 16, no. 3 (2013), 9–13.

39 Murphy, *Seizing the Means*, p. 168.

40 Kristin Luker, *Abortion and the Politics of Motherhood* (Berkeley, CA, 1984); Rickie Solinger (ed.), *Abortion Wars: A Half Century of Struggle, 1950–2000* (Berkeley, CA, 1998); Johnson and Hopwood, 'Modern Law and Regulation'.

41 Heather Munro Prescott, *The Morning After: A History of Emergency Contraception in the United States* (New Brunswick, NJ, 2011), p. 94.

42 Nelly Oudshoorn, *The Male Pill: A Biography of a Technology in the Making* (Durham, NC, 2003), pp. 52–68; Jessika van Kammen, 'Representing users' bodies: The gendered development of anti-fertility vaccines', *Science, Technology, & Human Values* 24 (1999), 307–37.

43 Oudshoorn, *Male Pill*, p. 80.

the Catholic gynaecologist John Rock, as an abortifacient.[44] Less expensive than a daily regime, especially for the uninsured, the morning-after pill promised to reduce health risks at a time when the safety of oral contraception was increasingly scrutinized. In 1968, Chang predicted that a variety of 'morning-after', 'week later', 'second-thought', 'abortion' and 'night before' pills 'would be a boon for couples who wanted 100 per cent effectiveness in preventing pregnancy'.[45] But FDA approval proved elusive, and pharmaceutical companies had little incentive to market a potentially controversial drug intended for infrequent, 'emergency' use.

College physicians who provided the synthetic oestrogen diethylstilbestrol (DES) off-label to 'girls unprepared for the night before' were forced to look elsewhere when longer-term use for other indications was linked to a rare form of vaginal cancer in daughters of women who had taken the drug during pregnancy. Canadian gynaecologist Albert Yuzpe's method of punching out four tablets of oral contraception was authorized in the early 1980s in Britain and West Germany, but not Canada or the United States, where feminists took matters into their own hands by distributing Yuzpe regimen dosages at rape crisis and student health centres. In the late 1990s, the FDA approved the Yuzpe method; a small New Jersey-based company marketed Preven, a combined oestrogen and progestin pill, as 'emergency contraception'; and feminists founded their own corporation to market Plan B (two progestin-only pills taken twelve hours apart).[46] In 2010, the FDA approved ellaOne (ulipristal acetate), which extended the window of use from seventy-two hours to five days, and, in 2013, the Obama administration announced it would allow over-the-counter sales of emergency contraception to girls and women of all ages.

Less ambiguous and more controversial than emergency contraception, the 'abortion pill' was first marketed in France in 1988 by Roussel-Uclaf, a company jointly owned by the French government and Hoechst, a major West German firm. Intended for use in early pregnancy (typically up to seven weeks) in combination with a prostaglandin, currently misoprostol, that causes uterine contractions, mifepristone or RU486, as it was then called, is an antiprogestin that alters the uterine lining to disrupt the attachment of a fertilized egg. Not as simple as popping a pill, 'medical abortion' initially required three or four clinical visits: for confirmation of pregnancy, usually by ultrasound; for abortion counselling and to swallow three tablets of RU486 under medical supervision; for an injection or suppository of misoprostol and to wait in the clinic to abort; and finally for a post-abortion check-up, usually also by ultrasound.[47] It was rapidly caught in America's abortion wars.

44 Prescott, *Morning After*, p. 7. 45 Quoted in ibid., p. 19.

46 Ibid., pp. 35, 101; on DES: Jean-Paul Gaudillière, 'Sex Hormones, Pharmacy and the Reproductive Sciences', Chapter 35, this book.

47 Adele Clarke and Theresa Montini, 'The many faces of RU486: Tales of situated knowledges and technological contestations', *Science, Technology, & Human Values* 18 (1993), 42–78.

Threatened with international boycotts by US anti-abortion groups, Roussel initially suspended distribution, but then resumed under orders from the French health minister who declared that RU486 was 'the moral property of women'.[48] When George H. W. Bush's administration banned importation in 1989, American abortion-rights groups campaigned for access. On the twentieth anniversary of *Roe v. Wade* in 1993, the newly elected President Bill Clinton lifted the ban, by which time Britain, China and Sweden had also passed the drug. Roussel transferred the US patent to the Population Council and the FDA granted tentative approval in 1996, but no major pharmaceutical company dared claim the commercial rights for fear of reprisals. Finally Danco, a small New York company with an unlisted phone number and address, was established with the sole purpose of marketing RU486 in the United States, where it debuted in September 2000 as Mifeprex.[49]

FDA authorization did not end the controversy, which continued when China announced that a Shanghai-based company would supply the raw compound to Danco. By then RU486 had been approved in over a dozen countries; hundreds of thousands of women in Europe and millions more in China had used it. In the United States, non-surgical providers were allowed to offer the drug as long as they could 'assess the duration of pregnancy accurately' and had made back-up arrangements for a surgical provider. Unusually for a drug of which the safety was not in question, physicians were obliged to sign a 'provider's agreement' stating that they had met the above requirements and would report all adverse events to Danco. Patients too were required to sign a detailed agreement.[50] Today, its use internationally remains subject to a host of restrictions that are not grounded in clinical need.[51]

Conclusion

The pill was a highly successful, even revolutionary drug. By 1989, it had been taken by over 75 per cent of women born in Britain between 1945 and 1959.[52] Yet many of them surely also used other methods and stayed on the pill for variable durations.[53] When the pill was first marketed in the 1960s, men and women had long controlled their fertility. New hormonal and surgical methods increased women's share of responsibility

48 Quoted in Prescott, *Morning After*, p. 79.

49 Carole Joffe and Tracy A. Weitz, 'Normalizing the exceptional: Incorporating the "abortion pill" into mainstream medicine', *Social Science & Medicine* 56 (2003), 2353–66.

50 Ibid.

51 Sally Sheldon, 'British abortion law: Speaking from the past to govern the future', *Modern Law Review* 79 (2016), 283–316.

52 Hera Cook, 'The English sexual revolution: Technology and social change', *History Workshop Journal* 59 (2005), 109–28, on 109.

53 Fisher, *Birth Control*, p. 242.

and control, but male methods persisted. Health concerns about the pill inspired 'vasectomania' in the 1970s, condoms made a comeback with the global AIDS crisis of the 1980s, and withdrawal was still 'a major, widespread method' in the 1990s.[54] Despite the failure of the pharmaceutical industry to produce a 'male pill', men and women collaborated in homes and clinics, variously combining male and female methods, contraception and abortion, new and old technologies. Though the sexual revolution did not see the sharp break in behaviours that is sometimes imagined, heated public debates around the pill, sterilization, abortion, women's health and population control engendered a mainstream culture that featured contraceptive technologies more prominently than ever.[55]

Though contraceptive use has generally risen, the resulting pattern has left few commentators satisfied. Today, critics complain of over-reliance on sterilization in Asia, but underuse of IUDs in the United States, where half of all pregnancies are 'unplanned'. Some feminists champion oral contraception as liberatory, while others criticize doctors for pushing women to go on the pill. Vasectomy, though cheaper and safer than female sterilization, is uncommon in most countries. Self-abortion persists where legal access is limited; in the United States, prominent arrests involving the off-label use of misoprostol, available as an ulcer drug, have reignited old debates.[56]

Corporations, states and NGOs have created and met demand for technologies of contraception and abortion from doctors, patients and consumers. This chapter has charted some of the major trajectories. While there is still much to discover, focusing on 'the pill' has clearly obscured a richer story in which not only American innovators and industrialists but also their state-supported counterparts in China and in France played leading roles in producing today's strikingly various cultures of fertility control.

54 Deborah Rogow and Sonya Horowitz, 'Withdrawal: A review of the literature and an agenda for research', *Studies in Family Planning* 26 (1995), 140–53, on 149.

55 Weeks, *Sex, Politics and Society*, pp. 334–5.

56 Tiana Bakić Hayden, 'Private bleeding: Self-induced abortion in the twenty-first century United States', *Gender Issues* 28 (2011), 209–25.

37 Hospital Birth

Salim Al-Gailani

You were probably born in a hospital. Exceptional around 1900, when the vast majority of women gave birth at home, within three generations institutional deliveries were the norm in most industrialized countries. The sharpest growth in hospital births occurred after World War II, as pronatalist western governments expanded health-care spending during reconstruction, but in some places the shift was already well under way. The United States, where the proportion of women delivering their babies in hospital leapt from 37 per cent in 1935 to almost 79 per cent in 1945, is only the best-known case. Although resource-rich nations led the way, the trend was not confined to the west. The Soviet Union claimed, like the United States, that by the late 1960s practically all births were in hospitals.[1]

Visible by the last third of the twentieth century even in low-income countries, the 'relocation of birth to the hospital' was first defined as a historical phenomenon in the western world, especially in the United States and Britain. New technologies for monitoring the fetus and intervening in labour, together with the mid-century decline in maternal mortality, sustained obstetric specialists' claims that hospitals were the only appropriate place to give birth. But by around 1970, among wider critiques of medical authority, women and their partners in both countries were systematically questioning hospital-based, high-technology obstetrics. Emboldened by the second-wave feminist call for women to control their own bodies, activists campaigned against professional paternalism and for greater choice in maternity care. During the so-called birth wars of the mid-1970s and early 1980s, some rejected hospital obstetrics altogether.

History and the Birth Wars

The same movement that pushed women's health, including maternity care, to the centre of the political stage in the United States and Britain also transformed understandings of the history of childbirth. In the 1960s, obstetricians' accounts of hospitalized birth as the triumphant end-point of a story of medical and technological progress that

1 Joint Study Group of the International Federation of Gynaecology and Obstetrics and the International Confederation of Midwives, *Maternity Care in the World: International Survey of Midwifery Training and Practice* (Oxford, 1966), p. 9.

began with the forceps went largely unchallenged.[2] Then second-wave histories reinterpreted the postwar trend towards near-universal hospital birth as the takeover by male medicine of a traditionally women's affair. In this view, the first lying-in institutions founded in the eighteenth century were instruments for diminishing female autonomy, of a piece with the maternity hospitals that many of these authors and their readers encountered first-hand.

For the activists, regaining autonomy meant 'returning' to a 'woman-centred' golden age and, for some, to the home deliveries that had mostly disappeared in the industrialized world.[3] Drawing on general critiques of paternalistic medical power, much new writing on childbirth framed modern obstetrics as a strategy for the surveillance and control of women's bodies; what British sociologist Ann Oakley termed 'the captured womb'.[4] Feminist critiques of institutionalized maternity care were bolstered by research in epidemiology and historical demography that challenged the assumption that hospital births were or ever had been statistically safer than delivery at home.[5] Social scientists researched birth cultures in countries that bucked the western trend; the Netherlands, where more than half of confinements still took place at home around 1970, boasted one of the lowest maternal and perinatal mortality rates in the world.[6]

Widely read during the birth wars, these studies not only informed the activism of the 1970s and 1980s, they also shaped social scientific and humanities scholarship on childbirth, including in the emerging field of social history of medicine. While taking up second-wave concerns with shifting power relations in the birthing room, much historical writing from the mid-1980s criticized the previous generation's portrayal of women as inert 'victims' of obstetrics. In step with the wider challenge to the concept of 'medicalization' as a pernicious collaboration of experts and state authority imposed from above, historians of childbirth stressed the key role of women's decision-making in driving change.[7]

2 But see Mary E. Fissell, 'Man-Midwifery Revisited', Chapter 22; and also Ludmilla Jordanova, 'Man-Midwifery Dissected', Exhibit 22, this book.

3 Monica H. Green, 'Gendering the history of women's healthcare', *Gender & History* 20 (2008), 487–518. I focus on writing about modern times; on the middle ages and early modernity: Katharine Park, 'Managing Childbirth and Fertility in Medieval Europe', Chapter 11; Lauren Kassell, 'Medieval Birth Malpresentations', Exhibit 10; Lea T. Olsan, 'A Medieval Birth Girdle', Exhibit 11; Sandra Cavallo, 'Pregnant Stones as Wonders of Nature', Exhibit 17; Fissell, 'Man-Midwifery Revisited'; Lianne McTavish, 'A Birthing Chair', Exhibit 18, this book.

4 William Ray Arney, *Power and the Profession of Obstetrics* (Chicago, IL, 1982); Ann Oakley, *The Captured Womb: A History of the Medical Care of Pregnant Women* (Oxford, 1984).

5 Sheila Kitzinger and John A. Davis (eds.), *The Place of Birth: A Study of the Environment in which Birth Takes Place with Special Reference to Home Confinements* (Oxford, 1978).

6 Brigitte Jordan, *Birth in Four Cultures: A Crosscultural Investigation of Childbirth in Yucatan, Holland, Sweden, and the United States* (Montreal, 1978).

7 Judith Walzer Leavitt, *Brought to Bed: Childbearing in America, 1750 to 1950* (New York, NY, 1986), p. 196.

Delving into letters, diaries, autobiographies, newspapers, magazines and hospital case notes, and conducting oral history interviews, social historians recovered abundant evidence of women's agency, both in resisting male authority and in supporting the medicalization of birth through consumer choice. Seeking to do justice to women's experiences of childbearing, historians also emphasized how decision-making over birth defined and was defined by gender, class and race, as well as identities as mothers, fathers and professionals. Others took issue with some activists' 'romanticizing' of home birth in the past, and the too crude contrast with the technocratic and alienating experiences assumed to be characteristic of the modern hospital.[8] This research has challenged linear explanations of the 'origins' and 'rise' of institutionalized maternity care, but midwifery, pregnancy and birth are still usually treated as having their own distinctive history, set apart from the major general transformations in medicine. By contrast, this chapter seeks to place changes in the management of childbirth within larger shifts in hospitals as institutions.

Lying-In Charities

Products of broader eighteenth-century hospital reform, specialist establishments for 'lying-in' care provided a new institutional context for both charitable support to the pregnant poor and midwifery instruction. Established across continental Europe as the rational and humanistic ideals of the Enlightenment redefined economic, fiscal and military strength in terms of a large and healthy population, lying-in hospitals were promoted as saving the lives of mothers and babies through improved midwifery (Fig. 37.1). There were earlier prototypes, notably the renowned *salle des accouchements* of the Hôtel-Dieu in Paris, which had accepted mostly female students for instruction on the wards since at least the early seventeenth century. A few urban midwives also offered care in private maternity homes.[9] Yet around 1800, when lying-in charities could be found in most major European cities, hospital deliveries remained incidental. Childbirth was in all but exceptional cases a domestic event.

Some histories have represented lying-in hospitals as extreme versions of the Foucauldian clinic, turning socio-economically vulnerable women into objects of emerging obstetrical science that male physicians could examine with impunity and use for instruction and research. These institutions have also been analysed as drivers of man-midwifery. They bolstered the professional identities of its practitioners and

8 Charlotte Borst, *Catching Babies: The Professionalization of Childbirth, 1870–1920* (Cambridge, MA, 1995); Wendy Mitchinson, *Giving Birth in Canada, 1900–1950* (Toronto, 2002); Judith Walzer Leavitt, *Make Room for Daddy: The Journey from Waiting Room to Birthing Room* (Chapel Hill, NC, 2009); Angela Davis, *Modern Motherhood: Women and Family in England*, c. *1945–2000* (Manchester, 2012).

9 Doreen Evenden, *The Midwives of Seventeenth-Century London* (Cambridge, 2000), p. 183.

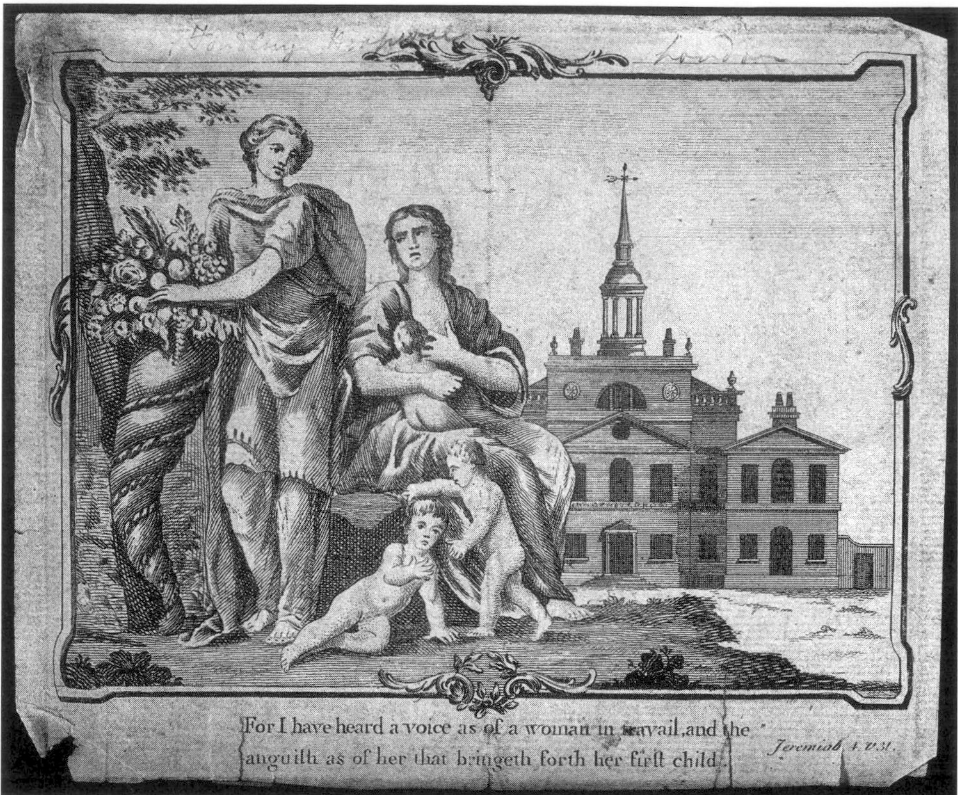
For I have heard a voice as of a woman in travail, and the
anguiſh as of her that bringeth forth her firſt child.
Jeremiah 4. v.31.

Figure 37.1 Engraving, mid-eighteenth to early nineteenth century, promoting the City of London Lying-In Hospital. Founded in 1750, this institution accepted only married women until rules were relaxed around 1900. The horn of plenty and the breast-feeding mother symbolically linked the work of the lying-in hospital with the Enlightenment concerns of charity, fertility, infant health and economic prosperity. Border 11 × 15 cm. Wellcome Library, London.

gave them control of a hierarchy that mostly subordinated female midwives. In addition, institutional care offered man-midwives access to pregnant and parturient women and contact with wealthy benefactors who were also potential patients. By the early nineteenth century, hospital practice began to demarcate a class of obstetric specialist not only from midwives, but also from the general practitioners for whom attending births became central to family practice.[10]

Yet lying-in hospitals neither necessarily undermined the status of female midwives nor led to unrestricted male control. Hospitals in fact typically gave midwives responsibility for normal births, while confining male practitioners to emergency work. Many continental

10 Margaret Versluysen, 'Midwives, medical men, and "poor women labouring with child": Lying-in hospitals in eighteenth-century London', in Helen Roberts (ed.), *Women, Health and Reproduction* (London, 1981), pp. 18–49; Bronwyn Croxson, 'The foundation and evolution of the Middlesex Hospital's lying-in service, 1745–86', *Social History of Medicine* 14 (2001), 27–57.

European lying-in hospitals trained midwives, either alone or alongside male medical students. Rather than facilitating the male monopoly of birth attendance, hospitals mostly consolidated existing arrangements.[11] Moreover, at the independent voluntary institutions more common in Britain and the United States, medical staff were socially subordinate to the lay, often female, philanthropists who founded and ran them. Regardless of the birth environment, before the twentieth century it was still largely women's expectations and wishes that set the parameters for obstetric intervention. Physicians had to adapt.[12]

Even where teaching staff intended to turn pregnant and parturient women into practice dummies for their students, hospital patients themselves neither were powerless nor necessarily perceived these institutions as oppressive. Many women set limits on medical control; for instance, by refusing to be examined, resisting operative interference, insisting on the presence of a female midwife, or by simply arriving at the hospital too late in labour for students to witness the birth or leaving before being delivered. Others undoubtedly welcomed medical attendance and accepted doctors' authority. For pregnant and often single women of the lower classes – some in desperate personal situations – hospitals were attractive because they offered free accommodation, food and support.[13]

Medicalizing Maternity

Charity and the moral revival of patients remained central goals of the nineteenth-century hospital. But as institutional priorities shifted to education and research, hospitals presented themselves as medical rather than charitable establishments. This was also true of lying-in or now more commonly 'maternity' hospitals, which were promoted as catering to those patients in need of specialist obstetric care and not just shelter. If the development of a separate nursing profession, the introduction of anaesthesia and antisepsis, and the associated growth in surgery consolidated the 'medicalization' of the general hospital in the late nineteenth century, similar trends shaped inpatient maternity care.[14]

Pharmaceutical pain relief would define the experience of hospitalized childbirth in the twentieth century, but anaesthesia was fiercely contested before it became routine around 1900. Arguments over the safety, efficacy and ethics of obstetric ether

11 Adrian Wilson, *The Making of Man-Midwifery: Childbirth in England, 1660–1770* (Cambridge, MA, 1995), pp. 145–58; see also Lucia Dacome, 'A Crystal Womb', Exhibit 21, this book.

12 Leavitt, *Brought to Bed*, p. 85; Virginia A. Metaxas Quiroga, *Poor Mothers and Babies: A Social History of Childbirth and Child Care Hospitals in Nineteenth-Century New York City* (New York, NY, 1989).

13 Nancy Schrom Dye, 'Modern obstetrics and working-class women: The New York Midwifery Dispensary, 1890–1920', *Journal of Social History* 20 (1987), 549–64; Jürgen Schlumbohm, '"The pregnant women are here for the sake of the teaching institution": The lying-in hospital of Göttingen University, 1751 to *c.* 1830', *Social History of Medicine* 14 (2001), 59–78.

14 Charles E. Rosenberg, *The Care of Strangers: The Rise of America's Hospital System* (Baltimore, MD, 1987); Guenter B. Risse, *Mending Bodies, Saving Souls: A History of Hospitals* (New York, NY, 1999); Alison Nuttall, '"Because of poverty brought into hospital ...": A casenote-based analysis of the changing role of the Edinburgh Royal Maternity Hospital, 1850–1912', *Social History of Medicine* 20 (2007), 263–80.

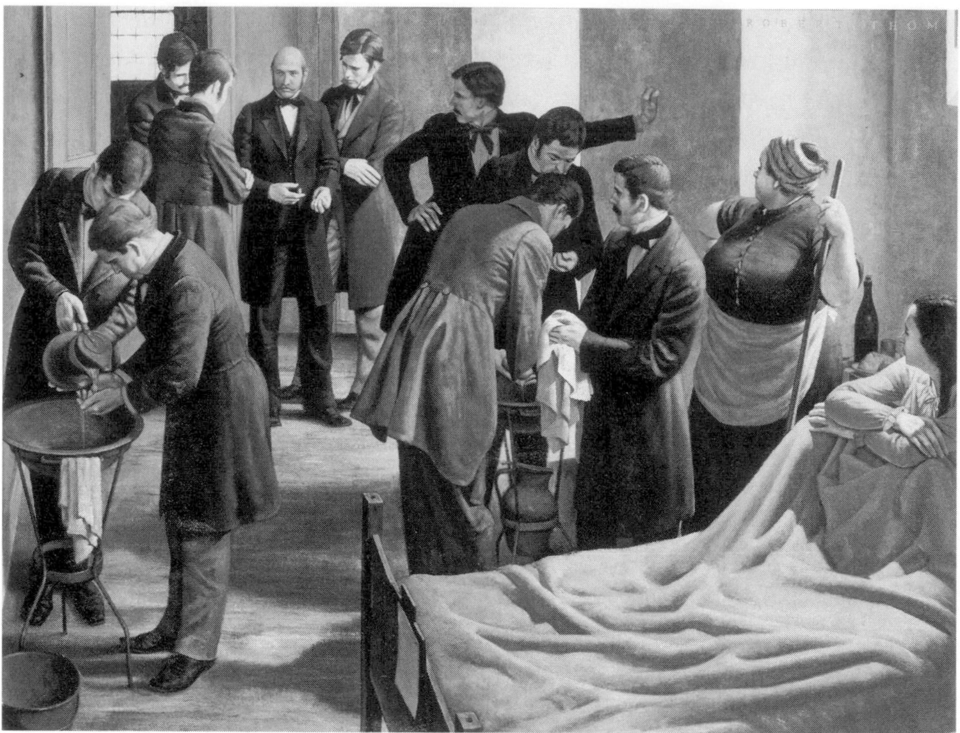

Figure 37.2 Oil painting celebrating Ignaz Semmelweis as the conqueror of maternal mortality. In this 1950s commission from the American pharmaceutical firm Parke, Davis & Company, he is shown training younger colleagues. Reproductions were mailed to physicians as posters and used in advertisements and books. 117 × 145 cm. From the collection of the University of Michigan Health System, gift of Pfizer, Inc., UMHS.26.

and chloroform were part of wider debates about surgery, and complicated by gender and religion. Some doctors and clergymen opposed anaesthesia on the grounds that pain was both God's curse upon Eve and necessary for the progression and management of labour. But specialists, pushed by the expectations of their private, paying clientele for pain-free births, came to agree on the value of anaesthesia in the delivery room. Since new drugs, such as scopolamine or 'twilight sleep', required specialist expertise and greater vigilance, women's demands for anaesthesia helped to drive childbirth into the hospital in the early twentieth century.[15]

This transformed the experience, but the danger of puerperal fever remained. In 1848, Ignaz Semmelweis of Vienna had suggested that doctors and medical students carried infection from autopsy room to maternity ward and from patient to patient, but that thorough hand-washing could largely prevent childbed fever (Fig. 37.2). This

15 Leavitt, *Brought to Bed*, pp. 116–41; Jacqueline H. Wolf, *Deliver Me From Pain: Anesthesia and Birth in America* (Baltimore, MD, 2009), pp. 44–72.

intervention fed into the nineteenth-century debate about the salubrity of hospitals. Commentators invoked alarming mortality statistics that pointed to rising 'hospitalism', or hospital-originated disease, and singled out lying-in institutions as the worst offenders. Suggestions that women giving birth at home were safer than their counterparts in institutions led a minority of critics, including the influential sanitarian and nursing reformer Florence Nightingale, to call for the abolition of large urban hospitals.[16] Fighting to protect them from closure, doctors ultimately accepted calls for reform, including by harnessing the sanitary ideal along with other procedural changes to banish infection from wards. The movement for hospital reform set the scene for the gradual acceptance and integration of antiseptic routines into surgery and obstetrics after the 1870s.[17] Demands for scrupulous cleanliness in the delivery room – practically impossible, specialists insisted, against the mortality data, in birthing women's own homes – underpinned arguments for the expansion of in-hospital maternity care.

There was no straightforward relationship between technical innovation and transformations in hospital practice, but anaesthesia and antisepsis did encourage surgeons to expand the range of interventions, to which patients were ever more willing to submit.[18] Late nineteenth-century obstetricians similarly embraced a more interventionist approach to managing labour in difficult cases. Specialists argued that such procedures as the caesarean section could be performed more safely, improving the chances of children as well as mothers. From the 1860s, confidence in surgical technique generated calls, especially from Catholic doctors, to abolish procedures that destroyed the living fetus in cases of obstructed delivery. In tandem with an emerging emphasis on the value of the 'unborn individual', the trend towards the more active management of birth in turn increased demands on the hospital.[19]

By 1900, renewed pleas for learning by doing combined with full-time clinical teaching and research to bind hospitals more tightly to academic institutes, particularly in the reformed American schools that were taken as the international model for medical education in the twentieth century. Amid ever-louder appeals for more practical training, including in obstetrics, medical schools established connections with lying-in institutions to give their students first-hand access to deliveries.[20] New knowledge about disease transmission by microorganisms and the explosion of bacteriological studies not

16 Florence Nightingale, *Introductory Notes on Lying-In Institutions; Together with a Proposal for Organising an Institution for Training Midwives and Midwifery Nurses* (London, 1871).

17 Irvine Loudon, *Death in Childbirth: An International Study of Maternal Care and Maternal Mortality, 1800–1950* (Oxford, 1992), pp. 196–203.

18 Sally Wilde, 'Truth, trust, and confidence in surgery, 1890–1910: Patient autonomy, communication, and consent', *Bulletin of the History of Medicine* 83 (2009), 302–30.

19 Joseph G. Ryan, 'The chapel and the operating room: The struggle of Roman Catholic clergy, physicians, and believers with the dilemmas of obstetric surgery, 1800–1900', *Bulletin of the History of Medicine* 76 (2002), 461–94; Sara Dubow, *Ourselves Unborn: A History of the Fetus in Modern America* (New York, NY, 2011).

20 Lawrence D. Longo, 'Obstetrics and gynecology', in Ronald L. Numbers (ed.), *The Education of American Physicians: Historical Essays* (Berkeley, CA, 1980), pp. 205–25.

only boosted reformers' calls for midwifery students to share in the benefits of laboratory training, but also emphasized the need to make the lying-in room a sterile environment.

The Chicago Lying-In, built by obstetrician Joseph DeLee from a small outpatient dispensary in 1895 into an 'exquisitely equipped' teaching hospital in 1917, came to symbolize the ultimate in maternity services the world over. DeLee's dismissal of midwives as 'relic[s] of barbarism' was characteristic of American obstetricians' confrontational attitudes to female practitioners, especially compared with their better-established European counterparts. European obstetric specialists, even in Britain, generally accepted that midwives should continue to attend normal births. DeLee railed against the 'old prejudice', in fact more of an old debate, that parturition was a 'physiologic act'; he argued instead that every labour had a 'pathologic dignity' which required significant amounts of surgery and drugs.[21] With the ideal of laboratory control ever more central to the identity of modern surgery, hospitals became the default setting for such interventions. Specially designed and equipped wards offered obstetricians both a base from which to build prestige for their discipline and a space in which they could aspire to control every aspect of childbirth.[22]

Supply and Demand

Even as specialists began to construct hospitals as temples of obstetric progress, institutional maternity care stayed negligible. The vast majority of births were still attended at home by a midwife around 1900, but the trend towards the hospital had set in by the interwar years in many countries, most strikingly in the United States. Private nursing homes became popular with the well-to-do, and the 'private-patient revolution' around World War I opened up American hospitals in general to an expanding proportion of fee-paying patients. Now, more than ever, growing numbers of middle-class women sought an institution for their confinements. Federal support for hospital building and the mid-century expansion of medical insurance schemes put the cost of hospitalization within most Americans' reach.[23]

For much of the twentieth century, obstetricians and social scientists alike framed discussions of the place of confinement in terms of government policy, especially the availability of maternity beds, the provision of statutory antenatal care and the quality of housing. While most historians now agree that the state played an important role in

21 Joseph B. DeLee, 'Progress toward ideal obstetrics', *American Journal of Obstetrics and Diseases of Women and Children* 73 (1916), 407–15; for a recent reassessment: Carolyn Herbst Lewis, 'The gospel of good obstetrics: Joseph Bolivar DeLee's vision for childbirth in the United States', *Social History of Medicine* 29 (2016), 112–30; for European colonists' similar attitudes to midwives: Philippa Levine, 'Imperial Encounters', Chapter 33, this book.

22 Thomas Schlich, 'Surgery, science and modernity: Operating rooms and laboratories as spaces of control', *History of Science* 45 (2007), 231–56.

23 Rosenberg, *Care of Strangers*, pp. 237–61.

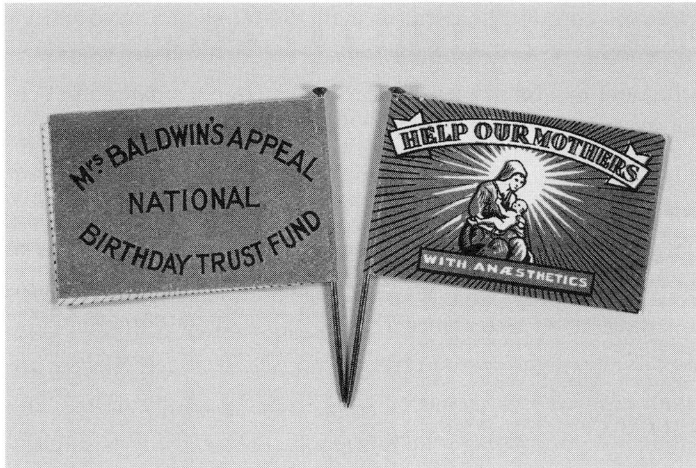
Mrs BALDWIN'S APPEAL
NATIONAL
BIRTHDAY TRUST FUND
HELP OUR MOTHERS
WITH ANÆSTHETICS

Figure 37.3 Flag pins from 1930 promoting one of many campaigns by the National Birthday Trust Fund for improvements in the British maternity services. Philanthropist Lucy Baldwin, wife of Conservative Prime Minister Stanley Baldwin, led the fund's efforts to increase access to obstetric anaesthesia with speeches, broadcasts and fundraising. She and other activists framed pain relief as a woman's right. Wellcome Library, London: National Birthday Trust Fund Archive, SA/NBT/G.6/1.

consolidating the transition to the hospital, not least in postwar European welfare states, social policies typically accelerated rather than instigated change. State interventions were felt unevenly, with access to medical services continuing to depend on class and race, and huge variations within and between countries. Pronatalist population policies and health-care spending worked in complex relations with other social and economic changes, including housing conditions, the centralization of medical care in hospitals, the relative status of obstetricians and midwives and, not least, the attitudes and expectations of birthing women and their families.[24] What drove them to choose hospital birth?

Publicity given to persistently horrifying rates of maternal mortality in the 1920s and 1930s exacerbated long-standing fears about the dangers of childbirth, and moved women to seek to improve their maternity experiences. Hospital births, contemporary observers recognized – and historians later confirmed – were still no safer and probably more dangerous than confinements at home. At precisely the time when more women began to choose to give birth in hospital, maternal mortality rates remained stationary, and in many urban centres increased.[25] Yet growing faith in hospitals as models of cleanliness, efficiency and expertise made institutional maternity care synonymous with 'safety'. The mystique of bacteriology and anaesthetics enhanced the appeal.[26]

As obstetricians developed routines for managing childbirth that incorporated systematic pain-relieving drugs and methods for inducing labour, women learned that they could plan when and how they would have their babies. Middle-class campaigns for more maternity beds went hand-in-hand with demands for access to anaesthesia, more available in hospitals although by no means routine (Fig. 37.3). The values of

24 For international comparisons: Loudon, *Death in Childbirth*; Signild Vallgårda, 'Hospitalization of deliveries: The change of place of birth in Denmark and Sweden from the late nineteenth century to 1970', *Medical History* 40 (1996), 173–96.

25 Loudon, *Death in Childbirth*, pp. 240–53, 365–95.

26 Leavitt, *Brought to Bed*, p. 174.

precision and control promoted through hospital-based technology had implications for the infant, as well as the mother. From around 1900, and especially after World War II, hospital specialists linked the incubator and specialist neonatal care with the programme of modern obstetrics.[27]

While the allure and promise of 'scientific' maternity care made medical institutions increasingly attractive, the growth of hospital confinement can be understood only in relation to the material conditions of women's lives. In an ever more industrialized, urbanized and mobile world, women could rely far less on the social networks on which delivery at home depended. New work rhythms imposed by industrial capitalism and women's greater involvement in wage labour made traditional lying-in unfeasible. If previous generations of women called on wide circles of family, friends and neighbours to help with the birth and manage the household, physical and psychological isolation made home confinements logistically difficult. The overcrowded rented accommodation, which many urban working-class families inhabited across the industrialized world, was a further disincentive to deliver at home. Hospitals may also have appealed as gateways not only to medical expertise, but also to an alternative 'collective subculture of the hospital ward': fellow mothers sharing the experience of giving birth and (typically female) caregivers familiar with lying-in women's needs.[28]

In interwar Britain, feminist and labour organizations such as the Women's Co-operative Guild, along with more conservative maternal and child welfare groups including the National Birthday Trust Fund, campaigned to make hospital beds and good medical care available to the poorest women. Historians have interpreted women's leadership in these organizations, from the ground-level work of health visiting through campaigning for access to pain relief to political lobbying for increased support for mothers, as evidence against the claim that hospitalization of birth was imposed by the medical profession or the state. Testifying to the extreme hardship and discomfort of childbearing in the early twentieth century, letters from working-class women published by the guild in 1915 expressed the wish to give birth in hospital.[29] In many urban areas of Britain, women's demand for institutional maternity care outstripped supply.[30] Women were not 'duped by obstetricians' into the hospital, Linda Bryder has written, 'but rather had their own ideas about the kind of services they

27 Jennifer Beinart, 'Obstetric analgesia and the control of childbirth in twentieth-century Britain', in Jo Garcia, Robert Kilpatrick and Martin Richards (eds.), *The Politics of Maternity Care: Services for Childbearing Women in Twentieth-Century Britain* (Oxford, 1990), pp. 116–32; Jeffrey P. Baker, *The Machine in the Nursery: Incubator Technology and the Origins of Newborn Intensive Care* (Baltimore, MD, 1996).

28 Wilson, *Making of Man-Midwifery*, pp. 204–6.

29 *Maternity: Letters from Working-Women, Collected by the Women's Co-operative Guild* (London, 1915).

30 Jane Lewis, *The Politics of Motherhood: Child and Maternal Welfare in England, 1900–1939* (London, 1980).

wanted … based primarily on the public esteem of science and professionalism in the early to mid-twentieth century'.[31]

Hospital Birth in the Consumer Age

The growing dominance of the 'corporate' system of mass health care, animated by a managerial concern for efficiency, consolidated the expansion of interventionist obstetrics before any demonstrable improvement in safety. Only from the 1930s did falling maternal mortality justify the more complete relocation of birth to the hospital. Maternal deaths declined across the industrialized world as a result of rising living standards, the availability of sulpha drugs and blood transfusion services, and better access to maternity care. Yet even as childbirth became statistically safer and institutional deliveries the norm, growing numbers of people expressed discontent with hospital obstetrics.[32]

The development of the organized consumer movement in the 1950s and 1960s increasingly shaped attitudes to public services. Groups such as the Patients Association, founded in Britain in 1963, argued that recipients of health care were 'consumers', with the right to determine their own fates.[33] Fostered by a postwar cult of motherhood, the international popularity of 'natural childbirth' techniques promoted by the reforming obstetricians Grantly Dick-Read and Fernand Lamaze helped to kindle interest in alternatives to highly drugged, physician-controlled maternity care.[34] By the early 1960s, disillusionment with 'assembly-line' hospital confinements had erupted into a sustained consumer challenge to obstetric authority. Pressure groups such as the National Childbirth Trust and the Association for Improvements in the Maternity Services, founded in Britain in the late 1950s, promoted low-technology obstetrics and campaigned to reform hospital care, including allowing pain relief without pharmaceuticals and permitting fathers into the labour room.

If consumer groups initially set out to reform maternity care within the hospital, the 1960s counterculture and not least the women's liberation movement radicalized many activists' goals. Readers of the Boston Women's Health Book Collective

31 Linda Bryder, '"What women want": Childbirth services and women's activism in New Zealand, 1900–1960', in Janet Greenlees and Bryder (eds.), *Western Maternity and Medicine, 1880–1990* (London, 2013), pp. 81–98, on p. 98.

32 Leavitt, *Brought to Bed*, pp. 194–5.

33 Alex Mold, 'Repositioning the patient: Patient organizations, consumerism, and autonomy in Britain during the 1960s and 1970s', *Bulletin of the History of Medicine* 87 (2013), 225–49.

34 Paula A. Michaels, *Lamaze: An International History* (New York, NY, 2014); Rebecca Jo Plant, *Mom: The Transformation of Motherhood in Modern America* (Chicago, IL, 2010), pp. 118–45.

handbook, *Our Bodies, Ourselves*, first published commercially in 1971, learned that women's personal experiences of medicine had political significance. Working to challenge the medical profession and health-care industries as instruments of patriarchal oppression, women's health activists targeted obstetrics.[35] As ongoing controversy over the safety of the contraceptive pill intensified feminist critiques of medical technology, and obstetric monitoring became ever more routine, birth activists focused on the alienating and disempowering effects of modern maternity care. Some came to see the obstetric armamentarium of fetal heart-rate monitors, ultrasound scanners and amniocentesis as instruments of 'torture', used to 'pressurize and frighten' mothers into consenting to hospital confinements and invasive interventions.[36]

When the interest of readers and publishers in pregnancy and childbirth, nurtured by a culture of self-help, produced a 'baby book boom' around 1980, the 'birth wars' moved from academic journals, activist newsletters and feminist magazines into the mainstream. Exposés of factory-like maternity wards in British tabloids and on television provoked public outcries, and thousands attended rallies (Fig. 37.4).[37] Middle-class housewives chose intervention-free deliveries in midwife-led birth centres. While the President of the American College of Obstetricians and Gynecologists declared out-of-hospital birth the 'earliest form of child abuse', others sought midwives willing to 'move mountains' by assisting them at home.[38]

For all the activism, the trend towards obstetric intervention intensified as corporate ideals of enhanced productivity became ever more entrenched. Caesarean rates skyrocketed, nearly tripling in US hospitals in the 1970s.[39] Through the twentieth century and most appreciably after the 1960s, obstetricians portrayed themselves as fetal advocates. Technologies for monitoring and intervening in pregnancy consolidated the sub-specialty of perinatal medicine, culminating in the emergence, by the 1980s, of experimental intrauterine surgery. Hailed in the media as pushing the frontiers of medicine, extremely invasive and high-risk though still comparatively rare, fetal surgery has

35 Wendy Kline, *Bodies of Knowledge: Sexuality, Reproduction, and Women's Health in the Second Wave* (Chicago, IL, 2010), esp. pp. 127–56; Kline, '*Our Bodies, Ourselves*', Exhibit 35, this book.

36 *Association for Improvements in the Maternity Services Quarterly Newsletter* (Summer 1981), 10; Oakley, *Captured Womb*, pp. 236–49; on the pill: Jesse Olszynko-Gryn, 'Technologies of Contraception and Abortion', Chapter 36; on prenatal diagnosis: Ilana Löwy, 'Prenatal Diagnosis, Surveillance and Risk', Chapter 38, this book.

37 Jane Feinmann, 'Standing up for birth rights', *Medical News* 14 (28 Oct. 1982), 16–19.

38 Quotations from Oakley, *Captured Womb*, p. 219; and Reva Kline, 'Birth: Home or hospital?', *Spare Rib* 98 (1980), 22–5, on 24. See also Wendy Kline, 'Communicating a new consciousness: Countercultural print and the home birth movement in the 1970s', *Bulletin of the History of Medicine* 89 (2015), 527–56.

39 Barbara Bridgman Perkins, *The Medical Delivery Business: Health Reform, Childbirth, and the Economic Order* (New Brunswick, NJ, 2004).

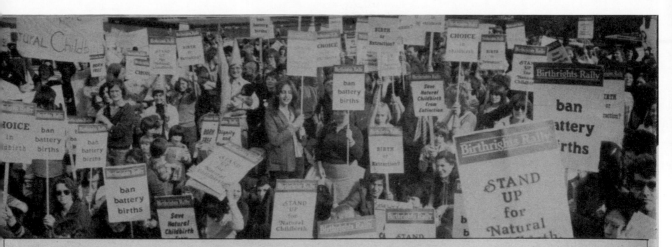

Standing up for birth rights

Jane Feinmann reports on a movement that looks set to make obstetricians reconsider their procedures in the delivery room

SHEFFIELD Health Authority has booked a bus to send its obstetric department down to London to attend the first International Conference on Active Birth on Saturday.

The Sheffield contingent is only one of several health authority groups travelling to the Wembley Conference Centre - along with hundreds of midwives and dozens of GPs and obstetricians - to learn about one of the swiftest

don, the foundations laid by Leboyer and Sheila Kitzinger, and by himself with National Childbirth Trust teacher, Janet Balaskas, who with her husband Arthur pioneered active childbirth

"unbelievable" interest.

Janet Balaskas, who is organising the Wembley Conference, found that after the initial announcement in August, applications poured in – and continue to

with Professor Ian Craft, of the Royal Free Hospital until he resigned, apparently partly over the row about active birth, being selected as the chief bogey man by the active childbirthers.

But that, too, looks like changing. Last week, the Royal College of Obstetricians and Gynaecologists confirmed its approval of the trend towards active childbirth - or at least "accommodating the pregnant woman's

Figure 37.4 Photograph in *Medical News*, a weekly magazine for health professionals, of the 'Birthrights Rally' on London's Hampstead Heath in April 1982. More than 5,000 people assembled to campaign for natural childbirth and against 'battery births'. The slogans on the placards expressed activists' dissatisfaction with the prevailing model of obstetric care in Britain. *Medical News* (28 Oct. 1982), 16.

reinforced feminist concern about the trend to reduce pregnant women to passive vessels for 'unborn patients'.[40] Yet partly as a result of consumer campaigns for more female physicians to care for their reproductive health needs, the gender balance in women's health care began to shift. The very procedures that feminists had denounced as subjecting pregnant women to professional male hegemony were ironically delivered increasingly by female doctors. In the United States, the proportion of women in residencies in obstetrics and gynaecology rose from 15 per cent in 1975 to 70 per cent in 2000.[41]

40 Monica J. Casper, *The Making of the Unborn Patient: A Social Anatomy of Fetal Surgery* (New Brunswick, NJ, 1998).

41 W. H. Pearse, W. H. Haffner and A. Primack, 'Effect of gender on the obstetric-gynecologic work force', *Obstetrics & Gynecology* 97 (2001), 794–7.

By the 1980s, women in the western world had become more assertive in demanding 'choice' in childbirth. Amid wider efforts to encourage lay involvement in medicine, governments and official bodies gave consumer groups a more active role in developing maternity policy and designing future services. As consumers, women came to expect more choice in their delivery options. Activist pressure led to modest revivals of home birth even in the United States, where malpractice insurance and legal restrictions devastated out-of-hospital midwifery in the 1980s and 1990s.[42] Yet the more significant worldwide trend has been towards shorter hospital stays as administrators, grappling with the challenges of shrinking budgets, staff shortages and capacity constraints, embrace strategies of 'managed care' and strive to cut costs.[43] 'Drive-by deliveries' and 'conveyor-belt maternity units' are aspects of this broader phenomenon.

Activists in the 1970s and 1980s argued that hospitalized obstetrics, with its cornucopia of instruments, interventions and pharmaceuticals, 'warped' the experience of maternity and that women's dissatisfaction resulted from their loss of autonomy, as mothers and as midwives, in the birthing room. In formulating alternatives to medicalized childbirth, from 'natural' pain relief in hospitals and birthing centres to 'holistic' and 'humane' deliveries at home, activists constructed 'hospital birth' as antithetical to 'woman-centred' care. The legacies of that activism can be seen not only in polarized present-day debate – every new statement on the relative risks of home versus hospital provokes heated controversy – but also in the major issues in the history of childbirth: questions of agency, control and choice.

42 Marian F. MacDorman, T. J. Mathews and Eugene Declercq, 'Home births in the United States, 1990–2009', *National Center for Health Statistics Data Brief* 84 (2012), www.cdc.gov/nchs/data/databriefs/db84.htm.

43 Oona M. R. Campbell *et al.*, 'Length of stay after childbirth in 92 countries and associated factors in 30 low- and middle-income countries: Compilation of reported data and a cross-sectional analysis from nationally representative surveys', *PLoS Medicine* 13 (3) (2016), e1001972, http://dx.doi.org/10.1371/journal.pmed.1001972.

38 Prenatal Diagnosis, Surveillance and Risk

Ilana Löwy

The Rise of the Supervised Fetus

Prenatal diagnosis – the practice of monitoring fetal development and spotting potential problems – has radically changed the experience of pregnancy for tens of millions of women worldwide. In the 1960s and 1970s, prenatal diagnosis was an exceptional approach, offered only to women at high risk of giving birth to a malformed child. Since then, it has been transformed into a routine screening technique that is part of the supervision of pregnancy in many industrialized countries. Screening made fetuses accessible to the medical gaze, and pregnant women became more aware of the risks of fetal malformation – knowledge that can generate stress.[1]

Before prenatal diagnosis, the birth of healthy children was promoted through the selection of partners and regimen. Nearly all known cultures have prescribed specific activities for pregnant women and prohibited others.[2] However, the effects of these interventions could not be observed till birth. For centuries, palpation was the only medical means of assessing the presence of a fetus. In the nineteenth century, doctors began also to listen to the fetal heart, and in the twentieth, as antenatal examination became more common, X-rays were occasionally used. Embryologists and gynaecologists investigated miscarried and aborted fetuses, while most of those depicted in Lennart Nilsson's famous 1965 *Life* magazine photographs of 'life before birth' were dead.[3] Until the 1970s, many women had variable and indeterminate images of the unborn. The

1 Ilana Löwy, 'How genetics came to the unborn: 1960–2000', *Studies in History and Philosophy of Biological and Biomedical Sciences* 47, part A (2014), 154–62; Löwy, 'Prenatal diagnosis: The irresistible rise of the "visible fetus"', ibid., 47, part B (2014), 290–9.

2 Salim Al-Gailani, 'Making birth defects "preventable": Pre-conceptional vitamin supplements and the politics of risk reduction', ibid., part B, 278–89; Clare Hanson, *A Cultural History of Pregnancy: Pregnancy, Medicine and Culture, 1750–2000* (Basingstoke, 2004). On earlier times: Maaike van der Lugt, 'Formed Fetuses and Healthy Children in Scholastic Theology, Medicine and Law', Chapter 12; Lauren Kassell, 'Fruitful Bodies and Astrological Medicine', Chapter 16, this book.

3 Barbara Duden, Jürgen Schlumbohm and Patrice Veit (eds.), *Geschichte des Ungeborenen. Zur Erfahrungs- und Wissenschaftsgeschichte der Schwangerschaft, 17.–20. Jahrhundert* (Göttingen, 2002); Karin Ekholm, 'Pictures and Analogies in the Anatomy of Generation', Chapter 15; Ekholm, 'A Placenta Painted and Engraved', Exhibit 15; Nick Hopwood, 'Images of Human Embryos', Exhibit 23; Solveig Jülich, '"Drama of Life before Birth"', Exhibit 34; see also Salim Al-Gailani, 'Hospital Birth', Chapter 37, this book.

development of prenatal diagnosis contributed to popularizing scientific representations of life in the womb and extended the capacity of medicine to study live fetuses and detect fetal malformations.[4] In a limited number of cases, the malformation can be corrected, either in utero or immediately after birth, but diagnosis of a severe malformation usually leads to a decision to terminate the pregnancy. This is historically unprecedented. Abortion is a very old method of fertility regulation, but only with the development of prenatal diagnosis have women had the option not to give birth to a child with specific traits.[5]

The present form of prenatal diagnosis resulted from the coming together of four technical innovations – the development of amniocentesis, the study of human chromosomes, the description of 'markers' of fetal anomalies in maternal blood and the invention of obstetric ultrasound – with an important social innovation, the liberalization of abortion. The initial stimulus was the wish to prevent the birth of children with hereditary pathologies. In the 1970s and 1980s, the widespread diffusion of this approach was driven by the desire to reduce the incidence of Down syndrome, a condition newly prominent as a public health problem. In the late twentieth century, the improved resolution of obstetric ultrasound favoured the direct observation of numerous fetal anomalies, but also the identification of 'risk markers', morphological changes that indicate an increased probability of fetal impairment.[6] In the early twenty-first century, genomic techniques again expanded the possibilities for studying the living fetus, opening new questions and creating new dilemmas.

Investigating the Living Fetus, 1950s–1970s

A PubMed search suggests that the term 'prenatal diagnosis' was already in use in the 1940s to refer, for example, to the prediction of haemolytic disease resulting from rhesus factor incompatibility between pregnant woman and fetus, but before 1968 it appeared in only a few article titles a year. The expression gained currency from 1971, when it

4 Rayna Rapp, *Testing Women, Testing the Fetus: The Social Impact of Amniocentesis in America* (New York, NY, 2000); Lorna Weir, *Pregnancy, Risk and Biopolitics: On the Threshold of the Living Subject* (London, 2006).

5 Sociologists, anthropologists and historians have studied various aspects of prenatal diagnosis; see, for instance: Barbara Katz Rothman, *The Tentative Pregnancy: Prenatal Diagnosis and the Future of Motherhood* (New York, NY, 1986); Rapp, *Testing Women*; Peter S. Harper, *First Years of Human Chromosomes: The Beginnings of Human Cytogenetics* (Bloxham, 2006); and Malcolm Nicolson and John E. E. Fleming, *Imaging and Imagining the Fetus: The Development of Obstetric Ultrasound* (Baltimore, MD, 2013). By contrast, the only systematic history of prenatal diagnosis is Ruth Schwartz Cowan's *Heredity and Hope: The Case for Genetic Screening* (Cambridge, MA, 2008).

6 On the rise of risk medicine: Robert A. Aronowitz, *Making Sense of Illness: Science, Society, and Disease* (Cambridge, 1998); Deborah Lupton, *Risk* (London, 1999); William G. Rothstein, *Public Health and the Risk Factor: A History of an Uneven Medical Revolution* (Rochester, NY, 2008).

became possible to study fetal cells in the amniotic fluid. This possibility originated in two independent technical innovations: the development of amniocentesis and the description of links between chromosomal anomalies and birth defects.

In the late nineteenth century, gynaecologists learned to drain an excess of amniotic fluid from the pregnant uterus with a hollow hypodermic needle, a technique first named 'amniotic tap' and later 'amniocentesis'. Women with diabetes tend to develop this condition, polyhydramnios, which can endanger the fetus. When insulin treatment allowed many diabetic women to survive to adulthood, the number of polyhydramnios cases went up. An additional stimulus for the development of the 'amniotic tap' in the 1950s was the wish to know whether the fetus suffered from haemolytic disease, in which antibodies produced by the pregnant woman (especially against rhesus antigens) destroy fetal red blood cells. When this condition was suspected – usually because the woman already had an affected child – the physician sampled her amniotic fluid. If the fluid was yellow – strongly indicating the destruction of fetal red cells – physicians induced an early birth and replaced the newborn's blood with blood devoid of harmful maternal antibodies.[7]

In 1948, a Canadian anatomist, Murray Barr, described a microscopical marker (the 'Barr body') present in female but not male cells. The fetal cells that float in the amniotic fluid could now be studied to determine fetal sex.[8] In countries such as Denmark, which had legalized abortion in cases at risk of severe hereditary diseases (so-called eugenic abortions), prenatal detection of sex opened the way to selective abortion of fetuses at risk of haemophilia, an X-chromosome-linked disease that male children born to a female carrier have a 50 per cent chance of inheriting. In 1960, two Danish researchers, Povl Riis and Fritz Fuchs, applied this method to determine the sex of the fetus of a woman carrying the haemophilia gene. Her previous child, a boy, had died hours after birth. When she discovered that she was pregnant again she opted for a 'eugenic' abortion, then heard of the possibility of finding out the sex of the fetus. She underwent amniocentesis, learned that the fetus was female, and gave birth to a healthy girl.[9]

The legalization of abortion in most western countries in the late 1960s and 1970s (1967 in the United Kingdom, 1973 in the United States and 1975 in France) was in part a result of doctors' campaigns for professional autonomy and in part a success of the argument of the women's liberation movement that women have a right to decide whether they wish to become mothers. In addition, changes in abortion laws were precipitated by the thalidomide disaster of 1961–2 and the German measles (rubella)

7 D. C. A. Bevis, 'The antenatal prediction of hæmolytic disease of the newborn', *Lancet* 1 (1952), 395–8.

8 Fiona Alice Miller, '"Your true and proper gender": The Barr body as a good enough science of sex', *Studies in History and Philosophy of Biological and Biomedical Sciences* 37 (2006), 459–83.

9 Povl Riis and Fritz Fuchs, 'Antenatal determination of fœtal sex in prevention of hereditary diseases', *Lancet* 2 (1960), 180–2.

epidemic of 1962–4. In 1961 the tranquillizer, thalidomide, widely prescribed for morning sickness in pregnant women, was found to be responsible for the appearance of severe birth defects in children, especially the absence of limbs.[10] This was closely followed by an epidemic of German measles, a disease which, when contracted early in pregnancy, produces severe fetal malformations.[11] These two events transformed lay and professional attitudes towards abortion. Before 1960, abortion, while widespread, had frequently been presented as a deviant practice associated with marginal social groups and loose sexual mores. After thalidomide and the German measles epidemic, abortion became identified also with the plight of 'blameless' middle-class women like the TV presenter from Arizona, Sherri Finkbine, who took thalidomide early in her pregnancy and, unable to obtain a legal abortion in the United States, travelled to Sweden to terminate her pregnancy.[12] The publicity increased the pressure to legalize abortion, and led to the establishment of regional, national and international registries of fetal malformations, primarily in order to identify potential environmental causes. These registries promoted the perception of birth defects as a public health problem and the development of a new branch of epidemiology dedicated to the surveillance of reproductive outcomes.[13]

In 1959 and 1960, scientists had found that the presence of an abnormal number of chromosomes (an aneuploidy) produces birth defects. 'Mongolism', now called Down syndrome, was linked to the presence of three copies of chromosome 21, or 'trisomy 21'. In the following years, researchers identified additional conditions that correlated with an abnormal chromosome number.[14] In the mid-1960s, they developed a method for studying the chromosomes of fetal cells in the amniotic fluid, opening the way to prenatal diagnosis of chromosomal anomalies and of hereditary diseases that produce metabolic changes in the cell (Fig. 38.1).[15] In the 1970s, amniocentesis induced miscarriage in 3–5 per cent of cases. Nevertheless, women who knew that they and/or

10 Ann Dally, 'Thalidomide: Was the tragedy preventable?', ibid., 1 (1998), 1197–9.

11 The link between German measles and fetal malformations was first reported in 1941: N. McAlister Gregg, 'Congenital cataract following German measles in the mother', *Transactions of the Ophthalmological Society of Australia* 3 (1941), 35–46.

12 Linda Greenhouse and Reva Siegel (eds.), *Before* Roe v. Wade: *Voices that Shaped the Abortion Debate before the Supreme Court's Ruling* (New York, NY, 2010), pp. 63–7; Leslie J. Reagan, *Dangerous Pregnancies: Mothers, Disabilities, and Abortion in Modern America* (Berkeley, CA, 2010), pp. 85–9; further on abortion-law reform: Martin H. Johnson and Nick Hopwood, 'Modern Law and Regulation', Chapter 40, this book.

13 Jennie Kline, Zena Stein and Mervyn Susser, *Conception to Birth: Epidemiology of Prenatal Development* (New York, NY, 1989), pp. 305–38.

14 Harper, *First Years.*

15 Henry L. Nadler, 'Antenatal detection of hereditary disorders', *Pediatrics* 42 (1968), 912–18. 'Hereditary diseases' are transmitted in families while the more general term 'genetic modifications' refers to all changes in the hereditary material of the cell, including those, such as Down syndrome, that are nearly always produced by a new mutation.

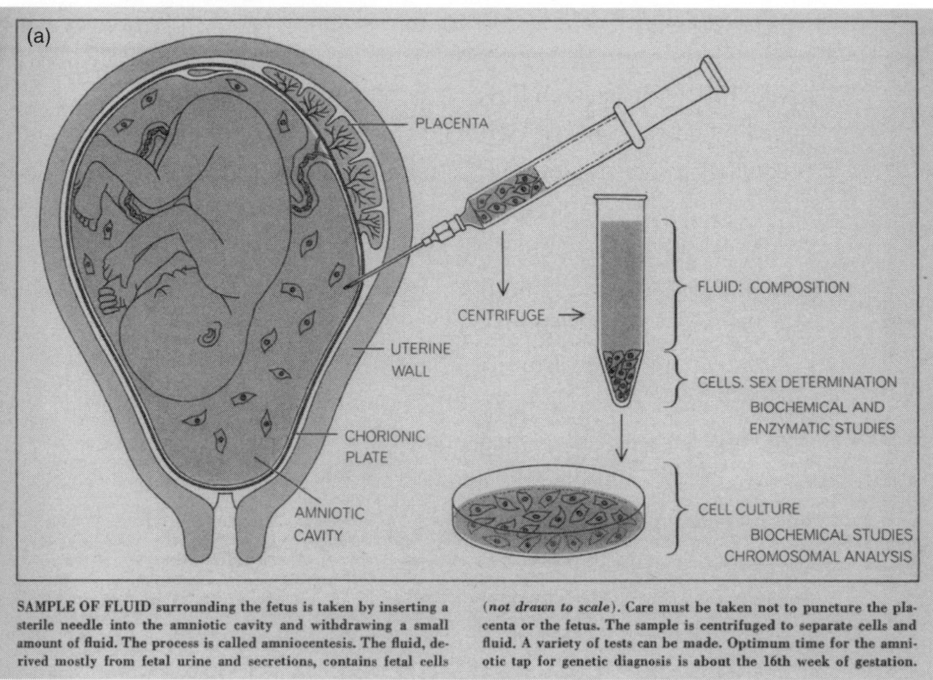

SAMPLE OF FLUID surrounding the fetus is taken by inserting a sterile needle into the amniotic cavity and withdrawing a small amount of fluid. The process is called amniocentesis. The fluid, derived mostly from fetal urine and secretions, contains fetal cells (*not drawn to scale*). Care must be taken not to puncture the placenta or the fetus. The sample is centrifuged to separate cells and fluid. A variety of tests can be made. Optimum time for the amniotic tap for genetic diagnosis is about the 16th week of gestation.

(b)

tive abortion were practiced. Such age criteria, however, do not apply in many genetic disorders.

achieved in the incidence of some recessive diseases. If the screening program could detect each family in which both

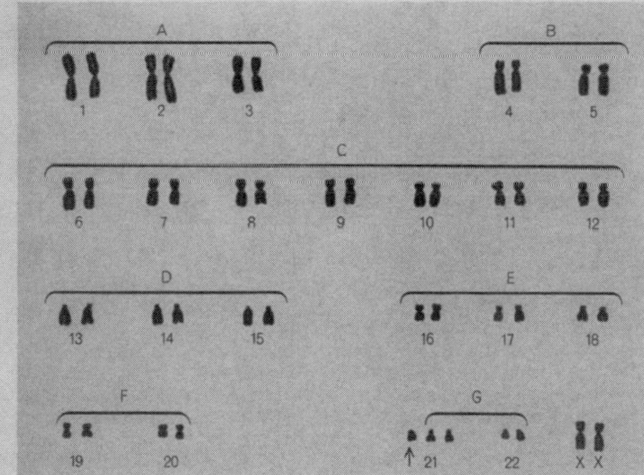

CHROMOSOMAL ANALYSIS of cells obtained by amniocentesis can determine if the developing embryo has Down's syndrome. This karyotype prepared by O. W. Jones shows that the girl has an extra No. 21 chromosome and will have the stigmata of mongolism.

the benefit. Is it only black figures in th ledger instead of red? Economic con siderations are undeniably importan but it seems a dangerous precedent t justify screening and selective abortio programs solely on the basis of compar ing their cost with the economic burde to families and to society. One coul argue cogently that we should be mor willing to spend money for the elimina tion of disease even if it proves to b uneconomical.

Recently some geneticists, notabl Arno G. Motulsky of the University o Washington School of Medicine an James V. Neel of the University of Mich igan, have become concerned with th possibility that large-scale genetic ma nipulations such as prenatal detectio and abortion might lead to detrimenta changes in the quality and the diversit of the human gene pool. Such change might be the inadvertent result of pr grams to eliminate disease or the delib erate consequence of eugenic program to eliminate certain undesirable gene from the population.

Motulsky and Neel have recentl shown that programs of prenat detection and selective abortion migh

38

Figure 38.1 Prenatal diagnosis explained in a *Scientific American* article. (a) Diagram of amniocentesis, focused on the fetus and its cells; (b) ordered photographs of chromosomes, showing trisomy 21. Panel (a) by Eric Mose and (b) prepared by Oliver Jones, from Theodore Friedmann, 'Prenatal diagnosis of genetic disease', *Scientific American* 225, no. 5 (Nov. 1971), 34–42, on 35 and 38.

their partners carried a hereditary disorder were often willing to run that risk when faced with the much higher risk of having a child with that condition (50 per cent if this was dominant, 25 per cent if recessive).[16]

In the 1980s, the use of ultrasound to guide amniocentesis increased safety. As a consequence, some professionals started systematically to offer amniocentesis also to older pregnant women (usually over 35), who had a higher chance of having a child with Down syndrome (about 0.5 per cent at the age of 37, 1.2 per cent at age 40). Obstetricians and geneticists who promoted early prenatal diagnostic techniques argued that they were responding to demand from women. This was often the case for women aware of a severe hereditary disorder in their family, but less true for risks linked to maternal age. Experts knew that the probability of giving birth to a Down syndrome child went up with age, but very few pregnant women were aware of this fact in the early 1970s.[17] Doctors and the media taught women to recognize age as a risk factor for Down syndrome.

Obstetric ultrasound not only facilitated the diffusion of amniocentesis, this medical visualization technology also became an independent and powerful means of diagnosing fetal malformations. Already in the early twentieth century, doctors had used X-rays to observe major fetal anomalies, and in 1916 they diagnosed fetal anencephaly (the absence of a brain) in this way.[18] Moreover, in the 1950s and 1960s, obstetricians increasingly employed X-rays to detect potential difficulties in childbirth, and to diagnose selected fetal problems including hydrocephalus (accumulation of liquid in the head) and skeletal malformations.[19] But X-ray diagnosis had a limited scope and exposed the fetus to risky radiation.[20] Obstetric ultrasound made it safer to observe the fetus directly. In the late 1950s, a Glasgow group led by the professor of midwifery Ian Donald employed this technology to diagnose gynaecological disorders. Later, they applied it to pregnancy, first to visualize twin pregnancies and those with a high risk of miscarriage, then to establish the stage of pregnancy, to make amniocentesis safer and to visualize possible obstacles to birth (Fig. 38.2).[21]

16 D. A. Christie and E. M. Tansey (eds.), *Genetic Testing: The Transcript of a Witness Seminar Held by the Wellcome Trust Centre for the History of Medicine at UCL, London, on 13 July 2001* (London, 2003).

17 The effect was first observed in 1933: L. S. Penrose, 'The relative effects of paternal and maternal age in mongolism', *Journal of Genetics* 27 (1933), 219–24.

18 Robert G. Resta, 'The first prenatal diagnosis of a fetal anomaly', *Journal of Genetic Counseling* 6 (1997), 81–4.

19 Ann Oakley, *The Captured Womb: A History of the Medical Care of Pregnant Women* (Oxford, 1984), pp. 95–107.

20 Alice Stewart *et al.*, 'Preliminary communication: Malignant disease in childhood and diagnostic irradiation in utero', *Lancet* 2 (1956), 447; Sarah Dry, 'The population as patient: Alice Stewart and the controversy over low-level radiation in the 1950s', in Thomas Schlich and Ulrich Tröhler (eds.), *The Risks of Medical Innovation: Risk Perception and Assessment in Historical Context* (London, 2006), pp. 116–32.

21 Nicolson and Fleming, *Imaging and Imagining the Fetus*.

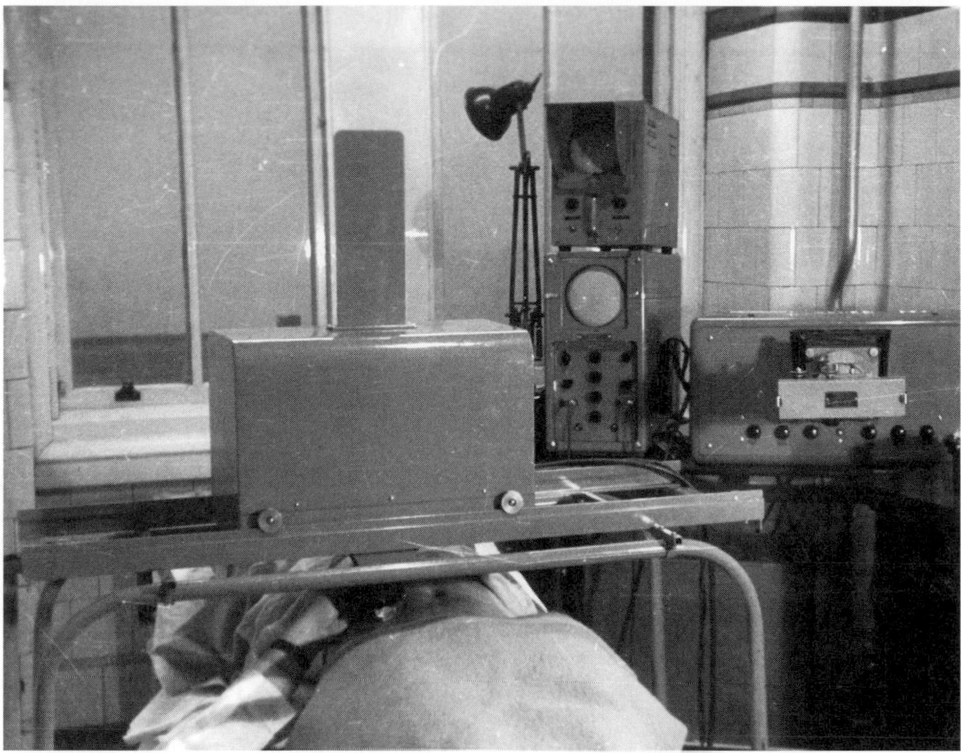

Figure 38.2 The 'bed-table scanner', with which engineer Thomas Brown pioneered two-dimensional ultrasound, at the Western Infirmary, Glasgow, in 1956, two years before Ian Donald and colleagues described its use to diagnose pregnancy. (The arm visible on the left may or may not be Donald's.) Though the patient's body is, typically, obscured by the large machine, Donald believed in treating the whole woman. Photograph from Donald's personal papers, NHS Greater Glasgow and Clyde Archives, reference HB110/3/29.

In the early 1970s, obstetricians employed ultrasound to detect major malformations of the fetal neural system, such as spina bifida (incomplete closure of the neural tube). A few years later, the introduction of linear array scanning improved the resolution of ultrasound images. The higher resolution led to quasi-recreational use: 'showing the baby' to pregnant women and their families, producing 'baby's first photograph' and announcing the fetal sex. In societies with no strong preferences for sons, knowing the future child's sex has emotional importance for many women and their partners. In societies which value daughters less, prenatal sex determination often leads to selective elimination of female fetuses.[22]

The perfection of obstetric ultrasound raised doctors' ability to monitor fetal development closely. Physicians observed numerous fetal structural malformations,

22 Janelle S. Taylor, *The Public Life of the Fetal Sonogram: Technology, Consumption, and the Politics of Reproduction* (New Brunswick, NJ, 2008); Richard M. Smith, 'Marriage and Fertility in Different Household Systems', Chapter 24, this book.

some of them relatively minor. They also identified 'ultrasound risk markers': morphological changes that indicate a higher possibility of birth defects; for example, they correlated increased 'nuchal translucency' (the accumulation of liquid behind the fetal neck), and a short nasal bone, with Down syndrome (Fig. 38.3). At the same time, biochemists showed that abnormal levels of several fetal and placental proteins in a pregnant woman's blood indicate a higher than average probability of carrying a fetus with Down syndrome.[23] Taken together, these safer and cheaper techniques opened the way to mass screening of pregnant women for 'Down syndrome risk'.[24] This made all pregnancies potentially risky, and turned all fetuses into supervised entities.

Prenatal Screening, 1980s–2010s

In the early 1970s, two US-based epidemiologists, Zena Stein and Mervyn Susser, first proposed that all pregnant women who wished it should be tested for fetal Down syndrome.[25] In the past, Stein and Susser argued, the majority of children with Down syndrome had died young, but thanks to medical progress, most by then survived to adulthood. New educational methods and better care had greatly improved their quality of life, but they continued to live in a state of permanent dependence that imposed a severe burden on their families and society. This 'burden' could be alleviated if all pregnant women – and not only those over 35 – were offered a prenatal test.[26]

In the 1970s, the only way for a woman to verify that she was carrying a fetus with Down syndrome was amniocentesis, but this was far too risky for general use. A young woman had a much higher chance of miscarrying following amniocentesis than of giving birth to a trisomic child. Yet specialists knew that many such children were born to young women.[27] So in the 1990s these experts welcomed the possibility of shifting to individualized evaluation of probabilities. Women in numerous industrialized

23 David J. H. Brock, 'Maternal serum alpha-fetoprotein as screening test for Down syndrome', *Lancet* 1 (1984), 1292; N. J. Wald *et al.*, 'Serum screening for Down's syndrome between 8 and 14 weeks of pregnancy', *British Journal of Obstetrics and Gynaecology* 103 (1996), 407–12.

24 In 'intermediary' countries, the situation may be very different. In Brazil (where abortion is illegal unless the life of the woman is endangered or the pregnancy results from rape) and in Vietnam (where abortion for fetal indications is often encouraged by the state and physicians), the main pathway for the detection of fetal anomalies is the widespread and unregulated use of obstetric ultrasound: Lilian Krakowski Chazan, *'Meio quilo de gente': Um estudo antropológico sobre ultra-som obstétrico* (Rio de Janeiro, 2007); Tine M. Gammeltoft, *Haunting Images: A Cultural Account of Selective Reproduction in Vietnam* (Berkeley, CA, 2014).

25 On Down syndrome: David Wright, *Downs: The History of a Disability* (Oxford, 2011).

26 Zena Stein and Mervyn Susser, 'The preventability of Down's syndrome', *HSMHA Health Reports* 86 (1971), 650–8; Stein, Susser and Andrea V. Guterman, 'Screening programme for prevention of Down's syndrome', *Lancet* 1 (1973), 305–10. The term 'burden' was used by Stein and Susser, who were concerned by the plight of poor families with severely disabled children.

27 Al-Gailani, 'Making birth defects "preventable"'.

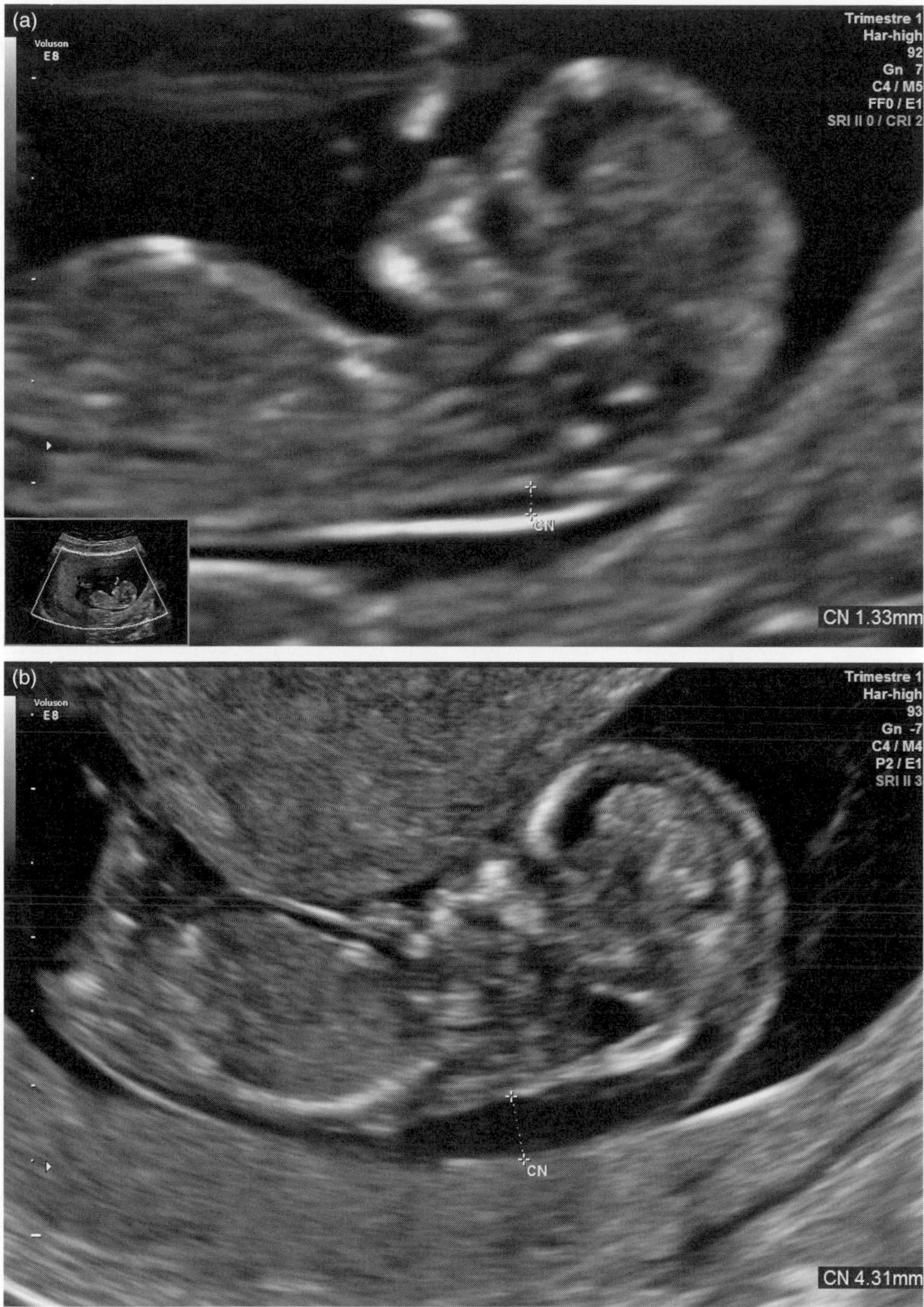

Figure 38.3 Increased nuchal translucency as a risk marker. The sonograms, taken in Paris in 2015, show this measurement (CN) in (a) a normal fetus, and (b) a fetus with abnormal chromosomes. Courtesy of Dr Véronique Mirlesse.

countries are today invited at the end of the first trimester of pregnancy to undergo screening for their 'Down risk'. They are given a diagnostic ultrasound and a test for Down-related serum markers, then receive an individualized 'risk number' calculated by a computer program. If a woman's risk of having a child with Down syndrome is greater than her risk of miscarrying following amniocentesis, her health-care providers offer her the chance to learn whether the fetus has a normal chromosome number.

The main goal of an analysis of fetal chromosomes (the karyotype) is to identify fetuses with Down syndrome, but this method also detects other conditions produced by an abnormal number. Some, such as Patau syndrome (trisomy 13) or Edwards syndrome (trisomy 18), have very poor prognoses. Others, including an abnormal number of sex chromosomes, produce minor functional anomalies (although some people contest the description of these anomalies as minor). As a consequence, pregnant women who believe that they know what they will do if they learn that a fetus has Down syndrome may face unanticipated and difficult choices.

Women screened for Down during the first trimester also often have a diagnostic ultrasound during the second trimester. Some women whose ultrasound was normal early in pregnancy have suspicious findings during the second or even third trimester. In these cases, their doctor often proposes amniocentesis to study fetal DNA. Few women who have just learned that something may be wrong with a future child decline the offer. When the aim of studying fetal cells is not to find out whether the fetus has two or three copies of chromosome 21 but to uncover what might have gone wrong, it is reasonable to go beyond simple observation of stained chromosomes to a newer, more refined technique, chromosomal microarrays or comparative genomic hybridization.[28] This allows the detection of numerous changes in the genetic material of the cell. Some variations are linked with specific pathological conditions. Others, labelled 'variants of unknown significance', may be either normal variations or linked in as yet unidentified ways with human diseases. Advocates argue that since comparative genomic hybridization can detect more genetic anomalies than visual inspection of chromosomes, it should be offered to all pregnant women.[29] It is highly unlikely that this proposal will be accepted, because amniocentesis is still too expensive and risky, and because a new diagnostic method, devoid of risk to the fetus – the study of fetal DNA in the maternal blood – will probably gradually replace the older technique.

Scientists have known since the 1970s that fetal cells and fetal DNA 'leak' into the maternal circulation. The first attempts to use this genetic material to detect fetal problems were unsuccessful; it was too difficult to separate the small signal (fetal DNA)

28 Lisa G. Shaffer *et al.*, 'Detection rates of clinically significant genomic alterations by microarray analysis for specific anomalies detected by ultrasound', *Prenatal Diagnosis* 32 (2012), 986–95.

29 Ronald J. Wapner *et al.*, 'Chromosomal microarray versus karyotyping for prenatal diagnosis', *New England Journal of Medicine* 367 (2012), 2175–84.

from the large noise (maternal DNA).[30] In the early twenty-first century, advances in molecular biology made this possible; the approach was named non-invasive prenatal testing, or more recently, screening (NIPT/NIPS).[31] Initially, commercialized NIPT looked for abnormal numbers of chromosomes in the fetus. The result is indicative only, and has to be confirmed by amniocentesis, but because NIPT detects conditions such as Down syndrome with high probability, only a small number of women need undergo the costly, risky and stressful amniocentesis. The new technique, its promoters have argued, is merely a safer replacement of the existing screening method, a technical improvement not a conceptual revolution.[32]

Future uses of NIPT may be very different. In spring 2014, commercial producers of non-invasive tests introduced testing for genetic syndromes linked with deletions of chromosome fragments. This testing is expected soon to be extended to a greater number of chromosomal anomalies, in several of which genetic data alone cannot predict the severity of the consequences of the observed deletion for the future child. Some people with these deletions are classified as 'normal', while others suffer severe physical and intellectual disability.[33] Experts predict that in the not too distant future, pregnant women could be offered a risk-free 'reading' of the entire fetal DNA.[34] Pregnant women and their partners who undergo a 'simple blood test' may receive a flood of confusing and potentially destabilizing information about the possible problems of their future child, and face difficult decisions about the continuation of the pregnancy.[35] As the anthropologists Tine Gammeltoft and Ayo Wahlberg put it, 'Rather than producing a brave new world of reproductive mastery, [selective reproductive technologies] throw their users into social worlds of contingency, ambivalence, and disorientation, worlds in which they must grapple with new and perhaps intensified reproductive anxieties and uncertainties.'[36]

30 Leonard A. Herzenberg *et al.*, 'Fetal cells in the blood of pregnant women: Detection and enrichment by fluorescence-activated cell sorting', *Proceedings of the National Academy of Sciences of the USA* 76 (1979), 1453–5.

31 Attie T. J. I. Go, John M. G. van Vugt and Cees B. M. Oudejans, 'Non-invasive aneuploidy detection using free fetal DNA and RNA in maternal plasma: Recent progress and future possibilities', *Human Reproduction Update* 17 (2011), 372–82.

32 Diana W. Bianchi, Dick Oepkes and Alessandro Ghidini, 'Current controversies in prenatal diagnosis 1: Should noninvasive DNA testing be the standard screening test for Down syndrome in all pregnant women?', *Prenatal Diagnosis* 34 (2014), 6–11.

33 Diana W. Bianchi *et al.*, 'In case you missed it: The *Prenatal Diagnosis* section editors bring you the most significant advances of 2013', ibid., 1–5.

34 Ilana R. Yurkiewicz, Bruce R. Korf and Lisa Soleymani Lehmann, 'Prenatal whole-genome sequencing – Is the quest to know a fetus's future ethical?', *New England Journal of Medicine* 370 (2014), 195–7.

35 Henry T. Greely, 'Get ready for the flood of fetal gene screening', *Nature* 469 (2011), 289–91.

36 Tine M. Gammeltoft and Ayo Wahlberg, 'Selective reproductive technologies', *Annual Review of Anthropology* 43 (2014), 201–16, on 208. This is true also of preimplantation genetic diagnosis in the context of in vitro fertilization: Sarah Franklin and Celia Roberts, *Born and Made: An Ethnography of Preimplantation Genetic Diagnosis* (Princeton, NJ, 2006); Nick Hopwood, 'Artificial Fertilization', Chapter 39, this book.

Conclusion: Prenatal Diagnosis and Risky Pregnancies

The rise of prenatal diagnosis was directly linked to the huge decrease in maternal, perinatal and child mortality in industrialized countries in the twentieth century. Once the survival of newborn children was taken for granted, the death or severe disability of a newborn baby, previously viewed as an almost unavoidable hazard of pregnancy, became far more traumatic. Professionals who developed ways to scrutinize the fetus were driven by a wish to reduce the incidence of such events.

Making the living fetus accessible to the medical gaze has produced a major shift in the management of pregnancies in industrialized, and increasingly also in 'intermediary', countries.[37] Despite its far-reaching consequences, the generalization of prenatal diagnosis has been, in the main, a silent revolution. The paucity of public debate about this technology may stem from its seemingly self-evident aspect. Pregnant women wish to be reassured about the normal development of a future child, and health professionals, public health experts and politicians wish to decrease the number of babies born with serious birth defects. They hope that the sum of individual decisions to terminate pregnancies with severely affected fetuses will provide a private solution to a public problem.

The low public visibility of prenatal diagnosis may also result from the fact that change, especially in obstetric ultrasound, has been incremental. A technique for detecting possible problems during childbirth was gradually transformed into a highly efficient tool for scrutinizing the fetus. Women who do not undergo formal 'prenatal screening' for 'Down risk' still frequently face some informal variant thereof during a routine ultrasound examination. Few pregnant women are fully aware that the celebratory production of 'baby's first picture' can become the beginning of a stressful medical trajectory.[38] Investigations that follow the observation of 'suspicious ultrasound findings' may lead to the detection of a specific problem or just to a period of uncertainty and anxiety, which can last during the whole pregnancy and sometimes well beyond.[39] Women who are finally told that the 'positive finding' of an ultrasound examination (in the topsy-turvy world of prenatal diagnosis, 'positive' always means bad news) is a false positive, may still experience stress and depression.[40] The question, 'Madam, do you want to know if your baby is all right?', may be less innocuous than it sounds.

In the 1960s, women who had German measles or used thalidomide early in pregnancy believed that they should be allowed to have an abortion. Professionals and

37 Barbara Duden, *Disembodying Women: Perspectives on Pregnancy and the Unborn*, trans. Lee Hoinacki (Cambridge, MA, 1993).

38 Annika Åhman *et al.*, 'Ultrasonographic fetal soft markers in a low-risk population: Prevalence, association with trisomies and invasive tests', *Acta Obstetricia et Gynecologica Scandinavica* 93 (2014), 367–73.

39 Jane Fisher, 'First-trimester screening: Dealing with the fall-out', *Prenatal Diagnosis* 31 (2011), 46–9.

40 Sylvie Viaux-Savelon *et al.*, 'Prenatal ultrasound screening: False positive soft markers may alter maternal representations and mother–infant interaction', *PloS One* 7 (1) (2012), e30935, https://doi.org/10.1371/journal.pone.0030935.

laypeople often agreed. Although many of these women gave birth to normal children, the serious risk of a disastrous outcome was increasingly viewed as a sufficient reason for a termination.[41] The logic behind the introduction of prenatal diagnosis in the 1970s and 1980s was different: to replace a probabilistic evaluation of risk with a firm diagnosis of an existing problem. Accordingly, this diagnostic technique was initially offered only to women who, in their doctors' assessments, had a higher than average chance of giving birth to a sick or disabled child. In the late twentieth century, however, prenatal diagnosis was transformed in many industrialized countries into population-based screening. Every pregnancy, many professionals believed, was potentially risky. This trend may be amplified in the future by the diffusion of new genomic techniques and invitations to pregnant women to become 'rational managers of fetal risks'.[42] Meanwhile, the rise of epigenetics is expanding the range and timeline of potential threats.[43]

People who live in the industrialized world often look in horror at past statistics of maternal mortality and pregnancy-related morbidity. Antibiotics, blood transfusions and improved obstetrics have vastly reduced the risks of pregnancy and childbirth, at least in countries where the vast majority of women have access to adequate health care. Yet the advances of modern medicine have not transformed pregnancy into a stress-free event. Pregnant women in industrialized and 'intermediary' countries no longer worry that childbirth will put their life and well-being at risk, but may still be apprehensive about the health of the future child. The possibility of studying the living fetus, a development that has helped limit birth defects, may paradoxically have heightened anxieties. In the twenty-first century, pregnant women may still share with those who expected a child in earlier periods the experience of living with fear.

41 One may assume that more fetuses were affected, but many of these aborted spontaneously.

42 Silja Samerski, 'Genetic counseling and the fiction of choice: Taught self-determination as a new technique of social engineering', *Signs* 34 (2009), 735–61.

43 Tatjana Buklijas, 'Developmental Origins of Health and Disease', Exhibit 39, this book.

39 Artificial Fertilization

Nick Hopwood

The modern expansion of non-reproductive sex and sexless reproduction was mostly about contraception, but techniques for promoting conception by manipulating sperm, eggs and embryos have gained prominence over the past hundred and especially the past forty years. Artificial insemination (AI), in vitro fertilization (IVF) and embryo transfer have not only produced such sensations as cattle sired by bulls on the other side of the world and women giving birth to their own grandchildren; with some half-million embryo transfers in cattle per year and about five million IVF children since Louise Brown's birth in 1978, these methods are also common enough that sexual intercourse can appear 'the old-fashioned way' of making babies.

A focus on fertilization risks privileging high-tech aspects of complex social arrangements and exaggerating their power. IVF is named after the step which takes place outside the bodies of the women who work hardest for a procedure still likely to fail. Yet artificial fertilization, always shaped by and shaping a wider world of reproductive labour, has generated major industries, new professions, legal frameworks and various ways of life. Mid-twentieth-century agriculture embraced AI as an aid to factory farming, but 'assisted reproduction' came into its own in a consumerist age. Clinics reinforced the nuclear family and then, by radicalizing the disaggregation of parenthood into social, genetic and gestational roles, also facilitated new family forms: lesbian couples and single women now use donor insemination; gay men may commission egg donors and surrogate mothers.

These innovations are often called 'historic', but we lack synthetic histories.[1] This selective survey explores the making of AI between the eighteenth century and the twentieth, charts the postwar rise of embryo transfer and IVF, and reflects on the generalization of assisted reproduction in the last few decades.[2] By grouping technologies

1 But see Gena Corea, *The Mother Machine: Reproductive Technologies from Artificial Insemination to Artificial Wombs* (London, 1985); Naomi Pfeffer, *The Stork and the Syringe: A Political History of Reproductive Medicine* (Cambridge, 1993); and Margaret Marsh and Wanda Ronner, *The Empty Cradle: Infertility in America from Colonial Times to the Present* (Baltimore, MD, 1996).

2 On infertility: Christina Benninghaus, 'Modern Infertility', Chapter 31; on regulation: Martin H. Johnson and Nick Hopwood, 'Modern Law and Regulation', Chapter 40; for a global perspective: Hopwood, 'Globalization', Chapter 43; on earlier times: Katharine Park, 'Managing Childbirth and Fertility in Medieval Europe', Chapter 11; Peter Murray Jones, 'Generation between Script and Print', Chapter 13; Lauren Kassell, 'Fruitful Bodies and Astrological Medicine', Chapter 16, this book.

and species, the chapter brings out general features, compares the manipulation of eggs and of sperm, and explores exchange, typically via research laboratories, between infertility clinics and animal breeding. Aims have differed in hospitals and on farms – the individual human pregnancy versus maximizing offspring from valuable animals (as many as 50,000 annually from one bull) – but the similarities have mattered, too.[3]

Some 'new reproductive technologies', as these were categorized in the 1980s, have strong claims to novelty, but replacing an act dependent on two parents' bodies and minds with a mechanical process was already debated in the late eighteenth century. The most potent vision of separating sexual desire from rational reproduction, Aldous Huxley's novel *Brave New World*, has shadowed the field since 1932, but we have never come close to growing babies in bottles to term. An adequate history should not only bring male and female techniques, humans and other animals into one frame; it should also encompass the fantasies and the firsts, while recognizing the greater significance of everyday use.

Artificial Insemination

Artificial fertilization is easier in animals in which the process is naturally external; by the mid-nineteenth century, fish farmers often mixed milt and roe, but only in 1827 was the definitive mammalian ovum even seen. Transferring the more accessible male semen into the cervix or uterus was easier, and did not depend on modern understandings of spermatozoa.[4] Histories of AI begin with 1322, when an Arab chief is alleged to have stolen horse semen from a neighbouring tribe, and rarely fail to mention the 1780 experiment on a spaniel by the professor and priest Lazzaro Spallanzani, or the 1799 report of anatomist John Hunter's assistance to a linen draper with severe hypospadias, a malformation in which the urethra opens in the perineum.[5] Among French revolutionary proposals for physical and moral regeneration, Spallanzani inspired fictions of medically supervised reproduction from 'great men' by means of 'huge collections of animalcules'. In *Pauliska*, the libertine novel of sexual cruelty, a feminist collective imagines exploiting his invention to propagate while avoiding contact with such beasts as the man they have captured and caged.[6] But it took another century and a half of debate and innovation for AI, previously called 'artificial impregnation' and 'artificial fecundation', to become reliable and routine, even in agriculture and especially by a human donor not married to the woman involved.

3 Sarah Wilmot (ed.), 'Between the farm and the clinic: Agriculture and reproductive technology in the twentieth century', *Studies in History and Philosophy of Biological and Biomedical Sciences* 38 (2007), 303–530; Wilmot, 'Breeding Farm Animals and Humans', Chapter 27, this book.

4 On which see Florence Vienne, 'Eggs and Sperm as Germ Cells', Chapter 28, this book.

5 Hermann Rohleder, *Test-Tube Babies: A History of the Artificial Impregnation of Human Beings …* (New York, NY, 1934); F. N. L. Poynter, 'Hunter, Spallanzani, and the history of artificial insemination', in Lloyd G. Stevenson and Robert P. Multhauf (eds.), *Medicine, Science, and Culture: Historical Essays in Honor of Owsei Temkin* (Baltimore, MD, 1968), pp. 97–113; Fig. 1.4, this book.

6 Joël Castonguay-Bélanger, *Les écarts de l'imagination: Pratiques et représentations de la science dans le roman au tournant des Lumières* (Montreal, 2008), pp. 195–204, quoting from *La philosophie de nos jours* (1788), p. 75.

The American gynaecologist J. Marion Sims claimed the first human success in 1866, by collecting sperm from the vagina after marital intercourse and injecting it into the uterus using a syringe. Masturbation being taboo and storage impossible, he lurked outside the bedroom; 'friction specimens' were not discussed for decades. Sims also announced that since another fifty-four attempts on six women had failed, he was giving up. He favoured surgery on the cervix, but some patients preferred injection. A spate of reports by French doctors provoked speculation in 1870 that it needed only a preservation method for 'a club of onanists' to advertise semen '[f]rom a 30-year-old blond with black eyes' and for its use to rejuvenate declining races.[7] After a court condemned artificial fecundation, the Medico-Legal Society of Bordeaux stated in 1883 that an 'honourable' doctor should neither propose nor withhold the 'operation'. With the potential to raise the low birth-rate, it was part of French gynaecology, but contested; the Paris faculty refused Jules Gérard a doctorate two years later. His activities having already inspired a novel, *Le faiseur d'hommes* (The man-maker), this harsh treatment ensured his own advice book a tenth edition (Fig. 39.1).[8] Prompted by the French debate, the Vatican condemned the practice in 1897, a milestone in articulating a Catholic discourse that engaged with interventions in reproduction earlier and more uncompromisingly than other religions.[9]

In the now dominant German medicine, artificial fertilization was still embarrassing; many also doubted uncontrolled one-off experiments. That mood changed following public discussion around 1912 and in response to the shortage of men after World War I.[10] Chiming with commitments to technology, eugenics and the nuclear family, the United States embraced AI most. In 1920, members of the American Gynecological Society heard its president recommend they study artificial impregnation by husbands.

If the profession kept its distance still, with many treating AI by donor (AID) as tantamount to adultery, individual practitioners selected married couples who fitted their gender norms; organized donation, ideally by young married doctors who had fathered healthy children and shared some paternal characteristics; and enforced secrecy. Even more than adoption, AI was supposed to have neighbours saying the child looked just like the doting dad, his masculinity restored. The press reported large numbers of 'test-tube babies', and World War II increased demand for semen to substitute for killed

7 'Gedanken über die Konsequenzen der künstlichen Befruchtung', *Wiener Medizinische Presse* 11 (1870), 449–50.

8 Caroline Arni, 'Menschen machen aus Akt und Substanz. Prokreation und Vaterschaft im reproduktionsmedizinischen und im literarischen Experiment', *Gesnerus* 65 (2008), 196–224, on 206.

9 Emmanuel Betta, *L'altra genesi: Storia della fecondazione artificiale* (Rome, 2012).

10 Iris Semke, *Künstliche Befruchtung in wissenschafts- und sozialgeschichtlicher Sicht* (Frankfurt am Main, 1996); Christina Benninghaus, 'Great expectations: German debates about artificial insemination around 1912', *Studies in History and Philosophy of Biological and Biomedical Sciences* 38 (2007), 374–92. On myths and realities of AI under National Socialism: Antje Kampf, 'Tales of healthy men: Male reproductive bodies in biomedicine from "Lebensborn" to sperm banks', *Health* 17 (2012), 20–36; Andreas Bernard, *Kinder machen: Neue Reproduktionstechnologien und die Ordnung der Familie. Samenspender, Leihmütter, künstliche Befruchtung* (Frankfurt am Main, 2014), pp. 230–47.

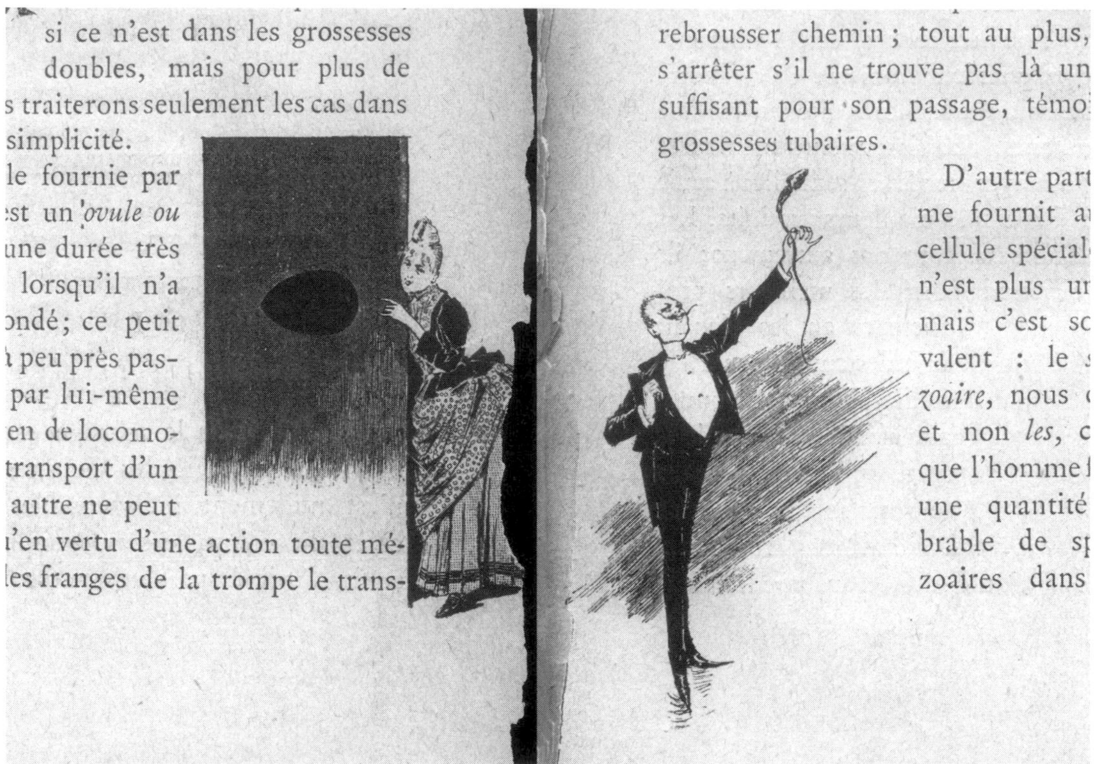
si ce n'est dans les grossesses
doubles, mais pour plus de
s traiterons seulement les cas dans
simplicité.
le fournie par
st un *ovule ou*
une durée très
lorsqu'il n'a
ondé; ce petit
peu près pas-
par lui-même
en de locomo-
transport d'un
autre ne peut
en vertu d'une action toute mé-
les franges de la trompe le trans-

rebrousser chemin ; tout au plus,
s'arrêter s'il ne trouve pas là un
suffisant pour son passage, témo
grossesses tubaires.
D'autre part
me fournit a
cellule spécial
n'est plus u
mais c'est s
valent : le
zoaire, nous
et non *les*, c
que l'homme
une quantité
brable de s
zoaires dans

Figure 39.1 Woman with egg and man holding sperm. Jules Gérard suggested that 'allegory shocks the eyes much less than the brutal reality of a purely anatomical plate'. Engravings by José Roy from *Nouvelles causes de stérilité dans les deux sexes: Fécondation artificielle comme moyen ultime de traitement*, édition définitive (Paris: Marpon & Flammarion, [1888?]), pp. 2–3. 18.5 × 22 cm.

or injured men (Fig. 39.2).[11] In Britain, pioneering doctors had quietly offered AID, while the birth controller Marie Stopes advised couples to arrange things themselves.[12] Faith was growing in the power of intervention, knowing the timing of ovulation improved the odds, and successes in animals had boosted confidence in the technique.[13]

Support from the Russian imperial studs had overcome fears that the costly procedure could lead to degeneration, and allowed the biologist Il'ya Ivanovich Ivanov to inseminate nearly seven thousand horses and over a thousand sheep by 1914. He also

11 Kara W. Swanson, 'Adultery by doctor: Artificial insemination, 1890–1945', *Chicago-Kent Law Review* 87 (2012), 591–633; Carolyn Herbst Lewis, *Prescription for Heterosexuality: Sexual Citizenship in the Cold War Era* (Chapel Hill, NC, 2010), pp. 113–43. On adoption: Ellen Herman, 'Technologies of Adoption Matching', Exhibit 33; and Benninghaus, 'Modern Infertility', this book.

12 Pfeffer, *Stork and Syringe*, pp. 110–41; Angus McLaren, *Reproduction by Design: Sex, Robots, Trees, and Test-Tube Babies in Interwar Britain* (Chicago, IL, 2012), pp. 109–33; Hayley Andrew, 'The reluctant stork: Science, fertility, and the family in Britain, 1943–1960', unpublished PhD thesis, York University, Toronto (2016).

13 On faith in intervention: Benninghaus, 'Modern Infertility'; on the menstrual cycle: Martina Schlünder, 'Menstrual-Cycle Calendars', Exhibit 31, this book.

May 5 1945 JOHN BULL 7

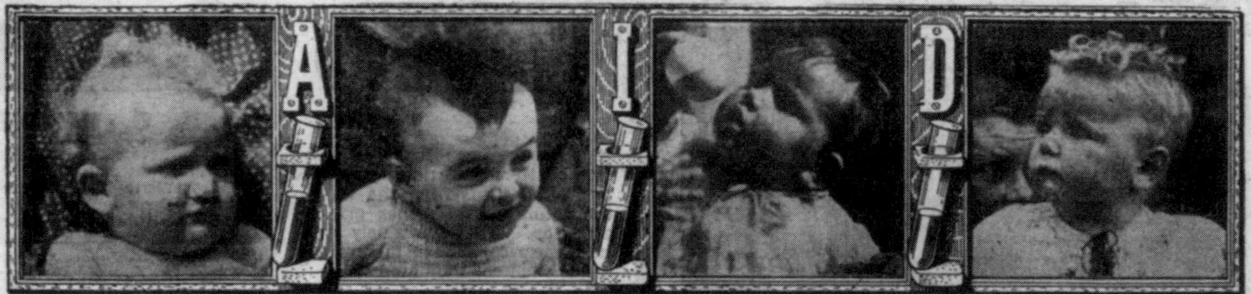

What do they look like—the children now being produced by artificial insemination? No different than the "normal" babies pictured above. And below—

Four experts help you to make up your mind about

TEST-TUBE BABIES

Civilisation faces a new and vital problem. JOHN BULL believes its readers will welcome these authoritative statements of the issues involved

DOCTOR

THE SUDDEN BLAZE of publicity thrown on artificial insemination has been out of all proportion to its immediate importance.

The technique has been used by breeders of cattle for many years as a means of increasing the usefulness of approved sires. Among human beings isolated experiments have been carried out over a considerable time both in this country and elsewhere.

In America, artificial insemination from a "donor"—that is, a man unknown to either husband or wife—is an established practice, and, in isolated cases, human semen has been successfully transported for long distances by 'plane. There are also reports of official experiments in the U.S.S.R.

In this country a few doctors have experimented with the technique in individual cases, but until recently there has been little or no scientific literature on the subject.

Active opposition is to be expected, mainly from certain religious bodies whose particular tenets reject the practice, or from lawyers and others chiefly concerned with inherited privilege and entailed property.

But whatever views are held about the ethics of artificial insemination, the problem of irremediable male sterility is too pressing to be ignored. Further research will perhaps help to reduce this condition; it can hardly expect to abolish it altogether.

tific experiment, but this honest searching after truth will be constantly hampered if it is allowed to become the target of ill-informed criticism.

ROMAN CATHOLIC PRIEST

THERE IS NOTHING MORE fundamental in human relationships than the union of the sexes. The Church, as our moral guide, helps us to know its exact nature. The medical profession deals with the mechanics of human reproduction, but has no right or qualification to give moral rulings.

The sexual union of man and woman is not the same as the reproductive relation of animals. The potentially reproductive act in man is the loving physical union between husband and wife. Reproduction procured in any other manner is contrary to man's nature, and therefore immoral.

Hence, as between husband and wife, artificial insemination is prohibited by the Catholic Church because insemination should be, not a medical operation, but the climax of the physical expression of love in actual and full sexual union.

As to "donor" insemination, that is immoral

Neither husband nor wife would be allowed to give evidence of non-intercourse, and the doctor would be under a bond of professional secrecy.

There is nothing in the law which would enable one partner in a marriage to insist on the use of artificial insemination, least of all from a donor, in order to produce children. If, however, a wife obtained a child by artificial insemination from a donor without her husband's consent, he could regard that as a serious matrimonial offence, entitling him to leave his wife, but he could not ask for divorce on the grounds of adultery—an offence inseparable from intercourse.

This means the husband might have little chance of adequate legal redress: his best protection lies in the scrupulous observance by the medical profession of the rule that the operation must never be performed without the husband's clear consent.

Finally, even if a donor's identity were known, he could never become liable for maintenance of the child. Such liability is inseparable from intercourse with the mother.

PSYCHOLOGIST

THE USE OF artificial insemination from a donor is too new as yet for us to do any more than guess at the psychological factors involved.

American doctors say that the wife undergoing the treatment is apt to be depressed at first—especially if the process is prolonged. But successful pregnancy brings her happiness.

Figure 39.2 'Test-tube babies', part of a 'sudden blaze of publicity' about AI. On 5 May 1945, the high-circulation British Sunday newspaper *John Bull* reproduced photographs of 'normal' babies above reassuring statements by an anonymous doctor, barrister and psychologist. But a priest opposed even AI by husband, because it was not 'the climax of the full expression of love in actual and full sexual union'. Picture strip 22 cm wide. Reproduced by permission of the Advertising Archives.

hybridized exotic species. Spallanzani had experimented with hybrids, and maverick evolutionists fantasized about using AI to demonstrate human–ape kinship. The extraordinary conditions of the Soviet Union allowed Ivanov to transgress. In French West Africa in 1927, he inseminated female chimpanzees with human sperm, a test supported at the Pasteur Institute in Paris and reported in the press. When this failed and the Soviet Academy of Sciences condemned it, the Communist Academy and the Society of Materialist Biologists backed Ivanov's plans for the reverse experiment with orangutan sperm and women 'volunteers'. Yet before he could perform it, the same cultural revolution that had created this opportunity exiled him as a counter-revolutionary specialist.[14]

Seen from Britain, a bastion of resistance, AI might appeal in centralized agricultural systems – also Japan and Argentina – that needed rapidly to improve and expand stock from a few stud animals. British farmers, breeders and officials valued 'competitive individualism, craft skills, breed variety and pedigree' and feared standardization, but demand for milk drove mass production. From 1920, a Livestock Improvement Scheme favoured pedigree bulls and licensing of those that stood for 'public service'. This established state intervention and paved the way to AI. Though Cambridge scientists had already researched methods, only during World War II did the Agricultural Research Council fund field trials in cattle. By 1960, 60 per cent of British cows were born by AI. Sperm had already been transported on ice; freezing and thawing, achieved with glycerol at the National Institute for Medical Research in 1949, further separated ejaculation and insemination.[15]

AI in livestock fed dreams and nightmares of industrializing human reproduction. In 1935, the socialist American geneticist Hermann Muller had imagined speeding up evolution. 'How many women, in an enlightened community', he mused, 'would be … proud to bear and rear a child of Lenin or of Darwin!' Such views remained marginal, but physicians did select donors for their genetic health; avoiding hereditary diseases became a significant motivation for AID.[16]

From 1953, the freezing of human semen allowed storage of what, like blood before the Spanish Civil War, had always been provided fresh. The first sperm banks were set up in the early 1970s. A Californian millionaire promised semen from Nobel laureates; more typical facilities let well-off men keep their 'fatherhood on ice' after a vasectomy. Plagued by low demand and failures with frozen semen, these businesses were saved by switching in the 1980s from holding deposits for men to selling to women. Testing reduced the risk of transmitting HIV and eased medical approval for direct-to-consumer marketing.[17]

The law had long withheld recognition, but in 1960 a UK government committee approved AI by husband, and in the 1970s restrictions broke down. AI was accepted

14 Kirill Rossiianov, 'Beyond species: Il'ya Ivanov and his experiments on cross-breeding humans with anthropoid apes', *Science in Context* 15 (2002), 277–316.

15 Sarah Wilmot, 'From public service to artificial insemination: Animal breeding science and reproductive research in early twentieth-century Britain', *Studies in History and Philosophy of Biological and Biomedical Sciences* 38 (2007), 411–41, on 418.

16 H. J. Muller, *Out of the Night: A Biologist's View of the Future* (London, 1936), pp. 152–3; Martin Richards, 'Artificial insemination and eugenics: Celibate motherhood, eutelegenesis and germinal choice', *Studies in History and Philosophy of Biological and Biomedical Sciences* 39 (2008), 211–21.

17 Kara W. Swanson, *Banking on the Body: The Market in Blood, Milk, and Sperm in Modern America* (Cambridge, MA, 2014), pp. 198–237; on vasectomy: Jesse Olszynko-Gryn, 'Technologies of Contraception and Abortion', Chapter 36, this book.

into medicine to support conventional marriage, but the feminist health movement promoted access for women without male partners. Going beyond the turkey baster, the market in reproductive services provided anonymized sperm banks and physician supervision to anyone who could pay.[18] By this time, however, 'test-tube babies' generally meant children born after IVF.

In Vitro Fertilization and Embryo Transfer

The prototype for mammalian IVF, technically and in its high media profile, was less the isolated late nineteenth-century reports of fertilization that histories have presented as failed precursors than two other experiments. In the 1890s, the Cambridge embryologist Walter Heape surgically transferred rabbit embryos from an Angora doe to a Belgian Hare who gave birth to Angora offspring as well as her own. Concluding that the foster-mother had no power of modifying the breed, he advertised uses in studying heredity.[19] In 1900, the German-born American biologist and materialist Jacques Loeb induced sea urchin eggs to undergo parthenogenesis: development without sperm. Newspapers reported that he had 'created life in a test tube'. In a prophecy to the Cambridge Heretics Society in 1923, J. B. S. Haldane drew on Heape to imagine 'ectogenesis', or development fully outside the womb, and so inspired the Central London Hatchery in *Brave New World*.[20] These fictions framed attempts to achieve the more limited goal of mammalian in vitro fertilization followed by embryo transfer within networks established for AI and population control.[21]

In the mid-1930s, the physiologist Gregory Pincus made in vitro fertilization a prominent line of work. He came from Harvard to the Agricultural Research Council-funded Animal Research Station in Cambridge to try parthenogenesis for mammals. Fertilization, at first the control, became a challenge in its own right. Joining his interest in culturing eggs with the local tradition of embryo transfer and concern to prolong the life of sperm, Pincus claimed success in rabbits in 1934. The *New York Times* wrote of 'test-tube babies' in this sense in 1941. Animal-breeding scientists sought to

18 Gayle Davis, 'Test tubes and turpitude: Medical responses to the infertile patient in mid-twentieth-century Scotland', in Janet Greenlees and Linda Bryder (eds.), *Western Maternity and Medicine, 1880–1990* (London, 2013), pp. 113–27; Swanson, *Banking on the Body*; Laura Mamo, *Queering Reproduction: Achieving Pregnancy in the Age of Technoscience* (Durham, NC, 2007).

19 J. D. Biggers, 'Walter Heape, FRS: A pioneer in reproductive biology: Centenary of his embryo transfer experiments', *Journal of Reproduction and Fertility* 93 (1991), 173–86.

20 Jon Turney, *Frankenstein's Footsteps: Science, Genetics and Popular Culture* (New Haven, CT, 1998), pp. 64–120; see also Susan Squier, *Babies in Bottles: Twentieth-Century Visions of Reproductive Technology* (New Brunswick, NJ, 1994).

21 For the networks: Wilmot, 'Public service', 430–3; Alison Bashford, 'World Population from Eugenics to Climate Change', Chapter 34, this book.

complement AI by controlling the female genetic contribution too, and America's leading fertility doctor, John Rock, envisaged 'conception in a watch-glass'.[22]

Working with Rock, Pincus's former assistant Miriam Menkin received eggs from ovaries removed in operations just before ovulation, matured them by incubation in the patient's serum and mixed them with sperm left over from AI. In 1944, she obtained two- and three-cell embryos and wide publicity.[23] Yet standards tightened as reproductive scientists organized in societies, conferences and journals. By 1951, leading laboratories doubted that anyone had ever fertilized mammalian eggs in vitro. They reinterpreted Pincus's results as really due to sperm sticking to the eggs transferred to the host, Menkin and Rock's as not fertilization but degenerative segmentation. In 1959 Pincus's Cambridge-trained Chinese colleague Min Chueh Chang finally announced a convincing demonstration in rabbits at a conference sponsored by the Population Council and the Planned Parenthood Federation of America; the system also had potential for testing contraceptives.[24]

Extended to rodents in the 1960s, IVF was not reported in a farm animal until 1981. Control over the female input was achieved in livestock by transferring embryos produced in vivo instead. The Cambridge station and two private American research foundations worked on superovulation (stimulation of the ovaries to produce extra eggs) and embryo transfer in cattle from the 1940s, with a Wisconsin team claiming a live birth in 1951, and the Soviet Union firsts in sheep and pigs. The breakthroughs came with technical improvements by Cambridge station researcher L. E. A. (Tim) Rowson: from 1972 his courses trained enthusiasts who built a $20 million North American industry by 1980 (Fig. 39.3). An incentive was to multiply offspring from valuable mothers that disease-regulating governments had made it more expensive to import. From this platform, sexing, cloning and IVF were added. Chilling allowed embryo culture long enough to fly hundreds of miles; viability after freezing and thawing was shown when the British vet who had pioneered IVF in mice collaborated with cryobiologists at Oak Ridge National Laboratory in Tennessee. In 2001, half of all transfers were from frozen, but only about 6 per cent with embryos produced in vitro. In IVF, the farm followed the clinic.[25]

A live birth after in vitro fertilization posed far more severe challenges in humans than rabbits or mice. It took scientific, clinical, ethical and public relations work and

22 Christine Schreiber, *Natürlich künstliche Befruchtung? Eine Geschichte der In-vitro-Fertilisation von 1878 bis 1950* (Göttingen, 2007).

23 Margaret Marsh and Wanda Ronner, *The Fertility Doctor: John Rock and the Reproductive Revolution* (Baltimore, MD, 2008), pp. 104–10.

24 Nick Hopwood, 'Proof and publicity in claims to human in vitro fertilization', in preparation.

25 Keith J. Betteridge, 'A history of farm animal embryo transfer and some associated techniques', *Animal Reproduction Science* 79 (2003), 203–44; on cloning: Christina Brandt, 'Cloned Frogs', Exhibit 37, this book.

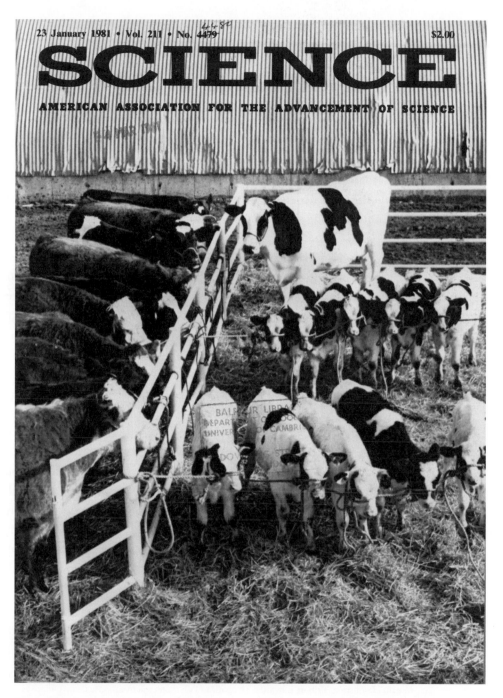

Figure 39.3 Cover of *Science*, one of the leading general science journals, advertising an article on 'Superovulation and embryo transfer in cattle'. 'The dairy cow (upper right) is the genetic mother of the ten calves. She was superovulated, and the embryos were recovered from her uterus', cultured in vitro and 'transferred to the uteri of the ten recipient cows (left) for gestation'. Reprinted with permission from John Messineo and AAAS.

depended on larger shifts in practice and opinion. From the 1950s to the mid-1960s, maverick clinicians, well placed to secure oocytes for maturation, publicized claims to have produced embryos and even babies. The Columbia gynaecologist Landrum B. Shettles, a mass-market advocate of a dubious sex selection method, rejected reproductive biologists' stringent standards also in his fertilization work.[26] By contrast, the successful team combined commitment to these norms with extraordinary access to clinical material. The two leaders might look like outsiders, but physiologist Robert Edwards had trained in leading centres and gynaecologist Patrick Steptoe helped to develop laparoscopy or keyhole surgery, which though initially controversial became routine.[27] The work depended on a British culture permissive of innovation and specifically on Cambridge reproductive physiology and the National Health Service in Oldham near Manchester.

Edwards had relied on clinicians for pieces of ovary, from which he matured oocytes in vitro for fertilization with his own sperm. From 1968, when he began collaborating with Steptoe, his own interests expanded from genetic selection to infertility. In 1969, using a new medium to treat sperm, they announced that they had produced early stages of fertilization in vitro. Widely reported, the work was criticized on moral and religious grounds and by specialists either unimpressed with results seemingly less advanced than Shettles's or still doubtful that fertilization had occurred. The following year, the British team showed later stages, now from oocytes recovered by laparoscopy (Fig. 39.4), and Steptoe led a media fightback that framed in vitro fertilization as hope for the infertile at last.[28]

In 1971, the UK Medical Research Council turned down a major grant application from Edwards and Steptoe. The referees insisted on more experimentation on other primates first; saw alleviating infertility as low priority or worse; and were alienated by the publicity.[29] The work proceeded nevertheless, thanks to support from the Oldham District and General Hospital and funding from the Ford Foundation and the San Francisco TV station owner Lillian Lincoln Howell – female philanthropy played a key role, like for the contraceptive pill.[30] Because from 1974 the US government enforced a

26 Robin Marantz Henig, *Pandora's Baby: How the First Test Tube Babies Sparked the Reproductive Revolution* (Boston, MA, 2004).

27 Mainly for sterilization: Olszynko-Gryn, 'Technologies of Contraception and Abortion'.

28 Robert Edwards and Patrick Steptoe, *A Matter of Life: The Story of a Medical Breakthrough* (London, 1980); Martin H. Johnson, 'Robert Edwards: The path to IVF', *Reproductive BioMedicine Online* 23 (2011), 245–62; Turney, *Frankenstein's Footsteps*, pp. 160–87.

29 Martin H. Johnson *et al.*, 'Why the Medical Research Council refused Robert Edwards and Patrick Steptoe support for research on human conception in 1971', *Human Reproduction* 25 (2010), 2157–74.

30 K. Elder and M. H. Johnson, 'Symposium: The history of the first IVF births', *Reproductive BioMedicine and Society Online* 1 (2015), 1–70, on 58–70.

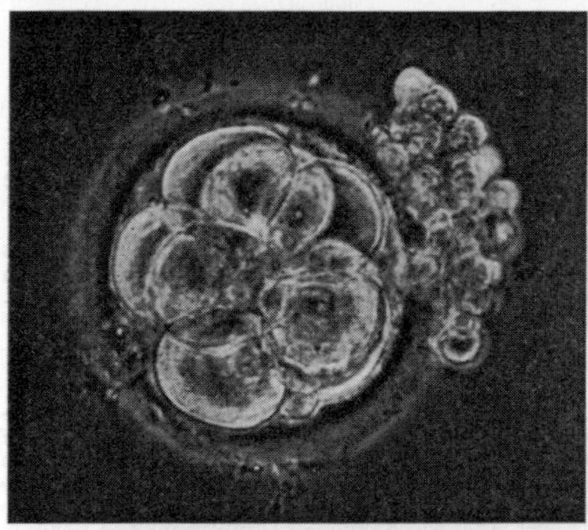

Figure 39.4 An '8-celled egg' developed from a human oocyte recovered by laparoscopy, fertilized and taken through early cleavage in vitro. An advance on the 'early stages of fertilization' reported previously, this still did not satisfy all sceptics. Reprinted by permission from Macmillan Publishers Ltd from R. G. Edwards, P. C. Steptoe and J. M. Purdy, 'Fertilization and cleavage in vitro of preovulator human oocytes', *Nature* 227 (26 Sept. 1970), 1307–9.

de facto moratorium on research on embryos or fetuses, the only serious competitors were two rival teams in Melbourne, Australia.

Oldham gave the charismatic Steptoe much freedom to build a programme. The nurses donated long hours, while other practitioners referred at least 282 patient volunteers who together went through some 495 cycles of laparoscopic oocyte recovery between 1969 and 1978 (Fig. 39.5). By December 1971, Steptoe and Edwards were confident enough that any children would be normal to begin embryo transfer. Having warned the patients that the work was experimental, they used only the husbands' sperm and required agreement to amniocentesis and a termination were any abnormality found. They won over a British Medical Association professional standards committee.[31]

Yet even sympathetic colleagues worried that the pair were going too fast. The news media carried the objections, but also reinforced the sense that alleviating infertility justified 'implants'. With population control in retreat, and a dearth of babies for adoption now that contraception and abortion were increasingly taken for granted, IVF chimed with the new health consumerism.[32] The press construction of desperateness for a child, and its resolution by a 'technomedical adventure', critiqued in and for the 1980s, was built for IVF through the 1970s; the more general view of reproduction as

31 Ibid., 9–18, 34–57.

32 Turney, *Frankenstein's Footsteps*, pp. 166–81; Michael Mulkay, *The Embryo Research Debate: Science and the Politics of Reproduction* (Cambridge, 1997), pp. 6–19.

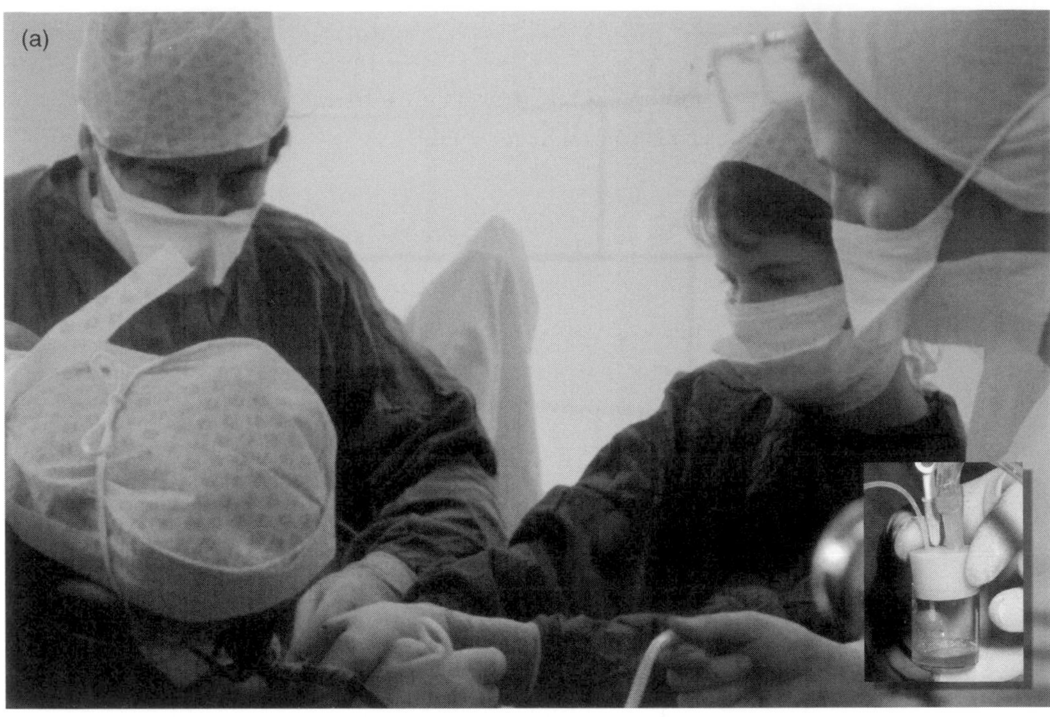

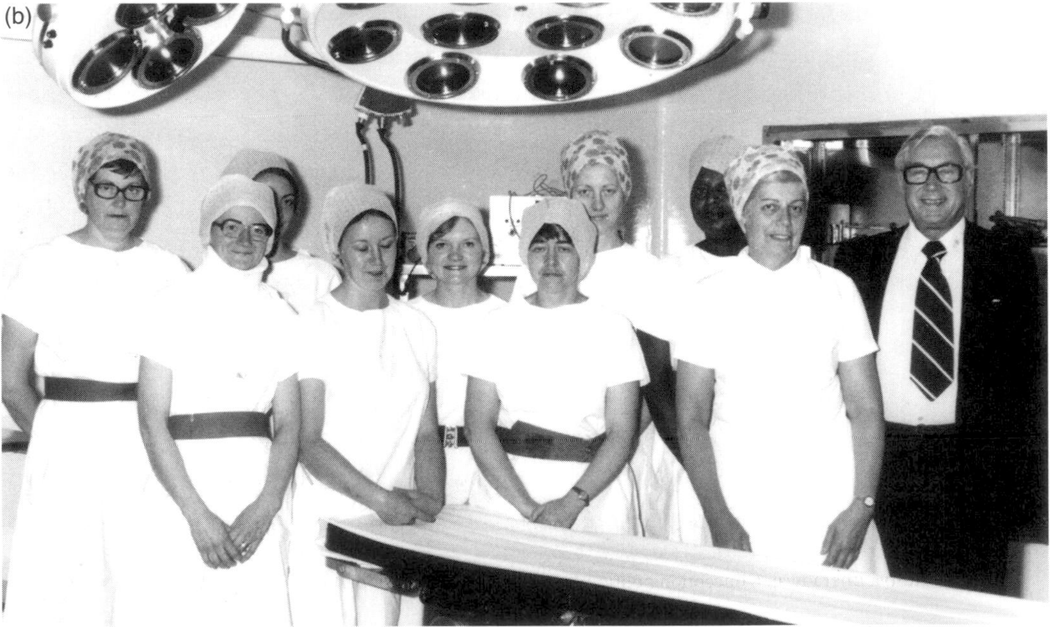

Figure 39.5 The gendered division of labour at Dr Kershaw's Hospital, Oldham. (a) Steptoe (head down) performing a laparoscopy, assisted by Edwards (who more typically worked in the next-door laboratory) and probably a junior doctor and nurse, in about 1970–2; the patient is hardly visible. Inset: the chamber into which the oocytes were aspirated. (b) The nursing team and Steptoe, summer 1978. Photographs courtesy of John Fallows.

needing intervention went back to around 1900.[33] When news of a pregnancy leaked out in April 1978, the method could thus count on support – provided all went well. Steptoe monitored the mother and the world's press tried to monitor him. Born on 25 July, Louise Brown was hailed as a miracle child.[34]

Assisted Reproduction

Front-page photos were one thing; clinical routine was quite another. For several years, attention focused on replication and reliability. After a contested Indian report, it took Edwards's closest American collaborators three years to gain permission, repeat the work and achieve a birth.[35] Some complained that the Oldham team – preoccupied with Steptoe's retirement and setting up a clinic and unsure what, after so many failures, accounted for their success – delayed publishing the details; others thanked them for advice. The British had seen natural cycles as key; the delivery of several IVF babies in quick succession in Melbourne made chemical stimulation of ovulation standard.[36] In a climate friendly to private enterprise, a hundred clinics had opened in a dozen rich countries by 1984, and a biomedical industry had taken off.

This brought transformation, because distinguishing 'genetic' from 'gestational' motherhood was unprecedented, and because the expansion of services reconfigured existing technologies. IVF facilitated larger social changes and prompted those involved to revisit issues long discussed for adoption and AI. Journalists, clinicians, academics and lawyers debated the implications of assisting nature. Reports of using donor eggs, to allow a 59-year-old woman to give birth to twins on 25 December 1993 and a black woman to bear a white child, heightened the sense that 'postmodern' reproduction overcame all constraints.[37]

Some Christian groups rejected the commodification of life and the separation of reproduction from marital sex. Some feminists had welcomed IVF, but the Feminist International Network of Resistance to Reproductive Technologies and Genetic

33 For the critiques: Mulkay, *Embryo Research Debate*; Sarah Franklin, *Embodied Progress: A Cultural Account of Assisted Conception* (London, 1997); for antecedents: Lisa Hope Harris, 'Challenging conception: A clinical and cultural history of in vitro fertilization in the United States', unpublished PhD thesis, University of Michigan (2006), p. 43; McLaren, *Reproduction by Design*, pp. 1–2; Benninghaus, 'Modern Infertility'.

34 Nick Hopwood, '"It's a Girl"', Exhibit 38, this book.

35 Aditya Bharadwaj, 'Conception politics: Medical egos, media spotlights, and the contest over test-tube babies in India', in Marcia C. Inhorn and Frank van Balen (eds.), *Infertility around the Globe: New Thinking on Childlessness, Gender, and Reproductive Technologies* (Berkeley, CA, 2002), pp. 315–33; on the United States: Harris, 'Challenging conception'.

36 John Leeton, *Test Tube Revolution: The Early History of IVF* (Clayton, Victoria, 2013).

37 José Van Dyck, *Manufacturing Babies and Public Consent: Debating the New Reproductive Technologies* (Basingstoke, 1995), p. 1.

Engineering objected to the demands placed on and the risks borne by the women involved. Criticism of safety and success rates, profit-seeking and multiple births, by contrast, implied that all would be well if only methods could be improved, a regulatory framework developed and access expanded. Within a few years the question, in countries without a strong Catholic opposition or difficult historical legacy, was no longer whether, but how.[38]

Regulation was an issue from the start, especially the frozen storage of and (non-reproductive) experimentation on 'spare' embryos. Controversy ran in tracks worn by the abortion debates, with outcomes dependent on nationally specific ways of knowing, or 'civic epistemologies'.[39] In Britain, a committee report followed by much parliamentary debate and lobbying led to the Human Fertilisation and Embryology Act 1990, which established a licensing regime and permitted experiments for the first fourteen days. IVF was allowed in the United States, but a moratorium on federal funding reduced government leverage and left reproductive services a 'wild West'.[40] National differences have combined with a globalized trade in services to promote travel for reproduction.[41] From 1998, IVF clinics also controversially provided embryos for the derivation of human embryonic stem cells.[42] By then, IVF was a platform for other techniques. From its initial construction as a procedure for older, white, professional women – the best free-market consumers – exotic methods have attracted more attention than equitable access.[43]

A mere six years after the first birth, *Time* magazine looked forward to variations on 'old-fashioned IVF'.[44] Intracytoplasmic sperm injection (ICSI), invented in Brussels in 1992, bypassed much male-factor infertility, though only by women's undergoing the rigours of IVF.[45] Building on an earlier demonstration in rabbits, human preimplantation genetic diagnosis (PGD) to avoid (sex-linked) muscular dystrophy by selecting female embryos was achieved in London in 1990, just before the UK parliament voted on embryo research.[46] Though often debated in terms of 'designer babies' and 'saviour

38 Ibid.; Harris, 'Challenging conception'.

39 Sheila Jasanoff, *Designs on Nature: Science and Democracy in Europe and the United States* (Princeton, NJ, 2005), pp. 247–71.

40 Mulkay, *Embryo Research Debate*; Harris, 'Challenging conception'; Johnson and Hopwood, 'Modern Law and Regulation'.

41 Hopwood, 'Globalization'.

42 Herbert Gottweis, Brian Salter and Catherine Waldby, *The Global Politics of Human Embryonic Stem Cell Science* (Basingstoke, 2009).

43 Harris, 'Challenging conception'.

44 Quoted in ibid., p. 179.

45 Françoise Laborie, 'Gender-based management of new reproductive technologies: A comparison between in vitro fertilization and intracytoplasmic sperm injection', in Ann Rudinow Saetnan, Nelly Oudshoorn and Marta Kirejczyk (eds.), *Bodies of Technology: Women's Involvement with Reproductive Medicine* (Columbus, OH, 2000), pp. 278–303.

46 Anastasia A. Theodosiou and Martin H. Johnson, 'The politics of human embryo research and the motivation to achieve PGD', *Reproductive BioMedicine Online* 22 (2011), 457–71.

siblings', for those involved PGD has remained a demanding way of avoiding genetic disease; use for 'family balancing' and to increase IVF success rates is more contested.[47] The 2008 revision to the Human Fertilisation and Embryology Act defined a 'permitted embryo' as one with unaltered DNA. Since then, mitochondrial replacement therapy has gained ground and genome editing is being discussed.

IVF has made other conceptive technologies more acceptable and visible, including their use by gay people; the revised act struck down the requirement that clinics take account of a child's 'need for a father'. Though ICSI reduced heterosexual demand for donor insemination, this was consolidated for lesbian couples. By the late 1980s, eggs were donated too, but where sperm donation was like a job paid on a piece rate, the more invasive egg donation, for a higher fee, was framed as an individual gift.[48] In the early 2000s, debate focused on the commodification of donated gametes, and the question, familiar from adoption, of donor tracing and a child's right to know his or her parents' identities.

Conclusion

The American zoologist F. R. Lillie wrote in 1919 about 'the union of the germ cells in the act of fertilization' that 'this supreme event' 'gathered' 'all the strands of the webs of two lives … in one knot'.[49] How quaint that 'two' seems, a hundred years and many moral and physiological experiments later! Today a child may have as many as five progenitors: two social parents, a gestational (surrogate) mother, a biological (sperm) father and a biological (egg) mother – some see mitochondrial donation in terms of parenthood too – while the social parents may be man and woman, both women or both men.

Certain general features of change are clear. Taking fertilization apart has increased control and selection, and both AI and IVF have served as platforms for other techniques. There has been a bias towards intervening in female bodies, but the accessibility of semen let male methods develop earlier and on a larger scale.[50] Transfers between humans and other animals were crucial. The farm often led the clinic, but human IVF came first; exchanges via laboratory animals went both ways.

This adds up to a revolutionary change, yet the timelines are long. When Lillie wrote, AI was already being performed, albeit still inefficiently and secretly in humans,

47 Sarah Franklin and Celia Roberts, *Born and Made: An Ethnography of Preimplantation Genetic Diagnosis* (Princeton, NJ, 2006).

48 Rene Almeling, *Sex Cells: The Medical Market for Eggs and Sperm* (Berkeley, CA, 2011).

49 Frank Rattray Lillie, *Problems of Fertilization* (Chicago, IL, 1919), p. 31.

50 Male similarly preceded female contraceptives, but the latter became more common: Olszynko-Gryn, 'Technologies of Contraception and Abortion'.

and many issues had been aired. A burst of publicity in the 1860s–80s followed a slow build-up of experience since the late eighteenth century; the 1930s–40s and the years around 1980 saw the most rapid transformations. Only in the last few decades has the natural/artificial distinction finally broken down. Once all reproduction potentially needed assistance, artificial fertilization was artificial no more.

40 Modern Law and Regulation

Martin H. Johnson and Nick Hopwood

Far more than the law has regulated reproduction.[1] Statutes often failed to grasp or change practice, and few cases came to court; popular attitudes, and community pressure, shaped behaviours. Yet disciplinary norms have operated in part through common-law restrictions and a swelling flood of legislation. Formal regulation, however effectively eluded or unevenly enforced, has incited subversion, provoked challenge and offered a yardstick for international comparison.

The major modernizations of legal systems in much of the world in the nineteenth century defined the bourgeois family and brought reproduction within an official framework. Patchworks of laws yielded to single codes for nation-states, which also took over residual legal functions from the Christian churches. For example, the Code Napoléon of 1804, which was emulated especially in Europe and the Middle East, made civil marriage primary and subordinated even aristocratic women to their husbands. In England and Wales, with their system of common or judge-made case law that was influential through the British Empire, the Matrimonial Causes Act 1857 moved divorce from the ecclesiastical to the civil courts and opened it to the middle class, but still favoured men. Laws also defined national populations through obligations to report births, marriages and deaths and complete census forms. Some states obstructed the distribution of contraceptives and criminalized practices that threatened the norm of procreative marital sex, notably abortion and homosexuality.

Early twentieth-century governments legislated more directly to raise population quantity and quality with measures from child tax allowances to compulsory sterilization. They typically proceeded cautiously on such contentious matters, and increasingly deferred to medical practitioners who were themselves often more concerned for their own status. But especially by the 1960s, states and medicine controlled reproduction to such an extent that their paternalism was the chief target of feminist and other reform campaigns. As rights to privacy were recognized and new reproductive technologies introduced, regulators with lay representation came to monitor large medical markets in conception and contraception.[2]

This chapter reviews some roles of law in reproduction since around 1800, mainly for the United Kingdom and the United States with their shared emphasis on common law

1 For the related case of sexuality: Jeffrey Weeks, *Sex, Politics and Society: The Regulation of Sexuality since 1800*, 3rd edn (Harlow, 2012).

2 On medicine and the law: Michael Clark and Catherine Crawford (eds.), *Legal Medicine in History* (Cambridge, 1994).

rather than civil codes. Leaving family and population on one side, the focus is on the prevention of births by contraception, sterilization and abortion, the most contested issue, and on their promotion by the techniques of assisted conception for which current regulatory regimes were introduced.[3] The expansion of the state and the medical profession into the market, challenges to their power and the rise of arm's-length regulation provide the central themes.

States, Doctors, Laws

Important early laws governed abortion not because of any public outcry, but because medical professionals and lawyers mobilized against it. In England and Wales, the common law had presumed that before quickening, when the woman felt a child move inside her, abortion was no offence and only a 'misdemeanour' thereafter. Lord Ellenborough's Act 1803 made attempted abortion by poisoning of 'any woman, then being quick with child', a capital crime, and criminalized the action of causing a miscarriage before quickening by 'any instrument or other means whatsoever' as a felony punishable by transportation. Pressing their claims to authority over pregnancy, doctors criticized the legal recognition of quickening, there being no 'sudden revolution or change' during gestation; 'what is called quickening, is merely the motions of the child becoming sensible to the mother'. An 1828 amendment outlawed the use of instruments at any stage, while an 1837 act abolished all reference to quickening and removed the death penalty to make conviction easier. Regular medical practitioners agitated to protect women from hazardous treatments, to safeguard the fetus and, not least, to block competition from irregulars ('quacks'). Two sections of the Offences Against the Person Act 1861 recognized these concerns by making it a felony punishable by a life of penal servitude to attempt to procure an abortion. This law also applied to a woman 'being with Child', who tried to 'procure her own Miscarriage', as well as anyone else, who used instruments or poison with the same intent, whether the woman was pregnant or not. Supplying these means became a misdemeanour.[4]

3 We know no survey history of reproduction and the law, but Andrea Tone (ed.), *Controlling Reproduction: An American History* (Wilmington, DE, 1997) excerpts legal documents among others. On topics not covered here: Stephen Cretney, *Family Law in the Twentieth Century: A History* (Oxford, 2005); Keith Breckenridge and Simon Szreter (eds.), *Registration and Recognition: Documenting the Person in World History* (Oxford, 2012); Lesley A. Hall, 'Movements to Separate Sex and Reproduction', Chapter 29; Jean-Paul Gaudillière, 'Sex Hormones, Pharmacy and the Reproductive Sciences', Chapter 35; Jesse Olszynko-Gryn, 'Technologies of Contraception and Abortion', Chapter 36; and for comparison with classical times: Tim Parkin, 'The Ancient Family and the Law', Chapter 6, this book.

4 Angus McLaren, *Reproductive Rituals: The Perception of Fertility in England from the Sixteenth to the Eighteenth Century* (London, 1984); John Keown, *Abortion, Doctors and the Law: Some Aspects of the Legal Regulation of Abortion in England from 1803 to 1982* (Cambridge, 1988), 1810 quotation on quickening on p. 31. On abortion in earlier times: Marie-Hélène Congourdeau, 'Debating the Soul in Late Antiquity', Chapter 8; Maaike van der Lugt, 'Formed Fetuses and Healthy Children in Scholastic Theology, Medicine and Law', Chapter 12, this book.

Other European countries and the United States passed similar legislation. The first American laws, from the 1820s–40s, aimed to regulate medicine for public safety and confirmed the acceptability of abortion before quickening. The rate and visibility of abortion increased between 1840 and 1880, especially among Protestant middle- and upper-class married women. In 1857, regular physicians launched an anti-abortion crusade, in part to attack the irregulars and discipline their peers, in part from moral and scientific objections and in part for fear of being outbred by Catholics. Between 1860 and 1900, all US states enacted a new kind of law, which made abortion a crime at any stage, including by the woman concerned.[5]

American social purity campaigners allied with physicians to bring about the 1873 federal Act for the Suppression of Trade in, and Circulation of, Obscene Literature and Articles of Immoral Use, which forbade the mailing of contraceptives and abortifacients, among other items. State-level laws further restricted their sale and, in Connecticut, even use. Made a special agent of the US Post Office, the law's chief proponent, Anthony Comstock, arrested sellers and abortionists (Fig. 40.1). Like British impediments to contraceptive advertising and sale, held to be obscene and immoral, it failed to stop a thriving business. The more important shift was in the mid-1930s, when the Food and Drug Administration (FDA) began to inspect condoms for efficacy, primarily as prophylactics against disease, and the 1936 appellate court ruling *U.S. v. One Package* gave doctors the right to purchase and prescribe contraceptives. FDA seizures sent small manufacturers of unreliable items to the wall, but many clinics, pharmacies and department stores provided birth control.[6]

As studies of many societies have shown, prohibition does not stop abortions, just makes them less safe and access more unequal, more dependent on the abortionists' goodwill or greed. Through the decades of illegality in Britain and the United States, abortion remained common and widely accepted, if hidden; prosecutions were rare unless a woman died and regular practitioners had little to fear. Physicians referred women to colleagues and midwives, but American doctors also aided the state by pressuring victims of botched operations to sign 'dying declarations' incriminating the abortionists. Though prised apart by doctors and jurists, contraception and abortion were often conflated, especially by lower-class women, who did not see taking pills for menstrual regulation as abortion at all, let alone as an illegal operation.[7]

5 James C. Mohr, *Abortion in America: The Origins and Evolution of National Policy, 1800–1900* (New York, NY, 1979).

6 Andrea Tone, *Devices and Desires: A History of Contraceptives in America* (New York, NY, 2001); Melanie Latham, *Regulating Reproduction: A Century of Conflict in Britain and France* (Manchester, 2002), pp. 25–6; Hall, 'Movements to Separate Sex and Reproduction'; Olszynko-Gryn, 'Technologies of Contraception and Abortion'; James M. Edmonson, 'Condoms', Exhibit 28, this book.

7 Barbara Brookes, *Abortion in England, 1900–1967* (London, 1988), pp. 2–9; Leslie J. Reagan, *When Abortion Was a Crime: Women, Medicine, and Law in the United States, 1867–1973* (Berkeley, CA, 1997).

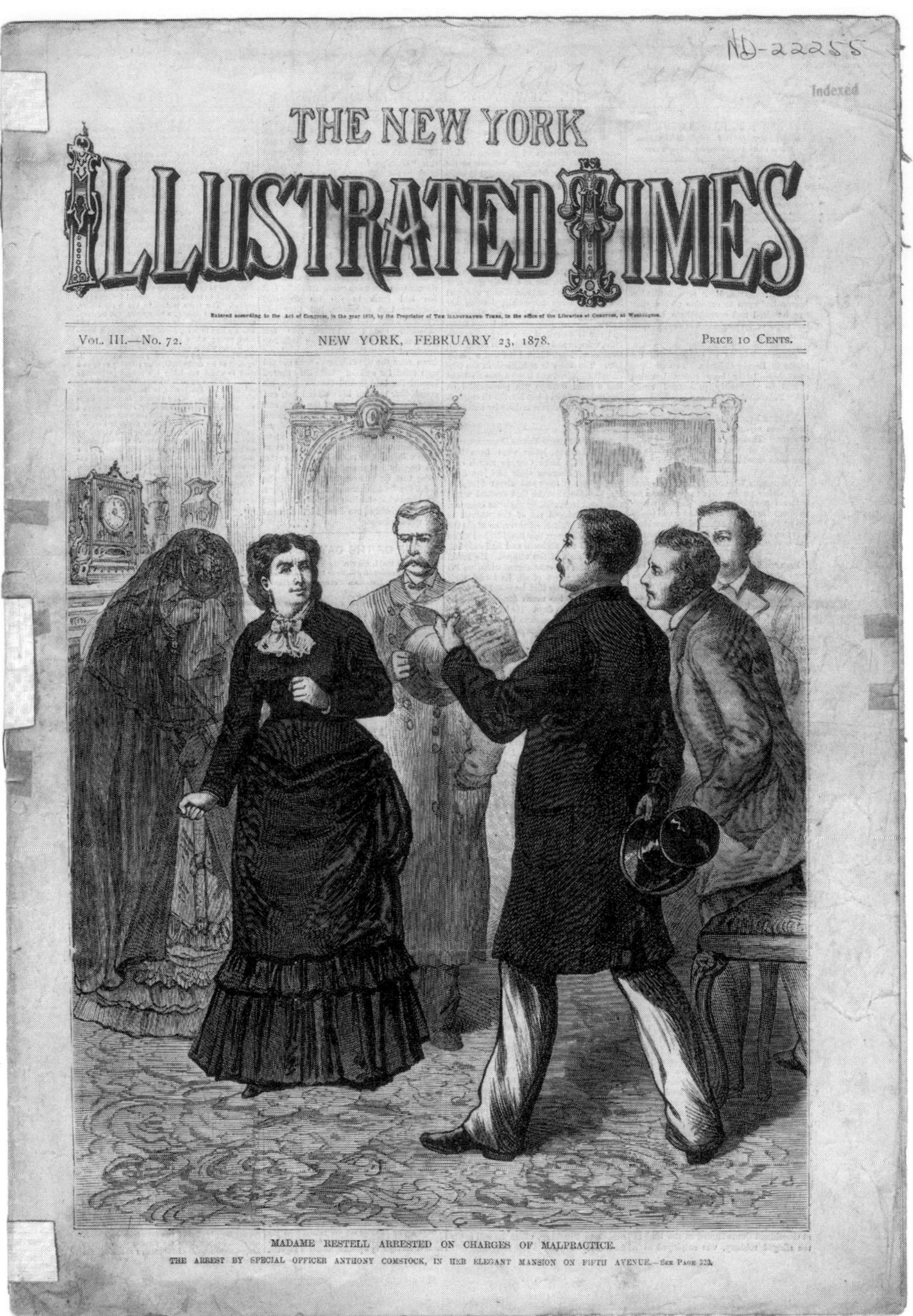

THE NEW YORK ILLUSTRATED TIMES

Entered according to the Act of Congress, in the year 1878, by the Proprietor of The Illustrated Times, in the office of the Librarian of Congress, at Washington.

Vol. III.—No. 72. NEW YORK, FEBRUARY 23, 1878. Price 10 Cents.

MADAME RESTELL ARRESTED ON CHARGES OF MALPRACTICE.

THE ARREST BY SPECIAL OFFICER ANTHONY COMSTOCK, IN HER ELEGANT MANSION ON FIFTH AVENUE.—See Page 323.

Figure 40.1 Cover engraving of Anthony Comstock arresting the abortionist Madame Restell at her Fifth Avenue mansion. He has entrapped her into selling an abortifacient, thus interrupting her aid to the crying woman. Restell, protected for decades by her society connections, committed suicide on the morning of her trial. From *New York Illustrated Times* 3 (23 Feb. 1878). Children's Literature Research Collections, University of Minnesota Libraries.

As birth-rates plummeted around 1900 and bodies politic cried out for regeneration after World War I, governments responded to pronatalist and eugenic campaigns with laws to raise the quantity and quality of their working, fighting populations. Legislation supported the production of healthy children in respectable families of the right race. France outlawed the provision of contraceptive information in 1920.[8] Eugenic measures included family tax allowances in Britain and sterilization of the 'unfit' in the United States.[9] Then the Depression raised the pressure on families to cut costs by preventing births, and increased sympathy for poor women denied access to safe abortions.

The other major change was in the position of women. Soviet Russia, a beacon or warning to the world, depending on one's politics, emancipated women, integrated them into the workforce and legalized abortion between 1920 and 1936.[10] In interwar Britain, as women slowly gained the vote and led more independent lives, the 1923 modification of the 1857 act made it marginally easier for them to petition for divorce on grounds of infidelity. Feminists founded the Abortion Law Reform Association (ALRA) in 1936.[11] Government bodies were unresponsive, but some progress was achieved by case law, especially *Rex v. Bourne* in 1938. This followed the introduction of the Infant Life (Preservation) Act 1929, which protected fetuses in the process of being born – covered by neither the 1861 act nor the law of murder – but made an exception of their destruction in good faith to preserve the woman's life. The 1929 act assumed that the capacity for life was acquired at twenty-eight weeks, medically defined limits of viability replacing quickening as the key boundary within pregnancy. In the test case, a 14-year-old girl, pregnant after rape by five soldiers, had been aborted by the respected gynaecologist Aleck Bourne, practising openly and without fee at St Mary's Hospital, London, all of which details Mr Justice Macnaghten contrasted with the typical case of the 'professional abortionist'. The judge relied on the wording of the 1929 act to flesh out what might be considered a lawful procurement of miscarriage. Thus, he reasoned, the Crown had to prove beyond reasonable doubt that the operation 'was not performed in good faith for the purpose only of preserving the life of the mother'; he ruled that this criterion could be interpreted to mean that 'the probable consequence of the continuance of the pregnancy would be to make the patient a physical and mental wreck'. Bourne's acquittal expanded access while tightening the medical monopoly by

8 Latham, *Regulating Reproduction*, pp. 24–52.

9 Philip R. Reilly, *The Surgical Solution: A History of Involuntary Sterilization in the United States* (Baltimore, MD, 1991); Paul Weindling, 'Pedigree of a "Schizophrenic Family"', Exhibit 29, this book.

10 Susan Gross Solomon, 'The Soviet legalization of abortion in German medical discourse: A study of the use of selective perceptions in cross-cultural scientific relations', *Social Studies of Science* 22 (1992), 455–85.

11 Lesley A. Hall, *Sex, Gender and Social Change in Britain since 1800*, 2nd edn (London, 2013); Hall, 'Movements to Separate Sex and Reproduction'.

demonizing 'backstreet abortionists', some of whom exploited and harmed their clients, while others did their best to meet a real demand.[12]

Medical Power and Social Reform

After World War II, countries set up or extended welfare states and health-care systems that reached far more people than ever before; childbirth completed its move into the hospital in most of the industrialized world. Biomedicine – medicine integrated with biological research in laboratories, industry and clinics – gained unprecedented status, including through the oral contraceptive pill. Then, major reforms of the 1960s and 1970s to laws affecting reproduction critiqued the state control and medical authority that had expanded in the previous hundred years, but also drew on agendas for change within the professions, and sometimes strengthened medical power.

Widely flouted restrictions on contraception were repealed amidst fears of global overpopulation and continued efforts to restrict the reproduction of people on welfare, including by sterilization. Arguments from a right to privacy, important in the *Griswold v. Connecticut* decision of the US Supreme Court in 1965, and its extension to unmarried couples by *Eisenstadt v. Baird* (1972), struck down the last of the Comstock laws. In Britain (and France) by 1974, thanks to feminist activism, the opportunity of National Health Service reorganization and a more liberal climate, contraception was supposed to be made available free of charge. But feminists found it problematic that the medical profession still controlled access to the pill.[13] Contraceptives were developed more for population control than individual empowerment; users embraced some, but others proved ineffective, harmful or both. With varying degrees of success, women sued the manufacturers, who then blamed the cost of liability insurance and government regulation for stifling innovation.[14]

Contraception benefited from the argument that it would reduce abortions; abortion itself was always a trickier topic. In Britain, where governments would not lead in such a sensitive area, private members' bills were the vehicles for reform. One became the Abortion Act 1967, part of the raft of 'permissive' legislation that also partially decriminalized homosexuality and facilitated divorce. These liberal reforms under a Labour government broke with authoritarian moralism, but sought more to reduce harm and strengthen institutions than to expand private freedoms.[15] The act made abortion

12 Barbara Brookes and Paul Roth, '*Rex v. Bourne* and the medicalization of abortion', in Clark and Crawford, *Legal Medicine*, pp. 314–43; Sally Sheldon, *Beyond Control: Medical Power and Abortion Law* (London, 1997), pp. 79–81.

13 David J. Garrow, *Liberty and Sexuality: The Right to Privacy and the Making of* Roe v. Wade (Berkeley, CA, 1998); John W. Johnson, Griswold v. Connecticut: *Birth Control and the Constitutional Right to Privacy* (Lawrence, KA, 2005); Latham, *Regulating Reproduction*, pp. 24–81.

14 Olszynko-Gryn, 'Technologies of Contraception and Abortion'.

15 Weeks, *Sex, Politics and Society*, pp. 344–7.

more public to stamp out backstreet operations and Harley Street racketeering, and formalized medical control to protect doctors as well as ensure parliamentary support. Reports of malformations after a recent German measles (rubella) epidemic and the thalidomide disaster bolstered public backing. The model was the liberal regime run by the Regius Professor of Midwifery at Aberdeen, Dugald Baird, who took advantage of the fact that in Scotland abortion had remained a common-law offence requiring 'criminal intent'.[16]

The act allowed termination by a registered medical practitioner if two practitioners held 'in good faith' that 'continuance of the pregnancy would involve risk to the life of the pregnant woman, or of injury to [her] physical or mental health … or any existing children of her family, greater than if the pregnancy were terminated', or if there was 'a substantial risk' of serious handicap in any child born. A doctor could act alone in an emergency, and there was a conscientious objection clause. The 1861 law stayed on the books, but medical practitioners – throughout Britain, though not in Northern Ireland – were now protected from prosecution.

The 1967 act came to be described as balancing the rights of fetus and woman, but feminists charged that it primarily reinforced those of physicians. Separate 'social' clauses, which (doctors feared) might have compelled them to perform abortions after rape or where the woman's capacity as a mother would be overstrained by the care of a child, were rejected in favour of medical criteria that include mental health and allow doctors to take account of the woman's environment. These requirements seem anomalous now that physicians are supposed to respect patients' rights to decide their own treatment, and can delay access.

Yet the courts' and parliament's respect for medical judgement has acted as a bulwark against external pressures. The act itself has withstood over twenty parliamentary challenges with the only major revision in 1990. This wrote a time limit of twenty-four weeks into the Abortion Act for those terminations performed on the basis of comparative risk to the woman's mental or physical health (but not on the other grounds). Medical support for reform notwithstanding, abortion, unlike homosexuality and divorce, has been too contested to benefit from further liberalizations since the late 1990s. But medicalization has helped to depoliticize the procedure in Britain – unlike in the United States.[17]

In Depression-era America, with abortion more needed and more visible in the hospitals, some pressure had built for reform, but traditional gender roles were reasserted in the 1940s. In a kind of pronatalist McCarthyism, therapeutic abortion committees

16 Gayle Davis, 'The medical community and abortion law reform: Scotland in national context, *c.* 1960–1980', in Imogen Goold and Catherine Kelly (eds.), *Lawyers' Medicine: The Legislature, the Courts and Medical Practice, 1760–2000* (Oxford, 2009), pp. 143–65.

17 Sheldon, *Beyond Control.*

limited doctors' legal room to manoeuvre; meanwhile, septic wards filled with those whose poverty or race had denied them access to procedures that should have been safe but accounted for ever higher proportions of maternal deaths. This repressive, discriminatory system provoked a reform movement among physicians and lawyers, while fear of rubella spurred the first mass efforts to decriminalize abortion. Then women's liberation groups went further, and by the late 1960s the medical profession – once cheerleading for criminalization – was agitating for repeal not reform. Physicians, their status now at a peak, disliked the infringement of their autonomy, while most of the public saw abortion, like contraception, as a private matter. More than in Britain a few years before, legal challenges drew on feminism and population control, but the key judgement also concerned a physician's freedom to practise.[18]

Campaigners brought two cases to the Supreme Court, which on 22 January 1973 struck down the state anti-abortion laws as unconstitutional. In *Roe v. Wade*, an appeal against the Texas law that allowed abortion only 'to save the life of the mother', the court recognized it as a fundamental right within the right of privacy, but subject to limitations defined by the end of the first trimester and fetal viability. The majority opinion declared that during the first trimester, when abortion was safer than childbirth, 'the attending physician, in consultation with his patient, is free to determine, without regulation by the State, that, in his medical judgment, the patient's pregnancy should be terminated'. Thereafter the state could intervene to protect 'maternal health', and after viability the state's interest in protecting 'potential life' became 'compelling'. The same day, in an appeal against the more liberal Georgia law, the court declared invalid the restrictions imposed by the medical committees.[19]

Roe v. Wade is a landmark in the histories of reproduction and of the United States. It did not give feminists all they wanted, but is credited, at least, with a steep fall in maternal mortality. As abortion moved to the centre of American politics and its culture wars, *Roe* also became one of the court's most vilified decisions (Fig. 40.2). Yet it did not do half the things for which both sides blame it – campaigners did. Anti-abortionists later criticized *Roe* as 'judicial activism', but first focused on a fetal rights amendment. When that failed, the majority swung behind an 'incrementalist' approach to hollowing out the freedoms granted in 1973: legal challenges, influencing elections, swaying judicial appointments. By knitting these strategies together in the late 1970s, the New Right ensured that abortion would dominate reproductive politics wherever

18 Reagan, *When Abortion Was a Crime*; Leslie J. Reagan, *Dangerous Pregnancies: Mothers, Disabilities, and Abortion in Modern America* (Berkeley, CA, 2010); also Garrow, *Liberty and Sexuality*; Sara Dubow, *Ourselves Unborn: A History of the Fetus in Modern America* (New York, NY, 2011).

19 *Roe v. Wade*, 410 U.S. 113 (1973), www.law.cornell.edu/supremecourt/text/410/113; *Doe v. Bolton*, 410 U.S. 179 (1973), www.law.cornell.edu/supremecourt/text/410/179.

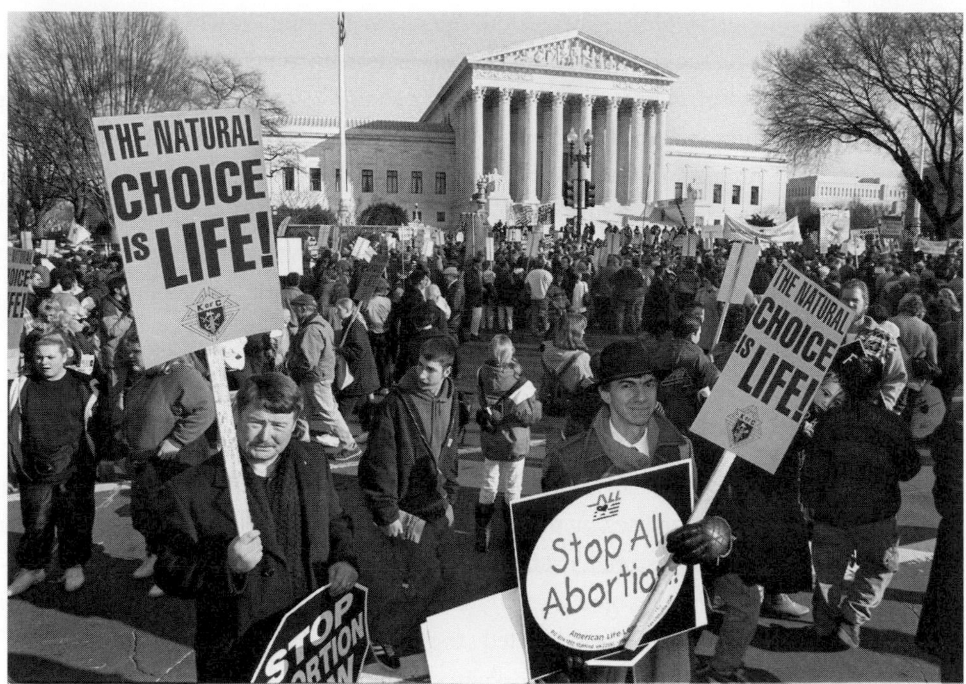
THE NATURAL CHOICE IS LIFE!
THE NATURAL CHOICE IS LIFE!
Stop All Abortion
STOP ABORTION

Figure 40.2 Abortion opponents march in front of the Supreme Court during a 1996 rally to mark the twenty-third anniversary of *Roe v. Wade*. In the foreground, the protesters hold placards by Catholic organizations, the Knights of Columbus and the American Life League; in the background, the west façade of Cass Gilbert's 1935 building bears the motto 'Equal justice under law'. AP Photo / Doug Mills, Rex Features.

in the world US influence was felt, especially through the 1973 Helms and 1976 Hyde amendments banning federal funding. Nor did *Roe* block feminist efforts to dissociate abortion from population control and craft a wider agenda for reproductive rights, which some did pursue through the mid-1970s; but following anti-abortionist successes, and in a neoliberal climate, 'choice' resonated more than equality. The meaning of *Roe* changed as debates polarized further, with the Supreme Court acting almost as a regulator, determining the acceptability of state laws.[20] Today, depending on where she lives and her resources, a woman in America may find that abortion is barely available, although a legal right.

Yet more has been at stake in the legal history of fertility control even than access to safe products and procedures, as the US history of sterilization shows. From 1971, the Association for Voluntary Sterilization, Zero Population Growth and the American

20 Mary Ziegler, *After Roe: The Lost History of the Abortion Debate* (Cambridge, MA, 2015), p. 201; also Johanna Schoen, *Abortion after Roe* (Chapel Hill, NC, 2015); Solveig Jülich, '"Drama of Life before Birth"', Exhibit 34, this book.

Civil Liberties Union supported 'Operation Lawsuit', in which white women succeeded in winning the right to voluntary sterilization, by then a simple laparoscopic procedure, by extending the privacy argument. By contrast, the many suits brought by poor black, Latina and Native American women for redress after forced sterilizations under government programmes from the 1960s mostly failed. Victory in the extreme case of *Relf v. Weinberger*, concerning black sisters of 12 and 14 sterilized without their knowledge in 1973, led a few years later to federal guidelines banning sterilization of minors and mandating informed consent for adults, but also restricting voluntary access to the procedure (Fig. 40.3).[21]

Regulating Infertility Services

More generally during the 1970s, revelations of infringements of reproductive rights, and other medical abuses by professional and state power, shook regulatory regimes. Medicine sought to restore trust by accepting some lay input into professional self-regulation, and by recognizing bioethics, which emerged as a distinct field in the United States in the 1970s and, with a more restricted scope, in the United Kingdom in the 1980s.[22] Alongside transplant surgery, euthanasia, vivisection and genetics, the most debate was provoked by research on gametes and embryos, and the resulting treatments for infertility.

Medico-legal commentators after World War II perceived a need to regulate new, or newly common, procedures. Artificial insemination had featured in court since the nineteenth century, but began seriously to exercise lawyers only now that insemination by donor was more widely reported. Although the practice was never criminalized in the United Kingdom, entering the husband's name on the birth certificate was illegal, but the law typically became involved only in divorce, illegitimacy or inheritance cases. In Britain in 1960, the government-appointed Feversham Committee recommended discouraging what the Christian churches condemned as adultery, but the medical establishment and the Anglican church gradually became more accepting. Donor insemination was legally recognized within the Family Law Reform Act 1987, the debate having been transformed by in vitro fertilization (IVF).[23]

21 Rebecca M. Kluchin, *Fit to Be Tied: Sterilization and Reproductive Rights in America, 1950–1980* (New Brunswick, NJ, 2009), pp. 114–83.

22 M. L. Tina Stevens, *Bioethics in America: Origins and Cultural Politics* (Baltimore, MD, 2000); Duncan Wilson, *A History of British Bioethics* (Manchester, 2014).

23 Kara W. Swanson, 'Adultery by doctor: Artificial insemination, 1890–1945', *Chicago-Kent Law Review* 87 (2012), 591–633; Naomi Pfeffer, *The Stork and the Syringe: A Political History of Reproductive Medicine* (Cambridge, 1993), pp. 112–41; Martin Richards, 'The development of governance and regulation of donor conception in the UK', in Susan Golombok *et al.* (eds.), *Regulating Reproductive Donation* (Cambridge, 2016), pp. 14–36; Christina Benninghaus, 'Modern Infertility', Chapter 31; Nick Hopwood, 'Artificial Fertilization', Chapter 39, this book.

Sterilization: Newest

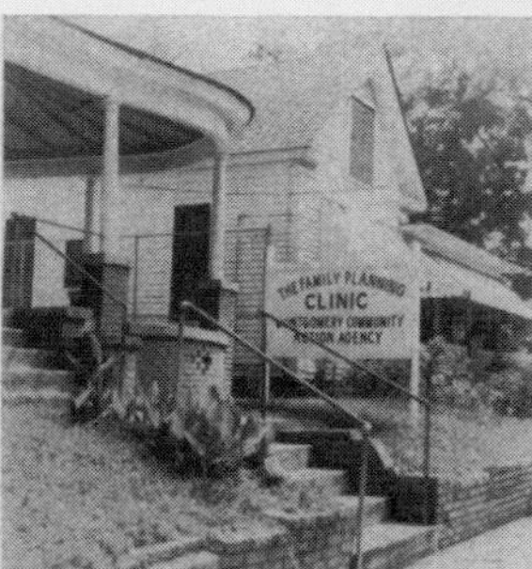

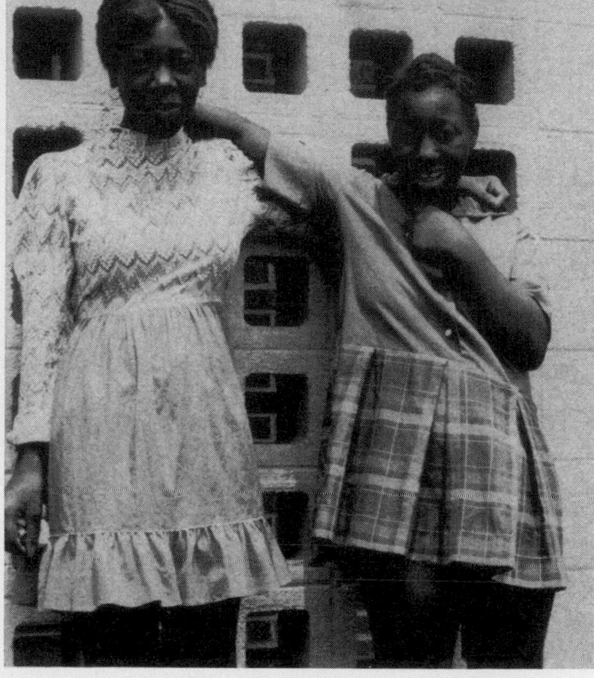

Looking deceptively harmless, Montgomery Family Planning Clinic (above) has nevertheless authorized numerous sterilizations of black minors such as Relf sisters (right), Mary Alice (l.), 14, and Minnie Lee, 12. Below is Joseph Levin, attorney for Relf family.

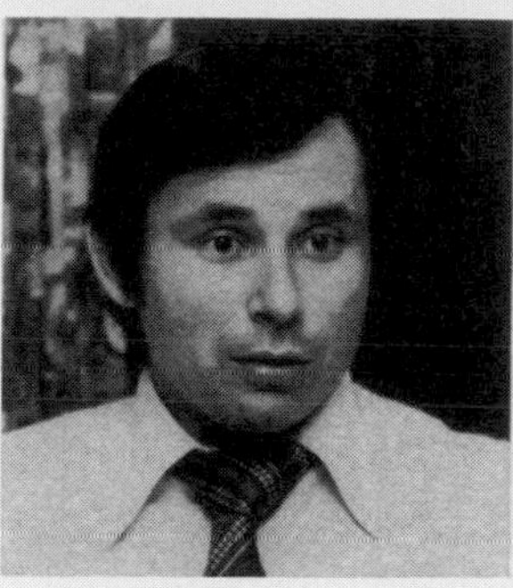

THIS is a story about a crime and a special kind of death in the land of equal opportunity. Last June, on a warm, unsuspecting morning in Montgomery, Ala., two young black girls were wheeled into a hospital operating room and rendered sexually sterile by tubal ligation because, somewhere in their neighborhood, somewhere on their block, so the authorities said, "boys were hanging around." Later it was learned that the girls and their parents were on welfare and that their welfare status had some direct connection with the sterilizations.

Four months have passed since that June morning, yet it is still difficult to comprehend fully the enormity of what actually happened to those young girls—difficult to digest the news of other sterilization cases reported in the nation, or the latest revelations that since 1964 more than one thousand American women, most of them black and all of them poor, have been forced to submit to involuntary sterilization. It is difficult even to understand what such a crime supposes itself to be saying, what it presumes itself to be wanting, what circumstances would permit it or what it portends.

Here are a few details:

• On June 13, two representatives of the federally financed Montgomery Community Action Agency called on Mrs. Minnie Relf, an illiterate welfare mother of four, to tell her that her two youngest daughters, Mary Alice, 14, and Minnie Lee, 12, needed some shots. (Agency officials, incidentally, have claimed that young Minnie Lee Relf is mentally retarded.) The nature of the shots, according to Mrs. Relf, seemed to be uncertain; but, believing that the agency had the best interests of her daughters' health in mind, Mrs. Relf consented—and subsequently signed an informed consent release. "I put an X on a paper," she said later. And, armed with that "X", the agency, which operates a family planning clinic also federally supported, affected its own version of population control—ostensibly because of those "boys . . . hanging around." (After the Relf case came to light, it was discovered that for the past 15 months, federally sponsored birth control clinics around the nation have sterilized at least 80 other minors.)

• In July, at a crowded press conference in New York City, Nial Ruth Cox, an angry, unwed black mother, accompanied by her lawyer from the American Civil Liberties Union (ACLU), revealed that eight years earlier, when she was pregnant with her only child, she too had been forced to undergo permanent sterilization in New Bern, N. C. Miss Cox, who is 26 years old, had agreed to the sterilization, she said, because she had been told it would be a temporary measure and also because she had been warned that if she did not agree, her family would cease to receive welfare payments. After a New York doctor recently told her she could never have another

150

Figure 40.3 The case of Mary Alice and Minnie Lee Relf, reported in the African-American magazine *Ebony*. This page shows the sisters, the clinic where they were sterilized, '[l]ooking deceptively harmless', and their lawyer, Joseph Levin of the Southern Poverty Law Center in Montgomery, Alabama. Jack Slater, 'Sterilization: Newest threat to the poor', *Ebony* (Oct. 1973), 150–6, on 150, 34 × 25 cm, courtesy Ebony Media Operations, LLC.

From the late 1960s to the late 1970s, general ethical questions dominated the transatlantic controversy over reports of progress with IVF, especially from the British team led by Robert Edwards, Patrick Steptoe and Jean Purdy. Their achievement of a live human birth in 1978 opened the possibility of government funding for further research and made it urgent to regulate clinics. While private-sector IVF within a traditional social and moral order exemplified the free-enterprise ideals of Margaret Thatcher's Conservative administration, a mission gained ground to discipline the professions, rejecting self-regulation by scientists and insisting on external oversight to safeguard consumer choice. In 1982, the government established a Committee of Inquiry into Human Fertilisation and Embryology. This embodied outside control in its lay chair, the moral philosopher Mary Warnock, together with three lawyers and two social workers, a theologian and a matron administrator with eight doctors and scientists, only one of whom had specialist embryological expertise.[24]

Warnock's 1984 report recommended allowing infertility treatment by IVF as well as egg and sperm donation within an assumed framework of (heterosexual) marriage, and research on human embryos up to fourteen days, subject to 'active regulation and monitoring' by a 'statutory licensing authority'. In a move unprecedented in British medicine, the committee proposed that this body, chaired by a layperson and with 'substantial lay representation' and the support of an inspectorate, should license treatment and research and offer guidance and advice. Different minorities on the committee dissented from the exclusion of gestational surrogacy from the remit and objected to embryo experiments.

The medico-scientific establishment responded to parliamentary criticism of Warnock's main recommendation by setting up a Voluntary Licensing Authority with a lay chair and lay majority. The government delayed action on most of the Warnock proposals, but did legislate in two areas of general agreement: to outlaw commercial surrogacy agencies (1985) and to recognize the partner of a woman inseminated with donor sperm as the father of the child, while removing the rights and duties of parenthood from the donor (1987). On embryo research, there ensued six years of public and parliamentary controversy, structured by battles over abortion and challenges to and defences of 'traditional' families. Scientists and doctors mobilized to stop the Unborn Children (Protection) Bill 1985, which would have allowed use of embryos for implanting only and required a separate licence for each one; researchers and clinicians instead built a consensus behind what became the Human Fertilisation and Embryology Act 1990. This implemented most of Warnock's recommendations by establishing a Human Fertilisation and Embryology Authority (HFEA) with a lay chair and 'at least one-third but fewer than half' of its members medical practitioners or persons 'concerned with keeping or

24 Hopwood, 'Artificial Fertilization'; Wilson, *History of British Bioethics*, pp. 140–86.

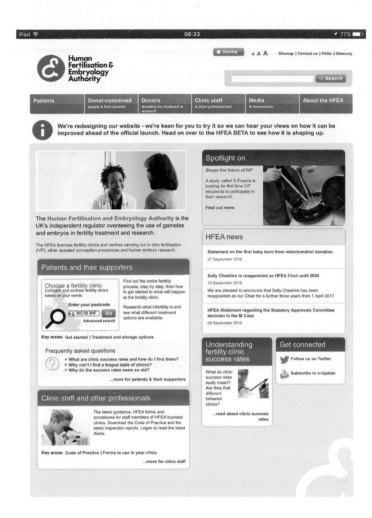

Figure 40.4 The website of the Human Fertilisation and Embryology Authority. The regulator presents itself as serving patients, children, donors, professionals, the media and researchers; as approachable and supportive; and as working in a fast-moving field in which there is much recent news. Screenshot of www.hfea.gov.uk, 14 July 2016.

using gametes and embryos outside the body'. The HFEA was charged with regulating and advising on infertility treatment, embryo storage and research (Fig. 40.4).[25]

Some practitioners have resented the stringent regulation, but the system inspires public confidence still. It represents a period 'when the emphasis on oversight, public accountability and rights complemented widespread demands for audit and consumer choice'. Statutory regulation of a medical specialty by a lay body, according to bioethical ideals, subsequently served as a model for the Human Tissue Authority and a reformed General Medical Council.

25 R. L. Cunningham, 'Legislating on human fertilization and embryology in the United Kingdom', *Statute Law Review* 12 (1991), 214–27; Jennifer Gunning and Veronica English, *Human in Vitro Fertilization: A Case Study in the Regulation of Medical Innovation* (Aldershot, 1993); Martin H. Johnson and Anastasia A. Theodosiou, 'PGD and the making of the "genetic embryo" as a political tool', in Sheila A. M. McLean and Sarah Elliston (eds.), *Regulating Pre-implantation Genetic Diagnosis: A Comparative and Theoretical Analysis* (Abingdon, 2013), pp. 37–70; Michael Mulkay, *The Embryo Research Debate: Science and the Politics of Reproduction* (Cambridge, 1997).

Critics of the neoliberal 'audit society' have fought back with claims that external oversight on behalf of supposedly empowered consumers has paradoxically corroded public trust, but the HFEA has survived attempted merger and abolition.[26] The authority has lasted in part because it has taken flexible and permissive approaches to new technologies, and because key laws have changed. Since 2004, donor-conceived offspring have had the right, from the age of 18, to be told the donor's identity. The 2008 revision of the HFE Act removed the requirement that clinics take account of a child's 'need for a father' and permitted two women each to be recognized as parents on a birth certificate. Calls are becoming louder to bring surrogacy more within the scope of regulation.

While the trend towards external regulation is international, other countries have adopted different approaches, shaped by national histories and stakeholders' strategies. In a globalized world, UK doctors take advantage of legal variations to operate clinics in other jurisdictions, and likewise patients travel for surrogacy, egg donation and anonymous sperm donation.[27] International directives, notably from the European Union on Tissues and Cells and on Patient Mobility, shape the law in member countries. So do judgements of the European Court of Human Rights, for example, against the refusal of states to recognize children born abroad after procedures illegal in the home country, and upholding governments' right to restrict treatments available elsewhere in the EU.[28]

The United States contrasts to the highly regulated United Kingdom. Medical and scientific opposition to IVF was strong in the early 1970s, especially from American bioethicists. The anti-abortion movement then made federal funding of embryo research politically impossible. IVF nevertheless took off in the early 1980s, and today the reproductive services industry generates revenue of several billion dollars a year. Mostly in the private sector, it is regulated by little more than market forces and private contract law. The 1992 Fertility Clinic Success Rate and Certification Act requests reporting, there are federal guidelines for clinic and laboratory quality, and FDA inspections screen for disease, the reliability of tests and the adequacy of data collection. Some states have legislated, for example, for the extent of insurance coverage, though most exclude IVF. The American Society for Reproductive Medicine promulgates standards of professional practice, but these are widely ignored. While abortion politics constrain state-financed human embryo and stem-cell research, payment for egg donation is generally permitted, anonymous sperm donation is standard and all kinds of procedures are exploited, also by travellers from other jurisdictions, in ways that would be illegal elsewhere.[29]

26 Martin H. Johnson, 'HFEA reprieved: For the moment!', *Reproductive BioMedicine Online* 26 (2013), 303–4; Wilson, *History of British Bioethics*, pp. 243 (quotation), 262–3.

27 Nick Hopwood, 'Globalization', Chapter 43, this book.

28 Golombok *et al.*, *Regulating Reproductive Donation*.

29 Deborah Spar, *The Baby Business: How Money, Science and Politics Drive the Commerce of Conception* (Cambridge, MA, 2006); Lisa Hope Harris, 'Challenging conception: A clinical and cultural history of in

Conclusion

Over the past two centuries, an increasing volume of ever more detailed statute and case law has not just prohibited activities but regulated practice and recognized reproductive rights – albeit often precariously and without linking these to a more comprehensive guarantee of gender equality. Legislation has shaped who could start a family and redefined what abortion and contraception meant. State and medical power has risen, but if states are now withdrawing from the market, reproduction is more medicalized than ever, although with laypeople involved in its regulation.

People have often ignored legislation. They have subverted or evaded the law through under-the-counter sales or underground referrals and by travelling to other countries or ordering items from abroad. Just as important, the daily workings of the legal and medical systems have changed even when the texts of laws did not: abortion was less available in 1950s America than in the 1920s, although the law on the books was the same. Yet laws have mattered enough to make them prime targets of reform campaigns and symbols of successful change.

vitro fertilization in the United States', unpublished PhD thesis, University of Michigan (2006); Thomas Banchoff, *Embryo Politics: Ethics and Policy in Atlantic Democracies* (Ithaca, NY, 2011).

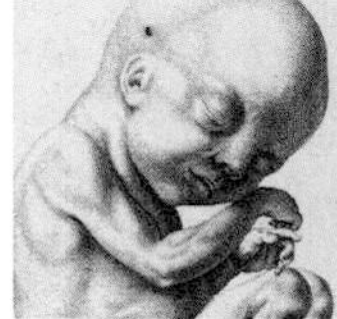

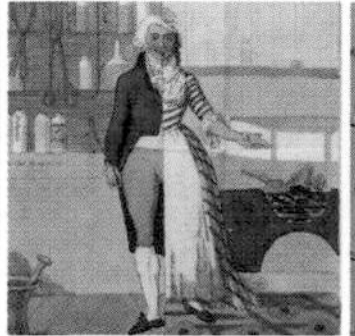

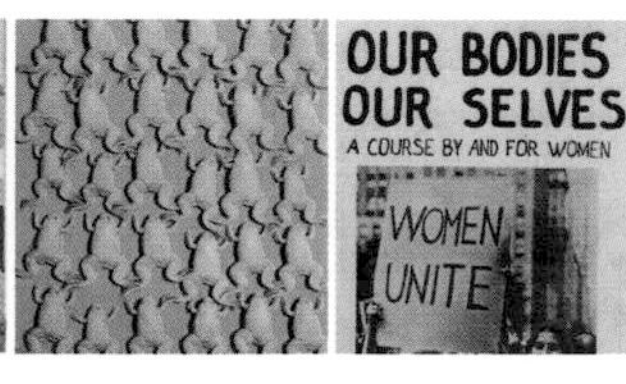

Exhibits 20–40

Exhibit 20

A Microscopical Salon

Mary Terrall

In the 1740s, Georges-Louis Leclerc de Buffon, director of the King's Garden in Paris, was working on a theory of reproduction based on controversial claims about the capacity of organic matter to organize itself. Rejecting the notion of pre-existing germs created by God, Buffon speculated that living beings form at each conception from mixtures of organic molecules in male and female fluids. Driven to combine by 'penetrating forces' analogous to gravity, these bits of organic matter would then build themselves into offspring resembling the parents, with no need for divine intervention.

This vignette opens the second volume of Buffon's massive *Natural History, General and Particular*, where he introduced his contentious theory to the public. The only image in the many tomes of the lavishly illustrated work to represent identifiable individuals doing experiments, it emphasizes the empirical justification for radical conjectures about self-organizing matter. Buffon enlisted the English naturalist and Catholic priest John Turberville Needham, and Louis-Jean-Marie Daubenton, curator of collections at the royal garden, as witnesses to his observations of seminal fluids. Using a state-of-the-art microscope belonging to Needham, all three agreed that they saw 'moving bodies', which Buffon took to be the organic molecules required by his theory, in fluids from both sexes.

The men are working in an ad hoc laboratory, a repurposed dining room or parlour still furnished with the amenities of an aristocratic home: armchairs, clock, carved wall panels and paintings in ornate frames. On the table, a screen decorated in the fashionable Chinese style – note the parasol and conical hat – directs candlelight onto the microscope stage. The screen also demarcates the messy work of the young assistant at left, reaching into the dissected uterus of a recently killed female dog to extract 'seminal liquid', from the elegantly dressed gentlemen who can observe the animal fluids without dirtying their hands. The central figure, probably Daubenton, peers into the microscope at samples from one of the animal carcasses unceremoniously strewn across the furniture. Seated at right, Needham (in clerical collar, facing us) and Buffon converse animatedly about what they have seen, foreshadowing conversations about theories of reproduction among readers of this provocative book.

This portrait of an experiment in progress also displays the intertwined elements necessary to knowledge-making: the skilled hands of the dissector, the trained eye of the microscopist and the ideas traded in spirited conversation, where empirical evidence fed theoretical speculation. By placing the light at the very centre of the image, the artist suggests a more emblematic reading as well: the reflected illumination and the microscope evoke the secular light of knowledge rooted in the senses. Ironically, despite the literary success of Buffon's *Natural History*, these observations proved difficult for others to replicate, and his theory of reproduction – the first to be so labelled – attracted very few adherents.

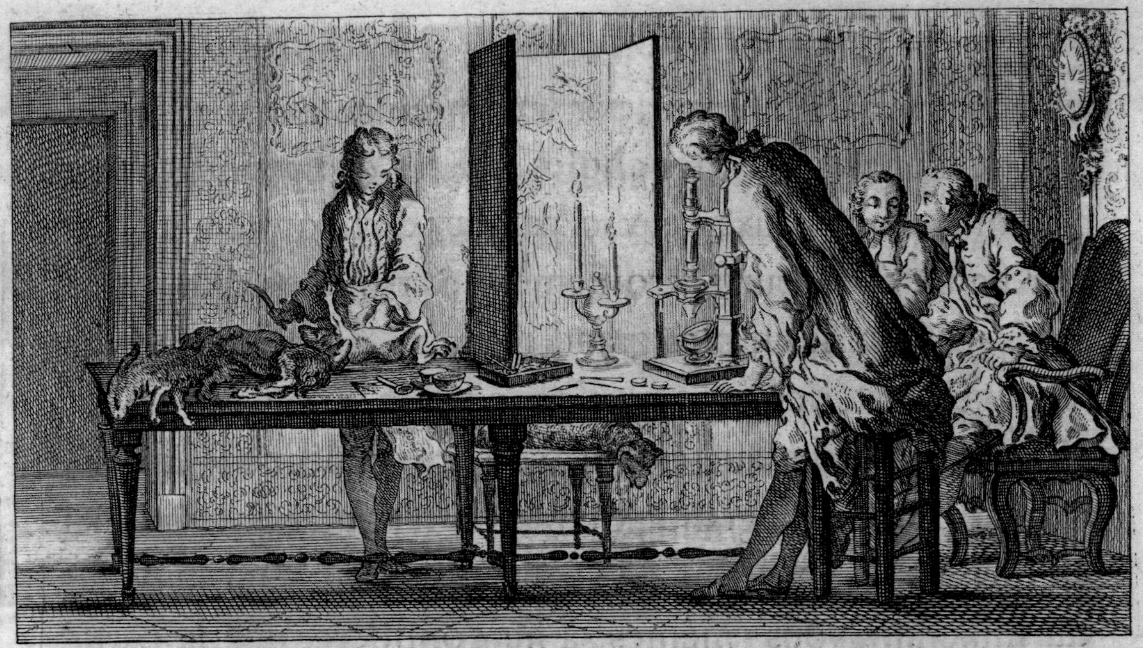

Title vignette, drawn by Jacques de Sève and engraved by François Antoine Aveline, from Georges-Louis Leclerc de Buffon, *Histoire naturelle, générale et particulière, avec la description du Cabinet du Roy*, vol. 2, 2nd edn (Paris: Imprimerie royale, 1750). Vignette 6.7 × 12 cm. Cambridge University Library.

FURTHER READING

Chapters 20, 26 and 28 and Exhibits 16, 22, 23, 26 and 32, this book.

Marc J. Ratcliff, *The Quest for the Invisible: Microscopy in the Enlightenment* (Aldershot, 2009).

Shirley A. Roe, 'John Turberville Needham and the generation of living organisms', *Isis* 74 (1983), 159–84.

Mary Terrall, 'Speculation and experiment in Enlightenment life sciences', in Staffan Müller-Wille and Hans-Jörg Rheinberger (eds.), *Heredity Produced: At the Crossroads of Biology, Politics, and Culture, 1500–1870* (Cambridge, MA, 2007), pp. 253–75.

Exhibit 21

A Crystal Womb

Lucia Dacome

This model is part of a midwifery collection gathered by the eighteenth-century surgeon and man-midwife Giovanni Antonio Galli in Bologna, Italy. It was one of several 'machines' supposed to mimic the female body in pregnancy and childbirth. The collection also included specimens of the pelvis, wax anatomies and numerous clay models of the gravid uterus. The model seen here is attributed to Antonio Cartolari, a Bolognese wood-carver, designer and mechanic. It consists of a wooden base, which represents a schematic anatomical section through a woman's life-size body from the abdomen to the sawn-off thighs, and an openable crystal ball depicting the womb at full term. A circular cavity replaces the external genitals. Midwifery trainees were supposed to reach in and extract a folding puppet from the crystal womb.

First displayed in Galli's residence, in 1757 the collection was purchased by Pope Benedict XIV, who donated it to the Institute of the Sciences, the Bolognese temple of natural knowledge, in the premises of which it can still be seen today. Here Galli continued to offer midwifery classes to midwives in training and medical students from the city and beyond. Visitors, including grand tourists – those members of the elite who travelled Europe for pleasure, health and education – also viewed the collection.

The models engaged users' senses in various ways. For lay visitors, they mainly addressed the eyes, eliciting a sense of wonder as they unveiled the elusive world of generation and pregnancy. For trainees, different models tutored the senses differently. Although midwifery was associated with manual dexterity, early modern midwives used both sight and touch. In Galli's collection, fragile wax models engaged the eyes through the systematic visualization of internal body parts, while clay models could also be examined manually. However, when trainees worked with the crystal model, they were blindfolded and forced to employ only their hands. The use of crystal presented the gravid uterus as an allegedly transparent object of knowledge, but the students had to extract the puppet without using their eyes. Galli, meanwhile, visually inspected their manual skills through the crystal ball. The scene staged an act of training and surveillance as well as an impressive spectacle.

Before Galli, other man-midwives, such as Richard Manningham in London, had used glass models and machines in their midwifery courses. After Galli, glass continued to feature in midwifery collections like the one his pupil Luigi Calza assembled in Padua. Midwifery machines, also called 'phantoms' or 'mannequins', still conjured up the performance of childbirth, sometimes in theatrical demonstrations. Realized in various materials such as leather, fabric, wood and wax as well as glass, they aimed to train practitioners 'without risk to the living'. Yet, as observation and the senses became integral to training in lying-in hospitals, the bodies of poor, unmarried women were sometimes turned, as the Göttingen man-midwife Friedrich Benjamin Osiander controversially put it, into 'living phantoms': materials to teach students alongside models and machines.

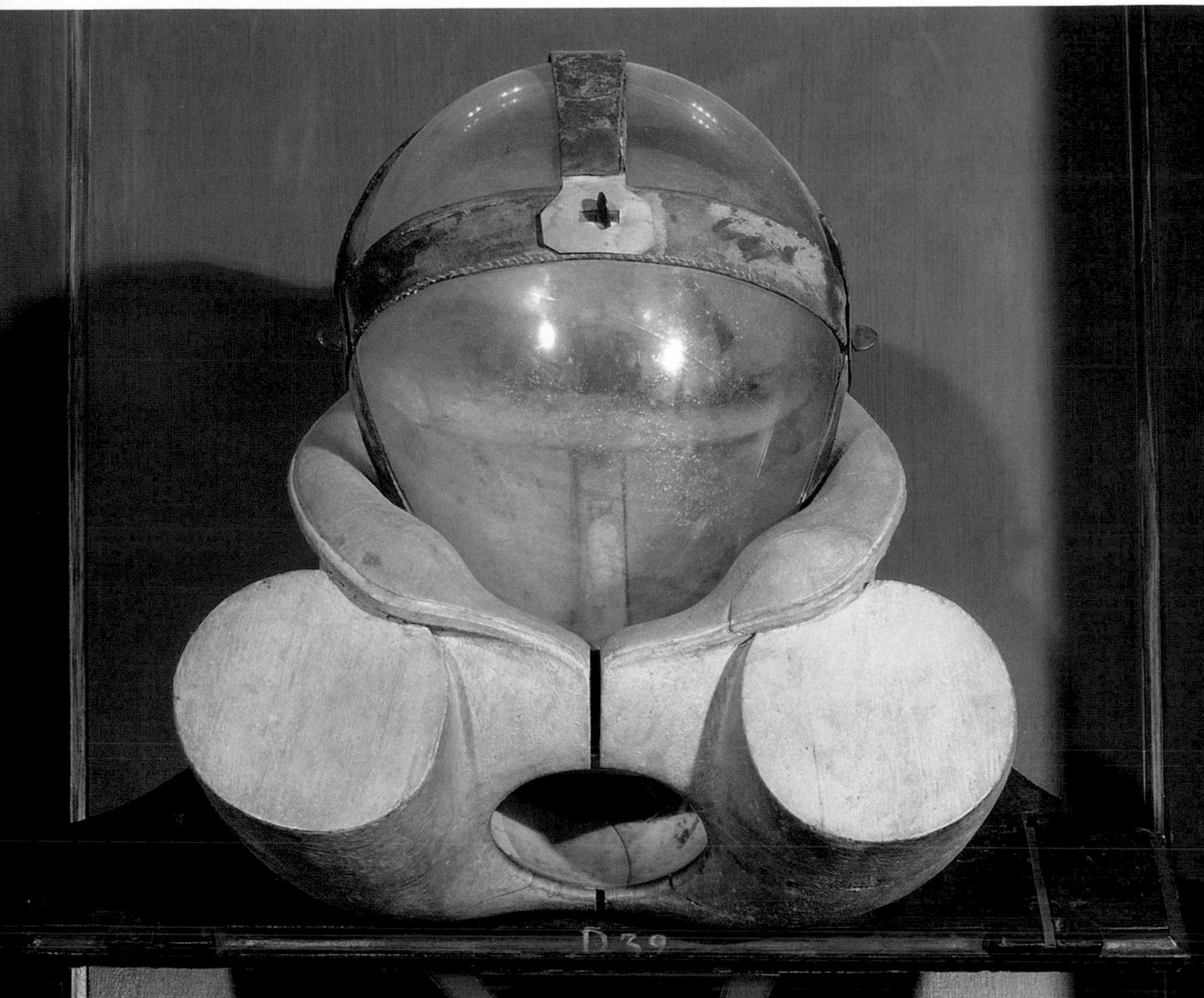

Antonio Cartolari, 'Abdomen and pelvis with crystal womb' in glass, wood and metal. Courtesy of Museo di Palazzo Poggi, Università di Bologna. 64 × 50 × 40 cm.

FURTHER READING

Chapters 15, 22 and 37 and Exhibit 22, this book.

Marco Bortolotti *et al.*, *Ars obstetricia bononiensis: Catalogo ed inventario del Museo ostetrico Giovan Antonio Galli* (Bologna, 1988).

Lucia Dacome, *Malleable Anatomies: Models, Makers, and Material Culture in Eighteenth-Century Italy* (Oxford, 2017).

Ambre Murard, 'La rappresentazione del corpo femminile nell'ostetricia settecentesca: "Le macchine" di Giovan Antonio Galli', in Claudia Pancino (ed.), *Corpi: Storia, metafore, rappresentazioni fra Medioevo ed età contemporanea* (Venice, 2000), pp. 41–54.

Exhibit 22

Man-Midwifery Dissected

Ludmilla Jordanova

This image has been reproduced so many times that its distinctiveness has been lost. The bisected figure originally appeared as the frontispiece to *Man-Midwifery Dissected*, an attack on men delivering babies, and as a stand-alone print. The book, first published in 1793, consists of fourteen letters to Alexander Hamilton, professor of midwifery in the University of Edinburgh, who was embroiled in disputes with other medical men about the management of childbirth. The author was named as John Blunt – the pseudonym of Samuel Fores, a successful printseller and publisher. The plate, possibly by Isaac Cruikshank, a well-known painter and caricaturist with whom Fores often worked, was subsequently hand-coloured. The fierce debates about who should assist women in childbirth gave the etching one context; the outpouring of satirical images that criticized every aspect of life in Georgian Britain provided another.

Social critique is expressed through a representation that looks innocuous at first sight. The standing figure, one side male, the other female, is decorous, lacking distorted body parts or grotesque facial expressions. The two halves match perfectly; Fores thereby stressed how deceptively dangerous male practitioners were. The instruments and potions in the background on the male side, with their sexual connotations, 'love water', for instance, provide a clue, but the words beneath the figure hold the real venom. They refer to the man-midwife as a monster, a specimen to be classified like any new species of animal. In 1793, the language of monstrosity was familiar in British culture as people struggled to come to terms with events in revolutionary France. Fores alluded to these when he presented the practices he abhorred as 'invented at Paris', while ironically invoking the famous French naturalist Buffon, recently deceased.

Fores plays with the word 'mid' by placing it precisely below the vertical line to reinforce his point about the artificiality of man-midwives, who are neither properly male nor female. Satirical prints had used bisected figures before; some even combined male and female faces to criticize women's supposedly unnatural participation in politics. The author here insisted on evidence and example to condemn 'obstetric butchery' as 'a personal, a domestic, and a national evil'. He opposed secrecy and instruments; childbirth was a 'process in nature' about which all adults should be well-informed.

Viewers of Fores's plate would have appreciated its satirical intent, and grasped that it attacked men encroaching on women's territory. We cannot know how many people saw the image, nor their reactions, but the book was small, accessible and relatively cheap. Deeming what happened in the delivery room, or was luridly imagined to go on there, to be of general interest, it testifies to the cultural idioms available to represent the intense feelings that man-midwifery provoked. It reveals awareness of what we call 'gender', and alarm at the blurring of boundaries between the sexes. The concern about men violating birthing women was no less heartfelt for all the elegance and simplicity of this composite monstrosity.

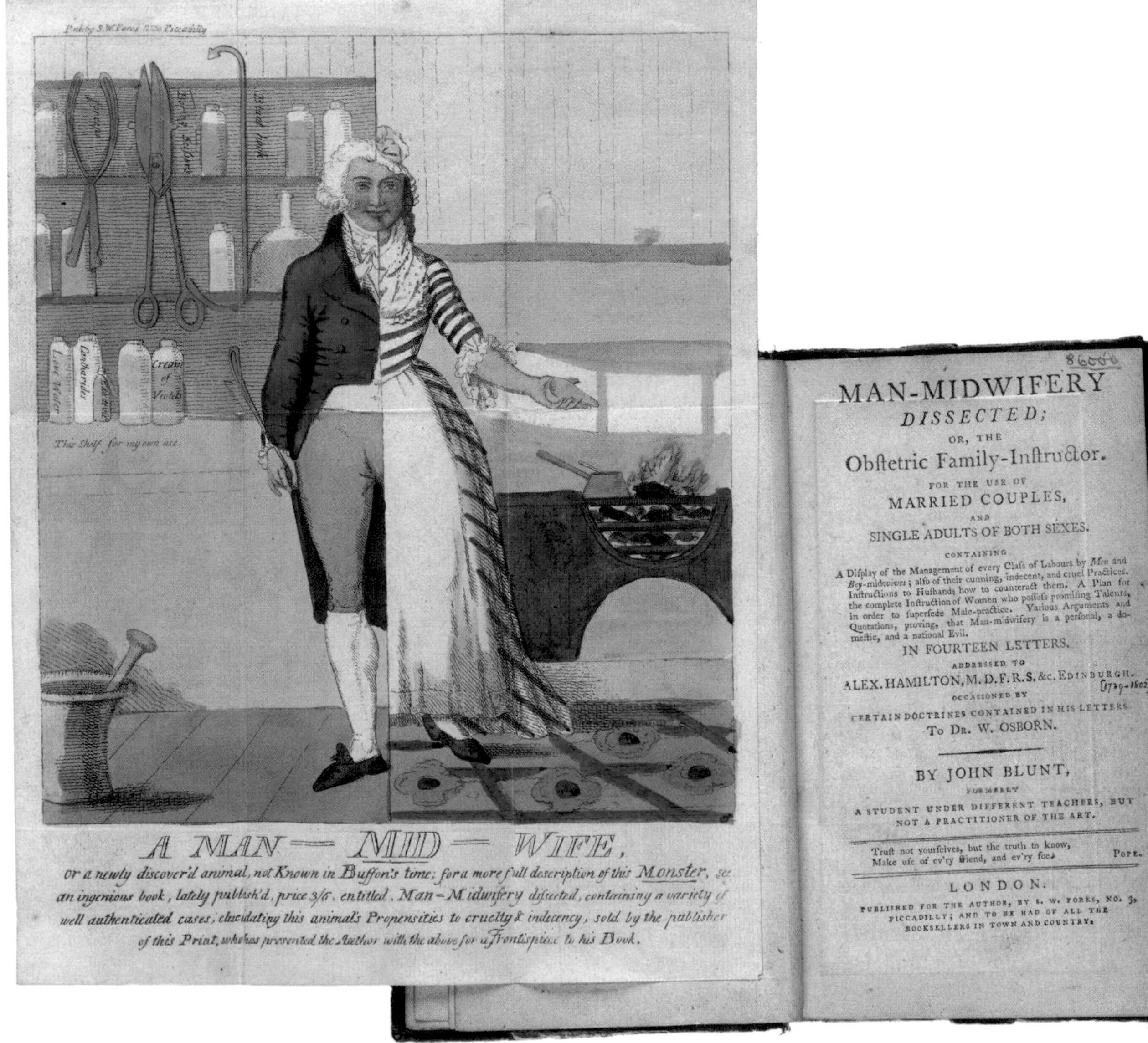

MAN-MIDWIFERY
DISSECTED;
OR, THE
Obstetric Family-Instructor.
FOR THE USE OF
MARRIED COUPLES,
AND
SINGLE ADULTS OF BOTH SEXES.
CONTAINING
A Display of the Management of every Class of Labours by *Men* and *Boy-midwives*; also of their cunning, indecent, and cruel Practices. Instructions to Husbands how to counteract them. A Plan for the complete Instruction of Women who possess promising Talents, in order to supersede Male-practice. Various Arguments and Quotations, proving, that Man-midwifery is a personal, a domestic, and a national Evil.
IN FOURTEEN LETTERS.
ADDRESSED TO
ALEX. HAMILTON, M. D. F. R. S. &c. EDINBURGH. [1729–1802]
OCCASIONED BY
CERTAIN DOCTRINES CONTAINED IN HIS LETTERS
TO DR. W. OSBORN.

BY JOHN BLUNT,
FORMERLY
A STUDENT UNDER DIFFERENT TEACHERS, BUT NOT A PRACTITIONER OF THE ART.

Trust not yourselves, but the truth to know,
Make use of ev'ry friend, and ev'ry foe. POPE.

LONDON:
PUBLISHED FOR THE AUTHOR, BY S. W. FORES, NO. 3, PICCADILLY; AND TO BE HAD OF ALL THE BOOKSELLERS IN TOWN AND COUNTRY.

Fold-out frontispiece (26 × 19 cm) and title-page (17 × 10 cm) to John Blunt [S. W. Fores, pseud.], *Man-Midwifery Dissected* (London: S. W. Fores for the author [1795?]). Wellcome Library, London, 22920/B.

FURTHER READING

Chapters 22 and 37 and Exhibits 13, 20, 21 and 25, this book.
Lisa Forman Cody, *Birthing the Nation: Sex, Science, and the Conception of Eighteenth-Century Britons* (Oxford, 2005).
Diana Donald, *The Age of Caricature: Satirical Prints in the Reign of George III* (New Haven, CT, 1996).
Ludmilla Jordanova, *Nature Displayed: Gender, Science and Medicine, 1760–1820* (London, 1999), pp. 23–7.

Exhibit 23

Images of Human Embryos

Nick Hopwood

Serial images of embryos and fetuses became the dominant representations of human origins only during the past hundred years, but visions of development have been traced back to a late eighteenth-century innovation. In 1799, the German anatomist Samuel Thomas Soemmerring authored 'images of human embryos': two large copper plates with ten pages of Latin text. Reproduced here, the first plate depicts 'embryos' between the third week and the fourth month of pregnancy in seventeen steps. It is generally regarded as the first connected series showing not just growth, but also an increase in complexity through human development.

Though earlier anatomists drew the uterus in ever greater detail, its contents had remained emblematic in drawings of children to come or about to be born. A scattered literature also contained studies of embryos, but Soemmerring complained that laypeople, judging by an adult standard of perfection, tended to reject them all 'with the greatest disgust as something malformed'. Insisting, by contrast, that some were most shapely, he wanted criteria appropriate to each age. We appreciate the rose in bloom, he wrote, but 'do not despise the bud'. He set out to offer the best series he could.

Soemmerring worked on collections of preparations that mostly originated in items that miscarrying women had brought to physicians. Reinterpreting these as embryos and fetuses, the collectors had usually dissected away the membranes, and with them traces of connection to the women. He and his artist Christian Koeck measured with a pair of compasses to produce a distanced and idealized effect. Soemmerring arranged the drawings in order of 'growth and development' and had those 'distinguished by beauty' engraved.

A controversial advocate of the innateness of human inequality, Soemmerring portrayed individuals as well as a series. Having recently drawn an adult female skeleton as distinct from the male throughout, he pointed out sex differences in embryonic chests, heads and extremities as well as genitals, and variations in character too. Looking along the bottom row, surely one male showed 'a certain innate (*nativam*) weakness' (fig. XV) and another 'strength' (XVI), and was there not already 'a certain innate friendliness' in the 'clear brow' of his favourite 'girl' (XVII)?

In the 1990s, the historian Barbara Duden presented Soemmerring's images as a novelty that heralded the 'public fetus'. Duden sketched how pregnancy, previously uncertain, precarious and of variable duration, became determinate and staged; and how doctors sought to replace quickening, that moment when the pregnant woman herself felt a child move, with independent testimony for use in paternity, infanticide and abortion trials. Today, there remains much evidence that pregnancies could be doubtful even into the twentieth century, but some historians find more certainty in the past. It has also been denied that Soemmerring's series is truly developmental, though the magnified outlines in the top row clearly change shape. Like so much else around 1800, these embryos were the culmination of an eighteenth-century tradition and began to map out a new terrain that others would cultivate, expand and contest.

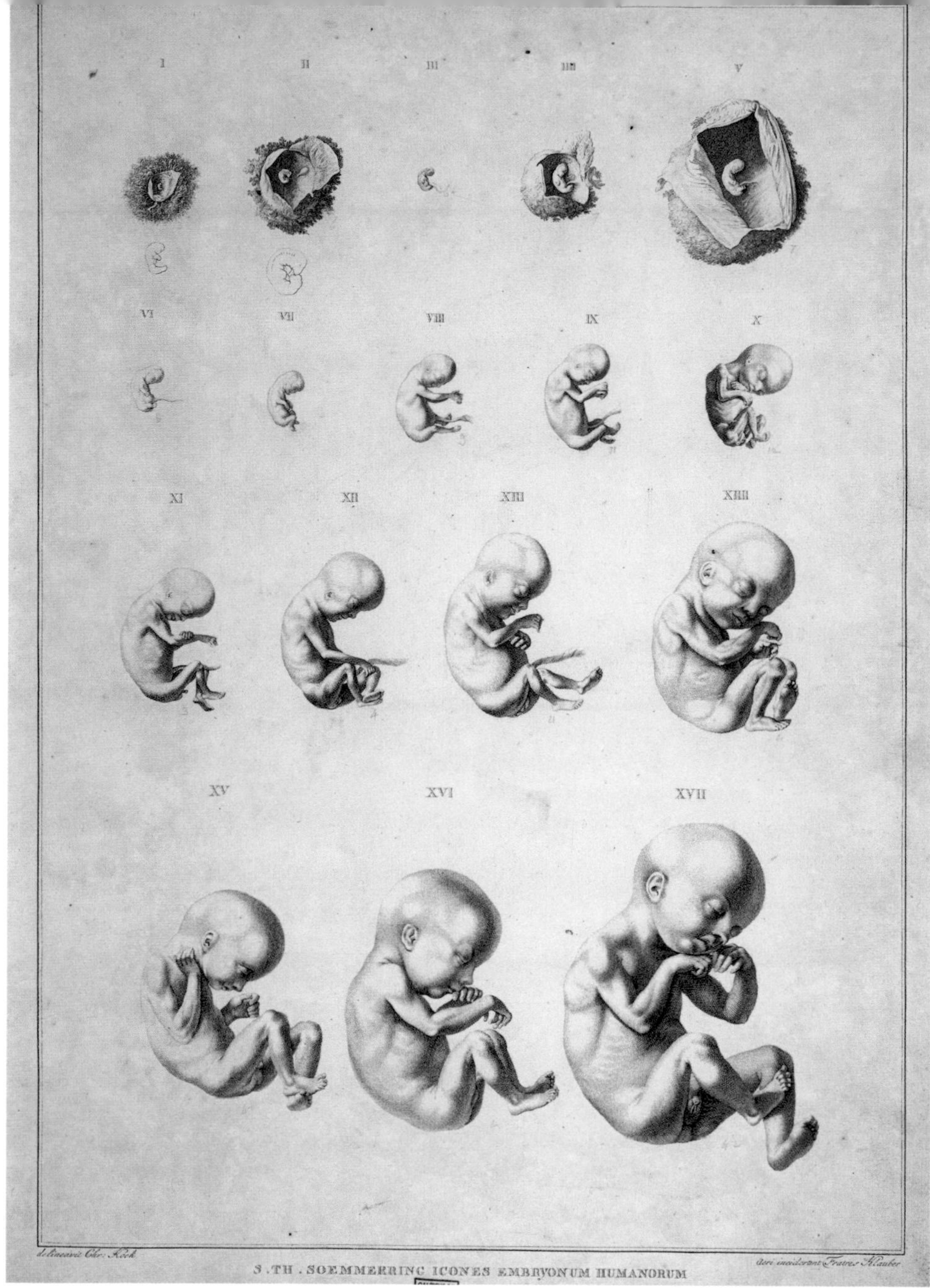

Copper engraving by the Klauber brothers, after drawings by Christian Koeck, from Samuel Thomas Soemmerring, *Icones embryonum humanorum* (Frankfurt: Varrentrapp und Wenner, 1799), plate I. 64 × 46 cm. Cambridge University Library.

FURTHER READING

Chapters 15, 16, 28, 38 and 39 and Exhibits 10, 15, 16, 32, 34 and 39, this book.

Tatjana Buklijas and Nick Hopwood, *Making Visible Embryos*, an online exhibition, www.hps.cam.ac.uk/visibleembryos/ (2008–10).

Barbara Duden, Jürgen Schlumbohm and Patrice Veit (eds.), *Geschichte des Ungeborenen. Zur Erfahrungs- und Wissenschaftsgeschichte der Schwangerschaft, 17.–20. Jahrhundert* (Göttingen, 2002).

Samuel Thomas Soemmerring, *Schriften zur Embryologie und Teratologie*, ed. Ulrike Enke, trans. Ferdinand Peter Moog (Basel, 2000).

Exhibit 24

Population in the South Sea

Rebecca Flemming

The British Admiralty instructed Captain James Cook, during his voyages of exploration in the late 1760s and 1770s, to survey and record the situation, nature and contents of the lands he encountered, to collect minerals and plants, and 'to observe the genius, temper, disposition, and number of the natives and inhabitants, where you find any'. While generally obedient to these orders, and contributing to the growing culture of quantification in many respects, Cook's published journals variously note the scarcity of people, or that his party was met by an immense crowd, but venture only a few counts of overall population.

Impressed by the quantity of men and war-canoes mustering in the bay at Oparee in 1774, Cook made an unusually detailed estimate of the total inhabitants of Tahiti, already famed as a paradisiacal island in the salons of Europe. He calculated the population based on the military manpower displayed, reckoning the numbers of canoes from each district, and their average crew, multiplying the resulting figure by three to account for women and children, and concluding that this territory, 'not forty leagues in circumference', supported at least 204,000 people, proof of its 'richness and fertility'. The episode appeared in the official account of the voyage, handsomely illustrated with engravings based on the work of the expedition artist William Hodges. This image emphasizes the crowding of the canoes in the bay, their complex construction and the exotic headdress of the warrior on the raised fighting platform.

Preparing their own expedition to the South Sea, members of the new Missionary Society eagerly read Cook's journals. Having his figure in mind, they were surprised, on landing in Tahiti in 1796, that an initial tour suggested a population of at most 50,000. Undertaking a fuller survey, Captain Wilson traversed the island asking, through an interpreter, about the numbers in each settlement, and recording the answers in the local units of principal and other households connected by worship at a shared 'morae' (*marae*). Allowing six persons to each unit, Wilson tabulated the results for a total of only 16,050. His approach was more systematic than that employed in the first census of Britain in 1801.

Travellers' accounts like these excited the interest of Thomas Robert Malthus. He was keen to bolster his *Essay on the Principle of Population*, much criticized on its initial appearance in 1798, with more data, and produced a 'very much enlarged' second edition of 1803. Tahiti, with its exuberantly fertile reputation and plummeting number of inhabitants, made an excellent case study. The 'great checks to increase' which Malthus identified from earlier descriptions as 'the vices of promiscuous intercourse, infanticide and war', aided by the ravages of European diseases, had clearly operated 'with most extraordinary force' since Cook's time, though Malthus considered Wilson's count excessively low. Yet unless the violence of European contact intervened, Malthus expected numbers to recover to their 'natural level'. These 'marked oscillations in … prosperity and population' were, and would continue to be, just as should be supposed 'from theory'.

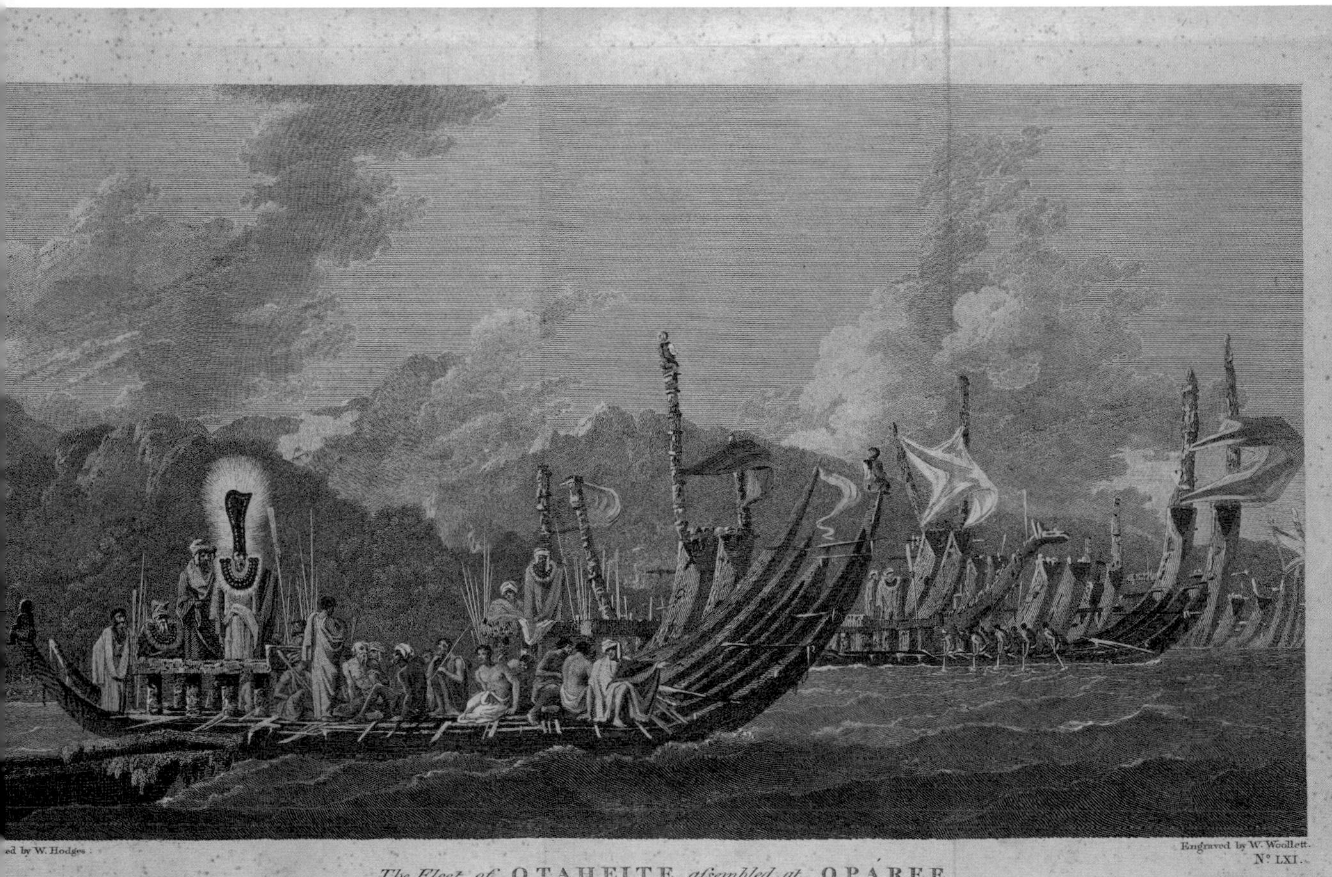

William Woollett after William Hodges, *The Fleet of Otaheite assembled at Oparee*, in Malthus's copy of James Cook, *A Voyage towards the South Pole, and round the World. Performed in His Majesty's Ships the* Resolution *and* Adventure, *in the years 1772, 1773, 1774, and 1775* (London, 1777), vol. 1, plate lxi, by permission of the Master and Fellows of Jesus College, Cambridge. 22 × 38 cm.

FURTHER READING

Chapters 18, 23, 24, 25, 33 and 34 and Exhibits 30 and 36, this book.

Alison Bashford and Joyce E. Chaplin, *The New Worlds of Thomas Robert Malthus: Rereading the* Principle of Population (Princeton, NJ, 2016).

Harriet Guest, *Empire, Barbarism and Civilisation: James Cook, William Hodges, and the Return to the Pacific* (Cambridge, 2007).

Nicholas Thomas, *Islanders: The Pacific in the Age of Empire* (New Haven, CT, 2010).

Exhibit 25

Aristotle's Masterpiece

Mary E. Fissell

The woman in this picture had not always looked as innocent as she appears here, in the frontispiece to an 1820s edition of *Aristotle's Masterpiece*, the bestselling manual of advice about generation. Something like a fly in amber, this book preserved various early modern ideas into the nineteenth and even the twentieth centuries, such as the importance of female pleasure for conception, or techniques for choosing a baby's sex. This history reminds us of the very long continuities that the conservatism of oral and written advice could produce.

Aristotle's Masterpiece began in 1684, when an anonymous writer pasted together bits of two sixteenth-century books. The printer added woodblock images of monstrous figures that had originally graced an English edition of the works of the French surgeon Ambroise Paré, and so launched a bestseller. It was usually a small-format book, cheaply produced, with a layout designed for novice readers. By the mid-eighteenth century, the total number of editions had outstripped those of all other midwifery books aimed at lay audiences in English.

Like covers today, frontispieces served to tempt buyers. The 1684 frontispiece was illustrated with two figures, a hairy woman and a black toddler. By 1710, these two were pictured walking into the study of the philosopher Aristotle that you see here. Iconographically, the image is like a medical consultation, with Aristotle in the practitioner's role. By the late eighteenth century, the black toddler was often omitted. Even more startling, the hairy woman had shed her hair. What had happened?

The original image showed the effects of the maternal imagination, the idea that what a pregnant woman looked at or desired could be impressed upon the plastic form of her unborn child. The hairy woman's mother had prayed to a small image of St John the Baptist in his desert years, clad in camel-skin, and this had imprinted on her frail female mind and turned her baby hairy. Similarly, the black toddler had been born to white parents when the mother's gaze fell on a painting of a black man in the marital bedroom at just the wrong moment. An artist in late sixteenth-century France combined the two in one woodblock, and they remained together for centuries. There are hundreds of variants; the image became a kind of trademark for the book, and printers frequently had it recut.

In the late eighteenth century, the black toddler dropped out of the picture, and the woman lost her hair, becoming nude or toga-clad, perhaps to represent Nature or Truth. She was posed modestly in the philosopher's study, which was filled with other natural curiosities and somewhat outdated technologies. In this 1820s version, however, the printer has added verses from John Milton's *Paradise Lost* that recast her as Eve. From a monstrous woman whose body bore witness to her mother's frailty, she has become a symbol of original sin. The text in the book remained the same, but the frontispiece had been transformed. Continuity and change are braided together in reproductive advice.

FRONTISPIECE.

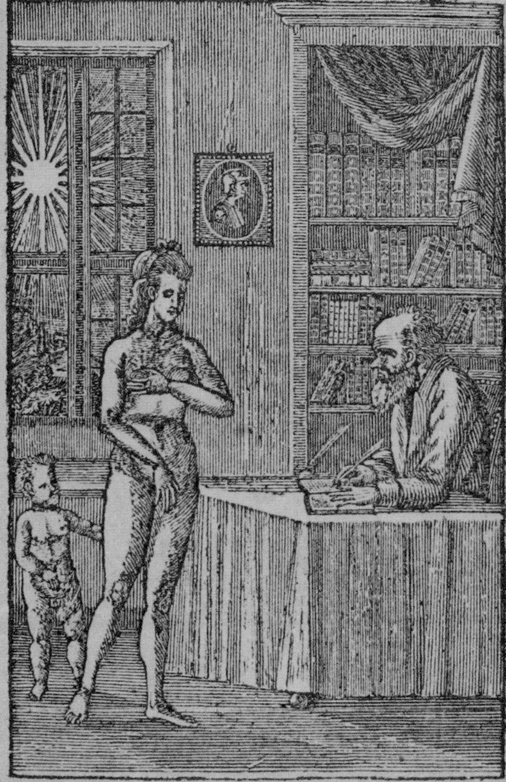

O fairest of creation, last and best,
Of all God's works, creature in whom excell'd
Whatever can to sight or thought be form'd
Holy, divine, good, amiable, or sweet!

MILTON.

THE
WORKS
OF
ARISTOTLE.

IN FOUR PARTS.

CONTAINING,

I. His COMPLETE MASTER-PIECE; displaying the Secrets of Nature in the Generation of Man. To which is added, The FAMILY PHYSICIAN, being approved Remedies for the several Distempers incident to the Human Body.

II. His EXPERIENCED MIDWIFE; absolutely necessary for Surgeons, Midwives, Nurses, and Child-bearing Women.

III. His BOOK of PROBLEMS; containing various Questions and Answers relative to the State of Man's Body.

IV. His LAST LEGACY; unfolding the Secrets of Nature respecting the Generation of Man.

FOURTH EDITION,
EMBELLISHED WITH SEVERAL FINE ENGRAVINGS.

LONDON:
PRINTED FOR THE BOOKSELLERS.
1822.

The Works of Aristotle in Four Parts ..., 4th edn (London: Printed for the Booksellers, 1822). 14 × 9 cm (closed book). Dittrick Medical History Center, Case Western Reserve University.

FURTHER READING

Chapters 13, 16, 26 and 32 and Exhibits 13, 22 and 35, this book.

Mary E. Fissell, 'Hairy women and naked truths: Gender and the politics of knowledge in *Aristotle's Masterpiece*', *William and Mary Quarterly* 60 (2003), 43–74.

Exhibit 26

Spontaneous Generation and the Triumph of Experiment

James A. Secord

Maggots arise from rotting meat; microorganisms appear in sealed, sterile flasks: the generation of life from non-living matter has fascinated philosophers since Aristotle. In textbook stories, superstitions of spontaneous generation are defeated by heroic scientists armed with the experimental method and especially by Louis Pasteur, the French savant who delivered the death blow. The epitome of the warrior scientist, he is shown here in a double-page spread from the weekly *Le monde Parisien* (The Parisian world) for 12 January 1884. Microscope slung like a gun over a shoulder, pen in hand, Pasteur sits astride a flask – the chemist's traditional attribute and symbol of his triumph over the myth of spontaneous generation.

Yet the history of spontaneous generation has never really involved simple victories. Pasteur was a brilliant experimentalist, and is famous for the germ theory of disease and the invention of anthrax and rabies vaccines, but his success depended equally on mastery of the mass media and association with the 'party of order' in the French Second Empire. When this lithograph was published soon after his sixty-second birthday, Pasteur had been a national celebrity for decades. The accompanying text recalls his battle in the early 1860s with the naturalist Félix Pouchet. In Pouchet's experiments, microorganisms had appeared in boiled hay infusions exposed to chemically generated oxygen under a layer of mercury to keep out dirty air. Pasteur pointed to the mercury as a potential source of contamination, and to rule it out designed flasks open to the air, but with necks so long, narrow and sinuous that they would catch any contaminating particles. This intervention was calculated to create a newspaper sensation and demonstrate that final victory had been achieved.

Le monde Parisien held conservative, monarchist views similar to Pasteur's own and followed his doings closely. Like many of the illustrated satirical periodicals that flourished during the nineteenth century, it often featured celebrity portraits. This one was commissioned from the Spanish emigré artist Manuel Luque de Soria, in a series including politicians, novelists and musicians. Luque recyled the design later that same year in another weekly magazine, *La caricature*. Issued in connection with a scientific congress in Copenhagen, that version highlights Pasteur's diplomatic skills. His face is patient, firm but calm, and the hand that once wielded a pen now carries a top hat. Tellingly, the emblematic flask has been reversed, its neck no longer rising suggestively between the great man's legs, but instead demurely drooping behind like a tail.

For all Pasteur's efforts, spontaneous generation never went away, and remains important today in discussing the origins of life on Earth and other planets. As Pasteur recognized, it was impossible to anticipate all possible circumstances in which life might arise; in opposing the idea, he could only reveal flaws in particular instances. Convinced that larger issues were at stake, he did not consider it important to repeat Pouchet's work precisely. Had Pasteur ever used hay infusions, heat-resistant spores would probably have produced life in his flasks too.

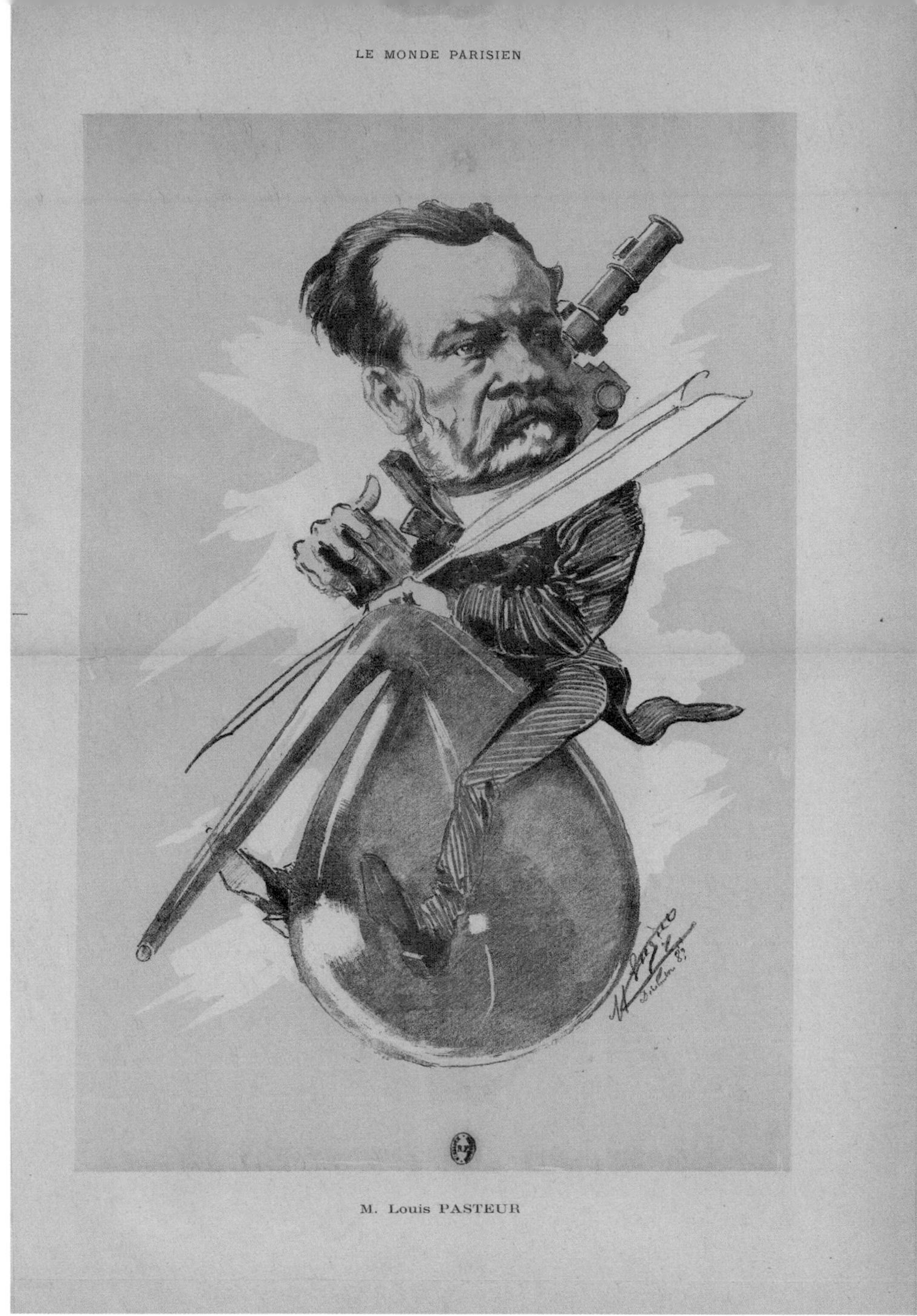

'M. Louis Pasteur', *Le monde Parisien* (12 Jan. 1884), between 5 and 6; see also 'Notre grande charge', ibid., 2. 54 × 35 cm. Bibliothèque nationale de France.

FURTHER READING

Chapters 20 and 26 and Exhibits 20, 32, 37 and 38, this book.
Noël Barbe *et al.*, *Caricaturer Pasteur* (Dole, 2014).
John Farley, *The Spontaneous Generation Controversy from Descartes to Oparin* (Baltimore, MD, 1977).
Gerald L. Geison, *The Private Science of Louis Pasteur* (Princeton, NJ, 1995), pp. 110–42.

Exhibit 27

'Pity the Poor Mother!'

Siân Pooley

In this British cartoon from 1907, experts crowd the poor, modestly dressed mother. She clutches her baby protectively to her breast, but is depicted as child-sized compared with the towering men and women who throng around. Charles Darwin is portrayed in the second row frowning at this representative of the species, while the body-builder, Eugen Sandow, displays his muscular physique. A wealthy lady thrusts forward an ugly doll, a sour-faced, Cambridge-educated spinster proffers instruction in making baby clothes, and the doddering 'bachelor' is similarly devoid of practical experience of 'the young' on whom his book claims professional expertise. William Haselden, the *Daily Mirror* cartoonist, sketched natural motherhood as surrounded by its opposite – childless, desiccated caricatures who ruled with their 'contrivances' in the 'age of science'.

Since the early modern period, European visual representations of 'neglectful' mothers and 'wanton' women had critiqued politics and morality. From the 1870s, however, newspapers appealed directly to an increasingly literate and female mass reading public; and as printing technologies allowed more illustrations, everyday foibles and fashions became central to humorous visual commentaries. In this cartoon, the disproportionately working-class, female and southern readers of the halfpenny *Daily Mirror* were expected to sympathize with the 'poor mother'. Reproduction was understood as besieged by scientific authority, but it was not assumed that the modern instructors would win.

An article on the foundation of the philanthropic St Pancras 'school for mothers' in North London prompted Haselden's cartoon. By promoting scientifically justified and medically informed working-class motherhood, such clinics sought to reduce infant mortality rates and improve the people's health. This was part of a larger 'maternalist' movement across Europe and the wider western and imperial world. States and voluntary institutions pioneered new approaches to infant and maternal welfare, often led by women philanthropists, physicians and campaigners. These interventions were prompted partly by eugenic and sometimes also imperial concerns that people who educated Europeans considered physically and racially 'fit' to reproduce were bearing fewer children. Western elites feared the ever greater demographic dominance of the poor, degenerate and ill-reared.

Importantly, the duties of working-class fathers were also represented as increasingly demanding. In the associated *Daily Mirror* article, one 'scientific reformer' urged that 'schools for husbands' be founded instead, while within two years the St Pancras school introduced paternal evening classes on housework and childcare. This burdensome model of parenthood encouraged fathers and mothers from all socio-economic backgrounds to limit their fertility, so as to avoid bearing and rearing many closely spaced children. Appreciation of the power of reformed parenthood not only to reduce human suffering but also to realize 'modern' aspirations for an idealized two-parent, two-child nuclear family became culturally dominant and socially normative as British birth-rates fell to a low point in 1933. Understandings of the natural, the scientific and the social were intertwined in these newly prominent – but always contested – public discussions of reproduction.

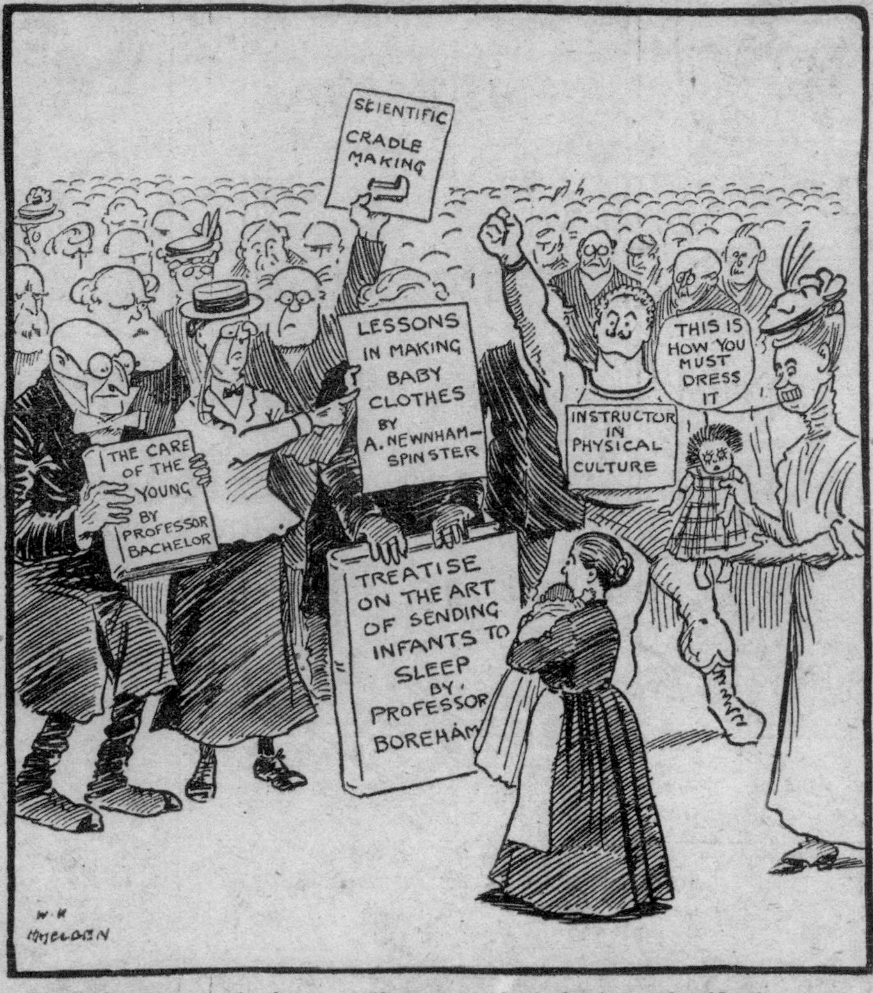

W. K. Haselden, 'Pity the poor mother!', *Daily Mirror* (6 June 1907), 7. Inner border 14 × 12 cm. © Mirrorpix.

FURTHER READING

Chapters 30, 31 and 33 and Exhibits 19 and 38, this book.

Anna Davin, 'Imperialism and motherhood', *History Workshop Journal* 5 (1978), 9–65.

Siân Pooley, 'Parenthood, child-rearing and fertility in England, 1850–1914', *History of the Family* 18 (2013), 83–106.

Ellen Ross, 'Mothers and the state in Britain, 1904–1914', in John R. Gillis, Louise A. Tilly and David Levine (eds.), *The European Experience of Declining Fertility, 1850–1970: The Quiet Revolution* (Cambridge, MA, 1992), pp. 48–65.

Exhibit 28

Condoms

James M. Edmonson

Condoms have long been morally ambiguous. Do they serve to prevent the spread of sexually transmitted diseases, or are they for birth control? Either or both. Some variants date to ancient times, but condoms flourished only with the spread of syphilis after 1500. Early models, fashioned of linen, sheep gut or fish bladders – a nineteenth-century animal membrane condom is the first shown here – thus became associated with venereal disease and prostitution. Euphemisms included 'safes', 'armour', 'machines' and 'French letters', while the French called them '*redingotes anglaises*' (English riding coats) and '*capotes anglaises*' (English capes). In America before 1840, condoms cost a dollar when a week's pay was fourteen dollars, effectively discouraging use to prevent either disease or conception.

A revolution in rubber processing changed everything. Charles Goodyear began vulcanizing in 1839, and the first rubber condom appeared a decade later. Manufacturers made 'rubbers' by chemically curing strips of raw rubber wrapped around a mold. Prices fell and use proliferated. In Germany in 1912, Julius Fromm further improved manufacture by dipping glass moulds into a solution of raw rubber. Latex, or rubber suspended in water, came in 1920 and, needing fewer solvents, proved safer to produce, as well as stronger and thinner, and had a shelf life of five years rather than three months.

The American Comstock Act of 1873 classified contraception manuals as obscene and banned mail-order condom sales, but barbers, hotel clerks and street pedlars grew a lively black-market trade. Equivalent laws were passed in France and Germany, in 1882 and 1900 respectively, but seldom led to prosecution; in interwar Europe condoms sold openly, and anonymously, from vending machines. Such outlets thrived in Britain, where working-class households favoured the condom over female appliance methods (cap, pessary and diaphragm). The London Rubber Company dominated the business, introducing the Durex brand ('durability, reliability, excellence') in 1929.

The 1918 Crane decision legalized condoms for disease prevention in the United States, lending them respectability and adding apothecary sales. After 1920, Schmid (Ramses and Sheik brands) and Youngs (Trojan brand) made fortunes selling condoms in metal tins featuring virile imagery from silent films, including Rudolph Valentino in *The Sheik* (1921). In the 1930s, with mass-produced latex models and government-mandated quality control, daily output reached one-and-a-half million. Large-scale wartime use promoted wide acceptance. Lubrication, introduced by Durex in the 1950s, was clearly intended for pleasure rather than disease prevention.

Although international sales grew after World War II, female methods ultimately eclipsed the condom in America and Europe. Market share among contraceptives in the United States declined from 27 per cent in 1955 to 19 per cent in 1965. Condom sales waned in the era of the pill, only to soar again with HIV/AIDS. Advertisements in mainstream magazines appeared in the mid-1980s, marketing condoms to both men and women. In the United States, TV commercials debuted in 2005, breaking a long taboo, while male teen use rose from 21 per cent in 1979 to 58 per cent in 1988; in 2011, 80 per cent of boys used one the first time they had sex. The condom is back.

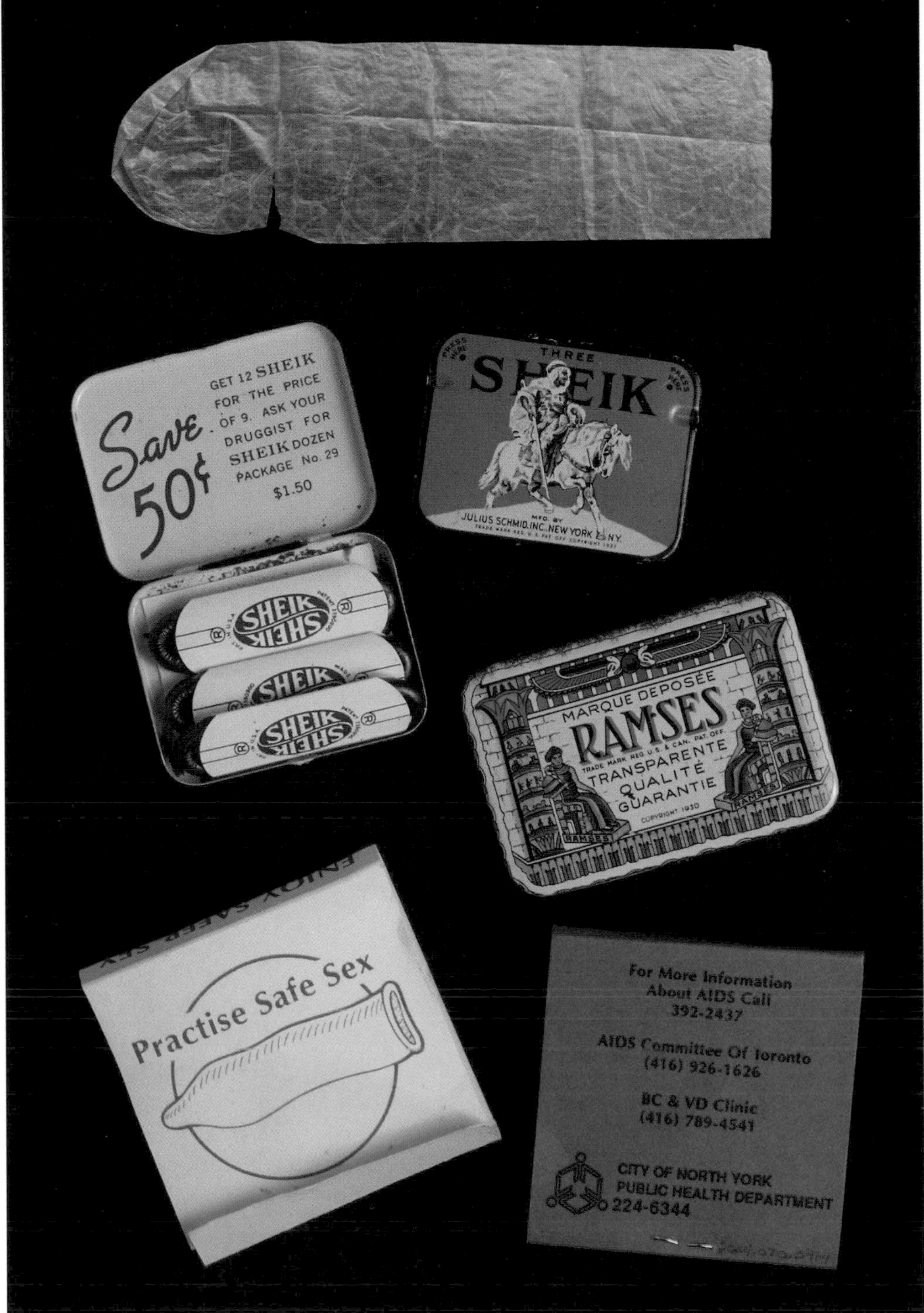

Selection of condoms. Dittrick Medical History Center, Case Western Reserve University.

FURTHER READING

Chapters 29, 30, 32, 36 and 40 and Exhibits 31 and 36, this book.

Joshua Gamson, 'Rubber wars: Struggles over the condom in the United States', *Journal of the History of Sexuality* 1 (1990), 262–82.

Robert Jütte, *Contraception: A History*, trans. Vicky Russell (Cambridge, 2008).

Andrea Tone, *Devices and Desires: A History of Contraceptives in America* (New York, NY, 2001).

Exhibit 29

Pedigree of a 'Schizophrenic Family'

Paul Weindling

Genetics adapted pedigrees from genealogy and animal breeding and used them to explain, to predict and sometimes to control inheritance in individuals and populations. This 1934 pedigree of a 'schizophrenic family' was compiled from genealogies collected by the psychiatrists Ernst Rüdin and Johannes Lange. Schizophrenic family members, the so-called schizoid, manic depressives and epileptics are indicated by the variously shaded symbols that, unlike in traditional pedigrees, represent heredity from female as well as male. The healthy appear as carriers of mental disorders deemed a threat to collective racial health. In Nazi Germany, such diagrams were used to justify wide-ranging genetic surveillance of the population, especially before marriage, as well as a colossal programme of coercive sterilization.

This programme sought a biological solution to social problems and to purify the race. The Swiss-born Rüdin had applied Gregor Mendel's rediscovered laws of heredity to schizophrenia and went on, with colleagues at the Kaiser Wilhelm Institute for Psychiatry in Munich, to pursue 'genealogical-demographic' research. An ardent racial hygienist, Rüdin advocated systematic screening of populations over generations for diseases and defects. Vivid pictograms communicated the supposed genetic risks to the wide audiences for hygiene exhibitions.

In July 1933, the Nazis passed legislation for compulsory sterilization of those presumed hereditarily sick and disabled. Modelled on a draft Prussian bill of 1932, the law added the element of compulsion that characterized earlier measures in America, Scandinavia and Switzerland. It imposed surgical sterilization on schizophrenics, the 'feebleminded', sufferers from Huntington's chorea, persons deemed to be hereditarily blind and deaf, so-called mental defectives and chronic alcoholics. This pedigree comes from a book about the law that Rüdin, the Nazi public health official Arthur Gütt and the jurist Falk Ruttke prepared for doctors and administrators. Over two hundred 'Genetic Health Courts', tribunals of two doctors and a lawyer, mandated the usually surgical sterilization of over 400,000 people. Most of these operations were carried out before 1940. The Nazi physicians' leader Gerhard Wagner opposed the law as insufficiently racial, and the outbreak of war saw a shift to the forced killing of an estimated 220,000 mentally ill and disabled people.

After the war, neither the German medical profession nor the state authorities offered survivors surgical reversal of sterilization, and the allies failed in their efforts to prosecute the doctors involved. A one-off compensation payment of 5,000 DM was granted from 1980, and a pension supplement from 1988, but the German state has not made a full apology. Coerced sterilization continued in Sweden and some other countries until the mid-1960s and found an echo in nominally voluntary population control programmes during the Cold War. Since then, global population thinking has shifted towards less extreme interventions, and from the 1960s and 1970s sterilization of men and women by vasectomy and laparoscopy respectively became the most common methods of contraception in some countries.

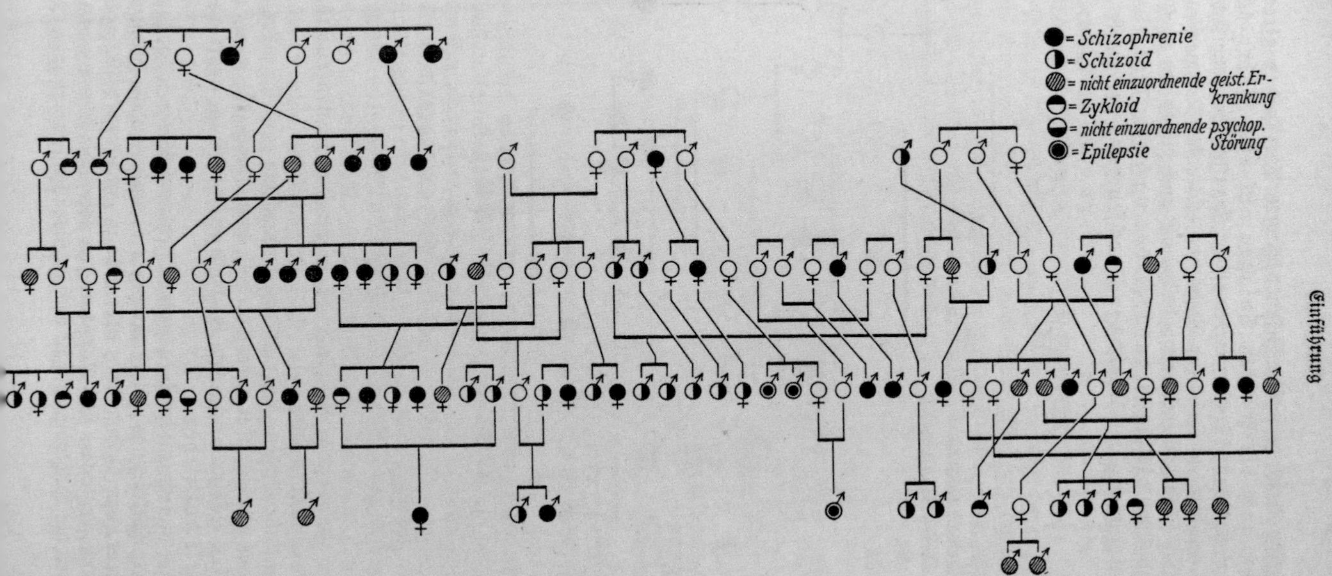

Pedigree of a 'schizophrenic family', from Ernst Rüdin, Arthur Gütt and Falk Ruttke, *Gesetz zur Verhütung erbkranken Nachwuchses vom 14. Juli 1933* (Munich: Lehmann, 1934), p. 41. 13 × 24 cm. Cambridge University Library.

FURTHER READING

Chapters 12, 17, 27, 29, 34, 36 and 40 and Exhibits 8, 30 and 39, this book.

Gisela Bock, *Zwangssterilisation im Nationalsozialismus. Studien zur Rassenpolitik und Frauenpolitik* (Opladen, 1986).

Robert G. Resta, 'The crane's foot: The rise of the pedigree in modern genetics', *Journal of Genetic Counseling* 2 (1993), 235–60.

Paul Weindling, *Health, Race and German Politics between National Unification and Nazism, 1870–1945* (Cambridge, 1989).

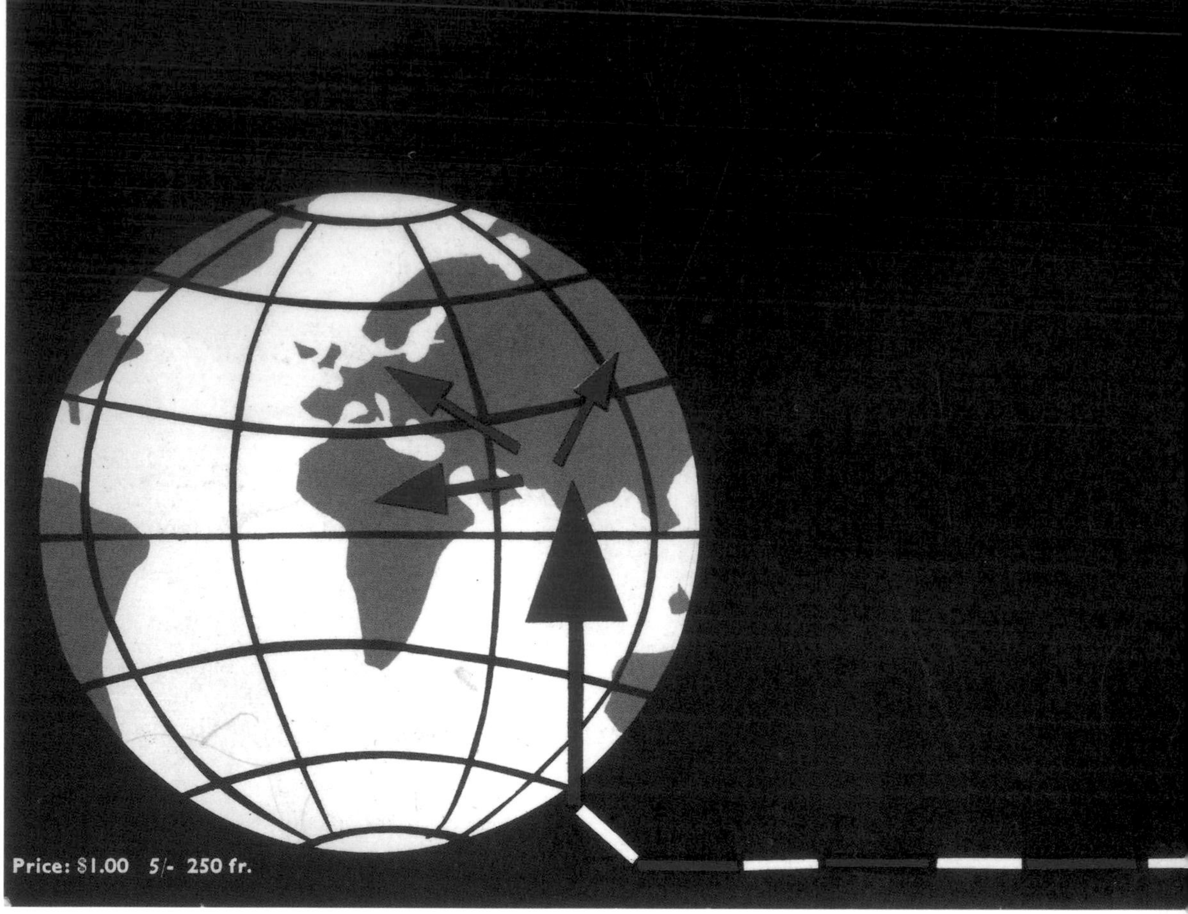

Exhibit 30

Populations, Genetics and Race

Jenny Bangham

As objects of international political scrutiny in the turbulent mid-twentieth century, human populations were central to public health, family planning, food production, ecology, international relations and the sciences of race. When the United Nations Educational, Scientific and Cultural Organization (UNESCO) launched a high-profile campaign to undermine the racial prejudice that had led to the Nazi concentration camps, 'populations' carried the message that the study of race could be scientific and non-discriminatory. These figures are from *What Is Race? Evidence from Scientists*, a picture book published by UNESCO in 1952 to explain the implications of population genetics to schoolchildren around the world. Its message was that races are not fixed, but dynamic and continually changing.

These claims were based on recent advances in mathematical techniques for modelling genetic change in populations, and on the vast accumulation of human blood-group data from the wartime and postwar expansion of blood transfusion. Rebutting Nazi notions of race purity, the picture overleaf, 'Melting Pot of Peoples in Europe before the Twelfth Century', offered a revised view of Europe's racial composition. Abstract figures dance across an

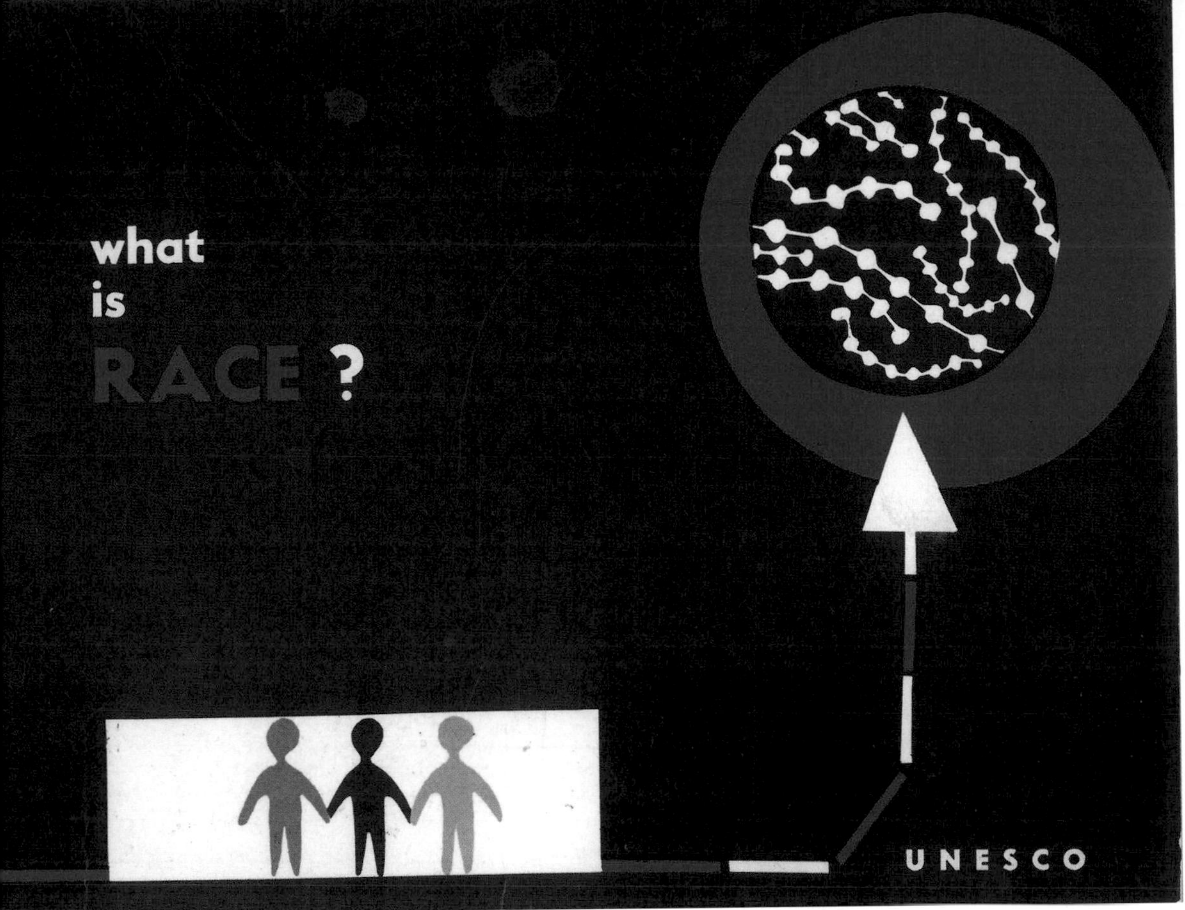

Diana Tead, *What Is Race? Evidence from Scientists* (Paris: UNESCO, 1952), back and front covers and (overleaf) p. 40 (all 15.6 × 21.5 cm), used by permission of UNESCO.

outline map, representing 'successive waves' of migration across Europe. It argues that the continent had long been home to a mixture of races, represented here in shades of grey.

Deeply political, these contentions of population genetics symbolized UNESCO's endorsement of science as a transparent, universal social remedy. Linking levels of explanation from chromosomes to populations, the front and back covers of *What Is Race?* (shown above) aligned genetics with the organization's commitment to 'unity in diversity'. The text was compiled by Diana Tead of the UNESCO Department of Mass Communication, which produced books, films and broadcasts to promote 'peace and human welfare'. The book's illustrator – painter and magazine artist Jane Eakin – used bold, abstracted shapes and a restricted colour palette that resemble the clear-cut, regular forms of Isotype, the 'International System Of TYpographical Picture Education' conceived in the 1920s as a means of conveying social information in graphical form. Confident in the power of pictures as a universal language, UNESCO designed the book for distribution in all UN-member countries, although the prose appeared in English and French only. The images took on lives of their own in a range of other media, including a filmstrip, a *Life* magazine article and a live broadcast on BBC television.

The postwar ideal of population genetics as a neutral science of human difference endures today. Now more than ever, it is expected to ground stories about ancestry and

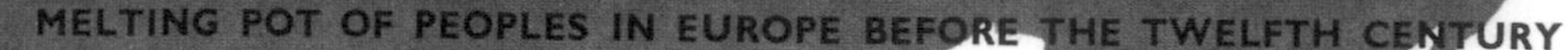

migrationary history. But as the authority of genetics has expanded, that neutrality has become more contested. Much-studied Indigenous communities have questioned who benefits from population genetics. Social scientists have pointed to the cultural frames through which geneticists define and sample populations. Advocacy groups have complained that direct-to-consumer genetic ancestry testing reinforces the notion that race and ethnicity is rooted in our genes. Genetics is powerful, but ancestral histories of human populations are still entangled in struggles over race.

40
MELTING POT OF PEOPLES IN EUROPE BEFORE THE TWELFTH CENTURY
Arrows give a general idea of the movements, mixing and cross-mixing of different peoples. For example, Britain had a Celtic-speaking population in the Iron Age, was invaded in historical times by the Belgae, another Celtic group, then the Romans, the Angles, the Saxons, the Jutes, the Vikings and the Normans. Across central Europe came genes from the East brought by Huns, Avars, Hungarians, and Turks. From the South some Negro genes mixed with those of Mediterranean peoples.
Red circles indicate centres of settlement where invaders mixed with natives or replaced them, usually moving on, after a certain period to blend with others. The results of these early migrations can still be seen among Europeans today, and make peoples in the Caucasoid group extremely difficult to classify into races.

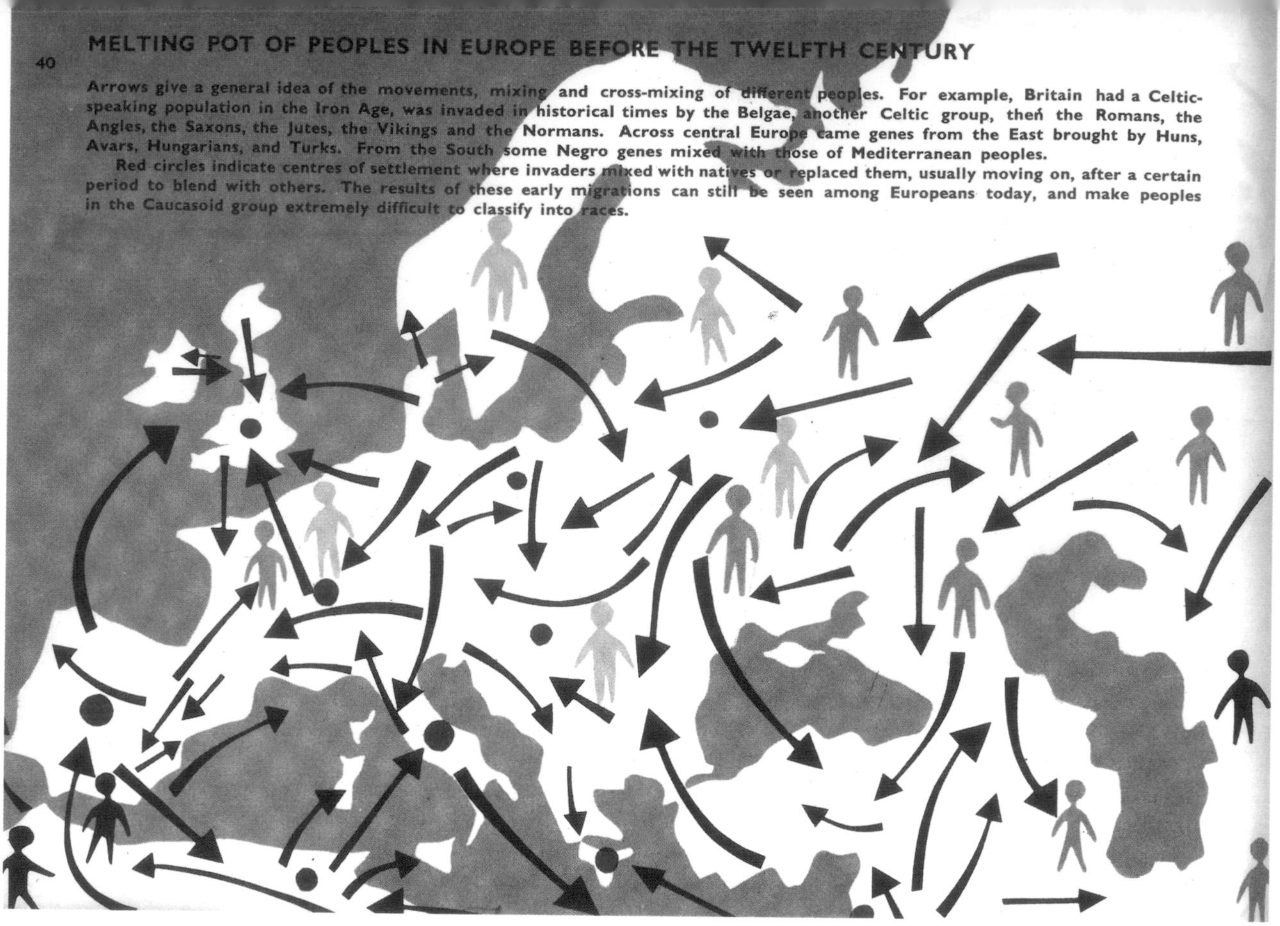

FURTHER READING

Chapters 25, 27, 33 and 34 and Exhibits 24, 29 and 39, this book.

Jenny Bangham, '*What Is Race?* UNESCO, mass communication and human genetics in the early 1950s', *History of the Human Sciences* 28, no. 5 (2015), 80–107.

Deborah A. Bolnick *et al.*, 'The science and business of genetic ancestry testing', *Science* 318 (2007), 399–400.

Jenny Reardon, *Race to the Finish: Identity and Governance in an Age of Genomics* (Princeton, NJ, 2005).

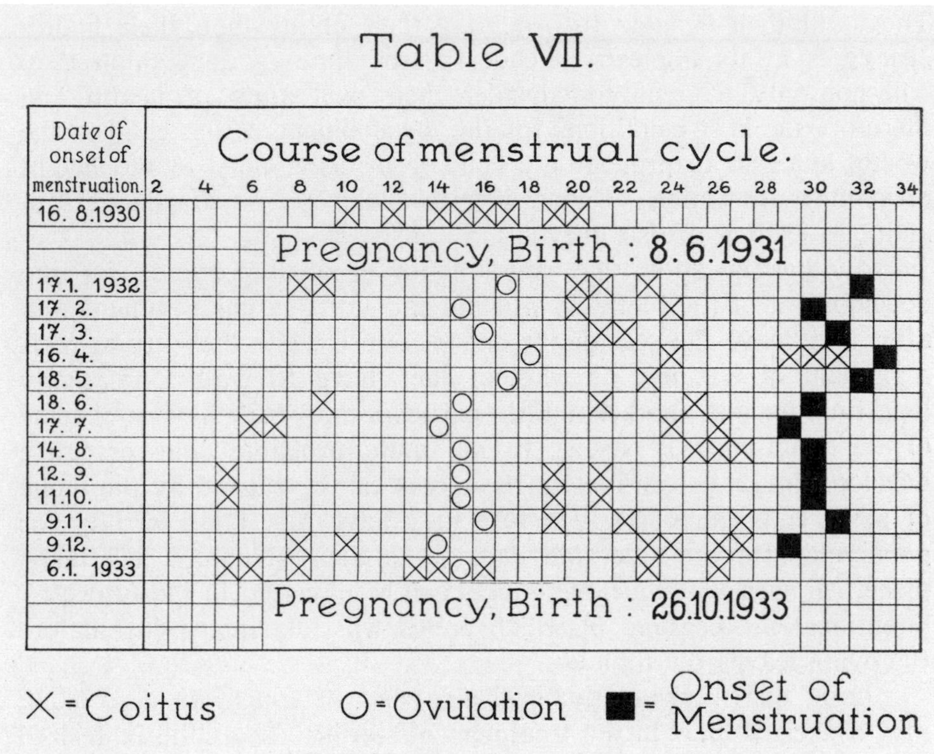

Hermann Knaus, *Periodic Fertility and Sterility in Woman: A Natural Method of Birth Control*, trans. D. H. Kitchin and Kathleen Kitchen (Vienna: Maudrich, 1934), p. 103. Table 7 × 12 cm.

Exhibit 31

Menstrual-Cycle Calendars

Martina Schlünder

The monthly recurrence of bleeding as a sign of womanhood and its disappearance as an indicator of pregnancy have been familiar for centuries. Yet modern scientific medicine had no physiological explanation for the phenomenon until the concept of the menstrual cycle was established in the early twentieth century, thus marking the beginning of reproductive physiology. What in the nineteenth century had been considered a periodic sickness, which weakened the female body through nervousness and anaemia, was reframed as a normal process caused by and following ovulation. Attempts to control fertility – to promote or prevent conception – focused on ovulation, but this lay hidden in the ovaries, while menstruation was visible. Women had long recorded their periods, but specially designed menstrual calendars now became scientific tools for inferring the time of ovulation. These did not merely continue simple calendar marking, but rather translated the reproductive time of the cycle into everyday time.

Chart, wheel and chart plus wheel from T. S. Welton, *Rhythm Birth Control: The Modern Method of Birth Control* (New York, NY: Grosset & Dunlap, 1960). Chart page 18.5 × 12 cm.

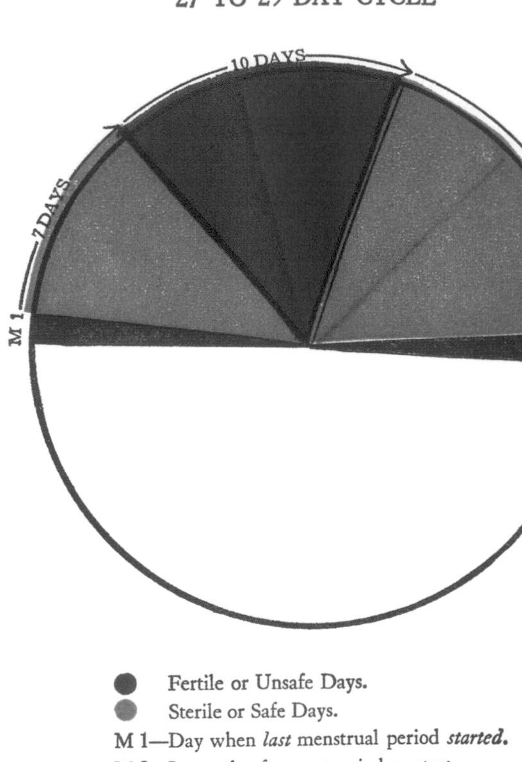

The Austrian gynaecologist Hermann Knaus produced such tools in the 1930s by using statistics and a formula for calculating the day of ovulation based on his endocrinological research. He postulated that the second half of the cycle, between ovulation and menstruation, always comprised 15 days in healthy women. By self-observation for a year, any woman could calculate her fertile days using the probabilistic 'Knaus formula': the interval between the shortest cycle (28 days in the chart shown) minus 15 days minus 2 days as a safety margin (28 − 15 − 2 = 11) and the longest cycle in a twelve-month period (32 days) (32 − 15 + 2 = 19) indicated the fertile period (here from the eleventh to the nineteenth day of the cycle). Sexual intercourse during this interval would lead to pregnancy, Knaus claimed, while avoiding those days would work better than a mechanical contraceptive. Women could mark the onset of menstruation by filling a square, and use a cross to mark days when they had sex. But the exact day of ovulation could only be calculated after the next menstruation and was then marked with an 'O'.

Knaus offered the calendar or 'rhythm method' to the women's movement of the Weimar Republic and to the Nazi regime, which gave the calendars an important role in its pronatalist policies, and after the war to the Catholic church. Other capitalist societies

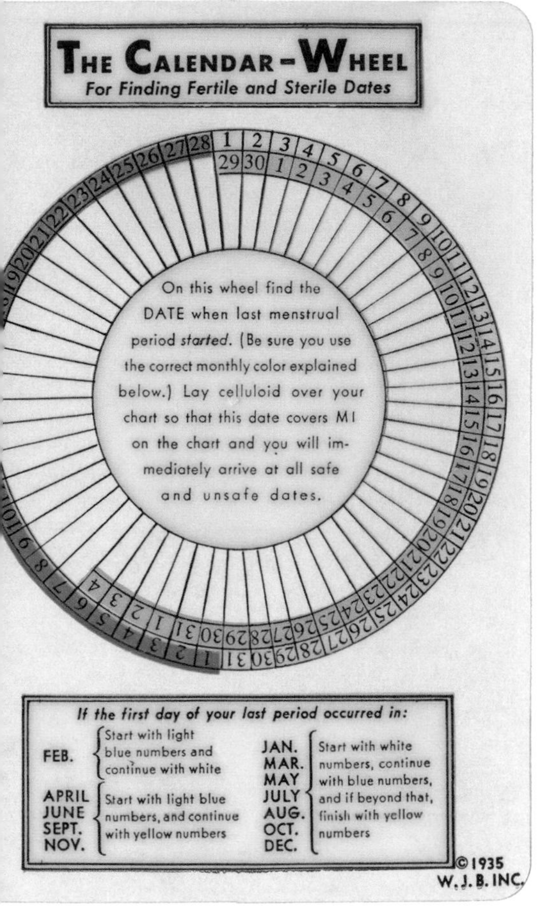

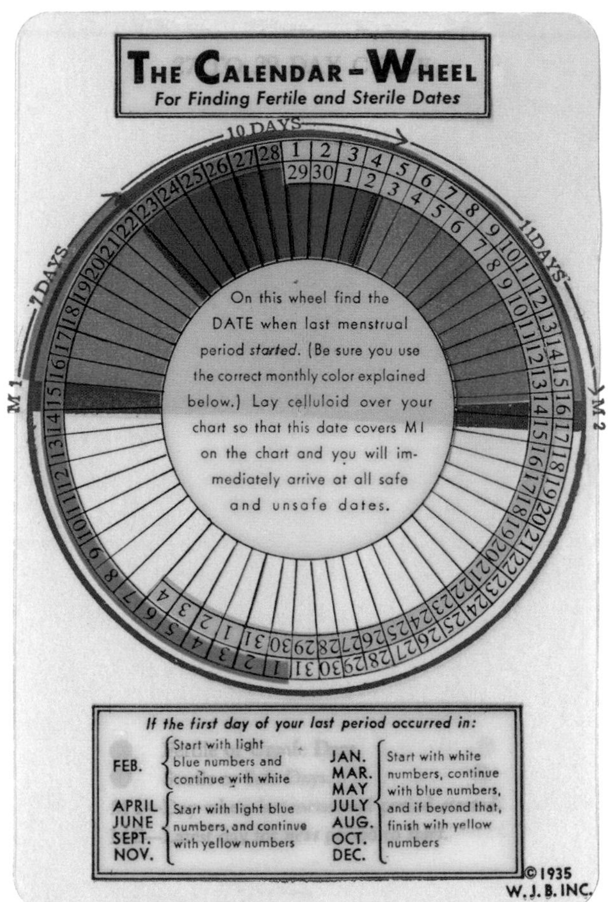

developed consumer technologies such as the calendar-wheels shown here. Women aligned reproductive time with everyday time by recording menstruation data for a year, choosing the chart that fitted their data from a collection of charts, and placing a transparent plastic calendar-wheel over it to align (in)fertile days with dates in the month. The rhythm method lost much of its significance as a contraceptive tool with the marketing of the pill. It reappeared in the 1970s with the feminist health movement as a side-effect-free, though much less reliable contraceptive. Today, timing devices play a major role in fertility treatments such as in vitro fertilization, for which monitoring the cycle is essential.

FURTHER READING

Chapters 16, 36 and 39 and Exhibits 14 and 32, this book.

Martina Schlünder, 'Die Herren der Regel/n? Gynäkologen und der Menstruationskalender als Regulierungsinstrument der weiblichen Natur', in Cornelius Borck, Volker Hess and Henning Schmidgen (eds.), *Maß und Eigensinn. Studien im Anschluß an Georges Canguilhem* (Munich, 2005), pp. 157–95.

Paula Viterbo, 'I got rhythm: Gershwin and birth control in the 1930s', *Endeavour* 28 (2004), 30–5.

Exhibit 32

Pregnancy Testing with Frogs

Jesse Olszynko-Gryn

On 17 December 1952, the *Chicago Sun-Times*, a respectable daily tabloid, illustrated the short article, 'Convening doctors see speedy pregnancy test', with a cropped version of this photograph. Taken at an obstetrics and gynaecology convention at the historic Palmer House hotel, it shows 'medical technician Mrs Donald Simerson' (left), microscope at the ready, looking on admiringly as the 'comely Minnesota doctor' Jane Hodgson – who in 1970 would become known for publicly challenging the abortion law in her state – injects a male frog with a female patient's urine. Laid out before them are test tubes, droppers, reagents, a funnel, pH paper, pipettes and frogs in jars. Coyly avoiding mention of sperm, the caption explains: 'If patient is pregnant, male frog cells will appear in frog's urine within a matter of hours.' Worlds away from the privacy of today's home tests, the transgressively gendered frog test implicated at least two other males (Donald and a potential father) and three women: doctor, technician and patient.

Though uroscopy for pregnancy detection goes back centuries at least, animals were first used in the 1920s, when Berlin gynaecologists Selmar Aschheim and Bernhard Zondek invented a 'biological' pregnancy test. Mice or rabbits were injected with urine, then killed and dissected to read the hormone-induced changes in the ovaries. After World War II, laboratories worldwide adopted amphibians as living pregnancy tests that could be reused. Imperial Britain imported South African clawed toads, *Xenopus laevis*, from Cape Town for use in three centres that performed tens of thousands of tests every year. Pregnant women's urine caused the females to extrude their large, easily visible eggs. In the United States, many doctors like Hodgson preferred locally abundant and commercially available male frogs, which could be conveniently stored in a state of induced hibernation. As the *Sun-Times* article explains, the frog test 'merely requires the services of a nurse-technician, a few simple instruments, and a supply of male frogs with a refrigerator to house them'.

These bioassays were not pregnancy tests in our sense of self-monitoring tools. In the 1960s, commercial laboratories started using immunological test kits to serve women as 'clients'; before then, diagnostic services were accessible only indirectly to 'patients'. Doctors had typically sent samples not to confirm or exclude pregnancy in healthy, married women, but rather when it was medically indicated to differentiate between a normal pregnancy and, for instance, a tumour.

'Predictor', the first reliable do-it-yourself test, debuted in 1971 and resembled a small chemistry set. Only after Unilever launched 'Clearblue One Step' in 1988 did a younger generation of consumers embrace home tests in their currently dominant form: a plastic 'wand' displaying blue or pink lines. Today women still factor in bodily signs of pregnancy, including a missed period and morning sickness, but self-testing has become the norm. Though doctors are no longer in control, the purchase of an over-the-counter retail product is often a first step in an elaborate and controversial monitoring regime – from routine ultrasound to prenatal genetic screening.

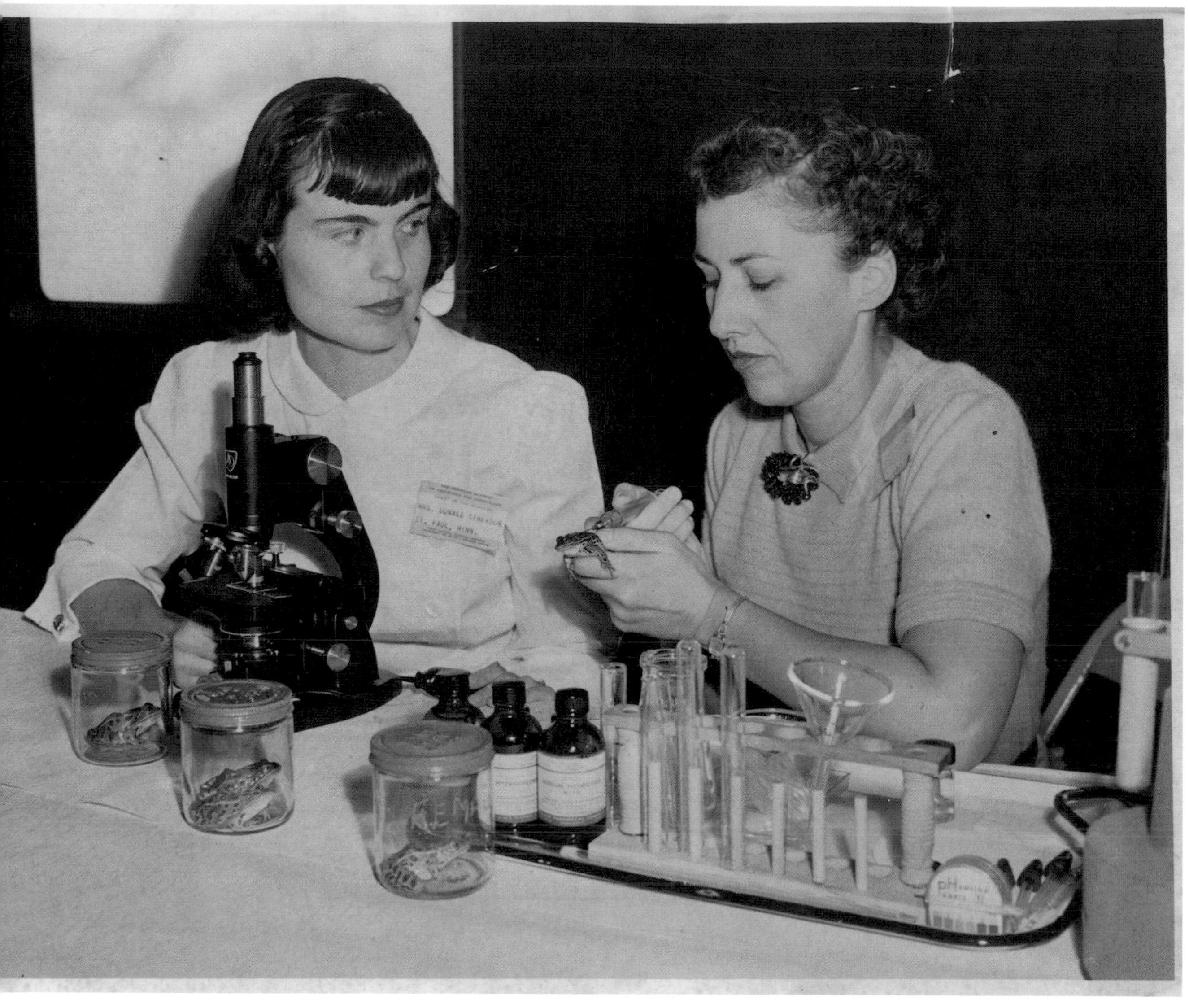

'Pregnancy Test', press photograph by Paul Olsen, 16 Dec. 1952. 20 × 25 cm. Courtesy of Sun-Times Media.

FURTHER READING

Chapters 16, 35 and 38 and Exhibits 14, 26, 31 and 37, this book.

Jane E. Hodgson, 'Office use of the frog test for pregnancy', *Journal of the American Medical Association* 153 (1953), 271–4.

Sarah A. Leavitt, '"A private little revolution": The home pregnancy test in American culture', *Bulletin of the History of Medicine* 80 (2006), 317–45.

Jesse Olszynko-Gryn, 'The demand for pregnancy testing: The Aschheim-Zondek reaction, diagnostic versatility, and laboratory services in 1930s Britain', *Studies in History and Philosophy of Biological and Biomedical Sciences* 47 (2014), 233–47.

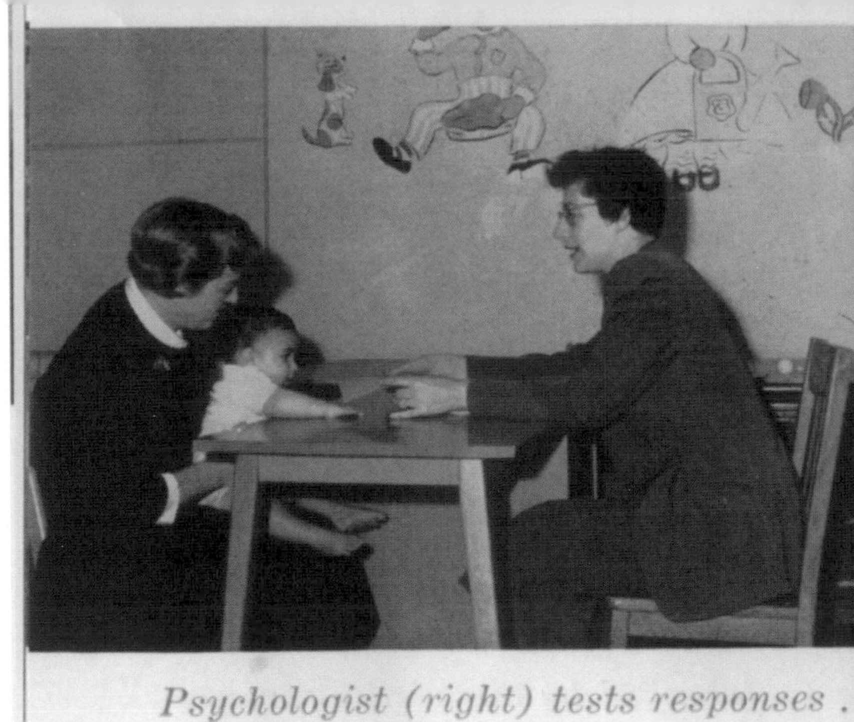

Psychologist (right) tests responses .

Exhibit 33

Technologies of Adoption Matching

Ellen Herman

Matching, the philosophy that governed adoption during much of the past century, emphasized physical resemblance, intellectual similarity, and racial and religious continuity between parents and children. Matching stood for sameness and sameness stood for safety. Difference in families, it was believed, spelled trouble.

Matching made modern adoption historically novel. Before the twentieth century, individuals engaged in placing children with new parents did not try to match them, nor did adoption necessarily sever relationships between children and natal kin. American adoption laws originated in the mid-nineteenth century, putting the United States well ahead of western Europe in legalizing adoption, but matching was a twentieth-century practice. Promoted by transnational networks of female policy professionals determined to put children's needs above adult desires, it was firmly established in many countries by 1950. Matching aimed to join unrelated adults and children so skilfully that the resulting adoptions were undetectable. In America after 1917, state laws sealed original birth records, an example of utilizing social means to secure natural appearances.

Mental and developmental tests, such as the one pictured in this promotional brochure for Louise Wise Services in New York City, were key matching technologies. Many agencies tested children. The psychologist measured the child's motor, vocal and social responses to objects and pictures, comparing the results with population norms. By claiming to predict development and educational potential, scores became as indispensable in matching children with parents as skin and hair colour, body type and other features related to heredity. Especially when little was known about a child's origins, tests promised to decrease risk, increase certainty and transform family-making into a safe, scientific operation.

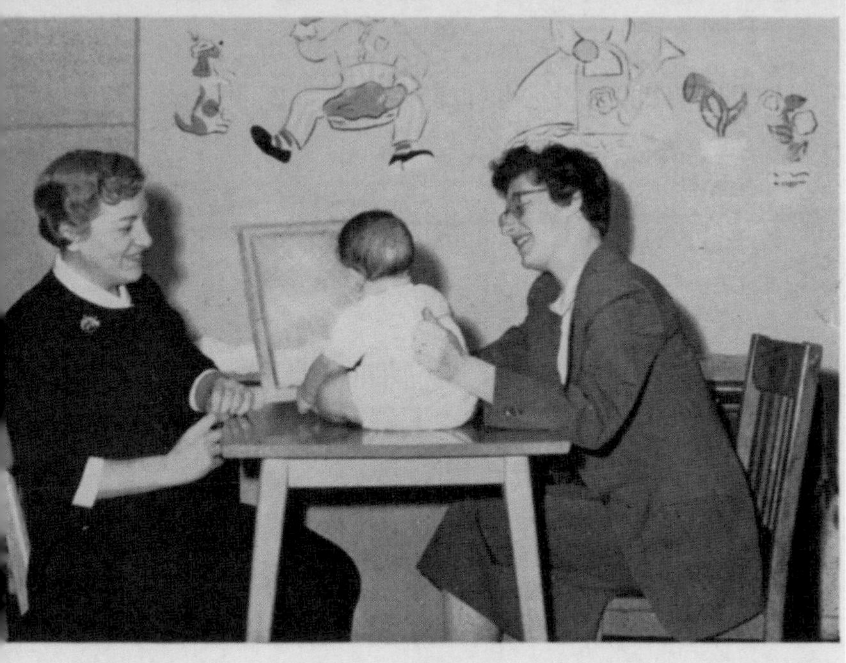

Photographs from Louise Wise Services brochure (1955), Viola W. Bernard Papers, Archives & Special Collections, Columbia University Health Sciences Library. Right-hand photo 6 × 8.5 cm.

In theory, matching substituted one family for another so completely as to render the birth family invisible. In practice, adoptive parents were supposed to be married heterosexual couples who looked, felt and behaved as if they had conceived their own children – even though adoption was understood as compensation for reproductive failure. Between 1920 and 1970, matching was especially popular among infertile couples; many agencies insisted on infertility as a qualification for adoption. When blood meant belonging, the central challenge was making kinship without blood. Matching met this challenge with paradoxical results. It strengthened the conviction that blood was thicker than water, the very ideology that made adoption an inferior option, while seeking to valorize adoptive families. Proponents believed that well-designed adoptions could deliver exclusive, authentic and permanent – in other words, natural – kinship.

Matching still has ardent defenders today, especially with regard to race. Since 1970, however, the consensus has crumbled. Movements opposing confidentiality and sealed records, advocating openness and encouraging reunions between adoptees and natal relatives have all criticized matching. Transracial and transnational adoptions flout matching by making families visibly formed across lines of race, ethnicity and nation. Today's adoption reformers acknowledge truths that matching concealed. Adoptive kinship is a purposeful social achievement. Birth families do not simply disappear. A person can have more than one mother, one father and one family.

FURTHER READING

Chapters 6, 31 and 39 and Exhibits 27 and 38, this book.
Laura Briggs, *Somebody's Children: The Politics of Transracial and Transnational Adoption* (Durham, NC, 2012).
Linda Gordon, *The Great Arizona Orphan Abduction* (Cambridge, MA, 1999).
Ellen Herman, *Kinship by Design: A History of Adoption in the Modern United States* (Chicago, IL, 2008).

Exhibit 34

'Drama of Life before Birth'

Solveig Jülich

On 30 April 1965, a stunning colour image of a 'Living 18-week-old fetus' by the Swedish photographer Lennart Nilsson featured on the glossy cover of *Life*, the leading news magazine in the postwar United States. Enveloped in the white amniotic sac, and set against a dark background, the fetus was depicted as an astronaut floating in a starry sky. These were the years of the space race. The magazine promised to reveal, for the first time, the 'Drama of life before birth', and Nilsson's photo-essay included close-ups of fertilization as well as embryos and fetuses of various ages. This story of human reproduction sparked so much interest that the entire print run of eight million sold out in only four days and publication in the *Sunday Times*, *Paris Match* and *Stern* caused sensations too.

Embryos and fetuses had been displayed before. In the late seventeenth century, the Dutch anatomist Frederik Ruysch put allegorical tableaux composed of fetal skeletons on public show. With the making of human embryology and a large audience for science in the nineteenth century, not just atlases and textbooks but also popular anatomy museums, advice books and periodicals showed developmental series of human embryos and fetuses. As the market for ever more highly illustrated magazines expanded through the twentieth century, photographs of human development proliferated. Some had previously appeared in *Life*. Unlike earlier images, Nilsson's purported to portray life in the womb, complete with amniotic sac, umbilical cord and placenta, and in full colour. Yet this was an illusion: the fetuses were in fact dead or dying.

Most of Nilsson's photographs were made possible through surgical interventions following miscarriages or ectopic pregnancies or through legal abortions. After such operations, the fetus was immersed in a tank containing saline solution, and lit softly from behind and the sides. If done sufficiently quickly, enough blood still circulated to register in the colour photographs. The fetus on the cover of *Life* was thus floating in glass, not a body, and the star-like details were bubbles and bits of placenta.

It is not widely known that Nilsson's images came out of a gynaecologists' campaign against the liberal Swedish abortion law. Beginning in the early 1950s, he collaborated for many years with physicians at women's clinics, and his pictures appeared in illustrated magazines in Sweden, in articles opposing abortion. The *Life* essay did not have that frame, and over the years, the cover picture has acquired various and contradictory meanings, including in Nilsson's bestselling advice book *A Child Is Born*. In some places, especially Sweden, it became closely associated with sex education in schools. Elsewhere, in particular in the United States, anti-abortion activists appropriated it for their campaigns, while feminists have critiqued it for devaluing the role of women's bodies during pregnancy. Nilsson's photograph is today a contested icon at the intersection of diverse politics of reproduction.

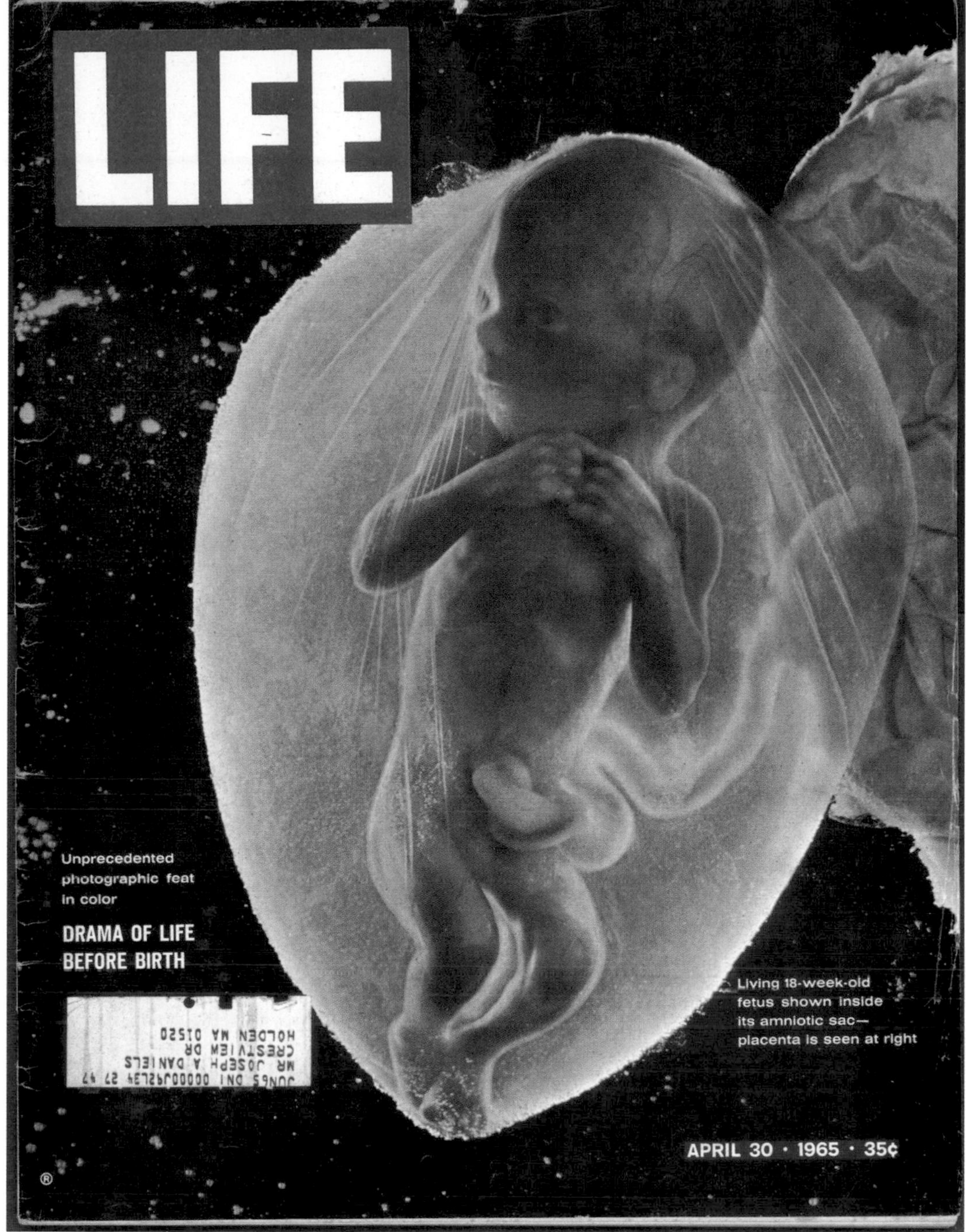

LIFE
Unprecedented photographic feat in color
DRAMA OF LIFE BEFORE BIRTH
Living 18-week-old fetus shown inside its amniotic sac—placenta is seen at right
APRIL 30 · 1965 · 35¢

Cover of *Life* 58, no. 17 (30 Apr. 1965). 35 × 27 cm. *LIFE* logo and cover design © Time Inc., image © TT News Agency.

FURTHER READING

Chapters 15, 38, 39 and 40 and Exhibits 15 and 23, this book.

Barbara Duden, *Disembodying Women: Perspectives on Pregnancy and the Unborn*, trans. Lee Hoinacki (Cambridge, MA, 1993).

Solveig Jülich, 'The making of a best-selling book on reproduction: Lennart Nilsson's *A Child Is Born*', *Bulletin of the History of Medicine* 89 (2015), 491–525.

Lynn M. Morgan, *Icons of Life: A Cultural History of Human Embryos* (Berkeley, CA, 2009).

Exhibit 35

Our Bodies, Ourselves

Wendy Kline

'INFORMATION INSPIRES ACTION', reads the website of *Our Bodies, Ourselves*. Complete with a blog ('Our Bodies, Our Blog'), resources on sexuality and reproductive health, and reader stories, the twenty-first-century version of the women's health handbook bears little resemblance to the original stapled newsprint edition that was circulated by hand in 1971. The singular black-and-white photograph of two women carrying a handwritten 'WOMEN UNITE' sign, exhibiting diversity in age but little else, was replaced on the 2011 cover by over fifty colour headshots of women of numerous cultures, races, ages and nationalities.

Before it was a book or a website or a blog, *Our Bodies, Ourselves* was a series of papers written in 1970 by Boston-area women frustrated at their experiences with doctors, nearly 97 per cent of whom were male. 'We are considered stupid, mindless creatures unable to follow instructions', they wrote, '[while] the doctor preserves his expertise and powers for himself.' Twelve women who had met at a women's liberation conference in 1969 researched female bodies and sexuality, then offered the findings in courses called 'Women and Their Bodies' the following year. Participants chimed in with their own personal experiences, some of which were incorporated into the book. 'Including the personal anecdotes and individual feelings about all these issues – now, that was very powerful', remembered one reader. *Our Bodies, Ourselves* presented personal stories as a crucial – and overlooked – component of women's health, and stressed that 'in an age of professionals, women are the best experts on themselves'. This radical assertion, marketed by Simon and Schuster to a captive audience of budding feminists, helped to revolutionize the doctor–patient relationship and women's health. Many recall their awe as they opened the cover. Historian Estelle Freedman, who received the book when she was 25 from her best friend from childhood, 'immediately sat and read through [it] … and felt a shift in my world view'. Twelve chapters, ranging from 'Women, Medicine, and Capitalism' to abortion and pregnancy, underscored the message that knowledge equals power.

It is because *Our Bodies, Ourselves* involved readers that it has remained a vibrant and bestselling source of information about female health and sexuality for over forty years. While a group of white, 20-something, college-educated women living in Boston penned the papers that became the first edition, they sought to reach a far more diverse audience, from whom they welcomed feedback. In response, readers chastised the collective for failing to include material they perceived as relevant. 'I'm a Lesbian, which means that only about 1/3 of the book applies to me', wrote Maggie in 1982. 'Now I'm sure you've had it suggested many times before that the rest of the book should integrate lesbianism more thoroughly.' Maggie was one of hundreds of women who requested more attention to homosexuality in the text, which underwent a major revision in 1984. There were also fierce battles over race. By demanding the inclusion of diversity, ordinary readers ensured that generations of women worldwide would continue to read *Our Bodies, Ourselves*.

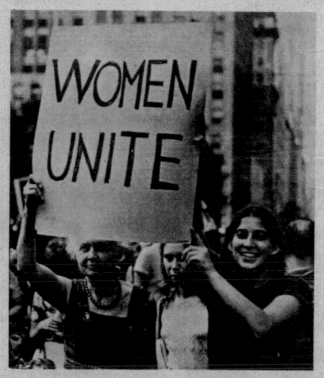

Boston Women's Health Course Collective, *Our Bodies, Our Selves: A Course By and For Women* (Boston, MA: New England Free Press, 1971). 28 × 22 cm.

FURTHER READING

Chapters 29, 41 and 42, this book.

Kathy Davis, *The Making of* Our Bodies, Ourselves*: How Feminism Travels across Borders* (Durham, NC, 2007).

Wendy Kline, *Bodies of Knowledge: Sexuality, Reproduction, and Women's Health in the Second Wave* (Chicago, IL, 2010).

Exhibit 36

Z.P.G.

Patrick Ellis

Accompanying the paradoxical tag line for the 1972 film *Z.P.G.* – 'The time is tomorrow and there's no time left' – this poster includes a cluster of enigmatic vignettes. Against the backdrop of a crowded planet, bell-bottomed residents of the future resist apprehension by a giant dome; one child is being pointed to, while another is about to be thrown; drones circle above. These curious images, akin to science-fiction paperback covers, are a visual précis of the film. Many people would have spotted the poster in newspapers, on billboards and at movie theatres; for most, it was their first encounter with the concept 'Z.P.G.': Zero Population Growth.

Zero Population Growth began as an ideal for environmentalists in the 1960s. Responding to predictions of a catastrophic rise in human population, this ethic of replacement-level family planning demanded two children, and no more, for two parents as the only way to defuse the so-called population bomb. The principle was purveyed by Paul Ehrlich, professor of biology at Stanford University, and taken as a title by his band of activists.

Concerned environmentalist and first-time film director Michael Campus, adapting the screenplay *The First of January*, came to an agreement with Ehrlich's group, which approved the title *Z.P.G.* The plot, however, exaggerated the meaning of Zero Population Growth: in an overpopulated, polluted year 2000, the World Deliberation Council issues an edict mandating that, for the next thirty years, any childbirth shall be a capital crime. ('The penalty for birth is death', the poster announces.) To fulfil maternal desires, women are sold facsimile, robot babies; but the protagonists, played by Geraldine Chaplin and Oliver Reed, conceive a secret child. Ultimately, the defiantly reproductive heroes are discovered, and flee into a contaminated region, where the film ambiguously ends.

Generically, the story is a 'demodystopia': those dark fictions that present scenarios wrought by great demographic change, from H. G. Wells's *The Time Machine* (1895) to *Children of Men* (2006). *Z.P.G.* is not as memorable as the key demodystopia of its decade, *Soylent Green* (1973), which presented the Swiftian solution of cannibalism to the Malthusian problem of overpopulation and became a cult metaphor. *Z.P.G.* is instructive for its intersection with activism.

Campus intended *Z.P.G.* as a warning, advocating voluntary action now, lest government enforce change later. He saw draconian policy as inevitable, and support from his technical advisor, a Danish demography professor, allowed him to claim that *Z.P.G.* was 'not science fiction, it is science fact'. But the facts, as Ehrlich wished them to be understood, were confused along the way. Audiences overwhelmingly came away with the idea that Zero Population Growth meant having zero children.

Ehrlich's group commissioned a survey that evidenced this, and petitioned to have the title changed. The studio that distributed the film, Paramount, denied them; so, too, did a California judge. Ehrlich's group resorted to picketing cinemas and writing letters, but soon realized there was little need. *Z.P.G.* fared poorly at the box office, and was negatively reviewed – 'The film is a miscarriage', *Cue* magazine punned.

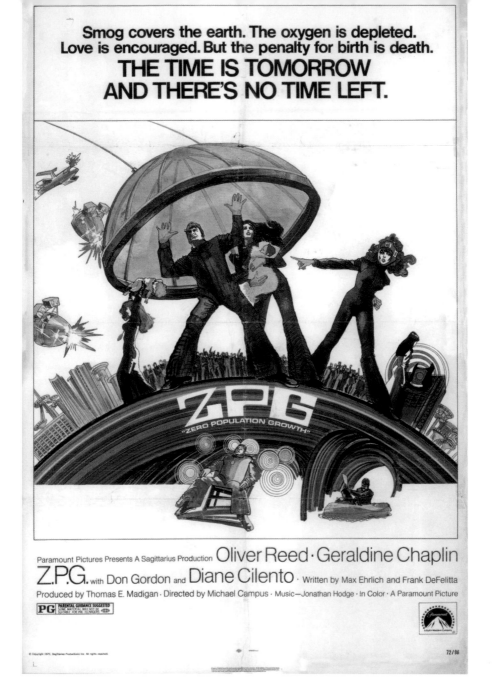

Z.P.G. poster. 104 × 69 cm. © Paramount Pictures Corp. All rights reserved.

FURTHER READING

Chapters 34, 36 and 43 and Exhibit 28, this book.

Andreu Domingo, '"Demodystopias": Prospects of demographic hell', *Population and Development Review* 34 (2008), 725–45.

Jesse Olszynko-Gryn and Patrick Ellis, 'Malthus at the movies: Science, cinema, and activism around *Z.P.G.* and *Soylent Green*', *Cinema Journal* 57 (2018), in press.

Jesse Olszynko-Gryn, Patrick Ellis and Caitjan Gainty (eds.), 'Reproduction on film', special issue, *British Journal for the History of Science* 50, no. 3 (2017).

Exhibit 37

Cloned Frogs

Christina Brandt

In 1977, John Gurdon, a staff scientist at the Medical Research Council Laboratory of Molecular Biology in Cambridge, published this photograph of a clone of South African clawed frogs in a review article based on a prestigious lecture. The thirty albino offspring had developed from the enucleated eggs of a wild-type female into which he had transplanted cell nuclei from an albino embryo, itself obtained by mating two albino parents. The presence of the mutation proved that the genetically identical frogs originated from the donor nuclei only. Displaying both the power of cloning and much experimental virtuosity, the picture was the result of over two decades of research.

Working in Michaïl Fischberg's laboratory at the University of Oxford, Gurdon had first cloned frogs around 1960 because 'it is often desirable to conduct biological experiments with genetically identical animals', something otherwise impossible in vertebrates. This was a spin-off of a research programme to answer a question that had engaged embryologists since the late nineteenth century: does the nucleus change irreversibly during cell differentiation or is it just differently controlled? The frog clones, especially those made from differentiated cells, provided physical evidence that these still contain a full complement of genetic information and thus that differentiation depends only on changes in gene expression. Gurdon had previously identified frogs using a microscopically visible chromosomal mutation, but now employed a new genetic marker. The obvious lack of pigment in the albinos confirmed the older work and made a more striking image for a prize lecture.

In the 1970s, debates about reproductive medicine, genetic engineering and embryo research converged in public, cloning became highly controversial and Gurdon's frogs represented a first step 'toward the clonal man' (James D. Watson, 1971). By 1978, when an American popular science book asked if *The Cloning of Man* was *A Brave New Hope … or Horror?* the 'Oxford' frogs symbolized the power of the new science of reproduction. In Germany, the current affairs weekly *Der Spiegel* as well as the science magazine *bild der wissenschaft* reprinted pictures of Gurdon's albino frogs in articles that conflated research on in vitro fertilization with visions of the production of human doubles. The aesthetics of the image seemed designed to feed fears about a science of human cloning. Though a close look revealed differences in size, probably as a result of rearing conditions, the series of all-female frogs, lined up in rows, and the artificial cream colour of the animals, reinforced science-fiction clichés of unnatural replication generating the horror of endless similarity.

Gurdon's group went on to search for molecules that regulate and can 'reprogramme' gene activity, but for a long time scientists assumed that mammals could not be cloned. Then, at the end of the century, the step from laboratory to farm, from embryology to reproduction, was taken. In the form of Dolly, the sheep cloned in 1996, the techniques developed on frogs began to reshape both scientific interventions and public debate.

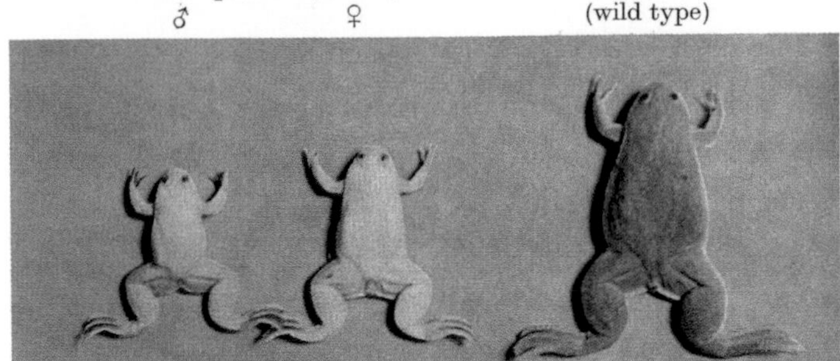

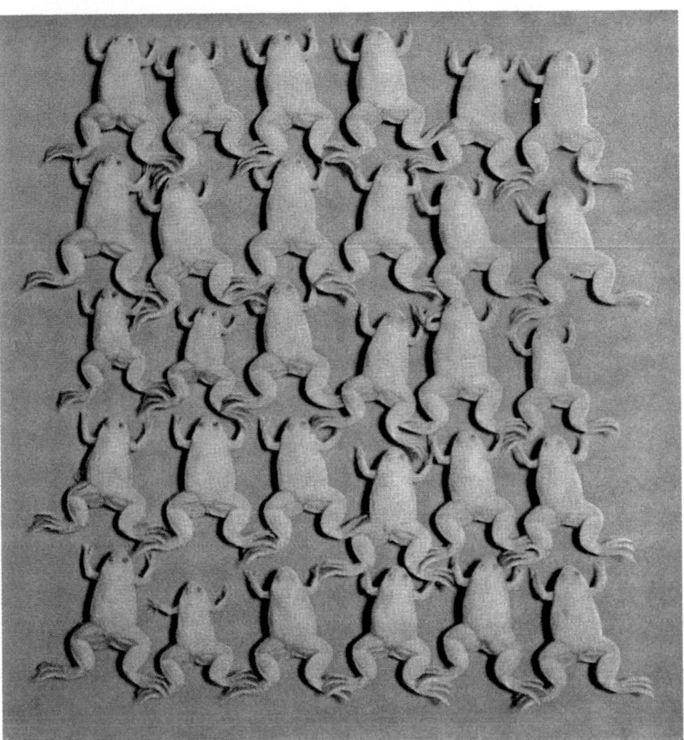

Nuclear transplant clone

FIGURE 5. A clone of frogs (*Xenopus laevis*) produced by nuclear transplantation. A single tail-bud embryo (stage 18) was obtained from a cross between two albino a^p/a^p mutants (donor parents). Its cells were dissociated and their nuclei transplanted into u.v.-enucleated unfertilized eggs of the wild-type female (recipient) shown. The group of 30 frogs (nuclear-transplant clone) shown are all female and albino; they were obtained from a total of 54 nuclear transfers. All were products of a first transfer experiment (see figure 3).

'Nuclear transplant clone' from J. B. Gurdon, 'The Croonian Lecture, 1976: Egg cytoplasm and gene control in development', *Proceedings of the Royal Society of London B* 198 (1977), 211–47, plate 2, by permission of the Royal Society. 24 × 16 cm.

FURTHER READING

Chapters 12, 27, 28 and 39 and Exhibits 13, 32, 38 and 39, this book.

Sarah Franklin, *Dolly Mixtures: The Remaking of Genealogy* (Durham, NC, 2007).

Sir John B. Gurdon, 'The egg and the nucleus: A battle for supremacy. Nobel Lecture, 7 Dec. 2013', Nobel Media AB 2014, www.nobelprize.org/nobel_prizes/medicine/laureates/2012/gurdon-lecture.html.

John B. Gurdon and Nick Hopwood, 'The introduction of *Xenopus laevis* into developmental biology: Of empire, pregnancy testing and ribosomal genes', *International Journal of Developmental Biology* 44 (2000), 43–50.

Exhibit 38

'It's a Girl'

Nick Hopwood

Broadsides and prodigy books once classified unusual nativities as natural, demonic or divine; in modern newspapers science makes the most miraculous births. This front page announced the arrival of the 'world's first test tube baby' at 11.47 the previous evening, Tuesday 25 July 1978. She was conceived when an egg and sperm from 'happy parents' Lesley and John Brown were mixed in a dish. She was born with what *Newsweek* called 'a cry . . . round the brave new world'. John ran the hospital corridors telling everyone, 'It's a girl.'

The birth brought to fruition a decade-long collaboration between Cambridge physiologist Robert Edwards and gynaecologist Patrick Steptoe from Oldham near Manchester. They fertilized eggs from infertile volunteers in vitro, then in 1971 began implanting embryos and trying to maintain pregnancies. Newspapers and television carried occasional reports and debated their progress: 'hope for the childless' or, as the Catholic church and the new bioethicists argued, biology out of control? Even supportive scientists worried that the team might cut corners in the race to be first, and that the slightest blemish would end any prospect of medical use. Edwards had gained confidence from experiments in laboratory animals that no serious abnormality would survive to term, and Steptoe monitored Lesley Brown, but no one really knew how healthy her baby would be.

The *New York Post* discovered the pregnancy in April 1978. When journalists besieged the Oldham hospital where Steptoe was keeping Lesley under observation, he brokered a deal with the *Daily Mail*, a conservative tabloid with many women readers. Annoyed rivals were left training their cameras on a ward window, while the *Mail* – itself previously ambivalent – framed the event as 'a mother's dream come true'. The moment of birth was so secret, and the hour so late, that even the *Mail* reporters discovered the sex only just in time for this final edition in the early hours of 26 July. The doctors had long known, but Lesley had chosen to preserve the surprise – and the *Sun* had stated that she was carrying a boy. Using an existing shot of the parents, the *Mail* lauded 'a triumph of research' and a much-wanted addition to what they represented as an ordinary, working-class family. The next day came the name to caption the real exclusive: a photograph of 'the lovely Louise', a miracle of normality.

The news was still controversial, and a few scientist competitors levelled accusations of failure to publish properly. The top American science journal gave the 'tempest in [a] test tube' two sentences, then sneered: 'For longer renditions of these facts, see any newspaper or magazine.' With Edwards and Steptoe extremely busy, and unsure what accounted for success after hundreds of failures, it took six months for a symposium to reveal the details and two years for the full articles to appear. By then, more births had validated the *Mail*'s claim: that girl had 'made' 'medical history' and reproduction would never be quite the same again.

Daily 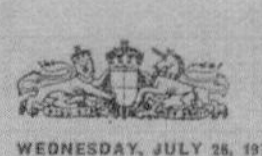 **Mail**

WEDNESDAY, JULY 26, 1978

8p (CHANNEL ISLANDS 9p)

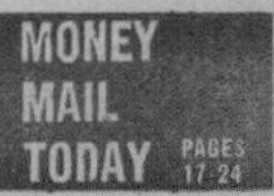

First test-tube baby is born and medical history made as a mother's dream comes true

IT'S A GIRL

Daily Mail Reporters

THE world's first test tube baby was born last night–a 5lb. 12oz. girl.

She was nine days premature and delivered by caesarian section at 23.47

For medicine, it was a moment of history. For gynaecologist Patrick Steptoe, it was a triumph of research.

But for 30-year-old Lesley Brown, the tiny bundle at Oldham General Hospital was nothing less than a miracle.

After nine years, she had the baby she longed for, thanks to the breakthrough by Mr Steptoe and Cambridge physiologist Dr Robert Edwards. Their achievement was to create life outside the womb—fertilising an egg with the husband's sperm in the laboratory and then returning it to the mother for a successful pregnancy.

Mr Steptoe had decided to operate as soon as tests had shown the baby was supporting her own life. Lesley was unconscious during the five to ten-minute operation.

Chain-smoking

With Mr Steptoe was his medical team and Dr Edwards. Lesley's husband John waited outside the delivery room, anxiously going through the expectant-father's chain-smoking ritual.

Mrs Brown, confined to her small room in the maternity unit of Oldham General for six weeks, was told only hours beforehand of the operation. The wait had become more tense, more nerve-racking, by the day. She had not been expected to give birth until August 2 and had to live with the knowledge that she was the first test-tube mother.

The wait had become quite unbearable for John, who had been spending most of his time at her bedside. Yesterday he was out shopping to buy Lesley a present for her 31st birthday next Monday.

He arrived back at the house where he is staying with Sharon, the 17-year-old daughter of his first

Turn to Page 2, Col. 1

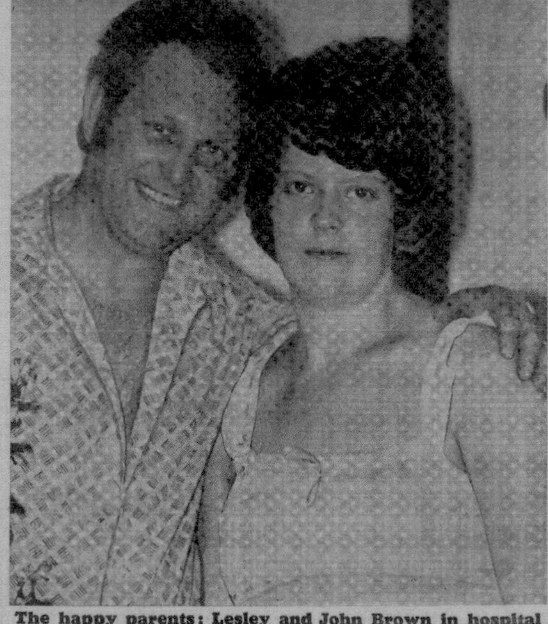

The happy parents: Lesley and John Brown in hospital

INSIDE: Lynda Lee-Potter 7, Femail 12, City 18-19, Classified Adverts 18, 32-34, TV 26-27, Theatre Guide 28, Prize Crossword 29, Letters and Strips 30

Daily Mail, 26 July 1978 (final edition), p. 1. 39 × 29 cm.

FURTHER READING

Chapters 31 and 39 and Exhibits 13, 26, 27 and 37, this book.

Lesley and John Brown with Sue Freeman, *Our Miracle Called Louise: A Parents' Story* (London, 1979).

K. Elder and M. H. Johnson, 'Symposium: The history of the first IVF births', *Reproductive BioMedicine and Society Online* 1 (2015), 1–70.

Jon Turney, *Frankenstein's Footsteps: Science, Genetics and Popular Culture* (New Haven, CT, 1998).

SMR SIGNIFICANTLY HIGH, IN TOP TENTH
SMR SIGNIFICANTLY HIGH, NOT IN TOP TENTH
SMR NOT SIGNIFICANTLY HIGH, IN TOP TENTH
OTHER AREAS
SMR NOT SIGNIFICANTLY LOW, IN BOTTOM TENTH
SMR SIGNIFICANTLY LOW, NOT IN BOTTOM TENTH
SMR SIGNIFICANTLY LOW, IN BOTTOM TENTH

ISCHAEMIC HEART DISEASE
MEN, 1968–78
BY LOCAL AUTHORITY AREA

Exhibit 39

Developmental Origins of Health and Disease

Tatjana Buklijas

The idea that events between conception and early infancy are important in shaping susceptibility to disease was once controversial, but has found wide acceptance over the past three decades. In 1984, the Medical Research Council Environmental Epidemiology Unit at the University of Southampton published a compendium of maps that used colour to show differences in mortality (strictly, the standardized mortality ratio, or SMR) from selected diseases across England and Wales between 1968 and 1978. The death-rate from ischaemic heart disease appeared highest (bright red) in poor areas and lowest (deep green) in rich

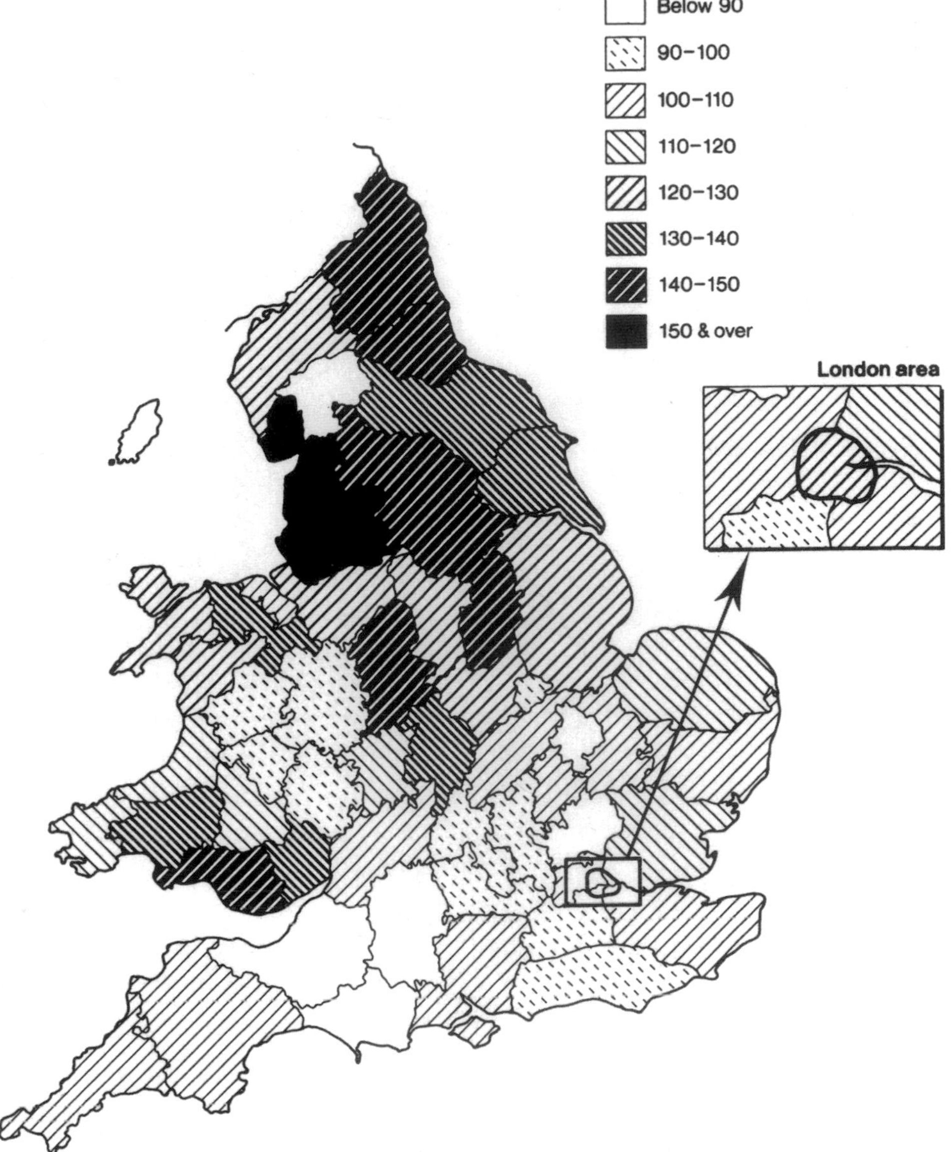

Left: M. J. Gardner, P. D. Winter and D. J. P. Barker, *Atlas of Mortality from Selected Diseases in England and Wales, 1968–1978* (Chichester: Wiley, 1984), p. 18. Courtesy of Paul Winter. 27 × 25 cm.
Right: D. J. P. Barker, *Mothers, Babies, and Disease in Later Life* (London: BMJ Publishing Group, 1994), p. 4, based on map included in the *Registrar General's Statistical Review of England and Wales, 1901–1910*. Courtesy of John Wiley & Sons. 14 × 12 cm.

ones (left map). This finding opposed the received view, which ascribed the modern 'epidemic' of cardiovascular disease to affluent lifestyles.

David Barker, the clinical epidemiologist at the Southampton unit, took early life conditions to explain adult risk. This approach was shaped by his PhD research, under Thomas McKeown at the Department of Social Medicine at the University of Birmingham in the 1960s, on 'prenatal influences and subnormal intelligence'. At Southampton, working with the statistician Clive Osmond, Barker observed a strong geographical correlation between ischaemic heart disease mortality in 1968–78 and infant mortality in the early twentieth century. He would eventually represent the latter as a map (right). In 1986, the *Lancet* published the first in a series of essays arguing that 'poor nutrition in early life increases susceptibility to the effects of an affluent diet'.

From 1990, Barker's observation grew into a field known first as 'fetal origins of adult disease', then 'developmental origins of health and disease'. Epidemiological observations were tested in clinical studies and animal experiments, but early critics found the developmental model lacking a mechanism of disease causation. By the early 2000s, however, proponents had found an ally in epigenetics – the study of modifications in gene expression patterns heritable through cell division without change in DNA sequence – a field buoyed by dissatisfaction with reductionist genetics. Epigenetics helped to explain how cues acting even before conception could set physiological pathways along pathological routes. At the same time, the developmental model offered a fresh start to policymakers who had failed to halt the rise of obesity by modifying adult lifestyles. Not only what a mother ate or cried about, but – through the epigenetic marking of primordial germ cells – also the experiences of fathers and grandparents are now seen as sources of risk and sites for medical intervention.

This pair of maps symbolizes the 'Barker hypothesis', one depicting adult cardiovascular mortality, the other infant mortality. Maps have a long history in thinking about populations, but in the much-cited early journal articles, Barker relied on other genres of medical figure such as graphs. He reserved maps for communication with wider audiences, in books and lectures and on websites. Yet journalists, researchers and Barker's obituarists have all assigned 'the serendipitous discovery' of 'the striking resemblance between maps' a key place in the history of the field. Providing vivid arguments for the developmental model, these maps anchor individuals in the worlds into which they were born.

FURTHER READING

Chapters 17, 27 and 38 and Exhibits 29, 30 and 37, this book.

D. J. P. Barker and C. Osmond, 'Infant mortality, childhood nutrition, and ischaemic heart disease in England and Wales', *Lancet* 1 (1986), 1077–81.

P. D. Gluckman, M. A. Hanson and T. Buklijas, 'A conceptual framework for the developmental origins of health and disease', *Journal of Developmental Origins of Health and Disease* 1 (2010), 6–18.

Tom Koch, *Disease Maps: Epidemics on the Ground* (Chicago, IL, 2011).

Exhibit 40

The Room of the Ribbons

Jessica Hughes and Rebecca Flemming

The walls of the *Sala dei Fiocchi* ('Room of the Ribbons'), within the shrine of Saint Gerard Majella in Materdomini, a hamlet some hundred kilometres east of Naples, are crammed with photographs of infants and mothers (see overleaf). The ceiling drips with ribbons, many tied in bows or attached to the small fabric cushions with which Italian families mark a baby's birth: blue for a boy, pink for a girl. Alongside recent colour photos, there are thousands of black-and-white images from the early twentieth century onwards. The upper floors of the shrine display more traditional metal votives, representing parents and children, body parts and religious commitment, together with painted tablets and processional banners from diaspora communities. Elsewhere in Campania, ancient sanctuaries have yielded rich finds, including terracotta infants and other ex-votos associated with generation. Ritual practices to secure divine support for producing healthy children go back over two millennia here.

Some things have changed. Expectant, hopeful and thankful parents now bring ribbons and photos to the shrine, putting them in the container beneath the large painting of St Gerard that is the focal point of the room. Some post their offerings, with letters that the sanctuary magazine may publish. Gender is now more strictly demarcated, with offerings predominantly in pink or blue. The theology of the transaction has also shifted. The reciprocity of the classical ex-voto – summed up in the Latin phrase, *do ut des*, 'I give so that you may give' – has been replaced by the more asymmetrical relationship between humans and the divine expressed in the Italian votive formula, *per grazia ricevuta* (PGR), 'for grace received'. Yet doctrinal distinctions blur as offerings commemorating requests for conception and safe delivery are presented alongside objects giving thanks for healthy children.

Gerard himself was an early member of the society of missionary priests, the Redemptorists, founded in 1732, and active around Naples in the 1750s. The story is recounted of how a handkerchief he dropped during a visit later saved one of the daughters of the house and her baby from death during childbirth; and his connections with maternity and children strengthened since then. His protection of childbirth was mentioned during his beatification process in 1893; Pope Pius X canonized him in 1904. The *Sala dei Fiocchi* demonstrates the increasing importance of this aspect of his activities, as do churches dedicated to him worldwide, especially in North America.

Globalized and modernized, Gerard is one of several Catholic saints who, on the internet as well as at local shrines, offer support for those seeking to conceive, maintain a pregnancy and safely give birth. Reproduction has been medicalized, but there is still space for appeal to higher powers, in ways that invite reflection on continuity and change. Terracotta infants were remade in wax and metal, and have since been joined by baby photos and feasts of pink and blue. The precise combination of request and thanks has altered, yet much remains the same: people call on all available resources to help them have healthy children.

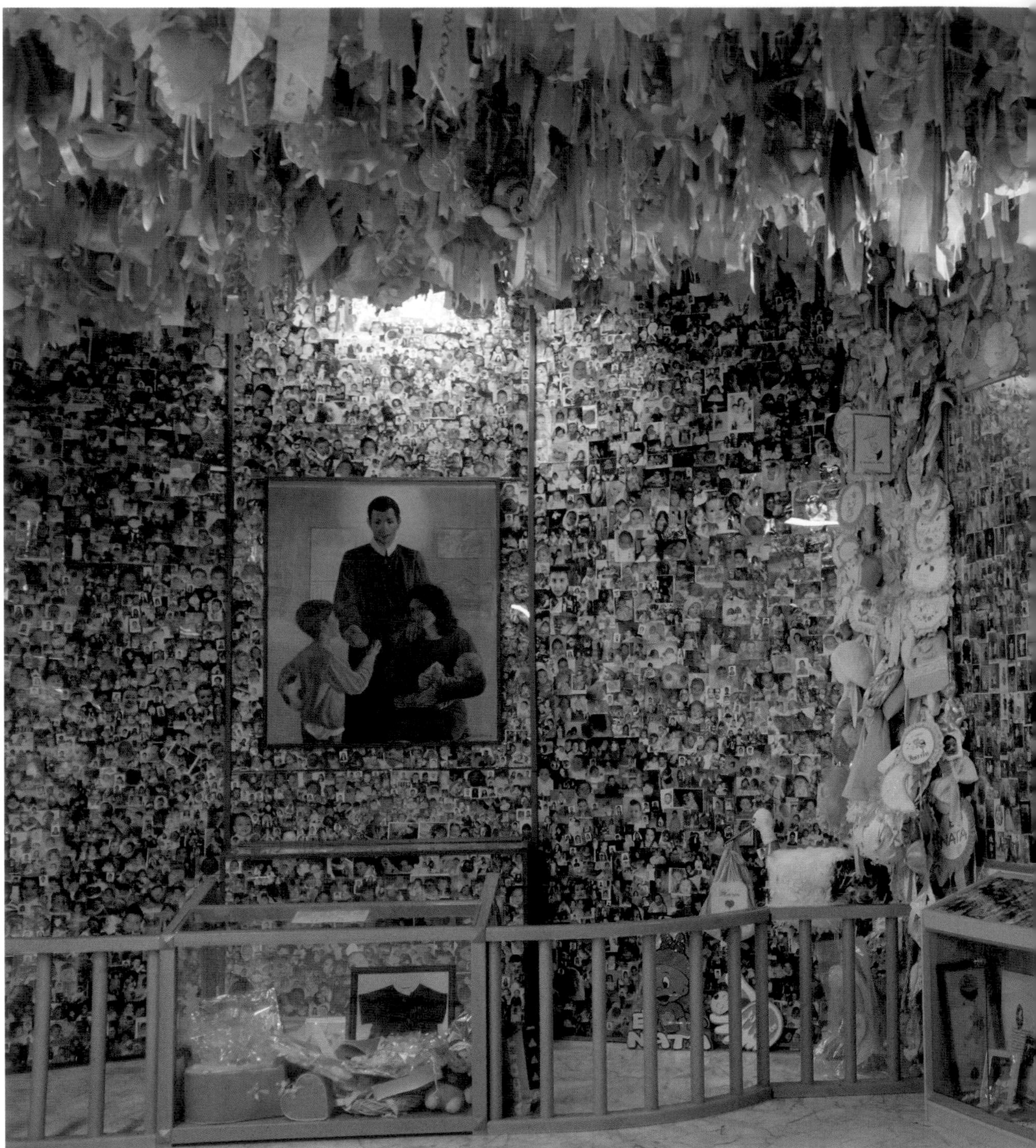

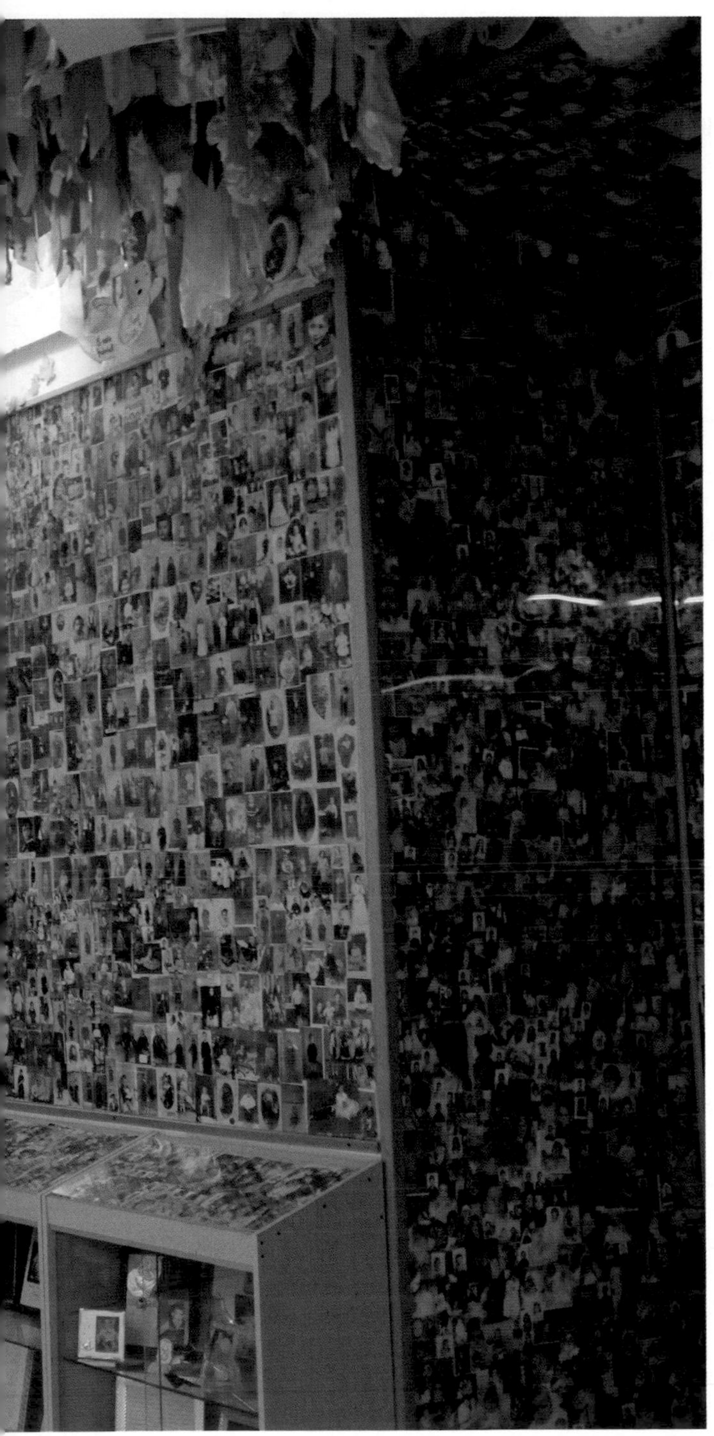

Sala dei Fiocchi (Room of the Ribbons), shrine of St Gerard Majella in Materdomini, 2017. Photo: Jessica Hughes.

FURTHER READING

Chapters 3, 31 and 43 and Exhibits 1, 4 and 38, this book.

Marion Bowman, '"He's my best friend": Relationality, materiality, and the manipulation of motherhood in devotion to St Gerard Majella in Newfoundland', in Terry Tak-ling Woo and Becky R. Lee (eds.), *Canadian Women Shaping Diasporic Religious Identities* (Waterloo, ON, 2016), pp. 3–34.

Pietro Caggiano, Michele Rak and Angelo Turchini, *Sweet Mother* (Pompeii, 1990).

Ittai Weinryb (ed.), *Ex Voto: Votive Giving across Cultures* (New York, NY, 2016).

41 Sex, Gender and Babies

John Forrester

'Sexuality came into being as part of a progressive differentiation of sex from the exigencies of reproduction.'[1] Thus Anthony Giddens glossed the influential theses of Michel Foucault. The speculative analysis in the first volume of *The History of Sexuality* has for forty years offered the important hypothesis that modernity is characterized by a dynamic relationship between 'reproduction', 'sex' and 'sexuality'. This chapter examines the relevance of this argument to the period 1960–2015.

Foucault aimed to upset what he saw as the liberal consensus about sex in the twentieth century. He questioned the self-congratulatory view that contrasted the censorship and repudiation of sexuality assumed to typify the nineteenth century with the twentieth-century pretension that the freeing of sexuality would lead to general social reform, even revolution, since sex, the core of our being, was always on the side of truth and opposed to power.

Foucault's polemic qualified the supposed interdiction and silencing constitutive of conventional, progressive views of Victorian sexuality with what he asserted was 'a regulated and polymorphous incitement to discourse' characteristic of the place of sexuality in the west for nearly two hundred years.[2] Foucault's most stinging gibes were directed at those for whom talking about sex is a prophecy of the 'enlightenment, liberation, and manifold pleasures' which the lifting of centuries of repression will bring about, and those who, unique to western civilization, 'are paid to listen to all and sundry impart the secrets of their sex' (p. 7).

The two motors driving these various discourses of sexuality were, Foucault posited, the traditional 'apparatus (*dispositif*) of alliance' and the modern 'apparatus of sexuality'. Every society has an apparatus of alliance, specifying and governing unions of blood and lineage, legitimacy and illegitimacy, natural and unnatural relations.[3] The anomalous and innovative feature of western societies is the use, since the eighteenth century, of a non-prohibitive, inciting and controlling system governing 'sexuality'.

1 Anthony Giddens, *The Transformation of Intimacy: Sexuality, Love, and Eroticism in Modern Societies* (Stanford, CA, 1992), p. 27.

2 Michel Foucault, *The History of Sexuality*, vol. 1: *An Introduction* (New York, NY, 1978 [French original, 1976]), p. 34. Further references to this work are given as page numbers in brackets in the text.

3 In French, 'alliance' has strong political and family connotations; one meaning is 'wedding ring'.

From 1850, four figures of sex emerged as key nodes: 'the hysterical woman, the masturbating child, the Malthusian couple, and the perverse adult' (p. 105). From the hysterical woman there are connections to the development of psychopathology and psychoanalysis through to the emergence of shell shock and its successor, post-traumatic stress disorder. The masturbating child was since the late eighteenth century a focus of popular scares and medical preoccupation, with teachers, doctors and psychologists mobilized to confront the dangers of premature, self-abusing sexuality, along the way enlisting (and thus colonizing) the family into the struggle; this preoccupation was then inverted and extended in the alarming figure of the sexually abused child who emerged in the 1960s.[4] The Malthusian couple is recognizable in the development of demography and eugenics, allied to medico-political battles over contraception and fears of overpopulation, underpopulation and the fate of the state. And the figure of the pervert, without which sexology might never have been invented, is familiar in the Long March from the medical invention of the 'homosexual' in 1870 to the victory of gays and their allies over the institutions of psychiatry in the 1970s.

'Sexuality' was part of Foucault's revisionist account of 'disciplinary', 'carceral', 'surveilling' or 'biopolitical' power (p. 83).[5] In contrast with sovereign, legal power, its mechanisms are local, 'micro-', or capillary, and its sources dispersed, such as in relations between doctors and patients. In Foucault's analysis, the medieval field of flesh and penance that once governed 'sex' was dispersed into an array of modern discourses and practices in demography, biology, medicine, psychiatry, psychology, ethics, pedagogy and political criticism (p. 33). Yet the rump of the unitary field still remains in late capitalist western societies, centred on descent ('ancestors', 'antecedents', 'progeny', 'descendants') linked to property relations and a skeleton of the old patriarchal family. Not only that: the apparatus of sexuality gains traction from its connection to the traditional family, taken as constituting legitimate reproductive sex – the 'hinge' between the anatomo-politics of the individual body and the biopolitics of the social body (p. 139).[6]

Two regimes – the apparatuses of alliance and sexuality. Four figures – the hysteric, the masturbating child, the Malthusian couple, the pervert. The new disciplinary practices associated with biopower interlinked with the older regime of sovereignty and alliance through the hinge of the family. Do Foucault's analytic categories adequately cover the disparate and spectacular transformations of the field of the sexual in the second half of the twentieth century, or do they lose their grip? Can one renew his four figures by positing that the hysterical woman became the feminist, the homosexual the

4 Ian Hacking, 'The making and molding of child abuse', *Critical Inquiry* 17 (1991), 253–88.

5 Andrea Rusnock, 'Biopolitics and the Invention of Population', Chapter 23, this book; Thomas Lemke, *Biopolitics: An Advanced Introduction*, trans. Eric Frederick Trump (New York, NY, 2011).

6 For 'hinge': Michel Foucault, *Psychiatric Power: Lectures at the Collège de France, 1973–1974*, ed. Jacques Lagrange, trans. Graham Burchell (Basingstoke, 2006), pp. 80–1.

gay activist, and the Malthusian couple the bearer of legal reproductive rights and agent of planned parenthood, while the masturbating child morphed into the abused, traumatized child? Or does this list, riddled with political sensitivities and even implausibilities, not indicate that the 'apparatus of sexuality' was unstable and indeed fragmenting under the pressure of the very forces that provoked Foucault's historical revisionism in the 1960s and 1970s? To put this another way: did the contraceptive revolution, the neutering of the term 'perversion', the irruption of the gay and feminist movements, and the success of assisted reproductive technologies and the concept of 'gender' leave in tatters whatever plausibility his analysis ever had?[7]

To address these questions, let us consider a number of historical changes since 1960: in masturbation, contraception, new reproductive technologies, and the politics of sex and gender.

The Ascendancy of Masturbation

It is a commonplace of the history of sexuality that from the eighteenth to the mid-twentieth centuries masturbation was uniformly regarded as dangerous to body and mind, and acutely so in childhood, when it caused permanent damage and was even a principal sign and cause of a degenerate constitution. From 1950, the position of masturbation changed in significant and telling ways. The first phase of sexology had been preoccupied with pathology: general, special and criminal, and in particular what Richard von Krafft-Ebing called the 'contrary sexual instinct'. Now the American sexologists Alfred Kinsey, and William Masters and Virginia Johnson, sought not only to reveal the secrets of sex, but also to promote a guilt-free ideology, the self-described 'permissive society' of the 1960s and 1970s.[8] Kinsey's reports declared masturbation universal amongst males and widely practised amongst females, and increasingly so as they become more sexually experienced. With Masters and Johnson's laboratory investigations, masturbation became the default mode of 'human sexual response'. At the heart of the sexological statistics and laboratory protocols of mid-century America is the solitary individual in orgasm – engaged in a sexual act with an indefinitely variable, but fundamentally optional, other (Fig. 41.1).

Second-wave feminism reconfigured the sexual life of women according to the principle of independence from men in all things, including sexuality: 'A woman needs a man like a fish needs a bicycle.' Exhortations to wrest control from doctors through disseminated knowledge, self-discovery and public disclosure found expression, for

7 Adele E. Clarke, *Disciplining Reproduction: Modernity, American Life Sciences, and 'the Problems of Sex'* (Berkeley, CA, 1998), p. 19.

8 Vern L. Bullough, *Science in the Bedroom: A History of Sex Research* (New York, NY, 1994); Thomas Maier, *Masters of Sex: The Life and Times of William Masters and Virginia Johnson* (New York, NY, 2009).

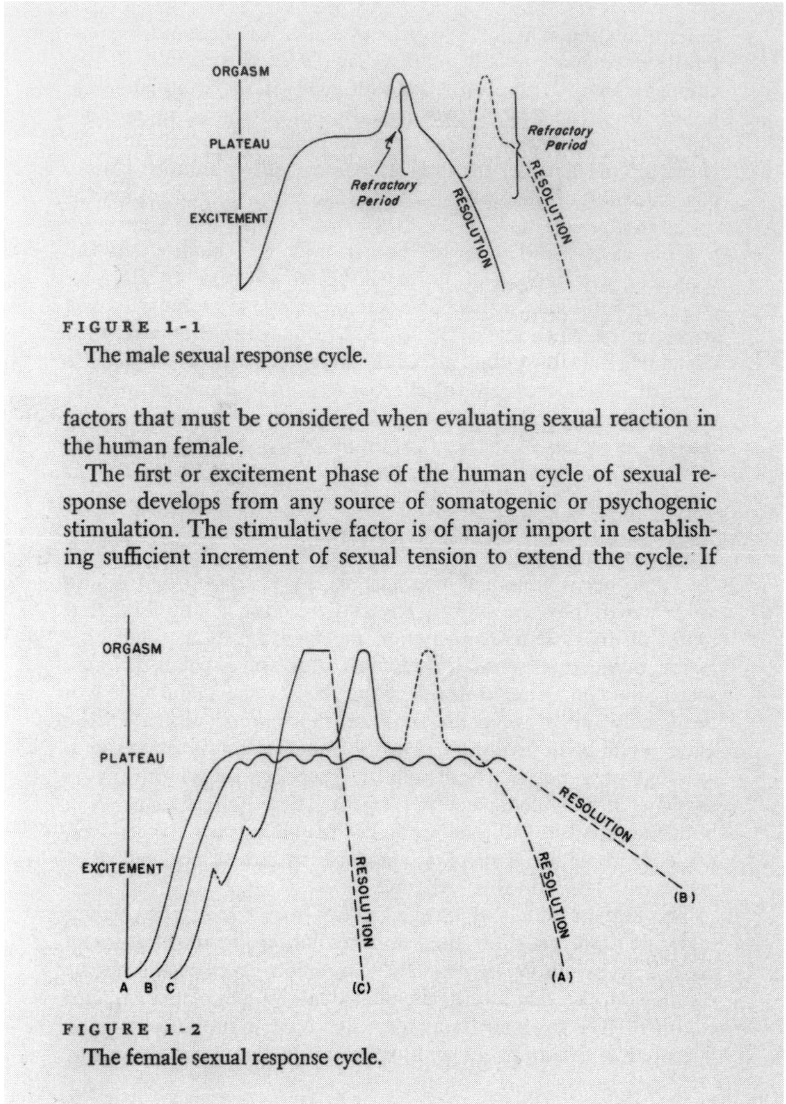

FIGURE 1-1
The male sexual response cycle.

factors that must be considered when evaluating sexual reaction in the human female.

The first or excitement phase of the human cycle of sexual response develops from any source of somatogenic or psychogenic stimulation. The stimulative factor is of major import in establishing sufficient increment of sexual tension to extend the cycle. If

FIGURE 1-2
The female sexual response cycle.

Figure 41.1 The male and female sexual response cycles according to Masters and Johnson. The graphs separated the varied female from the more uniform male response. These maps of sexual activity depicted individuals, never couples. From William H. Masters and Virginia E. Johnson, *Human Sexual Response* (Boston, MA: Little, Brown and Company, 1966), p. 5, by permission of Ishi Press International.

example, in the Boston Women's Health Course Collective's *Women and Their Bodies*, the forerunner of *Our Bodies, Ourselves* (1970–3), which focused on sex and reproduction (Fig. 41.2).[9] Masturbation as the exemplary sexual act within the sexological

9 Wendy Kline, '*Our Bodies, Ourselves*', Exhibit 35, this book.

30

FANTASIES

"I masturbated to this fantasy: an older woman whom I had never met entered a dressing room I was in. After a brief conversation, I placed her against the wall and explored her body with my mouth. First her breasts, then her vagina. As I fanta-sized this part, I had an orgasm. Afterwards, I felt very disturbed because making love to a woman had been so intensely pleasurable and I was afraid of being "homosexual", and because the woman I created was older and made me think of my mother. I would decide that it was a bad fantasy to have had, and that I was a little abnormal for having had it."

"I imagined I was sitting in a room. The walls were all white. There was nothing in it, and I was naked. There was a large window at one end, and anyone who wanted to could look in and see me. There was no place to hide. There was something very arousing about being so exposed. My heart started to pound and my stomach sort of pulsed in a very powerful way. I masturbated while having this fantasy, and afterwards I felt very sad. I thought---I must be so sick, so distorted inside that this image of myself could give me such intense sexual pleasure. It was more satisfying than making love.'

Figure 41.2 Excerpt from the Boston Women's Health Course Collective's *Women and Their Bodies: A Course* (1970), p. 30. Fantasy and masturbation were important topics in second-wave feminism, since freedom from shame about sexual experiences was seen as essential to acquiring independence and autonomy as a woman. Reproduced with permission of Our Bodies Ourselves, www.ourbodiesourselves.org. Schlesinger Library, Radcliffe Institute, Harvard University.

field conformed with the political ideal of autonomy within the personal-political sphere of sexuality. The feminist credentials of masturbation were echoed in the *Hite Report* (1976), which declared clitoral masturbation the most reliable route to female orgasm. Nancy Friday's *My Secret Garden* (1973), a miscellaneous confessional of women's first-person sexual fantasies employed in masturbation or in sexual intercourse, aimed to spread enlightenment and, in effect, create a community of proud masturbators. Alongside the transformation of contraceptive practices from 1960, the 'cordless electric vibrator' – packaged in 1969 for the self-help market – became a staple element, like the tampon, the diaphragm and the pill, in the array of a modern woman's sexual prosthetics.[10]

Both novel products, the vibrator and the pill, fed the emergence of the sexually independent woman who regarded her pleasure – with or without a partner – as a right, not a cause for embarrassment or shame. Young single women on the pill, close to

10 Rachel P. Maines, *The Technology of Orgasm: 'Hysteria', the Vibrator, and Women's Sexual Satisfaction* (Baltimore, MD, 1999), p. 166 n. 168.

80 per cent of those under 20 in West Germany in 1975–7, or married and single women with vibrators (over 50 per cent of American women used vibrators, and 20 per cent did so regularly, in 2009) – these women were newly dedicated to a sexual-pleasure-seeking lifestyle.[11]

Yet the largest trade in products related to masturbation was directed at men. The pornography industry exploded from strip clubs to *Playboy* in the 1950s and 1960s, through porn videos in the 1980s to DVDs in the 1990s and the saturation of the internet in the 2000s. The market in aids to men's masturbation was far larger than for the vibrator, which in turn was double that of the condom. Western culture had come a long way from the nineteenth-century invention of spiked penis rings to suppress masturbation to their routine sale along with a myriad other devices to promote sexual pleasure. One of the principal and enduring features of the mass dissemination of sexual images was the continuum between 'sex educational' products (often sponsored by governments), advertising and pornography, just as tele-sex work produced a continuum from decorative newsreaders to online pay-per-view porn. The young idealists and hedonists of the 1960s and 1970s promoted revolutions of desire; western culture had created 'an endless circuit of stimulus and arousal, display and looking': the 'onanization of sex'.[12]

Contraception

The 'Malthusian couple' may be a misleading term with which to capture the long history of contraception since the late nineteenth century.[13] But there is a line of development from that figure through eugenics, population policy and the transformation of the place of contraception in the second half of the twentieth century, including the abrogation of restrictive laws. In Britain, conservative doctors in the early 1960s had opposed prescribing the pill on the grounds that the possibility of pregnancy was not a medical condition and doctors had no right treating healthy patients; by 1974, NHS directives had converted its prescription into a first-rank medical duty.

The speed of these changes should alert us to the power of the transformative forces in play: it was the rapid uptake of the pill, initially amongst educated, increasingly single, young women, that was the symbol and part-motor of this change. In the 1960s and early 1970s, intense concerns about overpopulation and the excessive breeding of

11 For the German figure: Dagmar Herzog, *Sexuality in Europe: A Twentieth-Century History* (Cambridge, 2011), p. 139; for the American one: Debra Herbenick *et al.*, 'Prevalence and characteristics of vibrator use by women in the United States: Results from a nationally representative study', *Journal of Sexual Medicine* 6 (2009), 1857–66.

12 Herzog, *Sexuality in Europe*, pp. 139 ff., 206.

13 Lesley A. Hall, 'Movements to Separate Sex and Reproduction', Chapter 29; Jesse Olszynko-Gryn, 'Technologies of Contraception and Abortion', Chapter 36, this book.

the poor (often in the figure of the unmarried mother) may have fused older eugenic concerns with 'liberal' ideas of women's rights, and so produced government policies which, as in the United Kingdom, made contraceptives free and accessible to all.[14] The pill also became one of the first 'population-cohort' preventive drugs: medicines taken by a significant proportion of the relevant population to prevent life-threatening events (in 2012 in the United Kingdom, two million women took the pill; seven million men and women took statins).

Yet the success of the pill, like the cultural revolution in which it was born, was never complete. The most widely used modern contraceptive is surgical not pharmaceutical: sterilization. Hundreds of millions of women of childbearing age and their husbands have been sterilized, and some surprising countries are among those with the highest rates: in 2009 China, India, South Korea, Thailand, the United States, the United Kingdom and Switzerland all had figures for combined female and male sterilization between 40 per cent (China) and 22 per cent (Switzerland) of those using contraception. The pill rarely exceeds these levels of uptake (but does in Germany, at 53 per cent). Sales of the condom, the emblematic male contraceptive, declined with the dissemination of the pill, but bounced back after AIDS made preventing disease as important as avoiding pregnancy. In Japan, abortion is a far more prevalent form of contraception than the pill.[15] Longer-term pill usage depended less upon collective sexual ethics and more upon the economics of health care in different countries – whether it was supplied free, in a clinic or by a medical specialist – and other contingent local factors.

Biopolitics, from Malthus to Zero Population Growth, were always envisaged on a species scale.[16] It turned out that the best way to achieve macroeconomic effects was via the market for consumables, and the most efficent way of liberalizing this market was to medicalize it. The market was often combined with aggressive state population policies: 'Get sterilized and drive away in a Nano car!' declares promotional material from the Indian state Rajasthan – or end up in prison in Kerala if you are the father of a third child.[17]

One could posit that in place of the Malthusian couple there arose the contraceptive individual, in particular young women, at first (1955–65) mainly from the middle classes, who adopted 'a sexual lifestyle in which reproduction was separate from sexual

14 Lara V. Marks, *Sexual Chemistry: A History of the Contraceptive Pill* (New Haven, CT, 2001), p. 257.

15 United Nations, Department of Economic and Social Affairs, Population Division, 'World Contraceptive Use 2009', www.un.org/esa/population/publications/contraceptive2009/contracept2009_wallchart_front.pdf; Marks, *Sexual Chemistry*, pp. 243–5; Richard M. Smith, 'Marriage and Fertility in Different Household Systems', Chapter 24; Olszynko-Gryn, 'Technologies of Contraception and Abortion'; James M. Edmonson, 'Condoms', Exhibit 28, this book.

16 Alison Bashford, 'World Population from Eugenics to Climate Change', Chapter 34; Patrick Ellis, '*Z.P.G.*', Exhibit 36, this book.

17 'News section: Demography', *Journal of Global Health* 1 (2011), 127–8.

activity and marriage was no longer a marker of either'.[18] Combining the 'masturbating child', the 'Malthusian couple' and the 'hysteric', the late twentieth century produced a different figure: the orgasmic autonomous woman. She owed much to the 'sexual revolution' – a name for a set of moral, legal and social transformations, the exact depth and importance of which recent historians have debated. But simple and new or reconfigured technologies also played key roles: the pill, suitably packaged as the Dialpak, and the smooth plastic battery-driven vibrator, both straddling the border between the medical and the proprietary, both targeted at a large and rapidly expanding consumer market (Fig. 41.3).[19]

New Reproductive Technologies

The baby-boom generation was soon to have another series of life-transforming products: in vitro fertilization (IVF), the most prominent of the assisted reproductive technologies developed in the postwar period and a platform for others.[20] Modern miracles as these were, the social imagination had been well prepared: in the 1920s, the Cambridge biochemist J. B. S. Haldane projected a science-fiction future of 'ectogenesis' taking over from womb-conception and pregnancy in the supply of new human beings.[21] Haldane's artificial womb is not yet realizable in IVF, but surrogate mothers take on that function.

If the scientific imaginary had long primed us for IVF, its mode of biopolitical implantation was the surprise. Haldane and other early eugenicists always assumed that planning would drive the dissemination of technoscientific human reproduction. The rise of IVF was the opposite of planned: in the postwar era, a borderline respectable science and clinical practice was working uphill to alleviate the individual miseries of involuntarily childless couples against the grain of modernist fears of overpopulation; its eventual success owed more to the media and the consumer than public research programmes.[22] While ethical and political debate vacillated between admiration and horror, the rapid response by teams of embryologists and gynaecologists in various jurisdictions to the demands of childless couples ensured that, whatever the political and ethical decisions and prohibitions in any one country, there would now be a worldwide IVF industry. Instead of a global population policy, with or without accompanying eugenics, we now have a

18 Hera Cook, *The Long Sexual Revolution: English Women, Sex, and Contraception, 1800–1975* (Oxford, 2004), p. 337.

19 On Dialpak: Patricia Peck Gossel, 'Packaging the pill', in Robert Bud, Bernard Finn and Helmuth Trischler (eds.), *Manifesting Medicine: Bodies and Machines* (London, 1999), pp. 105–21.

20 Nick Hopwood, 'Artificial Fertilization', Chapter 39, this book.

21 J. B. S. Haldane, *Daedalus, or Science and the Future* (London, 1924).

22 Naomi Pfeffer, *The Stork and the Syringe: A Political History of Reproductive Medicine* (Cambridge, 1993).

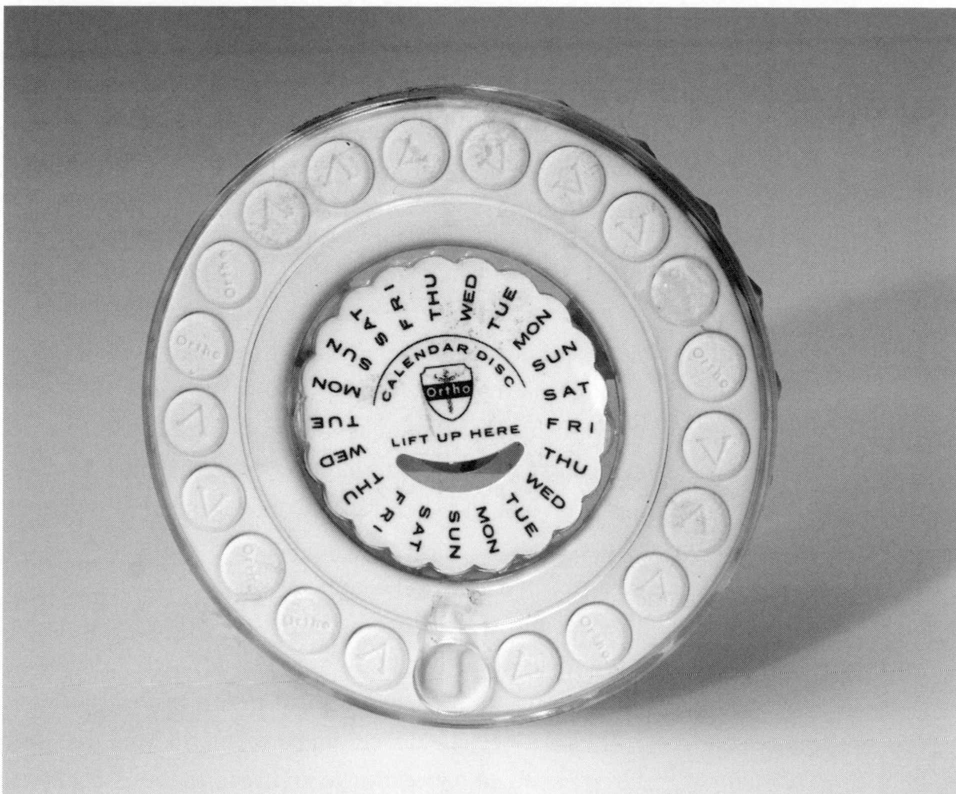

Figure 41.3 Dialpak dispenser for oral contraceptives. Ortho Pharmaceutical marketed this compliance packaging in Canada in 1961 and then in the United States to reinforce and simplify the daily routine of pill taking. In this early model, the plastic central disc had to be taken out and reinserted to show the correct first day. *c.* 6 cm diameter, Dittrick Medical History Center, Case Western Reserve University.

market in reproductive services, rapidly and increasingly globalized by the labyrinth of local medico-legal restrictions, responsive to the desperate desires and willingness to pay of the childless.[23] With changes in divorce law transforming property transmission, with the autonomous, single, sexually active, contraceptive-deploying woman linked to the demise of the nuclear family, with technologies of assisted reproduction ever more available, the 'apparatus of alliance' has, through the realization of science-fiction dreams and the revolution in the position of women, been transformed.

Is this the most important historical transformation of the postwar period: that like for other multifaceted novelties, such as flying, a liberalized market allowed mass access to desired 'sexual' products, from the vibrator to the pill, from pornography to IVF?

23 Marcia C. Inhorn and Frank van Balen (eds.), *Infertility around the Globe: New Thinking on Childlessness, Gender, and Reproductive Technologies* (Berkeley, CA, 2002).

Gender and Identity

Although strictly speaking the introduction of the term 'gender' can be dated to 1955, it is useful to delineate four phases in the development of the concept. In an early phase of 'incubation', from the 1930s to the mid-1950s, associated with anthropology (especially Margaret Mead) then sociology, inquiry into the distribution of functions and characteristics of individuals in different societies deployed the binaries 'male/female' and 'masculine/feminine' and then the concept of 'role'. Second, the Johns Hopkins paediatric psychologist John Money coined 'gender' (tied to 'gender role') in 1955, to give an account of intersexed, transsexual and transvestite patients, and the UCLA psychiatrist Robert Stoller introduced 'gender identity' in 1963 (and then 'core gender identity') to mean 'the sense of knowing to which sex one belongs, that is, the awareness "I am a male" or "I am a female"'.[24] Stoller promoted an influential psychoanalytic account of 'sex and gender' in his 1968 book of that title; the contrast with biological 'sex' gave the term 'gender' its weight. But, from the start, clinicians' and psychologists' usage wavered between ascribed social category ('gender role') and self-reported psychological datum.

In a third phase, feminist theorists, notably Kate Millett, Germaine Greer, Ann Oakley and Gayle Rubin, used 'gender' in the 1970s to advance the view that what had been regarded as biological and unchangeable was in fact historically variable and socially constructed. The term became disseminated very widely in academic and political discourse, its fortunes linked between 1970 and 1990 to the impact of second-wave feminism; it came to be seen as a fundamental category for historical, social and cultural description and analysis, on a par with 'class' and 'race'. Finally, re-evaluation, particularly from 'within' feminism, led by Judith Butler's influential *Gender Trouble* (1990) and also by queer theorists and transgender activists, criticized the concept for covertly reintroducing the contested essentialist elements it had been invented to oppose.[25] But the movement had been too successful: 'gender' was here to stay and became enshrined in laws such as the UK Gender Recognition Act 2004 as well as in a thriving and ever-growing academic and NGO industry of research and teaching ('gender studies', with its power base in the United States).

'Sex change' was made possible by the development of surgical techniques and hormone manufacturing. Initially surrounded by media sensationalism and always subject to ethical and aesthetic circumspection, these growing powers, though rarely entirely successful, supplemented the arts of fashion and changing dress codes to produce the desired 'sex' or 'gender'.[26] A handful of specialized medical centres (Charing

24 R. J. Stoller, 'A contribution to the study of gender identity', *International Journal of Psycho-Analysis* 45 (1964), 220–6, on 220.

25 Sarah Franklin, 'Feminism and Reproduction', Chapter 42, this book.

26 Joanne Meyerowitz, *How Sex Changed: A History of Transsexuality in the United States* (Cambridge, MA, 2002).

Cross, Los Angeles, Johns Hopkins) were established for sex change or gender reassignment, as it later came to be called. Ironically, a wider range of technical options for bodily fashioning and manipulation went hand in hand with increasingly accepted self-affirmations of the fundamental stability of a 'gender identity'. From the start, 'patients' played active parts, through looping effects, in establishing new categories and 'kinds of people'.[27] In 1980, this led to the entry of 'gender identity' and related categories ('gender dysphoria', 'gender identity disorder') into the now hegemonic *Diagnostic and Statistical Manual of Mental Disorders* (DSM-III), just as it jettisoned 'homosexuality'. Medical technology was essential; but the orchestrated demand for recognition of a newly achieved and long concealed stable identity was equally crucial. By the end of the twentieth century, demand for the social recognition of 'identity' coexisted with scientists' forgoing their authority to rule on the facts of that complex continuum of sexual orientations and gender identities – social, cultural, bodily, chromosomal – best summed up in the complicated politics of such acronyms as LGBTQ. But achieving the fixed identity took active social labour: what Harold Garfinkel had called 'passing', which for Butler was crystallized in the performative. Gender identity never lost its internal paradox as what is most fixed for an individual and most transparently socially and technologically constructed.

Yet the success of gender as a category owed more to its being treated as self-evident and fundamentally social. Gender analysis could draw in microeconomics, or the division of labour, controversies about psychological differences between 'the sexes' and modes of social organization. 'Gender' suddenly made visible what everyone always already knew. To feminists, it promised to separate biological 'sex' from the social domain of struggle; and to dispel the invisibility of divisions between men and women, boys and girls.

Abortion, contraception, pregnancy, childbirth, sexuality, sexual exploitation and violence: these were core issues for second-wave feminism. Enlightenment and the struggle to provide and access medical and paramedical services would remain key elements alongside agitation for the repeal of anti-women laws. What by the beginning of the twenty-first century could be called 'rights to sexual and reproductive self-determination' had been at the heart of the larger political movement of feminism since the late 1960s.[28] Concerns over population were 'trumped by the success of the feminist tradition of presenting reproductive rights as human rights'.[29] One might even chart the successes and failures of feminism through the uneven demography, changing legal status and clamorous politics of abortion. In the late twentieth century, abortion was surely the hinge where, as Foucault had put it, the anatomo-politics of the individual body met the biopolitics of

27 Ian Hacking, 'The looping effects of human kinds', in Dan Sperber, David Premack and Ann James Premack (eds.), *Causal Cognition: A Multidisciplinary Debate* (Oxford, 1995), pp. 351–83.

28 Herzog, *Sexuality in Europe*, p. 220.

29 Bashford, 'World Population'.

the social body – and where the politics of gender, the right to sexual pleasure and the regulation of reproduction intersected.[30]

A crucial attraction of the concept of gender for feminism, one it shared with many other movements gathered in the 1980s under the umbrella term 'politics of identity', was the sense that it is both conventionally political, in that individuals choose to belong to the identity group, and 'a choice predicated on the strongly held, intensely conceived belief that the individual has absolutely no choice but to belong to that specific group'.[31] Blacks, women and gays: these groups who had spearheaded struggles for rights and against discriminatory laws, found they had much in common – and yet much that separated them. The phrase 'politics of identity' names this uneasiness and points to its source: each group was defined by a simultaneously exclusionary and inclusionary biological or corporeal trait, which condemned members to membership, and yet their struggles were in the name of universalistic categories – freedom, rights, autonomy: part of the struggle consisted in converting non-volitional membership into a matter of pride and celebration ('black pride', 'gay pride'). The later theorizing of 'intersectionality', to deconstruct the too exclusive preoccupation with single group identities, was a response to this constitutive incoherence.

Both feminism and gay liberation were fundamentally attached to an ideal of sexual self-determination which required the separation of sex from reproduction, for both (lesbian and non-lesbian) women and (gay) men, whose sexuality would no longer be defined by the nineteenth-century definition of perversion as any act that separates sex from reproduction. About this 'normal' aim of the 'sexual instinct' sexology had virtually nothing to say: it was focused on sexual pleasure, but above all on its deviations, aberrations and perversions – from kissing to licking excrement. So, having defined 'normal sexuality' by its linkage with reproduction, sexological writings then rigorously shunned conception, pregnancy and childbirth in their studies of 'human sexuality'. Kinsey's mentioned pregnancy only in the phrase 'fear of pregnancy'. Masters and Johnson's physiology of sex bore few traces of Masters's own first expertise in infertility; their therapy was focused solely on 'sexual dysfunction'. Even when Viagra was introduced in 1998, successfully supplanting many other sexual dysfunction therapies, it was not for reproductive purposes but strictly for the 'sexual pleasure' market; effects on reproductive capacity (such as sperm count and viability) were barely considered.

The concept of 'gender identity' added a third force to those stemming from sexology and the campaign for contraception into the increasingly estranged relations between reproduction and sexuality. From 1970 to 2005 in the United Kingdom, the legal and administrative refusal to accept a MTF transsexual as a woman was based

30 On struggles over abortion law: Martin H. Johnson and Nick Hopwood, 'Modern Law and Regulation', Chapter 40, this book.

31 O. Patterson, 'The nature, causes, and implications of ethnic identification', in C. Fried (ed.), *Minorities: Community and Identity* (Berlin, 1983), pp. 25–50, on pp. 28–9.

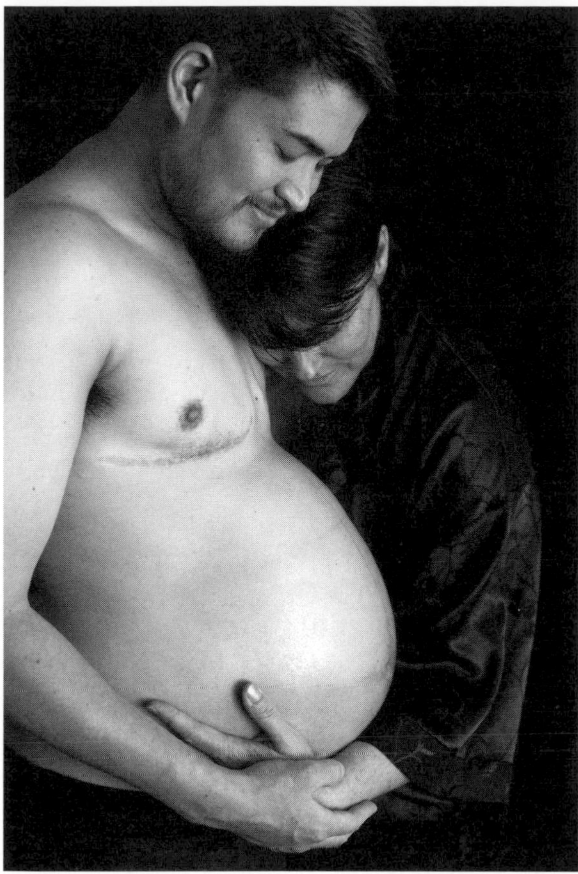

Figure 41.4 Photograph of Thomas and Nancy Beatie, widely publicized in 2008 to illustrate news stories about the 'pregnant man'. Transgender, legally male and pregnant, the American Thomas Beatie was emblematic of early twenty-first-century intersections of sex, gender, identity and reproduction. The Beaties publicly stressed the universal desire to reproduce. Kristian Dowling / TB, Getty Images.

on two assumptions: that 'sex' was determined biologically and could not change; and that 'sex' (not 'gender') was the relevant criterion for deciding on the validity of a marriage, assumed firstly to be 'ordained for the procreation of children' (Book of Common Prayer, 1662). The profound shift in the latter half of the twentieth century towards 'companionate marriage' ('the mutual society, help, and comfort, that the one ought to have of the other, both in prosperity and adversity') was crucial in the change in the law governing change of gender (whereby gender identity became legal sex) and in the widening of the concept of marriage to include 'same-sex' partners (in the UK Marriage [Same Sex Couples] Act 2013 and similar laws in other countries). Marriage was no longer essentially linked to reproduction. For social purposes, 'sex' was no longer tied to the capacity to reproduce; the laws governing the recognition of gender identity and same-sex marriage were the visible triumphs of this shift (Fig. 41.4).

Conclusion

The separation of sex from reproduction resulted from the confluence of three very different historical currents: successful campaigns, both ideological and technological, to infiltrate marriage with a contraceptive regime focused on and primarily servicing the needs of autonomous women; the detailed mapping of the diversity of sexual activities and the widespread acceptance of 'perversions' – by definition non-reproductive – followed by their normalization as the practices of all and sundry; finally, the victory of the category of 'gender' for analytic, civic and legal purposes over the 'biological' category of sex. The biomedical sciences had earlier vied with social scientific and ethico-religious competitors for ideological supremacy in the sphere of sex and reproduction; they had failed in many respects, but instead had ended the twentieth century as essential and profit-making technical services for the sexual and reproductive consumer.

Does Foucault's analysis of the '*incorporation of perversions* and a new *specification of individuals*' (pp. 42–3) do justice to these movements: seeing them as a continuation, by other means, of this individualizing and splintering effect of the apparatus of sexuality? One can, I reckon, only preserve this analysis by recognizing many other forces at work – not least the liberalization of moral codes in the postwar west and the liberalization of the market in medical and other goods which produced the autonomous sexual consumer of that era and eliminated the core element of the 'apparatus of alliance' – the production of descendants – from marriage, while preserving its capital-accumulating and elite-preserving functions. But these later fortunes of the 'apparatus of sexuality' also demonstrate the agency of those caught up in it to transform the relations of power, often through their explicit demands. Whether these are explicitly political and contestatory, as with gays, lesbians and feminists, or individualistic in the novel mode of the barely fettered consumer – as in the infertile and the orgasmic autonomous woman – the structure of the field of sexuality was transformed. Foucault's own conception of power – capillary, local, digressive – had offered the ingredients which could assimilate resistance, liberation and creative innovation; but the appearance of the orgasmic autonomous woman, the surrogate mother, the transsexual, the array of liberated gay and lesbian individuals and their communities, and the reconstitution of history and culture through the frame of gender was by no means apparent in Foucault's original dual analytics of alliance and sexuality with their four historical figures. Not only did he omit the pressure of consumer demand and the mass marketing of devices and desires alongside the consequences of activist ingenuity and the resultant archipelago of sexual communities; not only did he underestimate the political triumphs of the movements organized around these new figures; he also underestimated the sheer success of the sexual sciences and technologies and their integration into the medico-industrial complex of which sex became so full a part.

42 Feminism and Reproduction

Sarah Franklin

The histories and meanings of 'feminism' and 'reproduction' are so deeply intertwined that it is impossible to disentangle them from one another, or from the histories of sex and sexual inequality to which they are central. Both terms are fundamental also to the meaning of 'modernity'; yet, as feminist writers and activists have long argued, canonical accounts of modern life have excluded the radical transformations of reproduction and gender since the late seventeenth century. These opposing feminist emphases – on the crucial importance of gender and reproduction to all aspects of modernity, and their absence from social, political and economic analysis – combine to produce a dilemma of two halves. While feminists have sought to raise the profile of reproduction within accounts of social organization and political economy, they have at the same time worked to separate 'women' from their perennial association with reproductive labour and biology. Key to this effort have been consistent challenges to the reductive determinisms that have naturalized women, reproduction and 'the facts of life'. These determinisms include the privatization of domesticity that has separated the home, childcare and housework from the public sphere, and the individualization of citizenship that has equated personal freedom with autonomy.

'Reproduction'

Feminist scholars from several disciplines, and historians in particular, have long pointed to the difficulty of defining 'reproduction'.[1] In her account of the mid-eighteenth-century borrowing of this term to describe the generation of new life, Ludmilla Jordanova claimed that its introduction by authors such as Buffon reflected an abstraction and professionalization of knowledge about 'the process of producing new individuals of the same species'.[2] Similarly for Londa Schiebinger, the intersection of reproduction

1 Nick Hopwood, 'The Keywords "Generation" and "Reproduction"', Chapter 20, this book; Faye D. Ginsburg and Rayna Rapp, 'The politics of reproduction', *Annual Review of Anthropology* 20 (1991), 311–43; Sarah Franklin and Helena Ragoné, 'Introduction' to Franklin and Ragoné (eds.), *Reproducing Reproduction: Kinship, Power, and Technological Innovation* (Philadelphia, PA, 1998), pp. 1–14; Rene Almeling, 'Reproduction', *Annual Review of Sociology* 41 (2015), 423–42.

2 Ludmilla Jordanova, 'Interrogating the concept of reproduction in the eighteenth century', in Faye D. Ginsburg and Rayna Rapp (eds.), *Conceiving the New World Order: The Global Politics of Reproduction* (Berkeley, CA, 1995), pp. 369–86, on p. 372 (quoting the *OED*).

and the early life sciences marked a turning point in the development of the concept.[3] Barbara Duden had already noted that by around 1850 'reproduction' was moving to the centre of political economy. With an increasing emphasis on economic production, its use to describe the composite functions resulting in childbirth indexed the process through which the uterus came to be seen as both a workhorse of the body politic and 'living proof of the natural origin of economic concepts'.[4] In the nineteenth and especially the twentieth century, Adele Clarke argued, 'reproduction' became central to the science of biology – with a consequence that a process formerly linked to interdependence, fruitfulness and spirituality was depersonalized, professionalized and 'disciplined'.[5]

As Gillian Beer and Marilyn Strathern have noted, Darwin's strategic transfer of the generative idioms of reproduction and fertility into his radical account of nature as a single, law-like system of shared descent helped to familiarize his readers with the concept of evolution. Beer observed, following Marx, that Darwin's delight in reproductive imagery was a product of his time, its material conditions (the rapid growth of industrial technology) and political economy (the birth of industrial capitalism and the proletariat). Like the supercharged development of industrial machinery that so dominated the nineteenth-century imagination, reproduction under Darwin became an autonomous, protean force. 'The natural order produces itself, and through reproduction it produces both its own continuance and its diversity', commented Beer, in an echo of Marx's famous charge against Darwin of transferring the Malthusian theory of population to beasts and plants. According to Strathern, a further consequence of 'Darwin's loan' is that reproduction was newly naturalized, so that 'the emergence of personhood itself was taken to be … the outcome of biological development rather than the person's own moral standing or participation in relationships with other persons'.[6] As Duden stressed, 'reproduction' came to be used in the nineteenth century not only in natural history, but also in medicine, demography and political science, owing to the changing economy of commodity production as well as modern scientific epistemologies.[7]

3 Londa Schiebinger, *Nature's Body: Gender in the Making of Modern Science* (Boston, MA, 1993).

4 Barbara Duden, *The Woman beneath the Skin: A Doctor's Patients in Eighteenth-Century Germany*, trans. Thomas Dunlap (Cambridge, MA, 1991), pp. 205, 28–9.

5 Adele E. Clarke, *Disciplining Reproduction: Modernity, American Life Sciences, and 'the Problems of Sex'* (Berkeley, CA, 1998), pp. 5–11.

6 Gillian Beer, *Darwin's Plots: Evolutionary Narrative in Darwin, George Eliot and Nineteenth-Century Fiction* (London, 1983), p. 48; Marilyn Strathern, *Reproducing the Future: Essays on Anthropology, Kinship, and the New Reproductive Technologies* (New York, NY, 1992), pp. 16, 23.

7 Duden, *Woman beneath the Skin*, p. 28.

Modernity

The system of political economy associated with 'reproduction' is modern, and definitively so. Aided by the many fusions encompassed by the term, which combines the activities of humans, other animals and machines, production is the dominant value in modern society and in the lives of the metropolitan citizens to whose behaviour the term 'modernity' was applied.[8] Productivity is celebrated in myriad forms: as design, creativity and technological sophistication, and as the literally earth-shattering powers of industrial equipment such as steam engines, turbines and dynamite. Meanwhile, in contrast to the modern freedoms of style, movement and creativity associated with the masculinized public sphere, pregnancy and parturition stay in a prelapsarian state of nature. Despite the new importance of 'reproduction' as a public, professional and scientific concern, the bearing and raising of offspring was increasingly segregated within the private family home. The facts of life are antediluvian, and required to be: in the new industrial order, domesticity remains morally uncorrupted and innocent precisely as a respite from all that industrial production entails. This radical new division between productive and reproductive labour is crucial to the organization of modern industrial economies, but often overlooked in accounts of their emergence. It is one of the great conjuring tricks of modern history that some of its best-known analysts managed to neglect the great divide through which childcare and housework, the basic infrastructures of modern life, became private, 'uneconomic' activities.

The modern division of the domestic sphere from production is peculiar as well as recent. Despite the new dependence of the family on a salary, industrial capitalism was celebrated for the independence of incomes from families. Thus, in *Ancient Law* (1861), one of the formative descriptions of modernity, the legal theorist, Henry Maine, described 'the gradual dissolution' of an enforced system of dependence on family and kinship relations which was progressively succeeded by the free individual 'as the unit of which civil laws take account'. From a situation in which 'the relations of Persons are summed up in the relations of Family' emerged a new social order, Maine claimed, 'in which all these relations arise from the free agreement of Individuals' – a transformation he codified as the shift 'from Status to Contract'. 'Nor is it difficult to see', Maine argued, 'what is the tie between man and man which replaces by degrees those forms of reciprocity in rights and duties which have their origin in the Family. *It is Contract*.'[9] This autonomous modern individual, freed from the bondage of kinship, can enter a

8 Charles Baudelaire is credited with the first use of 'modernity' in this sense in his 1864 essay 'The painter of modern life'; see further Marshall Berman, *All That Is Solid Melts into Air: The Experience of Modernity* (New York, NY, 1988).

9 Henry Sumner Maine, *Ancient Law: Its Connection with the Early History of Society, and Its Relation to Modern Ideas* (London, 1861), pp. 168–9 (emphasis added).

contract by choice, and exchange his labour for wages in a free-market economy, as opposed to inheriting a familial status with its rigid constraints. Precisely because he has no familial status, he becomes the prototypical modern citizen – the fully enfranchised, rights-bearing, wage-earning worker, and a free individual under civil law. His birth, according to Maine, confirms the dawn of an era defined by the decreasing power and influence of kinship and family ties; freedom is now equated with autonomy.

Yet this purported loosening of traditional kinship obligations in the face of a new 'tie between man and man' had no such enfranchising effect on those members of society destined to become either wives or mothers: these roles became more not less restrictive. As the social critic and philosopher Mary Wollstonecraft pointed out in 1792, the privileges of modern freedom were not only segregated by sex, but increasingly defined what either sexes or societies could become.[10] The male citizen was distinguished by his emancipation from reproductive labour: his privileged access to education, waged employment and mobility separated him from his female counterpart, who took on the greater burden of domestic service. None of the freedom from 'the relations of family', nor access to individual rights, educational opportunity, autonomy of movement or contractual choice, could be enjoyed by those modern individuals tasked with the unwaged service of maintaining domestic family life.

From Contract to Contract

Far from gaining emancipation through new contractual freedoms such as wage labour, women of all classes remained subject to the all-important (and largely unaltered) contract of marriage – still today an institution in which the relation of status to contract remains highly sex-linked. With women more subject than their male counterparts to enforced marital servitude, conjugal bonds continued to restrict the horizons of 'the female sex' despite the notable autonomies that citizens of modern nation-states had won. Bound by marriage laws which made of them and their offspring precisely the form of private patriarchal property that Maine presented modern 'persons' as having escaped, 'women' were increasingly defined by their reproductive roles as industrial capitalism came to dominate the modern era. Nearly a century after Maine's proclamation of universal 'personal' liberty, Simone de Beauvoir concluded that marriage remained a premodern institution: 'in marriage woman was a ward, to be beaten, her conduct watched over in detail, and her fortune used at will'.[11] To modern feminism, then, reproduction, marriage and the family assumed greater political centrality as it became clear that few things compromise 'women' more severely than the ascribed status of wife or mother.

10 Mary Wollstonecraft, *A Vindication of the Rights of Woman: With Strictures on Political and Moral Subjects* (London, 1792).

11 Simone de Beauvoir, *The Second Sex*, ed. and trans. H. M. Parshley (New York, NY, 1974 [1953]), p. 114.

According to Christine Delphy, one of the twentieth century's leading feminist sociologists, marriage and the family have remained the 'main enemy' by enforcing and maintaining women's relegation to the domestic mode of production that is primarily defined by housework and childcare.[12] Gender inequality (the sexual division of labour) and the privatization of kinship and family (through the contractual institution of modern marriage) combine to keep (unpaid) domestic reproductive labour subordinated to the market and the state, while reproduction paradoxically provides the basic means of supplying and maintaining the productive economy.

In sum, then, the problem with reproduction is that its narrow scientific and medical modernization was not accompanied by a similar transformation of childcare or domestic labour. Instead, the roles of wife and mother remained status-defining and limiting for women, thus disabling their full participation in society. Further cementing this profound historic division is the naturalization of reproduction as a process linked to female biology – a circular ethos that obscures its own origin. The privatization, feminization and biologization of reproduction had become so pronounced by the mid-twentieth century that even Michel Foucault overlooked these changes almost completely.[13]

The Second Sex

According to Simone de Beauvoir, in her 1949 classic *The Second Sex*, the two primary impediments to women's emancipation are marriage – an institution she describes as a form of feudal bondage – and reproduction, or women's 'enslavement to the generative function', which is in her view 'the fundamental fact' of women's oppression (Fig. 42.1).[14] Notable is de Beauvoir's abiding interest in reproductive physiology and embryology, including reproductive technologies such as artificial insemination as well as contraception. She predicted hopefully that modern technological control would enable woman finally to leave behind 'the slavery of reproduction' and 'assume the economic role that is offered her and will assure her of complete independence' (p. 136).

Inspiring many other feminist writings, Chapter 1 of *The Second Sex* begins with a critical examination of 'The Data of Biology'. De Beauvoir reviews a variety of

12 Christine Delphy, *The Main Enemy: A Materialist Analysis of Women's Oppression*, trans. Lucy ap Roberts and Diana Leonard Barker (London, 1977).

13 Sarah Franklin, *Biological Relatives: IVF, Stem Cells, and the Future of Kinship* (Durham, NC, 2013), p. 47; Susanne Lettow, 'Population, race and gender: On the genealogy of the modern politics of reproduction', *Distinktion: Scandinavian Journal of Social Theory* 16 (2015), 267–82; further: John Forrester, 'Sex, Gender and Babies', Chapter 41, this book.

14 De Beauvoir, *Second Sex*, p. 132. Further references to this work are given as page numbers in brackets in the text.

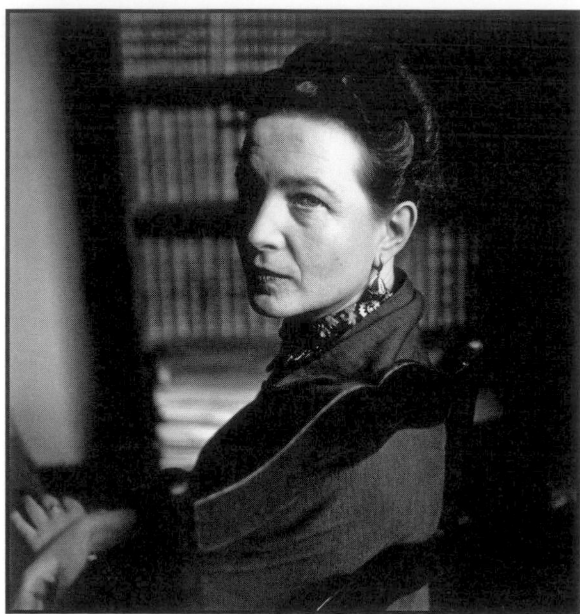

Figure 42.1 Simone de Beauvoir photographed in her apartment by Elliott Erwitt in 1949, the year Gallimard published *Le deuxième sexe* in two parts in Paris. Magnum.

reproductive arrangements in amoebae, sponges, worms, insects and vertebrates, including fission, budding, parthenogenesis and hermaphroditism. She then transitions from biology to philosophy, critiquing Plato, Aristotle, Merleau-Ponty, Sartre, Hegel and Heidegger for taking the division of species into male and female individuals for granted (pp. 3–7). These opening pages condense the central premise of de Beauvoir's existentialism, namely that '[t]here are two interrelated dynamic aspects of life: it can be maintained only through transcending itself, and it can transcend itself only on the condition it is maintained'. She continues:

> These two factors always operate together and it is unrealistic to try to separate them, yet now it is one and now the other that dominates. The two gametes at once transcend and perpetuate themselves when they unite; but in its structure the egg anticipates future needs, it is so constituted as to nourish the life that will wake within it. The sperm, on the contrary, is in no way equipped to provide for the development of the embryo it awakens.

In this passage, which explores biological reproduction as a model of both immanence and transcendence, we see the ambivalent and tautological consequences of fighting the fire of biological determinism with the extinguisher of biological fact. 'It would be foolhardy indeed to deduce from such evidence that woman's place is in the home', notes de Beauvoir, 'but there are foolhardy men', such as the philosopher Alfred Fouillée, who founded his definition of woman '*in toto* upon the egg' (pp. 14–15).

Yet de Beauvoir herself slipped into this kind of reasoning, arguing that feminine individuality is the greatest 'sacrifice to the species' a woman must make, unlike the male who 'even in his transcendence toward the next generation … keeps himself apart and maintains his individuality within himself' – a trait that, she adds, is 'constant' across all known species, 'from the insect to the highest animals' (p. 25). Thus, although de Beauvoir insists that '[b]iology is not enough to give an answer to the question that is before us: why is woman the *Other*?' (p. 17), she nonetheless grounds her philosophical interpretation of individual existence primarily within the physiology of reproduction.

Such is the prevalence of biological explanations for gender, sex and reproduction that the tendency to biologize ontology itself became the object of increasing study within feminism. The radical feminist theorist Shulamith Firestone described the situation of the modern female in *The Dialectic of Sex* (1970), a revolutionary manifesto for the burgeoning women's rights movement inspired by de Beauvoir:

> [T]he elimination of sexual classes requires the revolt of the underclass (women) and the seizure of control of *reproduction*: not only the full restoration to women of ownership of their own bodies, but also their (temporary) seizure of control of human fertility – the new population biology as well as all the social institutions of childbearing and childrearing … The reproduction of the species by one sex for the benefit of both would be replaced by (at least the option of) artificial reproduction: children would be born to both sexes equally, or independently of either … The tyranny of the biological family would be broken.[15]

Often misread as a technological determinist who overstated the role of biological sex differences in her call for 'control of human fertility', Firestone is more accurately understood as a theorist of consciousness (Fig. 42.2).[16] Among the first to articulate the principle that reproduction is neither outside history nor inside the body, Firestone argued that the social organization of reproduction, rather than biological destiny, determined not only female but human potential.

Inspired by *The Origin of the Family, Private Property and the State* (first published in German in 1884), in which Friedrich Engels charted changes to the sexual division

15 Shulamith Firestone, *The Dialectic of Sex: The Case for Feminist Revolution* (New York, NY, 1971), pp. 10–11.

16 Sarah Franklin, 'Revisiting reprotech: Firestone and the question of technology', in Mandy Merck and Stella Sandford (eds.), *The Further Adventures of* The Dialectic of Sex: *Critical Essays on Shulamith Firestone* (New York, NY, 2010), pp. 29–60.

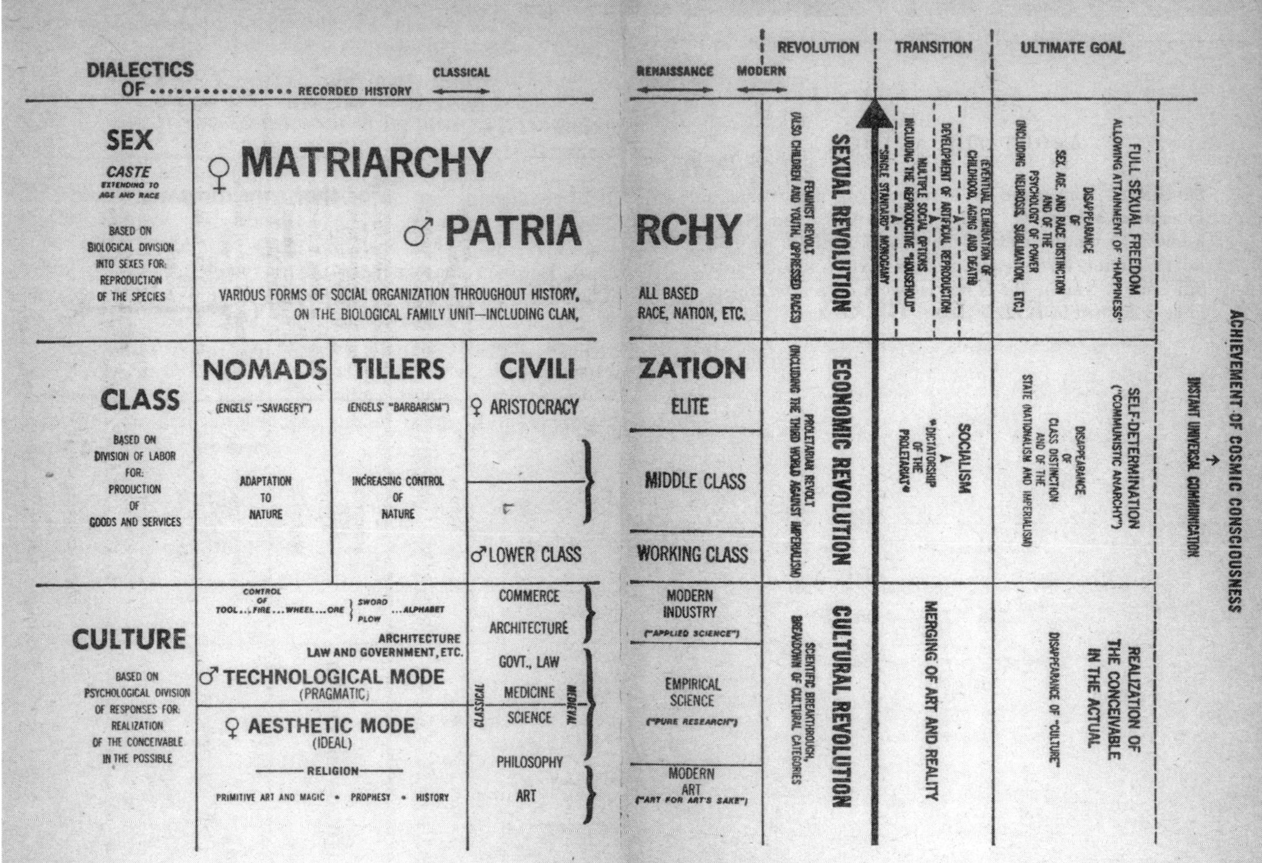

Figure 42.2 The concluding chart of '3-D revolution' in Shulamith Firestone's book, for 'that rare diagram freak'. It anticipated the revolutions, sexual, economic and cultural, that might achieve 'full sexual freedom', 'self-determination', 'the realization of the possible in the actual' and ultimately even 'cosmic consciousness'. From *The Dialectic of Sex: The Case for Feminist Revolution* (New York, NY: Bantam, 1971), pp. 244–5.

of labour through serial reorganizations of marriage, parenthood and property law, Firestone challenged the separation of the domestic and public spheres, and the supposed primacy of modern contractual freedom over the bonds of kinship. A range of feminist scholars further developed these themes in the 1970s, pointing not only to the continued interdependence between the family and the state, and domestic and market economies, but also the tyranny of biological determinism in justifying the sexual division of labour. As Donna Haraway put it in 1978, the gendered history of the modern sciences can itself be interpreted as a parable of reproductive physiology: '[t]he union of the political and the physiological' 'linked natural and political economy on multiple levels.'[17] Londa Schiebinger further noted that '[t]he opposition between science and femininity formed a cornerstone of the [Enlightenment] doctrine … that the sexes were not equals', thus ensuring that 'ancient prejudices against femininity were not overturned but merely translated into the language of modern science'.[18] The naturalization of reproduction as universal female biology is paradoxically a hallmark of modernity. 'Ever since the Enlightenment,' claims Duden, 'science and medicine have used the nature they deal with, [including] the inner body ("reproduction," "sexuality," and so on), to imply indirectly that whatever they conceptualize is immutably fixed.' This alleged immutability had become a primary concern of writers such as Wollstonecraft even before the term 'feminism' was coined in 1872, and continues in the present day. With the concept of 'nature', Duden concluded, modern reproductive determinism 'imposed its inescapable grid on everything it embraced'.[19] Far from becoming free individuals within a new economy of contractual labour, modern science and medicine reinforced women's subjugation to a sexual division of labour allegedly based in natural fact. Activities which have never been inherently debilitating – pregnancy is not a disease, childcare can be shared and maternity is not incompatible with paid employment – were redefined for many (not all) modern women in terms of biological destiny, thus justifying their sequestration as wives and mothers within the timeless sphere of domesticity.

The Separation of Reproduction from Sex

This problem for feminists – that there is no exit from the spiralling and interlocking logics of biological reproduction and sexual difference – received its definitive treatment in 1990 from the American feminist philosopher Judith Butler, a close reader of de Beauvoir and an astute diagnostician of the trouble with biological facts. Proposing that sexual dimorphism is a self-fulfilling prophecy, or 'felicitous self-naturalization', driven by the expectation that gender must materialize in a highly polarized form, Butler, like de Beauvoir, revisited biological accounts of early mammalian development and specifically gametogenesis.[20] Drawing on the work of developmental biologist Anne Fausto-Sterling, Butler examined how scientists at the Massachusetts Institute of Technology could recently have described Testis Determining Factor as encoded by the 'master gene' of sex binarism despite the fact that similar genes were located on both male and female sex chromosomes. In the prestigious

17 Donna Haraway, 'Animal sociology and a natural economy of the body politic, part I: A political physiology of dominance', *Signs* 4 (1978), 21–36, on 21.

18 Londa Schiebinger, *The Mind Has No Sex? Women in the Origins of Modern Science* (Cambridge, MA, 1991), pp. 233–4.

19 Duden, *Woman beneath the Skin*, p. 21.

20 Judith Butler, *Gender Trouble: Feminism and the Subversion of Identity* (New York, NY, 1990), p. 106.

journal *Cell*, the MIT team claimed to have found 'the binary switch upon which hinge all sexually dimorphic characteristics'.[21] This claim was especially contentious given that the research subjects included several intersexed individuals. Rather than confirming a primary biological mechanism of sexual dimorphism, the results revealed the reverse – that sex–gender variation exists as a biological continuum. Butler's critique – and her influential account of gender as 'performative' – catalysed the refusal of compulsory sex and gender binarism which has since come to dominate both popular culture and feminist politics.

Butler's intervention built on a substantial corpus of scholarship by feminist anthropologists, literary scholars and historians. The alternative to the presumption that reproduction can largely be explained in terms of biology, and that the logics of gender and sex are essentially reproductive, is the claim that had dominated feminist thinking for half a century: gender articulates a social logic. De Beauvoir had launched a version of what would become the feminist structuralist, and later post-structuralist, explanation of both sex and gender when she claimed that 'one is not born but rather becomes a woman' and asked if 'women still exist' (p. xv). Her critique drew on structuralist anthropology; in the introduction to *The Second Sex*, de Beauvoir thanked Claude Lévi-Strauss for lending her a proof copy of *The Elementary Structures of Kinship*. Despite his own apparent diffidence about the implications of his argument, his method for reading gender, kinship and marriage as components of a cultural grammar, or code, offered a model of reproductivity.[22] 'Women', Lévi-Strauss declared, are the 'valuables par excellence', and thus '[t]he emergence of symbolic thought must have required that women, like words, should be things that were exchanged'. Without the social grammar of organized exchange, reproduction would fail: the law of exogamy is 'the only means … of avoiding indefinite fission and segmentation which the practice of consanguineous marriages would bring about'. Such fragmentation would inevitably create 'so many closed systems or sealed monads which no pre-established harmony could prevent from coming into conflict'.[23]

In the 1970s, the political implications of the structuralist model – that kinship does not come 'after' biological reproduction any more than gender is 'based on' biological sex – grounded several now classic essays by feminist anthropologists including Sherry Ortner, Gayle Rubin and Nicole-Claude Mathieu.[24] From a feminist point of

21 David C. Page *et al.*, 'The sex-determining region of the human Y chromosome encodes a finger protein', *Cell* 51 (1987), 1091–104, on 1091.

22 'Reproductivity' refers to the capacity to reproduce of both an individual and a population. It is used here to mean the formation of reproductive capacity from many linked forces, including social organization through kinship, gender and marital systems.

23 Claude Lévi-Strauss, *The Elementary Structures of Kinship*, trans. James Harle Bell, John Richard von Sturmer and Rodney Needham (Boston, MA, 1969), pp. 481, 479.

24 Sherry Ortner, 'Is female to male as nature is to culture?', *Feminist Studies* 1, no. 2 (1972), 5–31; Gayle Rubin, 'The traffic in women: Notes on the "political economy" of sex', in Rayna R. Reiter (ed.), *Toward*

view, the possibility of theorizing identity, status, classificatory systems, kinship, ritual, language and group organization as social technologies offered the important possibility of accounting for reproductive causality by means other than physiology. This further bolstered de Beauvoir's early claims.[25] According to these theories, social organization not only plays a causal role in the determination of reproductive outcomes, but must be seen as constitutive of reproductivity itself.

From Status to Consciousness

According to the logic that insists that reproduction must be socially organized in order to become biologically viable, 'reproduction' can no longer simply refer to reproductive biology: 'reproduction' must instead include all aspects of society and consciousness. The reproduction of gender identities – or what de Beauvoir described as women's entrapment as '*the* sex' – must become the priority – as Firestone argued in *The Dialectic of Sex*. Butler stressed that it is the compulsory nature of gender binarism which must be challenged. The feminist case that society, rather than biology, produces fertility radically reverses the assumed causal primacy of reproductive mechanisms such as ovulation, fertilization and gestation, through which the primary causes of pregnancy and childbirth are commonly defined.

From this point of view, the separation of 'reproduction' in its narrow physical or physiological sense from its more general meaning as the establishment of structural conditions for human existence can only be interpreted as an effect of power. As Firestone argued, the political relation between gender and power is one of consciousness – and political resistance consequently begins with consciousness change. Revolutionary feminist transformation could only be achieved by shattering the seemingly unbreakable chains of causality linking women to childbirth, childbirth to sexual difference and sexual difference to nature. No one would ever truly be free until the compulsory structures of binary sex and gender were eliminated.

Theorists such as Firestone, Haraway and Butler thus challenge the assumption that feminism is primarily related to reproduction through campaigns for birth control, abortion rights or increased reproductive choice.[26] They propose rather that the intransigent and all-encompassing association of women with reproduction, and vice versa, is a self-perpetuating mythology. While it remains essential to acknowledge the significant political gains achieved through the reproductive rights movement, it

an Anthropology of Women (New York, NY, 1975), pp. 157–210; Nicole-Claude Mathieu, 'Man-culture and woman-nature?', *Women's Studies International Quarterly* 1 (1978 [French original, 1973]), 55–65.

25 Franklin, *Biological Relatives*.

26 On those campaigns: Lesley A. Hall, 'Movements to Separate Sex and Reproduction', Chapter 29; Martin H. Johnson and Nick Hopwood, 'Modern Law and Regulation', Chapter 40, this book.

is equally important to recognize that the close links between feminism and reproductive rights are symptomatic of the larger problem of perceiving gender, sex and reproduction as private, natural and biological. In the words of the activist and political theorist Rosalind Pollack Petchesky: 'Reproductive politics is in large part about language and the contestation of meanings.'[27] We can neither understand the feminist struggle for reproductive rights outside the wider political and economic context of modern industrial society, nor should we narrow the meaning of 'reproductive politics' to the struggle to ensure women's access to contraception and safe and legal abortion. These are only part of the much broader question of how reproductivity is organized, disciplined and activated.

The American feminist historian Linda Gordon argued powerfully in *Woman's Body, Woman's Right*, her pioneering study of the birth control movement in America, that no amount of technological advance could substitute for the politicization of consciousness necessary for truly feminist change in the realm of reproductive choice: 'If there is such a thing as "natural" human sexual behavior we do not and cannot know what it is; sexual behavior is always culturally regulated.'[28] Feminists have consistently contested the view that either sexuality or reproduction (or gender or kinship) emerge 'naturally' from a biological base and have instead sought the ultimate reproductive politics in the effects of such claims on consciousness and perception. For it is only through the forceful denial and repression of alternative models of reproduction and parenting that a narrow and exaggerated emphasis on female responsibility for these activities can be maintained.

Conclusion

The late twentieth-century introduction of new technologies of reproduction such as in vitro fertilization unsurprisingly recapitulated many of the struggles that feminist scholars and activists have long waged. The rise of alternative family structures and new kinships created through donor gametes, IVF, surrogacy, transnational adoption, cryopreservation – and various combinations of these techniques and practices aided by the internet – has been accompanied by a worldwide movement to enfranchise lesbian, gay and transgendered people. This has resulted in a new cycle of consciousness change: corporations and nation-states now use gay-friendly policies as a symbol of progressive tolerance. Traditional kinship formations, such as the nuclear family and

27 Rosalind Pollack Petchesky, 'The body as property: A feminist re-vision', in Ginsburg and Rapp, *Conceiving the New World Order*, pp. 387–406, on p. 387.

28 Linda Gordon, *Woman's Body, Woman's Right: A Social History of Birth Control in America* (New York, NY, 1976), p. 119. On conciousness-raising: Wendy Kline, '*Our Bodies, Ourselves*', Exhibit 35, this book.

biological reproduction, as well as traditional symbols of kinship such as genes, have been transformed in these scenarios into resources for individual and collective resistance to sexual, reproductive and gender norms. Sexual and reproductive divisions of labour are transformed in the making, for example, of lesbian families.[29] Here, in the reverse of the common Anglo-European pattern of biologizing reproduction in the service of affirming normative gender and kinship roles, biology is refashioned as a flexible resource with which to reinvent both reproduction and gender. Such examples demonstrate the rapid reorganization of reproductivity, though this can also remain entrenched within traditional norms.

These reinventions and restructurings of human reproductivity exemplify the feminist argument that society not biology produces fertility. Although historically linked in ongoing struggles over reproductive rights, the most important connection between feminism and reproduction should thus be in overturning the reductive and deterministic associations between women, pregnancy and childbirth. This potential, on which de Beauvoir and Firestone insisted, remains to be realized: 'reproduction' will need to be after 'women', just as 'women's' role in 'reproduction' will need to be reinvented in order for either to become fully valued and visible as vital components of any social community or polity.

29 Corinne P. Hayden, 'Gender, genetics, and generation: Reformulating biology in lesbian kinship', *Cultural Anthropology* 10 (1995), 41–63.

43 Globalization

Nick Hopwood

In the documentary *Google Baby* (2009), Indian women become pregnant for would-be parents in America and Israel, who go online to select gametes for fertilization, and embryos for freezing, shipping and implantation, then fly out to collect a child after nine months. Nor is it just in the travel disparaged as 'reproductive tourism' and appreciated as 'cross-border reproductive care' that reproduction has been globalized. Making and not making babies depends also on less obvious flows of people, policies, practices and products. In Northern Ireland, for example, abortion is currently still allowed only 'to protect the mother's life or health', but women unable to go to Britain for the procedure have ordered pills from India via a charity in Amsterdam.[1]

In 1995, anthropologists Faye Ginsburg and Rayna Rapp brought scholars together around the observation that 'seemingly distant power relations shape and constrain local reproductive experiences'. They further promoted Shellee Colen's concept of 'stratified reproduction' to analyse how, within and between countries, 'some categories of people are empowered to nurture and reproduce, while others are disempowered'.[2] After two centuries of increasingly dominant nation-states, the end of the Cold War prompted this recognition of transnational links. There had been earlier forms of globalization, but most historians accept that interaction intensified from around 1900 and again after 1980, in uneven, resisted and reversible, yet unmistakable trends.[3] By the 1890s, various agencies were starting to target reproduction, a phenomenon significant to humanity at large and peoples everywhere, through projects to universalize western norms. Following sometimes coercive population-control programmes in international development after World War II, reproduction was prominently reframed in the 1990s as a matter of individual choice, and has become a key issue in global health and a major sector of biomedical industry worldwide. This raises two main questions.

1 Juliette Jowit and Aparna Pallavi, 'From Nagpur to Northern Ireland: Pill pipeline helping women get round abortion laws', *Guardian*, 6 Jan. 2016.

2 Faye D. Ginsburg and Rayna Rapp (eds.), *Conceiving the New World Order: The Global Politics of Reproduction* (Berkeley, CA, 1995), pp. 272 (in Sharon Stephens's chapter), 3 (in the editors' introduction); also Carole H. Browner and Carolyn F. Sargent (eds.), *Reproduction, Globalization, and the State: New Theoretical and Ethnographic Perspectives* (Durham, NC, 2011).

3 A. G. Hopkins (ed.), *Globalization in World History* (London, 2002).

First, how did practices of procreation travel, and to what extent did the connections make reproduction the same? In the twentieth century, countries converged on medicalized childbirth (routine supervision by medical attendants leading to hospital delivery) and – with significant pronatalist exceptions – on birth control leading to smaller families. Almost all now have at least one IVF clinic. Yet they did not 'develop' along a single path. Various modernities rather coexisted and interacted; the periods of greatest change overlapped; and the metropoles, whose own modernity owed much to empire, imported colonial and postcolonial innovations.

Second, how have the most powerful influences changed and with what effects? Although international agencies often found reproduction too controversial, in some ways its history parallels that of colonial medicine and 'international', then 'global' health.[4] Narrow, crisis-oriented population control is equivalent to top-down, single-disease eradication programmes, the colonial approach reasserted for the 'American century' during decolonization after World War II. In the 1970s, critics charged both with ignoring long-term social and economic determinants. The 'global health' paradigm incorporated some of this critique and, in Cairo in 1994, the International Conference on Population Control and Development echoed the slogans of 'participation' and 'empowerment' as it broadened the agenda to 'reproductive health'. But at the same time the International Monetary Fund (IMF) and the World Bank imposed 'structural adjustment' – budget cuts, privatization and market reform that hollowed out public sectors and burdened women disproportionately. Still-targeted interventions achieved some reductions in infant and even maternal mortality, while private health care, including high-tech infertility treatments, boomed. If that is a fair sketch, then how, more specifically, to assess and explain the balance of continuity and change?

This chapter tackles aspects of these questions for three topics, beginning with childbirth, which changed fast through the mid-twentieth century but international agencies neglected and their historians have given short shrift.[5] For family planning, which by contrast dominates historical writing on reproduction in developing countries, a focus on policymaking in one particularly important nation, India, complements surveys of international debates and technologies.[6] Finally, a review of the global market in methods of assisted reproduction highlights the paradoxical centrality of nation-states.[7]

4 Randall M. Packard, *A History of Global Health: Interventions into the Lives of Other Peoples* (Baltimore, MD, 2016).

5 See also Philippa Levine, 'Imperial Encounters', Chapter 33; and Salim Al-Gailani, 'Hospital Birth', Chapter 37, this book.

6 Alison Bashford, 'World Population from Eugenics to Climate Change', Chapter 34; Jesse Olszynko-Gryn, 'Technologies of Contraception and Abortion', Chapter 36, this book.

7 See also Nick Hopwood, 'Artificial Fertilization', Chapter 39; Martin H. Johnson and Hopwood, 'Modern Law and Regulation', Chapter 40; and John Forrester, 'Sex, Gender and Babies', Chapter 41, this book.

Maternities and Modernities

Imperial administrations and nationalist governments were promoting maternal and child welfare by around 1900. Missionaries and colonial officials, the League of Nations Health Organization and the Rockefeller Foundation imported European medicine to combat maternal and infant mortality. They found allies in western-trained medical practitioners and nationalist leaders who shared the conviction, fostered by international comparisons, that reducing childbirth deaths was an important marker of the modern – even as people fought over what that meant.[8]

National differences began in pre-existing arrangements and the rejection of metropolitan assumptions: for example, that female birth attendants should be subordinate to male obstetricians. In nineteenth-century Egypt, the British reversed the reforms of the Ottoman viceroy Muhammad Ali by demoting women to assistants and carers and putting men in charge. In British India, by contrast, where the all-male indigenous medical practitioners had left birth to experienced female family members and hereditary midwives, women's dominance was justified as necessary to access spaces of seclusion. The lying-in hospitals thus employed British medical women without competing with the men or criticizing male primacy in European obstetrics.[9] Men were never likely to take the lead in China either. The Republic instructed a new cadre of midwives in western methods and retrained 'granny midwives' in antisepsis; after 1949, the communists extended the Republican model. Over the next half-century, the feminization of British and especially American obstetrics made the period of male dominance look anomalous, even within their own national histories.[10]

Childbirth changed most rapidly in the mid-twentieth century, and strikingly in the Congo, where medical supervision increased from 1 per cent of babies in 1935 to 43 per cent in 1958, when the country had the most extensive health infrastructure in Africa. Historians are only beginning to reconstruct the complexities, as Nancy Rose Hunt did for a British missionary station at Yakusu near Stanleyville/Kishangani in a forest region on the upper Congo River. From the 1920s, following the demographic disaster of King Leopold's murderous 'red rubber' regime, Belgian government pronatalism sought to replenish labour forces for plantations and mines – an extreme form of the widespread concern about African depopulation. Particularly after World War II, the

8 Valerie Fildes, Lara Marks and Hilary Marland (eds.), *Women and Children First: International Maternal and Infant Welfare, 1870–1945* (London, 1992).

9 Maneesha Lal, 'The politics of gender and medicine in colonial India: The Countess of Dufferin's Fund, 1885–1888', *Bulletin of the History of Medicine* 68 (1994), 29–66.

10 Hibba Abugideiri, *Gender and the Making of Modern Medicine in Colonial Egypt* (Farnham, 2010); Tina Phillips Johnson, *Childbirth in Republican China: Delivering Modernity* (Lanham, MD, 2011).

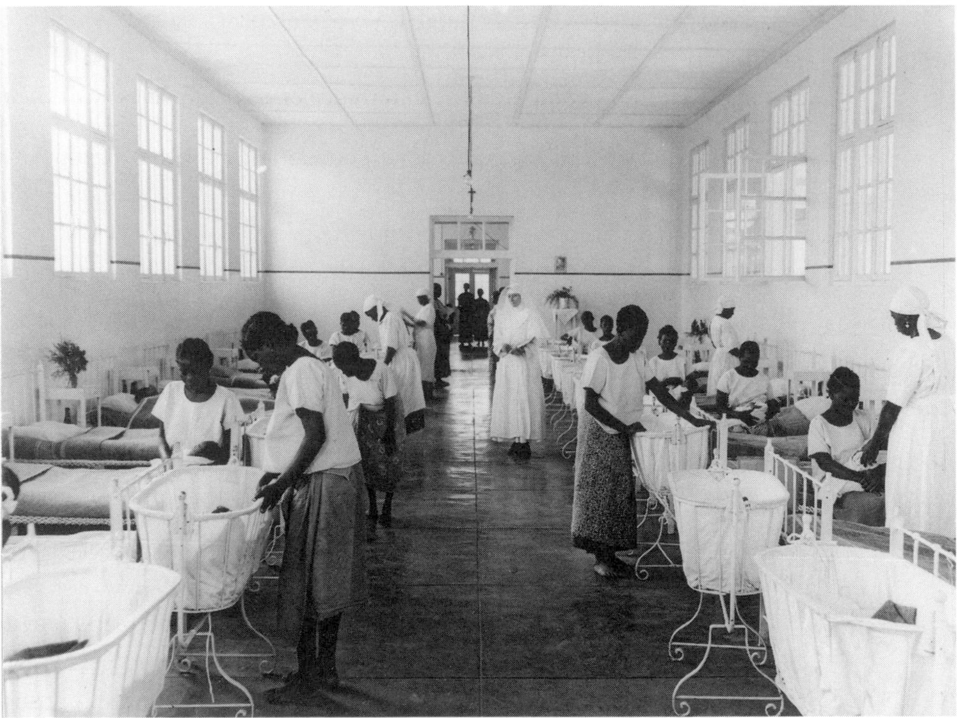

Figure 43.1 Maternity ward in the Mining Union Hospital for Natives at Elisabethville in the Belgian Congo (today Lubumbashi) in 1945. African mothers and nurses attend the babies under the supervision of a white sister. Congopresse photograph by Elja Lebied, who worked for Inforcongo, the information service of the colonial ministry. 18 × 24 cm. © Royal Museum for Central Africa, Tervuren, HP.1956.15.8793.

Yakusu station, though Baptist, enrolled in this Catholic maternalism; from 1950, there was even a specialized infertility clinic to the west at Befale.

Medicalization often brought hospitalization (Fig. 43.1). In Kishangani, a baptized local midwife and a flexible European nurse cajoled Congolese women to give birth in the hospital. These mediators translated medical hygiene into an indigenous idiom and adapted the institution to the patients. Improved maternal survival helped make the case. The hospital then became a place for more than emergencies with the training of African male midwives, the giving away of new baby clothes, bonuses for attendance by a 'State-recognized white person' and bureaucratic pressure to obtain certificates issued free only for hospital births. Going to hospital suited a mobile world of riding bicycles and seeing aeroplanes overhead, yet delivery remained a brief interlude in village traditions, from nourishing the unborn baby to postnatal seclusion.[11]

11 Nancy Rose Hunt, *A Colonial Lexicon: Of Birth Ritual, Medicalization, and Mobility in the Congo* (Durham, NC, 1999); on depopulation and the infertility clinic: Hunt, *A Nervous State: Violence, Remedies, and Reverie in Colonial Congo* (Durham, NC, 2016).

Even as birth practices converged, anthropologists evidenced humans' divergent constructions of a natural event. They pointed to the prominence of home birth in Dutch midwifery and compared the endurance of UK midwives with their American cousins' near-extinction. In the 1970s and 1980s, romanticized images of non-medical childbirth in Africa, Asia and South America countered equally one-dimensional representations of western women subjugated by medical men. Yet the 'natural' was 'cultural' too, and scientific medicine was appropriated in various ways.[12]

Psychoprophylactic techniques of pain management from the Soviet Union provide a vivid example. Stalinist Russia favoured an inexpensive method with a Pavlovian pedigree. Chinese communists briefly embraced this scientific, socialist tool for fighting 'the feudal cultural remnant' in midwifery while correcting the 'arrogance' of western-trained medical personnel; propaganda painted anaesthesia as capitalist and Soviet-style 'painless childbirth' as a model for serving the masses. The obstetrician Fernand Lamaze led import to the west through the French Communist Party. Prenatal instruction and husbands' involvement appealed in France and the United States, but French feminists later demanded the pharmacological pain relief that many American advocates of natural childbirth opposed.[13]

Use of biomedical services continued to be negotiated, however unequally. In Cecilia Van Hollen's ethnography of lower-class, lower-caste women in and near Madras (now Chennai), capital of Tamil Nadu in south India, during the mid-1990s, those seeking hospital birth set different priorities from most American women: they rejected painkillers, but wanted biomedical induction to speed labour more than the traditional drugs. This suited government hospitals in dire economic straits. Resistance to hospital births was also different; though the norm in cities, these then represented only 20 per cent of all deliveries nationally (today they are 50 per cent). Where western feminists targeted male-dominated, over-technologized and alienating experiences, Madras women objected to the terms of access to state facilities. They identified hospital birth with a desired modernity, but were treated as backward and made to pay; they dreaded being alone and mistreated and the disparagement of time-honoured postpartum practices. Some resisted this discrimination by employing a former public health worker who offered home birth plus hormonal induction and modern professionalism.[14]

12 Reviewed in Cecilia Van Hollen, *Birth on the Threshold: Childbirth and Modernity in South India* (Berkeley, CA, 2003), pp. 10–16.

13 Paula A. Michaels, *Lamaze: An International History* (Oxford, 2014); Byungil Ahn, 'Reinventing scientific medicine for the socialist republic: The Soviet psycho-prophylactic method of delivery in 1950s China', *Twentieth-Century China* 38 (2013), 139–55, on 144.

14 Van Hollen, *Birth on the Threshold*; further: Cecilia Van Hollen, *Birth in the Age of AIDS: Women, Reproduction, and HIV/AIDS in India* (Stanford, CA, 2013); Kalpana Ram and Margaret Jolly (eds.), *Maternities and Modernities: Colonial and Postcolonial Experiences in Asia and the Pacific* (Cambridge, 1998).

Medicalized childbirth was thus made global and local at the same time. Differences remain stark, within and between countries, as the standardized World Health Organization (WHO) figures display, though at the cost of homogenizing the diverse experiences that anthropologists have described. More resources having gone into child survival, international conferences in the late 1980s demanded action to reduce maternal mortality in its own right. 'Safe motherhood' became a prominent goal of global health, and mortality fell 43 per cent between 1990 and 2015 worldwide (neonatal mortality dropped 47 per cent) – but inequality increased because the countries with the highest death tolls improved least. About 2.7 million babies per year still died in the first month of life (with a similar number stillborn) and there are some 800 daily maternal deaths, two-thirds in sub-Saharan Africa. Challenges have included the difficulty of addressing the social determinants of health in a context of declining infrastructure, years of conflict and the introduction of user fees, and the need to go beyond generic, top-down, biomedical solutions (Fig. 43.2).[15] There is also the more general legacy that interventions have been less concerned to support maternity than to prevent births.

Family Planning and Poverty

Fear of world overpopulation has a long history, but dominated debates about reproduction and economic development only after 1945. Europe was the main worry until the Cold War, when US-led agencies, private then governmental and even international, promoted population control in the 'Third World' to stave off the Communist threat to American supplies of raw materials and markets for finished goods. Independent governments accepted that population growth would stymie efforts to lift people out of poverty, but framed family planning as nation-building. Some, like India, the major arena for international organizations, established programmes so big they rivalled total public spending on health.[16]

The last colonial census of India, in 1931, fed a discourse of overpopulation, but birth control and eugenics were too controversial to become a British priority. Indian advocates lamented the behaviour of the poor and asked the state to intervene, but 'breeding a better India' was left to the self-styled secular, scientific and modern middle

15 Carla AbouZahr, 'Safe motherhood: A brief history of the global movement, 1947–2002', *British Medical Bulletin* 67 (2003), 13–25; WHO, *Trends in Maternal Mortality: 1990 to 2015. Estimates by WHO, UNICEF, UNFPA, World Bank Group and the United Nations Population Division* (Geneva, 2015); WHO, 'Children: Reducing mortality', updated Sept. 2016, www.who.int/mediacentre/factsheets/fs178/en/; Hunt, *Colonial Lexicon*, pp. 281–319.

16 Matthew Connelly, *Fatal Misconception: The Struggle to Control World Population* (Cambridge, MA, 2008); Alison Bashford, *Global Population: History, Geopolitics, and Life on Earth* (New York, NY, 2014); Bashford, 'World Population'.

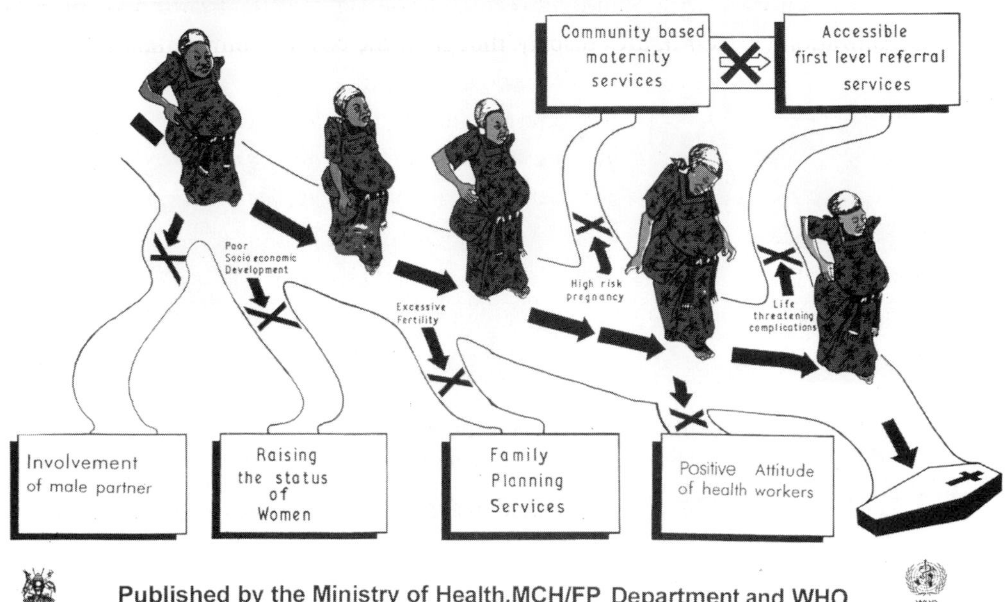

Figure 43.2 'The road to maternal death.' This diagram and others like it, presented in lectures and films and on posters around the world, has framed the 'Safe motherhood' movement. It presents the challenge as taking 'Mrs X', a universalized 'developing country' woman, off that fateful road by intervening to unblock the exits, the relative importance of which has been much discussed. Poster published by Ugandan Ministry of Health and WHO in the late 1990s. National Library of Medicine.

class. Notwithstanding religious opposition, Mahatma Gandhi's preference for self-restraint, and arguments that population would anyway fall with economic growth, influential nationalists came to see birth control as necessary to protect advances in productivity. While communalists in the 1940s wanted more Hindus or Muslims, war-time shortages and the Bengal famine may have strengthened the case for limitation.[17]

In 1952, independent India was the first country to make family planning government policy. Birth control still had a modest place, as a contribution to national strength and women's health, in the first Five-Year Plan, for 1951–6. Subsequent plans reversed priorities by presenting population growth as an independent variable to be reduced in quasi-military campaigns. US philanthropists, fresh from debates over occupied Japan and civil-war China, focused on India as the largest, poorest and most

17 Sarah Hodges, 'South Asia's eugenic past', in Alison Bashford and Philippa Levine (eds.), *The Oxford Handbook of the History of Eugenics* (Oxford, 2010), pp. 228–42; also Hodges, *Contraception, Colonialism and Commerce: Birth Control in South India, 1920–1940* (Aldershot, 2008); Sanjam Ahluwalia, *Reproductive Restraints: Birth Control in India, 1877–1947* (Urbana, IL, 2008).

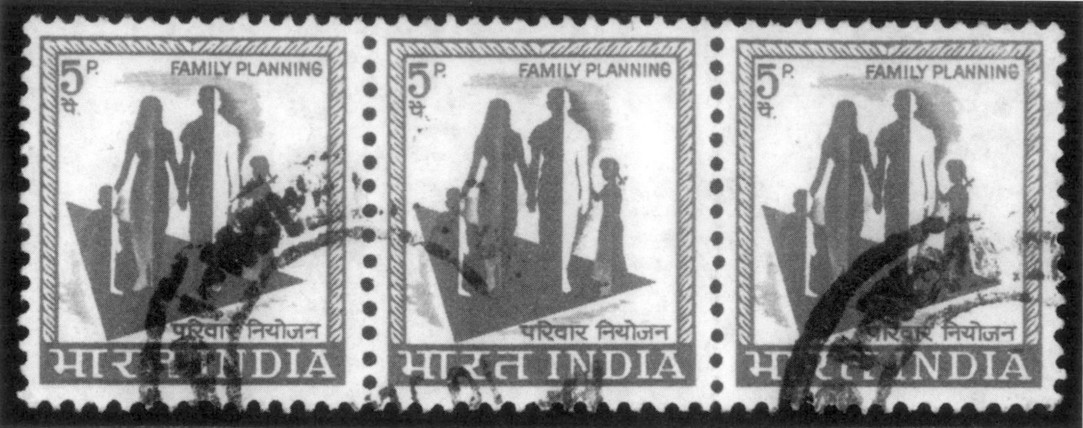

Figure 43.3 Indian 5 paisa stamps, issued in 1967 and perhaps the most used of many that have promoted family planning. The two-child family stands on the red triangle, symbol of contraception. When overprinted with 'refugee relief', this stamp was used to pay the surcharge levied on postal items to support Bengalis fleeing genocide and war in East Pakistan (soon Bangladesh). Compare the illustration on p. 498, this book. Each stamp 2.2 × 2.0 cm.

accessible population. The Indian National Congress accepted the policy as consistent with nationalist ideals.[18]

Family planning initially meant clinics, and then also education, long the most important intervention (Fig. 43.3). In 1960, the programme expanded from instruction in the rhythm method, and a few sterilizations, to mobile vasectomy camps. Foreign advisors allied with Indian bureaucrats against the health minister's prioritization of general health. Americans smuggled in intrauterine devices and set up a factory producing 20,000 a day. In the face of problems, including pain, bleeding and spontaneous expulsion, clients ('acceptors') and staff were pressured to carry on. Indira Gandhi, Congress prime minister from 1966, and Sripati Chandrasekhar, head of the renamed Ministry of Health and Family Planning, further stressed incentives and targets for procedures, while starving the health infrastructure of funds.[19]

Evidence of failure accumulated: women would not resort to birth control where infant mortality remained high, and structural factors not neo-Malthusianism explained any fall in the rate of population growth. In the United States itself, the 'Malthusian moment' passed: the domestication of foreign policy ('as we prescribe for Delhi, so must we take account of Detroit') entered a crisis after a fragile coalition collapsed and involuntary sterilizations of African-American welfare recipients, its own '"less

18 Nilanjana Chatterjee and Nancy E. Riley, 'Planning an Indian modernity: The gendered politics of fertility control', *Signs* 26 (2001), 811–45; Mohan Rao, *From Population Control to Reproductive Health: Malthusian Arithmetic* (New Delhi, 2004).

19 Connelly, *Fatal Misconception*, pp. 213–30.

developed" population', were exposed.[20] The World Population Conference in Bucharest in 1974 staged anti-imperialist criticism of the 'population establishment'. Some advocated more integrated development to confront poverty directly; others pushed harder for population control.

In 1975, Gandhi declared an Emergency to quell unrest and, with foreign support, focused the national anti-poverty strategy on coercive mass sterilization. Rehousing after slum clearance, for example, depended on a certificate of vasectomy. In 1977, after many deaths and the first electoral defeat of the Congress, the government shifted from the politically toxic vasectomy to female sterilization and long-acting injectables, and rebranded the programme 'family welfare'.[21] Population control was failing generally, but in 1979 China embarked on a radical campaign of 'birth planning', the one-child policy, which overcame peasant resistance and reduced numbers, but at great cost to individuals and families.[22]

In the 1980s and 1990s, western governments, led by the United States and the United Kingdom, let markets run free, exacerbating a global recession and putting indebted developing countries at the mercy of the IMF and the World Bank. Typically, in 1991 the Indian government cut budgets, privatized state enterprises and liberalized markets as conditions of an IMF loan. In this inauspicious context, feminist experts and activists at the 1994 Cairo conference organized against Catholic, conservative Islamic and some family planners' resistance. Under the banner of 'reproductive health', compulsion was to give way to 'choice', and single procedures to a life-course approach. India abolished central family-planning targets, but individual states still set method-specific quotas and ran unhygienic sterilization camps. The new policies emphasized girls' education – especially its economic benefits – and reducing child and maternal mortality, but the old population agendas distorted priorities while inequality worsened, the public health system withdrew and vaunting ambitions were reduced to interventions – however valuable – that NGOs could measure.[23]

20 Ford Foundation and Population Council reports quoted in Donald T. Critchlow, *Intended Consequences: Birth Control, Abortion, and the Federal Government in Modern America* (New York, NY, 1999), pp. 99, 86; also Thomas Robertson, *The Malthusian Moment: Global Population Growth and the Birth of American Environmentalism* (New Brunswick, NJ, 2012); Johnson and Hopwood, 'Modern Law and Regulation'; Patrick Ellis, '*Z.P.G.*', Exhibit 36, this book.

21 Connelly, *Fatal Misconception*, pp. 276–326.

22 Tyrene White, *China's Longest Campaign: Birth Planning in the People's Republic, 1949–2005* (Ithaca, NY, 2006); Susan Greenhalgh, *Just One Child: Science and Policy in Deng's China* (Berkeley, CA, 2008).

23 Betsy Hartmann, *Reproductive Rights and Wrongs: The Global Politics of Population Control*, rev. ed. (Boston, MA, 1995); Rao, *Population Control*; Connelly, *Fatal Misconception*, pp. 327–69; Mohan Rao and Sarah Sexton (eds.), *Markets and Malthus: Population, Gender and Health in Neo-Liberal Times* (Los Angeles, CA, 2010); Michelle Murphy, 'The girl: Mergers of feminism and finance in neoliberal times', *S&F Online* 11.1–11.2 (2012/13), http://sfonline.barnard.edu/gender-justice-and-neoliberal-transformations/the-girl-mergers-of-feminism-and-finance-in-neoliberal-times/.

Change, however partial, had come with population control in the 1950s and the new terms of engagement negotiated between the 1970s and the 1990s. Many celebrate 1994 as a break, but critics have found enduring coercion. The more significant continuities are neglect of social and economic conditions and of health systems. Large numbers of people nevertheless gradually internalized the right and responsibility to regulate their fertility around a small-family norm.[24] That change is most striking in China, where the government worries that even the universal 'two-child policy' implemented in 2016 will not raise the working-age population fast enough to support the elderly: for Chinese people with money, IVF has become an increasingly routine and acceptable option in fertility control.[25]

Reproscapes of IVF

With the rise of 'globalization' in the 1990s, those 'seemingly distant' effects on reproduction became obvious in the high-tech, free-enterprise world of IVF. Histories of assisted conception are sparse, but ethnographers have grappled with the cultural differences and transnational exchanges while aggregating the intensified flows of people, technologies, finance, media images and ideologies into 'reproscapes'.[26]

Since the first so-called test-tube baby was born in England in 1978, the groups and nations who experience most infertility have had least access to this expensive procedure and the techniques for which it is a platform. In the 1980s, entrepreneurs opened private facilities in rich nations. In the 1990s, middle-income countries boasted IVF babies as symbols of their advanced modernity; and between 2000 and 2010, IVF expanded to the global south, with 500 of the world's 4,000 to 4,500 clinics in India and one in Bamako, capital of impoverished Mali. Campaigners are today working to meet the potentially massive African demand with low-cost methods.[27]

Assisted conception went global after national pioneers adapted foreign standards and beat their own paths; reproductive medicine depended on assimilation to local traditions and on transforming them. Across Europe and the anglophone world, for example, a mosaic of legal regimes ranges from the laissez-faire United States through more

24 Bashford, *Global Population*, p. 351.

25 Ayo Wahlberg, 'The birth and routinization of IVF in China', *Reproductive BioMedicine and Society Online* 2 (2016), 97–107.

26 Marcia C. Inhorn, *Cosmopolitan Conceptions: IVF Sojourns in Global Dubai* (Durham, NC, 2015), pp. 22–6 (following Arjun Appadurai); Inhorn and Frank van Balen (eds.), *Infertility around the Globe: New Thinking on Childlessness, Gender, and Reproductive Technologies* (Berkeley, CA, 2002); Michi Knecht, Maren Klotz and Stefan Beck (eds.), *Reproductive Technologies as Global Form: Ethnographies of Knowledge, Practices, and Transnational Encounters* (Frankfurt am Main, 2012); Sarah Franklin and Inhorn (eds.), 'Symposium, IVF: Global histories', *Reproductive BioMedicine and Society Online* 2 (2016), 1–136.

27 Hopwood, 'Artificial Fertilization'; Inhorn, *Cosmopolitan Conceptions*, pp. 105–15.

or less permissive regulation (more in the United Kingdom and Spain, less in Sweden, Denmark and France) to Germany and Italy, which the Nazi past and present Catholic politics made the most prohibitive jurisdictions. Use of donor gametes, embryo freezing and gestational surrogacy are among the most forbidden activities, but France is not alone in outlawing assisted reproduction for gay couples and single people.[28]

The pronatalist Middle East embraced IVF. Israel, with its state commitment to maintaining a Jewish majority and much faith in technology, has the highest density of clinics in the world and the most government funding. Even conservative rabbis support IVF to be fruitful and multiply, alleviate suffering and keep families together. Orthodox rabbinic opinion tends to allow gestational surrogacy, provided a Jewish woman carries the pregnancy – the womb determines Jewishness – and donor insemination, if a Gentile donates the sperm, to avoid masturbation by a Jewish man and the risk of adultery or incest.[29] The Muslim countries have taken a more cautious approach, with differences between the Sunni-dominant and Shia-majority nations. Sunni clerics accepted IVF within marriage, but treated donor insemination as tantamount to adultery; this pushed Egyptians to Dubai and Turks to Northern Cyprus. The Supreme Leader of Shia Iran, Ayatollah Khamenei, issued fatwas in 1999 that were interpreted as allowing these procedures provided no forbidden touch or gaze was involved, notably by exploiting the Shia practice of 'temporary marriage'. The edicts left room for negotiation between religious teachings, biomedical authority and cultural imperatives to overcome the trauma of childlessness and maintain the male lineage.[30]

Overall, IVF has reinforced traditional marriage, and then in some countries also facilitated more varied family forms. Assisted reproduction trades on genetic, especially patrilineal relationships. By contrast, adoption, controversially organized across international borders since the 1930s, is stigmatized in many societies, including India and the Muslim Middle East.[31] Religions have debated one major challenge that distinguishes IVF as a field of high-tech medicine: its role in producing new humans, and helped with another: this 'hope technology' usually fails. In Hindu India as elsewhere, clients are asked to 'leave everything to God or your destiny'.[32] Yet there are not just different

28 Johnson and Hopwood, 'Modern Law and Regulation'.

29 Susan Martha Kahn, *Reproducing Jews: A Cultural Account of Assisted Conception in Israel* (Durham, NC, 2000); see also Rhoda Ann Kanaaneh, *Birthing the Nation: Strategies of Palestinian Women in Israel* (Berkeley, CA, 2002).

30 Marcia C. Inhorn and Soraya Tremayne (eds.), *Islam and Assisted Reproductive Technologies: Sunni and Shia Perspectives* (London, 2012); Miri Shefer-Mossensohn and Rebecca Flemming, 'Generation in the Ottoman World', Chapter 19, this book.

31 Ellen Herman, 'Technologies of Adoption Matching', Exhibit 33; Christina Benninghaus, 'Modern Infertility', Chapter 31, this book; Laura Briggs, *Somebody's Children: The Politics of Transracial and Transnational Adoption* (Durham, NC, 2012).

32 Clinic instructions quoted in Aditya Bharadwaj, *Conceptions: Infertility and Procreative Technologies in India* (New York, NY, 2016), p. 234.

national IVFs; every country's procedures are stratified by ability to pay, marital status and sexuality, and involve continual international exchange of biological materials, reagents, plasticware and people (Fig. 43.4).

It is often implied that reproductive travel began with IVF, but the infertile have journeyed to shrines and healers since antiquity. In the 1960s, women availed themselves of mass tourism to fly to territories that had passed more liberal abortion laws.[33] Yet conceptive technologies have a special relation to travel because, when combined with sperm and embryo freezing, they enable reproduction across time and space. People have gone to access services unavailable in their own countries, or avoid legal or religious prohibitions, high costs, long waits or safety concerns. In Europe alone, there are tens of thousands of cross-border IVF cycles a year.

Eggs freeze poorly, so must be aspirated where and when they are needed, in a relatively arduous procedure. Commercial donation began in the United States, it seems, on the model of recruitment for (traditional) surrogacy. In the absence of regulation, egg donation then developed into a stratified market in which youth and the supposed genetic benefits of beauty, sporting prowess or an Ivy League education justify higher prices. European restrictions on payment produced a flatter market with economic gradients. By the early 2000s, a few countries were emerging as hubs, with Spain and the Czech Republic favoured for oocyte donation by tourist infrastructure and enough compensation to incentivize financially precarious young women. Spain offered a cosmopolitan clientele a choice of eggs, including from Latin American and eastern European students and care workers, these last matching northern preferences for blond hair and blue eyes. Prague clinics, supplied from rural areas, promised whiteness more obviously.[34]

Reproductive services were more recently offshored to Thailand and India. Accessible via the internet, Indian IVF clinics proffered 'First World health care at Third World prices', doctors familiar from (and with) western medical systems, and procedures that were illegal in some other countries. Corporate medicine grew and the public sector shrank. These facilities were out of most Indians' reach; a few travelled instead to cosmopolitan Dubai, where they met elite Africans in search of more trusted care, British couples with demands unmet by the National Health Service and Middle Eastern Muslims circumventing restrictions. Though the sojourns depended on the

33 Christabelle Sethna, 'All aboard? Canadian women's abortion tourism, 1960–1980', *Women's History Magazine* 73 (2013), 29–37.

34 Sven Bergmann, 'Resemblance that matters: On transnational anonymized egg donation in two European IVF clinics', in Knecht, Klotz and Beck, *Reproductive Technologies*, pp. 331–55; Melinda Cooper and Catherine Waldby, *Clinical Labor: Tissue Donors and Research Subjects in the Global Bioeconomy* (Durham, NC, 2014), pp. 62–77.

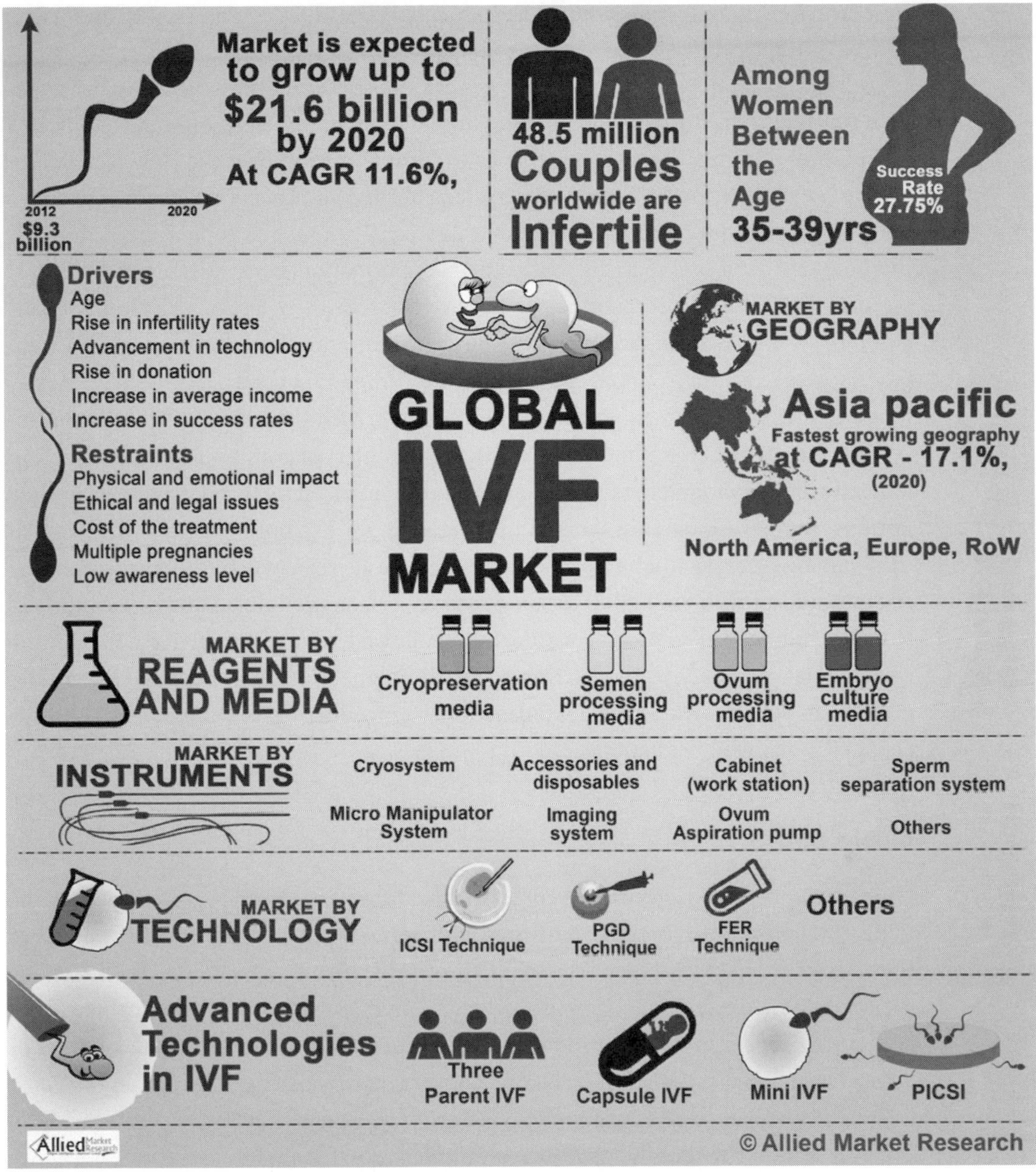

Figure 43.4 Diagram presenting an overview of the projected IVF devices and consumables market, from a January 2014 report by Debbie Shields for Allied Market Research in Portland, Oregon. The report predicted a compound annual growth rate of 11.6 per cent while highlighting drivers of and restraints on growth in world markets by reagents and media, instruments and technologies. Downloaded from http://uk.prweb.com/releases/in-vitro-fertilization/market/prweb11884411.htm, 19 Apr. 2016.

tourist industry, and some were marketed as holidays, few 'reprotravellers' described them as such.[35]

The most banned intervention is gestational surrogacy, in which would-be parents contract a third-party woman to be implanted with an embryo produced by IVF from donor gametes, carry the pregnancy to term and hand over the child. California, the early centre of the surrogacy industry, established contracts that advantage the intending parents, but by 2005 former Soviet states, Thailand and India were competing in a market that is less spatially limited than egg donation, because it leaves no ethnic trace. Nayana Patel performed her first surrogacy treatment in 2003 at the Akanksha clinic in Anand, Gujarat, and appeared on *Oprah* in 2007. For advocates, the western parents gained a much-wanted child and the destitute Indian surrogate received money that transformed her own family's prospects. For critics, this extreme exploitation involved intrusive disciplining and the most alienating act of commodification for rather less reward.[36] Ethnographers have painted a more nuanced picture. Given their limited options, some working-class women in Bangalore, for example – many of them sterilized having had two children of their own – chose surrogacy over the garment industry, but did not earn enough to escape precarity or compensate for the risks, pain and work, including of alienation.[37] In 2016, India followed scandal-hit Thailand in banning commercial surrogacy, while also reasserting the primacy of heterosexual marriage and of services for its own citizens. Transnational reproduction is vulnerable to sudden changes in national regulations.

Conclusion

Global connections have made reproduction everywhere more similar, yet not the same. Globalization has rather enriched and refracted the traditions this book has traced and those from other regions of the world. Insofar as some of the latter incorporated Greek and Islamic medicine, encounters outside Euro-America may have juxtaposed 'generation' and 'reproduction' in distinctive ways. Practices and concepts of 'reproduction' and 'population' facilitated convergence by privileging abstraction. Feminism and changed gender relations altered attitudes and actions around the world.[38]

In childbirth, family planning and infertility treatment, lines of continuity link arguments, practices and critiques, yet the constellation looks different in 1900, 1950 and today. Colonial projects were about ministries and missionaries converting

35 Inhorn, *Cosmopolitan Conceptions*.

36 Cooper and Waldby, *Clinical Labor*, pp. 78–87.

37 Amrita Pande, *Wombs in Labor: Transnational Commercial Surrogacy in India* (New York, NY, 2014); Sharmila Rudrappa, *Discounted Life: The Price of Global Surrogacy in India* (New York, NY, 2015).

38 On a US export and its reimport: Kathy Davis, *The Making of* Our Bodies, Ourselves: *How Feminism Travels across Borders* (Durham, NC, 2007).

practices framed as 'primitive', including traditional midwifery, into various modern forms. Postcolonial programmes sought to strengthen national populations and international institutions. Global reproductive health might be summarized as integrating clients in localities assumed equivalent into markets in which they are empowered to work harder, consume more – and produce the next generation of worker-consumers.[39] Nation-states have risen and fallen, but remained important even before Brexit and President Trump.

National laws drive reprotravel, while borders constrain those who cannot leave, but life is transnational, and not only with respect to high-tech interventions for global elites. When 'fertility chains' intersect with 'care chains' – when eastern European migrant workers look after elderly Spaniards, donate oocytes to German couples and remit wages to their own families back home in Moldova or the Ukraine – their labour reproduces households across large distances. Ethnographies have illuminated the movements of people, policies, practices and products; the historical challenge is to reflect more deeply on continuity and change.

39 Nicholas B. King, 'Security, disease, commerce: Ideologies of postcolonial global health', *Social Studies of Science* 32 (2002), 763–89; Vincanne Adams (ed.), *Metrics: What Counts in Global Health* (Durham, NC, 2016).

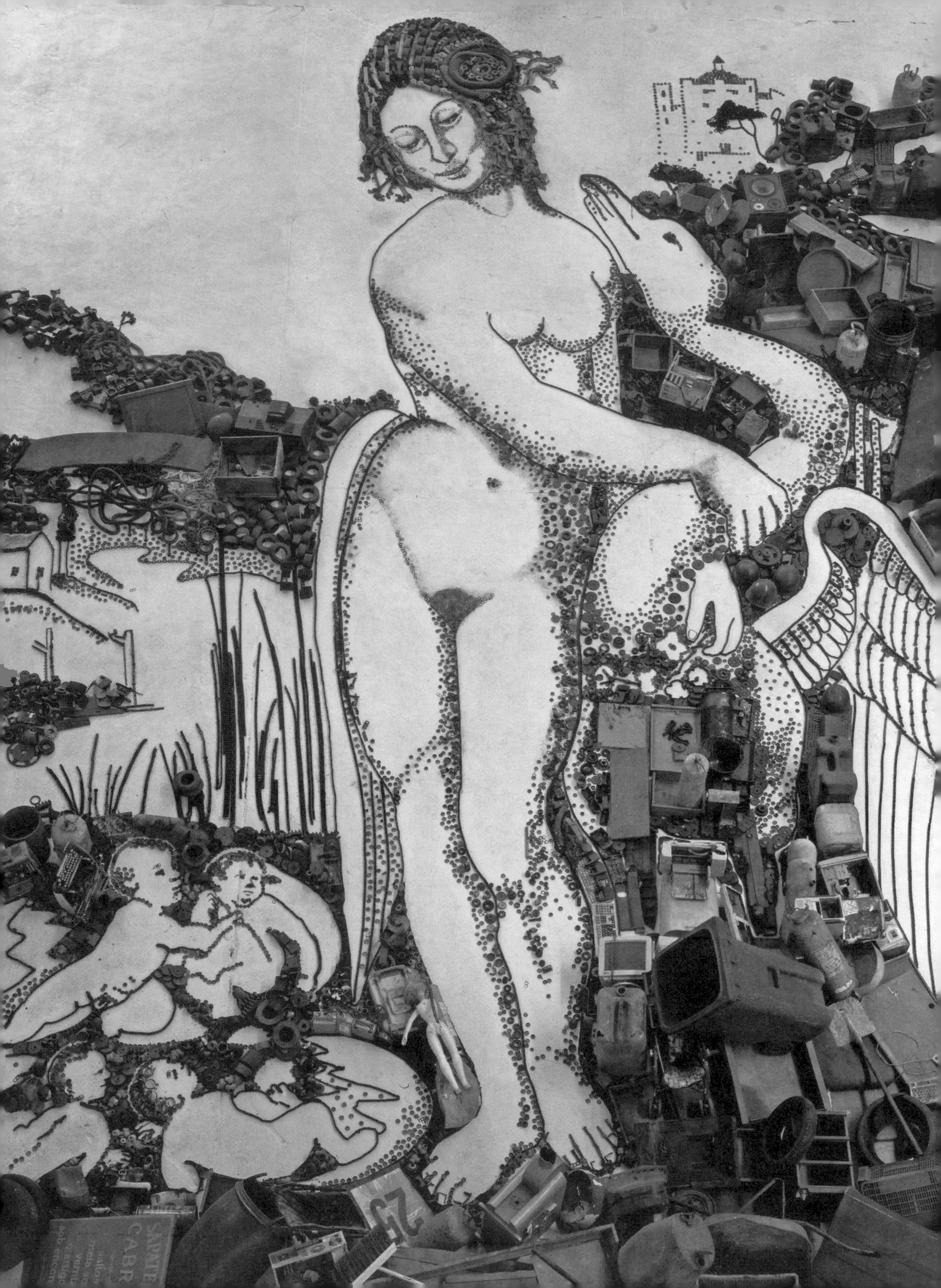

Epilogue

'Leda and the Swan, after Leonardo da Vinci'. In this version of the Greek myth, Zeus took the form of a swan to seduce Leda, Queen of Sparta. Subsequently she produced eggs, from which hatched two sets of twins: Castor and Pollux, Helen of Troy and Clytemnestra. Leonardo painted the subject in 1508, and an early copy of his lost original formed the basis of this 2009 reworking by Brazilian artist Vik Muniz. As part of his 'Pictures of Junk' series, Muniz used post-industrial waste to recreate mythological subjects painted by great masters, then photographed the assemblages. Most of the many modern Ledas focus on the seduction or rape, but in following Leonardo, Muniz retains the ancient trope of precocious infants hatched from giant eggs. Dye coupler print, 241 × 191 cm (mounted).

44 Concluding Reflections

Nick Hopwood, Rebecca Flemming and Lauren Kassell

Once inscribed in cuneiform script on a clay tablet from Babylonia, the idea that the time of birth shapes a person's life sells horoscopes today, though readers' expectations have been transformed. The arrivals of the monster of Cracow and of 'test-tube babies' all made international news, but in vastly different ways. And when a woman records her periods on a digital calendar, she does something like the Elizabethan mathematician who noted his wife's bleeding in a diary, yet revolutions in knowledge, technology and gender relations separate their actions. Long views reveal continuities we miss by focusing on a mere century or two, but the very similarities direct attention to the specifics of change.

This book has appraised established findings, revised received views, placed specialist insights in a wider frame and opened up new topics to produce a sustained long-term history of generation and reproduction. Different dimensions of these rich phenomena have shifted on multiple timescales and interacted in complicated ways. The pace and sometimes the direction of innovation have varied geographically even within our chosen regions, primarily the Mediterranean, western Europe, North America and their empires. Yet we can recognize broad outlines of endurance and alteration and identify a few concerted transformations.

These reflections proceed by way of three broad themes. First, we consider the different functions of the defining frameworks, reviewing the genesis and career of the old 'generation' – the active making of humans and beasts, plants and even minerals – and of the modern 'reproduction' – the more abstract process of perpetuating living organisms – and exploring how the stakes changed while the questions stayed much the same. Next we place the eighteenth-century emergence of population as an object of knowledge in relation to a longer history of multitudes and states. Then we reconstruct ideals and realities of control in the history of contraception and abortion, pregnancy and childbirth, asking what happened as coping with uncertainty gave way to managing risk. We end by pondering some challenges and opportunities of long views.

Generation and Reproduction

Whether 'generation' or 'reproduction', the frameworks defined the range and significance of debate in every period. It is thus important not just to engage with the notion that there was a shift 'from generation to reproduction' since the mid-eighteenth century, but also to examine the longer life of generation.

'Generation' was 'invented' when writers brought diverse ancient discourses in philosophy, medicine and agriculture together to grapple systematically with the problem of 'coming to be'. This discursive coalescence over many centuries was linguistically complex, but the Indo-European root *gen**, which gave Aristotle *genesis*, covered much of the semantic field. Enabled by growing wealth, expanding Mediterranean networks of exchange and settlement, and greater political diversity, the new conceptual repertoire drew on general explanatory models and responded to specific practical needs. Unlike in the ancient Near East and Egypt, which envisaged fertility as male, generation became a project shared – unequally, but with both male and female actively involved.

By designating the generative substance as 'seed', which could come from mother, father or both, ancient medical writings offered a flexible approach to explanations of how the fetus was formed and came to resemble its parents. Bodies and souls generated a child under the influence of the environment at the moment of conception and through pregnancy. The womb and menstrual material were vital, whether or not the woman produced seed, and whether or not her seed contributed to the embryo. In a creative, multistage process, pre-existing elements might also play a role. Within these constraints, generation was adaptable and open enough to accommodate opposing theories of matter and causation, divergent ideas of sex determination and family likeness, and commitments to the mortality or immortality of the soul.

This framework underwrote interventions at individual, family and state levels to affect the quantity and quality of offspring. Doctors and divinities assisted in having healthy and beautiful children; midwives managed births, infants and their mothers; laws eased divorce, remarriage and (adult) adoption, infant exposure and abortion. The fixed point was male superiority within a cosmic hierarchy of generation that stretched from the gods down through humans and animals to plants and stones. In these patriarchal societies, any female seed simply was inferior, so the relative inputs of women and men were mere details. Rome's vast empire spread and systematized concepts of generation, but did not use them to write distinctions between ruler and ruled on their bodies; location, climate, culture and laws determined the differences between peoples.

Thriving as the empire Christianized in the fourth century AD, this repertoire passed into the medieval successor states, Christian and Islamic. Building on Jewish tradition, the divine became a crucial participant in generation and the pre-eminent source of moral rules; the soul came to the fore as the basis of the human relationship with God. Christians broke most radically from a sexual ethics structured by gender, power and status. They argued, with increasing success from the sixth century, that the only legitimate sex was that intended to produce children within marriage.

Reframed, re-evaluated and entangled in webs of biblical and quranic exposition and exegesis, the framework of generation attained its greatest geographical range in the middle ages and achieved unparalleled hegemony in a Christian west now suffused with orthodoxy. In the early eleventh-century Islamicate world, Ibn Sina (Avicenna) laid the intellectual groundwork with an innovative synthesis of classical theories that travelled east and south, north and west. In the thirteenth century, Thomas Aquinas articulated Christian theology and (Avicenna's) Aristotelian philosophy, and this was matched by the institutional conjunction between the church and the newly established universities. Codified teachings on generation reached from episcopal thrones and professorial chairs to the street-preaching of friars and the practices of local physicians. Hierarchies and discourses aligned.

From the fourteenth century, an explosion of writing, and a fragmentation of authority, sparked a long, slow transformation in how procreative knowledge was understood and by whom. With the rise of vernaculars and the invention of printing, a broader array of people, including women and artisans as well as natural philosophers, physicians and poets, contested questions of generation. It was at issue in the debates over rank and family, body and soul, fate and predestination that proliferated in the Renaissance and the Protestant Reformation. Orthodoxy and heresy had always been locked in close embrace, but the division of Christendom politicized claims about nature and institutionalized opposing beliefs. Participants might deploy ancient concepts and echo medieval concerns, but played for higher stakes. The stronger associations of stances on generation with religious and political attitudes posed the alternatives more starkly, and by the eighteenth century a wider range of opinions could be expressed.

As naturalists explored colonized landscapes, their encounters with the unfamiliar denizens of the New World challenged, but did not defeat, received views. Mechanical, fermenting and nervous bodies vied with the ancient humoral model, but it dominated understandings of generation for a long time. While philosophers debated coming to be in general terms, the methods of collective, experimental, observational inquiry that constituted the so-called scientific revolution focused attention on the microscopic mysteries of procreation. The medical doctors and natural philosophers, who from the seventeenth century argued over the contributions of eggs and 'animalcules', pleasure and the soul, stayed initially within the generation framework, but would eventually push beyond it to 'reproduction'. Revisiting the protagonists' work in light of their medical consultations, such as advice on how to have children, could open up research to connect seemingly esoteric ideas and everyday routines.

The age of revolutions between the 1740s and the 1840s reorganized knowledge of generation. The traditional intellectual landmark, Buffon's 1749 adoption of the term 'reproduction' for the common power of organisms to propagate their species, excluded minerals and included plants. Unifying 'life', it all but banished the soul. A more abstract process linked individual and population, rendering it easier to see regularities and plan the betterment of family and species. Practical overlaps between medicine and agriculture have a long history, but in the generation framework, conceptual relations often operated by analogy and metaphor. Thinking in terms of reproduction facilitated more direct transfers of knowledge and technology between humans, other animals and even plants. Breeding for improvement went hand in hand with schemes for perfecting people. Conversely, by blaming nature for the plight of the poor, Thomas Robert Malthus exposed himself to censure that he belittled men as 'mere animals' and the labouring classes as 'stock'.

Yet there was no sudden switch to a regime of 'reproduction', not least because that word caught on slowly, while 'generation' acquired a new lease of life in the sense of a cohort born at the same time. Early population engineers, improving breeders, plant acclimatizers or man-midwives – even those bureaucrats of enlightened absolutism who drafted systems of medical administration from cradle to grave – did not necessarily march under the banner of reproduction. 'Population' gained political potency first. In ways that cry out for thorough scrutiny, a unified discourse of reproduction took much of the nineteenth century to appear, in part as materialism, transformism and evolutionism undermined the model of God's creation.

From mid-century, reproduction was consolidated as a coherent topic in science and medicine, consumer markets, early welfare states and expanding European and American empires. From the valorization of motherhood as 'bringing up reinforcements' in Britain during World War I to the radicalization of sterilization and euthanasia into genocide in Nazi-occupied Europe during World War II, reproduction had become a major target of state power. Scientifically trained professionals forged links between academic biology, agriculture, industry and medicine. They founded institutions for eugenics and laboratories that produced striking innovations, beginning with hormonal pregnancy tests. From the 1940s, livestock breeding incorporated artificial insemination and lobbies were organized for population control, driving the setting up of societies, journals and departments of demography and eventually of 'reproductive biology'. Neo-Darwinians influentially explained life in terms of differential reproductive success.

The postwar era, that acme of state intervention, communitarianism and professional authority, realized long-standing medico-scientific ambitions. Biological research and health-care systems combined in biomedicine; childbirth and contraception were more fully medicalized. The battles of the 1970s for civil and consumer rights, social reform and feminism inspired critiques of medical science and technology and defined key themes in reproductive debate. People now claimed 'reproductive rights', fought over 'reproductive technologies' and would soon be using 'reproductive medicine' while seeking 'reproductive health'. Yet the women's health movement also insisted on going 'beyond reproduction', and with growing success. Calls for 'reproductive justice' took account of intersecting forms of discrimination, such as by race and sexuality as well as gender, around the world.

The ancient seed models had competed for low political stakes among elite men writing in patriarchal societies. Approaches and voices diversified in the late middle ages and early modernity, with women more obviously included. Modern sciences have tended to dismiss other knowledge as simple ignorance. Yet telling the first mass audience about gonads and hormones, birth-rates and contraception expanded the options for divergent readings. On the one hand, the new facts of life established a dominion no theory of generation had ever enjoyed. Experience, religion and tradition may stake claims, but there is now no alternative to eggs and sperm. On the other hand, meanings are much contested, and it matters, for example, if depictions of the behaviour of sperm and eggs reinforce or challenge stereotypes of active male and passive female. 'Life', a new soul, is potent in debates over abortion independently of the warrant of science.

Modern reproduction is not just different from premodern generation; it is a framework of another kind. We see that in its abstraction and in a further modern characteristic – the potentially uncontrollable dynamic within the endless repetition – which has made reproduction central to modern societies and the challenges they face. The new reproduction might seem narrower than the old generation, if we take this to have broken down also into the study of development and of heredity. Yet not only is 'reproduction' used more broadly to include embryology, genetics and much more besides; the very abstraction of the concept has let it link individual bodies and bodies politic in distinctive ways through its association with population, and so to reconfigure that relationship for modern times.

States and Populations

'Population' became integral to the modern rise of reproduction as a way of seeing groups of organisms and as a mediator between individuals and states. The eighteenth-century innovations in the definition and management of populations were, however, only the most important in a sequence of changes in relations between states and peoples that reaches back into antiquity. It is not just that Plato had already limited the size of his ideal community or that Aristotle aimed for that smaller number which could optimize political life and general well-being, but 'be taken in at a single view'. This book has emphasized early concepts, notably 'multitude', that were loosely linked to generation. Recovering their relations will give 'population' a richer premodern history and throw the distinctive features of the modern notion into sharper relief.

Abstract ideas of multitude, and debates about the desirable proportions and composition of polities, were first recorded in the classical Mediterranean, which was also home to state practices of categorizing and counting people and encouraging marriage and childbearing within patriarchal households. The Romans' elaborate habits of census-taking survived the fall of the Western Empire to continue, with successive revisions, in the East; persisted to some extent in the more centralized kingdoms of the early medieval west; and were adapted by the Umayyad caliphs. Censuses enabled direct taxation, the most reliable state revenue, and codified social hierarchies. Both mattered in the administrative development of the medieval Islamic domains, while fiscal crisis motivated the Florentine *catasto* of 1427–30, a survey of wealth and income, age and household relationships that typified the return to a more systematic accounting of people and property.

Classical controversies over multitude were revived and reformulated in Christian Europe from the late twelfth century and in the writings of the North African historian Ibn Khaldun two hundred years later. Engagement with earlier scholarship and contemporary geopolitics shaped these reflections: the mid-fourteenth-century ravages of the second plague pandemic focused attention on numbers of people, while the fragmentation and restructuring of the Islamicate world posed questions about the roles of size and organization in the fates of dynasties and states.

In 18 BC and AD 9, the Emperor Augustus had enacted legislation penalizing the unmarried and the childless, and rewarding those with children, yet since Justinian repealed those laws five hundred years later, active political interventions in fertility had been scarce. The need for family continuity and the Muslim imperative to marry as part of leading a good life were enough. Islamic codes, more supportive of the male drive for progeny than either canon or medieval Christian civil law, enabled divorce, remarriage, polygyny (under certain conditions) and slave concubinage (to produce legitimate children). Sharia excluded the adoption of heirs, a key family strategy in ancient Greece and Rome, and adoption fell out of favour among Christians too, though fostering flourished.

The Christian churches' interest in tracking members, and regulating their religious lives, led to systematic parish records. Newly Protestant England and Wales required the registration of 'every wedding, christening and burying' from 1538; the Council of Trent ordered the Catholic world to follow suit in 1563. With interests as much civil as ecclesiastical, inheritance concerns and matrimonial rules coincided in their effects. In the seventeenth century, these delineations of communities and identities were exported to European colonies, which drew sharper lines between people of different status, and restricted marriage and legitimate procreation; plantation economies counted slaves and forced them to procreate. Political arithmetic was pursued more widely, but inquiries at the level of the whole population of a state had such subversive potential that governments tended to block access to the records through the eighteenth century.

Innovation then built on these practices to reconceptualize populations in the aggregate and as objects of more sustained management. Typically, Malthus reworked debates that engaged with classical antiquity – was the Roman Empire more populous than modern kingdoms? – while drawing also on biblical scholarship and Renaissance statecraft to frame world history and geography as a development through stages from hunter-gatherers to commercial civilization. But the synthesis was new, and modern states, though still levying taxes and raising armies, began to invest more positively in their human resources. From the 1830s onwards, comprehensive censuses and civil registers let statistical bureaux measure populations as phenomena defined in terms of fertility and mortality. Physicians claimed roles in managing populations onto which nationalists projected hopes and fears. 'Open', incommensurable, locally and hierarchically organized associations became, in theory, 'closed' groups of equivalent individuals. In fact, more than ever people both migrated overseas and were divided by race.

Around 1900, 'geopoliticians' argued that, after four centuries of European colonization of the Americas, Asia and Africa, the world itself was 'closed' again, now on a global scale. This claim set the stage for battles over living space, or food, fertility and migration. Demography, now measuring reproduction rates and defining mortality and fertility transitions, was touted as a key to human history, a route to peace and a weapon of war. Pressure groups used maps and graphs to teach European elites to fear the maldistribution of people and resources and relative declines in their own birth-rates; Germans heard that they were a '*Volk* without youth' as much as a '*Volk* without space'. Eugenicists peddled the fantasy that selective breeding would raise human quality, as they supposed it had improved their animals.

After World War II, western governments managed populations on an unprecedented scale through pronatalist welfare states, and covered labour shortages through immigration from southern Europe and the global south, while attention shifted to the rise in population in 'underdeveloped countries', many of which had once been considered underpopulated, too. With many more nations conducting censuses according to UN criteria, it was easier to compare growth rates. Against Catholic and communist opposition, US-led agencies enrolled postcolonial governments in population control. A brief consensus on defusing a 'population bomb' and preventing an ecological crisis fell apart soon after the first Earth Day, 22 April 1970. As governments ceded some influence to corporations, NGOs and supranational organizations, the end of the Cold War consensus made it still harder to press the case for state power. Today, reproduction and contraception are marketed in most places as individual duties and consumer choices. The threat of anthropogenic climate change has fed calls to rehabilitate population control, while old agendas surface where global inequalities run in parallel with worries about too few and too many.

The liberal logic of commensurability, of framing populations as collections of equivalent individuals, has been promoted and resisted, in the first place in relation to the family. External institutions and agencies have increasingly brought resources to bear on individual citizens directly, rather than through male heads of households; development aid often targets girls. But families are still economic as well as procreative units, and for women to combine having children with paid work has remained a basic, contested challenge in family strategies and public policy. Much of the reproductive biomedicine industry addresses the failure of a labour market that compels women to 'choose' to delay childbearing. Still caught in systems of male domination, they have been disproportionately disadvantaged by the worsening of public provision as welfare states have retreated.

Population and family intersect in the politics of race and of sexuality. Population genetics had struggled to replace racial typologies with gene frequencies even before direct-to-consumer genetic testing began fostering identity politics. Yet adoption, redesigned in the mid-twentieth century to create 'as-if natural' families, is now usually open – and conspicuously so in the transracial and inter-country variants that most explicitly transfer children towards wealth and whiteness. Attempts to buttress the heterosexual nuclear family still conflict with the principle of commensurability. Access to parenthood is extremely unequal, and lesbians and gay men may marry in few countries beyond the Americas and western Europe. But technologies of assisted conception, though founded on the promise of biological resemblance, have separated social, gestational and genetic parenthood and facilitated the creation of new family forms.

Control of Fertility, Pregnancy and Birth

Whether paired with 'population' or 'birth', 'control' became the controversial hallmark of modernity, its centrality assumed in what by the 1970s was the key question: 'Who controls reproduction?' Still disputed among policymakers and activists, doctors and patients, this issue has driven much historical scholarship, where 'control' is also problematic. While helpful in linking the prevention and promotion of procreation, the term may be too modern for centuries before the twentieth. People have always aimed to achieve certain objectives for family continuity and population size, individual health and happiness, but their conceptual and practical tools have changed. Uncertainty, with the strategies to mitigate it, has mostly turned into risk, with its expectations of quantitative decisions.

Before the fertility transitions, families strove above all to have healthy children. Though readily available in antiquity, contraceptive and abortive substances and techniques served to support the production of legitimate offspring within marriage. These aids were integral to prostitution, access to which was part of the male sexual prerogative, and permitted to protect a wife's health, especially her generative capacity, but condemned when concealing her adultery. Infanticide, exposure and adult adoption completed this system of paternal control, designed primarily to preserve patrimony.

Christians tried to break up the Roman sexual order and root out contraception, abortion and exposure. The medieval church transformed debate, but made fewer inroads into practices. Extra-marital sex still drove demand for the means to prevent or end pregnancies, and could lead to the abandonment of newborns. Contraception, abortion before quickening, and the giving up of children were tolerated as occasional requirements in marriage. Islam, too, prohibited infanticide, and brought fetal life under the remit of sharia, with theologians and jurists pondering the timing of ensoulment and the permissibility of abortion. But they took a more positive view of marital sexuality and contraception, and endorsed a more expansive approach to the production of heirs; this alignment with family strategies made the system more stable.

The modern politics of control came to be dominated by relations to doctors as well as states. In nineteenth-century Europe and America, and even in some Islamic countries, abortion at any stage of pregnancy was declared not only a sin (an affront to religious teaching) and a tort (a legally actionable harm), but also a crime (an offence against the community). Responding to medical vilification of unlicensed practitioners, governments criminalized abortion more fully; anxiety about falling birth-rates strengthened state resolve. As imperial legislation, the French and English laws were either binding on, or extended to, colonial holdings. Undoing these dictats has proved more complex; some postcolonial polities liberalized, while others imposed harsher restrictions. Yet abortion remained common everywhere; prohibition just made it more dangerous, particularly for those who could not afford discreet treatment.

Alongside their efforts to limit abortion and contraception, nation-states more successfully enacted laws to codify middle-class marriage. Yet the fertility transitions relied more on people using the old technologies of withdrawal, abstinence and condoms than on new methods. Only in the mid-twentieth century was birth control officially sanctioned as a social and moral good, thanks to feminism, eugenics and population control. From the 1960s, a more precarious legalization of abortion sought initially to safeguard physicians' autonomy, then to secure women's rights. In Japan, by contrast, abortion – sanctioned by the older practice of infanticide – was the main means of achieving a remarkable postwar fertility decline. From the 1970s, right-wing and religious opposition, channelled internationally through US foreign policy and the Catholic church, has made abortion the prime 'hinge' through which individual reproductive rights and population politics intersect and conflict.

For as long as physicians have advised on contraception and abortion, they have also treated infertility. Since Greek antiquity, this involved medicine as well as religion, with responsibility divided between the sexes, but intervention concentrating on women. Promoting healthy procreation was crucial to ancient and medieval physicians' prestige, and a foundation for professional expansion through early modernity. From around 1900, infertility differed primarily in a new sense that scientific medicine could help infertile couples as medical consumers in a culture of choice and design. Though sometimes successful, patients often found themselves poorer and still childless; or, especially after 1945, they adopted infants professionally matched to their social and intellectual profiles. Like contraception, infertility treatment created and responded to expectations of control.

As scientific medicine won state recognition and guided professional interventions into reproduction, it became pivotal to gendered struggles over the location of childbirth and the identities of the attendants. The twentieth-century move into the hospital built on a history of lying-in wards, which went back to the Enlightenment valorization of population, childhood and motherhood. These became more medical around 1900, with hospitalization facilitating the 'masculinization' of childbirth, but by 2000 most obstetricians training in the United States were women, as they always had been, for example, in British hospitals in India. Interventions still increased, and the return to home birth was small.

Nor had birth ever been an all-female domain. It was standard practice for women – friends, relatives, neighbours and midwives – to attend births, but male doctors were always possible additions, from classical Greece through imperial Rome to medieval societies that segregated the sexes. Learned gynaecology had flourished alongside community-recognized specialist midwives in the cities of the Roman Empire. Both lost out in the Christian west, and under early medieval Islam, and both revived by the thirteenth century. Contrary to assumptions framed by the twentieth-century United States, urban culture, expansive male medical discourse about female fertility and an established profession of midwifery generally went together.

Experiences of pregnancy illustrate changing expectations of safety and control, chance and risk. Premodern women might give birth or miscarry many times; in industrialized countries, mothers and babies eventually became far more likely to survive birth. Miscarriages remained frequent, but pregnancies were rarer events in women's lives and each one thus more significant. Nineteenth-century European hospitals worsened outcomes, but infant mortality fell decisively from 1900, though maternal in only a few countries before the 1930s. Pregnancy has become more predictable also in other respects. The ebb and flow of fluids, chiefly in menstruation, once shaped the lives of women of childbearing age. The stopping of the menses, even for several months, might indicate a child to come, but like the swelling of the belly, had other meanings too; feeling a 'kick' was only the most definite in a complex of uncertain signs. Some premodern women seem to have known soon that they were carrying a child, and a small number today remain unaware until they are in labour, but hormonal tests typically provide early diagnoses of a state that, among the globally wealthy, medicine monitors stage by stage.

There was no simple transition from privacy to publicity – the very distinction is modern, and the pregnancies of princesses and paupers have long been broadcast. But wombs have become more transparent, and fetuses now compete for attention. Since 1991, naked, pregnant models have occasionally featured on magazines, and in 2017, when Beyoncé announced twins by displaying her bulge on Instagram, she was 'liked' over six million times in eight hours. Publicity feeds a consumer market in prenatal accessories. The rich may host 'fetus parties' to welcome family members represented by 4-D sonograms and plastic models, or they may put under surveillance the surrogate mothers who carry fetuses for others. There is far more control over pregnancy, childbirth and fertility, but many do not experience it as such.

'Birth control', like its successor 'family planning', served divergent visions. Some obtained the freedom, and the duty, to control their own fertility; some were snared in others' plans. But the terms always implied that planning was better; universalizing a middle-class value, advocates equated 'planned' with 'wanted', while promoting rational choice and medical science. Even where control promised safety, risk culture was anxiogenic. Pregnancies became more precious and more certain – and tentative in new ways, thanks to prenatal diagnosis and the possibility of selective termination. Advanced technologies did not necessarily put either prospective parents or their doctors in charge; some methods offer little more than hope. Developing countries have reduced maternal mortality in recent decades, but the least powerful are still most likely to die; in this sense the politics of reproduction are all about control.

Long Views

'*Ex ovo omnia*' – everything from an egg. Compared with Aristotle's assumption that those eggs had to be laid, the words on William Harvey's frontispiece can sound modern although they were written in 1651. Yet his egg was not ours, but more like an embryo, and in many other ways he lived in a different world. As late as the mid-nineteenth century, microscopists still argued over whether the sperm had a role, and complained that the idea of such origins disgusted laypeople. Far from proving a fact, Harvey sparked debates that have resonated ever since.

These controversies are part of major changes in frameworks, populations and control which add up to a long, perhaps still incomplete revolution that endorses the notion of a shift 'from generation to reproduction'. Extending the timeline puts the change in perspective, but even if it took a couple of centuries for reproduction to gain its present prominence, this still represents a huge transformation. Exploring other themes, from the family and sexuality to inheritance and the law, would confirm as well as complicate this generalization.

We thus find little support for the suggestion that the recent history of reproductive medicine and population politics represents a return from modernity to a (less patriarchal but) in some ways premodern world. States have withdrawn from many functions. Rich parents – no longer viewed as mere vessels for genes or (if they ever were) as passive objects of medical power – are actively making their children again, albeit now as consumers. Nor is biology today the unchallenged substratum of social life, as IVF shows every time it assists nature. Yet late modern reproduction, with its potential for comprehensive surveillance, integrated infrastructures, risk management, precise molecular interventions and abortion wars – even its customized bodies and female obstetricians – is otherwise as unlike early modern generation as could be.

Looking over longer periods points the way to generalizations that make better sense. Modern historians cannot have all the contrasting premodern backdrops they might like, but historians as a whole can have the framework of generation, provided its own eventful history is recognized along with the complexity of the transition to reproduction. Historians of earlier centuries should resist the temptation to claim relevance by casually identifying ideas and practices with modern ones; the deeper layers of modernity require more nuanced excavation. Nor should ancient historians assume that nothing has changed or that every innovation is really a return – but some activities do have extremely long histories, and innovators invoke classical traditions even today. History highlights the freshness of some twenty-first-century arrangements, and how far others go back. Recognizing the mix of novelty and repetition underlines the challenge of causal explanation and the need for long views.

This cannot be a single view, as if one narrative could ever capture a subject as rich and contested as reproduction. It should involve a commitment to placing discussion of any past century in relation to earlier and later periods, with the appropriate timescale depending on the topic. The different ways the world has and has not been joined up are already part of this story of an expanding and shifting network of approaches. But accounts of the United States and western Europe remain dominant. We cannot and should not all become whole-planet historians; we should think globally when writing locally, so as to recognize the patterns of connection and exchange.

This book has shown how generation and reproduction, because they are so socially embedded, are fundamental to tackling a larger set of historical problems. Taking reproduction seriously is also a precondition for understanding current issues from environmental degradation to economic inequality, and perhaps for effecting real change. Long views of reproduction allow us to evaluate the past and grasp the future.

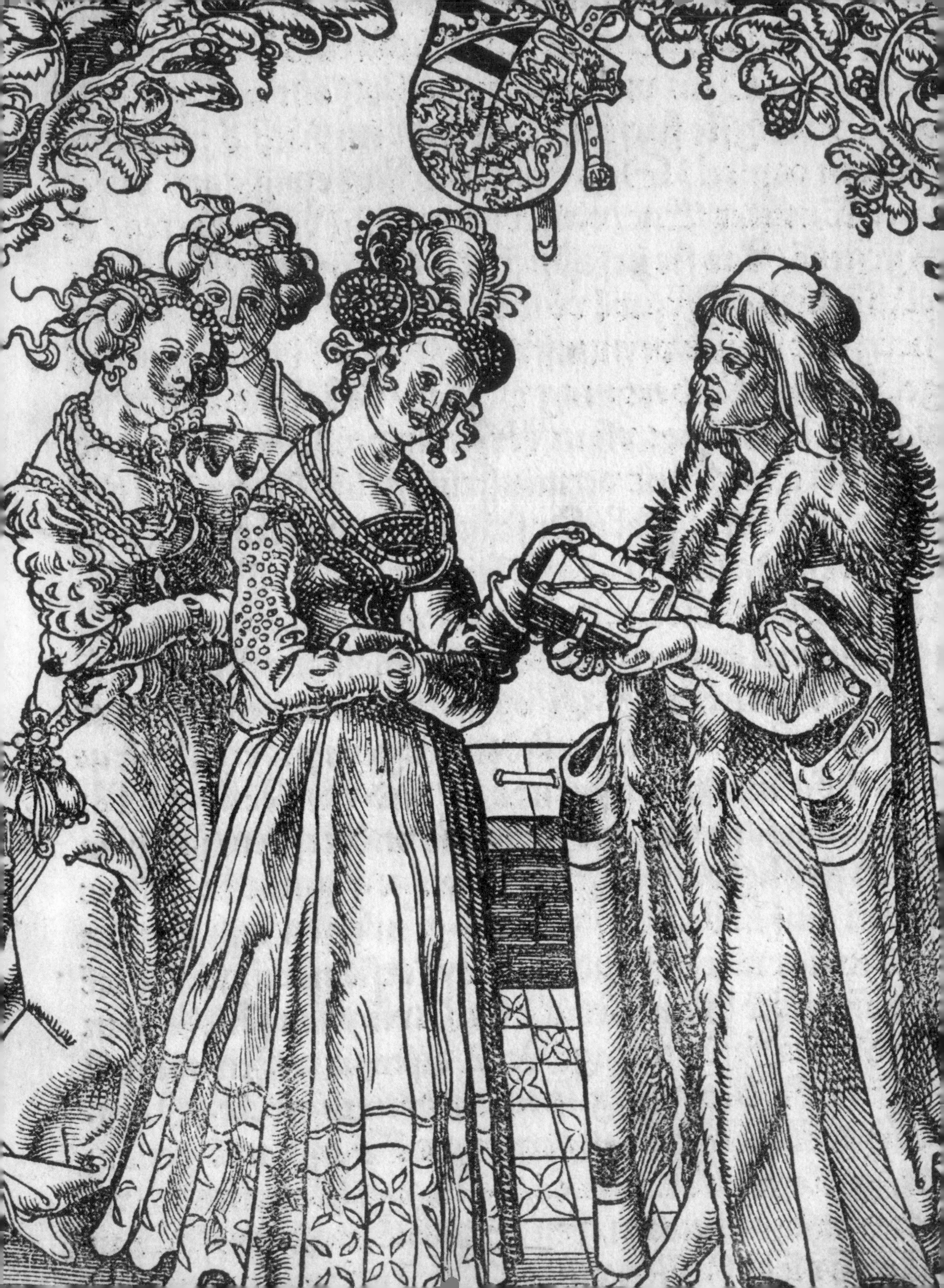

Select Bibliography

Eucharius Rösslin, physician to the city of Worms, presents *Der Rosengarten* (The rose garden), the first printed book on midwifery, to his pregnant patron, Katherine, Duchess of Braunschweig-Lüneburg. This frontispiece may play on the association between authoring books and birthing babies. Martin Caldenbach's woodcuts for the book, which also included a woman in labour, a birth chamber and a then already venerable sequence of birth presentations, have often featured in histories of midwifery (Figs. 1.2, 22.2 and Exhibit 10, this book). From *Der Swangern frawen vnd hebamme[n] roszgarte[n]* ([Hagenau]: [Gran], [1515]). 22 × 16 cm. Bayerische Staatsbibliothek, Rar. 1511, f. A3r.

This selective list gives access to the large literature in history of generation and reproduction from antiquity to the present day. While we have sought to represent a wider variety of topics and approaches even than are covered in the chapters and exhibits, we have prioritized books, and among these, the most synthetic and recent works.

General

Berthiaud, Emmanuelle, *Enceinte: Une histoire de la grossesse entre art et société* (Paris, 2013).

Borsay, Anne, and Billie Hunter (eds.), *Nursing and Midwifery in Britain since 1700* (Basingstoke, 2012).

Boswell, John, *The Kindness of Strangers: The Abandonment of Children in Western Europe from Late Antiquity to the Renaissance* (Chicago, IL, 1998).

Charbit, Yves, *The Classical Foundations of Population Thought: From Plato to Quesnay* (Dordrecht, 2010).

Dasen, Véronique (ed.), *L'embryon humain à travers l'histoire: Images, savoirs et rites. Actes du colloque international de Fribourg, 27–29 octobre 2004* (Gollion, 2007).

Davis, Gayle, and Tracey Loughran (eds.), *The Palgrave Handbook of Infertility in History: Approaches, Contexts and Perspectives* (London, 2017). (This volume was published after the present book went to press.)

Duden, Barbara, Jürgen Schlumbohm and Patrice Veit (eds.), *Geschichte des Ungeborenen. Zur Erfahrungs- und Wissenschaftsgeschichte der Schwangerschaft, 17.–20. Jahrhundert* (Göttingen, 2002).

Dunstan, G. R. (ed.), *The Human Embryo: Aristotle and the Arabic and European Traditions* (Exeter, 1990).

Dupâquier, Jacques (ed.), *Histoire de la population française*, 4 vols. (Paris, 1988).

Finucci, Valeria, and Kevin Brownlee (eds.), *Generation and Degeneration: Tropes of Reproduction in Literature and History from Antiquity through Early Modern Europe* (Durham, NC, 2001).

Fischer, Jean-Louis, *Monstres: Histoire du corps et de ses défauts* (Paris, 1991).

Fissell, Mary, Nick Hopwood, Peter Jones, Francis Neary and Jim Secord, *Books & Babies: Communicating Reproduction*, legacy website of exhibition, Cambridge University Library, www.lib.cam.ac.uk/exhibitions/Babies/ (2011).

Foyster, Elizabeth, and James Marten (eds.), *A Cultural History of Childhood and Family*, 6 vols. (Oxford, 2010).

Frydman, René, Émile Papiernik, Cédric Crémière and Jean-Louis Fischer (eds.), *Avant la naissance, 5000 ans d'images* (Le Havre, 2009).

Goody, Jack, *The Development of the Family and Marriage in Europe* (Cambridge, 1983).

Haines, Michael R., and Richard H. Steckel (eds.), *A Population History of North America* (Cambridge, 2000).

Hibbard, Bryan, *The Obstetrician's Armamentarium: Historical Obstetric Instruments and Their Inventors* (San Anselmo, CA, 2001).

Himes, Norman E., *Medical History of Contraception* (New York, NY, 1970).

Hinde, Andrew, *England's Population: A History since the Domesday Survey* (London, 2003).

Hopwood, Nick, Peter Murray Jones, Lauren Kassell and Jim Secord (eds.), 'Communicating reproduction', special issue, *Bulletin of the History of Medicine* 89 (2015), 379–556.

Hornuff, Daniel, *Schwangerschaft. Eine Kulturgeschichte* (Paderborn, 2014).
Huet, Marie-Hélene, *Monstrous Imagination* (Cambridge, MA, 1993).
Jackson, Mark (ed.), *Infanticide: Historical Perspectives on Child Murder and Concealment, 1550–2000* (Aldershot, 2002).
Johnson, Christopher H., Bernhard Jussen, David Warren Sabean and Simon Teuscher (eds.), *Blood and Kinship: Matter for Metaphor from Ancient Rome to the Present* (New York, NY, 2013).
Jütte, Robert (ed.), *Geschichte der Abtreibung. Von der Antike bis zur Gegenwart* (Munich, 1993).
King, Helen, *Midwifery, Obstetrics and the Rise of Gynaecology: The Uses of a Sixteenth-Century Compendium* (Aldershot, 2007).
The One-Sex Body on Trial: The Classical and Early Modern Evidence (Farnham, 2013).
Kingsbury, Noel, *Hybrid: The History and Science of Plant Breeding* (Chicago, IL, 2009).
Knibiehler, Yvonne, *Histoire des mères et de la maternité en Occident*, 3rd edn (Paris, 2012).
Knibiehler, Yvonne, and Catherine Fouquet, *Histoire des mères du Moyen-Age à nos jours* (Paris, 1977).
Kreager, Philip, Bruce Winney, Stanley Ulijaszek and Cristian Capelli (eds.), *Population in the Human Sciences: Concepts, Models, Evidence* (Oxford, 2015).
Laqueur, Thomas, *Making Sex: Body and Gender from the Greeks to Freud* (Cambridge, MA, 1990).
Lechner, Gregor Martin, *Maria gravida. Zum Schwangerschaftsmotiv in der bildenden Kunst* (Munich, 1981).
Lesky, Erna, *Die Zeugungs- und Vererbungslehren der Antike und ihr Nachwirken* (Vienna, 1951).
Livi-Bacci, Massimo, *A Concise History of World Population*, 6th edn (Chichester, 2017).
McLaren, Angus, *A History of Contraception from Antiquity to the Present Day* (Oxford, 1990).
Müller-Wille, Staffan, and Hans-Jörg Rheinberger, *A Cultural History of Heredity* (Chicago, IL, 2012).
(eds.), *Heredity Produced: At the Crossroads of Biology, Politics, and Culture, 1500–1870* (Cambridge, MA, 2007).
Noonan, Jr, John T., *Contraception: A History of Its Treatment by the Catholic Theologians and Canonists* (Cambridge, MA, 1965).
Omran, Abdel Rahim, *Family Planning in the Legacy of Islam* (London, 1992).
Pancino, Claudia, *Voglie materne: Storia di una credenza* (Bologna, 1996).
Pancino, Claudia, and Jean d'Yvoire, *Formato nel segreto: Nascituri e feti fra immagini e immaginario dal XVI al XXI secolo* (Rome, 2006).
Parnes, Ohad, Ulrike Vedder and Stefan Willer, *Das Konzept der Generation. Eine Wissenschafts- und Kulturgeschichte* (Frankfurt am Main, 2008).
Porter, Roy, and Lesley Hall, *The Facts of Life: The Creation of Sexual Knowledge in Britain, 1650–1950* (New Haven, CT, 1995).
Porter, Roy, and Mikuláš Teich (eds.), *Sexual Knowledge, Sexual Science: The History of Attitudes to Sexuality* (Cambridge, 1994).
Riddle, John M., *Contraception and Abortion from the Ancient World to the Renaissance* (Cambridge, MA, 1992).
Eve's Herbs: A History of Contraception and Abortion in the West (Cambridge, MA, 1997).
Sasson, Vanessa R., and Jane Marie Law (eds.), *Imagining the Fetus: The Unborn in Myth, Religion and Culture* (Oxford, 2009).

Schlumbohm, Jürgen, Barbara Duden, Jacques Gélis and Patrice Veit (eds.), *Rituale der Geburt. Eine Kulturgeschichte* (Munich, 1998).

Shail, Andrew, and Gillian Howie (eds.), *Menstruation: A Cultural History* (Basingstoke, 2005).

Shorter, Edward, *A History of Women's Bodies* (London, 1983).

Smith, Richard M., and Naomi Tadmor (eds.), 'Kinship in Britain and beyond from the early modern to the present', special issue, *Continuity and Change* 25, no. 1 (2010).

Speert, Harold, *Iconographia gyniatrica: A Pictorial History of Gynecology and Obstetrics* (Philadelphia, PA, 1973).

Staupe, Gisela, and Lisa Vieth (eds.), *Unter anderen Umständen. Zur Geschichte der Abtreibung* (Dresden, 1993).

Toulalan, Sarah, and Kate Fisher (eds.), *The Routledge History of Sex and the Body, 1500 to the Present* (London, 2013).

Walle, Etienne van de, and Elisha P. Renne (eds.), *Regulating Menstruation: Beliefs, Practices, Interpretations* (Chicago, IL, 2001).

Weigel, Sigrid, *Genea-Logik: Generation, Tradition und Evolution zwischen Kultur- und Naturwissenschaften* (Munich, 2006).

Woods, Robert, *Death before Birth: Fetal Health and Mortality in Historical Perspective* (Oxford, 2009).

Wrigley, E. A., *Population and History* (London, 1969).

Wrigley, E. A., and R. S. Schofield, *The Population History of England, 1541–1871: A Reconstruction*, new edn (Cambridge, 1989).

Zirkle, Conway, *The Beginnings of Plant Hybridization* (Philadelphia, PA, 1935).

Ancient

Bagnall, Roger S., and Bruce W. Frier, *The Demography of Roman Egypt* (Cambridge, 1994).

Bien, Christian G., *Erklärungen zur Entstehung von Mißbildungen im physiologischen und medizinischen Schriftum der Antike* (Stuttgart, 1997).

Boylan, Michael, 'The Galenic and Hippocratic challenges to Aristotle's conception theory', *Journal of the History of Biology* 17 (1984), 83–112.

Brisson, Luc, Marie-Hélène Congourdeau and Jean-Luc Solère (eds.), *L'embryon: Formation et animation. Antiquité grecque et latine, traditions hébraïque, chrétienne et islamique* (Paris, 2008).

Brown, Peter, *The Body and Society: Men, Women, and Sexual Renunciation in Early Christianity*, rev. edn (New York, NY, 2008).

Budin, Stephanie Lynn, 'Fertility and gender in the ancient Near East', in Mark Masterson, Nancy Sorkin Rabinowitz and James Robson (eds.), *Sex in Antiquity: Exploring Gender and Sexuality in the Ancient World* (New York, NY, 2015), pp. 30–49.

Images of Woman and Child from the Bronze Age: Reconsidering Fertility, Maternity, and Gender in the Ancient World (Cambridge, 2011).

Clarysse, Willy, and Dorothy J. Thompson, *Counting the People in Hellenistic Egypt*, 2 vols. (Cambridge, 2006).

Congourdeau, Marie-Hélène, *L'embryon et son âme dans les sources grecques (VIe siècle av. J.-C. – Ve siècle apr. J.-C.)* (Paris, 2007).

Connell, Sophia M., *Aristotle on Female Animals: A Study of the* Generation of Animals (Cambridge, 2016).

Couto-Ferreira, M. Erica, 'She will give birth easily: Therapeutic approaches to childbirth in 1st millennium BCE cuneiform sources', *Dynamis* 34 (2014), 289–315.

Cox, Cheryl Anne, *Household Interests: Property, Marriage Strategies, and Family Dynamics in Ancient Athens* (Princeton, NJ, 1998).

Dasen, Véronique, *Le sourire d'Omphale: Maternité et petite enfance dans l'Antiquité* (Rennes, 2015).

(ed.), *Naissance et petite enfance dans l'Antiquité: Actes du colloque de Fribourg, 28 novembre – 1er decembre 2001* (Fribourg, 2004).

Dean-Jones, Lesley, *Women's Bodies in Classical Greek Science* (Oxford, 1994).

'Clinical gynecology and Aristotle's biology: The composition of *HA* X', *Apeiron* 45 (2012), 180–99.

Demand, Nancy, *Birth, Death, and Motherhood in Classical Greece* (Baltimore, MD, 1994).

Dixon, Suzanne, *The Roman Mother* (London, 1988).

Eijk, Philip J. van der, 'On sterility ("*HA* X"): A medical work by Aristotle?', *Classical Quarterly* 49 (1999), 490–502.

Flemming, Rebecca, *Medicine and the Making of Roman Women: Gender, Nature, and Authority from Celsus to Galen* (Oxford, 2000).

'The invention of infertility in the classical Greek world: Medicine, divinity, and gender', *Bulletin of the History of Medicine* 87 (2013), 565–90.

Foucault, Michel, *The History of Sexuality*, vol. 2: *The Use of Pleasure*, trans. Robert Hurley (New York, NY, 1985).

The History of Sexuality, vol. 3: *The Care of the Self*, trans. Robert Hurley (New York, NY, 1986).

Gaca, Kathy L., *The Making of Fornication: Eros, Ethics, and Political Reform in Greek Philosophy and Early Christianity* (Berkeley, CA, 2003).

Gourevitch, Danielle, Anna Moirin and Nadine Rouquet (eds.), *Maternité et petite enfance dans l'Antiquité romaine: Catalogue de l'exposition, Bourges, Muséum d'histoire naturelle, 6 novembre 2003 – 28 mars 2004* (Bourges, 2003).

Grubbs, Judith Evans, and Tim Parkin (eds.), *The Oxford Handbook of Childhood and Education in the Classical World* (Oxford, 2013).

Hanson, Ann Ellis, 'The eight months' child and the etiquette of birth: *Obsit omen!*', *Bulletin of the History of Medicine* 61 (1987), 589–602.

'The medical writers' woman', in David M. Halperin, John J. Winkler and Froma I. Zeitlin (eds.), *Before Sexuality: The Construction of Erotic Experience in the Ancient Greek World* (Princeton, NJ, 1990), pp. 309–38.

Hardy, Gavin, and Laurence Totelin, *Ancient Botany* (London, 2016).

Harper, Kyle, *From Shame to Sin: The Christian Transformation of Sexual Morality in Late Antiquity* (Cambridge, MA, 2013).

Hin, Saskia, *The Demography of Roman Italy: Population Dynamics in an Ancient Conquest Society (201 BCE – 14 CE)* (Cambridge, 2013).

Kapparis, Konstantinos, *Abortion in the Ancient World* (London, 2002).

King, Helen, *Hippocrates' Woman: Reading the Female Body in Ancient Greece* (London, 1998).

Köves-Zulauf, Thomas, *Römische Geburtsriten* (Munich, 1990).

Laes, Christian, 'The educated midwife in the Roman Empire: An example of differential equations', in Manfred Horstmanshoff (ed.), *Hippocrates and Medical Education* (Leiden, 2010), pp. 261–86.

'Midwives in Greek inscriptions in Hellenistic and Roman Antiquity', *Zeitschrift für Papyrologie und Epigraphik* 176 (2011), 154–62.

Leick, Gwendolen, *Sex and Eroticism in Mesopotamian Literature* (London, 1994).

Lloyd, G. E. R., *Science, Folklore and Ideology: Studies in the Life Sciences in Ancient Greece* (Cambridge, 1983).

Marshall, C. W. (ed.), 'Wet-nursing and breastfeeding in Greece and Rome,' special section, *Illinois Classical Studies* 42 (2017), 183–265.

Mayhew, Robert, *The Female in Aristotle's Biology: Reason or Rationalization* (Chicago, IL, 2004).

Miller, Timothy S., *The Orphans of Byzantium: Child Welfare in the Christian Empire* (Washington, DC, 2003).

Nardi, Enzo, *Procurato aborto nel mondo greco romano* (Milan, 1971).

Nathan, Geoffrey S., *The Family in Late Antiquity: The Rise of Christianity and the Endurance of Tradition* (London, 2000).

Papaconstantinou, Arietta, and Alice-Mary Talbot (eds.), *Becoming Byzantine: Children and Childhood in Byzantium* (Washington, DC, 2009).

Parkin, Tim G., *Demography and Roman Society* (Baltimore, MD, 1992).

Parpola, S., and R. M. Whiting (eds.), *Sex and Gender in the Ancient Near East: Proceedings of the 47th Rencontre Assyriologique Internationale, Helsinki, July 2–6, 2001* (Helsinki, 2002).

Petersen, Lauren Hackworth, and Patricia Salzman-Mitchell (eds.), *Mothering and Motherhood in Ancient Greece and Rome* (Austin, TX, 2012).

Preus, Anthony, 'Galen's criticism of Aristotle's conception theory', *Journal of the History of Biology* 10 (1977), 65–85.

Rawson, Beryl (ed.), *A Companion to Families in the Greek and Roman Worlds* (Chichester, 2011).

Reeve, M. D., 'Conceptions', *Proceedings of the Cambridge Philological Society* 35 (1989), 81–112.

Roth, Ann Macy, 'Father earth, mother sky: Ancient Egyptian beliefs about conception and fertility', in Alison E. Rautman (ed.), *Reading the Body: Representations and Remains in the Archaeological Record* (Philadelphia, PA, 2000), pp. 187–201.

Saller, Richard P., *Patriarchy, Property and Death in the Roman Family* (Cambridge, 1994).

Skinner, Marilyn, *Sexuality in Greek and Roman Culture* (Malden, MA, 2005).

Steinert, Ulrike, 'Concepts of the female body in Mesopotamian gynecological texts', in John Z. Wee (ed.), *The Comparable Body: Analogy and Metaphor in Mesopotamian, Egyptian, and Greco-Roman Medicine* (Leiden, 2017), pp. 275–357.

Stol, M., *Birth in Babylonia and the Bible: Its Mediterranean Setting* (Groningen, 2000).

Totelin, Laurence, *Hippocratic Recipes: Oral and Written Transmission of Pharmacological Knowledge in Fifth- and Fourth-Century Greece* (Leiden, 2009).

Wilberding, James, 'The revolutionary embryology of the Neoplatonists', *Oxford Studies in Ancient Philosophy* 49 (2015), 321–62.

Forms, Souls, and Embryos: Neoplatonists on Human Reproduction (London, 2017).

Medieval and Early Modern

Adelmann, Howard B., *Marcello Malpighi and the Evolution of Embryology*, 5 vols. (Ithaca, NY, 1966).

Astbury, Leah, 'Breeding women and lusty infants in early modern England', unpublished PhD thesis, University of Cambridge (2016).

Baernstein, P. Renée, and John Christopoulos, 'Interpreting the body in early modern Italy: Pregnancy, abortion and adulthood', *Past & Present* 223 (2014), 41–75.

Bednarski, Steven, and Andrée Courtemanche, '"Sadly and with a bitter heart": What the Caesarean section meant in the Middle Ages', *Florilegium* 28 (2011), 33–69.

Bell, Rudolph M., *How to Do It: Guides to Good Living for Renaissance Italians* (Chicago, IL, 1999).

Berriot-Salvadore, Evelyne, *Un corps, un destin: La femme dans la médecine de la Renaissance* (Paris, 1993).

Bertoloni Meli, Domenico, *Mechanism, Experiment, Disease: Marcello Malpighi and Seventeenth-Century Anatomy* (Baltimore, MD, 2011).

Biller, Peter, *The Measure of Multitude: Population in Medieval Thought*, rev. edn (Oxford, 2000).

Blum, Carol, *Strength in Numbers: Population, Reproduction, and Power in Eighteenth-Century France* (Baltimore, MD, 2002).

Blumenfeld-Kosinski, Renate, *Not of Woman Born: Representations of Caesarean Birth in Medieval and Renaissance Culture* (Ithaca, NY, 1990).

Broomhall, Susan, '"Women's little secrets": Defining the boundaries of reproductive knowledge in sixteenth-century France', *Social History of Medicine* 15 (2002), 1–15.

Brundage, James A., *Law, Sex, and Christian Society in Medieval Europe* (Chicago, IL, 1987).

Bummel, Julia, 'Human biological reproduction in the medicine of the Prophet: The question of the provenance and formation of the semen', in Peter E. Pormann (ed.), *Islamic Medical and Scientific Tradition*, vol. 2 (London, 2011), pp. 332–41.

Bynum, W. F., and Roy Porter (eds.), *William Hunter and the Eighteenth-Century Medical World* (Cambridge, 1985).

Cabré, Montserrat, 'Women or healers? Household practices and the categories of health care in late medieval Iberia', *Bulletin of the History of Medicine* 82 (2008), 18–51.

Cadden, Joan, *Meanings of Sex Difference in the Middle Ages: Medicine, Science, and Culture* (Cambridge, 1993).

Caiozzo, Anna, and Anne-Emmanuelle Demartini (eds.), *Monstre et imaginaire social: Approches historiques* (Paris, 2008).

Cavallar, Osvaldo, 'Septimo mense: Periti medici e partorienti in Baldo degli Ubaldi', in Carla Frova, Maria Grazia Nico Ottaviani and Stefania Zucchini (eds.), *VI centenario della morte di Baldo degli Ubaldi, 1400–2000* (Perugia, 2005), pp. 365–460.

Cavallo, Sandra, and Simona Cerutti, 'Female honor and the social control of reproduction in Piedmont between 1600 and 1800', in Edward Muir and Guido Ruggiero (eds.), *Sex and Gender in Historical Perspective*, trans. Margaret A. Gallucci (Baltimore, MD, 1990), pp. 73–109.

Cislo, Amy, *Paracelsus's Theory of Embodiment: Conception and Gestation in Early Modern Europe* (London, 2010).

Cobb, Matthew, *The Egg & Sperm Race: The Seventeenth-Century Scientists Who Unravelled the Secrets of Sex, Life and Growth* (London, 2007).

Cody, Lisa Forman, *Birthing the Nation: Sex, Science, and the Conception of Eighteenth-Century Britons* (Oxford, 2005).

Corbet, Patrick, *Autour de Burchard de Worms: L'Église allemande et les interdits de parenté, IXème–XIIème siècle* (Frankfurt am Main, 2001).

Crawford, Katherine, *European Sexualities, 1400–1800* (Cambridge, 2007).

Crawford, Patricia, *Blood, Bodies and Families in Early Modern England* (Harlow, 2004).

Cressy, David, *Birth, Marriage and Death: Ritual, Religion, and the Life-Cycle in Tudor and Stuart England* (Oxford, 1997).

Dabhoiwala, Faramerz, *The Origins of Sex: A History of the First Sexual Revolution* (London, 2012).

Dallal, Ahmad, 'Sexualities: Scientific discourses, premodern: Overview', in Suad Joseph (ed.), *Encyclopedia of Women and Islamic Cultures*, vol. 3: *Family, Body, Sexuality and Health* (Leiden, 2006), pp. 401–7.

Daston, Lorraine, and Katharine Park, *Wonders and the Order of Nature, 1150–1750* (New York, NY, 1998).

Delaporte, François, *Nature's Second Kingdom: Explorations of Vegetality in the Eighteenth Century*, trans. Arthur Goldhammer (Cambridge, MA, 1982).

De Renzi, Silvia, 'The risks of childbirth: Physicians, finance, and women's deaths in the law courts of seventeenth-century Rome', *Bulletin of the History of Medicine* 84 (2010), 549–77.

Desan, Suzanne, and Jeffrey W. Merrick (eds.), *Family, Gender and Law in Early Modern France* (University Park, PA, 2009).

Donahue, Charles, *Law, Marriage, and Society in the Later Middle Ages: Arguments about Marriage in Five Courts* (Cambridge, 2007).

Dorlin, Elsa, *La matrice de la race: Généalogie sexuelle et coloniale de la nation française* (Paris, 2006).

Duden, Barbara, *The Woman beneath the Skin: A Doctor's Patients in Eighteenth-Century Germany*, trans. Thomas Dunlap (Cambridge, MA, 1991).

Eccles, Audrey, *Obstetrics and Gynaecology in Tudor and Stuart England* (Kent, OH, 1982).

Ekholm, Karin, 'Fabricius's and Harvey's representations of animal generation', *Annals of Science* 67 (2010), 329–52.

Elliott, Dylan, *Spiritual Marriage: Sexual Abstinence in Medieval Wedlock* (Princeton, NJ, 1993).

Evans, Jennifer, *Aphrodisiacs, Fertility and Medicine in Early Modern England* (Woodbridge, 2014).

Evenden, Doreen, *The Midwives of Seventeenth-Century London* (Cambridge, 2000).

Fancy, Nahyan, *Science and Religion in Mamluk Egypt: Ibn al-Nafis, Pulmonary Transit and Bodily Resurrection* (London, 2013).

Ferraro, Joanne M., *Nefarious Crimes, Contested Justice: Illicit Sex and Infanticide in the Republic of Venice, 1557–1789* (Baltimore, MD, 2008).

Fildes, Valerie A., *Breasts, Bottles and Babies: A History of Infant Feeding* (Edinburgh, 1986).

(ed.), *Women as Mothers in Pre-industrial England: Essays in Memory of Dorothy McLaren* (London, 1990).

Fioravanti, Gianfranco, 'Un trattato medievale di eugenetica: Il *Libellus de ingenio bone nativitatis*', *Mediaevalia: Textos e estudos* 21 (2002), 89–111.

Fischer-Homberger, Esther, *Medizin vor Gericht. Gerichtsmedizin von der Renaissance bis zur Aufklärung* (Bern, 1983).

Fissell, Mary E., 'Hairy women and naked truths: Gender and the politics of knowledge in *Aristotle's Masterpiece*', *William and Mary Quarterly* 60 (2003), 43–74.

Vernacular Bodies: The Politics of Reproduction in Early Modern England (Oxford, 2004).

Flandrin, Jean-Louis, *L'Église et le contrôle des naissances* (Paris, 1970).

Furth, Charlotte, *A Flourishing Yin: Gender in China's Medical History, 960–1665* (Berkeley, CA, 1999).

Gelbart, Nina Rattner, *The King's Midwife: A History and Mystery of Madame du Coudray* (Berkeley, CA, 1998).

Gélis, Jacques, *History of Childbirth: Fertility, Pregnancy and Birth in Early Modern Europe*, trans. Rosemary Morris (Cambridge, 1991).

Giglioni, Guido, '"Conceptus uteri/conceptus cerebri": Note sull'analogia del concepimento nella teoria della generazione di William Harvey', *Rivista di storia della filosofia* 48 (1993), 7–22.

'Immaginazione, spiriti e generazione: La teoria del concepimento nella *Philosophia sensibus demonstrata* di Campanella', *Bruniana & Campanelliana* 4 (1998), 37–57.

Giladi, Avner, *Infants, Parents and Wet Nurses: Medieval Islamic Views on Breastfeeding and Their Social Implications* (Leiden, 1999).

Muslim Midwives: The Craft of Birthing in the Premodern Middle East (Cambridge, 2014).

Gowing, Laura, *Common Bodies: Women, Touch, and Power in Seventeenth-Century England* (New Haven, CT, 2003).

'Secret births and infanticide in seventeenth-century England', *Past & Present* (1997), 87–115.

Green, Monica H., *Women's Healthcare in the Medieval West: Texts and Contexts* (Aldershot, 2000).

'Gendering the history of women's healthcare', *Gender & History* 20 (2008), 487–518.

Making Women's Medicine Masculine: The Rise of Male Authority in Pre-Modern Gynaecology (Oxford, 2008).

Greenfield, Susan C., and Carol Barash (eds.), *Inventing Maternity: Politics, Science, and Literature, 1650–1865* (Lexington, KY, 1999).

Harrington, Joel F., *The Unwanted Child: The Fate of Foundlings, Orphans, and Juvenile Criminals in Early Modern Germany* (Chicago, IL, 2009).

Harvey, Karen, *Reading Sex in the Eighteenth Century: Bodies and Gender in English Erotic Culture* (Cambridge, 2004).

Hirai, Hiro, *Medical Humanism and Natural Philosophy: Renaissance Debates on Matter, Life and the Soul* (Leiden, 2011).

Hoffer, Peter C., and N. E. H. Hull, *Murdering Mothers: Infanticide in England and New England, 1558–1803* (New York, NY, 1981).

Ingram, Martin, *Carnal Knowledge: Regulating Sex in England, 1470–1600* (Cambridge, 2017).

Innes, Joanna, 'Power and happiness: Empirical social enquiry in Britain, from "political arithmetic" to "moral statistics"', in Innes, *Inferior Politics: Social Problems and Social Policies in Eighteenth-Century Britain* (Oxford, 2009), pp. 109–75.

Ivinski, Patricia R., Harry C. Payne, Kathryn Calley Galitz and Richard Rand, *Farewell to the Wet Nurse: Etienne Aubry and Images of Breast-Feeding in Eighteenth-Century France* (Williamstown, MA, 1998).

Jackson, Mark, *New-Born Child Murder: Women, Illegitimacy and the Courts in Eighteenth-Century England* (Manchester, 1996).

Katz, Marion Holmes, 'The problem of abortion in classical Sunni *fiqh*', in Jonathan E. Brockopp (ed.), *Islamic Ethics of Life: Abortion, War, and Euthanasia* (Columbia, SC, 2003), pp. 25–50.

Katzew, Ilona, *Casta Painting: Images of Race in Eighteenth-Century Mexico* (New Haven, CT, 2004).

Kessler, Gwynn, *Conceiving Israel: The Fetus in Rabbinic Narratives* (Philadelphia, PA, 2009).

Kinzelbach, Annemarie, 'Women and healthcare in early modern German towns', *Renaissance Studies* 28 (2014), 619–38.

Klapisch-Zuber, Christiane, *Women, Family, and Ritual in Renaissance Italy*, trans. Lydia Cochrane (Chicago, IL, 1985).

Kruse, Britta-Juliane, *Verborgene Heilkünste. Geschichte der Frauenmedizin im Spätmittelalter* (Berlin, 1996).

Kueny, Kathryn M., *Conceiving Identities: Maternity in Medieval Muslim Discourse and Practice* (Albany, NY, 2013).

Lewis, Margaret Brannan, *Infanticide and Abortion in Early Modern Germany* (London, 2016).

Lugt, Maaike van der, *Le ver, le démon et la vierge: Les théories médiévales de la génération extraordinaire, une étude sur les rapports entre théologie, philosophie naturelle et médecine* (Paris, 2004).

Lugt, Maaike van der, and Charles de Miramon (eds.), *L'hérédité entre Moyen Âge et Époque moderne: Perspectives historiques* (Florence, 2008).

McLaren, Angus, *Reproductive Rituals: The Perception of Fertility in England from the Sixteenth to the Eighteenth Century* (London, 1984).

Maclean, Ian, *The Renaissance Notion of Woman: A Study in the Fortunes of Scholasticism and Medical Science in European Intellectual Life* (Cambridge, 1980).

McClive, Cathy, *Menstruation and Procreation in Early Modern France* (Farnham, 2015).

McClive, Cathy, and Nicole Pellegrin (eds.), *Femmes en fleurs, femmes en corps: Sang, santé, sexualités, du Moyen Âge aux Lumières* (Saint-Étienne, 2010).

McCormick, Ted, *William Petty and the Ambitions of Political Arithmetic* (Oxford, 2009).

McTavish, Lianne, *Childbirth and the Display of Authority in Early Modern France* (Aldershot, 2005).

Marland, Hilary (ed.), *The Art of Midwifery: Early Modern Midwives in Europe* (London, 1993).

Martínez, María Elena, *Genealogical Fictions: Limpieza de Sangre, Religion, and Gender in Colonial Mexico* (Stanford, CA, 2008).

Martorelli Vico, Romana, *Medicina e filosofia: Per una storia dell'embriologia medievale nel XIII e XIV secolo* (Milan, 2002).

Mazzolini, Renato G., 'Albinos, Leucoæthiopes, Dondos, Kakerlakken: Sulla storia dell'albinismo dal 1609 al 1812', in Giuseppe Olmi and Giuseppe Papagno (eds.), *La natura e il corpo: Studi in memoria di Attilio Zanca* (Florence, 2006), pp. 161–204.

Mazzolini, Renato G., and Shirley A. Roe, *Science against the Unbelievers: The Correspondence of Bonnet and Needham, 1760–1780* (Oxford, 1986).

Miller, Naomi J., and Naomi Yavneh (eds.), *Maternal Measures: Figuring Caregiving in the Early Modern Period* (Aldershot, 2000).

Mistry, Zubin, *Abortion in the Early Middle Ages,* c. *500–900* (Woodbridge, 2015).

Monti, Maria Teresa, *Spallanzani e le rigenerazioni animali: L'inchiesta, la comunicazione, la rete* (Florence, 2005).

Müller, Wolfgang P., *The Criminalization of Abortion in the West: Its Origins in Medieval Law* (Ithaca, NY, 2012).

Musacchio, Jacqueline Marie, *The Art and Ritual of Childbirth in Renaissance Italy* (New Haven, CT, 1999).

Musallam, B. F., *Sex and Society in Islam: Birth Control before the Nineteenth Century* (Cambridge, 1983).

Nachtomy, Ohad, and Justin E. Smith (eds.), *The Life Sciences in Early Modern Philosophy* (Oxford, 2014), part 3.

Nelson, William Max, 'Making men: Enlightenment ideas of racial engineering', *American Historical Review* 115 (2010), 1364–94.

Oren-Magidor, Daphna, *Infertility in Early Modern England* (London, 2017).

Oren-Magidor, Daphna, and Catherine Rider (eds.), 'Infertility in medieval and early modern medicine', special issue, *Social History of Medicine* 29 (2016), 211–359.

Pancino, Claudia, *La natura dei bambini: Cura del corpo, malattie e medicina della prima infanzia fra Cinquecento e Settecento* (Bologna, 2015).

Park, Katharine, *Secrets of Women: Gender, Generation, and the Origins of Human Dissection* (New York, NY, 2006).

'Medicine and natural philosophy: Naturalistic traditions', in Judith M. Bennett and Ruth Mazo Karras (eds.), *The Oxford Handbook of Women and Gender in Medieval Europe* (Oxford, 2013), pp. 84–100.

Pinto-Correia, Clara, *The Ovary of Eve: Egg and Sperm and Preformation* (Chicago, IL, 2007).

Pomata, Gianna, 'Legami di sangue, legami di seme: Consanguineità e agnazione nel diritto Romano', *Quaderni Storici* 86 (1994), 299–334.

Ragab, Ahmed, 'One, two, or many sexes: Sex differentiation in medieval Islamicate medical thought', *Journal of the History of Sexuality* 24 (2015), 428–54.

Rawcliffe, Carole, 'Women, childbirth, and religion in later medieval England', in Diana Wood (ed.), *Women and Religion in Medieval England* (Oxford, 2003), pp. 91–117.

Read, Kirk D., *Birthing Bodies in Early Modern France: Stories of Gender and Reproduction* (Farnham, 2001).

Resnick, Irven, 'Conjoined twins, medieval biology, and evolving reflection on individual identity', *Viator* 44 (2013), 343–68.

Robilliard, Gabrielle, *Tending Mothers and the Fruits of the Womb: The Work of the Midwife in the Early Modern German City* (Stuttgart, 2017).

Roe, Shirley A., *Matter, Life, and Generation: Eighteenth-Century Embryology and the Haller–Wolff Debate* (Cambridge, 1981).

Roger, Jacques, *Les sciences de la vie dans la pensée française du XVIIIe siècle: La génération des animaux de Descartes à l'* Encyclopédie (Paris, 1963); *The Life Sciences in Eighteenth-Century French Thought*, ed. Keith R. Benson, trans. Robert Ellrich (Stanford, CA, 1997).

Rublack, Ulinka, 'Pregnancy, childbirth and the female body in early modern Germany', *Past & Present* 150 (1996), 84–110.

Rusnock, Andrea A., *Vital Accounts: Quantifying Health and Population in Eighteenth-Century England and France* (Cambridge, 2002).

Russell, Nicholas, *Like Engend'ring Like: Heredity and Animal Breeding in Early Modern England* (Cambridge, 1986).

Sánchez, Magdalena S., '"I would not feel the pain if I were with you": Catalina Micaela and the cycle of pregnancy at the court of Turin, 1585–1597', *Social History of Medicine* 28 (2015), 445–64.

Sayed Gadelrab, Sherry, 'Discourses on sex differences in medieval scholarly Islamic thought', *Journal of the History of Medicine and Allied Sciences* 66 (2011), 40–81.

Schäfer, Daniel, 'Embryulkie zwischen Mythos, Recht und Medizin. Zur Überlieferungsgeschichte von Sectio in mortua und Embryotomie in Spätantike und Mittelalter', *Medizinhistorisches Journal* 31 (1996), 275–97.

Schiebinger, Londa, *Nature's Body: Gender in the Making of Modern Science* (Boston, MA, 1993).

Schiebinger, Londa, and Claudia Swan (eds.), *Colonial Botany: Science, Commerce, and Politics in the Early Modern World* (Philadelphia, PA, 2005).

Schlumbohm, Jürgen, *Lebendige Phantome. Ein Entbindungshospital und seine Patientinnen 1751–1830* (Göttingen, 2012).

Schmitt, Stéphane, 'Introduction à l'*Histoire générale des Animaux*', in Georges-Louis Leclerc de Buffon, *Œuvres complètes*, vol. 2: *Histoire naturelle, générale et particulière, avec la description du Cabinet du Roy* (1749), ed. Schmitt (Paris, 2008), pp. 9–58.

Schmugge, Ludwig, *Marriage on Trial: Late Medieval German Couples at the Papal Court*, trans. Atria A. Larson (Washington, DC, 2012).

Shackelford, Jole, 'Seeds with a mechanical purpose: Severinus' *semina* and seventeenth-century matter theory', in Allen G. Debus and Michael T. Walton (eds.), *Reading the Book of Nature: The Other Side of the Scientific Revolution* (Kirksville, MO, 1998), pp. 15–44.

Siena, Kevin P., *Venereal Disease, Hospitals and the Urban Poor: London's 'Foul Wards', 1600–1800* (Rochester, NY, 2004).

Simons, Patricia, *The Sex of Men in Premodern Europe: A Cultural History* (Cambridge, 2011).

Smith, Justin E. H. (ed.), *The Problem of Generation in Early Modern Philosophy* (Cambridge, 2006).

Spinks, Jennifer, *Monstrous Births and Visual Culture in Sixteenth-Century Germany* (London, 2009).

Stephanson, Raymond, and Darren N. Wagner (eds.), *The Secrets of Generation: Reproduction in the Long Eighteenth Century* (Toronto, 2015).

Stolberg, Michael, 'A woman's hell? Medical perceptions of menopause in preindustrial Europe', *Bulletin of the History of Medicine* 73 (1999), 404–28.

'The monthly malady: A history of premenstrual suffering', *Medical History* 44 (2000), 300–22.

Taglia, Kathryn, 'Delivering a Christian identity: Midwives in northern French synodal legislation, *c.* 1200–1500', in Peter Biller and Joseph Ziegler (eds.), *Religion and Medicine in the Middle Ages* (Woodbridge, 2001), pp. 77–90.

Terrall, Mary, 'Salon, academy, and boudoir: Generation and desire in Maupertuis's science of life', *Isis* 87 (1996), 217–29.

Terrall, Mary, *The Man Who Flattened the Earth: Maupertuis and the Sciences in the Enlightenment* (Chicago, IL, 2002).

Catching Nature in the Act: Réaumur and the Practice of Natural History in the Eighteenth Century (Chicago, IL, 2014).

Tu ttle, Leslie, *Conceiving the Old Regime: Pronatalism and the Politics of Reproduction in Early Modern France* (Oxford, 2010).

Ulrich, Laurel Thatcher, *A Midwife's Tale: The Life of Martha Ballard, Based on Her Diary, 1785–1812* (New York, NY, 1991).

Vann Sprecher, Tiffany D., and Ruth Mazo Karras, 'The midwife and the church: Ecclesiastical regulation of midwives in Brie, 1499–1504', *Bulletin of the History of Medicine* 85 (2011), 171–92.

Wilson, Adrian, *The Making of Man-Midwifery: Childbirth in England, 1660–1770* (Cambridge, MA, 1995).

Ritual and Conflict: The Social Relations of Childbirth in Early Modern England (Aldershot, 2013).

Worth-Stylianou, Valerie (ed.), *Pregnancy and Birth in Early Modern France: Treatises by Caring Physicians and Surgeons (1581–1625)* (Toronto, 2013).

Ze'evi, Dror, *Producing Desire: Changing Sexual Discourse in the Ottoman Middle East, 1500–1900* (Berkeley, CA, 2006).

Modern

Abugideiri, Hibba, *Gender and the Making of Modern Medicine in Colonial Egypt* (Farnham, 2010).

Ahluwalia, Sanjam, *Reproductive Restraints: Birth Control in India, 1877–1947* (Urbana, IL, 2008).

Al-Gailani, Salim, 'Teratology and the clinic: Monsters, obstetrics and the making of antenatal life in Edinburgh, *c.* 1900', unpublished PhD thesis, University of Cambridge (2010).

Al-Gailani, Salim, and Angela Davis (eds.), 'Transforming pregnancy since 1900', special issue, *Studies in History and Philosophy of Biological and Biomedical Sciences* 47, part B (2014), 229–310.

Allen, Ann Taylor, *Feminism and Motherhood in Western Europe, 1890–1970: The Maternal Dilemma* (Basingstoke, 2005).

Apple, Rima D., *Perfect Motherhood: Science and Childrearing in America* (New Brunswick, NJ, 2006).

Arney, William Ray, *Power and the Profession of Obstetrics* (Chicago, IL, 1982).

Baker, Jeffrey P., *The Machine in the Nursery: Incubator Technology and the Origins of Newborn Intensive Care* (Baltimore, MD, 1996).

Balsoy, Gülhan, *The Politics of Reproduction in Ottoman Society, 1838–1900* (London, 2013).

Banchoff, Thomas, *Embryo Politics: Ethics and Policy in Atlantic Democracies* (Ithaca, NY, 2011).

Bänziger, Peter-Paul, Stefanie Duttweiler, Philipp Sarasin and Annika Wellmann (eds.), *Fragen Sie Dr Sex! Ratgeberkommunikation und die mediale Konstruktion des Sexuellen* (Berlin, 2010).

Bard, Christine, and Janine Mossuz-Lavau, *Le planning familial: Histoire et mémoire, 1956–2006* (Rennes, 2007).

Bashford, Alison, *Global Population: History, Geopolitics, and Life on Earth* (New York, NY, 2014).

Bashford, Alison, and Joyce E. Chaplin, *The New Worlds of Thomas Robert Malthus: Rereading the* Principle of Population (Princeton, NJ, 2016).

Bashford, Alison, and Philippa Levine (eds.), *The Oxford Handbook of the History of Eugenics* (Oxford, 2010).

Baynton, Douglas C., *Defectives in the Land: Disability and Immigration in the Age of Eugenics* (Chicago, IL, 2016).

Beisel, Nicola, *Imperiled Innocents: Anthony Comstock and Family Reproduction in Victorian America* (Princeton, NJ, 1997).

Benn, J. Miriam, *The Predicaments of Love* (London, 1992).

Benninghaus, Christina, 'Beyond constructivism? Gender, medicine and the early history of sperm analysis, Germany 1870–1900', *Gender & History* 24 (2012), 647–76.

Betta, Emmanuel, *Animare la vita: Disciplina della nascita tra medicina e morale nell'Ottocento* (Bologna, 2006).

L'altra genesi: Storia della fecondazione artificiale (Rome, 2012).

Betteridge, Keith J., 'A history of farm animal embryo transfer and some associated techniques', *Animal Reproduction Science* 79 (2003), 203–44.

Bland, Lucy, *Banishing the Beast: English Feminism and Sexual Morality, 1870–1914* (Harmondsworth, 1995).

Bledsoe, Caroline H., *Contingent Lives: Fertility, Time, and Aging in West Africa* (Chicago, IL, 2002).

Bock, Gisela, *Zwangssterilisation im Nationalsozialismus. Studien zur Rassenpolitik und Frauenpolitik* (Opladen, 1986).

Bock, Gisela, and Pat Thane (eds.), *Maternity and Gender Policies: Women and the Rise of the European Welfare States, 1880s–1950s* (New York, NY, 1991).

Bongaarts, John, and Robert G. Potter, *Fertility, Biology, and Behavior: An Analysis of the Proximate Determinants* (New York, NY, 1983).

Bourbonnais, Nicole C., *Birth Control in the Decolonizing Caribbean: Reproductive Politics and Practice on Four Islands, 1930–1970* (New York, NY, 2016).

Brandt, Allan M., *No Magic Bullet: A Social History of Venereal Disease in the United States since 1880*, expanded edn (Oxford, 1987).

Brandt, Christina, Bettina Bock von Wülfingen, Susanne Lettow and Florence Vienne (eds.), 'Temporalities of reproduction', special issue, *History and Philosophy of the Life Sciences* 37 (2015), 1–120.

Briggs, Laura, *Reproducing Empire: Race, Sex, Science, and US Imperialism in Puerto Rico* (Berkeley, CA, 2002).

Somebody's Children: The Politics of Transracial and Transnational Adoption (Durham, NC, 2012).

How All Politics Became Reproductive Politics: From Welfare Reform to Foreclosure to Trump (Berkeley, CA, 2017).

Brodie, Janet Farrell, *Contraception and Abortion in Nineteenth-Century America* (Ithaca, NY, 1994).

Brookes, Barbara, *Abortion in England, 1900–1967* (London, 1988).

Buklijas, Tatjana, and Nick Hopwood, *Making Visible Embryos*, an online exhibition, www.hps.cam.ac.uk/visibleembryos/ (2008–10).

Bullough, Vern L., *Science in the Bedroom: A History of Sex Research* (New York, NY, 1994).

Buske, Sybille, *Fräulein Mutter und ihr Bastard. Eine Geschichte der Unehelichkeit in Deutschland 1900–1970* (Göttingen, 2004).

Casella, Laura (ed.), 'Generazioni familiari, generazioni politiche (XVIII–XX secc.)', special issue, *Cheiron*, no. 49 (2008 [2010]).

Casper, Monica, *The Making of the Unborn Patient: A Social Anatomy of Fetal Surgery* (New Brunswick, NJ, 1998).

Clarke, Adele E., *Disciplining Reproduction: Modernity, American Life Sciences, and 'the Problems of Sex'* (Berkeley, CA, 1998).

Cohen, Deborah, *Family Secrets: Living with Shame from the Victorians to the Present Day* (London, 2013).

Cole, Joshua, *The Power of Large Numbers: Population, Politics, and Gender in Nineteenth-Century France* (Ithaca, NY, 2000).

Comfort, Nathaniel, *The Science of Human Perfection: How Genes Became the Heart of American Medicine* (New Haven, CT, 2012).

Connelly, Matthew, *Fatal Misconception: The Struggle to Control World Population* (Cambridge, MA, 2008).

Cook, Hera, *The Long Sexual Revolution: English Women, Sex, and Contraception, 1800–1975* (Oxford, 2004).

Cooper, Melinda, and Catherine Waldby, *Clinical Labor: Tissue Donors and Research Subjects in the Global Bioeconomy* (Durham, NC, 2014).

Cooter, Roger (ed.), *In the Name of the Child: Health and Welfare, 1880–1940* (London, 1992).

Corbin, Alain, *Women for Hire: Prostitution and Sexuality in France after 1850*, trans. Alan Sheridan (Cambridge, MA, 1990).

Corea, Gena, *The Mother Machine: Reproductive Technologies from Artificial Insemination to Artificial Wombs* (London, 1985).

Cowan, Ruth Schwartz, *Heredity and Hope: The Case for Genetic Screening* (Cambridge, MA, 2008).

Critchlow, Donald T., *Intended Consequences: Birth Control, Abortion, and the Federal Government in Modern America* (New York, NY, 1999).

Daniels, Cynthia R., *Exposing Men: The Science and Politics of Male Reproduction* (Oxford, 2006).

Das Gupta, Monica, 'Kinship systems and demographic regimes', in David I. Kertzer and Tom Fricke (eds.), *Anthropological Demography: Toward a New Synthesis* (Chicago, IL, 1997), pp. 36–52.

David, Henry P. (ed.), *From Abortion to Contraception: A Resource to Public Policies and Reproductive Behavior in Central and Eastern Europe from 1917 to the Present* (Westport, CT, 1999).

Davidson, Roger, *Dangerous Liaisons: A Social History of Venereal Disease in Twentieth-Century Scotland* (Amsterdam, 2000).

Davidson, Roger, and Gayle Davis, *The Sexual State: Sexuality and Scottish Governance, 1950–80* (Edinburgh, 2012).

Davin, Anna, 'Imperialism and motherhood', *History Workshop* 5 (1978), 9–65.

Davis, Angela, *Modern Motherhood: Women and Family in England,* c. *1945–2000* (Manchester, 2012).

Davis, Gayle, *'The Cruel Madness of Love': Sex, Syphilis and Psychiatry in Scotland, 1880–1930* (Amsterdam, 2008).

Davis, Kathy, *The Making of* Our Bodies, Ourselves: *How Feminism Travels across Borders* (Durham, NC, 2007).

Dawson, Gowan, *Darwin, Literature and Victorian Respectability* (Cambridge, 2007).

De Barros, Juanita, *Reproducing the British Caribbean: Sex, Gender, and Population Politics after Slavery* (Chapel Hill, NC, 2014).

De Luca Barrusse, Virginie, *Les familles nombreuses: Une question démographique, un enjeu politique, France (1880–1940)* (Rennes, 2008).

Demel, Walter, 'Wie die Chinesen gelb wurden. Ein Beitrag zur Frühgeschichte der Rassentheorien', *Historische Zeitschrift* 255 (1992), 625–66.

Demirci, Tuba, and Selçuk Akşin Somel, 'Women's bodies, demography, and public health: Abortion policy and perspectives in the Ottoman Empire of the nineteenth century', *Journal of the History of Sexuality* 17 (2008), 377–420.

Desmond, Adrian, *The Politics of Evolution: Morphology, Medicine, and Reform in Radical London* (Chicago, IL, 1989).

Dienel, Christiane, *Kinderzahl und Staatsräson. Empfängnisverhütung und Bevölkerungspolitik in Deutschland und Frankreich bis 1918* (Münster, 1995).

Dittrick Medical History Center, *History of Birth Control*, an online exhibition, http://artsci.case.edu/dittrick/online-exhibits/history-of-birth-control/, last accessed 8 June 2017.

Domingo, Andreu, '"Demodystopias": Prospects of demographic hell', *Population and Development Review* 34 (2008), 725–45.

Dowbiggin, Ian, *The Sterilization Movement and Global Fertility in the Twentieth Century* (Oxford, 2008).

Doyle, Shane, *Before HIV: Sexuality, Fertility and Mortality in East Africa, 1900–1980* (Oxford, 2013).

Drayton, Richard, *Nature's Government: Science, Imperial Britain, and the 'Improvement' of the World* (New Haven, CT, 2000).

Drixler, Fabian, *Mabiki: Infanticide and Population Growth in Eastern Japan, 1660–1950* (Berkeley, CA, 2013).

Dubow, Sara, *Ourselves Unborn: A History of the Fetus in Modern America* (New York, NY, 2011).

Duden, Barbara, *Disembodying Women: Perspectives on Pregnancy and the Unborn*, trans. Lee Hoinacki (Cambridge, MA, 1993).

Edwards, Robert, and Patrick Steptoe, *A Matter of Life: The Story of a Medical Breakthrough* (London, 1980).

Elder, K., and M. H. Johnson, 'Symposium: The history of the first IVF births', *Reproductive BioMedicine and Society Online* 1 (2015), 1–70.

Engelman, Peter C., *A History of the Birth Control Movement in America* (Santa Barbara, CA, 2011).

Farley, John, *Gametes & Spores: Ideas about Sexual Reproduction, 1750–1914* (Baltimore, MD, 1982).

Fildes, Valerie, Lara Marks and Hilary Marland (eds.), *Women and Children First: International Maternal and Infant Welfare, 1870–1945* (London, 1992).

Filippini, Nadia Maria, *La nascita straordinaria: Tra madre e figlio, la rivoluzione del taglio cesareo (sec. XVIII – XIX)* (Milan, 1995).

Fisher, Kate, *Birth Control, Sex and Marriage in Britain, 1918–1960* (Oxford, 2006).

Fitzgerald, Deborah, *The Business of Breeding: Hybrid Corn in Illinois, 1890–1940* (Ithaca, NY, 1990).

Foucault, Michel, *The History of Sexuality*, vol. 1: *An Introduction*, trans. Robert Hurley (New York, NY, 1978).

Security, Territory, Population: Lectures at the Collège de France, 1977–1978, ed. Michel Senellart, trans. Graham Burchell (New York, NY, 2007).

Franklin, Sarah, *Dolly Mixtures: The Remaking of Genealogy* (Durham, NC, 2007).

Franklin, Sarah, and Marcia C. Inhorn (eds.), 'Symposium, IVF: Global histories', *Reproductive BioMedicine and Society Online* 2 (2016), 1–136.

Fryer, Peter, *The Birth Controllers* (London, 1965).

Gaudillière, Jean-Paul, 'Better prepared than synthesized: Adolf Butenandt, Schering AG and the transformation of the sex steroids into drugs (1930–1946)', *Studies in History and Philosophy of Biological and Biomedical Sciences* 36 (2005), 612–44.

'DES, cancer and endocrine perturbation: Ways of regulating, chemical risks and public expertise in the United States', in Soraya Boudia and Nathalie Jas (eds.), *Powerless Science? Science and Politics in a Toxic World* (New York, NY, 2014), pp. 65–94.

Gausemeier, Bernd, Staffan Müller-Wille and Edmund Ramsden (eds.), *Human Heredity in the Twentieth Century* (London, 2013).

Glass, D. V., and D. E. C. Eversley (eds.), *Population in History: Essays in Historical Demography* (London, 1965).

Gluckman, P. D., M. A. Hanson and T. Buklijas, 'A conceptual framework for the developmental origins of health and disease', *Journal of Developmental Origins of Health and Disease* 1 (2010), 6–18.

Golden, Janet, *A Social History of Wet Nursing in America: From Breast to Bottle* (Cambridge, 1996).

Message in a Bottle: The Making of Fetal Alcohol Syndrome (Cambridge, MA, 2006).

Goldman, Wendy Z., *Women, the State and Revolution: Soviet Family Policy and Social Life, 1917–1936* (New York, NY, 1994).

Gordon, Linda, *The Moral Property of Women: A History of Birth Control Politics in America* (Urbana, IL, 2007).

Pitied but not Entitled: Single Mothers and the History of Welfare (New York, NY, 1994).

Gorney, Cynthia, *Articles of Faith: A Frontline History of the Abortion Wars* (New York, NY, 1998).

Greenhalgh, Susan, *Just One Child: Science and Policy in Deng's China* (Berkeley, CA, 2008).

Greenhouse, Linda, and Reva Siegel (eds.), *Before* Roe v. Wade*: Voices that Shaped the Abortion Debate before the Supreme Court's Ruling* (New York, NY, 2010).

Greenlees, Janet, and Linda Bryder (eds.), *Western Maternity and Medicine, 1880–1990* (London, 2013).

Grossmann, Atina, *Reforming Sex: The German Movement for Birth Control and Abortion Reform, 1920–1950* (New York, NY, 1995).

Hagner, Michael, 'Enlightened monsters', in William Clark, Jan Golinski and Simon Schaffer (eds.), *The Sciences in Enlightened Europe* (Chicago, IL, 1999), pp. 175–217.

Hall, Lesley A., *Sex, Gender and Social Change in Britain since 1880*, 2nd edn (Basingstoke, 2013).

Literary Abortion, www.lesleyahall.net/abortion.htm, last accessed 9 June 2017.

Hall, Stephen J. G., and Juliet Clutton-Brock, *Two Hundred Years of British Farm Livestock* (London, 1989).

Hanson, Clare, *A Cultural History of Pregnancy: Pregnancy, Medicine and Culture, 1750–2000* (Basingstoke, 2004).

Haran, Joan, Jenny Kitzinger, Maureen McNeil and Kate O'Riordan, *Human Cloning in the Media: From Science Fiction to Science Practice* (London, 2008).

Harper, Peter S., *First Years of Human Chromosomes: The Beginnings of Human Cytogenetics* (Bloxham, 2006).

Harris, Lisa Hope, 'Challenging conception: A clinical and cultural history of in vitro fertilization in the United States', unpublished PhD dissertation, University of Michigan (2006).

Hartmann, Betsy, *Reproductive Rights and Wrongs: The Global Politics of Population Control*, rev. edn (Boston, MA, 1995).

Hartmann, Heinrich, and Corinna R. Unger (eds.), *World of Populations: Transnational Perspectives on Demography in the Twentieth Century* (New York, NY, 2014).

Harwood, Jonathan, *Europe's Green Revolution and Others Since: The Rise and Fall of Peasant-Friendly Plant Breeding* (London, 2012).

Haugeberg, Karissa, *Women against Abortion: Inside the Largest Moral Reform Movement of the Twentieth Century* (Urbana, IL, 2017).

Healey, Jenna, 'Rejecting reproduction: The National Organization for Non-Parents and child-free activism in 1970s America', *Journal of Women's History* 28, no. 1 (2016), 131–56.

Henig, Robin Marantz, *Pandora's Baby: How the First Test Tube Babies Sparked the Reproductive Revolution* (Boston, MA, 2004).

Herman, Ellen, *Kinship by Design: A History of Adoption in the Modern United States* (Chicago, IL, 2008).

The Adoption History Project, http://darkwing.uoregon.edu/~adoption/index.html, last accessed 8 June 2017.

Herzog, Dagmar, *Sexuality in Europe: A Twentieth-Century History* (Cambridge, 2011).

Hoberman, John, *Testosterone Dreams: Rejuvenation, Aphrodisia, Doping* (Berkeley, CA, 2005).

Hodges, Sarah, *Contraception, Colonialism and Commerce: Birth Control in South India, 1920–1940* (Aldershot, 2008).

(ed.), *Reproductive Health in India: History, Politics, Controversies* (New Delhi, 2006).

Hoff, Derek S., *The State and the Stork: The Population Debate and Policy Making in US History* (Chicago, IL, 2012).

Hogan, Andrew J., *Life Histories of Genetic Disease: Patterns and Prevention in Postwar Medical Genetics* (Baltimore, MD, 2016).

Hollen, Cecilia Van, *Birth on the Threshold: Childbirth and Modernity in South India* (Berkeley, CA, 2003).

Honegger, Claudia, *Die Ordnung der Geschlechter. Die Wissenschaften vom Menschen und das Weib 1750–1850* (Frankfurt am Main, 1991).

Hopwood, Nick, *Embryos in Wax: Models from the Ziegler Studio* (Cambridge, 2002).

Haeckel's Embryos: Images, Evolution, and Fraud (Chicago, IL, 2015).

Horowitz, Helen Lefkowitz, *Rereading Sex: Battles over Sexual Knowledge and Suppression in Nineteenth-Century America* (New York, NY, 2002).

Houlbrook, Matt, and Harry Cocks (eds.), *The Modern History of Sexuality* (Basingstoke, 2006).
Hull, Isabel V., *Sexuality, State, and Civil Society in Germany, 1700–1815* (Ithaca, NY, 1996).
Hunt, Nancy Rose, *A Colonial Lexicon: Of Birth Ritual, Medicalization, and Mobility in the Congo* (Durham, NC, 1999).
A Nervous State: Violence, Remedies, and Reverie in Colonial Congo (Durham, NC, 2016).
Hurlbut, J. Benjamin, *Human Embryo Research and the Politics of Bioethics* (New York, NY, 2017).
International Institute of Social History, *Neo-Malthusianism: Birth Control in the Netherlands* and *Le Néo-malthusianisme en France*, online exhibitions, www.iisg.nl/exhibitions/neomalthusianism/, last accessed 8 June 2017.
Jablonski, Nina G., *Living Color: The Biological and Social Meaning of Skin Color* (Berkeley, CA, 2012).
Jacob, François, *The Logic of Life: A History of Heredity*, trans. Betty E. Spillmann (New York, NY, 1973).
Jaffary, Nora E., *Reproduction and Its Discontents in Mexico: Childbirth and Contraception from 1750 to 1905* (Chapel Hill, NC, 2016).
Jensen, Robin E., *Dirty Words: The Rhetoric of Public Sex Education, 1870–1924* (Urbana, IL, 2010).
Johnson, Tina Phillips, *Childbirth in Republican China: Delivering Modernity* (Lanham, MD, 2011).
Jordanova, Ludmilla, 'Interrogating the concept of reproduction in the eighteenth century', in Faye D. Ginsburg and Rayna Rapp (eds.), *Conceiving the New World Order: The Global Politics of Reproduction* (Berkeley, CA, 1995), pp. 369–86.
Kaler, Amy, *Running after Pills: Politics, Gender, and Contraception in Colonial Zimbabwe* (Portsmouth, 2003).
Kent, Susan Kingsley, *Sex and Suffrage in Britain, 1860–1914* (London, 1990).
Keown, John, *Abortion, Doctors and the Law: Some Aspects of the Legal Regulation of Abortion in England from 1803 to 1982* (Cambridge, 1988).
Kertzer, David I., *Sacrificed for Honor: Italian Infant Abandonment and the Politics of Reproductive Control* (Boston, MA, 1993).
Kevles, Daniel J., *In the Name of Eugenics: Genetics and the Uses of Human Heredity* (New York, NY, 1985).
King, Laura, *Family Men: Fatherhood and Masculinity in Britain, c. 1914–1960* (Oxford, 2015).
Klausen, Susanne M., *Race, Maternity, and the Politics of Birth Control in South Africa, 1910–39* (Basingstoke, 2004).
Abortion under Apartheid: Nationalism, Sexuality, and Women's Reproductive Rights in South Africa (New York, NY, 2015).
Klein, Marian van der, Rebecca Jo Plant, Nichole Sanders and Lori R. Weintrob (eds.), *Maternalism Reconsidered: Motherhood, Welfare and Social Policy in the Twentieth Century* (New York, NY, 2012).
Klepp, Susan E., *Revolutionary Conceptions: Women, Fertility, and Family Limitation in America, 1760–1820* (Chapel Hill, NC, 2009).
Kline, Wendy, *Bodies of Knowledge: Sexuality, Reproduction, and Women's Health in the Second Wave* (Chicago, IL, 2010).
Kloppenburg, Jack Ralph, Jr, *First the Seed: The Political Economy of Plant Biotechnology*, 2nd edn (Madison, WI, 2005).

Kluchin, Rebecca M., *Fit to Be Tied: Sterilization and Reproductive Rights in America, 1950–1980* (New Brunswick, NJ, 2009).

König, Malte, 'Geburtenkontrolle. Abtreibung und Empfängnisverhütung in Frankreich und Deutschland, 1870–1940', *Francia* 38 (2011), 127–48.

Koerner, Lisbet, *Linnaeus: Nature and Nation* (Cambridge, MA, 1999).

Koven, Seth, and Sonya Michel (eds.), *Mothers of a New World: Maternalist Politics and the Origins of Welfare States* (New York, NY, 1993).

Krassnitzer, Patrick, and Petra Overath (eds.), *Bevölkerungsfragen. Prozesse des Wissenstransfers in Deutschland und Frankreich (1870–1939)* (Cologne, 2007).

Kuhn, Walther, and Ulrich Tröhler (eds.), *Armamentarium obstetricum Gottingense. Eine historische Sammlung zur Geburtsmedizin* (Göttingen, 1987).

Kuxhausen, Anna, *From the Womb to the Body Politic: Raising the Nation in Enlightenment Russia* (Madison, WI, 2013).

Lal, Maneesha, 'The politics of gender and medicine in colonial India: The Countess of Dufferin's Fund, 1885–1888', *Bulletin of the History of Medicine* 68 (1994), 29–66.

Langston, Nancy, *Toxic Bodies: Hormone Disruptors and the Legacy of DES* (New Haven, CT, 2010).

Latham, Melanie, *Regulating Reproduction: A Century of Conflict in Britain and France* (Manchester, 2002).

Layne, Linda L., *Motherhood Lost: A Feminist Account of Pregnancy Loss in America* (New York, NY, 2003).

Leathard, Audrey, *The Fight for Family Planning: The Development of Family Planning Services in Britain, 1921–1974* (London, 1980).

Leavitt, Judith Walzer, *Brought to Bed: Childbearing in America, 1750 to 1950* (New York, NY, 1986).

Make Room for Daddy: The Journey from Waiting Room to Birthing Room (Chapel Hill, NC, 2009).

Leavitt, Sarah A., '"A private little revolution": The home pregnancy test in American culture', *Bulletin of the History of Medicine* 80 (2006), 317–45.

Leavitt, Sarah A., *et al.*, *The Thin Blue Line: The History of the Pregnancy Test Kit*, an online exhibition, https://history.nih.gov/exhibits/thinblueline/ (2003).

Ledbetter, Rosanna, *A History of the Malthusian League, 1877–1927* (Columbus, OH, 1976).

Lee, James Z., and Wang Feng, *One Quarter of Humanity: Malthusian Mythology and Chinese Realities* (Cambridge, MA, 2001).

Lemke, Thomas, *Biopolitics: An Advanced Introduction*, trans. Eric Frederick Trump (New York, NY, 2011).

Le Naour, Jean-Yves, and Catherine Valenti, *Histoire de l'avortement (XIXe–XXe siècle)* (Paris, 2003).

Leon, Sharon M., *An Image of God: The Catholic Struggle with Eugenics* (Chicago, IL, 2013).

Leridon, Henri, Y. Charbit, P. Collomb, J. P. Sardon and L. Toulemon (eds.), *La seconde révolution contraceptive: La régulation des naissances en France de 1950 à 1985* (Paris, 1985).

Lettow, Susanne (ed.), *Reproduction, Race, and Gender in Philosophy and the Early Life Sciences* (Albany, NY, 2014).

Lewis, Jane, *The Politics of Motherhood: Child and Maternal Welfare in England, 1900–1939* (London, 1980).

Lewis, Milton, *Thorns on the Rose: The History of Sexually Transmitted Diseases in Australia in International Perspective* (Canberra, 1998).

Lewis, Milton, Scott Bamber and Michael Waugh (eds.), *Sex, Disease and Society: A Comparative History of Sexually Transmitted Diseases and HIV/AIDS in Asia and the Pacific* (London, 1997).

Lindee, Susan, *Moments of Truth in Genetic Medicine* (Baltimore, MD, 2005).

López, Raúl Necochea, *A History of Family Planning in Twentieth-Century Peru* (Chapel Hill, NC, 2014).

Lord, Alexandra M., *Condom Nation: The U.S. Government's Sex Education Campaign from World War I to the Internet* (Baltimore, MD, 2010).

Loudon, Irvine, *Death in Childbirth: An International Study of Maternal Care and Maternal Mortality, 1800–1950* (Oxford, 1992).

Mackensen, Rainer, Jürgen Reulecke and Josef Ehmer (eds.), *Ursprünge, Arten und Folgen des Konstrukts 'Bevölkerung' vor, im und nach dem 'Dritten Reich'. Zur Geschichte der deutschen Bevölkerungswissenschaft* (Wiesbaden, 2009).

Maienschein, Jane, *Embryos under the Microscope: The Diverging Meanings of Life* (Cambridge, MA, 2014).

Maienschein, Jane, Marie Glitz and Garland E. Allen (eds.), *Centennial History of the Carnegie Institution of Washington*, vol. 5: *The Department of Embryology* (Cambridge, 2004).

Maines, Rachel P., *The Technology of Orgasm: 'Hysteria', the Vibrator, and Women's Sexual Satisfaction* (Baltimore, MD, 1999).

Marks, Lara, *Sexual Chemistry: A History of the Contraceptive Pill* (New Haven, CT, 2001).

Marland, Hilary, *Dangerous Motherhood: Insanity and Childbirth in Victorian Britain* (Basingstoke, 2004).

Marland, Hilary, and Anne Marie Rafferty (eds.), *Midwives, Society, and Childbirth: Debates and Controversies in the Modern Period* (London, 1997).

Marsh, Margaret, and Wanda Ronner, *The Empty Cradle: Infertility in America from Colonial Times to the Present* (Baltimore, MD, 1996).

Martucci, Jessica, *Back to the Breast: Natural Motherhood and Breastfeeding in America* (Chicago, IL, 2015).

Matthews, Sandra, and Laura Wexler, *Pregnant Pictures* (New York, NY, 2000).

May, Elaine Tyler, *Barren in the Promised Land: Childless Americans and the Pursuit of Happiness* (New York, NY, 1995).

May, John F., *World Population Policies: Their Origin, Evolution, and Impact* (Dordrecht, 2012).

Mayhew, Robert J., *Malthus: The Life and Legacies of an Untimely Prophet* (Cambridge, MA, 2014).

Mazumdar, Pauline M. H., *Eugenics, Human Genetics and Human Failings: The Eugenics Society, Its Sources and Its Critics in Britain* (London, 1992).

McDonagh, Josephine, *Child Murder and British Culture, 1720–1900* (Cambridge, 2003).

McEwen, Britta, *Sexual Knowledge: Feeling, Fact, and Social Reform in Vienna, 1900–1934* (New York, NY, 2012).

McFalls, Jr, Joseph A., and Marguerite Harvey McFalls, *Disease and Fertility* (Orlando, FL, 1984).

McIntosh, Tania, *A Social History of Maternity and Childbirth: Key Themes in Maternity Care* (London, 2012).

McKeon, Michael (ed.), 'Sex: A thematic issue', *Signs* 37, no. 4 (2012).

McLaren, Angus, *Sexuality and Social Order: The Debate over the Fertility of Women and Workers in France, 1770–1920* (New York, NY, 1983).

Reproduction by Design: Sex, Robots, Trees, and Test-Tube Babies in Interwar Britain (Chicago, IL, 2012).

Meloni, Maurizio, *Political Biology: Science and Social Values in Human Heredity from Eugenics to Epigenetics* (Basingstoke, 2016).

Meyerowitz, Joanne, *How Sex Changed: A History of Transsexuality in the United States* (Cambridge, MA, 2002).

Michaels, Paula A., *Lamaze: An International History* (Oxford, 2014).

Moeller, Robert G., *Protecting Motherhood: Women and the Family in the Politics of Postwar West Germany* (Berkeley, CA, 1993).

Mohr, James C., *Abortion in America: The Origins and Evolution of National Policy* (New York, NY, 1978).

Moore, James, *Good Breeding: Science and Society in a Darwinian Age* (Milton Keynes, 2001).

Morgan, Jennifer L., *Laboring Women: Reproduction and Gender in New World Slavery* (Philadelphia, PA, 2004).

Morgan, Lynn M., *Icons of Life: A Cultural History of Human Embryos* (Berkeley, CA, 2009).

Morgan, Lynn M., and Meredith W. Michaels (eds.), *Fetal Subjects, Feminist Positions* (Philadelphia, PA, 1999).

Morgen, Sandra, *Into Our Own Hands: The Women's Health Movement in the United States, 1969–1990* (New Brunswick, NJ, 2002).

Moscucci, Ornella, *The Science of Woman: Gynaecology and Gender in England, 1800–1929* (Cambridge, 1990).

Mulkay, Michael, *The Embryo Research Debate: Science and the Politics of Reproduction* (Cambridge, 1997).

Muri, Allison, 'Imagining reproduction: The politics of reproduction, technology and the woman machine', *Journal of Medical Humanities* 31 (2010), 53–67.

Murphy, Michelle, *Seizing the Means of Reproduction: Entanglements of Feminism, Health, and Technoscience* (Durham, NC, 2012).

The Economization of Life (Durham, NC, 2017).

Nelson, Jennifer, *Women of Color and the Reproductive Rights Movement* (New York, NY, 2003).

More Than Medicine: A History of the Feminist Women's Health Movement (New York, NY, 2015).

Nguyen, Thuy Linh, *Childbirth, Maternity and Medical Pluralism in French Colonial Vietnam, 1880–1945* (Rochester, NY, 2016).

Nicolson, Malcolm, and John E. E. Fleming, *Imaging and Imagining the Fetus: The Development of Obstetric Ultrasound* (Baltimore, MD, 2013).

Niethammer, Lutz, and Silke Satjukow (eds.), *'Wenn die Chemie stimmt ...'. Geschlechterbeziehungen und Geburtenkontrolle im Zeitalter der 'Pille' / Gender Relations and Birth Control in the Age of the 'Pill'* (Göttingen, 2016).

Nordlund, Christer, *Hormones of Life: Endocrinology, the Pharmaceutical Industry, and the Dream of a Remedy for Sterility, 1930–1970* (Sagamore Beach, MA, 2011).

Norgren, Tiana, *Abortion before Contraception: The Politics of Reproduction in Postwar Japan* (Princeton, NJ, 2001).

Nye, Robert A., 'Love and reproductive biology in *fin-de-siècle* France: A Foucauldian lacuna?', in Jan Goldstein (ed.), *Foucault and the Writing of History* (Cambridge, MA, 1994), pp. 150–64.

Nyhart, Lynn K., 'Embryology and morphology', in Michael Ruse and Robert J. Richards (eds.), *The Cambridge Companion to the 'Origin of Species'* (Cambridge, 2009), pp. 194–215.

Oakley, Ann, *The Captured Womb: A History of the Medical Care of Pregnant Women* (Oxford, 1984).

Oliver, Kelly, *Knock Me Up, Knock Me Down: Images of Pregnancy in Hollywood Film* (New York, NY, 2012).

Olszynko-Gryn, Jesse, 'Pregnancy testing in Britain, *c.* 1900–67: Laboratories, animals and demand from doctors, patients and consumers', unpublished PhD thesis, University of Cambridge (2014).

Olszynko-Gryn, Jesse, Patrick Ellis and Caitjan Gainty (eds.), 'Reproduction on film', special issue, *British Journal for the History of Science* 50, no. 3 (2017).

Orland, Barbara (ed.), 'Sexualität und Fortpflanzung in den Medien des 20. Jahrhunderts', special issue, *zeitenblicke* 7, no. 3 (2008), www.zeitenblicke.de/2008/3/.

Oudshoorn, Nelly, *Beyond the Natural Body: An Archeology of Sex Hormones* (London, 1994).

The Male Pill: A Biography of a Technology in the Making (Durham, NC, 2003).

Parry, Manon, *Broadcasting Birth Control: Mass Media and Family Planning* (New Brunswick, NJ, 2013).

Patriarca, Silvana, *Numbers and Nationhood: Writing Statistics in Nineteenth-Century Italy* (Cambridge, 1996).

Paul, Diane B., and Jeffrey P. Brosco, *The PKU Paradox: A Short History of a Genetic Disease* (Baltimore, MD, 2013).

Pavard, Bibia, *Si je veux, quand je veux: Contraception et avortement dans la société française (1956–1979)* (Rennes, 2012).

Pedersen, Susan, *Family, Dependence, and the Origins of the Welfare State: Britain and France, 1914–1945* (Cambridge, 1993).

Perkins, John H., *Geopolitics and the Green Revolution: Wheat, Genes, and the Cold War* (New York, NY, 1997).

Pernick, Martin S., *The Black Stork: Eugenics and the Death of 'Defective' Babies in American Medicine and Motion Pictures since 1915* (New York, NY, 1995).

Pfeffer, Naomi, *The Stork and the Syringe: A Political History of Reproductive Medicine* (Cambridge, 1993).

Phillips, Denise, and Sharon Kingsland (eds.), *New Perspectives on the History of Life Sciences and Agriculture* (Cham, 2015).

Pooley, Siân, 'Parenthood, child-rearing and fertility in England, 1850–1914', *History of the Family* 18 (2013), 83–106.

Population Knowledge Network (ed.), *Twentieth Century Population Thinking: A Critical Reader of Primary Sources* (London, 2016).

Prescott, Heather Munro, *The Morning After: A History of Emergency Contraception in the United States* (New Brunswick, NJ, 2011).

Quinlan, Sean, 'Heredity, reproduction, and perfectibility in revolutionary and Napoleonic France, 1789–1815', *Endeavour* 34 (2010), 142–50.

Ram, Kalpana, and Margaret Jolly (eds.), *Maternities and Modernities: Colonial and Postcolonial Experiences in Asia and the Pacific* (Cambridge, 1998).

Rao, Mohan, *From Population Control to Reproductive Health: Malthusian Arithmetic* (New Delhi, 2004).

Rao, Mohan, and Sarah Sexton (eds.), *Markets and Malthus: Population, Gender and Health in Neo-Liberal Times* (Los Angeles, CA, 2010).

Ratmoko, Christina, *Damit die Chemie stimmt. Die Anfänge der industriellen Herstellung von weiblichen und männlichen Sexualhormonen 1914–1939* (Zurich, 2010).

Reagan, Leslie J., *When Abortion Was a Crime: Women, Medicine, and Law in the United States, 1867–1973* (Berkeley, CA, 1997).

Dangerous Pregnancies: Mothers, Disabilities, and Abortion in Modern America (Berkeley, CA, 2010).

(ed.), 'Reproduction, sex, and power', special issue, *Journal of Women's History* 22, no. 3 (2010), 7–238.

Reardon, Jenny, *Race to the Finish: Identity and Governance in an Age of Genomics* (Princeton, NJ, 2005).

Reed, James, *From Private Vice to Public Virtue: The Birth Control Movement and American Society since 1830* (New York, NY, 1978).

Reis, Elizabeth, *Bodies in Doubt: An American History of Intersex* (Baltimore, MD, 2009).

Richards, Evelleen, *Darwin and the Making of Sexual Selection* (Chicago, IL, 2017).

Richardson, Angelique, *Love and Eugenics in the Late Nineteenth Century: Rational Reproduction and the New Woman* (Oxford, 2003).

Richardson, Sarah S., *Sex Itself: The Search for Male and Female in the Human Genome* (Chicago, IL, 2013).

Ritvo, Harriet, *The Animal Estate: The English and Other Creatures in the Victorian Age* (Cambridge, MA, 1987).

Roberts, Dorothy E., *Killing the Black Body: Race, Reproduction, and the Meaning of Liberty* (New York, NY, 1997).

Robertson, Thomas, *The Malthusian Moment: Global Population Growth and the Birth of American Environmentalism* (New Brunswick, NJ, 2012).

Ronsin, Francis, *La grève des ventres: Propagande malthusienne et baisse de la natalité en France, XIXe–XXe siècles* (Paris, 1980).

Rosental, Paul-André, *L'intelligence démographique: Sciences et politiques des populations en France, 1930–1960* (Paris, 2003).

Destins de l'eugénisme (Paris, 2016).

Ross, Ellen, *Love and Toil: Motherhood in Outcast London, 1870–1918* (New York, NY, 1993).

Russett, Cynthia Eagle, *Sexual Science: The Victorian Construction of Womanhood* (Cambridge, MA, 1989).

Saetnan, Ann Rudinow, Nelly Oudshoorn and Marta Kirejczyk (eds.), *Bodies of Technology: Women's Involvement with Reproductive Medicine* (Columbus, OH, 2000).

Salesa, Damon Ieremia, *Racial Crossings: Race, Intermarriage, and the Victorian British Empire* (Oxford, 2011).

Sasson, Tehila, 'Milking the Third World? Humanitarianism, capitalism, and the moral economy of the Nestlé boycott', *American Historical Review* 121 (2016), 1196–224.

Satzinger, Helga, *Differenz und Vererbung. Geschlechterordnungen in der Genetik und Hormonforschung 1890–1950* (Cologne, 2009).

Sauerteig, Lutz D. H., and Roger Davidson (eds.), *Shaping Sexual Knowledge: A Cultural History of Sex Education in Twentieth-Century Europe* (London, 2009).

Schlünder, Martina, 'Die Herren der Regel/n? Gynäkologen und der Menstruationskalender als Regulierungsinstrument der weiblichen Natur', in Cornelius Borck, Volker Hess and Henning Schmidgen (eds.), *Maß und Eigensinn. Studien im Anschluß an Georges Canguilhem* (Munich, 2005), pp. 157–95.

Schneider, William, *Quality and Quantity: The Quest for Biological Regeneration in Twentieth-Century France* (Cambridge, 1990).

Schoen, Johanna, *Choice and Coercion: Birth Control, Sterilization, and Abortion in Public Health and Welfare* (Chapel Hill, NC, 2005).

Abortion after Roe (Chapel Hill, NC, 2015).

Schreiber, Christine, *Natürlich künstliche Befruchtung? Eine Geschichte der In-vitro-Fertilisation von 1878 bis 1950* (Göttingen, 2007).

Schrepfer, Susan R., and Philip Scranton (eds.), *Industrializing Organisms: Introducing Evolutionary History* (New York, NY, 2004).

Schwartz, Mary Jenkins, *Birthing a Slave: Motherhood and Medicine in the Antebellum South* (Cambridge, MA, 2010).

Schweber, Libby, *Disciplining Statistics: Demography and Vital Statistics in France and England, 1830–1885* (Durham, NC, 2006).

Secord, James A., *Victorian Sensation: The Extraordinary Publication, Reception, and Secret Authorship of* Vestiges of the Natural History of Creation (Chicago, IL, 2000).

Sengoopta, Chandak, *The Most Secret Quintessence of Life: Sex, Glands, and Hormones, 1850–1950* (Chicago, IL, 2006).

Sevegrand, Martine, *Les enfants du bon Dieu: Les catholiques français et la procréation au XXe siècle* (Paris, 1995).

Sharpless, John, 'World population growth, family planning, and American foreign policy', *Journal of Policy History* 7 (1995), 72–102.

Sheldon, Sally, *Beyond Control: Medical Power and Abortion Law* (London, 1997).

Shteir, Ann B., *Cultivating Women, Cultivating Science: Flora's Daughters and Botany in England, 1760 to 1860* (Baltimore, MD, 1999).

Silies, Eva-Marie, *Liebe, Lust und Last. Die Pille als weibliche Generationserfahrung in der Bundesrepublik, 1960–1980* (Göttingen, 2010).

Smith, Angela M., *Hideous Progeny: Disability, Eugenics, and Classic Horror Cinema* (New York, NY, 2011).

Smith, Jane S., *The Garden of Invention: Luther Burbank and the Business of Breeding Plants* (New York, NY, 2009).

Society for the History of Technology, *Technology's Stories: Reproductive Technologies*, www.technologystories.org/category/reproductive-technology/ (2016–).

Solinger, Rickie, *Pregnancy and Power: A Short History of Reproductive Politics in America* (New York, NY, 2005).

Solinger, Rickie, and Mie Nakachi (eds.), *Reproductive States: Global Perspectives on the Invention and Implementation of Population Policy* (Oxford, 2016).

Sollors, Werner (ed.), *Interracialism: Black–White Intermarriage in American History, Literature, and Law* (Oxford, 2000).

Soloway, Richard A., *Demography and Degeneration: Eugenics and the Declining Birth-Rate in Twentieth-Century Britain* (Chapel Hill, NC, 1990).

Spary, Emma C., *Utopia's Garden: French Natural History from Old Regime to Revolution* (Chicago, IL, 2000).

Squier, Susan, *Babies in Bottles: Twentieth-Century Visions of Reproductive Technology* (New Brunswick, NJ, 1994).

Staggenborg, Suzanne, *The Pro-Choice Movement: Organization and Activism in the Abortion Conflict* (New York, NY, 1991).

Stanley, Liz, *Sex Surveyed, 1949–1994: From Mass-Observation's 'Little Kinsey' to the National Survey and the Hite Reports* (London, 1995).

Staupe, Gisela, and Lisa Vieth (eds.), *Die Pille. Von der Lust und von der Liebe* (Dresden and Berlin, 1996).

Stead, Evanghélia, *Le monstre, le singe et le fœtus: Tératogonie et décadence dans l'Europe fin-de-siècle* (Geneva, 2004).

Stern, Alexandra Minna, *Eugenic Nation: Faults and Frontiers of Better Breeding in Modern America* (Berkeley, CA, 2005).

Telling Genes: The Story of Genetic Counseling in America (Baltimore, MD, 2012).

Stokes, Patricia R., 'Pathology, danger, and power: Women's and physicians' views of pregnancy and childbirth in Weimar Germany', *Social History of Medicine* 13 (2000), 359–80.

Swanson, Kara W., *Banking on the Body: The Market in Blood, Milk, and Sperm in Modern America* (Cambridge, MA, 2014).

Symonds, Richard, and Michael Carder, *The United Nations and the Population Question, 1945–1970* (London, 1973).

Szreter, Simon, 'The idea of demographic transition and the study of fertility change: A critical intellectual history', *Population and Development Review* 19 (1993), 659–701.

Fertility, Class and Gender in Britain, 1860–1940 (Cambridge, 1996).

Szreter, Simon, and Kate Fisher, *Sex before the Sexual Revolution: Intimate Life in England, 1918–1963* (Cambridge, 2010).

Takeshita, Chikako, *The Global Biopolitics of the IUD: How Science Constructs Contraceptive Users and Women's Bodies* (Cambridge, MA, 2012).

Thane, Pat, and Tanya Evans, *Sinners? Scroungers? Saints? Unmarried Motherhood in Twentieth-Century England* (Oxford, 2012).

Therborn, Göran, *Between Sex and Power: Family in the World, 1900–2000* (London, 2004).

Thomas, Lynn M., *Politics of the Womb: Women, Reproduction, and the State in Kenya* (Berkeley, CA, 2003).

Timm, Annette F., *The Politics of Fertility in Twentieth-Century Berlin* (New York, NY, 2010).

Tone, Andrea (ed.), *Controlling Reproduction: An American History* (Wilmington, DE, 1997).

Devices and Desires: A History of Contraceptives in America (New York, NY, 2001).

Turner, Sasha, *Contested Bodies: Pregnancy, Childrearing, and Slavery in Jamaica* (Philadelphia, PA, 2017).

Turney, Jon, *Frankenstein's Footsteps: Science, Genetics and Popular Culture* (New Haven, CT, 1998).

University of Michigan Library, *Birthing Reproductive Justice: 150 Years of Images and Ideas*, an online exhibition, www.lib.umich.edu/online-exhibits/exhibits/show/reproductive-justice, last accessed 8 June 2017.

Usborne, Cornelie, *The Politics of the Body in Weimar Germany: Women's Reproductive Rights and Duties* (Basingstoke, 1992).

Cultures of Abortion in Weimar Germany (New York, NY, 2007).

Vienne, Florence, *Une science de la peur: La démographie avant et après 1933* (Frankfurt am Main, 2006).

Walkowitz, Judith R., *Prostitution and Victorian Society: Women, Class and the State* (Cambridge, 1980).

Walton, John R., 'Pedigree and the national cattle herd, *circa* 1750–1850', *Agricultural History Review* 34 (1986), 149–70.

Watkins, Elizabeth Siegel, *On the Pill: A Social History of Oral Contraceptives, 1950–1970* (Baltimore, MD, 1998).

The Estrogen Elixir: A History of Hormone Replacement Therapy in America (Baltimore, MD, 2007).

Weeks, Jeffrey, *Sex, Politics and Society: The Regulation of Sexuality since 1800*, 3rd edn (Harlow, 2012).

Weinbaum, Alys Eve, *Wayward Reproductions: Genealogies of Race and Nation in Transatlantic Modern Thought* (Durham, NC, 2004).

Weindling, Paul, *Health, Race and German Politics between National Unification and Nazism, 1870–1945* (Cambridge, 1989).

Wellmann, Janina, *The Form of Becoming: Embryology and the Epistemology of Rhythm, 1760–1830*, trans. Kate Sturge (Cambridge, MA, 2017).

White, Tyrene, *China's Longest Campaign: Birth Planning in the People's Republic, 1949–2005* (Ithaca, NY, 2006).

Williams, Daniel K., *Defenders of the Unborn: The Pro-Life Movement before* Roe v. Wade (New York, NY, 2016).

Wilmot, Sarah (ed.), 'Between the farm and the clinic: Agriculture and reproductive technology in the twentieth century', special issue, *Studies in History and Philosophy of Biological and Biomedical Sciences* 38 (2007), 303–530.

Winter, Jay, and Michael Teitelbaum, *The Global Spread of Fertility Decline: Population, Fear, and Uncertainty* (New Haven, CT, 2013).

Wolf, Jacqueline H., *Don't Kill Your Baby: Public Health and the Decline of Breastfeeding in the Nineteenth and Twentieth Centuries* (Columbus, OH, 2001).

Deliver Me From Pain: Anesthesia and Birth in America (Baltimore, MD, 2009).

Wu, Yi-Li, *Reproducing Women: Medicine, Metaphor, and Childbirth in Late Imperial China* (Berkeley, CA, 2010).

Zelizer, Viviana A., *Pricing the Priceless Child: The Changing Social Value of Children* (New York, NY, 1985).

Ziegler, Mary, *After Roe: The Lost History of the Abortion Debate* (Cambridge, MA, 2015).

Zimmerman, Jonathan, *Too Hot to Handle: A Global History of Sex Education* (Princeton, NJ, 2015).

Index

Page numbers in italics are figures; with 'n' are notes; E1–E40 are exhibits.

A. H. Robins, 542
abandonment, 368
  See also exposure, infant; foundlings/orphans
Aberdeen Bestiary, E9
abortifacients, 49, 161–2, 169–70, 235, 431, 435–6, 481, 536, *537*, 549–50, *600*
abortion, xxvii, 138, 142, 144, 150, 161–6, 168–70, 235, 428–30, 502, *547*, 667–8
  abortifacients, 49, 161–2, 169–70, 235, 431, 435–6, 481, 536, *537*, 549–50, *600*
  and birth control, 435–6, 439–40, *440*
  and colonialism, 490
  early Christian teachings, 109, 118, 119
  and ensoulment, 118, 119
  and fetal abnormalities, 568, 569–70, 578–9
  in Islamic law, 276–9
  laws, 138, 278–9, 597–602, *600*
    Abortion Act 1967 (Britain), 501, 602–3
    Comstock Laws (1873) (US), 431, 538–9, 599, *600*
    Infant Life (Preservation) Act 1929 (England/Wales), 601–2
    Lord Ellenborough's Act 1803 (UK), 428–9, 598
    Offences Against the Person Act 1861 (England/Wales), 598
    Roe v. Wade (US), 547–8, 604–5, *605*
  medical science and women's experiences, 479–80
  Mohr, *Abortion in America*, 10
  in Northern Ireland, 603, 641
  pills for, 549–50
  Pliny the Elder, 83
  and politics of gender, 623–4
  technologies, 535–6, 543–51
  See also Abortion Law Reform Association; anti-abortionism
Abortion Act 1967 (Britain), 501, 602–3
Abortion Law Reform Association (ALRA) (UK), 439, *440*, 601
abstinence/celibacy, 177, 337, 360, 392, 538, 667
  in Catholic church, 337
  See also chastity
acclimatization, 283, 315
Action (magazine), *477*
Adam, 116–18
  and Eve, 35, 112, 142–3, 199, 291
  See also Eve
adoption
  in ancient Greece and Rome, 88, 93
  in China, 356
  international and transracial, 651, 666
  and Islamic law, 270, 651, 664
  matching, E33
  and modern childlessness, 395, 458, *459*, 465, 468–70
adultery, 82–3, 164, 179, 236, 238, 249–50, 307, 583, 606, 651, E2
advertisements, 188–9, 468, *474*, 531, 536, *537*, 599, E28
advice books, 13, 129, 468, *469*
  animal breeding, 398, 402
  Aristotle's Masterpiece, 193, 473, E25
  A Child Is Born (Nilsson), E34
  Die Ärztin im Hause (The woman doctor in the home) (Springer), *467*
  Examen de ingenios para las sciencias (*The Examination of Mens Wits*) (Huarte), 246–9, 246n11
  Hints to Mothers (Bull), 473, 476
  Nouvelles causes de stérilité (New causes of sterility) (Gérard), *15*, 583, *584*
  Our Bodies, Ourselves (Boston Women's Health Book Collective), 564, 616, *617*, E35
Aelian, *On Animals*, 54, 59
Aeschylus, *Eumenides*, 54
aetites (eagle-stone), E17
Africa, North
  late antique, 107, 111, 114–15, E10
  See also Egypt

Africa, sub-Saharan
birth control, 490, 535
birth-rates, 486
childbirth and midwives in, 326, *491*, 643–4, *644*
classification of people by colour, 361–2, 363–4, 364–6, *365*, 367
after colonialism, 487–8
experiments on human–ape hybrids, 585–6
IVF, 650, 652
maternal mortality and 'safe motherhood' campaigns, 646, *647*
matrifocal households (West Africa), 358
mothercraft and *gouttes de lait* (milk depots), 493, *494*, *495*, 495–6
South African clawed frogs/toads, E32, E37
and STIs, 451–2
agricultural societies, 399
agricultural writing, classical antiquity, 21, 53–66, *55*, *56*, *60*, *64*
agriculture. *See* agricultural societies; agricultural writing; botany; cattle breeding; horse breeding; livestock breeding
Agrippa von Nettesheim, Heinrich Cornelius, 190
AI. *See* artificial insemination
AI by donor (AID), 583, 586
Albert the Great (Albertus Magnus), 176, 185
See also Secretis Mulierum, De (*On the Secrets of Women*)
albinism, 364–6, *365*
Albucasis. *See* al-Zahrawi
alchemy, 188, 190, 204–5
and radical moisture, 199–203, *202*, 204–5
Aldobrandini, Naddino, 162–3
d'Alembert, Jean le Rond, 295, 298, 335n11
Alexis of Piedmont, 188
Allbutt, H. Arthur, *The Wife's Handbook*, 473
Alliance nationale pour l'accroissement de la population française (National Alliance for the Growth of the French Population), *390–1*, 431
alternation of generations, 302, *303*
American Birth Control League, 7, 434, 507
See also Planned Parenthood Federation of America
American Civil Liberties Union, 605–6
American Society for Reproductive Medicine, 610–11
amniocentesis, 568, 569–72, 574–6
amulets, *45*, 165
agnus dei, E17
eagle-stones, E17
in the Roman Empire, E7
to aid in childbirth, 156
See also charms
analogies. *See* metaphors/analogies
Anastasius II (Bishop of Rome), 118
anatomical museums, 481
'anatomo-politics', 9, 333–4
anatomy
of albinism, 364–6
Alexandrian, 99
early modern, 209–24, *214*, *217*, *218*, *219*, *221*, E15, E16
Galen's, 95–108
of hyena, E9
and midwifery, 323–4, E21
modern, 381–2, 413–26, E23
Ottoman, 271–6
See also one-sex/two-sex models
ancestors
and fertility, E1
See also kinship
ancient Greece, 20–1, 39–52, *75*, 195–7, 460, E2
art, xxvi, *18–19*, *40*, *45*, *55*
law, 81, 84, 88
mythology, 39–40, E2
poetry, 42, 54, 63
population, 68–75, 79–80
ancient Near East/Egypt, 25–38
ancient Rome, *19*, 21–2, *110*, 111, 660
agricultural writing, 21, 53–4, 60, 65–6
art, *56*, *92*, E5
census, *76*, 77–9
Christianization, 111
division of Empire into East and West, *110*, 111
embryo hooks, E6
law, 81–94, *82*, *86*, *90*, *92*, 174–6
midwifery, 157, 320
Pompeii wall-painting, E5
and population, 75–9, *76*, *78*, 79–80
surgical instruments, 12e
swaddling, E4
'Third-Century Crisis', 109–10
Andrieu, Pierre, *Golden Apple*, E10
anencephaly, 572
Anglican church, 292, 437, 606
Anglicus, Gilbertus, *Compendium medicinae* (Medical compendium), 187
Animal Breeding Research Department (Edinburgh), 409
Animal Research Station (Cambridge), 587, 588
animalcules, 291, 364, 413, 415, *416*, 582, 661, E16
Annunciation, xxvi, *120*, 121
al-Antaki, Dawud, 275
Memorial (*Tadhkirah*), 273–4
anti-abortionism, 439–40, 550, 599, 610, E34
See also Roe v. Wade

aphrodisiacs, 59, E22
Apostolic Constitutions, 119
apothecaries/chemists (shops)
early modern, 244, E17
medieval, 164
modern, 437, 481, *482*, 536, 538
apparatuses of alliance and of sexuality (Foucault), 613–15
al-Aqsara'i, Jamal al-Din, *Hall al-Mujaz* (Resolution of the epitome), 135–6, *136*
Aquinas, Thomas, 114, 661
Ara Pacis, *92*
Aranzio, Giulio Cesare, E15
Archelaus, 63
Arderne, John, E10
Aristotelians, on the soul, 111
Aristotle
and dissection, 212
on ensoulment, 113
and Hobbes, 255
on hyenas, E9
innate heat, 196
in the middle ages, 145–7, 170, 176
on nature, 54–5
radical moisture, 201
on Sparta, 80
use by Galen, 99–100
works
Ethics, 170
Generation of Animals (*GA*), 53, 55–7, 58–9, 61, 62–3, 65, 132, 260, 290
History of Animals (*HA*), 43–4, 59
On Generation and Corruption, 290
On the Length and Shortness of Life, 142, 143
Politics, 67–8, 72–3, 142, 170
See also Problemata (*Problems*)
Aristotle's Masterpiece, 473, E25
Arnald of Villanova, 199
Arnott, Neil, *Elements of Physics*, 382
artificial fertilization, 417, 581–96
See also artificial insemination; embryo transfer; in vitro fertilization
artificial insemination (AI), *15*, 394, 397, 410–12, 462–3, 581, 582–7, *584*, *585*, 595–6
regulation, 606
Aschheim, Selmar, E32
assisted reproduction, 427, 581, 593–5, 621, 642, 651–2
See also in vitro fertilization
association, 254–7
Association for Improvements in the Maternity Services (UK), 563
Association for Voluntary Sterilization (US), 605
astrological medicine, 225–40
astrology, 176
in Babylonia, E3
and John Dee, E14
and livestock breeding, 398
and medicine, 225–40
Athena, birth of, 39, *40*
Athenaeus, 103
Atomists, 111
Atrahasis (Mesopotamian tale), 30
Augustine
City of God, 174
ensoulment, 118, 119
Questions on the Heptateuch, 114
See also Questions and Answers on the Old and New Testament
Augustus (Roman emperor), 4, 83, 84, 88, 91–4, 664
Aurelius, Marcus, *96*
autonomy. *See* self-determination
autopsies. *See* dissection
'Autumn' (depiction of stage of life), *122–3*
Aveline, François Antoine, E20
Aveling, James, 321–2
Avicenna. *See* Ibn Sina
Ayscough, Lady, 191
ʿ*azl* (withdrawal), 270, 274, 277
Aztecs, 362–3

baby boom (generation), *xxxvi–1*, 302, 500
Bachofen, Johann Jakob, 7
Bacon, Francis, *History of Life and Death*, 205, 258–60
Bacon, Roger, 201
Baer, Karl Ernst von, 283, 417–19
Bakewell, Robert, 397, 403
Baldo degli Ubaldi, 176
Baldwin, Lucy, *561*
Ballard, Martha, 326
Balme, D. M., 63
bananas, 314, *315*
baptism, 160, 171–2, 174, 326
barbers
middle ages, 160, 164, 172
modern, 481, 538, E28
Roman, 160
Barker, David/Barker hypothesis, E39
Barr, Murray/Barr bodies, 569
barrenness. *See* infertility
Bartholin, Thomas, E16
Basil of Caesarea, 119
Bateson, William, 405
Bayezid II, 268, 271

Bayle, Pierre, 207–8
bean-counting, 145
Beatie, Thomas and Nancy, *625*
de Beauvoir, Simone, *The Second Sex*, 630, 631–3, *632*, 636
Beer, Gillian, 628
bees, 63–4, *64*
Benedetti, Alessandro, 210
Benedict XIV (pope), E21
Benjamin, Walter, 299
Bennett, Judith, 319
Bentham, Jeremy, 428
Berengario da Carpi, 212–13
Bernard de Gordon, *Lilium medicinae* (Lily of medicine), 187
Besant, Annie, 430
bestiality, 174–6, 388
bestiaries, 54, E9
Beveridge, William, 446
Bible, 23, 30–2, 35, 37
Bill & Melinda Gates Foundation, 516–17, 543
Biller, Peter, *The Measure of Multitude*, 67, 141–2
bills of mortality, 259, 263, 339
bioethics, 606, 609–10, E38
biology, 282–3, 287, 388
'biomedicalization', 503, 531–2
biomedicine, 500, 503, 602
biopolitics, 9, 10, 334–6, 344, 614, 619, 623–4
biopower, 284, 333–4, 614
birth. *See* childbirth
birth assistants/attendants, 643, 668
  ancient, *104*, E6
  colonialist critiques, 491–6
  early modern, *8*, E18
  medieval, 157, 159–60, *159*
  See also midwifery
Birth Control International Information Centre, 438, 511
birth control (term), 392, 434
  See also contraception
birth girdles, E11
birth trays, 155–6, *155*, *159*, 159–60
'birth wars', 553–5, 564, *565*
birth-rate, 67–8, 347–60, *390–1*, 407–8, 443–56, 486–90
  See also fertility transitions; population
birthing chairs/stools, *104*, 157, E18
birthing rooms, 157, 324–5, *328*, 554, 559, 560, 566
Black Death. *See* plague
Black, William, *Arithmetical and Medical Analysis of the Diseases …*, 338–40
Blacklock, Mary, 494–5
bladder stones, cutting for, 272
blood
  in animal breeding, 402, 406–7
  Aristotle on blooded and bloodless animals, 55–7
  bloodstone amulet, E7
  -clot in Islamic medicine, 132, 138
  groups and genetics, E30
  and haemolytic disease, 569
  in Hippocratic medicine, 44, 45, 205
  and the humours, 195–7, 198, 361
  and innate heat, 195–7
  Mesopotamian mythology, 35
  and radical moisture, 198, 206–7
  test, 577
  and uterine mole, 41
  See also livestock breeding; menstruation; paternity; race; ranking people
bloodletting, 324–5
Blum, Carol, 337
Blumenbach, Johann Friedrich, 366
  De generis humani varietate nativa (On the natural varieties of mankind), 369–72
Blunt, John (Samuel Fores), *Man-Midwifery Dissected*, E22
Boaistuau, Pierre, E13
Boas, Franz, 302
Book of the Dead of Sesu, 27, *28*
Boston Women's Health Book/Course Collective, *Our Bodies, Ourselves*, 564, 616, *617*, E35
botany, 305–18, *308*, *313*, *315*, *316*
Boudewinsz, Willem, 176
Bourdeille, Pierre de, Lord of Brantôme, E12
Bourgeois, Louise, 325, 327
Bourguet, Louis, *Lettres philosophiques* (Philosophical letters), 294
Bourne, Aleck, 601–2
Bourrit, Marc-Théodore, 365
Bowler, Peter, *Evolution: The History of an Idea*, 375
Boyd Orr, John, *Food: The Foundation of World Unity*, 512–13
Boyer, Jean-Baptiste, Marquis d'Argens, *379*
Boym, Michael, 195
Bradlaugh, Charles, 430
brain, *117*, *384*
  anencephaly, 572
  development, 102
  and professions, 247
  and 'white juice', 205–6
breast-feeding, 34, 493, *556*

Family Group with a Mother Feeding Her Children (van der Mij), E19
and fertility, 347, 356, 358, 487
See also milk
breeding. *See* cattle breeding; horse breeding; livestock breeding; plants
Britain
abortion and contraception, 436, 437, 535–51, *537*, *540*, *542*, 599–602, 602–4, E28
Abortion Law Reform Association (ALRA), 439, *440*, 601
Lord Ellenborough's Act 1803, 428–9, 598
the pill, 500–1, 541
artificial fertilization
AI, 584, *585*, 586–7, 606
Human Fertilisation and Embryology Acts 1990 and 2008, 594, 595, 608, 610
Human Fertilisation and Embryology Authority (HFEA), 608–9, *609*
IVF/embryo transfer, 590–3, *591*, *592*, 608–10
censuses/registration, 343, 360, 664, E24
childbirth, E22
hospital, 553–4, *556*, 562–3, *565*
See also man-midwifery
colonialism, 485–6, 495
communication about generation, reproduction and sex, 375–89, 471–84
fertility, *232*, 360
Gender Recognition Act 2004, 622
household systems, 350, *351*
livestock breeding, 397–412
Marriage (Same Sex Couples) Act 2013, 625
and neo-Malthusianism, 430–2
nuptiality valve, 353–5, 359–60
and population, 254–66, 284, 338–45, *341*, *342*
and STIs, 444–6, *447*, 453–4
Britannica (encyclopaedia), 299
Bromyard, John, 150
Brown, Lesley and John, E38
Brown, Louise, 581, 593, E38
Brown, Thomas, *573*
Browne, Stella, *439*
Browne, Thomas, 363–4
Bruni, Leonardo, 145–6
Bruno, Giordano, 367
Bryder, Linda, 562–3
Buffon (Georges-Louis Leclerc, Comte de), 4, 282, 285, 288, 294–5, *296*, 413, 661–2
and equality of sexes in reproduction, 424
Histoire Naturelle (Natural history), 294, *296*, 378–80, E20
and race, 364, 372
Bull, Thomas, *Hints to Mothers*, 473, 476
Bund für Mutterschutz (League for the Protection of Mothers), 433
Burgh, John, *The Eye of the Pupil* (*Pupilla oculi*), 150
Burke's Peerage, 399
burial, 168–70, 171, *173*, 338, 339, E6
See also bills of mortality
Butenandt, Adolf, 525
Butler, Judith, *Gender Trouble*, 622, 623, 635–6
Buzzi, Francesco, 366

Cadden, Joan, 153
Caelius Aurelianus, 106–7
Caesar, Julius, 88, 160, *161*
caesarean section, 160, *161*, 326, 559, 564
See also fetal excision
Cagnoli, Gérard, 163
Calcar, Jan van, *214*
Caldenbach, Martin, *672–3*
calendars, 536
menstrual, 125, E14, E31
pregnancy, *234*
Calza, Luigi, E21
cameralism, 314
Campbell, Dame Janet, 511
Camper, Petrus, 373–4
Campus, Michael, E36
Canaanite/Ugaritic mythology, 32, 35–6
Cangiamila, Francesco, *Embriologia sacra* (Sacred embryology), 326
Cannan, Edwin, 444
'captured womb' (Oakley), 554
Cardano, Girolamo, 190
cardiovascular disease, E39
caricature/satire, *465*, *474*, E22, E26, E27
Carlile, Richard, *Every Woman's Book; or, What Is Love?*, 428, *429*, 475
Carr-Saunders, Alexander, 512
Cartolari, Antonio, E21
casebooks, medical, 227–8, *232*
Cassiano dal Pozzo, E17
Cassius Dio, 89
caste system, Spanish, 368–73, *370–1*
Casti Connubii (Of chaste wedlock) (Pius XI), 509
catasto (Florence), 664
Catholic church, 664
and abortion, 163–4, 668
and AI, 463, 583, *585*

Catholic church (*cont.*)
biopolitical discourse, 395
and birth girdles, E11
and colonial caste system, 368–73
and contraception, 165, 430, 436, 437, 511, 538, E31
and eugenics, 509
and *experimenta*, 192
on IVF, E38
Montesquieu on, 337
and *Roe v. Wade* (US), *605*
and surgical techniques, 559
cattle breeding, 400, *401*, 407, *408*, 410–12
celibacy. *See* abstinence/celibacy
cell theory, 414, 419–22, 422–6, 423–4
Celsus, E6
censuses, 257, 333, 343, 405, 664
Census of Pedigree Livestock, 407
Fertility Census (1911) (UK), 359–60, *448*
Givry (France), 149
Roman, 77–9
See also parish records; sex ratio
cervix, 458, 462
dilation for abortion, 536, 546
seen through speculum, 466–8, *467*
Chamberlen family, 321–3
Chambers, Ephraim, *Cyclopaedia*, 290–1
Chambers, Robert, 385
Chambers's Encyclopaedia, 299, *303*
Chandrasekhar, Sripati, 509, 648
Chang, Min Chueh, 548–9, 588
character. *See* traits
charity, 162–3, 330–1, 494–6, 553–5, 557–60, 641, E19
charms, 156, 163, 182–3, 191, 192–3, E11
See also amulets
Chartres Cathedral, Tree of Jesse, E8
chastity, 47, 148, 153, 456, E19
Chauvin, Étienne, *Lexicon rationale*, 207
cheese as analogy for generation, *117*, 132
chick embryos
Fabrici d'Acquapendente on, 219–20, *221*
Harvey on, 223–4
Malpighi on, 223–4
in Réaumur, xxvi
chicken crest assay, *524*
child production, in mythology, 34–6
childbirth, xxvi, *19*
birth girdles, E11
colonial, 491–6, *491*
and eagle-stones, E17
equipment
birth trays, 155–6, *155*, 159–60, *159*
birthing chairs, *104*, E18
birthing stools, 157
embryo hooks, 272, 323, 546, E6
forceps, 320, 321–4, *322*
globalization, 643–6, *644*, *647*
in Hippocratic medicine, 50
home birth, 480, 555, 566, 645, 668
in hospital, *xxxvi–1*, 553–66, *556*, *558*, *561*, *565*, 643–6
middle ages, 153–66, *155*, *158*, *159*, *161*
obstructed, 153, 164–5n33, 323, 327, 559, E6
malpresentation, E10
pain relief, 331, 557–8, 561–2, *561*
Roman Empire, 87, 104–5, 146
rooms, 157, 324–5, *328*, 554, 559, 560, 566
See also hospitals; lying-in; midwifery
childlessness
voluntary, 464, 468
See also infertility
China
abortion pill, 550
contraception, 542, 543, 546, 619, 649
IVF, 650
joint household system, 356
medicine, 195
midwifery, 643
one-child policy, 4, 519
two-child policy, 650
chlamydia, 443
Christian II of Denmark, portrait of children, 241, *242*
Christianity, 22
Annunciation, xxvi, *120*, 121
and assisted reproduction, 593–4
and contraception, 430
and infanticide, 114, 118–19
middle ages, 124–5, 144, 153–66
and the soul, 22, 109–21, *110*, *117*, *120*, 168, 169, 171
See also Anglican church; Catholic church
chromosomes, and fetal abnormalities, 568, 569, 570–2, *571*, *575*, 576–7
Churchill, John, 381
Ciba, 527–9
Cicero, 91–2
Laws, 78–9
Republic, 78–9
Clark, Alice, 319, 331
Clark, Anna, 480
Clarke, Adele, *Disciplining Reproduction*, 290, 304, 409, 521–2, 526, 531, 628
class. *See* social class
classification
of animals and plants, 53–66, 305–18

anthropological, of practices, 9
of human populations, 253–66, 333–45
of humans by colour, 366–7
of humans by wealth, 76–9
of man-midwives, E22
Clement VII (pope), E12
Clifford, George, 314
climate change, 502, 519, 665–6
Clinton, Bill, 550
cloning, 412, E37
Coale, Ansley J., 449–51, *450*
Coale–Hoover model, 449, *450*
Cobbett, William, 299n35
Code Napoléon, 597
coitus interruptus (withdrawal), 47–8, 165, 270, 274, 277, 538, 551, 667
Coke, Thomas, 399, *400*
Colen, Shellee, 641
colonies/colonialism, 13, 284, 393, 654–5, 661, 667
and indigenous knowledge, 476
and racial theories, 361–74
and STIs, 451–2
and women, 485–97
colour, classification of humans by, 366–7
Columella, 53, 60, 65
commentaries
Arabic, 129–40, *136*, 269, 270, 277
and Jerome, 116
middle ages, 143, 145–7, 151, 170, 176
Committee of Inquiry into Human Fertilisation and Embryology (Warnock Committee) (UK), 608
Commodus, *96*
Commons Act 1908 (England/Wales), 407
communication, 13, 181–93, 375–89, 471–84
communism, xxvii, 501, 585–6, 643, 645, 665
anti-, 514, *518*, 646
See also China; Soviet Union
Comstock, Anthony, *600*
Comstock Laws (1873) (US), 431, 434, 538, 599, *600*, 602, E28
conception, technologies of, 581–96
See also in vitro fertilization
condoms, 481, *482*, 535, 538–9, 551, E28
Condorcet, Marquis de, 343, 427
Congo, childbirth in, 643–4, *644*
conjoined twins, 174, *175*
conservation, 517–19
See also environmentalism
Constantine (Roman emperor), 111
consumers/consumerism, *523*, 535, *542*, 551, 555, 626, 655, 662, 670, E31
and activism, 502, 533
after Comstock, 538–9
and artificial fertilization, 581–96, 620, 626
and choice, 608, 609–10, 665, 668
and contraception, 447, *450*
of *experimenta*, 183, 193
and genetic testing, 666, E30
home pregnancy tests, 478, E32
and hospital birth, 563–6
prenatal accessories, 669
Contagious Diseases Acts (England), 445
Contendings of Horus and Seth (Egyptian tale), 32–3
contraception, 163–6, 669
advice in the middle ages, 150
and the Bill & Melinda Gates Foundation, 516–17
histories of, 7, 47–8
and 'Malthusian couple', 618–20
movements for, 427–41
and poverty, 646–50
technologies of, 535–51
terminology, 392, 434
contraceptives, 161–2, 169–70
condoms, 481, *482*, 535, 538–9, 551, E28
diaphragms, 539
implants and injections, 542–3
intrauterine devices (IUDs), 535, 541–3, *542*, 551, 648
in Islamic medicine, 273–4
See also pills; rhythm method; sterilization
contracts
adoption, 458
and IVF, 610–11
marital, 630–1
See also marital debt
surrogacy, 654
'control', 666–9
See also birth control; population, control
Cook, Captain James, E24
cosmogony, 26–32, *28*
counselling
abortion, 502, *547*, 549
genetic, 180, 501
marital, 438
crayfish regeneration, 292, *293*
'creatianism', 116, 118
Crew, Francis, 407–8
Cruikshank, Isaac, E22
Cuvier, Georges, 298, 381
Czech Republic, 652

d'Alembert, Jean le Rond, 295, 298, 335n11
Dalkon Shield, 541–2
Dally, Eugène, 403

Danco, 550
Darwin, Charles, 284, 382–3, 385–8, *387*, 404–5, 628
  Descent of Man, 386–8
  in Haselden cartoon, E27
  On the Origin of Species, 385–6
Darwin, Erasmus
  Botanic Garden, 380
  Temple of Nature, 380
Daubenton, Louis-Jean-Marie, E20
Davis, Kingsley, 507, 512
Dawson, Gowan, 376
decorum. *See* modesty
Dee, John and Jane, E14
deformities/disabilities/monsters
  ancient Greece/Rome, 39, 44–5
    exposure/infanticide, 68–70, 76
  Aristotle's Masterpiece, E25
  Augustine on, 119, 174
  conjoined twins, 174, *175*
  in Linnaean botany, 312
  man-midwives as, E22
  and medieval law and theology, 168, 174–6
  Minotaur, E2
  'monster of Cracow', E13
  prevention of, 176–9, *178*, 567–79
  transmission of, 422
degeneration, 393, 432, 444–5
  in animal breeding, 398, 400–1, 406–7, 585
  and colonialism, 490, 497
  Linnaeus's fears of, 318
DeLee, Joseph, 560
delivery rooms. *See* birthing rooms
Delphy, Christine, 631
Demand, Nancy, 49
demodystopia, E36
Demographic Committee (League of Nations), 512
Demographic Transition Theory, 7, 443–4, 446–51, *450*, 451–2
demography, 7, 333, 335, 405, 665
  See also population
demons, 162, E7, E9, E13, E38
  See also witches/witchcraft
Depo-Provera, 542
depopulation, 67, 336–8
  and colonialism, 486–90
  and plague, 162
DES (diethylstilbestrol), 532–3, *532*, 549
Descartes, René, 291
Devay, Francis, 403
developmental origins of health and disease, E39
Deventer, Hendrik van, 327
diabetes, 569
diagnosis, prenatal, 567–79, *571*, *573*, *575*
Diagnostic and Statistical Manual of Mental Disorders (DSM-III), 623
Dialpak, 620, *621*
diaphragms, 539
Dick-Read, Grantly, 563
Didache, 118, 119
Diderot, Denis, 295
  Encyclopédie, 290, 298
diet. *See* food/diet
dietetics, 310
diethylstilbestrol (DES), 532–3, *532*, 549
Diodorus of Tarsus, 113
Dionysius of Halicarnassus, 77–8, *78*
Dioscorides, *Materia medica*, E17
disabilities, prevention of, 567–79
  See also deformities/disabilities/monsters
disease
  developmental origins of health and disease, E39
  'disease woman', *186*
  hereditary, 252, 310, 567–79, E29
  plague, 125, 149–50, 162
  See also sexually transmitted infections
dissection, 209, 211–12, 213–19, 223–4
  and Galen, 99, 104, 211
  in Hellenistic Alexandria, 99
  See also anatomy
divination, 192, 230, *487*, E3
  See also astrology
division of labour, 10, 631, 633–5
divorce, 660
  ancient Greece/Rome, 74–6, 84–5, 87
  and the church, 177, 337
  England/Wales, 597, 601, 602, 606
  and infertility in the Weimar Republic, 465–6
  Islamic law, 664
  and the Kinsey Report, *477*
  and STIs in West Africa, 358
doctors. *See* physicians; surgeons/surgery
Dolly (cloned sheep), E37
domesticity, 415, 485, 627, 635
Donald, Ian, 572
Douglas, James, 322–3
Down syndrome, 568, 570–2, 574–8, *575*
Drummond, Henry, *The Ascent of Man*, 389
Drysdale, Charles Robert, 430, 433, 506
Drysdale, George, 433, 506
  Physical, Sexual and Natural Religion (later *Elements of Social Science*), 430–1

du Coudray, Angélique, 329–30
  Abrégé de l'art des accouchements (Summary of the art of delivering children), *329*
du Mas, Monsieur, 365–6
Dubai, 651, 652
Dubois, Jacques, 210
Duden, Barbara, E23
  The Woman beneath the Skin, 289, 461, 628, 635
Dumas, Jean-Baptiste, 415–19, *416*, *418*
Dun, Finlay, 402
'Durex' condoms, 538, E28
'dying race' theory, 489

eagle-stones, E17
Eakin, Jane, E30
East, Edward, 506
Ebony (magazine), report on sterilization, *607*
economy, 295–8, *297*
  See also industry; '*oeconomia naturae*'; political economy; reproduction, in analysis of wealth
'ectogenesis', 587, 620
Edwards, Robert, 590–3, 608, E38
eggs, 669–70, E16
  analogies, 219–24
  Aristotle on, 43–4, 57, 61
  de Beauvoir on, 632
  chicken, 219–24, *221*
  and cloned frogs, E37
  compared to seed, 61–2
  dissection of, 211, 219–24
  donation, 610–11, 652–4
  Empedocles, 54
  as germ cells, 413–26, 663
  in Hippocrates, 44
  in mythology, xxvi, *656–7*
  ovism, 206, E16
  and pregnancy testing, E32
  sea urchin, 587
  and sexual desire, 311
  Theophrastus on, 61
  wind-eggs, 61–2, 223
  See also animalcules; artificial fertilization; assisted reproduction; in vitro fertilization
Egypt, xxvi, 22, *48*
  Alexandria
    Christian school, 22
    Hellenistic, 114
    medical education in, 99, 105
  ancient iconography (*Book of the Dead of Sesu*), 27, *28*
  ancient mythology, 26–8, *28*, *29*, 32–3, 34–5, 36–7
  fertility figurine, E1
  Mamluk, 134–9
  modern, 485, 493, 495–6, 643, 651
  Ottoman, 271, 273–4
  Roman, E7
Ehrenreich, Barbara, *Witches, Midwives, and Nurses*, 5–7, *8*, 320
Ehrlich, Paul R., 446
  Population Bomb, xxvii, 517, *518*
  and *Z.P.G.*, E36
Eisenstadt v. Baird (US), 539, 602
Eliot, George, 386
Ellis, Havelock, 9
embryo hooks, 272, 323, 546, E6
embryo transfer, 412, 581, 587–91, *589*, 595
embryogenesis, 417, *418*
embryology
  de Beauvoir and, 631
  communication of, *479*, E23, E34
  in Darwin, 386
  early modern, 219, 282–3, 291
  Embriologia sacra (Sacred embryology), 326
  and fertilization, 417, 424
  and frog clones, E37
  Geoffroy's studies, 381
  Heape on, 587
  Hippocratic, 98
  and human origins, 381
  images, *418*, *479*, *591*, E23, E34
  medieval, 171, 196–8, 201, 203, 206
  modern, 283, 386, 413, 417, 567, 620, 663, E37, E38
    making the modern science, 224, 300, 303
  and *Vestiges*, 384–5, *384*
  wax models, 481
  See also embryos; epigenesis; fetuses; Human Fertilisation and Embryology Acts; Human Fertilisation and Embryology Authority; pre-existence theory
embryos, E23, E34
  ancient terminology, 98
  chick, xxvi, 219–23, *221*, 223–4, 282–3, 382
  embryo transfer, 412, 581, 587–91, *589*, 595
  freezing, 641
  frog, *418*
  human, *591*, E23
  mangrove, *487*
  'permitted', 595
  research on, 591, 594–5, 606, 608–9
  'spare', 594
  See also embryology; fetuses; in vitro fertilization

embryotomy. *See* fetal excision
emmenagogues/menstrual regulators, 161–2, 235, 480–1, 500, 536–8, *537*, *540*, 599
Empedocles, 54
Encyclopaedia Britannica, 299
Encyclopédie (Diderot and d'Alembert), 290, 298
endocrinology, 521
Engelmann, George Julius, *Labor Among Primitive Peoples*, *491*, 492
Engels, Friedrich, *The Origin of the Family, Private Property and the State*, 4–5, 7, 633–4
English, Deirdre, *Witches, Midwives, and Nurses*, 5–7, *8*
Enki and the World Order (Sumerian hymn), 28–30, 33–4
Enlightenment, 11, 127, 294, 305, 321, 376–80, 388–9, E19
  and motherhood, 324, 327, 330–1, 332, 555, *556*, 668, E19
  and population, 333, 668
ensoulment. *See* soul
environmentalism, 502, 507–9, 517–19, *518*, E36
epidemiological transition, 443
epigenesis, 251–2, 291
epigenetics, 579, E39
episiotomy, 159
Erasistratus, 99
erotic art/writing, 294, 378, 380, 481, E12
  See also pornography
Esquire (magazine), *544*
estrogen. *See* oestrogen
'Ethiopians', 143, 363–4
eugenic abortions, 569
eugenics, 10, 180, 393, 464, 501
  animal breeding, 397–412, *404*
  and Aristotle, 72–3
  and birth control, 438
  and colonialism, 490, 497
  and neo-Malthusianism, 432–3, 514
  and Plato, 68–72, *69*
  and population control, 514–15
  See also hereditary disease; heredity; population
Eugenics Record Office (UK), 405
European Court of Human Rights, 610
European Fertility Project, 449
European Union, 610
Eve, 291, 557–8, E25
  See also Adam and Eve
evolution, 375–6, 386–9, 586, 628
  See also Darwin, Charles
experience. *See* knowledge
experimenta, 181–93, *186*, *192*
exposure, infant, 70, 73, 75, 109, 118
Fabrici d'Acquapendente, Girolamo, 204
  De formatione ovi et pulli (On the formation of the egg and chick), 219–20, *221*
  De formato foetu (On the formed fetus), E15
Falcucci, Niccolò, *Practica*, 166
fallopian tubes, 457, 463, E16
  ligation, 535, 543–6, *545*
Fallopius, Gabriele, E16
family, 666
  in classical antiquity, 74–5, 81–94, *82*, *86*, *90*, *92*
  and colonialism, 486–8
  history of the, 7–9
  Linnaeus's, 317–18
  new forms, 581, 638–9, 666
  nuclear, 487, *498–9*, 581, 621, 666, E27
  resemblance, 46, 104, 126, 182, 241–52, *242*, *243*, 424, E33
  traits, 241–52, *242*, *243*
  See also household systems
Family Law Reform Act 1987 (England/Wales), 606
family planning. *See* contraception
Family Planning Association (UK), 437, 438
Farley, John, 414
Farr, William, 393
Fasciculus medicinae (Bundle of medical treatises) (pseud. Johannes de Ketham), 185–7, *186*
fascism, 436
  See also Germany; National Socialism
fathers/fatherhood, E19
  in ancient Rome, 83–8, 90–1
  ancient writing on, 54
  duties of, E27
  hereditary material, 422, 423, 426
  Islamic commentaries, 135–6
  in the labour room, 563
  Linnaeus as, 317–18
  in mythology, 27, 28–30, 34, 35–6, 37–8
  'need for' in IVF, 595, 610
  presentation of baby to, 159, *175*
  resemblance of children, 241–52, *243*
  sperm donation, 583–4, 586–7, 595, 608
  See also adoption; paternity; resemblance, family; semen/seeds
Fausto-Sterling, Anne, 635
fear of pregnancy, 624
female semen, 132, *140*, 198–9, 203–6
femininity, 421, 635
feminism, xxvii, 4–5, 10, 282, 288–9, 502
  and assisted reproduction, 593–4
  and gender and identity, 622, 623–4, 627–39
  and history of women's medicine, 161–2
  law and reform, 597, 601, 602–6

and marriage, 630–1
and masturbation, 615–18, *617*
and modernity, 627–39
and neo-Malthusianism, 432
and reproduction, 627–39, *632*, *634*
and STIs, 445, 456
and technology, 440, 530, 533, 564, 565, 638, 645
See also Our Bodies, Ourselves
Feminist International Network of Resistance to Reproductive Technologies and Genetic Engineering (FINRRAGE), 593–4
Fénelon, François, 292–4
Fernel, Jean, *Physiologia*, 139–40, *140*, 204
fertility, 637
and AI, 410–12
Egyptian figurine, E1
enhancement of, 161–3
and household systems, 347–60
male, 25–38
and political arithmetic, 263–5, 266
regulation of services, 606–11, *609*
and STIs, 443–56, *447*, *455*
See also birth-rate
Fertility Census (1911) (UK), 359–60, 446, *448*
Fertility Clinic Success Rate and Certification Act (1992) (US), 610
fertility transitions, 14, 347, 446–51, 667–8
fertilization
sperm, role of, 413–26
See also in vitro fertilization
fetal excision (embryotomy), 160, 172, *173*, E6
See also caesarean section
fetal origins of adult disease, E39
'fetal patient', 502, 565
fetuses
anatomical images, E15, E23
ancient theories of development
early Christian, 109–21
Galenic, 97–105
Hippocratic, 43–4, 47, 50
in archaeological find, *173*
in consumer culture, 669
early modern anatomy, 209–24
formed/unformed, 167–80
medieval and early modern images, *117*, *276*, E10, E15
medieval and early modern Islamic theories, 131–9, 275
Nilsson's photographs, 567, E34
in obstetrics, 559, E6
personhood, 502
prenatal diagnosis, 567–79
See also abortion; embryos; soul
Feversham Committee (on AI), 606
fillets, *322*, 323
film, *447*, 641, E36
Finkbine, Sherri, 570
Fioravanti, Leonardo, *Capricci medicinali* (Medical caprices), 188–9
Firestone, Shulamith, *The Dialectic of Sex*, 633, *634*, 637
Fischberg, Michaïl, E37
Fischer-Dueckelmann, Anna, *The Wife as the Family Physician*, *469*
Fol, Hermann, *425*
follicles, Graafian, E16
Food and Agriculture Organization (FAO), 512
Food and Drug Administration (FDA) (US), 530, 539, *540*, 549–50, 599, 610
Food for Peace programme, 514
food/diet
and babies/fetuses, 134, 493, E39
and blood, 196–8
dietetics, 310
and disease, 523, E39
and family resemblance, 248–9
and fertility, 460, 468, 487
and generation, 180
non-naturals, 310
and philanthropy, 513–14
and population, 284, 343, 349, 506–7, 512–13, 515
and pregnancy, 50, 452n31
and radical moisture, 198–9
See also milk
forceps, 320, 321–4, *322*
Ford Foundation, 10, 501, 513, 590
Fores, Samuel, E22
Forman, Simon, 227–40
Fortpflanzung, 291, 299–300
fostering, 358, 468, 664
See also adoption
Foucault, Michel, 67, 73, 626
and biopolitics, 9, 10, 333–6, 344, 614, 619, 623–4
The History of Sexuality, 613–15
The Order of Things, 287
'power-knowledge', 9
'repression' of sexuality, 471
Fouillée, Alfred, 633
foundations, philanthropic, 513–17
foundlings/orphans, 270, 338, 339
France
abortion, 164, 549, 569
AI, *15*, 462–3, 582, 583, *584*
assisted reproduction for gay and single people, 651

France (*cont.*)
  Chartres Cathedral, E8
  Code Napoléon, 597
  contraception, 436, 542, 549, 601, E28
  fertility, 444, 506
  generation and reproduction, debates over, 287–304, 364–5, 381, E20, E26
  gouttes de lait (milk depots), 493
  horse breeding, 407
  kin marriage, 403
  maternal deaths, 340–1, *342*
  midwifery, 160, 325, 329–30, *329*, 555
    Lamaze method, 645
  Le monde Parisien (The Parisian world), E26
  Paris Academy of Sciences, 381
  pharmaceutical companies, 527, 549–50
  plague, 150
  and population, 146–8, 148–9, 149–50, 339, *390–1*
    demography, 343, 347, 350–2, 354, 446
Frankenstein (Shelley), 427–8
Freedman, Estelle, E35
Friday, Nancy, *My Secret Garden*, 617
frogs, 417, *418*, *420*, E32, E37
Fromm, Julius, E28
Fuchs, Fritz, 569

Gadelrab, Sherry, 130
Gaitskell, Debbie, 495–6
Galen of Pergamum, E15
  generation theories, 95–108, 197
  works
    Anatomical Procedures (*AA*), 96
    On the Anatomy of the Uterus (*Ut. Diss.*), 96
    On the Formation of the Fetus (*Foet. Form.*), 96, 102–3
    On Seed (*Sem.*), 96, 98, 103
    On Simple Drugs, *106*
    On the Usefulness of the Parts (*UP*), 96, 97–100
Galli, Gian (Giovanni) Antonio, 330, E21
Galton, Francis, 404–5, *404*, 410, 432
Gamble, Clarence, 516
Gandhi, Indira, 648–9
Gassendi, Pierre, 205
gay men. *See* homosexuality
Gay, Peter, 483
gender
  division of labour, 10, 631, 633–5
  equality of germ cells in reproduction, 413–26, *425*
  and feminism, 627–39
  and identity, 622–5, *625*
  and sex hormones, 522–6, *524*
  See also one-sex/two-sex models
gender reassignment/transsexuality, 622–3, 624–5, *625*
genealogies, E8
  Burke's Peerage, 399
  racehorse/cattle, 399
  'schizophrenic family', E29
  Tree of Jesse, E8
  See also patrilineal descent
generation
  as cohort, 23, 290–1, 300–2
  as framework, 4, 9–10, 13–14, 20–1, 124–8, 282, 285, 287–90, 659–63
  as keyword, 23, 287–304, *303*
'generation gap', 302
genesis (term), 290
genetic counselling, 501
genetics, 393, 666
  preimplantation genetic diagnosis (PGD), 594
  and race, E30
  See also eugenics; genealogies; hereditary disease; heredity
genitals. *See* cervix; hymen; penises; testes/testicles; vaginas
genocide, *648*, 662
Gentile da Foligno, 166
Geoffrin, Madame, 378
Geoffroy Saint-Hilaire, Étienne, 381–2
Gérard, Jules, 583
  Nouvelles causes de stérilité (New causes of sterility), *15*, *584*
Gerard, St, E40
germ cells, 413–26, *416*, *420*, *425*
  See also eggs; sperm
German measles, 569–70
Germany
  abortion and birth control, xxvii, 434–5, 538, 549, 618, 619, E28
  AI and assisted conception, 583, 651
  customary law, 164n30
  'generation' and 'reproduction', terms for, 291, 299–300
  horse breeding, 407
  hospitals, 330, 462, 463–4
  infertility, 457–8, 461–2, 466–70, *469*
  microscopy, 413–26
  National Socialism, xxvii, *1*, 393, 437, 501, 511, 518–19, E29
  pharmaceutical companies, 527–9
  population, 406, 665
  reaction to cloned frogs, E37
  universities, 145, 187, 251, 283, 381, 413–26

Gessner, Conrad, *Historiae animalium*, E9
gestation, 383–8, *384*
Aristotle on, 65
Ibn Sina on, 132
and the soul, 121
and *Vestiges*, 383–8, *384*
ghurra, 277–9
Giddens, Anthony, 613
Giffard, William, 324
Ginsburg, Faye, 641
globalization, 641–55
godparents, 171–2
Godwin, William, 343
Goethe, Johann Wolfgang von, 381
Goldsmith, Oliver, *History of the Earth and Animated Nature*, 298, 380
gonads. *See* ovaries; testes/testicles
gonorrhoea, 443, 445, 451–2, 453–4, 462
González Laguna, Francisco, 326
Goodyear, Charles, E28
Google Baby (documentary), 641
Gordon, Linda, *Woman's Body, Woman's Right*, 7, 638
Gossaert, Jan, *The Children of Christian II, King of Denmark* (painting), *242*
gouttes de lait (milk depots), 493, *494*
Graaf, Reinier de, 413, 415, 417n18
De mulierum organis, E16
Grant, Robert Edmond, 382–3
Graunt, John, 338
Natural and Political Observations upon the Bills of Mortality, 257–65, *259*, 338
Green, Monica, 161–2
Greer, Germaine, 622
Gregory the Great, 177–9
Gregory of Nyssa, *On the Making of Man*, 115–16
Griswold v. Connecticut (US), 539, 602
guilds, 325, 562
Gumilla, José, 369
Gurdon, John, E37
Gütt, Arthur, E29
gynaecology, *5–6*, 668
medieval and early modern, 184–5, 225
modern, 283, 284, 415, *467*, 525, E31, E32, E34
Ottoman, 271–6, *273*, *274*
and women practitioners, 565
See also experimenta; Hippocratic medicine; Soranus of Ephesus

Hackett, Jo Ann, 25
Hacking, Ian, 262, 344
hadith, 129, 134, 269
Haeckel, Ernst, *The Riddle of the Universe*, 389
Hajnal, John, 349–50
Haldane, J. B. S., 587, 620
Hales, Stephen, *Vegetable Staticks*, 312
Hall, Prescott, 'Immigration restriction and world eugenics', 508
Haller, Albrecht von, 251
Haly Abbas (al-Majusi), 131, 133
Hamilton, Alexander, E22
Hammond, John, 410
hands
and anatomical knowledge, E20
and health advice literature, 468
midwives', *322*, E6
Hanson, Ann Ellis, 46, 50–2
Haraway, Donna, 634–5, 637
Harley, Robert and Edward, E11
Hartlieb, Johann, 185
Harvey, William, 204, 205–7, 210–11, 291, 669, E15, E16
Exercitationes de generatione animalium (Anatomical exercitations concerning the generation of living creatures), xxvi, 206–7, 209, 220–3
Haselden, William, 'Pity the poor mother!' (cartoon), E27
Heape, Walter, 409, 587
The Breeding Industry, 409
heart
Aristotle on, 44
Ibn Sina on, 132
in chick eggs, 222
development of, 102, 206, 223, 275
disease, E39
fetal heart-rate monitors, 564
as symbol, E19
heat
and female bodies, 43, 61–2, 98, 100, 134–5
and fetal/child development, 43, 103–5, 247–8, 250–1
'in heat', 60, 397
innate, 61, 62–3, 195–7, 203, 204–8
and male bodies, 100, 134–5, 215–16
and racial theories, 367
and sexual pleasure, 195–6
Heberden, William, 338
Observations on the Increase and Decrease of Different Diseases …, 340, *341*
Helen of Troy, birth of, xxvi
Helmont, Johann Baptist van, 204, 205
Helms amendment (US), 547–8, 605
Henry, Louis, 347, 449–51

herbals, *60*, *158*
hereditary disease, 252, 402–5
  and AI, 586
  albinism, 364–6, *365*
  Linnaeus on, 310
  and prenatal diagnosis, 567–79
  'schizophrenic family', E29
heredity, 302, 402–5, 424
  and chromosomes, 568, 569, 570–2, *571*, *575*, 576–7
  family traits, 241–52, *242*, *243*
  germ cells as carriers of, 419–26
  and human varieties, 368–73, E30
  See also eugenics; genealogies; genetics; hereditary disease; livestock breeding
hermaphrodites, 174
  hyenas, E9
Herodotus, 58
Herophilus, 99–100
heterosexuality, 70, 666
  and adoption, E33
  and IVF, 595, 608
  and Linnaeus, 306, 309
  in mythology, 34, 35–6
  and surrogacy law, 654
Heyne-Heeren, Wilhelmine, 461
HFEA. *See* Human Fertilisation and Embryology Authority
Hidaya, 269–70, 277–8
Hildegard of Bingen, *117*
Himes, Norman, 7
Hippocratic medicine, 21, 39–52, *40*, *51*, 195–6
  treatises
    Airs, Waters, Places, 339
    Barrenness (*Mul. 3*), 47
    Diseases of Women 1 (*Mul. 1*), 42–3, 46, 52, 196
    Epidemics, 42
    Fleshes, 47
    Oath, 47, *48*
    On Ancient Medicine, 43
    On Generation/Nature of the Child (*Genit./Nat. puer.*), 41, 43–7, 98, 105, 195–6
    Physician, 47
    Regimen, 196
The Hite Report, 617
Hittites, 32
HIV/AIDS, E28
  and AI, 586
Hobbes, Thomas, *Leviathan*, 254–5, *256*
Hodges, William, E24
Hodgson, Jane, E32
Holweg, Walter, 528
home birth, 480, 555, 566, 645, 668
home pregnancy tests, 478
homosexuality, 4, 392, 427, 428, 441, 614, 638
  and assisted reproduction, 581, 595
  defences of, 428
  Ellis on, 9
  epistemology of the closet, 484
  and identity, 623
  and law, 433, 597, 602, 603, 625
  and marriage, 666
  in Linnaeus, 306, 307
  and *Our Bodies, Ourselves*, *617*, E35
hooks, embryo, 272, 323, 546, E6
Hoover, Edgar M., 449, *450*
Horace, 92–3
'horary' astrology, 228
hormone replacement therapy (HRT), 529–31
hormones. *See* sex hormones
Horne, Jan van, E16
'horned' uterus, 100, *101*, *214*, 218–19
horoscopes. *See* astrology
horse breeding, 59, 399, 407
Horse Breeding Act 1918 (UK), 407
hospitals
  childbirth in, 160, 284, 330–1, 553–66, *556*, *558*, *561*, *565*, 643–6
  lying-in, 284, 330–1, 340–1, *341*, 554, 555–9, *556*, 643, E21
household systems, marriage and fertility in, 347–60
Howell, Lillian Lincoln, 590
Huarte de San Juan, Juan, 246–9
human embryonic stem cells, 594
Human Fertilisation and Embryology Acts (UK)
  1990, 594, 608
  2008, 595, 610
Human Fertilisation and Embryology Authority (HFEA) (UK), 608–9, *609*
humanism, 140, 145, 247, 254, 255, E13
humanitarianism, 497, 505, 506, 514–15
Humboldt, Alexander von, *Essai politique sur le royaume de la Nouvelle-Espagne* (Political essay on the Kingdom of New Spain), 372
humour, sexual, *236*, 309, E12
humours, 195–7, 198, 361
Hunt, Nancy Rose, 643
Hunter, John, 582
Hunter, William, 323, 324
Huth, Alfred, *Marriage of Near Kin*, 405
Huxley, Aldous, *Brave New World*, 395, 582, 587
Huxley, Julian, 410, 512–13, 514–15
Huxley, Thomas Henry, 386
  Evidence as to Man's Place in Nature, 386

hybrids, *64*, 65–6, E2
  human under colonialism, 367–73, 374, 490
  human–ape through AI, 585
  plant, 312, 315
Hyde amendment (US), 605
hydra. *See* polyps
hydria (water jug), E2
hyenas, E9
hylomorphism, 197, 198, 203
hymen, 462
hysterical woman, in Foucault, 614

Ibn Hajar al-ʿAsqalani, 137, 139
Ibn Ilyas (Mansur), *Mansur's Anatomy* (*Tashrih-i Mansuri*), 275
Ibn Kathir, 137
Ibn al-Nafis, 131, 134–5, 137, 139
Ibn Nujaym, 274
Ibn Qayyim al-Jawziyya, 137–9
  Commentary on the Oaths of the Quran, 137–8
Ibn al-Quff, 135–7, 139
Ibn Sallum, 275–6
Ibn Sina (Avicenna), 131–4, 139, 170, 205, 271, 661
  Canon of Medicine, 130, 131, 132, 198–9, 201
  Healing, 131–2, 133
  on radical moisture, 198–9, 201
Ibn Taymiyya, 134
identity, 11
  and gender, 622–5, *625*
  and knowledge, 481–4
  occupational/professional/disciplinary, 157, 300, 555–6
  politics of, 624
ignorance
  men's, 182, 473
  midwives', 320, 324, 491–3
  modern, 471–84
  with respect to science, 663
  women's, 5, 46, 85, 233, 473, 493
ʿilm, 131
imagery, water, 26, 30–2
imagination, 363, 401
  and *Aristotle's Masterpiece*, E25
  and family resemblance, 126, 241, 248–52
  and health of offspring, 176, 180
imaging. *See* visualization technologies
Imberti, Antoni, 162
immigration/migration, 4, 257, 261, 263–4, 302, 353, 502, 507–9
  after World War II, 665, E30
  and colonialism, 361, 362, 406, 486–8, 489
  and the Ottoman Empire, 268
imperialism, 13, 485–97
  See also ancient Rome; Ottoman Empire; Persian Empire
implants, contraceptive, 542–3
impotence, E12
in vitro fertilization (IVF), 299, 470, 502, 581–2, 587–93, *591*, *592*, 593–6, 620–1
  and globalization, 650–4, *653*
  regulation, 606–11, *609*
inbreeding/in-and-in breeding, 402–5
  See also kin/cousin marriage
incest, 179
  Aristotle on, 59
  See also kin/cousin marriage
India, 485
  abandonment of mixed-race children, 368
  abortion, 359
  adoption, 651
  colonialism, 486–7, 494, 497, 643
  family planning/population control, 4, 449, *450*, 506–7, 513, 518, 545–6, 619, 642, 646–9, *648*
  hospital birth, 643, 645
  household systems, 355–6
  IVF, 650, 651, 652
  surrogacy, 654
industry/industrialization, 11, 298, 299, 628–9, 630
  in biomedicine, 500, 503, 602
  breeding, 397–412, 585–6, 588
  contraceptive manufacturing, 535–51, E28
  fears about, 586
  pharmaceutical, *12*, 521–34
  physiocrats on, 295–8, *297*
  pornography, 618
  reproductive biomedicine, 593–5, 610–11, 620–1, 650–4
  and sexual knowledge, 471–84
  STIs, effect on, 452
  surrogacy, 654
  See also artificial fertilization; livestock breeding; pharmaceutical companies
Infant Life (Preservation) Act 1929 (England/Wales), 601–2
infant mortality, 338–40, *341*, *342*, E39
  ancient Rome, 86
  and household systems, 355
infanticide, 68–70, 76, 154
  in ancient Greece/Rome, *75*, 76
  as capital offence, 164
  in China, 356
  and early Christianity, 114, 119
  infant exposure, 109, 118
  in Japan, 356–7, 667

infertility, 394–5, 668
in ancient Greece, 50, 52
in ancient Rome, 85, 88–93
in historical writing, 14, 460
in medieval and early modern Europe, 162–3, 184–5, 191, 235–8, 261–71, 275, 279
modern, 457–70, *459*, *469*, 587–93, 593–5, 606–11, 650–4
See also in vitro fertilization
injections, contraceptive, 542
innate heat, 44, 62–3, 128, 195–7, 203, 204–8
Innes, Joanna, 263
inoculation. *See* vaccination/inoculation
intellectual property, 528, 529
International Conference on Population Control and Development (Cairo, 1994), 515, 516, 642, 649
International Federation of Neo-Malthusian Leagues, 431
International Malthusian League, 432
International Neo-Malthusian Conference (1922), *439*
International Planned Parenthood Federation, *510*, 514
International Union for the Scientific Investigation of Population Problems, 511
internationalism, 506–7, 514
intersex, 66, 622, 636
See also hermaphrodites
intrauterine devices (IUDs), 535, 541–3, *542*, 551, 648
intracytoplasmic sperm injection (ICSI), 594, 595
Iran
assisted reproduction in, 651
See also Persian Empire
Isidore of Seville, 124
Islam, 124, 129–30, 269, 270, 277, 664, 667
and adoption, 270, 651, 664
commentaries, 129–40, *136*, *140*, 203, 269, 270, 277
and IVF, 651
law/regulation, 126, 267–79
legitimacy/illegitimacy, 664
and medicine, 129–40, 271–6
and the soul, 134–9
and twins, 271
two-seed concept, 133, 137–9, 275
See also Ottoman Empire
Israel, 651
Itaki, Şemseddin, *The Anatomy of the Body* (*Tashrih-i abdan*), 274–5
Italian Books of Secrets Database, 189
Ivanov, Il'ya Ivanovich, 585–6

Jacob, François, *La logique du vivant* (*The Logic of Life*), 9, 282, 287–8, 414
Jacobs, Aletta, 431, 434
James, William, 375
Japan, 356–7, 359, 489, 667
Jefferson, Thomas, 373
Jerome, on ensoulment, 114, 116, 118
Jews/Judaism, 118, 126, 165n39, 245, E7
Aztecs as descendants, 362–3
and heredity, 248
and IVF, 651
in the Ottoman Empire, 268, 271, 278
See also Bible
John Chrysostom, 113
Johnson, Virginia, 615, *616*, 624
Jordanova, Ludmilla, 289, 627
Joubert, Laurent, 191
Journal of Reproduction and Fertility, 300
Julian of Eclanum, 116–18
Julian (Roman emperor), 105
Junkmann, Karl, 528
Justinian (Roman emperor), *82*, 664

Kant, Immanuel, 367, 372
Karman, Harvey, 547
Keber, Ferdinand, 423
Kehrer, Ferdinand, 462, 466
Kertbeny, Karl-Maria, 428
Ketham, Johannes de. *See Fasciculus medicinae*
Key, Adriaen Thomasz, *Family Portrait* (painting), *243*
Khamenei, Ayatollah, 651
Khayr al-Din, 278
kin/cousin marriage, 177–9, *178*, 402–5, *404*
King, Gregory, 263–4
King, Helen, 216
Kinsey, Alfred, 615
Sexual Behavior in the Human Female, *477*, 624
kinship, 13–14, 81, 93, 190, 356, 359, 629–30
See also family; lineage; marriage
al-Kirmani, Nafis ibn ʿIwad, 135, *136*, 137
Knaus, Hermann, E31
knowledge
and modern ignorance, 471–84
natural, 127
science, claim to monopoly on, 394, 476, 663
through sight, 209
visual and haptic, 329–30, E21
Knowlton, Charles, *Fruits of Philosophy*, 428, 430
Knox, Robert, *The Races of Men*, 374
Koeck, Christian, E23
Kreager, Philip, 67, 72

laboratories, 3, 394, 615, 662
  and artificial fertilization, 581–2, 588–93, 595
  and biology, 388
  and cloning frogs, E37
  in the Enlightenment, *280–1*, E20
  and livestock breeding, 502
  in obstetrics, 559–60
  and pregnancy testing, E32
  regulation, 610
  and sex hormones, 522–6, *524*, 527–9, 531, 533, 534
  Wassermann test, 446
  and WHO, 548
Laboratory of Molecular Biology, Cambridge, E37
lactation, 189, E17
  and agriculture, 409–10
  See also milk
Lallemand, Claude François, 422–3
Lamarck, Jean-Baptiste, 298, 382–3
Lamaze, Fernand, 563, 645
The Lancet, 381
Lancilotto, Nicola, 368
Lange, Johannes, E29
Laqueur, Ernst, 527
Laqueur, Thomas, *Making Sex*, 11, 130, 216, 413
law/regulation, 667–8
  Abortion Act 1967 (Britain), 501, 602–3
  adoption, E33
  Augustan marriage
    lex Iulia, 88–9, 92–3
    lex Papia Poppaea, 88–9
  Code Napoléon, 597
  Commons Act 1908 (England/Wales), 407
  Comstock Laws 1873 (US), 431, 434, 538, 599, *600*, 602, E28
  Contagious Diseases Acts (England), 445
  Fertility Clinic Success Rate and Certification Act (1992) (US), 610
  Gender Recognition Act 2004 (UK), 622
  Horse Breeding Act 1918 (UK), 407
  Human Fertilisation and Embryology Acts (UK)
    1990, 594, 608
    2008, 595, 610
  Infant Life (Preservation) Act 1929 (England/Wales), 601–2
  Islamic, 126, 267–79
  Lord Ellenborough's Act 1803 (UK), 428–9, 598
  Marriage (Same Sex Couples) Act 2013 (UK), 625
  Matrimonial Causes Act 1857 (England/Wales), 597
  medieval, 170–1, 174–6
  modern, 597–611
  New Poor Law (1834, England/Wales), 430
  Offences Against the Person Act 1861 (England/Wales), 598
  Roman, 81–94, 174–6
  Unborn Children (Protection) Bill 1985 (England/Wales), 608
Lawrence, William, *Lectures on … the Natural History of Man*, 366, 403
League of National Life (UK), 436
League of Nations, 509–12
  See also United Nations
League for the Protection of Mothers (Bund für Mutterschutz), 433
Leavitt, Judith, 324–5, 331
Leclerc, Georges-Louis, Comte de Buffon. *See* Buffon
Leda, xxvi, *656–7*, E2
'Leechcraft' collection, 187–8
Leeuwenhoek, Antonie van, 223, 413, E16
legitimacy/illegitimacy, 606
  in ancient Greece, 81, 93–4
  and colonialism, 368–9, 664
  and family resemblance, 243, 244, 249
  Foucault on, 613
  and Islamic law, 664
  middle ages, 153, 235
  and nuptiality valve, 353–4
  in Ottoman Empire, 268, 270
  Roman, 71, 83–4, 86–9, 93–4
  See also paternity
Legitimation League, 433
Leiras Oy, 543
lekythoi, *45*
Lemnius, Levinus, *Occulta naturae miracula* (Secret miracles of nature), 181–2
Leonardo da Vinci, *656–7*
leprosy, 177, 363
lesbians. *See* homosexuality
Lesthaeghe, Ron, 350, 358
Lévi-Strauss, Claude, *The Elementary Structures of Kinship*, 636
Levine, Baruch, 37
lex Iulia, 88–9, 92–3
lex Papia Poppaea, 88–9
Life (magazine), *xxxvi–1*, E34
lifespan, 199
Ligue de la régénération humaine (League for Human Regeneration), 431
Lillie, F. R., 595
lineage, 126
  Tree of Jesse, E8
  See also genealogies; heredity; legitimacy; patrilineal descent

Linnaeus, Carl, 283, 305–18
on albinos, 365
Lapland journal, *316*
marriage/family, 317–18
sexual system, 283, 305–10, *308*, 318
works
Adonis Uplandicus, 307, *308*
Diaeta naturalis, 310–11
Genera plantarum, 316–17
Generatio ambigena, 311–12, *313*
Musa Cliffortiana, 314, *315*
Species plantarum, 317
Systema naturae, 305–6, 307–9, 318, 367
Linnaeus, Carl the Younger, 318
literacy, 41–2, 148, 182, 394
livestock breeding, 21, 397–412, 502, 582–3, 585–6, 588, *589*
Livi Bacci, Massimo, 352
Loeb, Jacques, 587
Lombard, Peter, *Four Books of the Sentences*, 142–3, 145, 147, 151
London Rubber Company, 538, E28
Lonie, Iain, 42, 43
Lopes, Odoardo, 363
Lord Ellenborough's Act 1803 (UK), 428–9, 598
Lord, Perceval, *Popular Physiology*, 382
Lotto, Lorenzo, *Venus and Cupid* (painting), E12
Louise Wise Services, E33
love magic, 162, E12
Lovejoy, Arthur O., *The Great Chain of Being*, 309, 375
Lucretius
De rerum natura, 375
on ensoulment, 116
Lull, Raymond, 201
Luque de Soria, Manuel, E26
luxury, and depopulation, 337
lying-in, 159–60, *159*, 562
and birth girdles, E11
hospitals, 284, 330–1, 340–1, *341*, 554, 555–7, *556*, 557–9, 643, E21
See also home birth

McCormick, Katharine Dexter, 539
machines
midwifery, E21
women as, 290
See also industry/industrialization
Maclean, Ian, 203
magic
fertility, 162
love, 162, E12
See also amulets; birth girdles; charms
Maine, Henry, *Ancient Law*, 629, 630
al-Majusi (Haly Abbas), 131, 133
Malpighi, Marcello, 223–4, 363
malpresentation, in childbirth, 159, 325, E10
See also childbirth, obstructed
Malthus, Thomas Robert, 7, 299, 300, 333, 444, 506–9, 662
effect of marriage practices on population, 348–50, 359–60
and the English poor law, 354
Essay on the Principle of Population, 284–5, 342–3, 348–9, 427, 506, E24
See also neo-Malthusians
Malthusian couple, in Foucault, 614–15
Malthusian League, 430
'Malthusian moment', 648–9
man-midwifery, 283–4, 319–32, 555–6, E21
Man-Midwifery Dissected (Blunt), E22
'mannequins' (in midwifery), E21
Mannheim, Karl, 'Das Problem der Generationen' (The problem of generations), 302
Manningham, Richard, E21
Mansur (Ibn Ilyas), *Mansur's Anatomy* (*Tashrih-i Mansuri*), 275
manufacturing. *See* industry/industrialization
Manuli, Paola, 49
manuscripts, and print, 127, 181–93
Mapondé, 364–5, *365*
Marcuse, Max, 468
al-Marghinani, Burhan al-Din, 269–70
Hidaya, 269–70, 277–8
marital debt, 125, 177
Marland, Hilary, 320, 496
marriage
ancient, 4, 74–6, 81–94, *86*
Aristotle on, 72–3, 146
Plato on, 68–72
and the church, 22, 125–6, 142–3, 167–8, 236, 242
and colonialism, 486–8
and feminism, 630–1
and gender, 625
and household systems, 347–60
and ideal age, 143, 146
kin/cousin, 177–9, *178*, 179, 402–5, *404*
laws on, 597, 667–8
Augustan, 88–9, 92–3
Islamic, 126, 268–70, 277
Linnaeus on, 317–18

Malthus on, 348–50, 359–60
Mongol, 144
Nicholas of Vaudémont on, 147–8
origins of, 9
and race, 373
same sex, 440, 625, 638–9
See also registration (births/marriages/deaths)
Marriage (Same Sex Couples) Act 2013 (UK), 625
Marsh, Margaret, 466
Marshall, Francis, 409–10
Physiology of Farm Animals, 409–10
Physiology of Reproduction, 300
Martin, Emma, 381–2
Masaccio, Tomasso, *155*
masculinity, 30, 584, E12
Masters, William, 615, *616*, 624
masturbating child, in Foucault, 614–15
masturbation, 26–8, 422–3, 583, 614–15, 615–18, *616*, *617*
matching, adoption, E33
maternal and child/infant welfare, 393, *479*, 485, 494–6, 562–3, 643–6, E27
See also infant mortality; maternal mortality; mothercraft
maternal impression. *See* imagination
maternal mortality, 154, 340–1, *341*, *342*, 355, 392–3, 500, 646, *647*
and hospital births, 554, 558, 561, 563
maternalism, E27
Mathieu, Nicole-Claude, 636
Matrimonial Causes Act 1857 (England/Wales), 597
Mattioli, Pietro Andrea, E17
Maupertuis, Pierre Louis de, 294, 364–5
Dissertation physique à l'occasion du nègre blanc (Physical dissertation occasioned by the white negro), 364
Vénus physique (Physical Venus), 364–5, 378
Maximus the Confessor, *On Difficulties in the Church Fathers*, 115–16
May, Elaine Tyler, 466
Meaux (France), 148–9
medical encounters, 46–8, 153–66, 225–40, 457–70, 471–84, E25
images of, *8*, *104*, *158*, *159*, *175*, *226*, *229*, *236*, *273*, *328*, *491*, *547*, *644*, E10, E25
'medicalization', 5, 491, 554, 557–60, 566, 644, 645–6, *647*, 668
Menkin, Miriam, 588
Mensinga, Wilhelm, 431, 434
menstruation, 44, 49–50, 98, 177, 238–9, 238, 660, E7, E14
and birth control, 536–8
calendars, 125, E14, E31
emmenagogues/menstrual regulators, 161–2, 235, 480–1, 500, 536–8, *537*, *540*, 599
See also female semen; *syllēpsis*
mercantilism, 298, 327
Merchant, Carolyn, *The Death of Nature*, 289
Mesopotamia, 28–30, *31*, 33–4, 35, 36, 37, E3
Messalina, 83
metaphors/analogies, 196, 662, E7, E17, E18, E36
in ancient Greece, 41, 42–6, 52, 53, 54–5, *55*, 61, 132, 196
Buffon's, to gravity, 295, E20
in demography, to bird territories, 351
early modern, 209–24
Harvey's, 220–2
in Islamic medicine, between formation of semen and milk, 137
lamp of life, 198
marriage in Linnaean botany, 307, 309
menstruation as 'flowers', E14
newborns moulded like wax, 72
between sperm and animals, 419, 426
between state and individual, 255
traits 'poured' between generations, 245
Metellus Macedonicus, Quintus, 83–4
microscopy, 223–4, 413, 415–19, 669–70, E16, E26
midwifery, 10, 12, *104*, 668
birthing chairs, *104*, E18
colonial, 491–3
man-, 283–4, 319–32, 555–6, 644, E21, E22
middle ages, 148–9, 154–6, 157–62, *158*, 320
modern, 319–32, 555–7, 560, 645
Ottoman Empire, 272
Roman Empire, 157, 320
Der Rosengarten (The rose garden) (Rösslin), 327, *328*, *672–3*, E10, E18
mifepristone (RU486), 549
migration. *See* immigration/migration
Mij, Hieronymus van der, *Family Group with a Mother Feeding Her Children* (painting), E19
milk
and breast-feeding, 105, 493, E19
breeding of dairy cattle, 406, 409, 410–12, *411*, 586
cow's, for babies, 493, *494*
formula, 502
gouttes de lait (milk depots), 493, *494*
Ibn al-Nafis on, 134–5, 137
See also lactation
Milk Marketing Board (UK), 410
Millett, Kate, 622

Milne-Edwards, Henri, 422–3
Minotaur (on water jug), E2
miracles, 163–4, 181–2, 593, E38
Mirena, 542
miscarriage, 169, 237, 459, E14
  and amniocentesis, 570
  amulets/recipes to prevent, 191, E17
  caused by fear, 278
  in Islamic law, 278–9
  Pliny the Younger on, 85–6
  See also abortion; stillborn children
misoprostol, 549–50
missionaries, 486, 487, 492–3, 495, 496, 643–4, 654–5, E24, E40
Mizauld, Antoine, 190
models
  crystal womb, E21
  wax, 330, 466–8, 481
modernity
  control as hallmark of, 666–9
  infertility in, 457–70
  and reproduction, 627–39
  and sexuality, 613–15
modernization theory, 449
modesty, 228–30, 321, 331, 536, E25
Moerbeke, William of, 145
Moheau, Jean-Baptiste, *Recherches et considérations sur la population de la France* (Research and considerations on the population of France), 339–40, 339
Mohr, James, *Abortion in America*, 10
molecules
  Buffon's organic, 295, *296*, 378–80, E20
  typified by hormones, 534
Le monde Parisien (The Parisian world), E26
Mondino de Liuzzi, 212
Money, John, 622
Mongolia, marriage in, 144
Mongols, 143–4
monogamy, 9, 59, 307, 309, 358, 488
'monster of Cracow', E13
monstrous births. *See* deformities/disabilities/monsters
Montesquieu, Charles-Louis de Secondat, Baron, 336–7
  Persian Letters, 333
Montyon, Antoine Auget de, 339
moon, E3, E14
Moore, Hugh, xxvii, 514
Moraea, Sara Lisa (wife of Linnaeus), 317–18
Morandi, Anna, 330
Morgan, Lewis Henry, 7–9
Morris, Sir William, 445
Morrison, Robert, 140
Morrow, Prince, 445
mortality
  bills of, 259, 263, 339
  See also infant mortality; maternal mortality
Morton Anderson, Charles, 488
mothercraft, and colonialism, 494–6, *495*
motherhood, 415, 421, 433, 491–6, 496–7, 563, E27
  and Egyptian goddesses, 25–38
  in the Enlightenment, 324, 327, 330–1, 332, 555–6, 668, E19
  genetic/gestational, 593
  as goal of women's existence, 421
  'safe', 646, *647*
  scientific, 464
  and the left, 437
  modern, 433, *515*
  See also surrogacy
mothers
  children taking status of (Virginia), 373
  goddesses in ancient Near East and Egypt, 25–38
  as needing information, 473, *479*
  slave, 270, 325–6, 485–6
  See also maternal and child/infant welfare; maternal mortality
Mudie, Robert, *Man, His Physical Structure and Adaptations*, 383
Mukerjee, Radhakamal, 506
mules, 65
Muller, Hermann, 410, 586
Müller, Johannes, 421–2
Müller-Wille, Staffan, 424
multitude. *See* population
Muniz, Vik, *656–7*
Musallam, Basim, 129–30
Muscio, *101*, 107, E10
museums, 466–8, 475, 481, E17
Musonius Rufus, 84–5
Mussolini, Benito, 436
mythology
  ancient Greece, 39–41
  ancient Near East and Egypt, 25–38

Napier, Richard, 227–40, *232*
nation-states, 67–8, 253, 284, 333, 597, 642, 655
  See also population
National Alliance for the Growth of the French Population (Alliance nationale pour l'accroissement de la population française), *390–1*, 431

National Birth Control Association (UK), 437
National Birthday Trust Fund (UK), 562
National Childbirth Trust (UK), 563
national herd, 405–7
National Institute for Medical Research (London), 411, 586
National Institute for Research in Dairying (Reading), 409
National Socialism, xxvii, *1*, 393, 437, 501, E29
natural childbirth, 563, 645
'natural fertility', 347, *348*, 359
natural history
  Buffon, 294, *296*, 378–80, E20
  of man, 362
  Pliny the Elder, 54, 57, 65–6, 83
natural particulars, 127, 227
natural selection, 284, 386
Nazism. *See* National Socialism
Needham, John Turberville, E20
Nelson, Gaylord, 541
neoliberalism, 500, 502, 605, 610
Neo-Malthusian League (Nieuw-Malthusiaansche Bond), 431
neo-Malthusians, 392, 427–32, *439*, 506–11
neoliberalism, 605, 610
Neoplatonism, 110, 112
  Porphyry, 112, 113, 114
The Netherlands, E19
  childbirth, 554
  colonialism, 361, 492–3
  midwifery, 492–3, 645
  neo-Malthusianism, 431, 506
  pharmaceutical companies, *12*, 527
Newsholme, Sir Arthur, 445
newspapers, 381, 468, *540*, *585*, E27, E38
Nicholas of Vaudémont, 147–8
Nicolaus of Damascus, 60
Nielsen, Folmer, 410
Nietzel, Dietrich, 314
Nieuw-Malthusiaansche Bond (Neo-Malthusian League), 431
Nightingale, Florence, 559
Nilsson, Lennart, 567, E34
  A Child Is Born, E34
Noeggerath, Emil, 462
non-governmental organizations (NGOs), 516–17
non-invasive prenatal testing (or screening) (NIPT/NIPS), 577
non-naturals, 310–11
Norplant, 542–3
Notestein, Frank, 447–9, 512
nuchal translucency, 574, *575*
nuptiality valve, 350–5, 359–60
Nuremburg Chronicle, *200*
nurses, *18–19*, 70, 433–4, *479*, 557, 559, 591, *592*, *644*, E32
  wet, 157, 337, E19, E32
nutrition. *See* breast-feeding; food/diet; milk

Oakley, Ann, 554, 622
obesity, 460, E39
obstetrics, *5–6*, 553–66, 668
  See also caesarean section; midwifery; prenatal diagnosis; technologies
Oceania, STIs in, 451–2
'*oeconomia naturae*', and Linnaeus, 312, 314
oestrogen, *12*, 524, 527
  DES, 532–3, *532*
  HRT, 529–31
Offences Against the Person Act 1861 (England/Wales), 598
Office of Population Research (Princeton), 7, 447–50, 512
one-sex/two-sex models, 11, 130, 215–16, *217*, 414
oocyte/egg donation, 595, 610–11, 652
'Operation Lawsuit', 606
Oresme, Nicole, 145–7
organic molecules (Buffon), 295, *296*, 378–80, E20
Organon, *12*, 527
orgasm, 26–7, 132, 460, 615–18, *616*, *617*
Oribasius, 105–7
Origen, on ensoulment, 115, 116
original sin, 116–18
origins, myths and theories, 26–32, 126, 375–89
orphans/foundlings, 270, 338, 339
Ortho Pharmaceutical, 548, *621*
Ortner, Sherry, 636
Osborn, Fairfield, *Our Plundered Planet*, 517
Osiander, Friedrich Benjamin, E21
Osler, Sir William, 445–6, 454
Osmond, Clive, E39
Ottoman Empire, 267–79
Oudshoorn, Nelly, 522–3, 524, 525, 527
Our Bodies, Ourselves (Boston Women's Health Book Collective), 564, 616, *617*, E35
ova. *See* eggs
ovaries, *5–6*, 283, 421, 462, E16
  Eve's, 291
  and IVF, 588–90
  and livestock breeding, 411–12
  and sex hormones, 523, 528
  transplantation, 458
  See also menstruation; testes/testicles, female

ovarium, 219–20
overpopulation, 74, 665–6
  and colonialism, 486–90
  in middle ages, 144
  and poverty, 646–50, *648*
ovism, 206, E16
ovulation
  agricultural terms, 397
  calendars, E31
  and menstruation, 464
  and the pill, 478
  stimulation, 463
  super-, 412, 588, *589*, 593
Owen, Robert Dale, *Moral Philosophy*, 428

pain relief
  in childbirth, 157–62, 331, 557–8, 561–2, *561*, 563, 645
Palladius, 54
  On Grafting, 65–6
pangenesis, 205–6
Pankhurst, Christabel, 454
  The Great Scourge, 445
Paolo da Certaldo, 180
Papinian, 84
Paré, Ambroise, 325, E13, E25
Paris. *See* France
parish records, 148–50, 263–5, 664
  See also censuses
Parke, Davis & Company, *558*
Parnes, Ohad, 302
Parran, Thomas, *455*, 456
Pascal, Blaise, 262, 292
Pasteur, Louis, E26
Patel, Nayana, 654
paternalism, and medical professionals, 553–4, 597
paternity, 86, 249–51, 271
  disputes, 233, 243, 249, 277
  See also fathers/fatherhood; legitimacy/illegitimacy
Pathfinder International, 516
patients
  activism, 531–2
  advice to physicians on seeing, 324
  ancient Greece, 39, 46–8
  compliance, 539
  early modern, 225–40
  empowerment, 440–1, 541
  'fetal'/'unborn', 502, 565
  and gender identity, 623
  and hospital birth, 553–66
  infertility (modern), 457–8, 463–6
  and knowledge, 466–70
  in the middle ages, 185
  'private-patient revolution' (US), 560
  and record-keeping, 344
  rights, 501, 603
  and technologies, 559, *573*
  See also consumers/consumerism; medical encounters; travel
Patients Association (UK), 563
patriarchy, 7, 37, 248, 614, 630–1, 660, 663
  ancient Egypt, E1
  and colonialism, 451
  and oppression, 564
patrilineal descent, 37, 153, 185, 355, 651
patrimony, 87, 357, 614, 667, E12
Paul of Aegina, 272
Pauliska (novel), 582
Paulus Macedonicus, Lucius Aemilius, 88
Pearson, Karl, 444–5
Pechlin, Johannes, 363
pedigrees. *See* genealogies
Pelagius, 116–18
pelvic inflammatory disease, 453–4
penises, 25–38, 216, *217*, E5, E9
Percival, Thomas, 264–5
Persian Empire, 20, 111
perversions/perversion, 615, 624, 626
  and Charles Darwin, *387*, 388
  in Linnaeus, 309
  in Foucault, 614–15, 626
pessaries, 274, 431, 434, 460, 462, 468
Petchesky, Rosalind Pollack, 638
Peter of Spain, *Thesaurus pauperum* (Treasury of the poor), 187
Petty, William, 338
Peyrère, Isaac La, 363
phantoms (obstetric), E21
pharmaceutical companies, 478–9, 521–34
  and abortion, 549
  and contraception, 548
  Leiras Oy, 543
  Organon, *12*, 527
  Ortho Pharmaceutical, 548, *621*
  Parke, Davis & Company, *558*
  Roussel-Uclaf, 527, 549–50
  Searle, 539
  See also pills
philanthropy, 453, 488, 513–17, 539, 557, *561*, 590, 647–8
  St Pancras 'school for mothers', E27
phlebotomy. *See* bloodletting

physicians
  and abortion, 435–6, 599, 603–4
  ancient Greece, 39–52
  astrological, 225–40
  Catholic, 559
  and contraception, 392–3, 430, 434, 436–7, 500, 535–51, 618–20
  and control, 666–9
  and infertility, 437, 457–70, 584, 668
  and the law, 597–611
  and midwives, 326, 491–6
  paternalism, 553–4, 597
  status loss, 503, *523*
  women, 565, 668
physiocrats, 294, 343
physiognomy, 249
  See also resemblance
physiology, reproductive, 300, 409–10, 526, 533, 590, 631, 634–5, E31
pills
  abortifacient, 435–6, 536, *537*
  abortion (mifepristone), 549–50, 641
  advertising, *474*, *537*
  contraceptive
    female ('the pill'), 478, 535, 539–41, 550–1, 564, 617–20, *621*
    male, 548
  morning after, 548–9
  Viagra, 624
Pincus, Gregory, 548–9, 587
pituitary gland, 526
'Pity the poor mother!' (Haselden cartoon), E27
Pius XI (pope), *Casti Connubii* (Of chaste wedlock), 437, 509
Place, Francis, 428
placenta, 157, 159, E15, E34
  and Down syndrome, 574
  and Vesalius, 213, *214*
plague, 125, 149–50, 162
Planned Parenthood Federation of America, 438, 518
  See also American Birth Control League
plants, 59–60, *60*, 61, 65–6
  fetuses as, 113
  Linnaeus on, 305–18
  and spontaneous generation, 62–3
  See also polyps
Plato
  Laws, 70–2
  Republic, 68–70, *69*, 112
Platonists, 111
pleasure, sexual, 427–8, 460, 618, 624, E12
  right to, 125, 624
Pliny the Elder, 88
  Natural History (*HN*), 54, 57, 65–6, 83
Pliny the Younger, 85–6, 87, 88, 90–1
Plotinus, 112
Ployant, Teresa, 327
Plutarch, 75
podalic version, 325, E10
political arithmetic, 254, 263–5, 338–41, *341*, *342*
  See also demography
political economy, 10, 289, 335, 342–4, 505–8, 627–9
politics
  of identity, 624
  and population, 505–19
  of reproduction, *1*, 4–5, 7, 500, 669, E34
polygamy, plant, 314
polygyny, 358, 487, 664
polyhydramnios, 569
polyps (hydra), *280–1*, 282–3, 292, 376–80, *377*
Pompeii, E5, E6
poor laws (England/Wales), 354, 430, 444
popular errors (genre), 191
population, 284, *390–1*
  in the ancient world, 21–2, 67–80
  and biopolitics, 333–45
  bombs, *518*, 519, 665, E36
    The Population Bomb (Ehrlich), xxvii, 517, *518*
  and colonialism, 486–90
  control, 7, 512–19, 641, 646–50, 665–6
    See also contraception; neo-Malthusians
  and different household systems, 347–60
  early modern and the state, 253–66
  and the environment, 517–19, *518*
  in the middle ages, 141–51
  'open' and 'closed', 67–8, 665–6
  and states, 663–6
  Tahiti, E24
  world, 505–19
Population Council, 514–17
pornography, 309, 481, 618, E5, E12
  See also erotic art/writing
Porphyry, 116
  To Gaurus On How Embryos Are Ensouled, 112, 113, 114
positive check (Malthus), 349
posters, *390–1*, *647*, E36

potions, 162, 164–5, 166, 274, E22
Pouchet, Félix, E26
poverty, 603–4, 646–50, *648*
  poor laws (England/Wales), 354, 430, 444
'power-knowledge', 9
prayer
  and childbirth in the Roman Empire, 146
  and infertility, 461
  in medieval childbirth, 156, 182–3, 192–3, E11
pre-Adamites, 363
pre-existence theory ('preformationism'), 251–2, 291, 364
pregnancy, 668–9
  duration of, 61, 169, *234*
  frequency of, 274, 436, 468, 668
  male, 32–4, *625*
  planned, 551
  and risk, 567–79
  signs of, 46–50, 226, 230–5, 324, 478, 536, E14, E31, E35
  testing, 478, E32
  and work, 151, 635
  See also IVF; quickening; twins
'pregnant stones', E17
preimplantation genetic diagnosis (PGD), 594
prenatal diagnosis, 567–79
preventive check (Malthus), 343, 348–50
Prévost, Jean-Louis, 415–17, *416*, *418*
Price, Richard, 264
printing, 127, *186*, 289, 298, 661
privacy, right to, 539, 597, 602, 604–6
Problemata (*Problems*) (pseud.-Aristotle), 187
'pro-life' activism. *See* anti-abortionism
progesterone, 524, 527, 529, 530
prognostications, 182–3, 188, 191
Progynon, 528
pronatalism, 392–3, 427, 500, 643–4
prophetic medicine, 134, 137
prostitution, 47–8, 249, 261, 307–9, 337, 667
  and STIs, 445, 489, E28
public health, 344, 345, 434, 443, *455*, 456, 489–90, 497, 568, 569–70, 649
publicity, 669, E23
  See also privacy, right to
puerperal fever, 344, 558–9
Puerto Rico, 516, 539, 542, 545–6
Purdy, Jean, 608
pygmies, 174

Quesnay, François, 282, 294, 295–8, *297*, 337
Questions and Answers on the Old and New Testament (pseud.-Augustine), 114
quickening, 41, 139, 230, *234*, E23
  and abortion, 429, 598–9
Quran, on generation, 129, 132–3

race
  and adoption matching, E33
  and eugenics/genetics, 393, E30
  purity of, 247–8
  'race suicide', 393, 445
  racism, 11, 373
  and sterilization, 606, *607*
  theories of, 361–74, 489
radical moisture, 195–208
Ramusio, Giovanni Battista, 366
ranking people, 244–6
rape, 388, 601, 603
  of Leda, xxvi, *656–7*, E2
  Seth and Horus, 32–3, 34
Rapp, Rayna, 641
al-Razi (Rhazes), 131
readers/reading, 13, 182–3, 189–90, 218–19, 386, 473, 481, 563–4, E35
Réaumur, René-Antoine Ferchault de, xxvi, 292, *293*
recipes
  to enhance fertility, 161–3
  See also experimenta; remedy-books
regeneration, 294–5, *296*
  of natural resources, 282, 303
registration (births/marriages/deaths), 149, 333, 345, 485, 606, 610, 664
regulation. *See* law/regulation
Relf v. Weinberger (US), 606, *607*
religion, 661
  and assisted reproduction, 651–2
  See also Anglican church; Catholic church; Christianity; Islam; Jews/Judaism
remedy-books, 187–8, 191–3, *192*
reproduction
  in analysis of wealth, 295–8, *297*
  as framework, 4, 9–10, 287–90, 392–5, 473, 659–63
  as keyword, 287–304
reproductive physiology, 409, 526, 533, 590, 631, 634–5, E31
reproductive sciences, 12, 300, 521–2, 527–8, 529, 533–4, 662
  and sex hormones/pharmacy, 521–34
resemblance
  family, 46, 104, 126, 182, 241–52, 424, E33
  See also imagination; paternity
Restell, Madame, *600*
resurrection of dead, 292, 295n26
Rex v. Bourne (Britain), 601

Rheinberger, Hans-Jörg, 424
rhythm method, 538, E31
Richards, Evelleen, 376
Richardson, Angelique, 376
Riddle, John, 49–50
rights
  human, 515–16, 623
  patients', 501, 603
  to privacy, 539, 597, 602, 604–6
  reproductive, 502, 506, 515, 605, 606, 611, 623, 637–8, 662–3
    and the Catholic church, 668
Riis, Povl, 569
risk
  hormones, 533
  pregnancies, 567–79, 666–9
  smallpox inoculation, 335
Robin, Paul, 431
Robins, A. H., 542
Rock, John, 549, 588
Rockefeller Foundation, 501, 513–14
Rockefeller, John D. III, 513–14
Roe v. Wade (US), 547–8, 604–5, *605*
Roger, Jacques, *Les sciences de la vie ...* (*The Life Sciences ...*), 288
Roman Empire. *See* ancient Rome
Ronner, Wanda, 466
'Room of the Ribbons' (*Sala dei Fiocchi*), E40
Rops, Félicien, 388
Rösslin, Eucharius, *Der Rosengarten* (The rose garden), *8*, 327, *328*, *672–3*, E10, E18
Rothman, Lorraine, 547
Rousseau, Jean-Jacques, E19
Roussel-Uclaf, 527, 549–50
Rousselle, Aline, 49
Rowson, L. E. A. (Tim), 588
Royal Commission on Venereal Diseases (UK), 445–6, *447*
rubella, 569–70
Rubin, Gayle, 622, 636
Rüdin, Ernst, E29
Rueff, Jakob, E13
Ruscelli, Girolamo, *I Secreti del Reverendo donno Alessio Piemontese* (Secrets of the Reverend Don Alessio Piemontese), 188
Russell, Nicholas, *Like Engend'ring Like*, 397–8
Ruttke, Falk, E29
Ruysch, Frederik, E34

Sabuco, Olivia, 205
Sabuncuoğlu, Şerefeddin, *Imperial Surgery* (*Cerrahiyetü'l-Haniyye*), 272, *273*, *274*
Sacra Rota, and paternity cases, 250–1
Sadler, John, *The Sicke Womans Private Looking-Glass*, *229*
St John, Lady Johanna, 191, *192*
St Pancras 'school for mothers', E27
Saint-Domingue, 325–6
saints, 156, 163, 192, 237, E11, E18, E40
Sala dei Fiocchi ('Room of the Ribbons'), E40
Saleeby, Caleb, 408
Sandow, Eugen, E27
Sanger, Margaret, 392, 433–7, 506, 507, *510*, 538–9
satire/caricature, *465*, *474*, E22, E26, E27
Schering, 527–9
Schiebinger, Londa, 306, 309, 627–8, 635
'schizophrenic family', E29
scholasticism, 167–80
Schwann, Theodor, 419–21
scientific revolution, 13,127, 661
Scragg, Roy, 452
sea urchins, 587
Seaman, Barbara, 530
  The Doctors' Case Against the Pill, 541
Searle, 539
Secretis Mulierum, De (*On the Secrets of Women*) (pseud.-Albertus Magnus), 185
secrets, 181–2, 188–91, 307–9, 321, 475, 480
'secrets of women' literature, 182, 184–5, 188–91, 472, E25
self-determination, 554, 566, 617, 623–4, 626, *634*
semen/seeds, *15*, 246, 660
  and AI, *411*, 582–7
  in ancient writings, 33
    Galen, 100–5, 107–8
    two-seed concept, 45–6, 95–6, 107–8
  Baer on, 283, 417–19
  Buffon on, 295, *296*
  female, 132, *140*, 198–9, 203–6, *296*
  Fernel on, 140
  Harvey on, 222
  and health of the fetus, 176, 180
  in the *Hidaya*, 271
  Ibn al-Nafis on, 134–5
  Ibn Qayyim al-Jawziyya on, 137–8
  Ibn Sina on, 132–4
  Lallemand on, 422
  and pangenesis, 205–6
  Treviranus on, 419, *420*
  urine conflated with, E12
  See also botany; sperm
Semmelweis, Ignaz, 344, 558
Seneca the Younger, 91

senses. *See* knowledge; touch; visualization technologies
separate spheres, 284, 485, 630
Sergius of Resaina, 105–6, *106*
Serres, Étienne, 381
Serres, Olivier de, 292
Servius Tullius, 77–8, 79
Sève, Jacques de, *296*, E20
'sex change', 622–3
sex determination
 questions about sex of children, 225, 230, E38
 theories of, 46, 103, 113, 635–6
sex education, 394, 471–84, 618, E34
sex hormones, 394, 521–34
 contraceptive injections, 542–3
 DES, 532–3, *532*
 and gender reassignment, 622
 HRT, 529–31
 and infertility, 463
 oestrogen, 524, 527
 progesterone, 524, 527, 529, 530
 testosterone, 524, 527
sex ratio, 144–5, 355, 359, 488
sex selection, 181–3, 193, *487*, 569, 573, 590, 594
sexology, 9, 614, 615, 624–5
sexual dimorphism, 635–6, E23
sexual health, 516
'sexual revolution', 11, 284, 500–1, 535, 536, 541, 551, 620
'sexual system', of Linnaeus, 283, 305–10, *308*, 318
sexuality
 Foucault on, 613–15
 Linnaeus on, 310–12
 male, in ancient Near East and Egypt, 26–32
 medieval Christian and Islamic norms, 165
 in period 1960–2015, 613–26
 See also heterosexuality; homosexuality; 'sexual revolution'
sexually transmitted infections (STIs), 443–56, *447*
 chlamydia, 443
 and colonialism, 486, 489–90
 and contraception, 539, E28
 and fertility, 443–56
 gonorrhoea, 443, 445, 451–2, 453–4, 462
 syphillis, 275, 451–2, *455*, 489–90, 497
shame, 46, 228, 617
Sharp, Jane, *The Midwives Book*, 230–1
Shelley, Mary, *Frankenstein*, 427–8
Shettles, Landrum B., 590
shrines, 163, 652, E1, E4, E40
Shteir, Ann, 306
Siegemund, Justine, 327, E18
Simerson, Mrs Donald, E32
Sims, James Marion, 462, 466, 583
slavery
 ancient, 71, 76
 de Beauvoir on women's 'enslavement', 631
 classification, 366, 368, 373
 colonial, 325–6, 361, 363, 485–6, 664–5
 in Islamic law, 268, 270–1
smallpox inoculation/vaccination, 335
Smellie, William, 323–4
 Treatise on the Theory and Practice of Midwifery, 323–4
Smith, Adam, *The Wealth of Nations*, 298
Smith, Ella T., *Exploring Biology*, *301*
social class, 289, *328*, 667–8, E27
 and abortion, 436–7, 570, 599
 and childbirth, *328*, 560, 561–3, 564, E18
 and contraception, 436–7, 446, 536–8, 539, 543, 669, E28
 and infertility, 447, 457
 and language, 289
 and Malthus, 427, 433, 436–7
 and marriage, 667–8
 and ranking people, 244–6
 and reading, 385, E27
 and reproductive knowledge, 381–2
social organization, 637–8
social purity movements, 431, 432, 599
socialism/socialists, 7, 381–2, 392, 393, 428, *439*, 586
 and neo-Malthusians, 430
 and sex education, 475
Society for Constructive Birth Control (UK), 434
Society for Promoting Christian Knowledge (UK), 382
Society for the Study of Fertility (UK), 410
Society for the Study of Reproduction (US), 300
Soemmerring, Samuel Thomas, *Icones embryonum humanorum* (Images of human embryos), E23
Solórzano Pereira, Juan de, *Politica Indiana*, 368–9
Sophocles, *Oedipus the King*, 43
Soranus of Ephesus, 106, E18
 Gynaecology, *101*, 103, 106–7, E4, E6, E10
soul, 660–3
 according to Aristotle, 54–5
 and Christianity, 109–21, *110*, *117*, *120*, 168, 171
 in Islamic law and medicine, 134–9, 278–9
Soviet Union
 abortion, 436, 439, 546, 601
 and AI, 585–6
 contraception, 546
 embryo transfer, 588
 hospital births, 553

pain relief in childbirth, 645
population, 513
surrogacy, 654
Soylent Green (film), 501, E36
Spain
caste system in colonies, 368–73, *370–1*
contraception, 436
IVF, 651
marital patterns, 352
midwifery, 330
oocyte donation, 652
purity of race, 247–9
resemblance and nobility, 247–9
Spallanzani, Lazzaro, 413, 582–3, 585
Sparta, 74–5, *75*, 79–80
speculum, 272, *273*, *274*, 461, 466–8, *467*
sperm, *15*, 223, 413–26
banks/donation, 583–4, 586–7, 608
'spermatozoa' (term), 417
Spiegel, Adriaan van den, E15
spontaneous generation, 62–4, 66, *301*, *303*, 379, 385, E26
Springer, Jenny, *Die Ärztin im Hause* (The woman doctor in the home), *467*
Stadius, Johannes, *Ephemerides*, E14
Stainpeis, Martin, *Liber de modo studendi … in medicina* (Book on the method of studying … medicine), 187
stamps, family planning, *498–9*, *648*
stars/planets as generative force, 176, 196
states. *See* nation-states; population; welfare states
statistics, 260–2, 333, 335, 345
Steen, Jan, *Doctor's Visit* (painting), *226*
Stein, Zena, 574
stem cells, human embryonic, 594
Steno, Nicholas, 223, E16
Steptoe, Patrick, 590–3, 608, E38
sterility. *See* infertility
sterilization
Catholic resistance, 509
as contraception, 535, 543–6, *544*, *545*, 551, 619
eugenic, 431, 436–7, E29
histories and critiques, 10, 516
Indian government campaigns, 518–19, 545–6, 619, 648–9
male, 543–6, *544*
in Nazi Germany, E29
and poverty, 648–9
and race, 606, *607*
Sterilization League (later Engender Health), 516
steroids, sex. *See* sex hormones
Stevenson, T. H. C., 446, *448*
stillborn children, 171–2, 237, 340, 646
Stöcker, Helene, 433
Stoff, Heiko, 523
Stoics, on ensoulment, 111, 113, 116
See also Athenaeus; Musonius Rufus
Stoller, Robert, 622
Stone, Sarah, 322
stones/minerals with fertility virtues, 156, E17
See also amulets
Stopes, Marie, 434–7
and AI, 584
Married Love, 434
Storch, Johann Peter, 461
Strathern, Marilyn, 628
Suetonius, 84, 89
Sumeria. *See* Mesopotamia
superovulation, 412, *589*, 593
surgeons/surgery
anatomists as, 213
caesarean section, 160, *161*, 326, 559, 564
and fertility treatments, 457–8, 462, 466, 583, 590–3
fetal excision, 160, 172, *173*
fetal surgery, 565
involvement in childbirth, 14, 323, 325–6, 557–60
and knowledge of women's bodies, E16, E21, E25
medieval, E10
by midwives, 159
and monsters, E13
Ottoman, 272
and sterilization, 535, 543–51, *544*
Surgeon-General (US), 456
veterinary, 410
See also abortion; embryo hooks; man-midwifery; sterilization
surrogacy, 25, 581, 595, 608–10, 620, 652–4
Susser, Mervyn, 574
al-Suyuti, Jalal al-Din, 137
swaddling
in Africa, 493–4
ancient Italy, 72, E4
middle ages, 156, 160, *328*
to show nobility, 248
Swammerdam, Jan, E16
Sweden, 343, 437, 453–4, 550, E29, E34
abortion, 570, E34
civil registration, 343
contraception and eugenics, E29
Linnaeus, 305–18
Nilsson's fetal photographs, E34
STIs, data on, 453–4

syllēpsis, 100–2, 107–8
syphilis, 275, 451–2, *455*, 489–90, 497
Szreter, Simon, 359–60

Tacitus, 89, 93
Tahiti, E24
Tassoni, Alessandro, 244, 245–6
Tead, Diana, *What Is Race?*, E30
technologies
  of adoption matching, E33
  conceptive, 470, 581–96, 650–4
  contraceptive and abortive, 535–51, E28
  feminist critiques, 530, 563, 645
  of hope, 466, 651–2
  hormones as, 535–51
  in midwifery and obstetrics, 5, *5–6*, 319–21, 321–4, *322*, 553–4, 563, E18
  new and old, 551, 582, 667, E18
  and risk, 529–32, 532–3
  technological determinism, 5, *5–6*, 633
  user agency, 13, 535
Teichmeyer, Friedrich, 251
telegony, 401
television, E28, E30, E38
Tenon, Jacques, 340–1, *342*
teratology, E13
Terentius Clemens, 89
Terrall, Mary, 376
Tertullian, 115, 118
  On the Soul, 114–15
'test tube babies'
  from AI, 584, *585*
  from IVF, 587, E38
  See also artificial insemination; in vitro fertilization
testes/testicles, 58, 140, 415, *416*
  female, 99–100, 104, 107, 216, *219*, 223, E16
testosterone, 524, 527
textbooks, 389, 521
  biology, 300, *301*
  on homosexuality, 9
  on male sterility, 462
  in medieval universities, 141–51
  of Ottoman law, 269
  veterinary, 409–10
  See also Aristotle; Justinian
Thailand, reproductive services, 652, 654
thalidomide, 569–70
Theodoret of Cyrus, 113
Theodosius I, 111
Theophrastus, 53, 57, 59–60, 61, 62, 63
Thérèse philosophe (Thérèse the philosopher), 378, *379*
'Third-Century Crisis', 109–10
Thompson, Warren, 506, *508*, 509
Thornton, Robert, 188
Tiedemann, Friedrich, *Systematic Treatise on Comparative Physiology*, 381
toads, E32, E37
Totelin, Laurence, 49
touch
  as analogy, 222
  and medical decorum/diagnosis, 153, 228, 463, 651
  and skill of midwives, 325, *329*, E18, E21
  as source of knowledge, 210, 222, E21
  Tournefort, Joseph Pitton de, 306–7
traducianism, 116–18
traits
  family, 241–52
  Galton on, 404–5
  species or individual, 302, 397–412
  transmission through semen, 422
  See also genetics; heredity
Trajan, 90
transmutation theory, 382–3, 385
transsexuality/gender reassignment, 622–3, 624–5, *625*
travel, reproductive, 570, 594, 610, 641, 652–4, 655, E4
Tree of Jesse, E8
trees of life, *31*, 199, *200*
Trembley, Abraham, *280–1*, 292, 376, *377*, 378
Treviranus, Gottfried Reinhold, 419, *420*, 426
Trota of Salerno, 156–7, 184
Trotula, 166, 184–5, *186*
Trussell, James, 449–51
twins, *341*, 593, 669
  conjoined, 174, *175*
  in Islam, 271
  mythology, 27, *92*, *656–7*
  in Paris after plague, 150
two-seed concept, 45–6, 107–8
  and Galen, 95–6, 203
  in Islamic medical texts, 133, 137–9, 275
two-sex/one-sex models, 11, 130, 215–16, *217*, 414

Ugaritic/Canaanite mythology, 32, 35–6
Ulpian, 86–7
Ulrich, Laurel Thatcher, 326
Ulrichs, Karl Heinrich, 428
ultrasound, 549, 568, 572–4, *573*, 576, 578
umbilical cord, 35, 43–4, 113, *120*, 159, 326, 493, E34
Unborn Children (Protection) Bill 1985 (England/Wales), 608
UNESCO (UN Educational, Scientific and Cultural Organization), 512, E30

United Kingdom. *See* Britain
United Nations, 512–17
  UNESCO, 512, E30
United States, 500
  abortion, 10, 501, 548–50, 569, 599, 603–4, E34
    Roe v. Wade, 501, 547–8, 604–5, *605*
  adoption, E33
  AI, 583
  census, 343
  childbirth, 324–5, 326, 331
    medicalization of, 559–60
  Comstock Laws (1873), 431, 434, 538, 599, *600*, 602, E28
  Demographic Transition Theory, 7, 446–51, *450*
  DES, 533
  embryo research, 590–1
  eugenics, 393
  family planning, 438, *498–9*, 500, 539, *540*, 541–3
    condoms, E28
    contraceptive pill, *621*
    IUDs, 541
    philanthropy, 501, 513–17
    population control, xxvii, 501, 513–17, 545–6, 646–50
    sterilization, 431, 543, *544*, 545–6, *545*, 605–6, *607*
  HRT, 529–32
  IVF, 610–11
  and Malthus, 508
  masturbation, 615–18, *616*, *617*
  pregnancy testing, E32
  race, 367, 373, 490, 606, *607*
  STIs, 443, *455*, 456
  U.S. v. One Package, 599
Universal Declaration of Human Rights, 515–16
universities, 143, 145–8, 167, 212, 283, 381, 413–26, 661
  Bologna, 166
  Cambridge, 409, 587, 590–3, E38
  Cologne, 145
  Edinburgh, 407–8, 409, E22
  Erfurt, 145
  Giessen (hospital), 462
  Göttingen (lying-in hospital), 251, 330
  Greifswald, 145
  Harvard, 375, 587
  Heidelberg, 145
  Krakow, 145
  Leipzig, 145
  Oxford, E37
  Padua, E15
  Prague, 145
  Princeton (Office of Population Research), 7, 447–50, 512
  Southampton, E39
  Stanford, E36
  Tübingen (hospital), 463–4
  University College London, 405
  Uppsala, Linnaeus's teaching at, 306–7, 310–11
  Vienna, 145, 187
urine, *12*, 231–3, E12, E32
U.S. v. One Package, 599
uterine mole, 41
uterus. *See* womb/uterus

vaccination/inoculation, 335–6, 344, 523, 548, E26
vaginas, 216, 462, E16
  and AI, *411*, 462–3
  childbirth, 157–9, 160
  and DES, 533, 549
  and the hermaphroditic hyena, E9
  as inside-out penises, 216, *217*
  ring to prevent conception, 162
Valignano, Alessandro, 368
Van Hollen, Cecilia, 645
Varro, 53, 63
vasectomies, 543–6, *544*
  See also sterilization
vectis, *322*, 323
Velleius Paterculus, 93
venereal diseases. *See* sexually transmitted infections
Venus
  in frontispiece to *Thérèse philosophe*, *379*
  models in anatomical museums, 481
  symbol of generative power, 375–6, 386–8
  Venus and Cupid (painting) (Lotto), E12
  Vénus physique (Physical Venus) (Maupertuis), 364–5, 378
Vesalius, Andreas, *De humani corporis fabrica* (On the fabric of the human body), 209, 210, 211–19, E16
Vestiges of the Natural History of Creation, 384–5, *384*
Vetti Priapus, E5
Veturia, 86
Viagra, 624
vibrators, 617–18, 620
Vickery, Alice, 430, 432
Virchow, Rudolf, 421
Virgil, 63–4
Virgin Mary, xxvi, *120*, 121, 127, 155, 192, 238, *328*, E8, E11, E19
Virginia (colonial America), 373
virginity, 143, 147–8, 188
visualization technologies, 209–24, 463, 478, 572–4
  See also ultrasound

vivisection, 99, 212–13, 215
Vogt, William, 518
  Road to Survival, 519
Voltaire, François-Marie, 364, 365, 376–8
Voluntary Licensing Authority (UK), 608
votive offerings, E4, E40
Vulgate, 23, 290

Wallace-Hadrill, Andrew, 91
Wagner, Gerhard, E29
Warnock, Mary/Warnock Committee, 608–9
Wassermann, August/Wassermann test, 446, 456
water imagery, 26, 30–2
Watkins, Elizabeth, 529–30
Wecker, Johann Jacob, *De secretis libri xvii …* (Seventeen books of secrets …), 189–90
welfare, maternal and child/infant. *See* maternal and child/infant welfare
welfare states, 253, 393, 457, 458, 470, 497, 500, 561, 602, 662, 665–6
  Australia, 489
  retreat of, 642, 666
  See also maternal and child/infant welfare; poor laws (England/Wales)
Wells, H. G., 392
  The Time Machine, 389
Wesley, John, 299
wet nurses/wet nursing, 157, 337, E19, E32
William of Moerbeke, 145
William of Paull, *The Eye of the Priest* (*Oculus sacerdotis*), 150
Williams, Raymond, *Keywords: A Vocabulary of Culture and Society*, 287
wills, ancient Rome, 87–8
Willughby, Percival, 323
Wilson, Adrian, 323
Wilson, Captain, E24
Wilson, Robert, *Feminine Forever*, 530
wind-eggs, 61–2, 223
witches/witchcraft, 7, 190, 191, 192, 237
  Witches, Midwives, and Nurses (Ehrenreich and English), 5–7, *8*, 320
withdrawal. *See* coitus interruptus
Wollstonecraft, Mary, 381–2, 630
womb/uterus, 25–6, 105, *120*, 660
  Aristotle on, 58
  in the Bible, 37
  'captured' (Oakley), 554
  crystal womb, E21
  'ectogenesis', 587, 620
  and ensoulment, 116, *117*
  in *experimenta*, 191
  Fabrici on, 219–20, E15
  in *Fasciculus medicinae* (Bundle of medical treatises), 185, *186*
  and fertility, 457–8, 462, 468, *469*
  Galen on, 96, 97, 98, 103–5
  Harvey on, 219–23
  Herophilus on, 99
  in Hippocratic medicine, 43, 44–5, 49, 50–2
  'horned' uterus, 100, *101*, *214*, 218–19
  Ibn Sina on, 132
  Mansur (Ibn Ilyas) on, 275, *276*
  and pregnant stones, E17
  Roman amulet, E7
  syllēpsis, 100–2, 107–8
  in Vesalius, *De humani corporis fabrica* (On the fabric of the human body), 215–19
  as votives, E4
  See also artificial insemination; fetal excision; menstruation
Women and Their Bodies: A Course (Boston Women's Health Course Collective), *617*, E35
Women's Cooperative Guild (UK), 562
women's health and liberation movements. *See* feminism
World Health Organization (WHO), 513, 548, 646, *647*
World League for Sexual Reform, 433
World Population Conferences
  1927 Geneva, *510*, 511
  1954 Rome, 513
  1974 Bucharest, 649
  1994 Cairo, 515, 516, 642, 649
Wyke, T. J., 453

yellow, as Chinese skin colour, 366
  'yellow peril' writings, 489
Youatt, William, 402
Yuzpe, Albert, 549

Zacchia, Paolo, 250–1, 252
Zadeh, Qadi, 277–8
al-Zahrawi (Albucasis), 272, *274*, E6, E10
Zedler, Johann Heinrich, *Universal-Lexikon*, 461
Zero Population Growth, 605–6, E36
Zeugung, 291, 299–300
Zieglerin, Anna, 190
Zondek, Bernhard, E32
Z.P.G. (film), E36
Zuccolo, Ludovico, 244–5